# HANDBOOK OF DRUGS
## for Nursing Practice

# HANDBOOK OF DRUGS
# for Nursing Practice

## Virginia Burke Karb, R.N., M.S.N.

Assistant Professor of Nursing,
School of Nursing,
University of North Carolina at Greensboro,
Greensboro, North Carolina

## Sherry F. Queener, Ph.D.

Professor of Pharmacology,
Indiana University School of Medicine,
Indianapolis, Indiana

## Julia B. Freeman, Ph.D.

Health Scientist Administrator,
National Institutes of Health,*
Bethesda, Maryland

*illustrated*

## The C. V. Mosby Company

St. Louis • Baltimore • Toronto • 1989

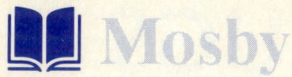

Editor: Don Ladig
Developmental editor: Robin Carter
Project manager: Mark Spann
Production editor: Mike Molloy
Designer: Susan E. Lane

**Printed in the United States of America**

The C. V. Mosby Company
11830 Westline Industrial Drive, St. Louis, Missouri 63146

**Library of Congress Cataloging-in-Publication Data**

Karb, Virginia Burke.
    Handbook of drugs for nursing practice/Virginia Burke Karb,
Sherry F. Queener, Julia B. Freeman.
        p.        cm.
    Bibliography: p.
    Includes index.
    ISBN 0-8016-2608-0
    1. Drugs—Handbooks, manuals, etc.   2. Nursing—Handbooks,
manuals, etc.   I. Queener, Sherry F.   II. Freeman, Julia B.
III. Title
    [DNLM: 1. Drug Therapy—nurses' instruction.   2. Pharmacology—
nurses' instruction.   QV 4 K18h]
    RM301.12.K37   1989
    615.5′8—dc19
    DNLM/DLC
    for Library of Congress                    88-23002
                                        CIP

TSI/TSI/D 9   8   7   6   5   4   3   2

# Consultants

**Donnie F. Booth, R.N., M.P.H.,**
Southeastern Louisiana University,
Hammond, Louisiana

**R. Keith Campbell, B.Pharm., R.Ph., M.B.A.,**
Washington State University,
Pullman, Washington

**Kathy Gutierrez, R.N., M.S.N.,**
Loretto Heights College,
Denver, Colorado

**Nancy Harms, R.N., M.S.N.,**
Midland Lutheran College,
Fremont, Nebraska

**Judith K. Holcombe, R.N., D.S.N.,**
University of Alabama,
Birmingham, Alabama

**Donna D. Ignatavicius, R.N., M.S.,**
DI Associates, Health Care Consultant,
Baltimore, Maryland

**Joan M. Jenks, R.N., M.S.N.,**
Thomas Jefferson University,
Philadelphia, Pennsylvania

**Ellen Lang, R.N., B.N.,**
Foothills Hospital School of Nursing,
Calgary, Alberta

**Edwina McConnell, R.N., M.S., Ph.D.,**
Nursing Consultant,
Madison, Wisconsin

**Maureen Osis, R.N., M.N.,**
Clinical Nurse Specialist and Consultant,
Calgary, Alberta

**Harry E. Peery, M.S., Ph.D. (candidate),**
Department of Pharmacology,
University of Toronto,
Toronto, Ontario

**Suzanne Philip, R.N., M.A.,**
Humber College,
Rexdale, Ontario

**Perle L. Slavik, R.N., M.A., Ph.D.,**
University of Iowa,
Iowa City, Iowa

**Mary L. Vande Berg, R.N.C., M.S.N.,**
Northern Michigan University,
Marquette, Michigan

**Mary Viergutz, R.N., M.S.N.,**
Carroll College/Columbia College,
Milwaukee, Wisconsin

**Patsy Wigodsky, R.N., M.S.N.,**
Methodist College of Nursing and Allied Health,
Omaha, Nebraska

**M. Carol Wild, R.N., B.N., M.Sc.N.,**
Foothills Hospital School of Nursing,
Calgary, Alberta

**Sheila Rankin Zerr, R.N., B.S., M. Ed.,**
University of Victoria,
Victoria, British Columbia

# Preface

*Handbook of Drugs for Nursing Practice* is designed to meet special needs of clinical instructors, students, practicing nurses, and nurses in retraining.

Clinical instructors will find the integration of pharmacological fact with nursing action to be a unique teaching tool. Relevance of the pharmacology is made clear by this device, and the student is helped to remember appropriate actions because the rationale is so clearly laid out. Instructors will also appreciate the overviews and drug summaries, which help the student learn drug categories rather than attempt to memorize information about a large number of unrelated drugs. The format of this handbook also emphasizes patient and family teaching. Guidance is given for involving the patient and the patient's family in the care plan. In this way clinical response, including expected or unusual side effects, may be evaluated more quickly and adjustments can be made.

Students will appreciate the consistent format and clear style of each drug monograph. The integration of pharmacological content with nursing activities helps the student bridge the gap between the classroom and the clinical setting.

The practicing nurse will find this book to be an easily accessible source of clinical information. A tab key for the Table of Contents allows immediate entry into specific units. A detailed index that includes names of generic, trade, and combination products contributes to the accessibility of specific information within chapters.

Practicing nurses, as well as students, will also find up-to-date information on the use of drugs in special patient populations. These categories include infants and children, the elderly, and patients with liver or kidney dysfunction. FDA pregnancy categories (p. 25) or pertinent clinical and animal data are listed for all drugs.

Finally, nurses in retraining will find this handbook especially well-suited to their special needs. Related drugs are covered in one place, and summary tables are included in many chapters to aid in comparing drugs within a class. Thus a nurse who has been out of the field for several years can quickly find the old, familiar drugs alongside the newer agents of the same type. This comparison, which is very difficult with an alphabetically arranged handbook, helps the nurse in retraining move quickly to a degree of familiarity with the new by building upon the old.

The authors wish to thank the editors and associates at The C.V. Mosby Company who have worked with us in the design and execution of the *Handbook:* Don Ladig, Julia Cardamon, Robin Carter, and Audrey Rhoades. Thanks also to Dr. H. R. Besch, Jr., Chairman of Pharmacology and Toxicology, for his support of this educational enterprise and to the colleagues who read, reviewed, critiqued, and strengthened our manuscript. These include Marilyn Evans, Ph.D., R.N., Rebecca Patterson, R.N., M.S.N., and Kenneth S. Karb, M.D.

Our goal in writing this handbook has been to put concrete and relevant drug information in the most useful form possible. As experienced teachers, we understand the process of learning and teaching, and we hope with this volume to have put a useful tool into the hands of the teacher, the student, and the practicing nurse. We welcome your comments on *Handbook of Drugs for Nursing Practice* so that we may improve future editions.

G.B.K.
S.F.Q.
J.B.F.

# Contents

# NURSING CONSIDERATIONS

**INTRODUCTION**   Chapter 1 introduces the special features of this handbook, highlighting the tab system and describing the formats for the drug entries.

Chapter 2 reviews the principles of pharmacology. The factors determining drug absorption, distribution, metabolism, and elimination (pharmacokinetics) are described. The relationships between the dose of the drug, the time intervals between drug administration, and the actions of a drug (pharmacodynamics) are presented. Drug interactions, an important topic, are discussed and include drug-drug, food-drug, and environmental factors–drug interactions.

Chapter 3 begins with Table 3-1, Summary of Major Routes for Systemic Administration of Drugs. The advantages and disadvantages of each route are summarized. The major routes of administration are then discussed in detail. Table 3-2, Forms of Medications, describes the common dosage forms. Figures 3-1 through 3-8 illustrate injection techniques and injection sites.

Chapter 4 presents drug administration and response in special patient populations. Biologic variation is discussed, and examples of how some genetic traits affect drug response are described. The very young and the very old have altered metabolic functions that must be considered when drugs are administered. Pregnant women and nursing mothers need special attention to limit exposure of their young to drugs. The FDA Pregnancy Categories are listed, and a list of medications contraindicated for nursing mothers is given.

# Chapter One

# How to use this book

Unit contents

Formats

**INTRODUCTION** The goal has been to develop an accurate, thorough, easy-to-use handbook for the student as well as the experienced nurse. The following features have been incorporated to accomplish this goal.

**UNIT CONTENTS** Drugs are presented in units (e.g., cardiovascular drugs), organized by chapters (e.g., antihypertensive agents), and subdivided into drug classes (e.g., centrally acting drugs) rather than presented as an alphabetical list. Presenting drugs in the context of units, chapters, and drug classes allows important overviews and comparisons to be presented. **Tabs** The number of units has been minimized in order to utilize page tabs. This allows the student or practitioner to locate a unit quickly. Unit 15, for example, can be easily located by using the tab. The first page of the unit lists the chapters covered in that unit with page numbers for the beginning of each chapter and sections within the chapters, followed by a brief description of each chapter. The first page of a chapter lists the drug classes and the individual drugs in each class. Each chapter and each drug class have an introduction to give a perspective for the material covered.

**FORMATS** A standardized format is used for the chapters, drug classes, and individual drugs. This provides the reader with information at each level. **Chapter format** Chapters begin with a *drug list* subdivided by drug classes. An *introduction* to the chapter describes the therapeutic roles of the drug classes covered. **Drug class format** Drugs are first presented by drug class with the features common to the class.

*Drug list*  Individual drugs for a given class are given.

*Drug combinations*  A list of the common drug combinations is given.

*Overview*  Background material relevant to the drug class is discussed.

*Mechanism of action*  Information is presented on how the drug class works biochemically or physiologically.

*Indications*  Major uses of the drug class are listed.

*Contraindications*  Major conditions that indicate avoidance or caution for the drug class are presented.

*Drug interactions*  Major drug interactions common to the drug class, for instance, the prohibition on combining drugs with CNS depressant activity, such as alcohol and tranquilizers, are listed.

*Diagnostic test interference*  This entry is made when applicable.

*Nursing considerations*  This entry is presented in three parts. The first category is *Side effects, toxicities, and associated nursing actions,* listed by body system (e.g., cardiovascular, central nervous system), with the nursing actions appropriate to avoid, monitor, or minimize these reactions. The second category, *Nursing intervention related to drug administration,* gives information for safe drug administration. The third category, *Patient and family education,* presents information for the nurse to review with the patient and family.

**Individual drug format** Each drug entry is complete, with some referral to the drug class for common information. The individual drug entry includes the following format.

*Generic name and type*  The common name of the drug is given with a pronunciation guide and with the drug category, e.g., antidepressant.

*Trade names and availability*  Canadian trade names are listed in addition to those of the United States. Names unique to Canada are indicated with a maple leaf. An *OTC* designation indicates an over-the-counter drug; no designation is given for prescription drugs. Drugs covered by the U.S. Federal Controlled Substances Act are designated by the schedule under which they fall: C-II, C-III, and C-IV.

*Mechanism of action*  This is an abbreviated entry; mechanisms are more fully discussed for the drug class.

*Indications*  A listing of the major therapeutic uses of the drug is presented.

*Contraindications*  Conditions that indicate avoidance or caution in the use of the drug are given.

*Dosage*  Dosages are listed by route and patient age group. A category is included for special patient populations, and information regarding dosage adjustment for age or health factors is included. Available information concerning the drug's use during pregnancy is also included.

*Preparations*    The forms under which the drug is sold (e.g., tablets, capsules) and the amount of drug in those forms are listed. If information about the stability or storage of the drug is important, it is mentioned here. Syringe incompatibilities are noted when applicable. If the drug is also marketed in a combination form, that is noted.

*Drug interactions*    Drug interactions documented or expected with the individual drug are presented.

*Diagnostic test interference*    This entry is made when applicable.

*Nursing considerations*    This is handled identically to the entry for the drug class, utilizing the same three categories: *Side effects, toxicities, and associated nursing action; Nursing interventions related to drug administration;* and *Patient and family education.* General information is repeated from the drug class along with information unique to the given drug. Specific requirements for the individual drug, e.g., to be given with food, are discussed here.

# Chapter Two
# Principles of pharmacology

**INTRODUCTION**    Drug therapy is only one aspect of the medical management of pain and disease. A healthy respect for the limitations of drug therapy requires a review of some of the basic principles of drug action.

**GENERAL PRINCIPLES**    Pharmacology is the study of the interaction of chemicals with living organisms to produce biologic effects. General principles of drug action that form the basis for understanding the action of specific drugs include the following considerations.

**Principle 1**    *Drugs do not create function but rather modify existing functions within the body.* The knowledgeable health professional has an understanding of what physiologic functions are altered by a given drug.

**Principle 2**    *No drug has a single action.* The *desired action* is the expected, predictable response. *Side effects* are actions or effects other than those for which the drug was originally given. Side effects may be harmful, beneficial, or of little consequence; most are predictable. For instance, morphine is effective in relieving severe pain; however, the patient may experience drowsiness that may or may not be beneficial, constipation that is usually not beneficial, and depressed respiration that may be harmful to some patients but beneficial to the patient with pulmonary edema.

   *Unpredictable reactions* occur less frequently than side effects and account for 25% to 30% of all drug reactions. Idiosyncratic reactions, unexpected reactions to a drug that are most often explained by a genetic difference between the patient and the general population, are unusual. A patient may experience a greatly exaggerated response or may have no response to a usual dose. For example, the muscle relaxant succinylcholine is normally rapidly degraded by the plasma enzyme pseudocholinesterase. Some individuals, however, genetically lack this enzyme and have a prolonged paralysis in response to small doses of succinylcholine.

   *Allergic reactions* may be triggered by the drug in its original form or by a metabolite of the drug. Allergic reactions do not occur unless the patient has been previously exposed to the agent or a chemically related compound. Previous exposure to the agent may take place without the patient's knowledge. For example, sensitization may result from the ingestion of a food product that contains a residue of the chemical. An allergic reaction may occur immediately after exposure to the offending agent or it may be delayed for hours or even days. *Urticaria* (or hives) is an allergic reaction characterized by raised, irregular-shaped patches on the skin, frequently accompanied by severe itching.

   *Anaphylaxis* is a life-threatening, acute allergic reaction marked by sudden contraction of the bronchiolar muscles and frequently by edema of the mouth and throat. The blood pressure falls, and the patient may go into shock. Other allergic reactions may include fever, enlarged glands, joint pains, hepatitis, or blood dyscrasias. Fortunately, drug allergies are uncommon, and, in general, a given drug is associated with a certain profile of potential allergic reactions.

**Principle 3**    *Drug action is determined by how the drug interacts with the body.* There are three general ways that drugs interact with the body. First, some drugs alter body fluids, for instance, the acidity of the stomach or urine. Second, drugs may interact nonspecifically with cell membranes, a property primarily found with the general anesthetics. Third, drugs may act through specific receptors; most drugs act through a receptor mechanism. **Receptor mechanisms** The concept of drug receptors is one of the major concepts in pharmacology. Most drugs seem to mimic a naturally occurring compound and interact with a specific biologic molecule to produce a biologic response. Receptors are those molecular entities capable of binding very specific compounds. The complex of receptor-compound alters cell functions to produce a biologic response. **AGONIST** Any compound, either natural or man-made, that binds to a specific receptor and produces a biologic effect by stimulating the receptor is called an agonist. For example, the neurotransmitter norepinephrine binds to specific sites in the heart called beta-1 adrenergic receptors. Stimulation of these receptors causes the heart to beat faster. The synthetic drug isoproterenol acts on the same receptors in the heart and produces the same effects. Both norepinephrine and isoproterenol are beta-1 adrenergic agonists. **ANTAGONIST** Some drugs produce their action not by stimulating receptors but by preventing natural substances from stimulating receptors. These drugs are called antagonists. For example, the drug propranolol blocks beta-1 adrenergic receptors and prevents agonists such as norepinephrine from stimulating the receptor normally. Propranolol is a beta adrenergic receptor antagonist. **AFFINITY AND EFFICACY** The ability to bind to the receptor and the capability of stimulating or preventing an action by the receptor are two different aspects of drug action. The ability to bind to the receptor is known as affinity. Drugs with high affinities have a great attraction to the receptor. The capability of stimulating the receptor to some action is efficacy. A drug may have high affinity but low efficacy, or vice versa.

**PHARMACOKINETICS** Pharmacokinetics is the study of how drugs enter the body, reach their site of action, and are removed from the body.

**Drug absorption from the enteral route** **DRUG DISSOLUTION** About 80% of the drugs used in clinical practice are administered orally. The drug may be given in liquid form, but most often it is given in a solid form such as a tablet or capsule. To achieve this solid form, the drug is usually mixed with other compounds that serve various functions. Starches and other compounds may be added as inert fillers, especially when the actual amount of drug required per dose is too small to be conveniently handled. Adhesive substances called *binders* may also be added to allow the tablet to hold together. Other compounds called *disintegrators* may be required to allow the tablet to absorb water and to break apart. The important feature of the formulation of a tablet or capsule is to allow dissolution of the drug so that it may be absorbed into the bloodstream. **CONTENTS OF THE GASTROINTESTINAL TRACT** The presence of food may interfere with dissolution and absorption of certain drugs. However, some drugs are so irritating to the stomach that food may be useful to dilute high local concentrations of the drug. There is considerable variation from person to person in gastric emptying times and, therefore, in the length of time the drug spends in the acid environment of the stomach. In addition, the amount of acid in the stomach varies with the individual and the time of day. The very young and the elderly have less stomach acid than middle-aged persons. Lower acidity may mean less drug is degraded and more is available for absorption. **CHEMICAL PROPERTIES OF THE DRUG** The chemical nature of the drug also determines how satisfactory oral administration will be. A drug must be a chemical that is not degraded to a large extent in the gastrointestinal system. To pass through the membrane lining of the gastrointestinal tract, a drug must be relatively *lipid soluble,* since the membranes themselves contain a high concentration of lipid. Charged (ionic) forms of drugs do not easily pass through those membranes. Once drugs are absorbed from the small intestine, they are transported by the portal circulation directly to the liver before entering the circulation to the rest of the body. The liver metabolizes a significant proportion of certain types of drugs before the drug can enter the general circulation. This process of absorption into the portal circulation with metabolism of the drug in the liver before the drug reaches systemic circulation is called the *first-pass phenomenon.* The first-pass phenomenon explains why oral doses of drugs that are readily metabolized by the liver must be much larger than would be given by other routes. The larger oral doses compensate for the drug lost through liver metabolism. The first-pass phenomenon may be avoided by using other routes of administration, such as *sublingual* (drug dissolved under the tongue), *buccal* (drug dissolved between the cheek and gum), and *rectal.* Drugs administered by these routes are absorbed directly across the mucous membranes and rapidly enter the systemic circulation.

**Drug absorption from parenteral routes** The parenteral routes of drug administration are primarily those that require injection of the drug into the skin, subcutaneous tissue, muscle, or blood. Injection necessarily involves breaking the skin, and sterile technique must be used to prevent bacteria from gaining entry. Special precautions often must be taken to avoid producing undue tissue damage with irritating drugs. **INTRADERMAL INJECTION** For diagnostic purposes and for determining sensitivity to injectable medications, intradermal injection (between the layers of skin) is used. **SUBCUTANEOUS INJECTION** For drugs that will be used in small volumes and for which slow absorption is desirable, subcutaneous injection (under the skin) is appropriate. **INTRAMUSCULAR INJECTION** When larger volumes of a drug must be injected, intramuscular injection (into a muscle) is appropriate. Absorption from intramuscular sites is faster than from subcutaneous sites, since the muscles are better supplied with blood vessels than is the skin. Absorption from either type of site can be enhanced by applying heat or massage to the site to accelerate blood flow. Absorption may be delayed with ice packs or by including epinephrine to constrict blood vessels. Insoluble forms of drug, called *depot* forms, can also be used to slow absorption. **INTRAVENOUS INJECTION** Special precautions are required for intravenous injection (directly into a vein). Drugs that are to be used intravenously must always be in solution and can contain no particular matter. Some drugs irritate the veins and cause thrombophlebitis if administered at too high a concentration. Other drugs must be injected slowly to avoid toxic concentrations of the drug reaching the heart or other vital organs. The intravenous route is valuable when large amounts of drug must be given or when drug concentrations must be maintained continuously, but this route has the disadvantage that potential harm to the patient is greater than by oral or other parenteral routes. **SPECIAL INJECTION ROUTES** For drug delivery at selective sites special injection routes are required. Examples include injection of local anesthetics into the spinal column for spinal anesthesia, injection of steroids into joints to relieve inflammation, or injection into arteries to localize the effect in a particular organ or tissue area. **INHALATION** For inhalation anesthetics and for many drugs used to treat asthma, inhalation is used.

**Drug distribution**    **MAJOR DETERMINANTS** Once a drug has entered the blood, several factors influence its distribution. Some drugs are *metabolized* by enzymes in the blood. *Blood flow* and *lipid solubility* determine how rapidly a drug enters a given tissue. Many drugs are not in free form in the blood but are *bound to blood protein*. Albumin, the most common blood protein, is the major carrier protein for blood-borne substances and frequently binds drugs as well. Drugs bound to albumin remain in the blood, since these proteins as a rule do not diffuse through capillary walls. Drug binding to albumin is a reversible process, and in the blood an equilibrium is established between drug bound to the protein and drug that is free in solution. Only free drug is able to diffuse into tissues, interact with receptors, and produce biologic effects. The same proportion of bound and free drug is maintained in the blood at all times. Thus when free drug leaves the blood, some drug is released from protein binding to reestablish the proper ratio between bound and free drug. The net effect of binding to albumin is to create a reservoir of the drug that is released to replenish free drug removed to other sites. In general, drugs that do not bind to plasma albumin remain in the body for shorter periods than do drugs that are tightly bound. A longer duration of action is thus one characteristic of drugs that are bound to plasma proteins.

**Drug metabolism**    **BIOTRANSFORMATION** Biotransformation is the ability of living organisms to modify the chemical structure of drugs. Most drugs are metabolized in the body in the liver, specifically by the microsomal enzyme system. These enzymes allow the body to metabolize potentially toxic compounds. Many types of chemical transformations are carried out, but in general these reactions create water-soluble compounds that can be eliminated from the body by the kidney. These enzymes have two important properties. First, the enzymes are relatively nonspecific; therefore many drugs may be metabolized by the same enzyme system. Second, the liver has the capacity to synthesize more enzymes in response to being exposed to higher than normal concentrations of certain drugs. This property means that the liver can increase its capacity to destroy a drug over a period of a few days. This increase in microsomal enzyme content in the liver is called *enzyme induction*. **BIOTRANSFORMATION IN TISSUES OTHER THAN LIVER** The liver is by far the most important site for biotransformation of drugs, but it is not the only site. Other sites for biotransformation include the kidney, which can make water-soluble conjugates of many drugs with sulfate or glucuronide, and the lung, which degrades prostaglandins.

**Drug elimination from the body**    There are three main routes by which drugs may be eliminated from the body. These routes involve the liver, kidney, and bowel.    **ELIMINATION IN THE URINE WITHOUT METABOLISM BY THE LIVER** Some drugs are not extensively metabolized anywhere in the body and are excreted unchanged in the urine. This excretion may take place in one of two ways. Some drugs are excreted by *passive diffusion* into glomerular fluid and are not extensively reabsorbed. Other drugs are *actively secreted* by specific systems in the renal tubule. These active processes lead to more rapid drug elimination and allow high urinary concentrations of drug to be achieved. Drugs that are normally eliminated unchanged in the urine will accumulate in the body when there is a loss of kidney function. Patients with kidney disease must frequently have drug dosages lowered to compensate for the reduced ability of the kidney to excrete various substances. Certain drugs are themselves nephrotoxic and may directly damage the kidneys and thereby interfere with their own excretion.    **ELIMINATION IN THE URINE AFTER METABOLISM BY THE LIVER** A second route of elimination involves the liver and the kidney. Common biotransformations of drug by the liver include formation of glucuronides, hydroxylations, and acetylations. The kidney is also capable of forming glucuronides and sulfates. All of these reactions tend to form water-soluble compounds that can be excreted by the kidney.    **ELIMINATION IN THE FECES** Another route involves uptake of the drug by the liver, release into bile, and elimination in the feces. However, drugs in the bile enter the small intestine, where they may be reabsorbed into the blood, returned to the liver, and again secreted into bile. This secretion and reabsorption process is called *enterohepatic circulation*. If the reabsorbed drug is in an active form, the duration of action of the drug is prolonged.    **OTHER ROUTES OF ELIMINATION** Although the most important routes of drug excretion are the kidney and the gastrointestinal tract, drugs may additionally be eliminated from the respiratory tract, in breast milk, and in saliva and sweat.

**PHARMACODYNAMICS**    Pharmacodynamics is the study of drug action at the biochemical and physiologic levels. Both the pharmacokinetics and the pharmacodynamics of a drug determine how a drug will be administered, how often it will be given, and what a dose will be. Some of the major factors influencing these parameters will be presented.

**Dose-response curve**    The relationship between the dose of a drug and the response to a drug is not a straight-line function, but an S-shaped curve (Figure 1-1). For a given response, there is a threshold dose, a minimum dose needed. Second, the drug-induced response will reach a plateau rather than increase indefinitely. A given drug may produce multiple predictable biologic effects, and for each of these effects a dose-response curve may be drawn. Increasing the amount of drug administered often produces undesired side effects to a greater degree than producing an increased therapeutic effect. These relationships are diagrammed in Figure 1-1.

**Time course of drug action**    Drugs may enter the body by a number of routes, but except for the intravenous route, some time will be required for the drug to enter the blood after administration. There is also a delay between the time the drug enters the blood and the time the drug reaches its site of action. If the response to a single dose of a drug is measured as a function of time, the pattern shown in Figure 1-2 is observed. The time for the *onset* of drug action is the time it takes after the drug is administered to reach a concentration that produces a response. As drug continues to be absorbed, higher concentrations of the drug reach the site of action, and the response increases. As the drug is being absorbed, it is also subject to the influences that tend to eliminate the drug from the body. Ultimately elimination dominates, and the actual concentration of the drug in the body begins to fall. As a result, the response also begins to diminish. The *time to peak effect* is the time it takes for the drug to reach its highest effective concentration. The *duration of action* of a drug is the time during which the drug is present in a concentration large enough to produce a response and is determined by the rate of absorption and the rate of elimination.    **DRUG HALF-LIFE OR ELIMINATION HALF-TIME** The time it takes for elimination processes to reduce the blood concentration of the drug by half is called drug half-life or elimination half-time. For example, if the elimination half-time of a drug is 2 hours, 50% would remain after 2 hours, 25% after 4 hours, 12.5% after 6 hours, and so forth. In each 2-hour period, the amount of drug in the body would be reduced by half.    **PLATEAU PRINCIPLE** When a drug is given repeatedly for therapy at fixed dosage intervals (e.g., 2 tablets every 4 hours), the concentration of drug in

**Figure 1-1. A,** A log dose-response curve. Percent of maximum biologic response is plotted on a linear scale on vertical axis. Dose of the drug is plotted on a logarithmic scale on horizontal axis. Threshold is the dose of drug required to cause a measurable response. Plateau is region of curve where increasing drug dose does not increase the biologic response.

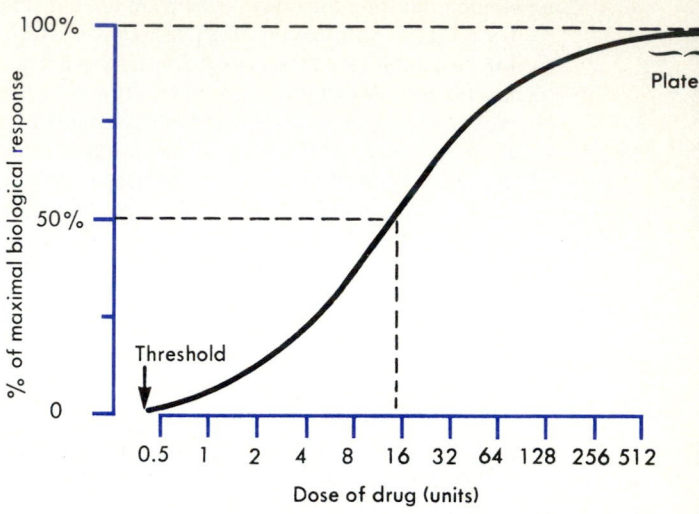

**B,** Log dose-response curves for effects of digitalis. In this example percent of patients responding to digitalis is plotted on vertical axis, and dose of digitalis is plotted on logarithmic scale on horizontal axis. *Curve A* represents strengthened force of contraction of the heart produced by digitalis; *curve B* measures nausea; *curve C* measures visual disturbances; *curve D* measures cardiac arrhythmias; and *curve E* measures ventricular fibrillation and death. These undesirable effects are all dose-related responses to digitalis. (From Clark JB, Queener SF, Karb VB: Pharmacological Basis of Nursing Practice, ed. 2, St. Louis, 1986, The C.V. Mosby Co.)

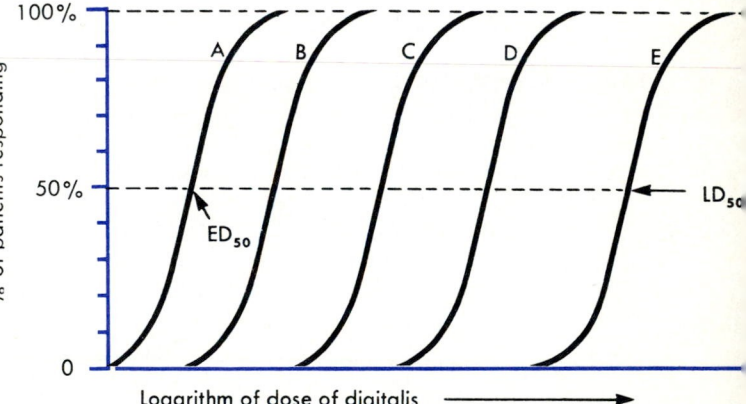

the blood reaches a *plateau* and is maintained at that level until either the dose or the frequency of administration is changed. The plateau principle states that the concentration of the drug in the blood fluctuates around a mean value, which approaches a plateau value after four elimination half-times have passed. This happens regardless of the dose or frequency of administration, as long as they are constant. In the example above in which the elimination half-time is 2 hours, the drug concentration would plateau after 8 hours.

**DRUG INTERACTIONS** A drug interaction is any modification of the action of one drug by another drug. Drug interactions may either potentiate or diminish the actions of the drugs involved. *Synergism* is a special drug interaction in which the effect of two drugs combined is greater than the effect expected if the individual effects of the two drugs acting independently were added together.

Drug interactions are commonly encountered in clinical practice and are sometimes actively sought as part of a therapeutic program. An excellent example is the treatment of moderate hypertension, which frequently involves several drugs, each amplifying the action of the others to lower the blood pressure.

The negative side of drug interaction is that the therapeutic result expected from a drug can be greatly distorted by the presence of other drugs. This negative side can be diminished when health care personnel are aware of the major drug interactions; are thorough in determining which drugs a patient is taking, including over-the-counter drugs, alcohol, and tobacco; and give careful instruction to the patients about which drugs will interact with their prescribed medication.

**Figure 1-2.** Time course of action of a single dose of a drug. Drug is administered at $T_0$. Time interval between $T_0$ and $T_1$ represents time of onset of action of the drug. Peak action occurs at $T_2$. Time interval between $T_0$ and $T_2$ represents the time for peak action. At $T_3$ drug response falls below the minimum required for clinical effectiveness. Time interval between $T_1$ and $T_2$ represents duration of action of the drug. (From Clark JB, Queener SF, Karb VB: Pharmacological Basis of Nursing Practice, ed. 2, St. Louis, 1986, The C.V. Mosby Co.)

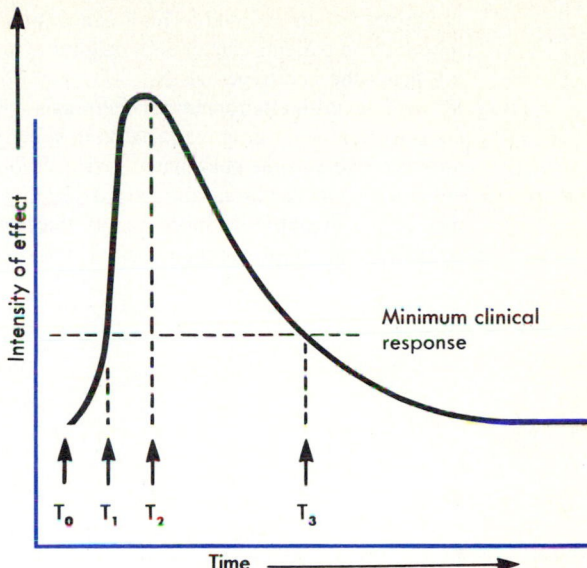

**Origin of drug interactions**    *Pharmacokinetic interactions* may arise when one drug alters the dissolution, absorption, protein binding, metabolism, or elimination of another drug. Drug interactions of the pharmacokinetic type are generally one sided, with one drug altering the pharmacokinetics of a second drug without its own pharmacokinetics being altered. The effect of the drug interaction is to change the actual concentration of the second drug in the blood and at its site of action.

   *Pharmacodynamic interactions* arise when two drugs have the same site of action. If two drugs have the same action, drug potentiation will result. A diminished result arises when two drugs are antagonists of each other.

   *Alcohol* is a frequent cause of pharmacodynamic drug interactions. As a central nervous system depressant, alcohol acts synergistically with the other drug classes that depress the central nervous system: antihistamines, sedative-hypnotics, antianxiety drugs, antidepressants, antipsychotics, general anesthetics, and the narcotic analgesics. At low doses the drowsiness characteristic of these drug classes is exaggerated by alcohol, although at higher doses respiration can be dangerously depressed. Alcohol may also interact with certain drugs to cause an intense reaction, including flushing of the face, palpitations, rapid heart rate (tachycardia), and low blood pressure (hypotension). This set of symptoms is called the *disulfiram reaction,* named for the chemical first shown to cause the reaction in persons taking alcohol. This reaction is occasionally observed in patients who ingest alcohol while receiving certain antibiotics, the sedative chloral hydrate, oral hypoglycemic agents, as well as other drugs.

**Food-drug interactions**    Foods may also interact with drugs and alter the effect of therapy, most obviously by altering the absorption of an orally administered drug. A few drugs are better absorbed or tolerated on a full stomach, but most drugs are absorbed more slowly or less completely when taken with food. A few of these interactions may significantly diminish the clinical usefulness of the drug. For example, the antibiotic tetracycline forms insoluble precipitates with calcium and magnesium in food. This interaction lowers absorption of the drug so that insufficient amounts of the antibiotic enter the blood, and therapy fails.    **ANTAGONISM** Some food-drug interactions directly antagonize the action of the drug in the body. For example, patients receiving a coumarin anticoagulant may lose the action of the drug if they ingest large amounts of leafy green vegetables and other foods high in vitamin K. Vitamin K directly antagonizes the action of the coumarins.

   Other food-drug interactions may arise when drugs interfere with normal mechanisms for removing noxious compounds from the body. For example, patients receiving monoamine oxidase (MAO) inhibitors have a diminished ability to metabolize catecholamines and related compounds such as tyramine. When exposed to high concentrations of tyramine from aged cheese, red wine, or other foods, these patients cannot eliminate the tyramine rapidly and the compound may accumulate, causing headache and hypertension.

**Drug interactions with environmental chemicals** Environmental chemicals are being recognized as agents causing significant drug interactions in some patients. For example, polycyclic hydrocarbons in cigarette smoke and the chlorinated hydrocarbons in pesticides are active inducers of liver microsomal enzymes. Persons chronically exposed to these chemicals metabolize drugs such as the antiasthmatic medication theophylline more rapidly than normal. In these persons the blood concentration of theophylline may be lower than desired unless dosage adjustments are made.

# Chapter Three
# Drug administration

**INTRODUCTION** The administration of medications requires care and thought. The nurse must remember the five "rights of medication administration": the right drug, to the right patient, for the right reason, via the right route of administration, in the right dose. The nurse should assess the patient before administering a drug and evaluate the patient, and the effects of the medication, after administering a drug. Individualized assessment must be done based on the medications administered. For example, it is customary to take the apical pulse for one full minute before administering a cardiac glycoside. The dose is withheld if the pulse rate in the adult is below 60 beats per minute.

As important as assessing, preparing, administering, and evaluating the patient and the medication effects is recording drug- related information. The nurse should record drug administration as soon as possible. Other notations dictated by current practice, agency policies or procedures, and common sense should also be made. These notations should include recording injection sites so that subsequent injections will not be made in the same site; recording blood glucose levels when insulin is administered; recording patient preference for liquid with which to take a medication; and recording effective nursing actions to get a child to take a medication. Other nursing responsibilities are discussed in greater length in pharmacology and fundamental nursing texts.

The actual techniques of administering drugs via the major routes are reviewed in the following sections. Table 3-1 summarizes the major routes for administration and the advantages and disadvantages of each route.

**ORAL ROUTE** The oral route is the most frequently used method of drug administration. Table 3-2 summarizes the major forms of medication, most of which are oral forms.

**Administration** After carefully checking and preparing the medication(s) ordered, the nurse identifies the patient, assists the patient to sit upright, if possible, and then hands the medication(s) and a glass of water or other preferred liquid to the patient. The patient then puts the pills, tablets, or capsules in the mouth and swallows them with the offered fluid. The patient should drink enough fluid to ensure that the medication reaches the stomach; approxiamately 4 ounces of fluid is usually sufficient. Patients who are not sitting upright may need additional fluid to help ensure that the medication has reached the stomach.

**Scheduling** The scheduling of medication must reflect such factors as whether the drug is best taken on an empty or full stomach and whether specific physiologic functions must be considered. For example, aspirin and other nonsteroidal antiinflammatory drugs irritate the stomach and are best taken on a full stomach. Diuretics cause the patient to urinate large volumes and are best given in the morning rather than at night when the diuretic action might distrub sleep. Glucocorticoids are normally given in high doses in the morning to mimic the natural circadian rhythm of the hormone.

**Multiple medications** When several medications must be taken simultaneously, the combination of drugs or the total amount of fluid needed by the patient to swallow the drugs may be nauseating. The nurse should try to ensure that the "more necessary" drugs are taken first. For instance, consider a patient receiving a cardiotonic, an antihypertensive, a diuretic, a potassium replacement, a vitamin,

Table
3-1.

## Forms of medications*

| Form | Description |
|------|-------------|
| Capsules | Solid dosage forms for oral use in which medication is enclosed in gelatin shell that dissolves in stomach or intestine. Gelatin of capsules is colored to aid in product identification. Various manufacturers have distinctive shapes for distinguishing their capsules from those of other companies. |
| Douche | Aqueous solution used as cleansing or antiseptic agent for part of body or body cavity. Douches are usually sold as powder or liquid concentrate to be dissolved or diluted before use. |
| Elixirs | Clear fluids designed for oral use and containing primarily water and alcohol with glycerin and sorbitol or another sweetener sometimes added. Alcohol content of these preparations varies. |
| Glycerites | Solutions of drugs in glycerin; they are primarily for external use. Solution must be at least 50% glycerin. |
| Pills | Solid dosage forms for oral use in which drug and various vehicles are formed into small globules, ovoids, or oblong shapes. True pills are rarely used; most have been replaced by compressed tablets. |
| Solution | Liquid preparations, usually in water, containing one or more dissolved compounds. Solutions for oral use may contain flavoring and coloring agents. Solutions for intravenous injection must be sterile and particle free. Other injectable solutions must be sterile. Solutions of certain drugs may also be used externally. |
| Suppositories | Solid dosage forms to be inserted into body cavity where medication is released as solid melts or dissolves. Suppositories frequently contain cocoa butter (cacao butter or theobroma oil), which is solid at room temperature but liquid at body temperature, or glycerin, polyethylene glycol, or gelatin, which dissolve in secretions from mucous membranes. |
| Suspension | Finely divided drug particles that are suspended in suitable liquid medium for injection or oral dosing. Suspensions must not be injected intravenously. |
| Sustained action | Form of medication that is altered so that dissolution is slow and continuous for extended period. Total dosage in sustained action medication is greater than for regular formulations, since drug is not all released at once but over extended period. |
| Syrups | Medication dissolved in concentrated solution of sugar such as sucrose. Flavors may be added to mask unpleasant taste of certain medications. |
| Tablets | Solid dosage forms, frequently shaped like disks or cylinders, that contain, in addition to drug, one or more of following ingredients: binder (adhesive substance that allows tablet to stick together), disintegrators (substances promoting tablet dissolution in body fluids), lubricants (required for efficient manufacturing), and fillers (inert ingredients to make tablet size convenient). |
| Enteric-coated tablets | Solid dosage forms intended for oral use. Medication in tablet form is coated with materials designed not to dissolve in stomach. Coatings do dissolve in intestine, where medication may be dissolved. |
| Press-coated or layered tablets | Preformed tablet has another type of material pressed on or around it. This practice allows incompatible ingredients to be separated and causes them to be dissolved at slightly different rates. |
| Tincture | Alcoholic or water-alcohol solutions of drugs. |
| Troches (also called lozenges or pastilles) | Solid dosage forms, frequently shaped like disks or cylinders, that contain drug, flavor, sugar, and mucilage. Troches dissolve or disintegrate in mouth, releasing medication such as antiseptic or anesthetic for action in mouth or throat. Troches dissolve more slowly than tablets. |

*From Clark JB, Queener SF, Karb VB: Pharmacological Basis of Nursing Practice, ed. 2, St. Louis, 1986, The C.V. Mosby Co.

| Table 3-2. | Summary of major routes for systemic administration of drugs* | | | |
|---|---|---|---|---|
| **Route** | **Description** | **Advantages** | **Disadvantages** |
| Oral | Drug swallowed; absorbed from stomach and/or small intestine | 1. Convenient<br>2. Nonsterile procedure<br>3. Economical | 1. Unpleasant taste may cause patient to discontinue medication<br>2. Irritation to gastric mucosa may induce nausea and vomiting<br>3. Patient must be conscious<br>4. Drug may be partly or completely destroyed by digestive juices<br>5. Absorbed drug enters portal circulation to liver, where drug may be destroyed. |
| Sublingual | Drug dissolved under tongue; absorbed across mucous membranes of mouth | 1. Convenient<br>2. Nonsterile procedure<br>3. Drug enters general circulation before passing through liver | 1. Route is not useful for drugs that taste bad<br>2. Irritation to oral mucosa may occur<br>3. Patient must be conscious<br>4. Only very lipid-soluble drugs are absorbed rapidly enough to be administered by this route |
| Buccal | Drug dissolved between cheek and gum; absorbed across mucous membrane of mouth | As for sublingual | As for sublingual |
| Rectal | Drug inserted into rectum; absorbed through mucous membranes of rectum | 1. May be used in unconscious or vomiting patient<br>2. Drug enters general circulation before passing through liver | 1. Route is inconvenient<br>2. Drug may irritate rectal mucosa<br>3. Drug must be made up into suppository |
| Inhalation | Drug inhaled as gas or aerosol | 1. Useful for drugs intended to act directly on lung<br>2. Useful for drugs that are gases at room temperature and very lipid-soluble (i.e., inhalation anesthetics) | 1. Absorption across membranes of lung is too slow to be useful for most drugs |
| Subcutaneous | Drug injected under skin | 1. Useful for drugs in soluble or relatively insoluble forms<br>2. May be used in unconscious or uncooperative patients | 1. Sterile procedures are necessary<br>2. Route produces relatively painful site, and patient may suffer irritation from drug |
| Intramuscular | Drug injected into muscle mass | 1. Relatively rapid absorption, since blood supply is good<br>2. Useful for drugs in soluble or relatively insoluble forms<br>3. May be used in unconscious or uncooperative patients | 1. Sterile procedures are necessary<br>2. Minor pain is present on injection for most drugs, but irritation and local reactions may occur |
| Intravenous | Drug injected directly into vein | 1. Allows direct control of blood concentration of drug<br>2. Most rapid attainment of effective blood levels | 1. Sterile procedures are necessary<br>2. Too rapid injection may produce transient, dangerously high blood concentrations of drug |

*From Clark JB, Queener SF, Karb VB: Pharmacological Basis of Nursing Practice, ed. 2, St. Louis, 1986, The C.V. Mosby Co.

and an iron supplement, all scheduled for 10 *am*. The cardiotonic, antihypertensive, diuretic, and potassium replacement are of greater priority. A solution would be to schedule the vitamin and the iron supplement at a time during the day when the patient is taking fewer drugs.

**Crushing medications** Many patients have difficulty in swallowing whole tablets or capsules. Some medications may be crushed or broken. However, the following should not be crushed: enteric-coated tablets, designed to provide an immediate, as well as sustained-release, action; tablets within tablets, usually of different colors, designed to have an immediate and a sustained-release effect; tablets designed for sublingual slow release; tablets containing speckled beads designed for sustained release; and capsules containing beads or pellets for slow release. Crushed medications are usually mixed with water or food and then swallowed by the patient.

**Liquid medications** Some medications are more readily taken in a liquid form. It is important to make substitutions carefully, often after consulting the physician and pharmacist. For example, a sustained-release form of a drug might be available in the tablet form, but the liquid preparation is not likely to be sustained release. The dosage frequency and amount of the liquid form would need to be changed.

## 🐚 NURSING CONSIDERATIONS

Liquids, especially suspensions, must be shaken thoroughly before the dose is poured. If the patient is taking the medication at home, this becomes especially important. The patient should be encouraged always to use the same spoon or other measuring device to avoid fluctuation in dosage. Liquid forms must frequently be stored in the refrigerator. If the taste is bad or the liquid might stain the teeth, the medication can be taken through a straw placed near the back of the mouth.

**Sublingual forms** Sublingual tablets are placed under the tongue and allowed to dissolve. The patient should be instructed to let the tablet dissolve under the tongue. The patient should not drink any fluid while the drug is dissolving. The most frequently prescribed sublingual drugs are the nitrates and nitrites taken for anginal heart pain.

**Buccal forms** Buccal tablets are designed to be held between the cheek and the gum and allowed to dissolve. The patient should be taught to alternate cheeks with each subsequent dose of medication to minimize the chance for irritation of the mucosa. Any oral irritation should be reported to the physician.

**Troches and lozenges** Troches and lozenges are solid dosage forms that should be allowed to dissolve slowly in the mouth. They are usually designed to exert a local antiseptic or anesthetic effect.

**Feeding tubes** Most medications can be administered via feeding tubes. Liquid preparations are preferred, but some medications can be finely crushed and mixed with sufficient water to ensure complete passage of the drug to the stomach. Before administering any drug via tube, the nurse must ascertain that the tube is in the correct place. If the drugs do not form a solid precipitate, they may be mixed together and administered. Otherwise, the drugs should be administered one at a time, each followed by approximately 15 ml of water to flush the drug through the tube and to help maintain the patency of the tube. After the last drug is administered, water should again be administered to clear the tube.

**PARENTERAL ROUTES** *Parenteral* means outside the intestines but in common usage means injections. There are many kinds of injections, and they are named by indicating the site at which the medication is deposited; thus there are *intradermal, intramuscular, intravenous,* and *subcutaneous* injections, all of which are given by the nurse in everyday practice. These injection types are illustrated in Fig. 3-1. Other injection sites that are usually given by the physician include *intracardiac* (usually reserved for resuscitation efforts), *intrathecal* (into the subarachnoid space via lumbar or ventricular puncture), and *intraarticular* (into a joint). The older term *hypodermic* is being replaced gradually by the term *subcutaneous*.

**Reconstitution** Many injectable medications are supplied as dry powders and must be reconstituted before administration. There may be restrictions on what fluid(s) may be used for this purpose, or a specific diluent may be supplied by the manufacturer. Many medications may only be used for a short period once they have been reconstituted. Once vials of medication have been reconstituted, they should be dated, the time of reconstitution noted, and the concentration labled. Many institutions also require that the nurse initial the vial and put the patient's name on it. Reconstituted medications must often be stored in the refrigerator.

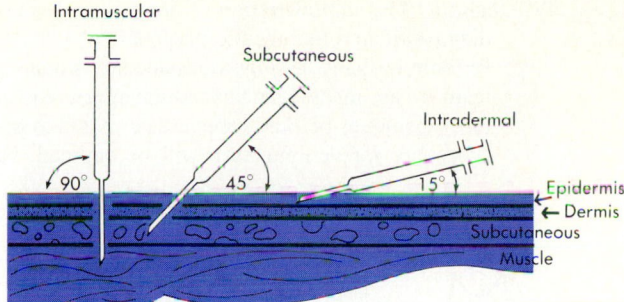

**Figure 3-1.** Comparison of angle of injection and location of deposition of medication for intramuscular, subcutaneous, and intradermal injections.

Some medications for injection are supplied in small glass ampules, from which a single dose is withdrawn and the ampule discarded. Other medications are provided in prefilled syringes.

**Intradermal injection**  An intradermal injection is made just below the epidermis, or outer layer of skin (Figure 3-1). It is used for allergy testing and for administration of local anesthetics. Usually a ⅜ to ½-inch 27 gauge needle is used with a 1 ml tuberculin syringe. The amount injected is usually small, less than 0.5 ml. The most frequently used sites for allergy testing are the medial surface of the forearm and the back.

**Administration** The chosen skin surface is cleansed with alcohol and the surface allowed to dry. The skin is held taut with one hand. With the other hand the needle is held bevel up, at a 10- to 15-degree angle, and the skin is gently but smoothly punctured until the bevel is completely under the skin surface. The needle is then rotated 90 degrees. The medication is injected, creating a raised wheal resembling a mosquito bite. If a wheal is not produced or the site bleeds, the needle was placed too deep, and the injection should be repeated. If several injections are being given in the same site (i.e., on the same forearm), the sites should be labeled with a pen, especially if the reaction is to be checked later.

**Subcutaneous injection**  A subcutaneous injection is used to place medication below the skin into the subcutaneous layer. A ½ or ⅝ inch, 23 or 25 gauge needle is used. The volume injected is usually less than 1 ml. The needle is inserted at a 45- to 90-degree angle, depending on the amount of subcutaneous tissue (Figure 3-1). Any body surface area with loose connective tissue not near major blood vessels or bones may be used. Common sites for subcutaneous injection are shown in Figure 3-2. The site chosen is cleansed with alcohol and allowed to dry. For deep subcutaneous injections, the skin is held taut and the needle inserted. If no blood can be aspirated, the medication is gently injected. Alternatively, the subcutaneous tissue is gently bunched between the thumb and index finger, and the needle is inserted, aiming for the ''pocket'' created between the subcutaneous tissue being bunched and the tissue below. The two medications most frequently administered via this route are heparin and insulin.

**Intramuscular injection**  Intramuscular injection is probably the method most familiar to students and patients because it is a method widely used for antibiotics and immunizations. Because the muscle layer is below the subcutaneous layer of skin, a longer needle is used, usually 1½ inches, and often of larger lumen size, such as 19 or 21 gauge. The needle is inserted at a 90-degree angle (Figure 3-1). The choice of needle is influenced by the viscosity of the medication to be injected, the muscle to be used, and the size and age of the patient.

**General technique** The four muscle areas most frequently used for intramuscular injection are described in Figures 3-3 to 3-6. The nurse assists the patient to assume a comfortable position and then identifies appropriate anatomic landmarks to help define the injection site. The nurse cleanses the skin, lets it dry, then holds the skin taut or gently pinches the skin, swiftly inserts the needle at a 90-degree angle, aspirates for blood, and, if no blood is present, gently but smoothly injects the medication. If after withdrawing the needle there is oozing of a little blood, the nurse applies gentle pressure and may apply a bandage. The patient is then repositioned to a comfortable position.

**IV injection**   The administration of drugs directly into the blood via the IV route is widely used today for diagnositic and therapeutic purposes.

**IV team** In many settings venipuncture is done only by members of an ''IV team.'' If no designated team exists, many agencies require special instruction, classes, and supervised practice in venipuncture techniques before nurses are permitted to perform this technique in their usual setting. A general procedure for venipuncture will be outlined, but it is important to remember that there are many

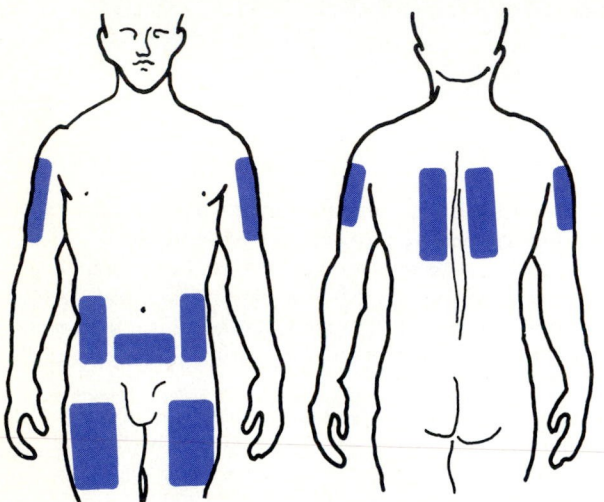

**Figure 3-2.** Commonly used subcutaneous injection sites.

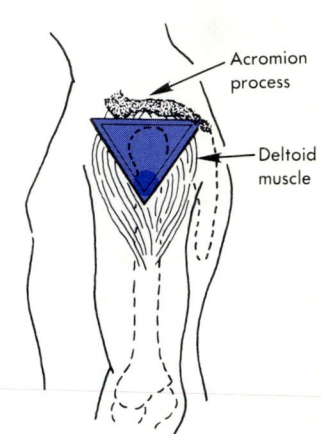

**Figure 3-3.** The deltoid muscle injection site forms an inverted triangle, with the acromion process as the base. The accessibility is the major advantage of the deltoid muscle. This muscle may be clearly visible in the muscular patient but is small in children, petite women, the elderly, and many men. This small size limits injection volumes to about 1 ml. The radial nerve is nearby, and needle and bruise marks are readily visible.

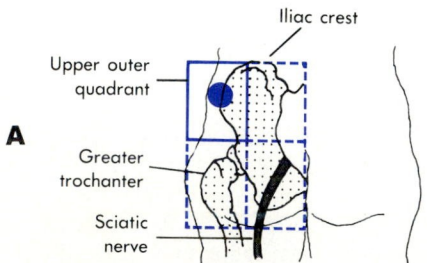
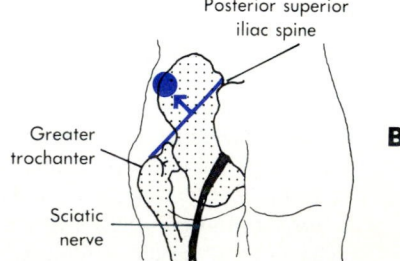

**Figure 3-4.** Two methods are used to define the dorsogluteal muscle. **A,** The patient's buttocks are divided on one side into imaginary quadrants. The center of the upper outer quadrant should be used as the injection site. **B,** The posterior superior iliac spine and the greater trochanter are located by palpation. An injection site up and out of the imaginary line between the two is used. The patient should be lying down, with the toes pointed inward, which helps foster muscle relaxation. In most ambulatory adults, this muscle can accommodate up to a 5 ml injection volume, although volume over 3 ml is generally uncomfortable. This site is not used in children under 3 years of age because the muscles are not yet well developed and because of the proximity of the sciatic nerve.

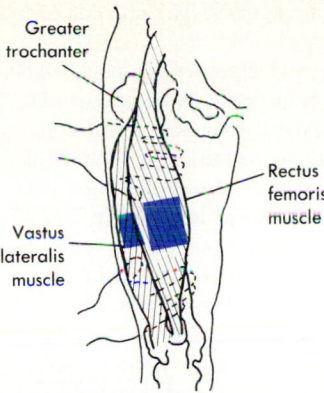

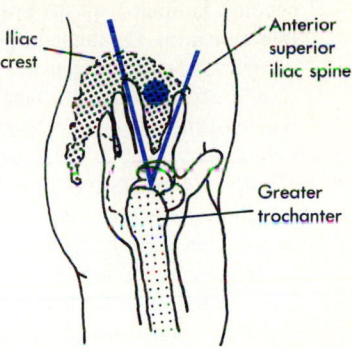

**Figure 3-5.** The vastus lateralis muscle and the rectus femoris muscle site are defined by placing one hand underneath, below the patient's greater trochanter, and one hand on top, above the knee. The space between the two hands defines the middle third of the underlying muscle. The rectus femoris is on the anterior thigh; the vastus lateralis is on the lateral thigh. The vastus lateralis muscle is the preferred injection site for children because it is well developed and has few major nerves present that could be injured. This site is also satisfactory for adults. The rectus femoris is most often the muscle chosen by adults who self-administer intramuscular injections because it is easily accessible. The acceptable volume for injection varies with age and with the size of the muscle. Up to 5 ml may be administered in a well-developed adult.

**Figure 3-6.** The ventrogluteal muscle injection site is located by placing the palm of one hand in the greater trochanter of the femur and making a V with the fingers of that hand. One finger runs from the greater trochanter to the anterior superior iliac spine, and the other finger runs from the greater trochanter to the iliac crest. This site is relatively free of large nerves and fat tissue. In the well-developed adult, the site can accommodate up to 5 ml.

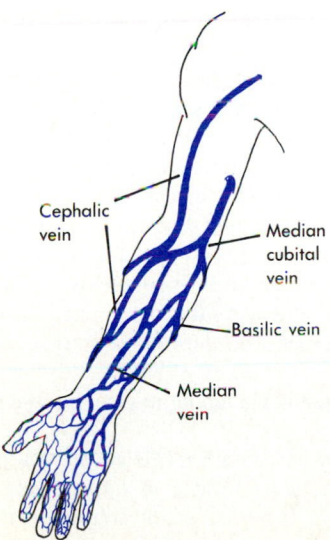

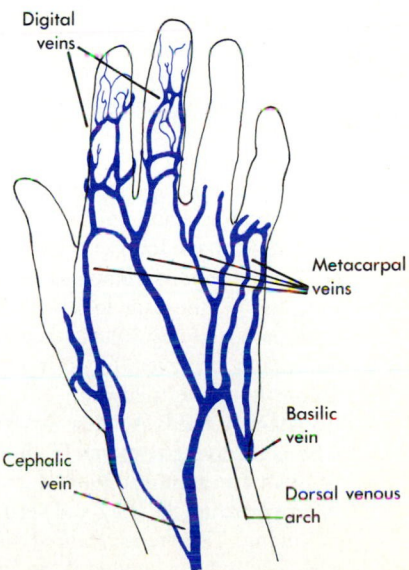

**Figure 3-7.** Veins of the medial aspect of the forearm commonly used for venipuncture.

**Figure 3-8.** Major veins of the dorsum of the hand.

variations in the way the steps are implemented in any specific agency. The nurse is encouraged to become familiar with the practices and policies of the agency.

**Injection sites** The nurse inspects the patient's forearms and dorsal aspect of the hand and chooses the venipuncture site. (Figures 3-7 and 3-8). If the patient is to have repeated venipunctures, the nurse should choose a distal rather than a proximal site. The rationale is that with each subsequent venipuncture the site should be moved more proximal, that is, closer to the major vessels of the chest. Other veins, such as those in the feet, are used only if absolutely necessary; their use may require a physician's order, and thrombophlebitis is more common. Scalp veins are used in infants.

**Injection** After choosing a site and preparing the necessary equipment (antiseptic, tourniquet, needle or catheter, tubing, blood collection devices, medication or infusion solution), the nurse applies a tourniquet several inches above the expected insertion site. The nurse dons gloves. The nurse palpates the vein to define further its location, then cleanses the skin with an antiseptic and allows it to dry. While the nurse uses one hand to stabilize the extremity and the vein, the other hand holds the venipuncture needle bevel up. The insertion site is approached at a slight angle, such as 10 degrees. The skin is punctured, then the vein. The experienced nurse can feel the vein wall being punctured. When blood appears in the tubing or syringe, the tourniquet is released. The medication is slowly injected into the vein, the blood is drawn, or the infusion device secured to the forearm, depending on the reason for the venipuncture.

**Treating the injection site** In removing any needle or tubing from a vein, the nurse carefully removes the tape and dressing and places a sterile sponge over the insertion site, applying gentle pressure. With the other hand the nurse swiftly withdraws the needle or catheter, pulling straight back from the angle of insertion; then firm pressure is applied for 2 to 5 minutes to prevent bleeding or bruising. A sterile dressing is then applied over the insertion site. If a medication has been administered, the nurse records the information, disposes of any needles and syringes, and again checks the patient. Further elaboration of these techniques can be found in fundamental nursing texts and agency procedure manuals. In addition, the Center for Disease Control in Atlanta has guidelines for preventing infections in venipuncture and IV infusions.

**Heparin lock** In some institutions IV medications are administered via a *heparin well* or *heparin lock*. This device consists of a needle attached to a short length of tubing capped by a piece of resealable rubber. The needle is placed in the vein and secured to the forearm. Its major advantage is that medication can be administered via the IV route without having the patient attached to continuous IV infusion. It can also eliminate the need for repeated venipunctures for multiple doses of medications. Heparin locks are particularly helpful in children needing IV medications without additional fluids because it allows children to be up and around.

One method for administering medications with intermittent infusion via heparin lock is described. The heparin lock is inserted, secured, and primed with 1 ml of a heparin solution. Solutions of 100 units per milliliter are available in prepacked syringes and multiple-dose vials, or they can be prepared by the pharmacy or nurse mixing the heparin with normal saline solution to achieve the desired concentration. Each time a drug is administered, the procedure is to (1) cleanse the rubber insertion site; (2) flush the lock with 1 to 2 ml of normal saline solution (this step may be omitted if the drug to be administered is compatible with heparin); (3) administer the prescribed medication via push or infusion; (4) flush the lock with 1 to 2 ml of normal saline solution; and (5) administer 1 ml of the solution containing 10 units heparin per milliliter. The purpose of leaving the heparinized solution in the lock is to prevent blood from clotting in the needle. The exact procedure of the individual institution should be followed.

**Constant IV fluids** Another way IV medications are administered is via tubing in place for the patient who is receiving constant IV fluids.

**IV push** The administration of a small amount of drug, usually less than 5 ml, is called ''IV push.'' After preparing the drug and verifying the patient's identity, the nurse locates an injection site on the IV tubing. The site is cleansed with an antiseptic solution; 2 ml of normal saline solution is injected (this step may be omitted if the IV push drug is compatible with the fluids infusing); and the ordered drug is administered, followed again by the saline solution. Generally, at least 1 minute is recommended for administering the drug. The ongoing infusion is then readjusted to provide the ordered rate. Most commercially available IV tubings have check valves (one-way valves) as part of the tubing. If one is not present, however, the nurse must clamp the tubing above the injection site before administering the drug as outlined above. If there is no check valve, or if the tubing is not clamped, the injected medication will go in the direction of lower pressure, which may be up toward the bag or bottle of fluid instead of down toward the patient. This is to be avoided. The problem with the medication going toward the large bag or bottle of fluid is that the patient does not receive the complete dose of drug until the bag is empty, and drugs administered after that dose may not be compatible with the drug remaining in the fluid line.

**Piggyback and volume-control burette** The administration of a bolus of medication, larger than the amount that would be administered in a single syringe and over a 15- to 30-minute period or longer, is usually accomplished with an infusion method. The drug is prepared and diluted in a larger volume of fluid of 50 to 250 ml. This volume can then be administered in several ways. One method is to add the volume to an in-line device such as a *burette* or *Volutrol.* The ongoing fluids are temporarily stopped, the bolus is allowed to infuse, then the ongoing fluids are continued. Another way is to use commercially available infusion tubing that has two ports for hanging IV bags or bottles. These tubing systems have an identified port for attaching the primary fluids and a secondary port for attaching (*piggybacking*) the intermittently administered bolus containing the drugs.

**OTHER ROUTES**   Other routes for drug administration include rectal, vaginal, skin, eye, nose, ear, and inhalation.

**Rectal medications**   Medication administered via the rectal route is an important alternative for patients who are nauseated or unable to swallow. Drugs administered via this route are usually in the form of a suppository or enema.

**Enema** The procedure for administering medication by enema is the same as for any enema. Usually, the goal is to have the patient retain the medication for as long as possible; therefore a small volume retention enema is administered. After preparing the medication and any necessary equipment, the nurse goes to the bedside, verfies the patient's identity, explains briefly what will be done, and draws the curtain for privacy. A protective covering should be placed on the bed. The patient is positioned on the left side, and the applicator or tubing tip is lubricated. Gloves are worn. The patient's buttocks are separated, and the patient is asked to take a deep breath; then the tubing or tip is inserted the desired distance. The medication is administered slowly to avoid stimulation and immediate expulsion. The applicator is withdrawn, and the buttocks are held gently together until the patient's immediate urge to defecate has subsided. The patient's buttocks are washed, and the patient is returned to a comfortable position. The patient is instructed to hold the medication for at least 30 minutes (or as indicated by the nature of the medication) if possible.

**Suppositories** Suppositories are medications that have been mixed with cocoa butter, glycerin, or other substances that allow them to remain solid at room temperature. Suppositories melt and release the medication when in contact with the warm rectal mucosa. Frequently suppositories are stored in the refrigerator to keep them firm. If a suppository is too soft to insert easily, run it under cold water (if foil wrapped) or place it in the refrigerator to help make it firm before administration. The general procedure for administration is similar to that described above for the enema. A finger cot or glove is worn and moistened with a water-soluble lubricant. The suppository should be inserted a finger's length in the adult, past the anal sphincter. Inserting the suppository blunt end first helps the patient retain the suppository, since the rectal muscles will close gently over the tapered end. If not inserted far enough, it will be uncomfortable for the patient and will be quickly expelled. It may be necessary to place a small gauze pad over the anus to absorb oozing medication after the suppository has been inserted. Unless the medication was prescribed to stimulate defecation, the patient should be cautioned to retain the suppository as long as possible and to report when it is expelled. If the suppository is administered to cause defecation, the patient may defecate as soon as the urge occurs.

**Vaginal medications**   Vaginal medications come in douches, creams, or suppositories.

**Douches** For best effect, douches should be administered with the patient lying down. The tip of the tubing or applicator should be moistened with water or a water-soluble lubricant. The applicator should be inserted about 2 inches initially, then advanced another 1 to 2 inches as the fluid is allowed to run in by gravity. The patient should keep her hips elevated for about 5 minutes before she sits and allows the fluid to drain into a bedpan.

**Suppositories** Vaginal suppositories are inserted by pushing the suppository high into the vaginal vault with a finger or with an applicator supplied by the manufacturer. For ease in insertion, vaginal suppositories may be lubricated with water or a water-soluble lubricant. The patient should remain lying down for a short period after administration of the suppository so that the medication will not be quickly lost. Generally, the patient should be instructed to continue the medication even during the menstrual period and to avoid the use of tampons while using vaginal medications. It is usually necessary for the patient to wear a sanitary napkin during the course of therapy.

**Vaginal creams** Vaginal creams usually come with an applicator supplied by the manufacturer. Guidelines outlined under vaginal suppositories also apply to vaginal creams. Creams are generally messier than suppositories and may not be as well accepted by the patient.

**Topical applications**    Many medications can be applied through the skin. Some topical preparations, such as emollients for dry skin, may be applied liberally as needed. Most, however, must be measured and applied as ordered to prevent the patient from receiving too much. The nurse should try to avoid direct contact with the medication to prevent sensitization and to avoid the effects of the medication. The nurse may wear gloves, apply the medication with applicators, gauze, or cotton balls, or make certain that the medication is applied directly to the measuring guide, as is done with topical nitroglycerin preparations. Depending on the medication, the nurse must also rotate application sites and avoid applying the medicine to abrasions, cuts, or other areas where the skin is no longer intact. Some topical preparations require dressings over them. If in doubt, the nurse should consult with the physician or pharmacist to determine the most effective method of administering the drug.

**New topical delivery system** A recent development in topical application is the single-dose, adhesive-backed delivery system. Examples include nitroglycerin preparations and a scopolamine preparation. The nurse should refer to the manufacturer's literature for guidelines about specific products because there are differences in application. Patient instruction sheets that provide illustrations and additional information are also supplied. Examples of information include the preferred location for application, frequency of changing, and whether contact with water will affect the delivery system.

**Eye medications**    Eye medications are available in the form of drops or ointments. The nurse and the patient should avoid contaminating the dropper, and each patient in an institutional setting should have a separate bottle of eye drops. The patient should be lying down or sitting with the head tilted back. With the hand holding the dropper, the nurse places the palm on the cheek or forehead to stabilize the hand and help prevent injury to the eye. The other hand gently pulls down the lower lid; it may be necessary to use a small gauze sponge or cotton ball to avoid contaminating the eye. The drops are carefully dropped into the lower conjunctival sac, never onto the eyeball. Eye ointments are applied much the same way as drops. A thin line of ointment is applied to the lower conjunctival sac, then the eye is closed and the eyelid gently rubbed to help distribute the dose.

**Patient education** Only medications labeled for ophthalmic use should be put into the eye. Patients should be cautioned to read labels carefully, especially on refilled prescriptions. Eye drops should be kept in a safe place, away from other similarly shaped containers. Occasionally patients have inadvertently put glue or other toxic substances in their eyes because they did not read the label or relied on touch to select the bottle or tube of medication. Many medications cause patients to have blurry vision briefly, so patients should not drive or engage in other dangerous activities immediately after using eye medications. Patients should be instructed that the use and misuse of eye medications can have serious consequences, so eye medications should be used only as prescribed.

**Sustained-release insert** A new drug form available for eye medications is the sustained-release insert. The insert is placed into the upper or lower conjunctival sac, and the medication is released slowly. Patients should be instructed to make sure that it is in place every morning, since the unit may fall out at night. Most units are designed to be replaced weekly.

**Nose drops and sprays**    For the application of nose drops, the patient's head should be tipped back and the nose drops applied into one or both nares, as indicated. The patient should remain in this position briefly, then, if possible, bend over into a head-down position to help distribute the drug. The patient should not blow the nose for several minutes so that the medication is not expelled.

**Nose sprays** require the patient to inhale through one nostril while occluding the other. The applicator should be removed from the nares before pressure is released to avoid pulling sensitive nasal mucosa to the applicator opening. The head should be upright or tilted slightly back. There are many OTC nose sprays available, especially the nasal decongestants. Patients should be cautioned to use these sprays only as needed, for as short a period as possible, and only as directed.

**Ear medications**    Most ear medications are in the form of drops. The patient should be lying down, with the affected ear up. The medication should be at body temperature. In the adult or the child over 3 years, the auricle (the top of the ear) should be pulled up and back to straighten the ear canal, then the prescribed number of drops gently dropped in. If the patient is a child under 3 years, the auricle should be pulled down and straight back. The patient should remain with the affected ear up for 10 minutes to allow the medicine to disperse. A medication-soaked cotton ball plug may be gently and loosely placed in the ear to prevent oozing; a dry cotton ball absorbs the medication. If necessary to treat the other ear, the procedure is repeated with the other ear after the 10-minute waiting period.

**Inhalation**    Perhaps the most difficult device to use is the inhaler. Inhalation requires a cooperative patient who can inhale deeply and can be taught to manage the psychomotor tasks of using the equipment and preparing the medication. In the institutional setting, inhalation therapy is used to deliver oxygen through a nasal cannula, nasal catheter, or face mask. Drugs may also be administered via intermittent positive pressure breathing (IPPB) machines. However, it is in the outpatient setting that the nurse faces the greatest challenge in ensuring correct use of inhalation therapy.

**Inhalation devices** Several inhalation drug delivery systems are available, such as metered-dose nebulizers and turbo-inhalers. Each has advantages and disadvantages. The nurse should make certain that the patient does a satisfactory return demonstration before concluding that the patient can use the prescribed drug correctly. Patients need to be reminded to keep hand-held nebulizers and other equipment clean to prevent contamination and infection. Patients also must be cautioned to use the product only as ordered to prevent side effects, drug overdose, and drug dependency.

**Other drug delivery systems**    There are other drug delivery systems available for specific drugs or specific purposes, such as pellets for subcutaneous implantation, which are designed for sustained release of the drug for up to 4 to 6 months. Frequently these are developed in response to a problem in patient compliance with the prescribed dosage regimen. Patients with limited vision, severe arthritis, or other medical conditions may have difficulty following prescribed therapy. When faced with a delivery system that is unfamiliar, the nurse should consult the manufacturer's literature and patient instruction sheet that accompany the dosage form.

# Chapter Four

# Drug administration and response in special patient populations

**INTRODUCTION**  Drug administration and response are not always as predictable as a textbook would seem to promise. Patients vary in their sensitivity to drugs. In addition to natural biologic variation and genetic effects, there are special aspects to drug response in the very young, the elderly, and the pregnant or lactating woman.

**EFFECTS OF BIOLOGIC VARIATION AND GENETIC TRAITS**  Not all patients respond to a set of drug dosage in the same way. Moreover, it is not always possible to predicts which patients will be more or less sensitive to a drug than normal. The term *normal* in this context really means average for the population.

**Biologic variation**  Biologic variation is based on subtle differences in physiologic functions that exist among people. For example, absorption of oral drug doses can be greatly influenced by stomach acidity, gastrointestinal motility, pancreatic function, and gastrointestinal microbiologic flora; however, these parameters vary greatly in normal people. Likewise, people vary in the sensitivity of certain tissue to drugs. This variation may be the result of differences in the number of drug receptors, differences in permeability barriers, or many other factors. These factors are all difficult to assess and yet greatly influence the magnitude of drug effects in patients.

In the clinical setting the causes of biologic variation are not usually known with any degree of certainty. Patients are observed for the proper response to a drug, and dosages are usually adjusted on the basis of clinical assessment of progress. Although the exact causes of biologic variation are not known for an individual patient, some general factors can be delineated that may influence patient responses to medications. These factors include age, sex, overall health status, and genetic background. Genetic background and age are the most important of these factors.

**Genetic traits**  **EXAMPLE OF GLUCOSE 6-PHOSPHATE DEHYDROGENASE DEFICIENCY** Some drug reactions can be clearly linked to a particular genetic trait that may be more prevalent in certain ethnic groups. For example, the enzyme glucose 6-phosphate dehydrogenase is abundant in the tissues of most people. In red blood cells this enzyme plays a role in generating nicotinamide adenine dinucleotide phosphate (reduced form, NADPH), a compound required to maintain active hemoglobin. As a result of a genetic alteration, some individuals lack adequate concentrations of this enzyme in their red blood cells; therefore NADPH is generated slowly. Under normal circumstances this alteration would not be critical. However, if a person with this trait is exposed to chemicals that enhance the conversion of hemoglobin to methemoglobin (a relatively inactive form of hemoglobin), serious problems can arise. Because of the lack of glucose 6-phosphate dehydrogenase, too little NADPH is present to fully reform active hemoglobin. When too much methemoglobin accumulates, the red blood cell is destroyed.  **DRUGS CONTRAINDICATED** Glucose 6-phosphate dehydrogenase deficiency is important for pharmacology because many drugs accelerate methemoglobin formation. Sulfonamides, antimalarial medications, and analgesic-antipyretic drugs (incluing aspirin) are in this category. In a person lacking adequate glucose 6-phosphate dehydrogenase activity, these drugs can cause life-threatening hemolysis (rupture of the red blood cells). The same drugs are relatively innocuous in the vast majority of the population who possess adequate glucose 6-phosphate dehydrogenase activity.  **POPULATIONS AT RISK** Certain populations have a high proportion of the gene that causes glucose 6-phosphate dehydrogenase deficiency. For example, 13% of black men and 20% of black women in the

United States may carry this gene. Sardinians also have an incidence of approximately 14%. More than half of the Kurdish Jews tested show glucose 6-phosphate dehydrogenase deficiencies. This genetic difference from most of the U.S. population places patients from these special populations at greater risk for serious reactions with the drugs mentioned. **DRUG ACETYLATION** The rate of drug acetylation in the liver is another genetically determined trait that may affect the incidence of certain drug reactions. Of persons in the United States, about half possess liver enzyme systems that acetylate drugs and other chemicals slowly, at rates less than half of those of the rest of the population. In contrast, slow acetylation is very rare in Eskimos and persons of Japanese ancestry. **ISONIAZID TOXICITY AND ACETYLATION** Isoniazid, a drug used to treat tuberculosis, illustrates how the genetically determined ability to acetylate a compound can influence the unwanted reactions that drug produces. Isoniazid is inactivated primarily by acetylation and eliminated by the kidney entirely as metabolites. In slow acetylation the half-life of the drug is about 3 hours, but in rapid acetylation it is only about 1 hour. Liver damage may be common in rapid acetylation because the concentration of a hepatotoxic acetylated metabolite is high. Slow acetylation may be more closely associated with dose-related toxicity (neuropathy, depression of liver biotransformation enzymes), since the untransformed drug may accumulate in persons with this trait. Therefore the effects of isoniazid vary with the genetic status of the patient. Those who acetylate rapidly require larger doses but are more prone to liver damage as a side effect. Those who acetylate slowly tend to accumulate the drug and experience dose-related toxicity. **SUCCINYLCHOLINE** About 1 in 2800 persons lacks the plasma pseudocholinesterase that rapidly inactivates the muscle relaxant succinylcholine. These persons will remain paralyzed for several hours following a standard dose, rather than for a minute or so and will probably require respiratory assistance.

## EFFECTS OF AGE ON DRUG RESPONSE

The age of a patient has predictable effects on drug response. These factors influence drug administration.

**Factors affecting the very young** **PREMATURE INFANTS AND NEONATES** may respond to medications differently than older children or adults because of differences in absorption, distribution, metabolism, and excretion of drugs. **GASTRIC PH** is less acidic in the neonate. Drugs such as nafcillin and penicillin G that are normally destroyed by acidic pH are better absorbed by the neonate. However, acidic drugs may not be as well absorbed in a less acidic environment, and milk tends to further decrease gastric acidity. Gastric emptying time and transit time through the small intestine tend to be greater in children and affect drug absorption. **THE LIVER** at birth lacks many of the metabolizing enzymes that enable the adult liver to biotransform certain types of compounds. Both microsomal and nonmicrosomal enzyme systems may be reduced. Before these activities increase to normal levels during the first weeks or months of life, the neonate is more vulnerable than the adult to chemicals requiring detoxification in the liver. Intrauterine exposure to certain drugs can induce early development of these detoxification enzymes, however. **THE KIDNEY** is also less efficient at birth than in adult life; therefore excretion of many compounds takes longer in the neonate than in the adult. The infant's kidneys are not as well perfused as the adult's kidneys; the glomerular filtration rate is lower, and there is a decreased ability to concentrate urine and to secrete or reabsorb substances. In addition, glucuronidation by the liver and kidney, a major mechanism of solubilizing drugs for excretion, is not well developed at birth. Failure to take into account this reduced excretory capacity can be important when certain drugs are administered to neonates. A prime example is the antibiotic chloramphenicol. Chloramphenicol is normally transformed to a glucuronide for excretion. A neonate will quickly accumulate toxic levels of chloramphenicol unless the dosage is reduced to below 25 mg/kg/day. **DRUG DISTRIBUTION** is also affected by the fact that neonates have a larger proportion of extracellular body fluid, a low proportion of body fat, and a decreased albumin concentration. These factors influence drug concentration and distribution, depending on the distribution properties of the drug.

**Factors affecting the elderly patient** **ELDERLY PATIENTS** also have physiologic changes that affect drug response. Body fat tends to be a greater proportion of body mass, and this affects drug distribution. The plasma concentrations of water-soluble drugs tend to increase, and those of fat-soluble drugs tend to decrease. Gastric acidity decreases, and gastrointestinal motility slows with age. The ability of the liver to metabolize drugs decreases, and the kidney is less able to excrete many drugs. Elderly patients are also more likely to be taking multiple medications, which increases the potential for drug interactions. Symptoms of adverse drug reactions such as confusion, weakness, and lethargy are likely to be attributed to old age or disease.

A good example of the type of drug likely to be most troublesome in elderly patients is an aminoglycoside antibiotic such as gentamicin. The aminoglycosides are excreted almost exclusively by the kidney. Therefore in elderly patients whose normal renal function is significantly lower than that of younger adults, aminoglycosides are excreted at reduced rates. If dosages are not carefully reduced to take this effect into account, the aminoglycosides will accumulate. One of the early signs of toxicity may be some loss of hearing or equilibrium. However, loss of hearing or an unstable gait in elderly patients may be mistaken for normal signs of aging. Therefore the older patient may suffer toxicity for a longer time than a younger patient, since in the latter the same signs would be recognized immediately as iatrogenic (caused by the drug).

## ❦ NURSING CONSIDERATIONS

**Drug administration and age**   **CHILDREN** can present some unique challenges to administering drugs. A child may be unable or unwilling to participate in taking prescribed medications. A developmental approach that takes the child's behavioral stage into account should be used. For instance, a 2-year-old is given simple directions, told of the procedure only shortly before administration (limited understanding of time), asked to take an oral dose alone (pride in performing well and feeding self), and given a limited choice of beverage (difficulty in making choices). The nurse is firm and consistent, following the same pattern with each administration (ritualistic).   **CONCERNS** Children vary in their ability to understand and accept the intrusive nature of some procedures. For example, the young child may be terrified of receiving ear drops because the child cannot see what the nurse is doing. Young children may fear that their insides will come out of the hole made by a needle and can be reassured by a bandage. Children are usually very concrete in their thinking until reaching the early teens. They may have difficulty, for instance, in understanding why an injection in the buttocks could help an earache. Children also have trouble understanding time relationships and thinking about long-term consequences.   **TECHNIQUES** Medications should not be diluted in a large volume of liquid or food. If the child does not finish all of it, the nurse does not know how much has actually been consumed. Medications should not be disguised in a favorite or essential food because the child may refuse to eat it again. The child should not be tricked. Drawings, stories, coloring books, and toys dealing with medications and hospitalization can be useful in explaining to children what is happening and allowing children to play out their feelings.   **THE ELDERLY PATIENT** can also present special situations. First, individual assessment and communication are essential. The patient may have several problems, each treated by a different practitioner without regard for other drugs that the patient may be taking. This may lead to drug interactions or toxicities. Sometimes drugs are no longer needed. The situation may arise in which a drug has been prescribed to treat the side effects of another drug but causes further problems of its own. Confusion or lack of memory should not be dismissed as a sign of aging but should be considered a possible drug side effect or drug toxicity. Patients who have failing vision and/or hearing may make errors in self-medication. The elderly may also be more sensitive to the frequently encountered side effect of nausea. If the patient must take a large quantity of drugs, this may compound the nausea. It may be necessary to readjust the dosage to spread out the prescribed medications over the course of the day.

**MEDICATIONS AND THE PREGNANT OR LACTATING WOMAN**   In the 1950s, the sedative thalidomide was widely prescribed in Europe for pregnant women. The result was an epidemic of deformed infants, usually missing arms or legs. This shocking tragedy led to an increased awareness of the potential for teratogenic (the production of physical defects in offspring in utero) effects of drugs and other substances. Furthermore, the infant nursing from the mother's breast is exposed to drugs the mother may be taking because of their excretion into breast milk. This section reviews the special concerns associated with drugs and the pregnant or lactating mother.

**Concerns during pregnancy**   The fetus is at special risk from exposure to harmful effects of drugs during the first and third trimester. During the first trimester, the fetal organs are developing, and this is the most sensitive period for drug-induced malformations. The general rule is that *no* drugs should be taken by the pregnant woman unless they are essential for maternal life. In fact, the woman trying to conceive should avoid medications, since organogenesis begins 13 days after conception, a time when many women do not yet realize they are pregnant. Although relatively few drugs have been proven teratogenic in humans, a number of drugs are highly suspect. The drugs for which a teratogenic effect in humans has been clearly documented include thalidomide, warfarin, isotretinoin, phenytoin, lithium, trimethadione, alcohol, penicillamine, diethylstilbesterol and other sex hormones, and antineoplastic drugs.

The last trimester is also regarded as a critical time for exposure of the fetus to maternal drugs. During this period the fetus is developed, but organ systems are not mature. As discussed earlier for neonates, the liver and kidney have not developed the enzyme systems at this stage to detoxify and eliminate foreign compounds. The fetal blood does not have abundant albumin, the protein that in adults binds many drugs to keep the concentration of effective drug low. The fetus does not have much body fat, a tissue that takes up many drugs in adults. The fetal circulatory system therefore carries a high concentration of free drug relative to the maternal system. The result of these differences in drug distribution and metabolism in the fetus is that toxic levels of drugs may be achieved even when the dose to the mother is well within a level safe for her. At the extreme, it is now well recognized that the excessive and prolonged maternal use of opiates and barbiturates during pregnancy to the time of delivery causes withdrawal symptoms in the infant after birth. Large doses of narcotic analgesics during labor depress the respiration of the infant at birth.

It is important that the pregnant patient be informed that OTC drugs, cigarettes, and alcohol all have demonstrated adverse effects on the unborn child. Aspirin products have an effect on blood coagulation. Cigarette smoking is associated with low birth weight of infants. Ingestion of as little as 3 ounces of alcohol a day has been associated with the ''fetal alcohol syndrome,'' which can include a small head, low-set ears, cardiac abnormalities, malformation of the female genitals, and growth and mental retardation. Excessive coffee (caffeine) consumption, greater than 7 cups a day, has been associated with a higher risk for miscarriage.

**FDA pregnancy categories** The FDA has established five categories of prescription drugs for use in pregnant women. All prescription drugs absorbed systemically or those known to have a potential for harm to the fetus are categorized according the level of risk. This information appears in the precautions section of the package insert for prescription drugs. The categories and their definitions are as follows. **FDA pregnancy category A** Controlled studies in women fail to demonstrate a risk to the fetus in the first trimester (and there is no evidence of a risk in later trimesters), and the possibility of fetal harm appears remote. **FDA pregnancy category B** Either animal reproduction studies have not demonstrated a fetal risk but there are no controlled studies in pregnant women, or animal reproduction studies have shown an adverse effect (other than decreased fertility) that was not confirmed in controlled studies in women in the first trimester (and there is no evidence of a risk in later trimesters). **FDA pregnancy category C** Either studies in animals have revealed adverse effects on the fetus (teratogenic, embryocidal, or other) and there are no controlled studies in women, or studies in women and animals are not available. Drugs in this category should be given only if the potential benefit justifies the risk to the fetus. **FDA pregnancy category D** There is positive evidence of human fetal risk, but the benefits for pregnant women may be acceptable despite the risk, as in life-threatening or serious diseases for which safer drugs cannot be used or are ineffective. An appropriate statement must appear in the warnings section of the labeling of drugs in this category. **FDA pregnancy category X** Studies in animals or humans have demonstrated fetal abnormalities, there is evidence of fetal risk based on human experience (or experience in both humans and animals), and the risk of using the drug in pregnant women clearly outweighs any possible benefit. The drug is contraindicated in women who are or may become pregnant. An appropriate statement must appear in the contraindications section of the labeling of drugs in this category.

**Concerns for the lactating mother** Approximately 50% of mothers breast-feed their infants. Because drugs are distributed to milk as well as other body fluids, the potential exists for drugs reaching the infant through the ingestion of breast milk. The factors that influence the distribution of drugs are the same for breast milk as for other fluids. Breast milk tends to be slightly more acid than plasma and is rich in protein and fat. It is estimated that up to 1% to 2% of the maternal dose of a drug is secreted in breast milk. The drug level in breast milk parallels the drug level in the body. Therefore when a medication is required, taking a medication after nursing rather than before nursing in general minimizes the amount of drug in the milk.   **Medications contraindicated for the lactating mother** Breast feeding should be suspended when one of the following medications is indicated for the mother:

antineoplastic drugs
chloramphenicol
dapsone
iodine-containing products
isoniazide
lithium
methimazole
nitrofurantoin
oral anticoagulants
phenindione
propylthiouracil
radioactive pharmaceuticals
sulfonamides (during the first 2 weeks postpartum)
tetracyclines.

# CARDIOVASCULAR DRUGS

II

**INTRODUCTION**   This unit covers drugs that are used primarily to alter cardiovascular function. Adrenergic drugs are prominent. Alpha adrenergic agonists are drugs used for counteracting the hypotension of spinal anesthesia and also for treating selected cases of shock. Beta-1 adrenergic agonists are drugs that stimulate the heart for treatment of selected cases of shock and congestive heart failure. Beta adrenergic blockers are a versatile class of drugs for the treatment of angina, hypertension, and additional selected indications. Newer blockers, including alpha-beta and alpha adrenergic blockers, are drugs used in the treatment of hypertensive conditions.

Cardiac glycosides are drugs that improve cardiac function in congestive heart failure. New miscellaneous inotropic agents have been introduced for the treatment of congestive heart failure. Antiarrhythmic drugs are available to treat disorders of pacing or conduction in the heart.

Current antihypertensive therapy uses a variety of drugs, including alpha and beta adrenergic blocking agents. Other drug types used in treating hypertension include centrally acting drugs, centrally and peripherally acting agents, ganglionic blocking drugs, vasodilators, and angiotensin antagonists.

Several drugs are used to improve blood flow. The antianginal nitrates are used for prophylactic and acute relief of angina. Calcium channel blockers are a new drug class, finding important uses in the treatment of angina and hypertension. Peripheral vasodilators are drugs of limited value for improving blood flow. Pentoxifylline is a new drug that improves blood viscosity.

# Chapter Five

# Cardiovascular drugs acting through alpha and beta adrenergic receptors

**Alpha adrenergic agonists**
epinephrine
mephentermine
metaraminol
norepinephrine
phenylephrine

**Beta-1 adrenergic agonists**
dobutamine
dopamine
ephedrine
(isoproterenol—see Chapter 52)

**Beta adrenergic blockers**
acebutolol
atenolol
esmolol
metoprolol
nadolol
pindolol
propranolol
timolol

**Alpha-beta and alpha adrenergic blockers**
labetolol
prazosin
phentolamine
phenoxybenzamine
terazosin

**INTRODUCTION**  The sympathetic nervous system plays a major role in controlling cardiovascular function. The overall cardiovascular effects on activating the sympathetic nervous system are increased blood pressure and increased cardiac output. On a cellular level, these responses are mediated by receptors on the surface of cells for the neurotransmitter of the sympathetic nervous system, norepinephrine, and the neurohormone, epinephrine. These adrenergic receptors fall into four classes: alpha-1, alpha-2, beta-1, and beta-2 receptors. These receptors mediate the biochemical responses of the sympathetic nervous system.

In this chapter, drugs acting through alpha-1 and beta-1 adrenergic receptors are presented. Drugs acting through alpha-1 adrenergic receptors are used to raise or lower blood pressure. Drugs acting through beta-1 receptors are used to modify cardiac function and are used in treating cardiac arrhythmias, cardiogenic shock, hypertension, and angina.

## Alpha adrenergic agonists

epinephrine ~ mephentermine ~ metaraminol ~ norepinephrine ~ phenylephrine

**OVERVIEW OF THE DRUG CLASS**  The alpha adrenergic drugs mimic the action of norepinephrine, the neurotransmitter of the sympathetic nervous system. Sympathomimetic drugs restore functions mediated through adrenergic receptors. A common use of sympathomimetic drugs is to overcome the hypotension secondary to spinal anesthesia. Spinal anesthesia blocks the sympathetic ganglia necessary for the control of blood pressure.

**MECHANISM OF ACTION**  Table 5-1 compares the sympathomimetic agents. Selected use of *direct-acting sympathomimetic amines* is made in treating certain types of shock by raising blood pressure by increasing peripheral resistance (activation of alpha-1 adrenergic receptors) and/or by increasing cardiac output (activation of beta-1 adrenergic receptors). *Indirect-acting sympathomimetic drugs* cause the release of norepinephrine from sympathetic neurons. The norephinephrine so released acts at alpha-1 and beta-1 adrenergic receptors, accounting for the activity of the drug.

**INDICATIONS**  **Shock** Adrenergic drugs may be used in addition to fluid administration to restore adequate circulation to tissues. Adrenergic drugs may increase blood pressure (alpha effect), increase cardiac output (beta effect), or increase renal circulation (dopaminergic effect).

**CONTRAINDICATIONS**  **Vascular collapse** Although drugs with an alpha effect raise arterial pressure, they may further reduce circulation to the kidney and brain through their nonselective vasoconstriction.

**Table 5-1.** **A comparison of sympathomimetic agents (alpha and/or beta-1 adrenergic receptor agonists)**

| Agent | Alpha receptor | Beta receptor | Major therapeutic indications |
|---|---|---|---|
| Dobutamine | 0 | +D | Cardiogenic shock, severe congestive heart failure |
| Dopamine | (+)I | (+)I | Shock (to maintain renal flow), congestive heart failure |
| Ephedrine | +I, D | +I, D | Hypotension, heart block, nasal congestion |
| Epinephrine | +D | +D | Anaphylactic shock, acute asthma attacks, prolong local Anesthesia |
| Mephentermine | +I, D | +I, D | Hypotension |
| Metaraminol | +I, D | +I, D | Hypotension |
| Norepinephrine | +D | +D | Hypotension |
| Phenylephrine | +D | 0 | Local vasoconstrictor |

**KEY: +, Significant (effect); (+), modest effect; D, direct effect; I, indirect effect.**

**Coronary artery disease** Patients with coronary artery disease may have cardiac function worsen when an adrenergic drug with a beta effect is used. • The beta effect may increase cardiac work without increasing myocardial oxygen.

**DRUG INTERACTIONS** **Beta blockers and guanethedine** enhance the pressor response of the direct-acting adrenergic drugs. **Tricyclic antidepressants** potentiate the cardiac action of direct-acting adrenergic drugs. **Tricyclic antidepressants** antagonize the cardiac action of the indirect-acting adrenergic drugs. **Oxytocic drugs** may cause severe persistent hypertension in women treated with alpha adrenergic drugs.

## ❦ NURSING CONSIDERATIONS

### Side effects, toxicities, and associated nursing actions

**CV** An excessive rise in blood pressure and/or cardiac arrhythmias may be seen even at therapeutic doses.
- Monitor the blood pressure and pulse every 2 to 5 minutes until stable. Excessive increases should be reported to the physician, and the rate of infusion slowed.
- The patient should be attached to a cardiac monitor. Be alert for the development of or worsening of arrhythmias.
- Monitor the central venous pressure or pulmonary capillary wedge pressure if these measurements are available.

**GU** Renal function may deteriorate with inadequate perfusion or oxygenation.
- Monitor intake and output. Urinary output should be measured every 30 to 60 minutes. The physician should be notified if the urine output falls below 30 ml per hour.
- Monitor the patient's weight daily.

**CNS** Transient side effects may include anxiety, fear, apprehension, and palpitations. In addition, patients who become markedly hypotensive may be anxious as a response to inadequate oxygenation of the brain and may have a sense of "impending doom."
- Monitor the respiratory rate.
- Provide calm reassurance to patients.
- Keep patients and family members informed of changes in the treatment plan.
- Do not leave patients unattended.

**Nursing interventions related to drug administration**
- Microdrip tubing and an infusion control device or electronic infusion monitor should be used for IV infusions.
- These drugs should not be added to infusions containing other drugs or blood.

**Patient and family education**
- Alpha adrenergic drugs for shock would rarely be used outside of the intensive care setting and would not be used for home management by the patient, except when used with an inhaler for treatment of bronchospasm. See also Chapter 52 for this use.

---

## epinephrine (adrenaline)  (ep-i-NEF-rin)                    sympathomimetic

- epinephrine (OTC): Bronkaid, Primatene, Susphrine
- epinephrine bitartrate (OTC): AsthmaHaler, Brontin Mist, Bronkaid Mist, Medihaler-Epi, Primatene Mist Suspension
- epinephrine hydrochloride: Adrenalin Chloride Solution (OTC), EpiPen Jr
- racepinephrine hydrochloride: Asthma Nefrin (OTC), Breatheasy, Dey-Dose, microNefrin, Nephron Inhalant, Vaponefrin

**MECHANISM OF ACTION**    Epinephrine acts directly at both alpha and beta adrenergic receptors. The beta adrenergic actions result in an increase in the heart rate and force of contraction and a relaxation of smooth muscle, particularly the bronchi. Mean blood pressure does not usually change because the vasoconstrictive alpha effect is counterbalanced by the beta-2 vasodilating effect.

**INDICATIONS**    **Anaphylactic shock** Epinephrine is the treatment of choice.    **Acute asthmatic attacks and hypersensitivity reactions** Epinephrine relaxes the bronchioles and raises the blood pressure.    **To prolong the action of intraspinal and local anesthetics** The vasoconstriction caused by epinephrine reduces systemic absorption of the anesthetic.    **To stop nasal bleeding** The vasoconstriction reduces blood flow.    **Chronic (wide angle) glaucoma** See Chapter 62.

**CONTRAINDICATIONS**    • Acute (narrow angle) glaucoma. • Shock not caused by anaphylaxis. • Labor. • With local anesthetics in fingers or toes. • Coronary insufficiency. • Elderly patients and patients with hyperthyroidism, angina, hypertension, or diabetes: use with caution.

**DOSAGE**    **To prolong local anesthetic effect:**    *Adults and children:* 0.2 to 0.4 ml of 1:1000 solution intraspinal or 1:500,000 to 1:50,000 mixed with local anesthetic.    **To reverse cardiac arrest:**    *Adults:* IV OR IC: 0.5 to 1 mg (0.5 to 1 ml of 1:1000 solution).    *Children:*    IV OR IC: 5 to 10 μ/kg (0.05 to 0.1 ml of 1:10,000/kg).    **Bronchospasm or anaphylaxis:**    *Adults:*    IM OR SC: 0.1 to 0.5 mg (0.1 to 0.5 mg of a 1:1000 injection) initially. SC doses may be repeated at 10- to 15-minute intervals in patients with anaphylactic shock and at 20-minute to 4-hour intervals in patients with severe asthma. A single dose should not exceed 1 mg nor should a patient receive more than 5 mg in 24 hours.    IV: In severe anaphylactic shock, an initial IV dose of 0.1 to 0.25 mg (1 to 2.5 ml of a 1:10,000 dilution) may be given over 5 to 10 minutes. This may be repeated in 5 to 15 minutes if necessary or may be followed by a continuous IV infusion of 1 μg/kg/min. This rate may be increased if necessary to a maximum of 4 μg/kg/min.    *Children:*    IM or SC: 0.01 mg/kg (0.01 ml/kg of a 1:1000 injection) or 0.3 mg/M$^2$ (0.3 ml/M$^2$ of a 1:1000 injection). A single dose should not exceed 0.5 mg. Repeat at 20-minute to 4-hour intervals, depending on the response. Alternatively, for a prolonged response, the 1:200 aqueous suspension is used in a single dose of 0.02 to 0.025 mg/kg (0.004 to 0.005 ml/kg) or 0.625 mg/M$^2$ (0.125 ml/M$^2$). The dose is repeated in 6 hours if necessary. A single dose should not exceed 0.75 mg in a child weighing less than 30 kg.    IV: In severe anaphylactic shock, an initial IV dose of 0.1 mg (10 ml of a 1:100,000 dilution) may be given over 5 to 10 minutes followed by a continuous IV infusion of 0.1 μg/kg/min. This rate may be increased if necessary to a maximum of 1.5 μg/kg/min.    **Oral inhalation as a bronchodilator:**    ADULTS AND CHILDREN: One inhalation via a metered aerosol (160 to 250 μg) repeated in 1 minute if necessary. Repeat after 4 hours if necessary. A hand-held nebulizer may be used to administer a solution of 1% epinephrine hydrochloride or 2.25%

racepinephrine hydrochloride. The dose is 1 or 2 deep inhalations repeated in 1 to 2 minutes if necessary. An IPPB apparatus may also be used to administer 0.03 ml (0.3 mg) of a 1% solution. **Topical hemostat:** ADULTS AND CHILDREN: A 0.002% (1:50,000) to 0.1% (1:1000) solution may be sprayed or applied to the skin, mucous membranes, or other tissues. *Special patient populations:* ELDERLY: Elderly patients are sensitive to the arrhythmic properties of epinephrine. PREGNANCY: Epinephrine is contraindicated during labor.

**PREPARATIONS**  Epinephrine: *suspension:* 1:200 (5 mg/ml); *aerosol:* 200, 250 μg per metered spray. Epinephrine hydrochloride: *solution (nebulization):* 1% (1:100); *solution (injection):* 0.1% (1:10,000), 0.5% (1:2000), 1% (1:1000) mg/ml. Racepinephrine hydrochloride: *solution (nebulization):* 1.83%, 2.25%. Protect solution from light, heat, and freezing. Do not use the solution if brown or if a precipitate is present. Solution should be clear, seal intact. The recommended diluent is 0.9% sodium chloride. Discard unused portion.

**DRUG INTERACTIONS**  **Other sympathomimetic drugs** administered concurrently with epinephrine will likely give additive effects and increased toxicity, especially serious cardiac arrhythmias.  **Digitalis, mercurial diuretics, and the anesthetics halothane and enflurane** are additional drugs that may sensitize the heart to arrhythmias.  **Tricyclic antidepressants, l-thyroxine, and antihistamines, especially diphenhydramine, tripelennamine, and chlorpheniramine** potentiate epinephrine.  **Propranolol and other beta blockers** may cause hypertension with epinephrine by blocking the beta adrenergic effects and thereby accentuating the alpha adrenergic effects.  **MAO inhibitors** place patients at risk for a persistent hypertensive response to epinephrine.  **Oxytocic drugs** should not be used in labor if epinephrine has been used to correct hypotension or in local anesthetic solutions because a severe and persistent hypertension may develop.  **Nitrites and alpha adrenergic blockers (phenoxybenzamine, phentolamine, prazosin, labetolol, trimazosin)** are vasodilators that counteract the vasopressive response to epinephrine.  **Guanethidine and guanadrel** Epinephrine can bypass the blockade of neuronal release of norepinephrine and thereby diminish the antihypertensive action of these drugs. **Alkalies and oxidizing agents such as reducible metals (especially iron), nitrites, chromates, permanganates, iodine, chlorine, bromine, and oxygen** are agents that destroy epinephrine.

**FATE**  Epinephrine is rapidly inactivated by the enzymes MAO and catechol-0-methyltransferase. Metabolites are further modified and conjugated as a sulfate or glucuronide for excretion in the urine. The urinary metabolite of epinephrine and other catecholamines is vanillylmandelic acid (VMA).

## ❦ NURSING CONSIDERATIONS

### Side effects, toxicities, and associated nursing actions
- See entry for drug class (p. 29).

**CNS** Transient and usually minor side effects include anxiety, fear, headache, or palpitations. Restlessness, throbbing headache, tremor, weakness, dizziness, pallor, and sweating are side effects that can be more severe. Nausea and vomiting can occur. Individuals with hyperthyroidism or hypertension are more prone to side effects

- The appearance of generalized side effects to an excessive degree (e.g., restlessness, dizziness, sweating, vomiting) may require a reduction in drug dosage or a switch to another drug. Notify the physician.
- Monitor blood glucose levels. Diabetic patients may require an adjustment in insulin dosage.

**CV** An excessive rise in blood pressure and/or cardiac arrhythmias may be seen even at therapeutic doses.

- See entry for drug class (p. 29).

**Other** Necrosis can result at sites of local injection of epinephrine.

- As with all injections, use aseptic technique to prevent contamination. Inspect injection sites carefully before use. Record and rotate injection sites.

### Nursing interventions related to drug administration
- Read labels carefully. Epinephrine preparations vary in strength. Not all preparations are safe for IV use.
- Use a tuberculin syringe for accurate measurement of small doses.
- For accidental overdosage or excessive hypertension, reduce the rate of infusion and notify the physician. In extreme cases, phentolamine, an alpha adrenergic blocking drug, or nitroprusside may be administered intravenously.

- Necrosis secondary to vasoconstriction can result at sites of local injection of epinephrine. Inspect IV infusion sites carefully for extravasation. If the drug is prescribed subcutaneously (as for anaphylaxis), inspect the injection site carefully for signs of necrosis.
- The rate of drug absorption from the injection site may be increased by massaging the site; in an emergency situation this may be desirable.

**Patient and family education**
- Selected patients with a history of anaphylactic reactions to identified allergens are appropriate candidates to be taught how to self-administer epinephrine. The patient and at least one family member should be taught how to prepare the correct dose or prepare the prepackaged syringe and administer the prescribed dose.

## mephentermine sulfate    (me-FEN-ter-meen)              sympathomimetic

- mephentermine sulfate: Wyamine Sulfate

**MECHANISM OF ACTION**    Mephentermine is an indirect-acting sympathomimetic amine, releasing norepinephrine to act primarily on alpha receptors and cardiac beta receptors. The overall effects are an increase in blood pressure, heart rate, and cadiac output.

**INDICATIONS** • Hypotension occurring with spinal anesthesia.

**CONTRAINDICATIONS** • Hypersensitivity. • Patients taking MAO inhibitors. • Hypotension caused by chlorpromazine.

**DOSAGE**    **Adults:**    **IM:** 30 to 45 mg. Onset of action is 10 to 20 minutes.    **IV:** 30 to 45 mg as a single injection or as an infusion of a 0.1% solution in 5% dextrose. To prepare the dilution, 20 ml of mephentermine (30 mg/ml) is added to 500 ml of 5% dextrose solution (actual concentration is 0.115%).    **Children:** **IM:** 0.4 mg/kg.    *Special patient populations:*    **ELDERLY:** Use with caution. Mephentermine may produce arrhythmias, AV block, or hypertension; the elderly are more sensitive to these effects. **PREGNANCY:** Safe use during pregnancy has not been established. Use with caution because of the possibility of causing fetal anoxia.

**PREPARATIONS**    *Solution (injection):* 15, 30 mg/ml.

**DRUG INTERACTIONS**    **Reserpine and guanethidine** may render therapy with mephentermine ineffective because these drugs deplete or inhibit norepinephrine stores.    **Digitalis, mercurial diuretics, or the halogenated anesthetics halothane and enflurane** may sensitize the heart to catecholamines, precipitating arrhythmias.    **Oxytocic drugs** A severe hypertensive response occurs when administered with mephentermine.    **MAO inhibitors** Patients are at risk for a persistent hypertensive response to mephentermine.    **Beta adrenergic blocking drugs** Mephentermine may reverse their effects.

**FATE**    Mephentermine is metabolized by the liver and excreted in the urine. An acidic urine increases the excretion of mephentermine.

## ❦ NURSING CONSIDERATIONS

**Side effects, toxicities, and associated nursing actions**    Side effects are minimum.

**CNS** Euphoria, nervousness, anxiety.

**CV** Cardiac stimulation (arrhythmias).

- See entry for drug class (p. 29).

**Patient and family education**
- See entry for drug class (p. 30).

## metaraminol bitartrate    (met-a-RAM-i-nole)              sympathomimetic

- metaraminol bitartrate: Aramine

**MECHANISM OF ACTION**   Metaraminol has both a direct effect, stimulating alpha adrenergic receptors, and an indirect effect, causing the release of stored norepinephrine. Metaraminol causes an increase in blood pressure, which causes a reflex slowing of the heart rate. These overall effects on heart rate and blood pressure are similar to those produced by norepinephrine but are more gradual in onset and longer in duration.

**INDICATIONS**   **Hypotension** Prevention and treatment of hypotension with spinal anesthesia and as adjunctive treatment when hypotension is caused by hemorrhage, medication reaction, surgical complications, and brain damage.   **Paroxysmal atrial tachycardia (PAT).**

**CONTRAINDICATIONS**   **Myocardial infarction, other heart disease, or hyperthyroidism** Patients may be especially prone to developing cardiac arrhythmias with metaraminol.   **Hypertension** Patients may be at risk for hypertensive episodes, especially because the effects of metaraminol are cumulative.

**DOSAGE**   **Adults:**   **IM OR SC:** 2 to 10 mg.   **IV INFUSION:** 15 to 100 mg in 500 ml sodium chloride or 5% dextrose, with infusion rate adjusted to maintain blood pressure.   **IV INJECTION:** 0.5 to 5 mg, followed by IV infusion, as above.   **Children:**   **IM OR SC:** 0.1 mg/kg.   **IV INFUSION:** A solution of 4 mg/100 ml 5% dextrose is infused to maintain blood pressure. Alternatively, begin with 5 $\mu$g/kg/min. Infusion rate can be calculated as follows: dilute 15 mg $\times$ wt (kg) in 250 ml 5% dextrose. Rate of infusion in $\mu$g/kg/min = rate in ml/hr.   **IV INJECTION:** 0.01 mg/kg.   *Special patient populations:*   **ELDERLY:** Use with caution. Mephentermine may produce arrhythmias, AV block, or hypertension; the elderly are more sensitive to these effects.   **PREGNANCY:** Safe use during pregnancy has not been established. May increase uterine contractions during the last trimester. Use with caution.

**PREPARATIONS**   *Parenteral:* 1% in 1 or 10 ml containers.

**DRUG INTERACTIONS**   **Digitalis, mercurial diuretics, or the anesthetics halothane and enflurane** may sensitize the heart to arrhythmias.   **Oxytocic drugs** may contribute to a severe hypertensive response when administered with metaraminol.   **MAO inhibitors** increase the risk for a persistent hypertensive response to metaraminol.   **Beta adrenergic blocking drugs** may be reversed by metaraminol.

**FATE**   *Onset* of action depends on the route of administration: 1 to 2 minutes IV, 10 minutes IM, 5 to 20 minutes SC. *Duration* of action varies from 20 to 90 minutes. Metaraminol is a noncatecholamine. Although the metabolism of metaraminol is not well characterized, noncatecholamines are not extensively metabolized and are excreted to a large degree unchanged in the urine.

## ☙ NURSING CONSIDERATIONS

### Side effects, toxicities, and associated nursing actions

- See entry for drug class (p. 29).

**CNS**   General side effects are those characteristic of sympathomimetic amines: headache, flushing, sweating, tremors, dizziness, nausea, and apprehension. Overdose may cause convulsions, cerebral hemorrhage, or cardiac arrhythmias.

**CV**   Sympathomimetic amines may cause arrhythmias, especially in patients with myocardial infarction.

**Other**   Because metaraminol acts primarily by releasing norepinephrine stores, repeated use may result in a decrease in sympathetic activity because of depletion of the neurotransmitter.

- Continue to monitor vital signs and blood pressure carefully throughout therapy with metaraminol.

### Nursing interventions related to drug administration

- Avoid extravasation; tissue necrosis and sloughing may occur. Ascertain that IV line is patent before administering. Inspect IV line and insertion site at regular intervals for redness, swelling, and signs of infiltration such as slowed infusion. If IV line has infiltrated, remove and restart in another vein.
- For accidental overdosage or excessive hypertension, reduce the rate of infusion and notify the physician. In extreme cases, an intravenous antihypertensive agent such as nitroprusside may be needed.

### Patient and family education

- See entry for drug class (p. 30).

---

## norepinephrine bitartrate   (nor-ep-i-NEF-rin)       sympathomimetic

- norepinephrine bitartate (noradrenaline, levarterenol): Levophed

**MECHANISM OF ACTION**   Norepinephrine is the naturally occurring sympathetic neurotransmitter. The primary effects seen after administration of a therapeutic dose of norepinephrine are (1) marked increase in blood pressure as a result of the increased peripheral resistance caused by vasoconstriction and (2) slowing of the heart rate as a result of the reflex vagal stimulation triggered by the increased blood pressure.

Because norepinephrine activates the beta receptors of the heart, the heart beat is strong (positive inotropic effect), although the expected beta adrenergic–mediated increase in heart rate is overcome by the reflex vagal stimulation. Cardiac arrhythmias may result from the increased conductivity (positive dromotropic effect) associated with beta adrenergic stimulation.

**INDICATIONS**   • Acute hypotensive states.

**CONTRAINDICATIONS**   **Poor tissue perfusion** as caused by blood volume depletion, severe peripheral or visceral vasoconstriction, decreased renal blood flow, or poor systemic blood flow.   **Thrombi** Particularly mesenteric or peripheral vascular thrombosis.   **Sensitization to arrhythmias** Halothane or enflurane anesthesia or patients with profound hypoxia, situations that predispose the heart to arrhythmias.

**DOSAGE**   **Adults:**   IV INFUSION: 2 to 3 ml/min of a 0.4 mg/100 ml solution and adjust rate to maintain a low normal blood pressure (80 to 100 mm Hg systolic). The solution is prepared by diluting a 4 ml ampule containing 4 mg into 1000 ml of a 5 percent dextrose solution.   **Children:**   IV DRIP: 0.1 μg/kg/min initially, titrate to attain desired perfusion. To calculate the rate: dilute 1.5 mg × wt (kg) in 250 ml 5 percent dextrose. Rate of infusion in μg/kg/min = 0.1 × rate in ml/hr.   *Special patient populations:* PREGNANCY: Safe use has not been established. A sympathomimetic drug may cause fetal anoxia.

**PREPARATIONS**   *Parenteral*: 1 mg/ml in 4 ml ampules. Store in a light–resistant container. Do not use discolored or precipitated solutions. Discard unused diluted solution.

**DRUG INTERACTIONS**   **Furosemide and thiazide diuretics** may diminish the effectiveness of norepinephrine to stimulate vasoconstriction.   **Guanethedine, reserpine, MAO inhibitors, or tricyclic antidepressants** may cause a prolonged hypertensive response because these drugs interfere with the reuptake of norepinephrine into neurons.   **Oxytocic drugs** may cause a severe hypertensive response.   **Digitalis, mercurial diuretics, or the halogenated anesthetics halothane and enflurane** may sensitize the heart to arrhythmias.   **Beta adrenergic blocking drugs** Effects may be reversed by norepinephrine.

**FATE**   Norepinephrine is rapidly metabolized by the enzymes MAO and catechol-O-methyltransferase, so norepinephrine must be continuously infused for proper effects.

☙ **NURSING CONSIDERATIONS**

**Side effects, toxicities, and associated nursing actions**

**CV** Slowing of the heart rate (bradycardia) may result from a vagal reflex if the increase in blood pressure is pronounced. Overdosage results in severe hypotension, reflex slowing of the heart rate, a marked increase in peripheral resistance, and a decreased cardiac output.

• See entry for drug class (p. 29).

**Patient and family education**

• See entry for drug class (p. 30).

---

# phenylephrine hydrochloride   (fen-ill-EF-rin)   sympathomimetic

• phenylephrine hydrochloride: Neo-synephrine (OTC), ♣Mydfrine

**MECHANISM OF ACTION**   Phenylephrine acts primarily at alpha-1 receptors with little effect at other adrenergic receptors. The predominant effect of phenylephrine administered systemically is a profound vasoconstriction that causes a rise in blood pressure. This pressor response can trigger reflex bradycardia. There is no direct effect on the heart to increase force or rate of contraction.

**INDICATIONS**   **Local vasoconstrictor** Phenylephrine is infused with a local anesthetic to prolong anesthesia by depressing its systemic absorption.   **Shock** Phenylephrine may be used to treat vascular failure in shock or shocklike states in which there is no blood loss, as in drug-induced hypotension, hypersensitivity reactions, or during spinal or general anesthesia.

**CONTRAINDICATIONS** • Hypersensitivity. • Severe hypertension. • Ventricular tachycardia. • Cardiac or vascular disease: Use with caution in patients with hyperthyroidism, slow heart rate, partial heart block, myocardial disease, or atherosclerosis. • Labor and delivery: may cause severe hypertension if used with oxytocin.

**DOSAGE** **Mild or moderate hypotension:** *Adults:* SC OR IM: Initial dose should be no more than 5 mg. The IM dose raises blood pressure for 1 to 2 hours. Thereafter, 1 to 10 mg, usually 2 to 5 mg. IV: Usual dose is 0.2 mg, range 0.1 to 0.5 mg. Injection should raise blood pressure for 15 minutes: do not repeat more often. *Children:* IV: 0.1 or 3 mg/M$^2$ initially; additional doses may be given in 1 to 2 hours if needed. **Severe hypotension and shock:** *Adults and children:* CONTINUOUS INFUSION: 10 mg is diluted to 500 ml with 5 percent dextrose or 0.9% sodium chloride solution. Infusion is begun at 100 to 180 drops/min and reduced to 40 to 60 drops/min when the blood pressure has stabilized to a low normal value. If a prompt increase in blood pressure is not obtained initially, the dose may be doubled by adding another 10 mg to the infusion bottle. **Hypotension of spinal anesthesia:** *Adults:* SC OR IM: 2 or 3 mg is injected 3 or 4 minutes before the spinal anesthetic is administered. *Children: SC or IM:* 0.5 to 1 mg/25 lb. **Prolongation of spinal anesthesia:** Two to 5 mg is added to the anesthetic solution. This usually doubles the duration of action of the local anesthetic. **Prolongation of regional anesthesia** One mg is added to 20 ml of the local anesthetic. *Special patient populations:* ELDERLY: Use with caution. Elderly patients are more likely to have cardiac or vascular disease, which are contraindications for phenylephrine use. PREGNANCY: May cause severe hypertension if used with oxytocin during labor and delivery.

**PREPARATIONS** *Parenteral:* 1% (10 mg/ml) in 1 ml ampules. Phenylephrine is also included as a decongestant in many oral combination drugs. These combination drugs are discussed in Chapter 53.

**FATE** Phenylephrine is not a catecholamine and is longer acting than epinephrine or norepinephrine. Phenylephrine does not readily cross the blood-brain barrier to act in the CNS. *Onset* of action is immediate with IV administration and 10 to 15 minutes after IM or SC drugs. *Duration* of action is 15 to 20 minutes after IV administration, 30 minutes to 2 hours after IM administration, and about 1 hour after SC administration.

**DRUG INTERACTIONS** **Halogenated hydrocarbon anesthetics enflurane and halothane** may cause cardiac arrhythmias when used with phenylephrine. **Oxytocin** may cause serious, persistent hypertension if used with phenylephrine **MAO inhibitors or tricylcic antidepressants** may potentiate phenylephrine. **Digitalis and beta adrenergic blocking drugs guanethidine or reserpine** may cause arrhythmias if administered with phenylephrine.

☙ **NURSING CONSIDERATIONS**

**Side effects, toxicities, and associated nursing actions**

**CNS** Headache, excitability, and restlessness.

**CV** Reflex bradycardia; rarely, arrhythmias.

• See entry for drug class (p. 29).

**Patient and family education**

• See entry for drug class (p. 30).

---

# Beta-1 adrenergic agonists

dobutamine ~ dopamine ~ ephedrine ~ (isoproterenol—see Chapter 52)

**OVERVIEW OF THE DRUG CLASS** Beta-1 adrenergic receptors mediate cardiac and metabolic effects. The pharmacologic use of beta-1 adrenergic agonists (drugs that stimulate the beta-1 adrenergic receptor) is to stimulate cardiac function. These drugs increase the force of contraction so that cardiac output increases. Blood flow to all organs is improved. A benefit in congestive heart failure is the improved blood flow to the kidneys, increasing urine production and aiding the clearance of edema. In addition to increasing the force of contraction (positive inotropic effect), other beta-1 cardiac effects include increased heart rate (positive chronotropic effect) and increased excitability.

In addition to beta-1 adrenergic effects, the beta-1 agonists frequently have beta-2, alpha-1, and/or dopaminergic agonist effects. Table 5-1 compares the sympathomimetic drugs. Stimulation of alpha-1 receptors in the vasculature causes vasoconstriction and elevated blood pressure. Stimulation of beta-2 receptors relaxes smooth muscle in various tissues. Isoproterenol and other drugs that are beta-2 adrenergic agonists are widely used for bronchiole dilation in the treatment of asthma and other respiratory diseases (see Chapter 52). Cardiovascular dopaminergic receptors are found principally in the renal vasculature. Stimulation of these dopaminergic receptors dilates the renal blood vessels, improving blood flow through the kidney. This is a desirable action in treating shock because it prevents kidney failure.

**MECHANISM OF ACTION**   Stimulation of the beta-1 class of adrenergic receptors activates adenylate cyclase, thereby increasing accumulation of cyclic AMP within cells. In the heart, cyclic AMP promotes the accumulation of the calcium required for contraction. As a result, cardiac contractility and rate are increased.

**INDICATIONS**   **Shock** Adrenergic drugs may be used in addition to fluid administration to restore adequate circulation to tissues. • Adrenergic drugs may increase blood pressure (alpha effect), increase cardiac output (beta effect), or increase renal circulation (dopaminergic effect).   **Congestive heart failure** The increased cardiac contractility and improved blood flow may be beneficial.   **Inotropic support after heart surgery.**

**CONTRAINDICATIONS**   **Coronary artery disease** The beta effect may increase cardiac work without increasing myocardial oxygen. Cardiac function may worsen in patients with coronary artery disease.   **Arrhythmias** Beta-1 agonists may exacerbate certain arrhythmias.   **Hypertension** These drugs can increase blood pressure.

**DRUG INTERACTIONS**   **Alpha-blockers, MAO inhibitors, sympathomimetics, diuretics, digitalis glycosides, and reserpine** can interact with the beta-1 agonists. See individual drug listings.   **Beta blockers** may prevent the cardiac actions of beta-1 agonists.   **Tricyclic antidepressants** potentiate the cardiac actions of drugs with beta-1 adrenergic activity and cause unacceptable high blood pressure from drugs with alpha adrenergic activity.   **Halogenated hydrocarbon anesthetics enflurane and halothane** sensitize the heart to the adrenergic action of dopamine. Cardiac arrhythmias may result.

## ☙ NURSING CONSIDERATIONS

### Side effects, toxicities, and associated nursing actions

**CV** Systolic blood pressure may rise excessively. Cardiac arrhythmias may be precipitated.
- Monitor the blood pressure every 2 to 5 minutes for IV preparations and every 15 minutes for oral preparations until blood pressure stabilizes. A rise of 10 to 20 mm Hg in systolic pressure is to be expected. Excessive increases should be reported to the physician, and the rate of IV infusion slowed.
- The patient should be attached to a cardiac monitor. Be alert for the development of or worsening of arrhythmias.
- Monitor the central venous pressure or pulmonary capillary wedge pressure if these measurements are available.
- Monitor the pulse when monitoring the blood pressure. An increase of 5 to 10 beats/min should be expected.
- The appearance of chest pain, arrhythmias, or shortness of breath requires medical evaluation.

**GU** The effects of renal function vary with the drug and the dose.
- Monitor the intake and output. Urinary output should be measured every 30 to 60 minutes. The physician should be notified if the urine output falls below 30 ml/hr.
- Monitor the weight daily.

**Other** Side effects such as anxiety, apprehension, and fear may result from the patient's emotional state, hypotension and associated decreased oxygenation of the brain, or the effects of the drug.
- Monitor the respiratory rate.
- Provide calm reassurance to patients.
- Keep patients and family members informed of changes in the treatment plan.
- Do not leave patients unattended.

### Nursing interventions related to drug administration
- Microdrip tubing and an infusion control device or electronic infusion monitor should be used for IV infusions.

- These drugs should not be added to infusions containing other drugs or blood.

**Patient and family education**
- When used for congestive heart failure or shock, these drugs are used only in the intensive care setting and are not used for home management by the patient.
- Keep the patient and family informed of changes in the patient's condition and treatment plan.

---

## dobutamine hydrochloride (doe-BYOO-ta-meen)    sympathomimetic

- dobutamine hydrochloride: Dobutrex

**MECHANISM OF ACTION**   Dobutamine acts primarily on myocardial beta-1 receptors. Dobutamine has little action on alpha receptors and no action on dopaminergic receptors. The overall effect of dobutamine is to improve cardiac output, accompanied by a modest increase in heart rate and blood pressure.

**INDICATIONS**   **Cardiogenic shock** Dobutamine supports cardiac and renal function.   **Chronic congestive heart failure** Dobutamine may be used intravenously for short-term improvement of cardiac output in severely ill patients.   **Cardiac surgery** Dobutamine may be used in the immediate postoperative period to improve contractility and cardiac output.

**CONTRAINDICATIONS**   **Idiopathic hypertrophic subaortic stenosis.**   **Atrial fibrillation** This arrhythmia may be converted to ventricular tachycardia because dobutamine improves AV conduction.   **Hypertension** Patient may have an exaggerated hypertensive response to dobutamine.   **Ventricular arrhythmias** Dobutamine is potentially dangerous to patients recovering from myocardial infarction because ventricular arrhythmias may be exacerbated.

**DOSAGE**   **Adults:**   IV INFUSION: 2.5 to 10 $\mu$g/kg/min. An infusion pump is used to adjust and control the rate of infusion. The rate is adjusted according to the response of the patient as indicated by the heart rate, blood pressure, urine flow, and presence of ectopic heartbeats. In facilities where central venous or pulmonary capillary wedge pressure and cardiac output can be monitored, these parameters are also used to adjust the rate of drug infusion.   **Children:**   IV INFUSION: 2.5 to 15 $\mu$g/kg/min. Rate can be calculated by the following: dilute 15 mg $\times$ wt (kg) in 250 ml 5% dextrose or normal saline solution. The rate of infusion in $\mu$g/kg/min = rate in ml/hr.   *Special patient populations:*   ELDERLY: Use with caution. Elderly patients are more likely to have cardiovascular disease. See Contraindications. PREGNANCY: Safe use has not been established. Use with caution.

**PREPARATIONS**   *Powder:* 250 mg vial. This is first diluted with 10 ml sterile water of 5% dextrose solution to dissolve the drug, and then to at least 50 ml (final concentration 5000 $\mu$g/ml). A final volume of 250 ml gives a concentration of 1000 $\mu$g/ml; 500 ml gives 500 $\mu$g/ml. The IV solution is stable for only 24 hours but should be discarded earlier if it is discolored or has a precipitate.

**DRUG INTERACTIONS**   **Nitroprusside** combined with dobutamine produces a higher cardiac output and a lower right ventricular (pulmonary wedge) pressure than either drug alone.   **Insulin** requirement may be increased for diabetics.   **General anesthetics** particularly the halogenated hydrocarbons halothane and enflurane sensitize the heart so that dobutamine may cause serious arrhythmias.   **Beta-blockers** may prevent the desired action of dobutamine on the heart.   **MAO inhibitors, tricyclic antidepressants, and oxytocic agents** may intensify the pressor effects of dobutamine to cause dangerous hypertension.

**FATE**   Rapidly metabolized to inactive compunds excreted in the urine. *Onset:* 1 to 2 minutes. *Peak:* 10 minutes. *Half-life:* 1 to 2 minutes.

### 🐾 NURSING CONSIDERATIONS

**Side effects, toxicities, and associated nursing actions**
- See entry for drug class (p. 36).

**CV** An increase in systolic pressure (10 to 20 mm Hg) and heart rate (5 to 15 beats/min) are usual. Nausea, headache, anginal pain, palpitations, or shortness of breath are experienced by 1% to 3% of patients.
- Monitor the blood glucose. Diabetics may need a change in insulin dosage.
- See entry for drug class (p. 36).

**Patient and family education**
• See entry for drug class (p. 37).

# dopamine hydrochloride   (DOE-pa-meen)                    sympathomimetic

• dopamine hydrochloride: Dopastat, Intropin, ✤Revimine

**MECHANISM OF ACTION**   Dopamine has dopaminergic, beta adrenergic, and alpha adrenergic actions. These effects are dose dependent. At small doses, 5 µg/kg/min or less, the effects are primarily dopaminergic, dilating the renal and splanchnic blood vessels. This maintains kidney function. At doses of 5 to 10 µg/kg/min, dopamine activates cardiac beta receptors to increase myocardial contractility. Doses greater than 20 µg/kg/min activate alpha receptors to increase peripheral resistance and thereby increase blood pressure.

**INDICATIONS**   **Shock** Maintenance of renal function and cardiac output in shock resulting from myocardial infarction, trauma, septicemia, open heart surgery, renal failure, or cardiac decompensation.   **Congestive heart failure** Improves cardiac output in patients with severe, refractory congestive heart failure. Peripheral vasoconstriction may increase blood pressure, which makes the drug especially useful in patients whose congestive heart failure is accompanied by hypotension.   **Cardiac surgery** Used postoperatively to increase cardiac output and support renal function.

**CONTRAINDICATIONS**   **Pheochromocytoma** Patients with this catecholamine-secreting tumor already suffer from an excess of catecholamines.   **Tachyarrythmias or ventricular fibrillation.**   **Occlusive vascular diseases** Circulation may be compromised by further vasoconstriction in patients with atherosclerosis, arterial embolism, Raynaud's disease, frostbite, diabetic endarteritis, or Buerger's disease.

**DOSAGE**   **Adults and children:**   IV INFUSION: 1 to 5 µg/kg/min is the usual initial rate of infusion. This is increased in increments of 1 to 4 µg/kg/min every 10 to 30 minutes until the desired response is obtained. Usual infusion rates are 20 to 50 µg/kg/min. An infusion pump is used to control and adjust the rate of flow.   *Special patient populations:*   ELDERLY: Use with caution. Elderly patients are more likely to have cardiovascular disease. See Contraindications.   PREGNANCY: Safe use has not been established. Use with caution.

**PREPARATIONS**   *Solution:* 40, 80, or 160 mg/ml in 5 ml vials. These are diluted with sterile sodium chloride solution or 5% dextrose solution for infusion. A 5 ml vial of 40 mg/ml (200 mg) diluted to 250 ml gives a concentration of 800 µg/ml; diluted to 500 ml gives a concentration of 400 µg/ml. Solutions or vials that are pink or violet should be discarded. Protect from light.

**DRUG INTERACTIONS**   See drug interactions characteristic of adrenergic drugs (p. 36).   **MAO inhibitors** Patients taking these need only 10% of the usual dose of dopamine. MAO inhibitors significantly reduce the metabolism of dopamine.   **Diuretics** may be potentiated by dopamine.   **Phenytoin** may cause seizures, hypotension, and slow heart rate when dopamine is also infused.

**FATE**   Dopamine is rapidly metabolized by MAO to an inactive metaboilte. *Onset:* 10 minutes. *Duration:* 10 minutes.

## ❦ NURSING CONSIDERATIONS

### Side effects, toxicities, and associated nursing actions
• See entry for drug class (p. 36).
**CNS** Headaches.
**CV** Ectopic heart beats, tachycardia, palpitations, anginal pain, and vasoconstriction. High doses can produce an excessively high blood pressure and constrict rather than dilate renal blood vessels.
**Respiratory** Difficulty in breathing.
• Monitor respiratory rate. Auscultate lung sounds.

### Nursing interventions related to drug administration
• For accidental overdosage or excessive hypertension, reduce the rate of infusion and notify the physician. In extreme cases, phentolamine, an alpha adrenergic blocking agent, may be administered intravenously.

• Avoid extravasation, which can cause tissue necrosis and sloughing. If extravasation occurs, infiltrate the area with subcutaneous injection of 5 to 10 mg of phentolamine diluted in 10 to 15 ml of normal saline solution. Notify the physician.

**Patient and family education**
• See entry for drug class (p. 37).

## ephedrine    (e-FED-rin)    sympathomimetic

- ephedrine: Same as generic
- ephedrine hydrochloride: Efedron
- ephedrine sulfate: Ectasule, Ephedsol, Vatronol

**MECHANISM OF ACTION**    Ephedrine acts as both a direct-acting and an indirect-acting adrenergic drug. As a direct-acting drug, ephedrine increases myocardial contractility, heart rate, and peripheral vascular resistance. As an indirect-acting drug, ephedrine releases norepinephrine from tissue stores. Ephedrine also produces CNS stimulation.

**INDICATIONS**    • Acute hypotension or spinal anesthesia. • Stokes-Adams syndrome with heart block: to increase ventricular rate. • CNS stimulant for narcolepsy. • Acute bronchospasm. • Nasal congestion. • Urinary incontinence.

**CONTRAINDICATIONS**    • Hypersensitivity. • Acute (closed angle) glaucoma. • Severe coronary artery disease, angina, or cardiac arrhythmias. • Hypertension or hyperthyroidism: may cause excessive pressor effects. • Prostate hypertrophy: may cause urinary retention.

**DOSAGE**    For orthostatic hypotension: *Adults:* IV, IM, SC: 25 mg, 1 to 4 times daily. *Children:* IM, SC: 3 mg/kg daily, divided into 4 to 6 doses. **As a bronchodilator or nasal decongestant:** *Adults:* PO: 25 to 50 mg every 3 or 4 hours. Alternatively, an extended-release preparation containing 15, 30, or 60 mg may be given every 8 to 12 hours. *Children:* PO: 2 to 3 mg/kg or 100 mg/M$^2$ in 4 to 6 divided doses daily. **To relieve severe, acute bronchospasm:** *Adults and children:* IM OR SC: 12.5 to 25 mg. **Nasal decongestion:** *Adults and children:* TOPICAL: Drops of a 0.5% to 1% solution every 4 hours. *Special patient populations:* ELDERLY: Elderly patients may be more sensitive to catecholamines. Use with caution. See Contraindications. PREGNANCY: Safe use has not been established. Do not use with oxytocic drugs during labor.

**PREPARATIONS**    Ephedrine hydrochloride: *nasal jelly:* 0.6%. Ephedrine sulfate: *nasal solution:* 0.5, 1%; *parenteral:* 25 mg/ml and 50 mg/ml; *capsules:* 25 and 50 mg; *extended-release capsules:* 15, 30, and 60 mg; *syrup:* 11 mg/5 ml and 20 mg/5 ml. The syrup contains alcohol. Ephedrine can oxidize and turn color. Protect against exposure to light and use only clear solutions. Discard unused portion. Ephedrine sulfate is widely used in combination with other drugs for the relief of colds and hay fever. These combination drugs are discussed in Chapter 53.

**DRUG INTERACTIONS**    See drug interactions characteristic of adrenergic drugs (p. 36). **Digitalis glycosides** sensitize the heart to sympathomimetic agents. **Alpha adrenergic blockers** reduce the hypotensive response. **Reserpine and methyldopa** may reduce the vasopressive action of ephedrine by depressing the amount of norepinephrine in nerve endings. **Guanethidine** The antihypertensive action is competitively blocked by ephedrine.

**FATE**    *Onset* within 1 hour after oral administration; *duration* about 4 hours. Not readily metabolized. Excreted largely unchanged in urine.

## 🐦 NURSING CONSIDERATIONS

**Side effects, toxicities, and associated nursing actions**

**CNS** Insomnia, headaches, nervousness, confusion, restlessness, delirium, anxiety, dizziness, and hallucinations. Irritability, suicidal behavior, personality changes, and convulsions are characteristic of toxic levels of ephedrine. Chronic use of ephedrine can cause tension and anxiety leading to psychosis.
• Perform careful mental status examination before therapy and repeat at regular intervals.

- Assess for signs of depression: withdrawal, lack of interest in personal appearance, insomnia, and anorexia.
- Caution patients to avoid driving or operating hazardous equipment until the effects of the medication can be evaluated.

**CV** Palpitations, tachycardia (fast heart rate), pain, and arrhythmias are occasionally experienced.
- See entry for drug class (p. 36).
- If this drug is given orally, changes in blood pressure and cardiac function usually occur more slowly than with IV preparations.

**GI** Nausea, vomiting, loss of appetite.
- Monitor weight.
- If GI symptoms are severe or persistent, notify physician.
- Review with patient the dosing schedule being followed. Patients may be inadvertently overdosing themselves to treat nasal congestion or other health problems.

**GU** Urination difficult or painful, especially in men with prostatic hypertrophy.
- Be especially alert for urinary retention in elderly men. Monitor intake and output. Instruct patients to report difficulty voiding or sense of incomplete emptying of the bladder.

**Patient and family education**
- See entry for drug class (p. 37).
- For a discussion of drugs used as nasal decongestants or to treat bronchospasm, see Chapters 52 and 53.

## Beta adrenergic blockers

acebutolol ~ atenolol ~ esmolol ~ metoprolol ~ nadolol ~ pindolol ~ propranolol ~ timolol

**DRUG COMBINATIONS**
- atenolol and chlorthalidone: Tenorectic.
- metoprolol and hydrochlorothiazide: Lopressor HCT.
- nadolol and bendroflumethiazide: Corzide.
- propranolol and hydrochlorothiazide: Inderide.
- timolol and hydrochlorothiazide: Timolide 10/25.

**OVERVIEW OF THE DRUG CLASS**   Table 5-2 compares the clinically used beta adrenergic receptor antagonists, commonly called beta blockers. Blocking the beta-1 adrenergic receptors of the heart decreases heart rate and force of contraction. A decrease in blood pressure follows. These actions decrease the work load of the heart and benefit coronary circulation, actions useful in treating hypertension and angina. Blockade of cardiac beta adrenergic receptors also prevents stimulation of repolarization and conduction velocity in the conducting tissue of the heart, a useful action in controlling certain arrhythmias and in preventing sudden death after a heart attack. Beta adrenergic blockers also inhibit production of renin by the kidney, thereby leading to a reduction in the amount of the vasopressor angiotensin II formed. This action is beneficial in treating hypertension.

**MECHANISM OF ACTION**   Beta adrenergic blockers bind to the beta adrenergic receptors on various tissues. The blockers are receptor antagonists, preventing the binding and action of the naturally occurring beta receptor agonists, the neurotransmitter norepinephrine and the neurohormone epinephrine.

Current beta adrenergic blockers are either *nonselective* or *cardioselective*. Nonselective blockers do not differentiate between the beta-1 and beta-2 adrenergic receptors. Cardioselective blockers are relatively selective, at therapeutic doses, for the beta-1 receptors of the heart. Beta-2 receptors mediate bronchiole dilation and glycogenolysis, among other functions. A beta blocker that is cardioselective is relatively safer for the patient with respiratory disease because the bronchiole dilation mediated by the beta-2 receptor is not blocked. A beta blocker that is cardioselective is also safer for the patient with diabetes because the breakdown of liver glycogen is not blocked. Liver glycogen is an important reserve of glucose when too much insulin is given and the patient becomes hypoglycemic.

**Table 5-2.**

## A comparison of beta receptor antagonists

| Agent | Cardioselective | Half-life (hrs) | Major therapeutic indications |
|---|---|---|---|
| Acebutolol | Yes | 3 − 4 | Cardiac arrhythmias, hypertension |
| Atenolol | Yes | 6 − 7 | Angina, hypertension |
| Esmolol | Yes | 10 min | Surgical tachycardia, surgical hypertension |
| Labetolol | No | 6 − 8 | Hypertension |
| Metoprolol | Yes | 3 − 7 | Angina, hypertension, myocardial infarction |
| Nadolol | No | 10 − 24 | Angina, Hypertension |
| ✱ Oxprenolol | No | 1.5 | Hypertension |
| Pindolol | No | 3 − 4 | Hypertension |
| Propranolol | No | 3 − 5 | Hypertension, angina, cardiac arrhythmias, hypertrophic subaortic stenosis, mycardial infarction, pheochromocytoma, migraine, anxiety |
| Timolol | No | 4 | Hypertension, glaucoma |

**INDICATIONS** **Hypertension** Beta adrenergic blockers are commonly used alone or in combination with other drugs, especially diuretics, for control of chronic hypertension. **Angina** Prophylactic use decreases the frequency of classic anginal attacks and reduces the requirements for nitroglycerin. **Myocardial infarction** The incidence of sudden death among patients who have survived a myocardial infarction is reduced by therapy for 6 months with a beta adrenergic blocker. • Metoprolol, propranolol, and timolol have been tested for this effect. **Anxiety** Because beta adrenergic blockers reduce the symptoms of sympathetic stimulation, the use of beta blockers for moderating anxiety attacks by reducing the symptoms is being tested.

**CONTRAINDICATIONS** **Respiratory diseases** Nonselective beta adrenergic blockers (propranolol, nadolol, timolol, and pindolol) are contraindicated for patients with allergic rhinitis, asthma, bronchospasm, or severe chronic obstructive pulmonary disease because these drugs compromise bronchial dilation. **Compromised cardiac function** Conditions in which the heart is already compromised and would be worsened with beta adrenergic blockers include sinus bradycardia, heart block greater than first-degree, cardiogenic shock, congestive heart failure, and right ventricular failure. **Diabetes mellitus or hypoglycemia** Beta adrenergic blockers may prevent the appearance of symptoms associated with acute hypoglycemia—increased pulse rate, tachycardia, and blood pressure changes.

**DRUG INTERACTIONS** **Reserpine** depletes catecholamines and may have an additive effect with beta adrenergic blockers. **MAO inhibitors** also decrease peripheral catecholamines and may have an additive effect with beta adrenergic blockers. **Digitalis** effectiveness in treating congestive heart failure may be decreased by beta adrenergic blockers. The toxic effect of digitalis may be increased by beta adrenergic blockers because of the further depression of AV conduction. **Calcium channel blockers** in combination with beta adrenergic blockers have both beneficial and adverse aspects. The combination of verapamil or nifedipine with beta adrenergic blockers is usually beneficial in the treatment of stable angina; however, this combination may lead to congestive heart failure or make some cases of angina worse. **Isoproterenol, norepinephrine, dopamine, and dobutamine** are drugs with beta adrenergic cardiac actions that antagonize the beta adrenergic blockers. **Phenytoin** a cardiac depressant, acts additively with beta adrenergic blockers. **Aminophylline** antagonizes the effect of beta adrenergic blockers. **Theophylline** Beta adrenergic blockers increase plasma levels of aminophylline, especially in smokers, who have an increased theophylline clearance. **Indirect-acting sympathomimetic drugs** Inotropic actions are inhibited by beta adrenergic blockers. **Prazosin** The acute postural hypotension seen with the first dose of prazosin may be intensified by beta adrenergic blockers.

## ☙ NURSING CONSIDERATIONS
### Side effects, toxicities, and associated nursing actions
**CNS** Dizziness, fatigue, mental depression, impaired concentration, disorientation, acute mental

changes, emotional lability. Symptoms of hypotension include dizziness, lightheadedness, weakness, and fainting.

- Obtain careful assessment of mental status and neurologic function before therapy and at regular intervals.
- Caution patients to avoid driving or operating hazardous equipment if CNS effects are prominent. Reassure patients that these side effects may lessen with continued use of the drug.
- Assess for signs of depression: withdrawal, insomnia, anorexia, lack of interest in personal appearance.

**CV** Symptoms of excessive cardiac depression, including bradycarida (slow heart rate), shortness of breath, worsening of angina, peripheral vascular insufficiency, edema, hypotension, and heart block. Discontinuing the drug abruptly may precipitate angina or lead to a myocardial infarction or ventricular dysrhythmia.

- Take the full-minute apical pulse before administering. If below 60 beats/min in an adult or below 90 to 110 beats/min in the child, do not administer and notify the physician.
- Monitor the blood pressure. Especially if the drug is being used to treat hypertension, monitor the blood pressure with the patient in lying, sitting, and standing positions. Hypotension is usually worse when patients begin therapy and during periods of dosage adjustment.
- Plasma levels do not correlate well with dosage.
- Monitor general parameters of cardiac and vascular functioning: intake and output, daily weight, and serum electrolyte level.
- Because many of these drugs accumulate in the presence of renal failure, monitor the BUN level.

**GI** Gastrointestinal disturbances.

- Instruct patients to take oral doses with meals or snacks to lessen gastric irritation.
- Instruct patients to notify physician if GI symptoms are severe or persistent.

**GU** Impotence and decreased libido.

- Assess patients tactfully about sexual problems; many patients are reluctant to discuss sexual difficulties. Sexual problems may prompt patients to discontinue medications. Provide emotional support as needed. Remind patients not to discontinue medications without notifying physician. Remind patients to take medications as prescribed for best effect. Consult physician for a change in drug or dosage.

**Metabolic** Beta blockade may mask symptoms of a hypoglycemic response to insulin.

- Observe diabetic patients carefully. Monitor blood glucose, urine sugar, and acetone levels (see individual drugs).

**Respiratory** Bronchospasm may be seen in susceptible individuals.

- Observe for signs of respiratory distress. Auscultate lung sounds and monitor respiratory rate.
- Encourage patients to report any unusual sign or symptom.

**Allergic** Skin rash, fever, sore throat, or unusual bleeding may indicate allergic reaction or depression of white blood cells.

- Instruct patient to report these or any new signs or symptoms.
- Monitor the complete blood count, white blood cell differential, and platelet count.

**Patient and family education**

- Review with patients anticipated benefits and possible side effects of drug therapy.
- Caution patients to consult with the physician before changing dosage or discontinuing the drug, especially because suddenly stopping the drug may precipitate angina or lead to myocardial infarction or ventricular dysrhythmia. Caution patients to check their supply of medications regularly to avoid running out.
- Teach patients the symptoms of hypotension: dizziness, lightheadedness, weakness, and syncope (fainting). If symptoms occur, instruct the patient to sit or lie down until symptoms pass and then to rise slowly. Hypotension is often worse in the morning and may be aggravated by long periods of standing, hot weather, hot showers or baths, ingestion of alcohol, and exercise.
- If appropriate, teach the patient how to take the full-minute pulse and instruct the patient to monitor the pulse at regular intervals (e.g., weekly). Determine with the physician the normal parameters for that patient and guidelines for when the patient should contact the physician.
- If appropriate, instruct patients to weigh themselves at home on a regular basis and to record these

weights. Weight gain in excess of 2 to 5 lb/week, or as directed by the physician, should be reported.

- Stress the importance of concomitant therapies, which might include diet therapy, weight reduction, sodium restriction, potassium replacement, diuretics, antihypertensives, and other medications.
- Many of these drugs cross the placenta and/or are excreted in breast milk (see individual drugs). Women of child-bearing age may wish to use a form of birth control during drug therapy. If a woman does conceive, she should notify the physician immediately.
- Caution diabetic patients that symptoms of hypoglycemia may be masked (see individual drugs).
- These drugs may be taken with or without food. Taking them with food may decrease GI distress, and absorption may be improved. Instruct patients to be consistent in the way the medications are taken, either with or without food.
- Careful and sympathetic questioning of patients taking these medications, particularly those patients exhibiting poor compliance, may help health care personnel to develop a more individualized care plan.

---

## acebutolol hydrochloride   (a-see-BYOO-to-lole)   beta blocker

- acebutolol hydrochloride: Sectral

**MECHANISM OF ACTION**   Acebutolol is a cardioselective beta blocker with mild partial agonist activity. The partial agonist activity lessens the depression of cardiac conduction and excitability characteristic of beta blockers.

**INDICATIONS**   **Hypertension** Alone or in combination with other drugs in the treatment of chronic hypertension.   **Antiarrhythmia** Taken chronically to control selected arrhythmias.

**CONTRAINDICATIONS**   **Cardiac failure** Especially patients on digitalis.

**DOSAGE**   **Adults:**   PO: Initially, 400 mg as a single dose or divided into two doses. Maintenance is 200 to 800 mg daily. Elderly patients should not receive more than 800 mg daily; others may require up to 1.2 g daily.   *Special patient populations:*   PREGNANCY: Safe use has not been established.

**PREPARATIONS**   *Capsules:* 200 and 400 mg.

**DRUG INTERACTIONS**   See entry for drug class (p. 41).

**FATE**   Acebutolol is only partially absorbed. The metabolite is active and has a longer *half-life* than the parent compound. About 35% of the drug is excreted unchanged in the urine.

### ☙ NURSING CONSIDERATIONS

#### Side effects, toxicities, and associated nursing actions
- See entry for drug class (p. 41).
   **Allergic** Hypersensitivity pneumonitis, pleurisy, and pulmonary granules.
- Monitor respiratory rate. Auscultate lung sounds.

#### Patient and family education
- See entry for drug class (p. 42).

---

## atenolol   (a-TEN-o-lole)   beta blocker

- atenolol: Tenormin

**MECHANISM OF ACTION**   Atenolol is a cardioselective beta adrenergic antagonist.

**INDICATIONS**   **Hypertension** Alone or in combination with other drugs for the treatment of chronic hypertension.   **Angina** Prophylactic therapy to decrease the incidence and severity of attacks.

**CONTRAINDICATIONS**   **Cardiac failure** Especially patients on digitalis.

**DOSAGE**   **Adults:**   PO: Initially, 50 mg once a day. After 2 weeks, the dosage may be increased to 100 mg once a day if needed.   *Special patient populations:*   PREGNANCY: Safe use has not been established. In general, beta blockers are excreted in milk, although only in trace amounts.

**PREPARATIONS**   *Tablets:* 50 and 100 mg. *Combinations: tablets:* 50 or 100 mg with 25 mg chlorthalidone.

**DRUG INTERACTIONS**   See entry for drug class (p. 41).

**FATE**   About 50% of the dose is absorbed. Atenolol is not metabolized by the liver and is excreted in the urine. Atenolol accumulates in patients with renal failure. Dosages are reduced by half in patients with mild renal failure, and in patients with severe renal failure this reduced dose is administered only every other day. Atenolol accumulates in breast milk.

## ❦ NURSING CONSIDERATIONS

### Side effects, toxicities, and associated nursing actions

**CNS** Atenolol does not cross the blood-brain barrier; therefore the CNS side effects characteristic of beta adrenergic blockers are not common.

• Side effects listed in the overview for CV, GI, GU, and Allergic are found with this drug also; see entry for drug class (p. 41).

### Patient and family education

• See entry for drug class (p. 42).

---

## esmolol   (es-MOE-lole)                                                        beta blocker

• esmolol: Brevibloc

**MECHANISM OF ACTION**   Esmolol is a cardioselective beta adrenergic antagonist.

**INDICATIONS**   **Supraventricular tachycardia** In emergency situations and during or following surgery. Esmolol also controls hypertension caused by excess adrenergic stimulation during surgery.

**CONTRAINDICATIONS**   **Heart conditions** Avoid in sinus bradycardia, heart block greater than first degree, cardiogenic shock, or overt heart failure.

**DOSAGE**   **Adults:**   IV INFUSION: 50 to 300 µg/kg/min during surgery controls the ventricular rate. To treat patients with supraventricular tachycardia, a loading dose of 500 µg/kg/min is infused for 1 minute, followed by a maintenance infusion of 50 µg/kg/min for 4 minutes. This procedure can be repeated if necessary.

**PREPARATIONS**   *Solution*: 2.5 gm in 10 ml (250 mg/ml). Do not mix with other drugs. Esmolol is not compatible with sodium bicarbonate solution.

**DRUG INTERACTIONS**   See entry for drug class (p. 41).

**FATE**   Esmolol is an ultrashort-acting drug. The *half-life* is 9 minutes. The *onset* of action is within minutes. Action may be readily terminated by discontinuing infusion.

## ❦ NURSING CONSIDERATIONS

### Side effects, toxicities, and associated nursing actions   Side effects are mild and transient. Symptomatic hypotension occurs in 12% of patients, and asymptomatic hypotension occurs in 25% of patients.

• See entry for drug class (p. 41).

### Nursing interventions related to drug administration

• See dosage above.

### Patient and family education

• This drug is not used for self-medication. Keep family informed of patient's condition.

• See entry for drug class (p. 42).

---

## metoprolol tartrate   (me-toe-PROE-lol)                                        beta blocker

• metoprolol tartrate: Lopressor

**MECHANISM OF ACTION**   Metoprolol is a cardioselective beta adrenergic antagonist.

**INDICATIONS**   **Hypertension** Alone or in combination with other drugs for the treatment of chronic hypertension.   **Myocardial infarction** Metoprolol has a protective effect against sudden death during the first 6 months of recovery.   **Angina** Prophylactic therapy to decrease the incidence and severity of attacks.

**CONTRAINDICATIONS** **Congestive heart failure** Especially patients on digitalis. **Diabetes mellitus and asthma** Although metoprolol is cardioselective, care should be used for patients with diabetes or asthma. **Impaired liver function** Dosage should be decreased.

**DOSAGE** **Adults** PO: Initially, 50 mg two times daily. If this is not adequate, the dosage may be gradually increased to no more than 450 mg daily divided in up to three doses. Absorption of metoprolol is enhanced when taken with meals. *Special patient populations:* PREGNANCY: Safe use has not been established. In general, beta blockers are excreted in milk, although only in trace amounts.

**PREPARATIONS** *Tablets:* 50 and 100 mg; *parenteral:* 1 mg/ml. *Combination:* metoprolol tartrate 50 or 100 mg and hydrothiazide 25 mg or metoprolol tartrate 100 mg and hydrochlorothiazide 50 mg.

**DRUG INTERACTIONS** See entry for drug class (p. 41). **Cimetidine** may increase the bioavailability of metoprolol.

**FATE** Metoprolol is well absorbed from the gastrointestinal tract. The bioavailability is limited by extensive degradation in the liver. Metoprolol accumulates in breast milk.

### ☙ NURSING CONSIDERATIONS

#### Side effects, toxicities, and associated nursing actions
- See entry for drug class (p. 41).

**CV** Metoprolol may aggravate peripheral vascular insufficiency, decrease HDL cholesterol, and increase serum triglyceride levels.

#### Nursing interventions related to drug administration
- IV doses may be administered by direct IV push. Monitor blood pressure and heart rate.

#### Patient and family education
- See entry for drug class (p. 42).

---

## nadolol (nay-DOE-lole) beta blocker

- nadolol: Corgard

**MECHANISM OF ACTION:** Nadolol is a nonselective beta adrenergic antagonist.

**INDICATIONS** **Hypertension** Alone or in combination with other drugs for the treatment of chronic hypertension. **Angina** Prophylactic therapy to decrease the incidence and severity of attacks.

**CONTRAINDICATIONS** **Congestive heart failure** Especially patients on digitalis. **Diabetes mellitus and asthma** Although metoprolol is cardioselective, care should be used for patients with diabetes or asthma. **Impaired liver function** Dosage should be decreased.

**DOSAGE** **Adults:** PO: Initially, 40 mg once a day. If this is not sufficient, the dosage may be increased by 40 to 80 mg. Usual maintenance dosage is 80 to 320 mg once a day. *Special patient populations:* **Pregnancy** Safe use has not been established. In general, beta blockers are excreted in milk, although only in trace amounts.

**PREPARATIONS** *Tablets:* 40, 80, 120 and 160 mg. *Combinations:* nadolol 40 or 80 mg and bendroflumethiazide 5 mg.

**DRUG INTERACTIONS** See entry for drug class (p. 41).

**FATE** Nadolol is slowly and incompletely absorbed from the gastrointestinal tract. Food does not markedly influence its absorption. Nadolol is excreted mainly in the urine but also in the feces. Nadolol is not metabolized and has a long serum half-life. The dosage interval must be increased for patients with renal failure. The dosage interval is determined by the degree of renal failure. Consult the physician.

### ☙ NURSING CONSIDERATIONS

#### Side effects, toxicities, and associated nursing actions
- See entry for drug class (p. 41).

#### Patient and family education
- See entry for drug class (p. 42).

## pindolol   (PIN-doe-lole)                                    beta blocker

- pindolol: Visken

**MECHANISM OF ACTION**   Pindolol is a nonselective beta adrenergic antagonist. Pindolol also has some intrinsic sympathetic activity so that it reduces cardiac output and heart rate less than other beta adrenergic blockers.

**INDICATIONS**   **Hypertension** Alone or in combination with other drugs for the treatment of chronic hypertension.   **Angina** Prophylactic therapy to decrease the incidence and severity of attacks.

**CONTRAINDICATIONS**   **Congestive heart failure** Especially patients on digitalis.   **Diabetes mellitus and asthma.**   **Impaired liver function** Dosage should be decreased.

**DOSAGE**   **Adults:**   **PO:** Initially, 10 mg two times daily or 15 mg three times daily. If the response is not sufficient, the dose may be increased every 2 to 3 weeks by 10 mg/day. The maximum dose is 60 mg daily.

**PREPARATIONS**   *Tablets:* 5 and 10 mg.

**DRUG INTERACTIONS**   See entry for drug class (p. 41).

**DIAGNOSTIC TEST INTERFERENCE**   Minor increases in serum transaminase levels have occurred in a few patients taking pindolol. This does not appear to be associated with liver damage.

**FATE**   Pindolol is well absorbed orally. It is excreted in the urine, and only about 50% is metabolized. Pindolol crosses the placenta and also appears in breast milk.

### ❧ NURSING CONSIDERATIONS

#### Side effects, toxicities, and associated nursing actions
- See entry for drug class (p. 41).

#### Patient and family education
- See entry for drug class (p. 42).

## propranolol hydrochloride   (proe-PRAN-oh-lole)            beta blocker

- propranolol hydrochloride: Apo-Propranolol, ♣Detensol, Inderal, ♣Novopranol, ♣Panolol

**MECHANISM OF ACTION**   Propranolol is a nonselective beta adrenergic antagonist.

**INDICATIONS**   Propranolol is the beta adrenergic blocker that has been used for the longest time and with the most approved indications.   **Hypertension** Alone or in combination with other drugs for the control of chronic hypertension.   **Angina** Prophylactic therapy to decrease the incidence and severity of attacks.   **Cardiac arrhythmias.**   **Thyrotoxicosis** To control cardiac effects.   **Hypertrophic subaortic stenosis.**   **Pheochromocytoma.**   **Migraine.**   **Anxiety** Propranolol controls excessive adrenergic symptoms.

**CONTRAINDICATIONS**   **Congestive heart failure** Especially patients on digitalis.   **Diabetes mellitus and asthma** Care should be used for patients with diabetes or asthma.   **Impaired liver function** Dosage should be decreased.

**DOSAGE**   **Hypertension:**   *Adults:*   **PO:** Initially, 40 mg two times a day. The dose is increased gradually until the desired decrease in blood pressure is obtained. Usual maintenance doses are 160 to 480 mg/day. Doses may be divided into three daily doses if the blood pressure tends to rise at the end of 12 hours. *Children:*   **PO:** Begin with 0.5 to 1 mg/kg/day. Increase slowly to a maximum of 2 mg/kg/day.   **Angina:**   *Adults:*   **PO:** Initially, 10 to 20 mg three or four times daily before meals and at bedtime. Dosage is increased if needed up to 320 mg/day.   **Arrhythmias:**   *Adults:*   **PO:** 10 to 30 mg three or four times daily at meals and at bedtime.   **IV:** For life–threatening arrhythmias or those occurring with the patient under anesthesia, 1 to 3 mg with ECG and blood pressure monitoring, given no faster than 1 mg/min. A second dose may be given after 2 minutes. No additional doses should be given for 4 hours.   *Children:*   **IV:** 0.01 to 0.1 mg/kg/dose to a maximum of 1 mg/dose by slow push.   **PO:** 0.5 to 1 mg/kg/day in three or four doses to a maximum of 60 mg/day.   **Hypertrophic subaortic stenosis:** *Adults:*   **PO:** 20 to 40 mg three or four times daily at meals and at bedtime.   **Pheochromocytoma**

(catecholamine secreting tumor): *Adults:* PO: 60 mg/day in four divided doses three days before surgery, given along with an alpha adrenergic blocker. **Migraine:** *Adults:* PO: Initially, 80 mg/day in three or four divided doses at meals and at bedtime. Gradually increase to an effective dose. The usual maintenance dose is 160 to 240 mg/day. **Thyrotoxicosis:** *Adults and children over 12 years:* IV: 1 to 3 mg/dose over 10 minutes. PO: 10 to 40 mg every 6 hours. *Neonates and children under 12 years:* PO: 2 mg/kg/day every 6 hours. *Special patient populations:* PREGNANCY: Safe use has not been established. In general, beta blockers are excreted in milk, although only in trace amounts.

**PREPARATIONS**   *Tablets:* 10, 20, 40, and 80 mg; *sustained–release capsules:* 80, 120, and 160 mg; *parenteral:* 1 mg/ml in 1 ml ampules. *Combinations:* *capsules (extended–release):* 80, 120, and 160 mg with 50 mg hydrochlorothiazide; *tablets:* 40 and 80 mg with 25 mg hydrochlorothiazide.

**DRUG INTERACTIONS**   See drug interactions characteristic of the beta adrenergic blockers (p. 41). **Lidocaine** clearance is impaired by propranolol. **Chlorpromazine, cimetidine, furosemide, and hydralazine** increase the plasma concentration of propranolol. **Smoking** reduces the plasma concentration of propranolol by increasing its clearance. **Indomethacin** may antagonize the hypertensive effects of propranolol.

**DIAGNOSTIC TEST INTERFERENCE**   Propranolol may elevate blood urea, serum transaminase, alkaline phosphatase, and lactic dehydrogenase levels.

**FATE**   Propranolol is rapidly and completely absorbed. It is readily metabolized by the liver, which limits the bioavailability of propranolol. Propranolol crosses the placenta and also accumulates in breast milk.

## NURSING CONSIDERATIONS

### Side effects, toxicities, and associated nursing actions
- See entry for drug class (p. 41).

### Nursing interventions related to drug administration
- See dosage.
- This drug is also administered intravenously. Before IV administration, attach patient to a cardiac monitor.
- Check doses carefully because the IV dose is much smaller than the oral dose.
- The IV dose may be given undiluted or diluted in 5% dextrose solution. Administer at a rate not exceeding 1 mg/min.

### Patient and family education
- See entry for drug class (p. 42).

---

## timolol maleate   (TYE-moe-lole)                                    beta blocker

- timolol maleate: Blocadren

**MECHANISM OF ACTION**   Timolol is a nonselective beta adrenergic antagonist.

**INDICATIONS**   **Hypertension** Alone or in combination with other drugs for the control of chronic hypertension. **Angina** Prophylactic therapy to decrease the incidence and severity of attacks. **Myocardial infarction** Timolol has a protective effect against sudden death during the first 6 months of recovery. **Chronic (wide-angle) glaucoma** See Chapter 62.

**CONTRAINDICATIONS**   **Congestive heart failure** Especially patients on digitalis. **Diabetes mellitus and asthma** Care should be used for patients with diabetes or asthma. **Impaired liver function** Dosage should be decreased.

**DOSAGE**   **Hypertension:** *Adults:* PO: Initially, 10 mg twice a day. The dosage may be increased once a week by 10 mg. Usual maintenance dosage is 20 to 40 mg/day, maximum 60 mg/day. **Myocardial infarction:** *Adults:* PO: 10 mg two times a day. *Special patient populations:* PREGNANCY: Safe use has not been established. In general, beta blockers are excreted in milk, although only in trace amounts.

**PREPARATIONS**    *Tablets:* 10 and 20 mg. *Combinations: tablets:* 10 mg with 25 mg hydrochlorothiazide.

**DRUG INTERACTIONS**    See entry for drug class (p. 41).

**DIAGNOSTIC TEST INTERFERENCE**    Timolol may produce slight increases in the BUN, serum potassium, and serum uric acid values. Hemoglobin may be slightly decreased.

**FATE**    Timolol is rapidly and completely absorbed from the gastrointestinal tract. Timolol is readily metabolized by the liver.

### ☙ NURSING CONSIDERATIONS

#### Side effects, toxicities, and associated nursing actions
- See entry for drug class (p. 41).

#### Patient and family education
- See entry for drug class (p. 42).

## Alpha adrenergic blockers

Alpha and beta adrenergic blocking drug ~ labetalol
Alpha adrenergic blocking drugs ~ phenoxybenzamine ~ phentolamine ~ prazosin ~ terazosin

**DRUG COMBINATIONS**
- prazosin and polythiazide: Minizide

**OVERVIEW OF THE DRUG CLASS**    The alpha adrenergic receptor antagonists prevent the changes in blood vessel tone important for maintaining blood pressure. Infusion of one of these drugs into a person with normal blood pressure produces little change in blood pressure as long as the person is lying down. However, any sudden shift to the upright position causes orthostatic (postural) hypotension because the blockade of the alpha-1 receptors prevents the vasoconstriction necessary to redistribute blood flow.

Alpha adrenergic blockers are effective antihypertensive agents for severe hypertension. Phenoxybenzamine and phentolamine are used to treat hypertensive emergencies; prazosin and labetalol are combined with other drugs for chronic antihypertensive therapy. (Drug combinations for antihypertensive therapy are described in Chapter 7.) Labetalol is the first of a new class of alpha blockers with beta blocking activity as well. The advantage of the beta receptor blockade is that the reflex increase in heart rate (reflex tachycardia) common with alpha blockade is eliminated.

**MECHANISM OF ACTION**    Norepinephrine is the sympathetic neurotransmitter that increases the tone of blood vessels and maintains blood pressure. Alpha adrenergic blockers bind to alpha adrenergic receptors on various tissues. The blockers are receptor antagonists, preventing the binding and action of the naturally occurring alpha receptor agonists, the neurotransmitter norepinephrine and the neurohormone epinephrine.

**INDICATIONS**    See individual drug.

**CONTRAINDICATIONS**    See individual drug.

**DRUG INTERACTIONS**    See individual drug.

### ☙ NURSING CONSIDERATIONS

**Side effects, toxicities, and associated nursing actions**    All drugs administered for the purpose of lowering blood pressure share the potential to cause the following.

**CV** Severe hypotension.
- Monitor the blood pressure and pulse before initiating therapy, at the start of therapy, and whenever dosage is changed.
- Monitor blood pressure with the patient in lying, sitting, and standing positions.
- The blood pressure in some patients varies significantly between arms. Occasionally check the pressure in both arms. If one arm differs from the other, note which arm is used for each blood pressure determination.
- If hypotension is severe, instruct the patient to sit or lie down.
- Monitor the intake, output, and weight.
- Supervise the ambulation of hospitalized patients to guard against injury should the patient become dizzy or faint. Use nightlights and bed side rails.

- The elderly are often more sensitive to hypotensive effects of drugs: monitor closely. The following side effects often occur with drugs in this class; see individual drugs.

  **GI** Dry mouth. Occasionally, nausea, vomiting, and diarrhea.

- For dry mouth, instruct patients to suck on ice chips or sugarless hard candy, or chew sugarless gum. Some patients may wish to try a commercially available saliva substitute.

- For constipation, instruct patients to increase daily fluid intake to 2500 to 3000 ml/day (if not contraindicated by other medical problems); increase dietary intake of fruit, fruit juices, and high-fiber foods; and increase daily exercise.

- If GI symptoms are persistent or severe, instruct patient to notify physician.

- If vomiting or diarrhea occurs, monitor intake, output, and weight. Monitor serum electrolyte levels.

  **Respiratory** Nasal congestion or stuffiness.

- Inform patients that this annoying side effect may decrease with continued use of the medication.

- Caution patients to avoid any medications, including OTC drugs, without prior approval of the physician.

  **GU** Sexual dysfunction.

- Assess patients tactfully for sexual dysfunction; some patients may be unwilling to discuss this. Sexual problems may prompt some patients to discontinue the medication without notifying the physician. Remind patients to take drugs as prescribed for best effect and not to discontinue the medication without notifying the physician. Consult physician about drug or dosage change. Provide emotional support as needed.

## Patient and family education

- Review with patients and families the anticipated benefits and possible side effects of drug therapy. Ask patients to report the appearance of any new sign or symptom.

- Postural hypotension is a common side effect, especially when the patient moves rapidly from a recumbent to a sitting or standing position. Symptoms include dizziness, lightheadedness, weakness, and syncope. If symptoms occur, instruct patients to sit or lie down until symptoms pass, then to rise slowly. Postural hypotension is often worse in the morning and may be aggravated by long periods of standing, hot weather, hot showers or baths, ingestion of alcohol, and exercise, especially if the exercise is followed by immobility. Hypotension is also worse at the start of therapy and during periods of dosage adjustment.

- Point out to patients that losing weight to reach ideal body weight, adhering to a low-sodium diet, avoiding smoking and excessive caffeine, and adhering to a regular exercise program may decrease the need for antihypertensive medications.

- If indicated, refer patients to a dietitian for instruction about sodium restriction. The need for sodium restriction depends on the patients' general medical condition, other medications, and usual dietary habits; consult the physician. Instructions should be directed to patients and to family members in the household who regularly cook.

- Selected patients may be instructed to record and monitor their weight at regular intervals at home. Weight gain in excess of 2 lb/day or 5 lb/week should be reported to the health care provider.

- Instruct patients taking antihypertensive medications to avoid other medications causing hypotension (e.g., alcohol, barbiturates, central nervous system depressants) or hypertension (e.g., sympathomimetics commonly found in cold remedies). Caution patients to avoid taking OTC medications without prior approval of the physician and to keep all health care providers informed of all medications being taken.

- Review with patients appropriate actions for missed doses. If the missed dose is remembered soon after it was due, it may be taken, and the usual schedule may resume. If the missed dose is remembered close to the time of the next dose, the patient should *not* double up or take two doses close together. Advise patients to seek clarification from the physician or nurse when in doubt about medication schedules.

- Remind patients to keep all medications out of the reach of children.

## labetalol hydrochloride    (la-BET-a-lole)    alpha-beta blocker

- labetalol hydrochloride: Normodyne, Trandate

**MECHANISM OF ACTION**   Labetalol has complex actions. It is both an alpha and a beta adrenergic antagonist but may have beta-2 agonist actions. Therapeutically, labetalol reduces peripheral vascular resistance (the alpha effect) with a decrease in heart rate (the beta effect). The beta effect is more prominent than the alpha effect.

**INDICATIONS**   **Hypertensive emergencies** Labetalol may be given intravenously. Mild to severe hypertension.

**CONTRAINDICATIONS**   Severe congestive heart failure. • Sinus bradycardia. • Severe chronic obstructive pulmonary disease.

**DOSAGE**   **Adults:**   **PO:** Initially, 100 mg twice a day. The dosage is increased if necessary. The usual maintenance dose is 200 to 800 mg/day, although patients with severe hypertension may require 1.6 to 2.4 g/day. Labetalol is usually added to diuretic therapy.   **IV:** 20 mg by slow injection over 2 minutes; at 10-minute intervals, additional injections of 40 or 80 mg can be added if necessary. The total dose should not exceed 300 mg.   *Special patient populations:*   **PREGNANCY:** Safe use has not been established. Labetalol does cross the placenta and is excreted in milk.

**PREPARATIONS**   *Tablets:* 100, 200, 300, and 400 mg; *parenteral:* 5 mg/ml solution in 20 ml vial.

**DRUG INTERACTIONS**   **Antihypertensive medications** Labetalol may cause paradoxical hypertension in patients receiving other antihypertensive medications.   **Cimetidine** increases the bioavailability of labetalol.

**DIAGNOSTIC TEST INTERFERENCE**   **Fluorometric and spectrophotometric methods of detecting catecholamines** Labetalol may interfere with these tests.

**FATE**   About 75% of an oral dose of labetalol is taken up immediately and metabolized by the liver (first-pass metabolism). Labetalol is conjugated and excreted in urine. In oral therapy, *peak* antihypertensive effects take 24 to 72 hours and in IV administration take 5 to 10 minutes.

### 🐦 NURSING CONSIDERATIONS

#### Side effects, toxicities, and associated nursing actions   See entry for drug class (p. 48).
**CNS** Fatigue and nervousness. Other side effects include lethargy, depression, and nightmares.
- Caution patients to avoid driving or operating hazardous equipment until the effects of the medication can be evaluated.
- Assess patients for signs of depression: anorexia, insomnia, neglect of personal appearance, withdrawal, and changes in mood or affect.
- Assess patients for the appearance of other signs or symptoms. If symptoms persist or are severe, it may be necessary to change drugs.

**CV** Flushed face. Orthostatic hypotension is sometimes seen at the beginning of therapy. Overdosage produces excessive slowing of the heart.
- Be especially alert for bradycardia if the patient is also receiving cardiac glycosides or other drugs that may slow the pulse.

**GI** Dry mouth and gastrointestinal disturbances.
**Respiratory** Nasal congestion.
**Allergic** Antinuclear antibody titer may increase; however, lupus syndrome is uncommon in patients taking labetalol.
- Remind patients to keep all physicians informed of drugs being taken.
**Other** Tingling of the scalp and muscle cramps; sexual dysfunction.

#### Nursing interventions related to drug administration
- Parenteral labetalol is usually administered as a bolus injection (see dosage).
- Drug may be further diluted to provide a constant infusion. For example, dilute 200 mg (40 ml) in 160 ml of diluent such as 5% dextrose solution to form a concentration of 1 mg/ml. Administer via microdrip tubing and use a volume or rate controlling device. Monitor blood pressure every 2 to 5 minutes until stable.

- During parenteral administration, keep patients supine. After administration of drug, monitor blood pressure every 15 to 30 minutes until stable. It may require several hours for blood pressure to stabilize sufficiently for patients to assume a sitting position.

### Patient and family education
- See entry for drug class (p. 49).
- Periodic eye examinations are recommended. The drug accumulates in the choroid, and the long-term effects of this are not known.
- Labetalol may mask cardiovascular symptoms of hypoglycemia (e.g., tachycardia). Caution diabetic patients of the effect and encourage them to be alert to possible signs of hypoglycemia: weakness, headache, and confusion.
- Sudden discontinuation of this drug may contribute to cardiac problems in susceptible individuals. Caution patients to take the drug as ordered. If the drug is discontinued by the physician, it is usually done gradually, over a 2-week period or longer.
- Inform patients that taking the drug with meals may reduce gastric irritation.

## phenoxybenzamine hydrochloride  (fen-ox-ee-BEN-za-meen)  alpha blocker

- phenoxybenzamine hydrochloride: Dibenzyline

**MECHANISM OF ACTION**  Phenoxybenzamine is an irreversible alpha blocker, acting at both alpha-1 and alpha-2 receptors. This blockade results in reduced peripheral vascular resistance and venous tone, decreased blood pressure, and reflex tachycardia.

**INDICATIONS**  **Hypertensive crises with pheochromocytoma** (an adrenal tumor producing excessive catecholamines).  **Vasospastic diseases** such as Raynaud's syndrome and frostbite aftereffects in which there is increased alpha adrenergic activity.

**CONTRAINDICATIONS**  **Cerebral or coronary atherosclerosis or kidney damage** Alpha adrenergic blockade may compromise circulation to these vital organs.  **Respiratory infections** Alpha adrenergic blockade may aggravate symptoms.

**DOSAGE**  **Adults:**  PO: Dosage must be individualized. Initially, 10 mg/day; after 4 days may be increased by 10 mg/day. Usual optimum doses are 20 to 60 mg/day.  *Special patient populations:*  **Pregnancy** Safe use has not been established.

**PREPARATIONS**  *Capsules:* 10 mg.

**DRUG INTERACTIONS**  **Sympathomimetic drugs** with alpha adrenergic effects are antagonized by phenoxybenzamine.  **Alcohol-induced vasodilation** is exaggerated; alcohol should be avoided.

**FATE**  Because phenoxybenzamine acts irreversibly, the drug must be started in low doses and increased gradually; up to 2 weeks may be required to titrate to the optimum dose. Effects last several weeks.

## NURSING CONSIDERATIONS
### Side effects, toxicities, and associated nursing actions  See entry for drug class (p. 48). Symptoms of adrenergic blockade common with phenoxybenzamine include the following.
**CV** Postural hypotension and increased heart rate.
- In cases of overdose, discontinue the drug and keep the patient lying down. Elevating the legs may improve circulation. In extreme cases it may be necessary to administer norepinephrine.

**CNS** Lethargy and shock, but only with overdoses.
- Caution patients to avoid driving or operating hazardous equipment until the effects of the medication can be evaluated.
- Assess for the appearance of other side effects.

**Respiratory** Nasal congestion.

**Ophthalmic** Miosis.

**Other** Inhibition of ejaculation.

**Patient and family education**
- See entry for drug class (p. 49).
- Instruct patients to take doses with meals or snacks to decrease gastric irritation.

## phentolamine mesylate   (fen-TOLE-a-meen)                    alpha blocker

- phentolamine mesylate: Regitine, ✤Rogitine

**MECHANISM OF ACTION**   Phentolamine blocks both alpha-1 and alpha-2 receptors. Total peripheral resistance and venous return to the heart are decreased.

**INDICATIONS**   **Hypertensive crises with pheochromocytoma** (an adrenal tumor producing excessive catecholamines).   **Treatment of dermal necrosis** secondary to extravasation of norepinephrine or dopamine during IV administration.   **Hypertensive crises** secondary to MAO inhibitor interaction with a sympathomimetic amine or to the rebound hypertension when clonidine or other antihypertensive drugs are withdrawn too abruptly.

**CONTRAINDICATIONS**   **Coronary heart disease:** myocardial infarction, coronary insufficiency, and angina. **Hypersensitivity** to phentolamine.

**DOSAGE**   **Prevention of hypertensive episodes in pheochromocytoma:**   *Adults:*   PO: 50 mg four to six times daily.   *Children:*   PO: 25 mg four to six times daily.   **Prevention and treatment of dermal necrosis following extravasation of IV norepinephrine:** *Prevention:* 10 mg is added to each liter of diluted norepinephrine. *Treatment:* inject 5 to 10 mg in 10 ml saline solution into the area within 12 hours. *Special patient populations:*   PREGNANCY: Safe use has not been established.

**PREPARATIONS**   *Tablets:* 50 mg; *parenteral:* 5 mg per vial for dilution.

**DRUG INTERACTIONS**   **Sympathomimetic drugs** Phentolamine antagonizes the alpha adrenergic effects of drugs with sympathomimetic activity.

**FATE**   Phentolamine is poorly absorbed orally. Phentolamine has a short *onset* and *duration of action.*

❦ **NURSING CONSIDERATIONS**

**Side effects, toxicities, and associated nursing actions**   See entry for drug class (p. 48).
    **CV** Hypotension—episodes may be acute or prolonged. Symptoms may include weakness, dizziness, flushing, and orthostatic hypotension.
- Caution patients to avoid driving or operating hazardous equipment if weakness, dizziness, or orthostatic hypotension are severe; notify physician.
- Hypotensive effects can be reversed with IV dopamine.
    **Respiratory** Nasal stuffiness.
    **GI** Nausea, vomiting, and diarrhea.

**Nursing interventions related to drug administration**
- For IV use, dilute each 5 mg with 1 ml of sterile water for injection. May be further diluted with 5 to 10 ml of sterile water for injection.
- Administer prepared doses immediately at a rate of 5 mg over at least 1 minute.
- Monitor blood pressure every 2 minutes until stable. Patient should be lying down. If patient has a history of heart disease, monitor ECG.

**Patient and family education**
- See entry for drug class (p. 49).

## prazosin hydrochloride   (PRA-zoe-sin)                    alpha blocker

- prazosin hydrochloride: Minipress

**MECHANISM OF ACTION**   Prazosin selectively blocks alpha-1 adrenergic receptors. This action dilates both arterioles and veins to reduce peripheral vascular resistance.

**INDICATIONS** **Moderate or severe hypertension** Prazosin is administered with a diuretic or with a diuretic and a beta-blocking drug. **Congestive heart failure.**

**CONTRAINDICATIONS** • No specific contraindications have been established.

**DOSAGE** Adults: PO: Initially, 0.5 to 1 mg two or three times daily. Doses may be gradually increased as necessary. Doses of 6 to 15 mg daily are common; doses larger than 20 mg daily are seldom required. *Special patient populations:* PREGNANCY: Safe use has not been established.

**PREPARATIONS** *Capsules:* 1, 2, and 5 mg. *Combinations:* 1, 2, or 5 mg with 0.5 mg polythiazide.

**DRUG INTERACTIONS** **Protein-bound drugs** may be displaced by prazosin, which is highly protein bound.

**FATE** About half of an oral dose of prazosin is absorbed. In the blood, over 90% of the drug is protein bound. Whereas the plasma *half-life* is about 3 hours, the *duration of action* is several hours. Prazosin is metabolized and excreted mainly in bile and feces.

**❦ NURSING CONSIDERATIONS**

**Side effects, toxicities, and associated nursing actions**

**CNS** Nightmares and lethargy.
- Caution patients to avoid driving or operating hazardous equipment until effects of the medication can be evaluated.
- Assess patients for signs of depression: anorexia, insomnia, neglect of personal appearance, withdrawal, and changes in mood or affect.

**GU** Sexual dysfunction.
- See entry for drug class (p. 48).

**Respiratory** Dry mouth and nasal congestion are common.

**Metabolic** First-dose effect: some patients react to initial therapy with marked orthostatic hypotension and fainting. Fluid retention: prazosin is commonly given with a diuretic.
- In the hospital, monitor blood pressure before administering dose and at regular intervals after dose until stable. Have patient remain supine until blood pressure is stable (see patient and family education below).
- Monitor weight. Instruct patients to report tight rings, shoes, or clothing. Instruct patients to monitor and record weight at home. Instruct patients to report weight gain in excess of 2 lb/day or 5 lb/week. Visually inspect patients for signs of edema.

**Patient and family education**
- See entry for drug class (p. 49).
- Patients beginning therapy, adding a diuretic to the drug regimen, or increasing the dose of prazosin are susceptible to the first-dose syndrome. Although characterized by hypotension, this syndrome can be severe enough to result in syncope and loss of consciousness. This hypotensive response usually occurs 30 to 90 minutes after the dose has been taken: it is more common with a first dose of 2 mg than 1 mg, so patients are usually started on the lower dose. Treatment is for the patient to lie flat; the condition is self-limiting. In rare cases the episode is preceded by tachycardia; heart rates up to 180 beats/min have been reported.
- Because first-dose syndrome effects may occur for a couple of days after initiating or changing the dose, caution patients to avoid activities in which a syncopal episode might be dangerous (driving or operating hazardous equipment).
- To minimize the possibility of the first-dose syndrome, instruct patients to take the first dose at bedtime and to remain lying down for at least 3 hours after the dose is taken.
- Review the hypotensive effects with families of patients receiving prazosin, both to allay anxiety should syncope occur and to ensure that the patient will receive correct treatment of the problem.

---

## terazosin hydrochloride (ter-AS-oh-sin) alpha adrenergic blocker

- terazosin hydrochloride: Hytrin

**MECHANISM OF ACTION** Terazosin is a long-acting alpha-1 adrenergic receptor blocker. This action results in a lowering of total peripheral resistance.

**INDICATIONS**   Mild to moderate hypertension.

**CONTRAINDICATIONS**   None known.

**DOSAGE**   PO:   ADULTS: Initially, 1 mg daily to avoid a severe hypotensive response; increase as needed and tolerated. Usual therapeutic range is 5 to 20 mg daily.   *Special patient populations:*   PREGNAN-CY: Safe use has not been established (pregnancy category C).

**PREPARATIONS**   *Tablets:* 1, 2, and 5 mg.

**DRUG INTERACTIONS**   **Antihypertensive drugs** Terazosin potentiates the action of other antihypertensive drugs.

**FATE**   *Peak* response is seen in 2 to 3 hours.

## NURSING CONSIDERATIONS

### Side effects, toxicities, and associated nursing actions

**CNS** Fatigue, headache.

- Obtain baseline evaluation of energy level. Assess for ability to maintain level of activities of daily living. If fatigue develops, notify physician.

**CV:** Dizziness, lightheadedness; marked hypotension with the first few doses; tachycardia, nasal congestion, edema.

- Instruct patients to avoid driving or operating hazardous equipment if dizziness or lightheadedness develops.
- See entry for drug class (p. 48).

**GI** Disturbances.

- See entry for drug class (p. 49).

**Eye** Blurred vision.

- Instruct patients to avoid driving or operating hazardous equipment if blurred vision develops; notify physician.

### Patient and family education

- See entry for drug class (p. 49).

# Chapter Six
# Drugs affecting cardiac strength and rhythm

**Cardiac glycosides**
deslanoside
digitalis glycosides
digitalis leaf
digitoxin
digoxin
digoxin immune Fab (see Chapter 26)
gitalin
ouabain

**Miscellaneous inotropic drugs**
amrinone
milrinone (investigational drug)

**Antiarrhythmic drugs**
amiodarone
bretylium
digoxin (see cardiac glycosides)
disopyramide
encainide
flecainide
lidocaine
mexiletine
phenytoin
procainamide
propranolol
quinidine
tocainide
verapamil

**INTRODUCTION**  When the heart muscle loses the ability to contract with normal strength, cardiac output falls. Three classes of drugs are used in congestive heart failure because they directly increase strength of contraction (positive inotropic effects). *Cardiac glycosides* increase contractility but may also slow heart rates and slow conduction through the AV node. *Beta-1 adrenergic receptor agonists* directly increase contractility but may also increase heart rates and blood pressure. The beta-1 adrenergic receptor agonists are discussed in Chapter 5 (p. 28). *Amrinone and milrinone* increase contractility by actions different from cardiac glycosides or beta adrenergic agents.

Cardiac function may be impaired by improper pacing or other arrhythmias. Because arrhythmias arise from many different causes, a variety of drug classes may be useful. Drugs such as *local anesthetics* may have greater effects on arrhythmias arising in ventricular tissues, but *beta adrenergic blockers* (Chapter 5) primarily affect arrhythmias arising from nodal tissue. *Calcium channel blockers* may be useful because they affect tissue dependent on calcium currents, which includes nodal tissue and ischemic tissue.

## Cardiac glycosides

deslanoside (desacetyl-lanatoside C)  ~  digitalis glycosides  ~  digitalis leaf  ~  digitoxin  ~  digoxin  ~  digoxin immune Fab (see Chapter 26)  ~  gitalin  ~  ouabain

**OVERVIEW OF THE DRUG CLASS**  Congestive heart failure arises when the pumping action of the heart is impaired, and cardiac output falls below venous return. Blood pools in the veins, increasing venous pressure, which may stretch cardiac fibers beyond normal limits and further damage their ability to contract with adequate strength. The low cardiac output may damage other organs. The kidneys receive insufficient blood flow to maintain salt and water balance, and fluid accumulates in the lungs and periphery. If cardiac output can be improved with drugs, many symptoms of congestive heart failure can be relieved.

**MECHANISM OF ACTION**  All cardiac glycosides inhibit $Na^+,K^+-ATPase$ and promote the accumulation within heart cells of the calcium required for contraction. These biochemical actions improve contractility, allowing cardiac output to increase. Increasing cardiac output improves blood flow to all organs. Improved blood flow to the kidneys increases urine production, aiding the clearance of edema.

**INDICATIONS**  **Congestive heart failure** Chronic therapy for congestive heart failure is with one of the oral preparations of cardiac glycosides. • IV preparations may be used in acute failure.  **Arrhythmias** Cardiac glycosides slow conduction through the AV node and protect the ventricles from excessive

| Table 6-1. | Summary of inotropic agents | | |
|---|---|---|---|
| **Drug** | **Route** | **Clinical use** | |
| Amrinone | IV | Acute refractory CHF* | |
| Deslanoside | IV, IM | Acute CHF | |
| Digitalis glycosides | PO | Chronic CHF, atrial arrhythmias | |
| Digitalis leaf | PO | Chronic CHF, atrial arrhythmias | |
| Digitoxin | PO, IV | Acute or chronic CHF, atrial arrhythmias | |
| Digoxin | PO, IV | Acute or chronic CHF, atrial arrhythmias | |
| Gitalin | wO | Chronic CHF, maintenance therapy in atrial arrhythmias | |
| Ouabain | IV | Acute CHF, acute therapy in atrial arrhythmias | |

*CHF, Congestive heart failure.

stimulation from atrial sites as may occur in atrial fibrillation, atrial flutter, or paroxysmal atrial tachycardia (Table 6-1).

**CONTRAINDICATIONS** **Ventricular fibrillation** Cardiac glycosides may worsen ventricular arrhythmias. **Hypokalemia, hypomagnesemia, alkalosis, hypoxia, or hypercalcemia** These electrolyte imbalances may increase the toxicity of cardiac glycosides toward the heart. **Impaired renal or hepatic function** Patients with these conditions tend to accumulate cardiac glycosides and therefore may be more prone to suffer toxic reactions; this category may include elderly or debilitated patients and neonates or premature infants. **Hypothyroidism and valvular heart disease** These conditions may increase the risk of toxicity with cardiac glycosides. **Acute myocardial infarction** Although cardiac glycosides have been used to help control pulmonary congestion following myocardial infarction, other drugs that improve contractility (e.g., dobutamine) are safer. • Cardiac glycosides can increase mortality if given during the first 48 hours following an acute myocardial infarction, apparently because cardiac glycosides can enhance ventricular automaticity.

**DRUG INTERACTIONS** **Antibiotics** may increase absorption of cardiac glycosides in the rare individuals (approximately 10% of the population) whose normal gastrointestinal flora significantly degrades cardiac glycosides. Toxic blood levels of the cardiac glycosides may result. **Antidiarrheal medications** (adsorbent suspensions), *antacids* (magnesium trisilicates), *neomycin*, and *anion exchange resins* (cholestyramine) may impair absorption of oral cardiac glycosides. Therapeutic effects of the cardiac glycosides are diminished. **Barbiturates, phenylbutazone, phenytoin, and rifampin** may decrease the effect of cardiac glycosides by stimulating enzymatic destruction of the glycosides in the liver. **Calcium salts, pancuronium, reserpine, succinylcholine, thyroid preparations, or sympathomimetics** can have additive effects with cardiac glycosides. Risk of arrhythmias is increased. **Potassium-wasting drugs** (e.g., thiazide and related diuretics, loop diuretics, corticosteroids, and amphotericin B) increase the risk of toxic reactions precipitated by hypokalemia. **Propantheline and diphenoxylate** may increase absorption of cardiac glycosides by reducing motility of the gut or prolonging transit time. Toxic blood levels of the cardiac glycosides may result. **Propranolol** may precipitate excessive bradycardia and cause heart block in patients receiving cardiac glycosides. **Quinidine and verapamil** block excretion of cardiac glycosides and lead to increased serum levels that may become toxic.

### ❦ NURSING CONSIDERATIONS
#### Side effects, toxicities, and associated nursing actions
**CV** Increased automaticity (irregular pulse, premature ventricular contractions, or other arrhythmias) and slowing of conduction through the AV node (bradycardia, partial or complete heartblock).
- Take the apical pulse for a full minute before administering. If the rate is below 60 beats/min in adults or below 90 to 110 in children, do not administer the dose and notify the physician. If the rhythm is abnormal (e.g., bigeminy), notify physician.
- Observe cardiac monitor or ECG tracings for possible effects: prolonged P-R interval, sagging S-T

segment, A-V block, atrial tachycardia, bigeminy, ventricular tachycardia, or premature ventricular contractions.

- Monitor serum electrolyte values with special attention to potassium. Hypokalemia predisposes to toxicity from cardiac glycosides. Symptoms of hypokalemia include weakness, thirst, depression, anorexia, nausea, vomiting, abdominal distention, postural hypotension, and hypoactive reflexes.
- Note that in infants and small children, changes in cardiac rate or rhythm may be the first signs of toxicity from the cardiac glycosides. Review this point with families and reinforce the importance of contacting the physician if there is a question.

**CNS** Stimulation of medullary centers leading to anorexia, nausea, and vomiting. Less commonly depression, confusion, drowsiness, or headaches arise.

**Metabolic** Fatigue is a common sign of toxicity from cardiac glycosides.

- Assess patient for symptoms that may accompany any chronic illness but which may be signs of drug toxicity: anorexia, nausea, depression, or fatigue. See CV side effects, above: toxicity in infants and children is more likely to present as changes in cardiac rate and rhythm, whereas toxicity in older children and adults is more commonly manifested as fatigue, anorexia, nausea, and vomiting.
- Monitor weight.
- Assess for signs of depression: change in mood or affect, lack of interest in personal appearance, anorexia, and difficulty sleeping.

**Ophthalmic** Blurred vision, color distortion, halos, or flashing lights are common signs.

- Assess for changes in vision.
- Instruct patients to avoid driving or operating hazardous equipment if visual changes occur; notify physician.

**GU** Renal failure may predispose to toxicity.

- Monitor weight, fluid intake and output, and blood pressure.
- Monitor blood urea nitrogen (BUN) and serum creatinine.

### Nursing interventions related to drug administration

- Check the name and dosage of medications carefully; there are several different drugs of this class with similar spellings.
- If the serum drug level has been ordered, check the value before administering. If the value is outside the limits of safety established for the particular drug and patient, withhold the dose and notify the physician.

### Patient and family education

- Review the anticipated benefits and possible side effects of drug therapy. Instruct the patient to notify the physician of any new sign or symptom.
- Instruct the patient to take the medication with or after meals to lessen gastric irritation.
- If appropriate, instruct the patient to take the apical pulse for a full minute before taking the drug. Ascertain that the patient can do this correctly. Determine with the physician the range that should be considered normal for each patient. Also determine when the patient should omit the dose and when the patient should contact the physician.
- If appropriate, instruct patients to weigh themselves regularly at home and to record these weights. Weight gain in excess of 2 to 5 lb/week indicates fluid retention and should be reported to the health care provider.
- Patients should avoid the use of OTC preparations unless first approved by the physician. Patients should keep all health care providers informed of all drugs being taken.
- Stress the importance of concomitant therapies, which might include diet therapy, weight reduction, sodium restriction, potassium replacement, diuretics, antihypertensives, and other medications.
- Teach patients taking the liquid form that even if the drug is supplied with a dropper, it should be taken orally.
- Teach patients that if a dose is forgotten, it should be omitted. Patients should not double up for missed doses. Tell the patient to notify the physician if doses for 2 or more days are missed.
- Instruct patients not to take other medications, including OTC preparations, without prior approval from the physician.

- Teach patients to avoid storing drugs in the bathroom, where moisture may cause the drug to break down. Store drugs away from light and heat.
- Suggest that patients wear a medical identification tag or bracelet indicating that they are taking a cardiac glycoside.
- Refer patients to a community-based nursing care agency if appropriate. Consult patient and physician.
- Remind patients to keep these and all medications out of the reach of children.

## deslanoside    (dez-LAN-oh-side)                                                 cardiac glycoside

- deslanoside (desacetyl-lanatoside C): Cedilanid-D

**MECHANISM OF ACTION**    Deslanoside is a cardiac glycoside derived from *Digitalis lanata*, the white foxglove. Deslanoside improves cardiac contractility, allowing cardiac output to increase.

**INDICATIONS**    **Congestive heart failure** Deslanoside is only for emergency IV therapy for congestive heart failure, to be replaced as soon as possible with one of the oral cardiac glycosides.

**CONTRAINDICATIONS**    **Ventricular fibrillation, ventricular tachycardia** Cardiac glycosides may worsen ventricular arrhythmias.    **Hypokalemia** may make a patient more sensitive to deslanoside and more likely to develop dangerous arrhythmias.    **Thyroid dysfunction** Hypothyroidism diminishes deslanoside excretion and may require a reduction in dosage. • Hyperthyroidism may increase resistance to deslanoside and may make the patient more prone to dangerous arrhythmias.

**DOSAGE**    **IV, IM:**    **ADULTS:** Initially, 0.8 mg repeated after 4 hours, or 1.6 mg in a single injection. The maximum dose is usually 2 mg total.    **CHILDREN:** Divide the following doses into two or three portions and administer at 3- or 4-hour intervals: newborns, 0.022 mg/kg; infants up to 3 years, 0.025 mg/kg; children over 3 years, 0.0225 mg/kg.    *Special patient populations:*    **PREGNANCY:** Safe use during pregnancy has not been established.    **RENAL FAILURE:** In renal failure the excretion of deslanoside is decreased, and doses may need to be adjusted downward.

**PREPARATIONS**    **Solution for injection:** 2 ml ampuls containing 0.2 mg/ml deslanoside; store between 15° and 30° C (59° and 86° F).

**DRUG INTERACTIONS**    Deslanoside is subject to the same drug interactions as other cardiac glycosides (see entry for drug class, p. 56).

**FATE**    Deslanoside is unreliably absorbed orally; *bioavailability* is usually unacceptably low. When deslanoside is given intravenously, the *onset* action is 10 to 30 minutes, with *peak* effect at 1 to 3 hours. The drug is excreted by the kidneys; however, the plasma *half-life* is 33 to 36 hours. The *duration* of action is 2 to 5 days.

### ❧ NURSING CONSIDERATIONS

#### Side effects, toxicities, and associated nursing actions
- See entry for drug class (p. 56).

#### Nursing interventions related to drug administration
- IM injection is painful; IV administration is preferred.
- Attach patient to a cardiac monitor before administering drug.
- Administer 0.2 mg (1 ml) or less over 1 minute. May be given undiluted. Do not mix with infusing IV fluids.

#### Patient and family education
- This drug is not used for self-administration.
- Keep patient and family informed of patient's condition.

## digitalis glycosides    (di-ji-TAL-iss)                                          cardiac glycoside

- digitalis glycosides: Digiglusin

**MECHANISM OF ACTION**   A refined mixture of cardiac glycosides from *Digitalis purpurea* with actions characteristic of the class (see entry for drug class, p. 55). This preparation is rarely used because better control can usually be achieved with one of the pure cardiac glycoside preparations.

**INDICATIONS**   **Chronic congestive heart failure or atrial arrhythmias (fibrillation, flutter, or paroxysmal atrial tachycardia)** Maintenance therapy only.

**CONTRAINDICATIONS**   See entry for drug class (p. 56).

**DOSAGE**   **Adults:**   PO: Loading dose, 2 digitalis units twice daily for 4 days, followed by maintenance doses of 0.5 to 3 units daily.   *Special patient populations:*   CHILDREN: Doses have not been established. PREGNANCY: Safe use during pregnancy has not been established.

**PREPARATIONS**   *Tablets:* the strength of this preparation is expressed in units rather than on a weight basis. Each tablet is formulated to contain one National Formulary (NF) unit of activity.

**DRUG INTERACTIONS**   See entry for drug class (p. 56).

   **FATE**   This preparation is similar to digitalis leaf (see below).

❦ **NURSING CONSIDERATIONS**
   **Side effects, toxicities, and associated nursing actions**
      • See entry for drug class (p. 56).
   **Nursing interventions related to drug administration**
      • See entry for drug class (p. 57).
   **Patient and family education**
      • See entry for drug class (p. 57).

---

## digitalis leaf   (di-ji-TAL-iss)                              cardiac glycoside

   • digitalis leaf: Same as generic (not available in Canada)

**MECHANISM OF ACTION**   A crude mixture of cardiac glycosides with actions characteristic of the class (see entry for drug class, p. 55), this preparation is not commonly used because better control can usually be achieved with one of the pure cardiac glycoside preparations.

**INDICATIONS**   **Chronic congestive heart failure** Maintenance therapy only.   **Atrial arrhythmias (fibrillation, flutter, paroxysmal atrial tachycardia)** Maintenance therapy only.

**CONTRAINDICATIONS**   See entry for drug class (p. 56).

**DOSAGE**   PO:   ADULT: The loading dose is 1.2 g total, given as several smaller doses every 6 hours. Maintenance doses range from 100 to 400 mg daily.   *Special patient populations:*   CHILDREN: Doses not established.   PREGNANCY: Safe use during pregnancy has not been established.

**PREPARATIONS**   *Tablets:* 32.5, 48.75, 65, and 100 mg. *Capsules:* 100 mg.

**DRUG INTERACTIONS**   See entry for drug class (p. 56).

   **FATE**   The *bioavailability* is adequate for oral administration. The *onset* of action is 2 to 4 hours, with a *peak* effect at 12 to 14 hours. The *duration* of action is 14 days. The major active ingredient is digitoxin.

❦ **NURSING CONSIDERATIONS**
   **Side effects, toxicities, and associated nursing actions**
      • See entry for drug class (p. 56).
   **Nursing interventions related to drug administration**
      • See entry for drug class (p. 57).
   **Patient and family education**
      • See entry for drug class (p. 57).

---

## digitoxin   (di-ji-TOX-in)                              cardiac glycoside

   • digitoxin: Crystodigin, De-Tone, Purodigin

**MECHANISM OF ACTION**   Digitoxin is a purified form of the primary active glycoside from *Digitalis purpurea,* the purple foxglove. Digitoxin inhibits Na$^+$, K$^+$-ATPase and promotes accumulation within heart cells of the calcium required for contraction. These biochemical actions improve cardiac contractility, allowing cardiac output to increase.

**INDICATIONS**   **Congestive heart failure** Oral maintenance therapy for congestive heart failure or parenteral therapy for acute control.   **Arrhythmias** Atrial fibrillation, atrial flutter, or paroxysmal atrial tachycardia may be controlled with digitoxin.

**CONTRAINDICATIONS**   **Ventricular fibrillation or ventricular tachycardia** Cardiac glycosides may worsen ventricular arrhythmias.   **Hypokalemia** may predispose a patient to dangerous cardiac toxicity with digitoxin.   **Hepatic dysfunction** may diminish metabolism of digitoxin and cause dangerous drug accumulation. • Renal impairment has little effect.   **Hypothyroidism** requires smaller doses and care in preventing toxic reactions.

**DOSAGE**   **PO:**   **ADULTS:** Loading doses may be 0.8 mg followed by 0.2 mg every 6 to 8 hours for 2 or 3 doses for rapid loading, or 0.2 mg twice daily for 4 days for slow loading. Maintenance doses range from 0.05 to 0.2 mg daily.   **CHILDREN:** Loading doses given below should be divided into at least 3 doses spaced 6 hours or more apart. Newborns receive 0.025 mg/kg; infants up to 1 year, 0.035 to 0.045 mg/kg; 1 to 2 years of age, 0.04 mg/kg; over 2 years of age, 0.02 to 0.03 mg/kg. The maintenance dose for children is approximately 10% of the loading dose.   **IV:**   **ADULTS, CHILDREN:** Loading doses as for the oral route.   *Special patient populations:*   **PREGNANCY:** Safe use in pregnancy has not been established.   **HEPATIC IMPAIRMENT:** Liver damage caused by alcoholism or other conditions may impair drug excretion and increase risk of accumulation to toxic levels.

**PREPARATIONS**   *Tablets:* 0.05, 0.10, 0.15, and 0.20 mg. *Solution for injection:* 1 ml ampuls contain 0.2 mg/ml with 49% alcohol.

**DRUG INTERACTIONS**   Digitoxin is subject to the same drug interactions as other cardiac glycosides. See entry for drug class (p. 56).

**FATE**   Digitoxin is almost completely absorbed orally, with an *onset* of action from 0.5 to 2 hours and a *peak* effect in 4 to 12 hours. High plasma protein binding (97%) and hepatic metabolism as the main route of excretion combine to give this drug a long serum *half-life* (5 to 7 days). The *duration* of action is approximately 14 days.

### ☙ NURSING CONSIDERATIONS

#### Side effects, toxicities, and associated nursing actions
• See entry for drug class (p. 56).

#### Nursing interventions related to drug administration
• IM injection is painful. IV administration is the preferred parenteral route.
• Before IV administration, attach patient to a cardiac monitor.
• Administer IV dose at a rate of 0.2 mg (1 ml) or less over 1 minute. May be given undiluted. Do not mix with infusing fluids.

#### Patient and family education
• See entry for drug class (p. 57).
• Purodigin brand may contain FD & C yellow #5 (tartrazine) and may cause allergic reactions in some individuals. This allergic reaction is seen more often in individuals with aspirin hypersensitivity.

---

## digoxin   (di-JOX-in)                                   cardiac glycoside, antiarrhythmic

• digoxin: Lanoxin, Lanoxicaps, ✽Novodigoxin

**MECHANISM OF ACTION**   Digoxin is a purified form of an active glycoside from *Digitalis lanata,* the white foxglove. Digoxin inhibits Na$^+$, K$^+$-ATPase and promotes the accumulation within heart cells of the calcium required for contraction. These biochemical actions improve cardiac contractility, allowing cardiac output to increase. Digoxin also lowers automaticity in the SA node and slows conduction through the AV node. These actions may be useful in controlling atrial arrhythmias.

**INDICATIONS**   **Congestive heart failure** Intravenously for acute control of congestive heart failure and orally for chronic control.   **Atrial fibrillation, atrial flutter, or paroxysmal atrial tachycardia** Intravenously for acute control or orally for chronic control of these conditions.

**CONTRAINDICATIONS**   **Ventricular fibrillation and ventricular tachycardia** Cardiac glycosides may worsen ventricular arrhythmias.   **Hypokalemia** Electrolyte disturbances and especially hypokalemia may predispose patients to dangerous cardiac toxicity with digoxin.   **Hypothyroidism** This condition requires smaller doses and care in preventing toxic reactions.   **Wolff-Parkinson-White syndrome** This form of paroxysmal tachycardia or atrial flutter responds atypically to digoxin and other cardiac glycosides.   **AV nodal blockade** Digoxin further slows AV conduction and may cause complete heart block.

**DOSAGE**   **PO with tablets:**   **ADULTS:** *Congestive heart failure,* loading dose initially 0.5 to 0.75 mg, with 0.25 to 0.5 mg following at 6- to 8-hour intervals for 2 or 3 doses for rapid loading. Maintenance dose also used for slow loading is 0.125 to 0.5 mg daily. *For supraventricular tachycardia,* the initial dose for a patient not already receiving a cardiac glycoside is 0.5 to 1 mg, with a second dose of 0.25 mg given 2 hours later. Daily doses thereafter are usually 0.25 to 0.5 mg/day.   **CHILDREN:** *For congestive heart failure,* loading doses given below should be divided and administered every 6 hours. Premature infants receive 0.02 to 0.03 mg/kg; newborns, 0.025 to 0.035 mg/kg; infants up to 2 years, 0.035 to 0.06 mg/kg; 2 to 5 years, 0.03 to 0.04 mg/kg; 5 to 10 years, 0.02 to 0.035 mg/kg; and over 10 years, 0.01 to 0.015 mg/kg. The maintenance dose for premature infants is 20% to 30% of the loading dose; for all other children, 25% to 35% of the loading dose.   **PO with capsule or IV:**   **ADULTS:** *For congestive heart failure,* loading dose of 0.25 to 0.5 mg followed by 0.25 mg two or three more times at 4- to 6-hour intervals. The maintenance dose ranges from 0.125 to 0.5 mg daily. For supraventricular arrhythmias, initial doses are 0.25 mg repeated at 1 hour and, if necessary, at 4 hours. Maintenance is with oral digoxin.   **CHILDREN:** *For congestive heart failure,* loading doses given below are divided and administered every 6 hours. Premature infants receive 0.015 to 0.025 mg/kg; newborns, 0.02 to 0.03 mg/kg; infants up to 2 years, 0.03 to 0.05 mg/kg; 2 to 5 years, 0.025 to 0.035 mg/kg; and 5 to 10 years, 0.015 to 0.03 mg/kg. The maintenance dose for premature infants is 20% to 30% of the oral loading dose; for all other children, 25% to 30% of the oral loading dose.   *Special patient populations:*   **ELDERLY:** Doses may be smaller than for younger adults, primarily because renal function is lower in the elderly, and they are more sensitive to cardiac glycosides.   **RENAL DYSFUNCTION:** Impaired renal function lowers excretion of digoxin and may cause dangerous drug accumulation.   **PREGNANCY:** Safe use during pregnancy has not been established.

**PREPARATIONS**   *Tablets:* 0.125, 0.25, and 0.5 mg. Tablets from various manufacturers have been noted to differ in bioavailability. *Elixir:* for oral use in pediatric patients, 0.05 mg/ml in 10% alcohol. *Solution for injection:* 1 or 2 ml ampuls, disposable syringe, or tubex containing 0.25 mg/ml or 0.1 mg/ml. *Solution in capsules:* 0.05 mg (red), 0.1 mg (yellow), or 0.2 mg (green) of digoxin. The trade name is Lanoxicaps.

**DRUG INTERACTIONS**   See entry for drug class (p. 56).

**FATE**   Oral absorption of digoxin is variable and depends on which preparation is used. *Bioavailability* of the tablets ranges from 60% to 80%, whereas that of the elixir or the rarely used IM form is 70% to 85%. Oral absorption of digoxin administered in capsules is essentially complete and is equivalent to IV dosing in terms of the total amount of drug absorbed. Digoxin given IV has an *onset* of 5 to 30 minutes and a *peak* effect in 1 to 4 hours. Orally administered digoxin takes effect in 0.5 to 2 hours and has *peak* action from 2 to 6 hours. The *duration* of action is 2 to 6 days for both routes. Plasma protein binding is 23%, and the plasma *half-life* is 32 to 48 hours. Digoxin is excreted by the kidneys.

## 🐦 NURSING CONSIDERATIONS

### Side effects, toxicities, and associated nursing actions
  • See entry for drug class (p. 56).

### Nursing interventions related to drug administration
  • See entry for drug class (p. 57).
  • IM injection is painful; IV administration is the preferred parenteral route.
  • Before IV administration, attach patient to a cardiac monitor.
  • Administer IV dose at a rate of 0.25 mg (1 ml) or less per minute. May be given undiluted. Do not mix with infusing fluids.

- Because bioavailability varies with oral form and manufacturer, do not switch oral forms without checking with pharmacy and physician; it may be necessary to adjust the dose or frequency of drug administration.

### Patient and family education

- See entry for drug class (p. 57).
- Because preparations from different manufacturers may vary in bioavailability, instruct patients not to switch brands of digoxin unless directed to do so by the physician.

---

## gitalin   (GI-tuh-lin)                                                      cardiac glycoside

- gitalin: Gitalignin

**MECHANISM OF ACTION**   A refined mixture of cardiac glycosides from *Digitalis purpurea* with actions characteristic of the class. See entry for drug class (p. 55). This preparation is not commonly used because better control can usually be achieved with one of the pure glycosides.

**INDICATIONS**   **Congestive heart failure** Maintenance therapy only.   **Atrial arrhythmias (fibrillation, flutter, paroxysmal atrial tachycardia)** Maintenance therapy only.

**CONTRAINDICATIONS**   See entry for drug class (p. 56).

**DOSAGE**   **PO:**   **ADULT:** Total loading dose of 6 to 9 mg given as a single daily dose of 1.5 mg for 4 to 6 days, or by initial dose of 2.5 mg followed by 0.75 mg every 6 hours up to the maximum dose. Maintenance doses range from 0.25 to 1.25 mg daily.   *Special patient populations:*   **CHILDREN:** Doses not established.   **PREGNANCY:** Safe use during pregnancy has not been established.

**PREPARATIONS**   *Tablets:* 0.5 mg. Tartrazine in the tablets may cause allergic reactions in sensitive patients.

**DRUG INTERACTIONS**   See entry for drug class (p. 56).

**FATE**   The *onset* of action of gitalin is 2 to 4 hours, with a *peak* effect at 8 to 12 hours. The *duration* of action is 12 days. The major active ingredient of gitalin is digitoxin.

### ☙ NURSING CONSIDERATIONS

#### Side effects, toxicities, and associated nursing actions

- See entry for drug class (p. 56).

#### Nursing interventions related to drug administration

- See entry for drug class (p. 57).

#### Patient and family education

- See entry for drug class (p. 57).
- Gitaligin brand may contain FD & C yellow #5 (tartrazine) and may cause allergic reactions in some individuals. This allergic reaction is seen more often in individuals with aspirin hypersensitivity.

---

## ouabain   (WAH-bain)                                                      cardiac glycoside

- ouabain (G-strophanthin): Same as generic

**MECHANISM OF ACTION**   Ouabain, a glycoside from *Strophanthus gratus*, inhibits $Na^+$, $K^+-ATPase$ and promotes the accumulation within heart cells of the calcium required for contraction. These biochemical actions improve cardiac contractility, allowing cardiac output to increase.

**INDICATIONS**   **Congestive heart failure** Acute control of congestive heart failure.   **Atrial arrhythmias (fibrillation, flutter, or paroxysmal atrial tachycardia)** Acute control of atrial arrhythmias.

**CONTRAINDICATIONS**   **Ventricular fibrillation, ventricular tachycardia** Cardiac glycosides may worsen ventricular arrhythmias.   **Hypokalemia** Hypokalemia may predispose a patient to dangerous cardiac toxicity with ouabain.   **Hypothyroidism** This condition requires smaller doses and care in preventing toxic reactions.

**DOSAGE**   IV:   ADULTS: The maximum dose is 1 mg in 24 hours. Initially, 0.25 to 0.5 mg may be given with an additional 0.1 mg added hourly, up to the maximum dose.   CHILDREN: 10 mg/kg body weight is the total dose. One half the dose is given initially, with the remainder divided into several small doses to be given at 30-minute intervals until response is achieved or the total dose is used up.   *Special patient populations:*   RENAL DYSFUNCTION: Impaired renal function lowers excretion of ouabain and may cause dangerous drug accumulation.   PREGNANCY: Safe use during pregnancy has not been established.

**PREPARATIONS**   *Solution for injection:* 2 ml ampuls contain 0.25 mg/ml ouabain with 2 mg potassium phosphate monobasic.

**DRUG INTERACTIONS**   Ouabain is subject to the same drug interactions as other cardiac glycosides (p. 56).

**FATE**   Ouabain is administered only intravenously. The *onset* of action is rapid, taking effect in 5 to 10 minutes, with *peak* effects at 0.5 to 2 hours. The plasma *half-life* is 21 hours, and the *duration* of action is 1 to 3 days. Ouabain is excreted by the kidneys.

### 🦌 NURSING CONSIDERATIONS
**Side effects, toxicities, and associated nursing actions**
- See entry for drug class (p. 56).

**Nursing interventions related to drug administration**
- See entry for of drug class (p. 57).
- This drug is for IV administration only.
- Before IV administration, attach patient to a cardiac monitor.
- Administer IV dose at a rate of 0.25 mg or less per minute. May be given undiluted. Do not mix with infusing fluids.

**Patient and family education**
- This drug is not used for self-administration.

---

# Miscellaneous inotropic agents

amrinone lactate  ~  milrinone (investigational)

**OVERVIEW OF THE DRUG CLASS**   Congestive heart failure is most often treated with cardiac glycosides (p. 55), diuretics (Chapter 9), and vasodilators (p. 114). When those therapies fail, amrinone or milrinone may be selected.

**MECHANISM OF ACTION**   Amrinone and milrinone inhibit phosphodiesterase and increase cyclic AMP in cardiac cells. This action increases calcium uptake and enhances the strength of contraction of the cells. Because this mechanism is different from that of other inotropic agents, amrinone and milrinone can have additive effects with cardiac glycosides.

**INDICATIONS**   Congestive heart failure Amrinone may be used in severe chronic heart failure resistant to cardiac glycosides, diuretics, or vasodilators.

**CONTRAINDICATIONS**   **Aortic or pulmonic valvular disease** Obstruction must be cleared before amrinone or milrinone can be given safely.   **Hypertrophic subaortic stenosis** Amrinone or milrinone may worsen outflow tract obstruction.

---

## amrinone lactate   (AM-ri-nohne)                                              inotropic agent

- amrinone lactate: Inocor

**MECHANISM OF ACTION**   Amrinone inhibits phosphodiesterase activity, thereby increasing strength of contraction of the heart muscle.

**INDICATIONS**   Congestive heart failure Severe chronic disease unresponsive to conventional therapy.

**CONTRAINDICATIONS**   See entry for drug class (above).

**DOSAGE** **Adults:** **IV:** Initially, 0.75 mg/kg as a bolus over 2 to 3 minutes; maintenance is with an infusion of 5 to 10 mg/kg/min. Total daily dose should not exceed 10 mg/kg. *Special patient populations:* **CHILDREN:** Doses have not been established. **PREGNANCY:** FDA pregnancy category C. **RENAL OR HEPATIC IMPAIRMENT:** Doses may need to be reduced.

**PREPARATIONS** *Solution for injection:* 5 mg/ml.

**DRUG INTERACTIONS** **Dextrose** solutions may chemically inactivate amrinone.

**FATE** Amrinone is used only intravenously because oral doses used chronically are not very effective. *Onset* of action occurs within 2 to 5 minutes, and *peak* effects are seen 10 minutes following IV doses. The *duration* of action is 0.5 to 2 hours. Amrinone is partially metabolized by the liver; unchanged drug and metabolites are excreted in urine.

## ❦ NURSING CONSIDERATIONS

### Side effects, toxicities, and associated nursing actions

**CV** Arrhythmias may occur in up to 3% of patients. Hypotension occurs in about 1.3%.
- Monitor ECG, blood pressure, and pulse.
- Keep patient in bed until vital signs are stable.
- Keep siderails up; supervise ambulation.

**Blood** Thrombocytopenia occurs in up to 2.4% of patients and may be dose dependent.
- Inspect patient for petechiae and bruising. Instruct patient to report the development of unexplained bleeding or bruising.
- Monitor the complete blood cell count and the platelet count.

**GI** Amrinone given intravenously causes nausea, vomiting, abdominal pain, or anorexia in less than 1.7% of patients. Oral amrinone causes severe GI side effects in many patients, preventing continued use of the drug by that route.
- Monitor weight.
- Assess for GI side effects.

**Liver** Liver enzyme concentrations may rise, and hepatocellular necrosis can occur. The effect may occur in some form in 0.2% of patients.
- Monitor liver function tests.
- Assess patient for jaundice, malaise, fever, right upper quadrant abdominal pain, and change in color or consistency of stools.

**Allergic** A severe reaction leading to liver and pulmonary failure is rare but has been seen with oral doses of amrinone given over 2 weeks.
- Instruct patient to report any difficulty breathing or the development of symptoms of liver dysfunction (see liver).
- Auscultate breath sounds and monitor respiratory rate.

**Local** Pain and burning at the injection site may occur in about 0.2% of patients.
- Assess patient for pain during drug administration. If pain occurs, slow infusion rate or further dilute drug (consult physician).

### Nursing interventions related to drug administration
- Attach patient to cardiac monitor before administering IV doses. Monitor blood pressure and pulse.
- May be given undiluted; administer dose slowly over 2 to 3 minutes.
- For infusion, dilute drug in 0.45% or 0.9% sodium chloride solution to a concentration of 1 to 3 mg/ml.
- Do not dilute with dextrose solutions, but drug may be administered into the tubing of a free-flowing IV line containing dextrose IV solution.

### Patient and family education
- Review with patients the anticipated benefits and possible side effects of drug therapy. Because this drug is rarely used outside of the acute-care setting, it is rarely self-administered. Keep patient and family informed of changes in the patient's condition.

## milrinone (MIL-ri-nohne)

- milrinone (investigational)

**MECHANISM OF ACTION** Milrinone, like amrinone, inhibits phosphodiesterase activity, thereby increasing strength of contraction of the heart muscle. In addition, milrinone has vasodilator activity.

**INDICATIONS** **Severe refractory congestive heart failure** Short-term improvement may occur, but long-term improvement or changes in mortality have not been proven.

**CONTRAINDICATIONS** See entry for drug class (p. 63).

**DOSAGE** **PO, IV:** Doses are not yet established.

### NURSING CONSIDERATIONS

#### Side effects, toxicities, and associated nursing actions

**CV** Tachycardia and other arrhythmias may occur. Myocardial ischemia may also be seen. Fluid retention worsens but may be alleviated with increased diuretic use.

- Monitor blood pressure and pulse before administering. Before IV use, attach patient to cardiac monitor.
- Monitor weight, and, if weight increases, monitor fluid intake and output. Instruct patient to monitor and record weight at home and to notify physician of weight gain in excess of 2 to 5 lb/week.
- Auscultate breath sounds. Assess for jugular venous distention and edema in dependent body parts.

**Other** Headache has been reported.

- Assess patient for headaches.

#### Nursing interventions related to drug administration

- Attach patient to cardiac monitor before IV administration.
- Consult manufacturer's literature for current guidelines regarding rate of administration and proper dilution.

#### Patient and family education

- Review anticipated benefits and possible side effects of drug therapy with patient. As this drug is more widely used, additional information will become available. Teach patients to notify physician of any new signs or symptoms that appear.

# Antiarrhythmic agents

amiodarone hydrochloride ~ bretylium tosylate ~ digoxin (p. 60) ~ disopyramide phosphate ~ encainide ~ flecainide acetate ~ lidocaine hydrochloride ~ mexiletine hydrochloride ~ phenytoin ~ procainamide hydrochloride ~ propranolol hydrochloride ~ quinidine sulfate ~ quinidine gluconate ~ quinidine polygalacturonate ~ tocainide hydrochloride ~ verapamil hydrochloride

**OVERVIEW OF THE DRUG CLASS** Arrhythmias are caused by disorders in initiating the heartbeat (pacing) or by disorders in conducting the impulse to beat through cardiac tissues. Disorders in heart pacing are often related to changes in automaticity of cardiac tissues, such as the SA node. Ectopic foci (automatic cells outside the SA node) may initiate beats, causing arrhythmias. Conduction disorders may either speed or slow the passage of impulses through the AV node to the ventricles; another common conduction disorder is called reentry, in which the impulse to beat cycles repeatedly through the same cells and prevents the entire heart from beating in concert.

**MECHANISM OF ACTION** Antiarrhythmic agents are drawn from several classes of drugs and have a variety of properties that make them useful for controlling arrhythmias. Antiarrhythmic agents have been classified according to mechanism of action. Class I antiarrhythmics include local anesthetics and other drugs that may alter cardiac cell membranes to change the sodium ion influx that allows cells to depolarize. Class II drugs block beta adrenergic activity in the heart, slow the rate at the SA node, and slow conduction through the AV node. Class III drugs prolong repolarization by mechanisms that are not completely understood. Class IV drugs block calcium channels, primarily changing the responses of cells highly dependent on the so-called slow calcium current, e.g., cells in the AV or SA nodes or in ischemic regions of heart muscle where ectopic beats may originate. The antiarrhythmic drugs are summarized by category in Table 6-2.

**INDICATIONS**   **Sinus tachycardia** Excessively rapid rates of firing at the SA node may respond to beta adrenergic blockade or to therapy aimed at the cause of the rapid rate, e.g., cardiac glycosides for congestive heart failure producing reflex tachycardia.   **Premature supraventricular complexes** These extrasystoles arising in the atria may respond to a variety of antiarrhythmic agents.   **Paroxysmal supraventricular tachycardia** Acute episodes are often terminated by IV verapamil. • A variety of agents may be used prophylactically.   **Atrial flutter and fibrillation** Digoxin or verapamil may prevent rapid ventricular rates secondary to atrial flutter or fibrillation. • Quinidine and other agents may prevent recurrences.   **Premature ventricular complexes** Usually benign, premature beats may be dangerous following myocardial infarction; a variety of agents may be used to prevent premature complexes. **Ventricular tachycardia** Because this rapid ventricular rate may lead to ventricular fibrillation, lidocaine or another antiarrhythmic agent may be required.

**CONTRAINDICATIONS**   Each agent in this diverse group may have specific contraindications. See the description of individual agents.

**DRUG INTERACTIONS**   Each agent in this diverse group may cause specific interactions. See the description of individual agents.

## ☙ NURSING CONSIDERATIONS
### Side effects, toxicities, and associated nursing actions
**CV** Arrhythmias (possible with all antiarrhythmics, especially at high doses); hypotension (all antiarrhythmics, especially when used intravenously); lowered contractility (quinidine, procainamide, disopyramide, propranolol, and verapamil therefore worsen congestive heart failure); slowed conduction through the AV node and AV nodal block (digoxin, quinidine, procainamide, propranolol, and verapamil are most likely to produce this effect).
- Monitor the vital signs and blood pressure. Although a change in the heart rate is frequently a desirable outcome of therapy, a heart rate less than 60 or greater than 120 beats/min (in an adult) should usually be avoided. Specific guidelines for an individual patient must be established in consultation with the physician.
- Monitoring the ECG is the best way to evaluate antiarrhythmic therapy. In the acute situation, continuous ECG monitoring should be done. The patient on maintenance therapy should have ECG tracings monitored at regular intervals. Assess for depression of cardiac activity: prolonged P-R interval, QRS complex, or Q-T interval.
- Monitor indicators of cardiovascular functioning as appropriate: blood pressure and pulse, intake and output, weight, heart and breath sounds, presence of edema (especially in dependent areas), and neck vein distention.

**Renal and liver** In the presence of renal or liver failure, these drugs may accumulate (see individual drugs).
- Monitor BUN and liver function studies.
- Monitor serum drug levels if available.

### Nursing Interventions related to drug administration
- For continuous infusion, microdrip tubing and an infusion control device or electronic infusion monitor should be used.
- These drugs should not be added to infusions containing other drugs or blood.
- Have emergency equipment and drugs available to counteract toxicity.

### Patient and family education
- Teach patients about the desired effects and common side effects of prescribed drugs. Tell patients to report the appearance of any unexpected sign or symptom.
- Review with patients the importance of taking medications as ordered. Antiarrhythmic drugs should not be taken on an "as needed" basis, but on a regular basis. If a dose is missed, patients should not "double up" on the next dose, unless instructed to do so by the physician. If the patient is having difficulty remembering to take the medication as ordered, the nurse should work with the patient to develop ways to improve compliance.

| Table 6-2. | Summary of antiarrhythmic agents | | |
|---|---|---|---|
| **Drug** | | **Route** | **Antiarrhythmic class\*** |
| Amiodarone | | PO, IV | III |
| Bretylium | | IV, IM | III |
| Disopyramide | | PO | IA |
| Encainide | | PO | IC |
| Flecainide | | PO | IC |
| Lidocaine | | IV, IM | IB |
| Mexiletine | | PO | IB |
| Procainamide | | PO, IV, IM | IA |
| Propranolol | | PO, IV | II |
| Quinidine | | PO, IV | IA |
| Tocainide | | PO | IB |
| Verapamil | | IV | IV |

\*Class I drugs change the sodium ion influx that allows cells to depolarize. Class IA drugs slow conduction and prolong refractoriness. Class IB drugs shorten the refractory period. Class IC drugs slow conduction without changing refractoriness. Class II drugs are adrenergic blockers. Class III drugs prolong refractoriness. Class IV drugs block calcium influx. See Mechanism of action for individual agents.

- Instruct patients not to discontinue antiarrhythmic medications without first discussing this with the physician.
- Stress the importance of concomitant therapies, which might include diet therapy, weight reduction, sodium restriction, use of potassium replacements, diuretics, antihypertensives, or other medications, limiting caffeine intake, and stopping smoking.
- The decision to have patients monitor the pulse, weight, intake and output, or other parameters on an outpatient basis must be made on an individual basis. Ascertain that the patient can perform the desired activity accurately before discharge.
- Suggest that the patient carry a medical identification tag or bracelet indicating that antiarrhythmic drugs are being used.
- Instruct patients to avoid the use of alcohol unless approved by the physician.
- Remind the patient to keep all health care providers, including dentists, informed of all medications being used.
- Remind patients to keep these and all medications out of the reach of children.
- Instruct patients not to store tablets or capsules in the bathroom, where heat or moisture may cause the drug to break down. Medicines should be stored in a dry place, away from heat or light.

## amiodarone hydrochloride   (AM-ee-oh-da-rone)   class III antiarrhythmic

- amiodarone hydrochloride: Cordarone

**MECHANISM OF ACTION**   Amiodarone alters function in all cardiac tissue. SA nodal firing is slowed, as is AV nodal conduction time; the refractory period is prolonged in AV node, ventricles, and atria.

**INDICATIONS**   **Refractory supraventricular or ventricular arrhythmias** Although amiodarone may be effective in many types of arrhythmias, it is currently indicated only for those that have failed to respond to other agents.

**CONTRAINDICATIONS**   **Severe sinus bradycardia** Amiodarone further slows heart rate by interfering with SA nodal firing.   **AV nodal blockade** Amiodarone further slows conduction through the AV node and may cause complete heart block. • The AV blockade produced by amiodarone is resistant to atropine.

**DOSAGE**   **Adults:**   **PO:** Initial daily doses may range from 600 to 1200 mg, divided into three doses. After a week, doses are reduced to 200 to 600 mg daily, divided into three doses.   **IV:** Doses up to 5 mg/kg may be given. Administer over a 5-minute period; do not repeat for at least 15 minutes. *Special patient populations:* CHILDREN: Doses have not been established. PREGNANCY: FDA pregnancy category C.

**PREPARATIONS** *Tablets:* 100 and 200 mg.

**DRUG INTERACTIONS** **Oral anticoagulants** are more effective in the presence of amiodarone. During therapy with amiodarone, the dose of oral anticoagulants should be reduced by about one half. **Digoxin and quinidine** concentrations in serum are increased by amiodarone. Toxicity may be triggered by drug accumulation. **Beta adrenergic blocking agents** may be potentiated by amiodarone, which is itself a weak nonspecific adrenergic blocker.

**FATE** Amiodarone has a long *onset* to action and is slowly eliminated from the body. The *half-life* of elimination is about 7 hours following a single dose, but during chronic therapy the *half-life* has been estimated at 29 days.

## ❧ NURSING CONSIDERATIONS

### Side effects, toxicities, and associated nursing actions

* See entry for drug class (p. 66).

**CNS** Tremor, headache, depression, insomnia, and hallucinations have occurred.

* Assess patient for the development of these side effects.
* Be alert for signs of depression: apathy, lack of interest in personal appearance, insomnia, and loss of appetite.

**GI** Anorexia, nausea, abdominal pain, and constipation.

* Assess for these GI side effects. Monitor weight.
* If constipation develops, suggest to patients that they increase fluid intake to 2500 to 3000 ml per day (if not contraindicated by the medical condition); increase dietary intake of fruit, fruit juices, and fiber; and increase level of exercise.

**Eye** Small corneal deposits that can impair vision may develop with long-term therapy. The deposits slowly disappear when the drug is discontinued.

* Obtain baseline assessment of vision before the start of therapy and reevaluate periodically. Suggest to patients who already wear glasses to continue periodic ophthalmic examinations. Instruct patients to report any changes in vision.

**Skin** Crystals may be deposited in the skin, causing light sensitivity and producing a bluish color.

* If photosensitivity develops (light sensitivity), instruct patients to avoid exposure to the sun or ultraviolet light, wear a wide-brimmed hat, keep extremities covered, and wear a maximum protection sunscreen containing zinc or titanium oxide on exposed skin surfaces.
* Warn patients about the possible skin side effects. Instruct them to notify the physician if these changes occur. The bluish skin color will fade after the drug is discontinued, but skin changes may require several months to resolve.

**CV** SA blockade, AV blockade, bradycardia, myocardial depression, and hypotension may occur. Severe AV nodal blockade, myocardial depression, and peripheral vasodilation would be expected with excessive doses of amiodarone.

* Monitor blood pressure and pulse. For IV administration, have patient attached to continuous cardiac monitoring.
* Keep patient supine after IV doses until vital signs are stable. Keep side rails up. Supervise ambulation. See Nursing interventions below.

**Lung** Pulmonary fibrosis or pneumonitis has been reported occasionally.

* Assess breath sounds and respiratory rate and for the presence of respiratory symptoms (shortness of breath, painful breathing) on a regular basis.

### Nursing interventions related to drug administration

* Note Dosage and CV side effects above. Administer IV dose over at least 5 minutes and do not repeat for at least 15 minutes. Monitor blood pressure and pulse every 5 minutes until stable.

### Patient and family education

* See entry for drug class (p. 66).
* Review anticipated benefits and possible side effects of drug therapy. Instruct patients to report the development of any new sign or symptom.

## bretylium tosylate   (bre-TILL-ee-um TOZ-ill-ate)   class III antiarrhythmic*

- bretylium tosylate: ✤Bretylate, Bretylol

**MECHANISM OF ACTION**   The antiarrhythmic effects of bretylium are not fully understood, although several actions of the drug are known. Bretylium initially releases catecholamines that increase sympathetic effects (tachycardia, rise in blood pressure), but these responses wane as peripheral adrenergic blockade becomes predominant (orthostatic hypotension). In animals bretylium alters electrophysiology of damaged or ischemic cardiac tissue but has less effect on normal tissue. If these same effects occur in humans they may explain the antiarrhythmic action of bretylium.

**INDICATIONS**   **Ventricular fibrillation** Short-term control or prevention of this potentially life-threatening condition.   **Ventricular tachycardia** Short-term therapy in patients who fail to respond to lidocaine, which is usually the drug of choice.

**CONTRAINDICATIONS**   **Aortic stenosis or pulmonary hypertension** Bretylium may cause dangerous hypotension in patients with severe aortic stenosis or severe pulmonary hypertension because these patients cannot increase cardiac output on demand. • If bretylium must be used, medical personnel should be prepared to treat acute hypotension.   **Arrhythmias induced by cardiac glycosides** Bretylium enhances toxicity of cardiac glycosides.

**DOSAGE**   **Adults:**   **IV:** 5 to 10 mg/kg may be given by rapid injection for life-threatening arrhythmias or over a period of 10 to 30 minutes for less critical arrhythmias. Doses are repeated as necessary for life-threatening arrhythmias but for other arrhythmias are usually repeated at intervals up to 6 hours. Bretylium may be given by constant infusion at a rate of 1 to 2 mg/min for continued suppression of arrhythmias. Daily doses rarely exceed 40 mg/kg.   **IM:** Undiluted drug may be injected at 5 to 10 mg/kg and repeated as often as hourly if needed. Injection sites should be rotated and intramuscular injection discontinued as soon as possible.   *Special patient populations:*   **ELDERLY:** Doses should be individualized; renal impairment requires that doses be reduced.   **CHILDREN:** Doses have not been standardized, although bretylium has been used occasionally in children.   **PREGNANCY:** Safe use has not been established.   **RENAL FAILURE:** Doses must be reduced when renal function is impaired.

**PREPARATIONS**   *Solution for injection:* 10 ml ampuls each containing 500 mg of bretylium tosylate in Water for Injection (USP). The pH of the solution has been adjusted as necessary with HCl or sodium hydroxide. The drug may be used undiluted for intramuscular injection or for rapid IV administration for life-threatening arrhythmias. For all other IV administration, bretylium should be diluted in Dextrose (5%) Injection (USP) or Sodium Chloride Injection (USP) to allow infusion of appropriate concentrations.

**DRUG INTERACTIONS**   **Cardiac glycoside** toxicity may be triggered by bretylium. Bretylium should not be administered to a patient suffering from an arrhythmia thought to be induced by a cardiac glycoside nor should a patient simultaneously be started on bretylium and a cardiac glycoside.

**DIAGNOSTIC TEST INTERFERENCES**   Urinary vanillylmandelic acid (VMA), epinephrine, and norepinephrine levels may increase when bretylium is administered.

**FATE**   Bretylium is variably absorbed orally and is not given by that route. The *onset* of antifibrillatory effects of bretylium occurs within minutes of IV administration; however, control of other ventricular arrhythmias may take longer. Bretylium is not metabolized. Unaltered drug is excreted by the kidneys. The elimination *half-life* is about 8 hours but may be increased by renal impairment. Bretylium is removed by dialysis.

### ☙ NURSING CONSIDERATIONS
#### Side effects, toxicities, and associated nursing actions
- See entry for drug class (p. 66).
  **CV** Temporary increases in blood pressure and possibly in the activity of ectopic pacemakers in the ventricle result from the initial increase in release of catecholamines caused by bretylium.
- Bretylium commonly causes a fall in supine blood pressure within an hour of IV administration; if

*Also adrenergic antagonist.

the pressure falls below 75 mm Hg, therapy with pressor agents may be required.

- Bradycardia or anginal attacks are sometimes induced.
- The use of this drug is usually limited to intensive care and coronary care units where continuous cardiac monitoring and equipment and personnel for emergency treatment and resuscitation are available.
- Monitor the vital signs, blood pressure, and ECG.
- Following IV administration, keep the patient lying down until the blood pressure stabilizes.
- With IV administration, monitor the blood pressure every 5 to 15 minutes until the blood pressure stabilizes.

**GI** Nausea and vomiting may occur if bretylium is given intravenously too rapidly.

- See Nursing interventions below.

**CNS** Vertigo, lightheadedness, and syncope may be caused by hypotension. Anxiety, confusion, and a variety of other emotional or psychiatric symptoms have occurred.

- Monitor blood pressure and pulse.
- Keep side rails up. Keep patients supine until blood pressure is stable, then supervise ambulation.
- Remain calm. Do not leave patient unattended until effects of drug can be evaluated. Reorient patient as needed.

### Nursing interventions related to drug administration

- See entry for drug class (p. 66).
- To lessen nausea and vomiting, dilute the drug and administer intravenously over at least 8 minutes.
- Review preparations. Although usually given intravenously, the drug can be given intramuscularly. No more than 5 ml should be administered at one intramuscular site at a time; rotate injection sites.
- For continuous infusion, dilute 1 g in 1000 ml of desired diluent to make a dilution of 1 mg/ml. Titrate the dose based on patient's response and within parameters established in consultation with the physician.

### Patient and family education

- Bretylium is rarely used for self-management. Keep the patient and family informed of the patient's condition and changes in the treatment plan.

## disopyramide phosphate   (dye-so-PEER-a-mide)                    class I antiarrhythmic

- disopyramide phosphate: Norpace, ✿Rythmodan

**MECHANISM OF ACTION**   Disopyramide slows the normally rapid depolarization of automatic cells in the heart by altering sodium ion flow across the cell membrane. The major effect is an increase in the action potential duration and an increase in the effective refractory period. These actions appear on the ECG as a widening of various intervals, such as the Q-T interval. Many of the actions of disopyramide resemble those of quinidine and procainamide. Disopyramide has little effect on alpha or beta adrenergic receptors but does produce noticeable anticholinergic effects resembling those of the muscarinic cholinergic receptor blocker atropine. Disopyramide is a potent negative inotropic agent (diminishes contractility of heart muscle). Unlike procainamide and quinidine, disopyramide does not cause vasodilation and in fact can set off reflex activities that may increase peripheral resistance.

**INDICATIONS**   **Premature (ectopic) ventricular contractions** Disopyramide limits activity of ectopic pacemakers.   **Ventricular tachycardia** Disopyramide is appropriate for controlling episodic ventricular tachycardia (rapid rate) but should not be substituted for DC cardioversion for persistent ventricular tachycardia.

**CONTRAINDICATIONS**   **Digitalis-induced arrhythmias** Disopyramide is not effective for these arrhythmias. **Preexisting second- or third-degree AV blockade** Ectopic pacemakers may be required to pace the heart in these conditions.   **Cardiogenic shock** Disopyramide tends to lower cardiac output.

**Glaucoma** The atropine-like effects of disopyramide may worsen glaucoma.    **Hypersensitivity** Patients known to be hypersensitive to disopyramide should not receive the drug again.    **Myasthenia gravis** The atropine-like effects of disopyramide may worsen this condition.    **Urinary retention** The atropine-like effects of disopyramide may worsen urinary retention.

**DOSAGE**    **PO:**    ADULTS: With the regular preparation for immediate release, doses of 100 to 150 mg every 6 hours are common. Daily doses may range from 400 to 800 mg if needed. An alternative schedule involves a loading dose of 300 mg initially, followed by 100 to 150 mg every 6 hours thereafter. Doses must be individualized and should be expected to be lower than the normal range for patients weighing less than 50 kg or for patients suffering from hepatic or renal impairment, cardiomyopathy, or congestive heart failure. These patients should not receive loading doses.    **CHILDREN:** Ages under 1 year, 10 to 30 mg/kg; 1 to 4 years, 10 to 20 mg/kg; 4 to 12 years, 10 to 15 mg/kg; and 12 to 18 years, 6 to 15 mg/kg.    **PO, sustained-release preparation:**    ADULTS: 300 mg every 12 hours is common; doses should be reduced to 200 mg every 12 hours for patients weighing less than 50 kg. The sustained-release preparation should not be used in patients with hepatic or renal dysfunction, cardiomyopathy, or congestive heart failure.    **CHILDREN:** The sustained-release preparation should not be used in children.    *Special patient populations:*    ELDERLY: Doses must be reduced for patients weighing less than 50 kg or for patients with cardiac, hepatic, or renal dysfunction; these conditions are more common in the elderly. The elderly are also more prone to suffer urinary retention. **PREGNANCY:** Disopyramide may initiate uterine contractions in pregnant patients. Experience with the drug in pregnant patients is limited.

**PREPARATIONS**    *Capsules:* 100 or 150 mg of disopyramide as the phosphate. *Suspension:* a suspension for pediatric use may be prepared by the pharmacist; the contents of regular capsules (not sustained-release) may be dissolved in cherry syrup NF to make a 1 to 10 mg/ml suspension. This suspension should be refrigerated and stored in an amber glass bottle with a child-proof closure. Under these conditions, the suspension may be stable up to a month. *Capsules, sustained-release:* 100 or 150 mg of disopyramide as the phosphate. The sustained-release preparations are marked ''Norpace CR'' and ''Rhythmodan LA.'' These preparations should not be used to make a pediatric liquid suspension.

**DRUG INTERACTIONS**    **Procainamide, quinidine, lidocaine, and propranolol** when used with disopyramide may cause serious negative inotropic effects (impairment of contractility) or may dangerously prolong conduction in the heart.    **Phenytoin, barbiturates, glutethimide, primidone, and rifampin** may induce enzymes in the liver that degrade disopyramide. As a result, elimination of disopyramide is increased, and the effective blood levels fall.

**FATE**    Disopyramide is absorbed rapidly and well on oral administration, achieving *peak* blood levels within 2 to 3 hours. Elimination of disopyramide is by renal and hepatic mechanisms, with 30% of a dose being eliminated as metabolites and about 50% appearing in the urine as unchanged drug. The elimination *half-life* is around 7 hours for normal adults but may be prolonged in renal failure or in patients with recent myocardial infarctions.

## ❦ NURSING CONSIDERATIONS

**Side effects, toxicities, and associated nursing actions**    Up to 70% of patients receiving disopyramide experience clinically significant side effects, and up to 20% may need to have the drug discontinued.

**CV** Congestive heart failure may be precipitated or worsened by disopyramide because of the negative inotropic effects of the drug. The incidence may be higher in patients who have in the past shown symptoms of congestive heart failure. Hypotension during disopyramide therapy may arise alone or in conjunction with congestive heart failure. Congestive heart failure and dangerous hypotension are usually associated with toxic levels of disopyramide. ECG changes are expected with disopyramide. Excessive widening of the QRS complex, excessive prolongation of the Q-T interval, bradycardia (slowing of the heart), disturbances of conduction in cardiac tissues, and asystole may arise with toxic levels of disopyramide.

• See entry for drug class (p. 66).

• Monitor the ECG. If widening of the QRS complex is greater than 25% of the original value or if prolongation of the Q-T interval or first-degree heart block develops, the drugs should be discontinued and the patient reevaluated.

- Monitor serum drug levels if available. Therapeutic levels are from 2 to 4 μg/ml or higher for severe arrhythmias.
- Monitor vital signs, weight, and fluid intake and output. Monitor serum electrolyte levels, especially potassium.

**CNS** Anticholinergic effects are observed in up to 40% of patients receiving disopyramide. Symptoms include dry mouth, urinary hesitancy, and constipation. Less commonly blurred vision and drying of mucous membranes may be observed. The anticholinergic effects of disopyramide are dose dependent; therefore at higher doses, anticholinergic effects become more common and more severe.

- Assess for anticholinergic side effects.
- If constipation develops, instruct patients to increase daily fluid intake to 2500 to 3000 ml (if not contraindicated by the medical condition); increase dietary intake of fruit, fruit juices, and fiber; and increase level of exercise as tolerated.
- If dry mouth develops, suggest that patients suck on sugarless hard candy or chew sugarless gum, suck on ice chips, and perform regular oral hygiene but avoid lemon-glycerin swabs or mouthwashes containing alcohol. Some patients may wish to try commercially available saliva substitutes.
- Question patients about urinary hesitancy: difficulty in starting voiding or a sense of inadequate emptying of the bladder. Palpate the bladder area if hesitancy is severe, and monitor intake and output.
- Instruct patients to avoid driving or operating hazardous equipment if blurred vision develops; notify physician.

**GI** Gastrointestinal side effects such as nausea, vomiting, bloating, or anorexia may occur in up to 9% of patients receiving disopyramide.

- Monitor weight.
- Be alert to the complaint of anorexia, which often accompanies chronic illness but which may be caused by medications.

**Metabolic** Disopyramide rarely has caused hypoglycemia. Alcohol may potentiate this effect.

- Instruct diabetic patients to monitor blood glucose levels frequently during periods of drug dosage adjustment; changes in diet or hypoglycemic medication may be necessary.
- Monitor blood glucose levels.
- Teach patients to avoid the use of alcohol while taking disopyramide.

**Other** Disopyramide causes nervousness, dizziness, insomnia, fatigue, or weakness in some patients.

- Instruct patients to avoid driving or operating hazardous equipment if dizziness develops.
- Supervise ambulation. Keep side rails up. Supervise smoking. Keep nightlights on.
- If insomnia is a problem, work with the patient and physician to adjust dosing schedule to make the last dose of the day earlier than at bedtime.

### Patient and family education

- See entry for drug class (p. 66).
- As noted under preparations, there are regular and sustained-release formulations of this drug. The two are not interchangeable without some adjustment of the dosing frequency. Instruct patients to be alert to the dosage form prescribed and to take it as ordered.
- Instruct patients taking sustained-release preparations to swallow tablets whole and not to crush or break them.
- Disopyramide is best taken on an empty stomach, 1 hour before or 2 hours after meals. Some physicians may instruct patients to take the doses with meals or snacks. Teach patients to take the doses in a consistent manner, either always with meals or always on an empty stomach.

---

## encainide   (en-CAY-nide)                                              class I antiarrhythmic

- encainide: Enkaid

**MECHANISM OF ACTION**   Encainide alters sodium ion influx and slows the rate of depolarization of cardiac cells. As a result of these biochemical actions, encainide prolongs conduction through various areas of the heart.

**INDICATIONS**   **Ventricular arrhythmias** Ectopic activity in ventricles is suppressed. Ventricular tachycardias resistant to other antiarrhythmics may respond to encainide.   **Supraventricular arrhythmias** Encainide may be effective for arrhythmias involving accessory pathways.

**CONTRAINDICATIONS**   **Ventricular tachycardia or fibrillation** Patients with a history of these arrhythmias seem especially vulnerable to having a serious ventricular arrhythmia induced by encainide. The drug may be used, but only with careful cardiac monitoring.

**DOSAGE**   **Adults:**   **PO:** Initially 25 mg every 8 hours; if needed, increase up to 35 mg every 8 hours after 3 to 5 days. Maximum doses for life-threatening arrhythmias are 300 mg daily, divided into 4 doses. *Special patient populations:*   **CHILDREN:** Doses have not been established.   **PREGNANCY:** FDA pregnancy category B.   **RENAL IMPAIRMENT:** Doses may need to be reduced.

**PREPARATIONS**   *Capsules:* 25, 35, and 50 mg.

**DRUG INTERACTIONS**   **Quinidine, procainamide, and disopyramide** would be expected to increase risk of heart block with encainide.

**FATE**   Encainide is well absorbed orally, but *bioavailability* is low in 90% of the population because rapid hepatic metabolism creates a first-pass effect; however, metabolites of encainide are also active as antiarrhythmics. In 10% of the population metabolism of encainide is less efficient, and bioavailability is high. The *onset* of effect is within 1 to 2 hours, and the *duration* of effect depends on metabolism because the active metabolites have *half-lives* ranging up to 11 hours. Elimination of encainide and its metabolites is by the kidney.

## 🐦 NURSING CONSIDERATIONS

### Side effects, toxicities, and associated nursing actions

**CV** Aggravation of ventricular arrhythmias occurs in up to 23% of patients, with the highest incidence in those patients with a history of ventricular fibrillation or tachycardia. Bradycardia and sinus pauses occur in 8% to 14% of patients.
- Monitor blood pressure and pulse. During IV administration, patient should be attached to continuous cardiac monitoring.
- See entry for drug class (p. 66).

**GI** Metallic taste is common (25%), with other GI effects less common.
- Monitor weight. Metallic taste can be very annoying. If patient is unable to tolerate this side effect, consult physician. Remind patient not to discontinue medication without consulting physician.
- Suggest that patients take ordered doses with meals or snacks to lessen GI side effects.

**CNS** Dizziness, visual disturbances, headache, or tremor have occurred in up to 60% of treated patients.
- Instruct patients to avoid driving or operating hazardous equipment if dizziness or visual changes develop; notify physician.

### Nursing interventions related to drug administration
- See CV side effects above. During IV administration, monitor blood pressure and pulse every 5 minutes until stable. Keep patient supine until vital signs are stable. Keep siderails up. Supervise ambulation.

### Patient and family education
- See entry for drug class (p. 66).

## flecainide acetate   (flee-CAY-nide)                                        class I antiarrhythmic

- flecainide acetate: Tambocor

**MECHANISM OF ACTION**   Flecainide alters sodium ion influx and hence impairs the ability of cardiac cells to depolarize. As a result of these biochemical actions, flecainide prolongs conduction through various areas of the heart. Conduction is especially slowed in the His-Purkinje system and the ventricles.

**INDICATIONS**   **Ventricular arrhythmias** Flecainide is indicated for symptomatic ventricular arrhythmias such as recurrent premature ventricular contractions and ventricular tachycardia.

**CONTRAINDICATIONS**   **Congestive heart failure** Flecainide may have some degree of direct depressant effect on cardiac contractility. • This action may worsen congestive heart failure.   **Heart block** Flecainide slows conduction through various structures in the heart and may worsen preexisting partial AV block.

**DOSAGE**   **Adults:**   PO: 100 mg twice daily. Dosage may be increased by 50 mg increments weekly up to a maximum dosage of 300 mg every 12 hours.   *Special patient populations:*   ELDERLY: The half-life of elimination is prolonged in elderly patients, but the significance of this finding has not been thoroughly evaluated.   CHILDREN: Doses not established.   PREGNANCY: FDA pregnancy category C.   CONGESTIVE HEART FAILURE: Doses may need to be reduced.   RENAL IMPAIRMENT: Patients may accumulate flecainide.

**PREPARATION**   *Tablet:* scored 100 mg tablet.

**DRUG INTERACTIONS**   **Verapamil, or disopyramide** can depress cardiac contractility and may cause unacceptable cardiac depression when given with flecainide.

**FATE**   Flecainide is well absorbed orally, with nearly 100% *bioavailability*. Metabolism of the drug occurs, but about one third of an oral dose is excreted unchanged. Excretion is primarily renal; renal failure results in accumulation of drug if doses are not adjusted. The elimination *half-life* of flecainide is about 20 hours in most patients, making twice daily administration feasible.

## ❦ NURSING CONSIDERATIONS

### Side effects, toxicities, and associated nursing actions
* See entry for drug class (p. 66).

**Eye** Changes in vision with dizziness and blurred vision caused by poor accommodation are common. Roughly one-third of patients receiving 400 mg total daily dose show these symptoms, which often resolve spontaneously.
* Assess patient for visual changes. Tell the patient that if blurred vision and/or dizziness occurs, the patient should refrain from driving or operating hazardous equipment and should notify physician.

**Other** Nausea, headache, anxiety, ataxia, and metallic taste have been reported but occur in less than 5% of treated patients.
* Instruct patients to report the appearance of any new sign or symptom.

### Patient and family education
* See entry for drug class (p. 66).
* Review anticipated benefits and possible side effects of drug therapy.

---

## lidocaine hydrochloride   (LIE-doh-cane)                    class I antiarrhythmic*

* lidocaine hydrochloride: Xylocaine, ♣Xylocard

**MECHANISM OF ACTION**   Lidocaine alters sodium ion influx and thereby impairs the ability of cardiac cells to depolarize. Lidocaine is relatively selective, suppressing automaticity at ectopic sites but having little effect on SA nodal automaticity or AV nodal function. Lidocaine has minimum effects on cardiac output, arterial pressure, heart rate, or contractility and does not interact with adrenergic receptors. Lidocaine usually causes no change in the ECG.

**INDICATIONS**   **Ventricular arrhythmias following myocardial infarction** Lidocaine may be given as a bolus injection for acute control and used as an infusion for continuous control during the immediate postinfarction recovery period.   **Ventricular arrhythmias following cardiac surgery** Lidocaine may control arrhythmias arising from the mechanical manipulation of the heart during surgery.   **Local anesthetic** See Chapter 46.

**CONTRAINDICATIONS**   **Known allergy to local anesthetics of the amide group** Lidocaine is chemically related to several other local anesthetics. • Patients allergic to one of these local anesthetics are allergic to all.   **Adams-Stokes syndrome** This syndrome is caused by heart block; lidocaine may be dangerous

---

*Also local anesthetic.

in these patients.    **Heart block** Lidocaine may suppress ectopic pacemakers that maintain cardiac function in certain types of heart block.    **Wolff-Parkinson-White syndrome** This syndrome may be aggravated by lidocaine.

**DOSAGE** **IV:** **ADULTS:** Only lidocaine without preservatives or catecholamines (e.g., epinephrine) should be used intravenously. Initial bolus injection may be 50 to 100 mg given at a rate of 20 to 50 mg/min; a second bolus of one half to one third the amount of the first may be given 5 minutes later if needed. Continuous infusion should be instituted to maintain constant therapeutic levels after the loading dose; the infusion rate should be 1 to 4 mg/min. No more than 300 mg of lidocaine should be given during an hour. Lidocaine is seldom given for longer than 24 hours; oral therapy is instituted with another agent as soon as possible.    **CHILDREN:** A bolus of 1 mg/kg followed by infusion of 3 µg/kg/min is recommended as a guideline, but the drug has not been thoroughly tested in children.    **IM:** **ADULTS:** As an emergency measure, 300 mg of lidocaine may be injected into the deltoid muscle. The patient should quickly be switched to IV therapy.    **CHILDREN:** Doses have not been established. *Special patient populations:*    **ELDERLY:** Dosages must be reduced in patients older than 60 years. **PREGNANCY:** Safe use has not been established.    **HEART OR HEPATIC FAILURE:** Dosages must be reduced in the case of heart or hepatic failure.

**PREPARATIONS** Lidocaine for use as an antiarrhythmic is marked Lidocaine HCl Without Preservatives or as Xylocaine HCl IV for Cardiac Arrhythmias. *Solution for injection:* 1% (10 mg/ml), 2% (20 mg/ml), 4% (40 mg/ml), and 20% (200 mg/ml) solutions are available in vials, ampuls, or syringes for bolus IV injection or preparing IV admixtures. For direct IV infusion, 0.2% (2 mg/ml) or 0.4% (4 mg/ml) solution in 5% dextrose. For IM injection, a 10% solution (100 mg/ml) in 5 ml ampuls is available.

**DRUG INTERACTIONS** **Propranolol** may impair blood flow to the liver and thereby interfere with the metabolism of lidocaine.    **Phenytoin** should not be given intravenously concurrently with lidocaine because of danger of excessive cardiac depression.    **Procainamide** and lidocaine may have additive neurologic effects.

**DIAGNOSTIC TEST INTERFERENCES** Creatinine phosphokinase (also called creatine kinase) levels may be elevated for 48 hours following IM administration of lidocaine. This effect can interfere with diagnosis of myocardial infarction.

**FATE** Lidocaine is administered only parenterally and primarily intravenously. IV doses are effective within a minute. The drug is subject to rapid hepatic metabolism. The *duration* of action of a single bolus dose is 10 to 20 minutes, but the effect of discontinuing an infusion is an even more rapid loss of action. Hepatic dysfunction may slow metabolism and prolong the *half-life*, but renal dysfunction is usually without effect.

## 🦆 NURSING CONSIDERATIONS

### Side effects, toxicities, and associated nursing actions

**CV** Hypotension, bradycardia, and cardiac arrest are possible.
- Continuous ECG monitoring should be done during lidocaine therapy. Monitor the blood pressure.

**Allergic** Urticaria, edema, cutaneous lesions, or anaphylactoid reactions indicate alllergy.
- If possible, question patient about history of possible allergy to local anesthetics before use of this drug. Have emergency drugs and resuscitation equipment available.

**CNS** Central nervous system effects are dose related, with drowsiness and dizziness occurring at the upper range for therapeutic concentrations. At plasma concentrations above 10 µ/ml, confusion, coma, and epileptiform seizures may occur. These reactions demand immediate cessation of lidocaine and treatment for the seizures.
- Monitor level of consciousness and mental status.
- Monitor serum lidocaine levels.

### Nursing interventions related to drug administration
- See entry for drug class (p. 66).
- Read labels carefully. For IV use, only lidocaine without preservatives or epinephrine should be used.
- Administer at the ordered rate or titrate to the patient's response, within guidelines established by the

physician (review Dosage). Most acute care settings have available guidelines for the usual dilutions used in that setting. Dilute 1 g of lidocaine in 1000 ml for a dilution of 1 mg/ml. Dilute 1 g of lidocaine in 500 ml for a dilution of 2 mg/ml.

- As noted, IM doses should be given in the deltoid muscle. Aspirate before injecting to avoid IV administration. The IM route can result in elevations of the serum creatinine phosphokinase (CPK) levels, thus reducing the value of this test in patients who may have myocardial damage.

### Patient and family education

- See entry for drug class (p. 66).
- This drug is rarely used outside of the hospital setting. Keep patient and family informed of changes in the plan of care.

## mexiletine hydrochloride    (mex-ILL-e-teen)    class I antiarrhythmic

- mexiletine hydrochloride: Mexitil

**MECHANISM OF ACTION**    Mexiletine has a mechanism of action similar to its chemical relative lidocaine. Mexiletine alters sodium ion flow in cardiac cells and shortens the action potential duration. Ventricular automaticity is diminished.

**INDICATIONS**    **Ventricular tachycardia** Mexiletine may be used alone, but more satisfactory results are often obtained when it is used in combination with other antiarrhythmic agents. • Mexiletine may be effective when other antiarrhythmics, including lidocaine, have failed.    **Ventricular ectopic activity following myocardial infarction** Mexiletine seems as effective as lidocaine.

**CONTRAINDICATIONS**    **Heart block or other conduction disorders** Although mexiletine does not slow conduction in normal patients, preexisting conduction disorders may be exacerbated. • The drug may be used with care.

**DOSAGE**    **Adults:**    **PO:** mg 3 times daily (10 to 15 mg/kg daily), given with food or antacids. Adjust dosage in 50 or 100 mg increments after 3 days as needed or as tolerated.    *Special patient populations:* **CHILDREN:** Doses have not been established.    **PREGNANCY:** FDA pregnancy category C. **HEPATIC FAILURE:** The half-life of the drug is prolonged when liver function is impaired.

**PREPARATIONS**    *Capsules:* 150, 200, and 250 mg.

**DRUG INTERACTIONS**    **Rifampin, phenytoin, phenobarbital, and primidone** induce enzymes in the liver that metabolize mexiletine. Mexiletine is eliminated more rapidly when these drugs are given.    **Cimetidine, chloramphenicol, isoniazid, dicumarol, and disulfiram** may inhibit hepatic enzymes metabolizing mexiletine, thereby increasing blood levels of mexiletine.

**FATE**    Oral *bioavailability* is 80% to 88%, making mexiletine a useful oral agent. *Peak* blood levels occur 2 to 4 hours after oral doses. Mexiletine is metabolized in the liver and excreted in urine. The elimination *half-life* is about 12 hours, but this value is increased following acute myocardial infarction.

### ☙ NURSING CONSIDERATIONS

#### Side effects, toxicities, and associated nursing actions    Up to 60% of patients receiving mexiletine may experience significant side effects, and up to 30% may require discontinuation of the drug.

- See entry for drug class (p. 66).

**CV** Bradycardia, hypotension, and transient AV blockade are more commonly seen following IV administration.

- Monitor pulse and blood pressure. Monitor ECG during IV administration. See Nursing interventions below.

**CNS** Tremors, nystagmus, diplopia, dizziness, confusion, and ataxia.

- Monitor patients for these side effects.
- Instruct patients to avoid driving or operating hazardous equipment if dizziness or visual changes occur; notify physician.

**GI** Dyspepsia, nausea, and vomiting may occur in 30% to 40% of patients.

- Monitor weight.
- Instruct patients to take ordered doses with meals or snacks to lessen GI side effects.

**Blood** Thrombocytopenia is rarely seen.

- Instruct patients to report the appearance of unexplained bruising or bleeding or the development of petechiae.
- Monitor complete blood count and platelet count.

### Nursing interventions related to drug administration

- Monitor blood pressure and pulse every 5 minutes until stable following IV administration. See CV side effects above. Keep siderails up, keep patient in bed until vital signs are stable, and supervise ambulation.

### Patient and family education

- See entry for drug class (p. 66).
- Review anticipated benefits and possible side effects of drug therapy with the patient. Instruct patient to notify physician of any new sign or symptom.

---

## phenytoin    (FEN-ee-toin)                                            anticonvulsant*

- phenytoin: Dilantin, ✽Novophenytoin

**MECHANISM OF ACTION**   Phenytoin is primarily used as an anticonvulsant (Chapter 39) but occasionally finds use as an antiarrhythmic agent. The drug suppresses spontaneous depolarization in ventricular tissues; this seems to be the primary action as an antiarrhythmic. Minor alterations in nodal function occur, and there are few changes in the ECG, with the exception of shortening the Q-T interval.

**INDICATIONS**   **Convulsant disorders** See Chapter 39.   **Digitalis-induced arrhythmias** Although phenytoin is not approved by the FDA as an antiarrhythmic drug, it has been used in restricted circumstances, usually involving digitalis toxicity.

**CONTRAINDICATIONS**   **Sino-atrial blockade, second- or third-degree AV nodal blockade, sinus bradycardia, and Adams-Stokes syndrome** Phenytoin lowers ventricular automaticity, which may be dangerous in these patients.

**DOSAGE**   **PO:**   **ADULTS:** Initial dose is 1 g, followed by 300 to 600 mg the second and third days; maintenance is with 300 to 400 mg daily divided in 1 to 4 doses.   **CHILDREN:** 10 to 15 mg/kg divided into 2 or 3 doses over the first 24 hours; maintenance is with 5 to 10 mg/kg daily divided into 2 or 3 doses.   **IV:** **ADULTS:** 100 mg every 5 minutes until arrhythmia is controlled or toxicity intervenes. The infusion rate should be less than 25 mg/min; the total dose should not exceed 1 g.   **CHILDREN:** Pediatric doses are not established.   *Special patient populations:*   **ELDERLY:** Elderly patients receiving phenytoin intravenously usually require smaller doses administered more slowly than for other adults. **HEPATIC IMPAIRMENT:** Smaller doses administered more slowly than normal may be required. **PREGNANCY:** Safe use has not been established.

**PREPARATIONS**   *Tablets:* 50 mg chewable tablets. *Oral suspensions:* 30 mg/5 ml or 125 mg/5 ml for pediatric use. *Capsules, prompt-release:* 30 or 100 mg. *Capsules, extended-release:* 30 or 100 mg capsules designated as Dilantin Kapseals.

**DRUG INTERACTIONS**   **Quinidine** serum levels may fall when phenytoin is also given, apparently because of the hepatic effects of phenytoin. Phenytoin may be involved extensively in drug interactions when the drug is used chronically as an anticonvulsant (Chapter 39). Many of these same interactions are possible if phenytoin is used beyond a few days as an antiarrhythmic agent.

**DIAGNOSTIC TEST INTERFERENCES**   See listing for phenytoin as an anticonvulsant (Chapter 39).

**FATE**   Phenytoin is absorbed erratically from the intestine, and *bioavailability* of preparations may differ. The *onset* of action may be 0.5 to 1 hour, and the effect may persist for up to 24 hours. The *half-life* of phenytoin ranges from 22 to 36 hours. Phenytoin is extensively metabolized by the liver, but metab-

*Also antiarrhythmic agent.

olism is highly variable among individuals; predicting plasma levels of phenytoin based on standard doses is difficult. Renal excretion of phenytoin is minimum.

## ❦ NURSING CONSIDERATIONS

### Side effects, toxicities, and associated nursing actions

- See entry for drug class (p. 66).
- See Chapter 39 for a detailed discussion of phenytoin used as an anticonvulsant.

**GI** Nausea and vomiting are common.

- These may signal toxic drug levels. Assess for GI symptoms. Monitor serum drug levels.
- If GI symptoms are severe, monitor intake and output and weight.

**CNS** Neurologic side effects are dose dependent and signal significant toxicity. Signs include fatigue, dizziness, nystagmus (rhythmic oscillation or movement of the eyeballs), and ataxia (lack of coordination).

- Monitor serum levels if available; effective therapeutic blood levels usually range from 10 to 20 $\mu$g/ml.
- Instruct patients to avoid driving or operating hazardous equipment if dizziness occurs.
- Monitor gait; monitor for other CNS signs.

**CV** Myocardial depression, bradycardia, hypotension, or even cardiac arrest may occur if phenytoin is administered intravenously at rates exceeding 25 mg/min.

- See Nursing interventions below.

**Skin** Pruritis and rash are common.

- Inspect patient for skin changes. If rash is severe or persistent, notify physician.

**Other** Hepatitis, blood dyscrasias, and pseudolymphoma may occur in rare patients.

- Monitor liver function tests and complete blood cell count.
- Instruct patient to report the development of signs of possible hepatitis: jaundice, fever, malaise, right upper quadrant abdominal pain, and change in the color or consistency of stools.
- Instruct patients to report the development of sore throat, unexplained bleeding or bruising, bleeding gums, and fatigue.

### Nursing interventions related to drug administration

- The IM route should be avoided because of erratic absorption with this route.
- Use only the diluent supplied by the manufacturer to dilute the powder. Do not add to IV infusions or mix with other drugs.
- Do not exceed an IV administration rate of 25 mg/min.
- Flush IV tubing before and after administration with normal saline solution, to avoid mixing the drug with the infusing fluids.
- The patient should be on a cardiac monitor; IV administration can cause cardiac arrest. Monitor pulse and blood pressure.
- When administering via nasogastric tube, do not mix with other medications, and flush tubing with water after administration to prevent clogging of the tube.

### Patient and family education

- See entry for drug class (p. 66).
- See Chapter 39 for a more detailed discussion of phenytoin.
- There is an oral suspension available. Shake the suspension vigorously before pouring the desired dose, and instruct patients and families to do the same. Failure to adequately resuspend the drug in the suspension can result in underdosage with doses from the top of the bottle and overdosage with doses prepared near the bottom of the bottle.
- Hyperplasia of the gums is common with chronic use of this drug. Instruct patients to perform regular, careful oral hygiene, including flossing, brushing, and daily use of a water-massage oral care device. Encourage patients to have regular dental care.

## procainamide hydrochloride    (pro-CAY-na-mide)    class I antiarrhythmic

- procainamide hydrochloride: Procan, Procan Sr, Pronestyl, Pronestyl SR

**MECHANISM OF ACTION**    Procainamide alters sodium ion influx and therefore slows the rate of depolarization of cardiac cells. The excitability of cells is lowered, and conduction is slowed through the heart.

The refractory period is lengthened, especially in the atria. As a result of these electrophysiologic changes, the QRS complex is usually widened in the ECG; P-R and Q-T intervals may also be prolonged. The actions of procainamide on the heart are very similar to those of quinidine.

**INDICATIONS**  **Ventricular tachycardia or premature ventricular contractions** Procainamide is often selected when lidocaine has failed.  **Paroxysmal atrial tachycardia or atrial fibrillation** Unlike lidocaine, procainamide causes useful changes in atrial tissue, which can be important in controlling atrial arrhythmias.  **Wolff-Parkinson-White syndrome** Procainamide lowers activity in accessory pathways that may contribute to this syndrome; as a result, procainamide, unlike many other antiarrhythmics, can aid in controlling the condition.

**CONTRAINDICATIONS**  **Allergy to procainamide or procaine** Procaine and related local anesthetics chemically resemble procainamide or its metabolites; hence the drugs are cross allergenic.  **AV nodal blockade** Procainamide slows conduction in some fibers and at high doses may contribute to AV nodal blockade. In patients with preexisting AV nodal blockade, complete heart block may result.  **Myasthenia gravis** Procainamide possesses a degree of anticholinergic activity that cannot be tolerated in these patients who already have limited cholinergic receptors.

**DOSAGE**  **PO:**  **ADULTS:** For ventricular tachycardia, a 1 g loading dose is followed by 50 mg/kg daily in divided doses administered every 3 hours. For premature ventricular contractions, the loading dose is omitted. For atrial fibrillation and paroxysmal atrial tachycardia, a 1.25 g loading dose is followed by 0.75 g 1 hour later. Doses of 0.5 to 1 g may be repeated every 2 hours until the arrhythmia is controlled or toxicity requires switching to another agent. Preventing recurrence of the atrial arrhythmias may be accomplished with 0.5 to 1 g every 4 to 6 hours. For maintenance therapy only, sustained-release preparations may be used; total dosage remains at 50 mg/kg daily, but the doses are administered every 6 hours.  **CHILDREN:** Children receive 50 mg/kg daily of the regular-release preparations divided into 4 to 6 doses.  **IV:**  **ADULTS:** Procainamide should be given no more rapidly than 25 to 50 mg/min until the arrhythmia is suppressed or up to a limit of 1 g of drug. Maintenance is with 2 to 4 mg/min.  **CHILDREN:** Doses have not been established.  **IM:**  **ADULTS:** 0.5 to 1 g may be administered to patients before surgery or to patients who are vomiting. The dose may be repeated at 4- to 8-hour intervals, but oral therapy should be substituted as soon as possible.  **CHILDREN:** Pediatric doses have not been established. *Special patient populations:*  **ELDERLY:** Geriatric patients are more prone to hypotension.  **PREGNANCY:** FDA pregnancy category C.

**PREPARATIONS**  *Tablets:* 250, 375, and 500 mg. All tablets sold in the United States under the trade name Pronestyl contain tartrazine (FD&C yellow #5), which can cause allergic reactions including bronchial asthma in rare patients. *Capsules:* 250, 375, and 500 mg. *Tablets, sustained-release:* Procan SR (250, 375, or 500 mg) or Pronestyl-SR (500 mg); these tablets do not contain tartrazine. *Solutions for injection:* 100 mg/ml (10 ml vial) or 500 mg/ml (2 ml vial). These solutions should be diluted in 5% dextrose solution before IV administration. Procainamide solutions are either colorless or very light yellow. If solutions become amber or show any other strong discoloration, they should be discarded. Store at between 50° and 87° F.

**DRUG INTERACTIONS**  **Lidocaine** may have additive neurologic side effects with procainamide.  **Cardiac glycosides** may have additive effects on the heart with procainamide that could lead to excessive toxicity.  **Antihypertensive agents** may have additive hypotensive effects with procainamide.  **Neuromuscular blocking agents** may produce excessive or prolonged blockade because of the neuromuscular blocking action of procainamide.

**DIAGNOSTIC TEST INTERFERENCES**  **Edrophonium tests** for myasthenia gravis may be unreliable because of the neuromuscular blocking action of procainamide.  **Alkaline phosphatase, bilirubin, lactic dehydrogenase (LDH), and serum aspartate aminotransferase (AST)** levels may all be increased by procainamide.

**FATE**  Oral procainamide takes effect within 0.5 hour, and *peak* blood levels occur by 1 hour. Absorption is excellent. Procainamide is metabolized in the liver to n-acetylprocainamide (NAPA) at variable, genetically determined rates. NAPA also has effects on the heart. About 50% of an administered dose of procainamide is excreted unchanged in the urine. Plasma *half-life* is 2.5 to 4.5 hours for procainamide and about 6 hours for NAPA. Renal failure increases the half-life. Following IV or IM administration the *onset* of action is rapid. *Peak* plasma concentrations of procainamide appear at 15 to 60 minutes following IM doses.

## ❦ NURSING CONSIDERATIONS

**Side effects, toxicities, and associated nursing actions**  Up to 60% of patients treated with procainamide develop significant toxicity, and up to 50% require discontinuation of the drug.

**Allergic** Procainamide given over a long period is commonly associated with the development of a lupuslike syndrome. Positive antinuclear antibody (ANA) tests are an early sign. Later signs include arthritis, polyarthralgia, pleuritic pain, myalgia, skin lesions, and fever. The syndrome is usually reversible when procainamide is discontinued, but steroid therapy is occasionally required. Fever, rash, urticaria, agranulocytosis, pancytopenia, and nephrotic syndrome may also signal allergy to procainamide in the absence of lupus.

- Monitor ANA tests. Question patients about signs and symptoms suggesting an allergic response. Instruct patients to report the development of fever, sore throat, unexplained bleeding or bruising, malaise, joint pain, muscle pain, or skin changes.
- Question patients about history of allergy to local anesthetics before use. Have emergency drugs and resuscitation equipment available to treat an acute allergic reaction.
- Monitor serum drug levels if available. Therapeutic blood levels range between 4 to 10 µg/ml, but higher levels may occasionally be required (17 to 34 µmole/1).

**GI** Anorexia, nausea, and vomiting may occur.

- Monitor weight. Assess for GI symptoms. This drug is best taken on an empty stomach either 1 hour before or 2 hours after meals. Suggest that the patient take the dose with a full glass of water to lessen GI symptoms. If GI symptoms are intolerable, the physician may suggest that the patient take the ordered doses with meals or a snack. Instruct patients to take doses consistently, either always with meals or always on an empty stomach.

**CV** Hypotension can be a serious reaction to high doses of procainamide but is more common with IV doses. Hypotension arises from the vasodilating effects of procainamide in the periphery. Widening of the QRS complex is common with procainamide, but if the widening is greater than 50%, serious toxicity may be indicated. Unless the drug is discontinued, AV nodal blockade, asystole, or ventricular fibrillation may follow.

- See Nursing interventions below.
- Monitor ECG tracings at regular intervals. During IV administration, continuous ECG monitoring should be done.

**Nursing interventions related to drug administration**

- Dilute before IV administration. For direct infusion, dilute 100 mg with 10 ml of 5% dextrose in water or sterile water for injection. For constant infusion, add 1 g to 500 ml 5% dextrose in water for a dilution of 2 mg/ml.
- The rate of IV infusion should not exceed 25 to 50 mg/min.
- Monitor the blood pressure during IV infusion. If a drop of greater than 15 mm Hg occurs, stop the infusion and notify the physician. Keep the patient supine.
- Do not mix with other drugs or infusions.
- The antidote for hypotension is phenylephrine or levarterenol.

**Patient and family education**

- See entry for drug class (p. 66).
- Review with patients the anticipated benefits and possible side effects of drug therapy. Point out the importance of reporting symptoms that may indicate an allergic response, and review these symptoms with patients (see above).
- Regular preparations and sustained-release preparations cannot be interchanged without changes in dosing frequency. Instruct patients to read labels carefully and to be aware of the form prescribed.
- Instruct patients taking sustained-release preparations to swallow the tablets whole, without crushing or breaking them.
- Pronestyl brand contains FD & C yellow #5 (tartrazine) and may cause allergic reactions in some individuals. This allergic reaction is seen more often in individuals with aspirin hypersensitivity.

## propranolol hydrochloride  (pro-PRAN-oh-lole)  class II antiarrhythmic*

- propranolol hydrochloride: Inderal

**MECHANISM OF ACTION**  Propranolol is a nonselective beta adrenergic antagonist. Because propranolol blocks the action of catecholamines in the heart, the drug slows AV nodal conduction while suppressing automaticity of cells. Propranolol effects on the ECG include prolonging the P-R interval and sometimes shortening the Q-T interval.

**INDICATIONS**  **Supraventricular and ventricular tachyarrhythmias** Unless the ventricular tachyarrhythmias are caused by excess catecholamines, these conditions are less likely to respond to propranolol than are atrial arrhythmias.  **Atrial flutter and atrial fibrillation arising from digitalis toxicity** These conditions often respond to discontinuation of digitalis and correction of electrolyte imbalances. • If these measures fail, oral propranolol may be effective.  **Arrhythmias caused by increased catecholamines** These arrhythmias may be caused by exercise, thyrotoxicosis, or pheochromocytoma.  **Hypertension, angina, hypertrophic subaortic stenosis, and migraine** See Chapter 5 for full discussion of these indications.

**CONTRAINDICATIONS**  **Congestive heart failure** Catecholamines may be the primary support of cardiovascular function in these patients; by removing catecholamine effects propranolol could dramatically worsen heart failure.  **Sinus bradycardia** Propranolol may further slow the heart.  **AV nodal blockade** Propranolol may further slow conduction and cause heart block.  **Bronchial asthma, bronchospasm, severe chronic obstructive pulmonary disease** Propranolol promotes constriction of the bronchioles by blocking beta-2 adrenergic receptors.  **Diabetes mellitus** Propranolol may cause hypoglycemia.

**DOSAGE**  **PO:**  **ADULTS:** 10 to 30 mg three or four times daily at meals and bedtime.  **CHILDREN:** 0.5 to 1 mg/kg daily in 3 or 4 doses, to a maximum of 60 mg/day.  **IV:**  **ADULTS:** For life-threatening arrhythmias 1 to 3 mg with ECG and blood pressure monitoring, given no faster than 1 mg/min. A second dose may be given after 2 minutes, but no further doses should be given for 4 hours.  **CHILDREN:** 0.01 to 0.1 mg/kg daily to a maximum of 1 mg/dose by slow push. Dosages for other indications are given in Chapter 5. *Special patient populations:*  **ELDERLY:** Geriatric patients have unpredictable responses to propranolol.  **PREGNANCY:** FDA pregnancy category C.  **RENAL OR HEPATIC IMPAIRMENT:** These patients may require lower doses.

**PREPARATIONS**  *Tablets:* 10, 20, 40, 60, 80, 90, and 120 mg. *Capsules:* 80, 120, and 160 mg for sustained release. *Solution for injection:* 1 mg/ml in 1 ml ampuls. This preparation may be stored at room temperature.

**DRUG INTERACTIONS**  See the drug interactions characteristic of beta adrenergic blockers (p. 41).  **Lidocaine** clearance is impaired by propranolol.  **Chlorpromazine, cimetidine, furosemide, and hydralazine** increase the plasma concentration of propranolol.  **Smoking** reduces the plasma concentration of propranolol by increasing the clearance.  **Phenytoin** administered intravenously may produce additive cardiac depressant effects with propranolol.

**DIAGNOSTIC TEST INTERFERENCES**  Propranolol may elevate levels of blood urea, serum transaminase, alkaline phosphatase, and lactic dehydrogenase.

**FATE**  *Bioavailability* of propranolol is limited by hepatic metabolism of the drug. Nevertheless, the *onset* of action following oral administration is about 0.5 hour, and the *duration* is 3 to 5 hours. Little propranolol is excreted by the kidneys. The elimination *half-life* is 2 to 6 hours.

## ☙ NURSING CONSIDERATIONS
### Side effects, toxicities, and associated nursing actions
- See entry for drug class (p. 66).
- See Chapter 5 for additional information about propanolol.

**CNS** Dizziness, fatigue, mental depression, impaired concentration, disorientation, acute mental changes, and emotional lability.
- Instruct patients to avoid driving or operating hazardous equipment if dizziness or disorientation occurs; notify physician.

*Also antianginal, antihypertensive, antithyroid, antidyskinetic.

- Be alert to signs of depression: lack of interest in personal appearance, change in appetite, apathy, and insomnia.

**GI** Symptoms including nausea, vomiting, and intestinal discomfort may vary among patients.

- Assess for GI side effects. Monitor weight. Suggest that patients take ordered doses with meals or snacks to reduce gastric irritation.

**GU** Impotence and decreased libido have been reported.

- Assess tactfully for changes in sexual functioning. Provide emotional support as needed. Remind patients not to discontinue this medication without prior discussion with the physician. Consult physician.

**Metabolic** Propranolol may intensify hypoglycemic reactions in diabetics, masking early symptoms of onset of the reaction.

- Review this side effect with diabetic patients. Instruct diabetic patients to monitor blood glucose frequently, especially during periods of propranolol dosage adjustment, as changes in diet or dose of hypoglycemic agent may be necessary.
- Monitor blood glucose.
- Instruct patients that propranolol may cover up usual signs of hypoglycemia such as changes in pulse rate.

**CV** Propranolol may excessively depress cardiac function. Symptoms include bradycardia, shortness of breath, worsening of angina, peripheral vascular insufficiency, edema, hypotension, and heart block.

- Monitor pulse and blood pressure before each dose. Monitor weight. Assess for other CV side effects.

**Lung** Propranolol at high concentrations or in sensitive patients can cause bronchospasm that may require therapy with a specific beta-2 agonist or with aminophylline.

- Auscultate breath sounds and monitor respiratory rate.
- Question patient about history of breathing problems or asthma before administering doses.

### Nursing interventions related to drug administration

- Monitor ECG continuously and blood pressure and pulse every 5 minutes during IV administration.
- For IV administration, may give undiluted or dilute each 1 mg in 10 ml of 5% dextrose in water. Administer at a rate of 1 mg over at least 1 minute. Drug may also be diluted in 50 ml of normal saline solution for infusion; administer over 10 to 15 minutes.
- Dose may be repeated after 2 minutes, but no further doses should be given for 4 hours (see Dosage).
- Keep patient supine until vital signs are stable. Supervise ambulation. Keep side rails up.

### Patient and family education

- See entry for drug class (p. 66).
- See Chapter 5 for more information about beta adrenergic blockers.

---

## quinidine   (KWIN-i-deen) class I antiarrhythmic

- quinidine sulfate: Cin-Quin, Quinora, Quinidex
- quinidine gluconate: Quinaglute Dura-Tabs, Quinalan, Quinatime, Quin-Release
- quinidine polygalacturonate: Cardioquin

**MECHANISM OF ACTION**   Quinidine alters sodium ion influx and therefore slows the rate of depolarization of cardiac cells. The excitability of cells is lowered, and conduction is slowed through cardiac tissues. The refractory period is lengthened, especially in the atria. As a result of these electrophysiologic changes, the QRS complex is usually widened in the ECG; P-R and Q-T intervals may also be prolonged. The actions of quinidine in the heart are very similar to procainamide.

**INDICATIONS**    **Atrial flutter or fibrillation** Quinidine is used primarily to maintain sinus rhythm after these arrhythmias have been converted by other means.    **Premature atrial and ventricular contractions** Quinidine controls ectopic sites.    **Paroxysmal atrial fibrillation** Quinidine may be more useful for this condition than for established continuous atrial fibrillation.    **Paroxysmal ventricular tachycardia** Quinidine is not used in patients with this condition who also have complete heart block.

**CONTRAINDICATIONS**    **Allergy to quinidine** A history of allergic or idiosyncratic reactions to quinidine is reason to withhold the drug.    **AV nodal blockade** Quinidine slows conduction in some fibers and at high doses may contribute to AV nodal blockade. • Patients with preexisting AV nodal blockade may suffer complete heart block.    **Digitalis toxicity manifested as AV blockade or arrhythmias** Quinidine may worsen the AV nodal blockade produced by toxic levels of digitalis.    **Myasthenia gravis** Quinidine has anticholinergic activity that cannot be tolerated in these patients who already have limited cholinergic receptors.    **Renal disease** Quinidine should not be used if marked azotemia is present as a result of renal disease. Renal tubular acidosis is also a contraindication.

**DOSAGE**    **PO:** *Adults:* **QUINIDINE SULFATE** (Cin-Quin, Quinidex) is usually given at doses of 200 to 400 g every 6 hours. Higher doses may be required for certain arrhythmias. *Children:* 6 mg/kg every 4 to 6 hours. **QUINIDINE POLYGALACTURONATE** (Cardioquin) doses are 275 mg every 8 to 12 hours. *Children:* Pediatric doses have not been established. **QUINIDINE GLUCONATE** (Duraquin, Quinaglute) doses are 324 to 972 mg (1 to 3 tablets) given every 8 to 12 hours. *Children:* Doses have not been established. **IV:** *Adults:* **QUINIDINE SULFATE** is available as a 200 mg/ml solution in 1 ml ampules. This solution should be diluted in 5% dextrose solution and administered at rates not exceeding 10 mg/min. **QUINIDINE GLUCONATE** is available for injection in 80 mg/ml solutions in 10 ml vials. IV injection is only for hospitalized patients being fully monitored; 200 to 400 mg diluted in 5% dextrose solution may be administered at rates not exceeding 10 mg/min. *Children:* Doses have not been established. *Special patient populations:* **ELDERLY:** Elderly patients require lower doses. **PREGNANCY:** FDA pregnancy category C. **ORGAN FAILURE:** Patients with renal insufficiency, impaired hepatic function, or congestive heart failure may require lower doses.

**PREPARATIONS**    **Quinidine sulfate** preparations contain 83% anhydrous quinidine alkaloid. *Tablets, regular-release:* 100, 200, or 300 mg. *Tablets, sustained-release:* 300 mg (Quinidex Extentabs). *Capsules:* 200 and 300 mg. *Solution for injection:* 200 mg/ml.    **Quinidine gluconate** preparations contain 62% anhydrous quinidine alkaloid. *Tablets, sustained-release:* 330 or 324 mg. *Solution for injection:* 80 mg/ml.    **Quinidine polygalacturonate** preparations contain 60% anhydrous quinidine alkaloid. *Tablets:* 275 mg.

**DRUG INTERACTIONS**    **Other antiarrhythmic agents** may cause additive cardiac depression when given with quinidine because of the negative inotropic effects of quinidine.    **Anticholinergic agents and neuromuscular blocking agents** may be potentiated by quinidine because of the anticholinergic action of quinidine.    **Digoxin** levels in the serum may be increased by quinidine.    **Acetazolamide, thiazide diuretics, sodium bicarbonate and certain antacids** can alkalinize the urine, slowing elimination of quinidine and allowing accumulation of the drug.    **Coumarin anticoagulants** can be potentiated by quinidine, occasionally leading to frank hemorrhage.

**FATE**    Quinidine is well absorbed orally. *Peak* concentrations in blood appear at 1 to 1.5 hours for quinidine sulfate and at 3 to 4 hours for quinidine gluconate; *peak* levels are slightly lower for gluconate and polygalacturonate salts. Quinidine is eliminated primarily by metabolism in the liver, with only 20% of the drug being excreted unchanged in urine. The elimination *half-life* is about 6 hours. In the elderly and in patients with congestive heart failure or hepatic insufficiency, elimination of quinidine is delayed.

☙ **NURSING CONSIDERATIONS**

   **Side effects, toxicities, and associated nursing actions**    Up to 40% of patients treated with quinidine develop significant toxicity, and as many as 20% have to discontinue the drug.

   • See entry for drug class (p. 66).

   **GI** Nausea, vomiting, abdominal pain, and diarrhea are common side effects of quinidine therapy.

   • Instruct patients to take doses on an empty stomach with a full glass of water, 1 hour before or 2 hours after meals or snack. If GI side effects are common, suggest that patients take doses with meals

or snack. Teach patients to take drug in a consistent fashion, always on an empty stomach or always with meals or snack.
- Monitor weight and serum electrolyte level.

**CV** Cardiovascular side effects may include widening of the QRS complex on the ECG. Cardiovascular function is dangerously altered by excessive concentrations of quinidine. AV nodal blockade may occur, as well as depression of cardiac contractility. Arrhythmias may develop. Hypotension may require therapy with norepinephrine or other pressor agents.
- Monitor blood pressure and pulse. Use continuous ECG monitoring during IV administration. See Nursing interventions below.
- Quinidine effectiveness is reduced in the presence of hypokalemia. Monitor the serum electrolyte level.
- Monitor serum drug levels if available.

**Blood** Rarely, dyscrasias such as hypoprothrombinemia, thrombocytopenia, and acute hemolytic anemia have been reported.
- Assess patient for pallor and fatigue. Monitor complete blood cell count, platelet count, and prothrombin time.
- Instruct patients to report the appearance of petechiae, bruising, or any unexplained bleeding.

**CNS** Central nervous system effects include headache, mood changes, altered consciousness, and a variety of visual changes, which may include optic neuritis. CNS depression may develop, even in the presence of convulsions. For this reason, CNS depressants should not be part of therapy in quinidine overdose.
- Obtain baseline mental status examination and repeat regularly.
- Instruct patients to avoid driving or operating hazardous equipment if visual changes develop; notify physician.

**Skin** Some patients report rash and urticaria with quinidine. Photosensitivity may also occur.
- If photosensitivity occurs, instruct patients to avoid exposure to the sun or other sources of ultraviolet light, wear a wide-brimmed hat, keep extremities covered, and use a maximum protection sunscreen on exposed skin surfaces.
- Assess for other skin changes. If severe or persistent, notify physician. Skin changes usually disappear after the medication is stopped, but it may take several weeks.

**Liver** A few patients have developed granulomatous hepatitis.
- Instruct patients to report the development of right upper quadrant abdominal pain, fatigue, malaise, fever, change in the color or consistency of stools, or jaundice.
- Monitor liver function tests.

**Other** Symptoms of cinchonism may occur in sensitive patients, occasionally after only a single dose. Symptoms include ringing in the ears, headache, nausea, and/or changes in vision.
- It is recommended that a test dose of 1 tablet or 200 mg intramuscularly always precede full-dose administration to test for idiosyncrasy.
- Review the symptoms of cinchonism with patients, and instruct them to notify the physician if they occur.
- If possible, continuous cardiac monitoring should be done when therapy is initiated.

### Nursing interventions related to drug administration
- Read labels carefully; do not confuse quinidine with quinine.
- Oral and IM routes are preferred over IV.
- For IV administration, dilute 10 ml (800 mg) in 40 to 50 ml of 5% dextrose in water. Do not add to IV solutions or mix with other drugs in a syringe.
- Administer intravenously at a rate not to exceed 1 ml (10 mg) per minute. Monitor blood pressure and pulse every 5 minutes until stable, and monitor ECG tracing. Keep patient in bed until vital signs are stable. Supervise ambulation. Keep side rails up.
- IM injections are painful, increase serum creatinine phosphokinase (CPK) levels, and are erratically and incompletely absorbed.

### Patient and family education
- See entry for drug class (p. 66).

- Review anticipated benefits and possible side effects of quinidine therapy with patient.
- Instruct patients taking sustained-release preparations to swallow tablets whole, without crushing or breaking them.
- Instruct the patient to report the appearance of fever, sore throat, infection, or bleeding or bruising, as these may represent hematologic side effects.
- Diarrhea occasionally occurs when therapy is initiated. Caution the patient to report the presence of diarrhea, and monitor the patient carefully for electrolyte imbalance.

## tocainide hydrochloride    (toe-CAY-nide)    class I antiarrhythmic

- tocainide hydrochloride: Tonocard

**MECHANISM OF ACTION**    Tocainide has electrophysiologic actions like those of lidocaine; sodium ion influx is altered, and the ability of cardiac cells to depolarize is impaired. Also like lidocaine, tocainide has minimum effects on cardiac output, arterial pressure, heart rate, contractility, or ECG.

**INDICATIONS**    Ventricular arrhythmias Tocainide may be useful in a variety of ventricular arrhythmias, including about 60% of ventricular arrhythmias that do not respond to quinidine, procainamide, disopyramide, or propranolol. • Arrhythmias that do not respond to lidocaine are unlikely to respond to tocainide.

**CONTRAINDICATIONS**    **Known allergy to local anesthetics of the amide group** Tocainide is chemically related to lidocaine and other similar local anesthetics. • Patients allergic to one of these local anesthetics will be allergic to tocainide as well.    **Heart block** Tocainide may suppress ectopic pacemakers that maintain cardiac function in certain types of heart block.

**DOSAGE**    **Adults:**  PO: 400 mg every 8 hours. Doses must be individualized, according to patient responses. *Special patient populations:*  ELDERLY: The elderly are more prone to dizziness and hypotension unless doses are reduced.  CHILDREN: Doses have not been established.  PREGNANCY: FDA pregnancy category C.  **RENAL OR HEPATIC FAILURE:** Dosage reduction is required.

**PREPARATIONS**    *Tablets:* 400 mg oval film-coated tablets.

**DRUG INTERACTIONS**    **Metoprolol** has additive effects with tocainide on the cardiac index.

**FATE**    Tocainide is an effective oral agent, unlike its chemical relative lidocaine; *bioavailability* is nearly 100%. Food slows absorption but does not lower the total amount absorbed. *Peak* blood levels occur within 0.5 to 2 hours. First-pass degradation in the liver is negligible. About 40% of a dose is excreted unchanged in urine. The average elimination *half-life* is 15 hours.

## ✽ NURSING CONSIDERATIONS

### Side effects, toxicities, and associated nursing actions

- See entry for drug class (p. 66).

**CNS** Central nervous system effects are common and include lightheadedness, vertigo, paresthesias, quivering, confusion, altered mood, visual disturbances, or ataxia. Central nervous system symptoms are dose related. Dizziness, numbness, or tremor may be early signs. Later signs are convulsions and respiratory depression.

- Instruct patients to avoid driving or operating hazardous equipment if dizziness, visual disturbances, or lightheadedness develop; notify physician.
- Assess for development of CNS side effects.

**GI** Gastrointestinal effects are also common, with up to 15% of patients reporting nausea, with or without vomiting and other symptoms.

- Suggest that patients take ordered doses with meals or snacks to lessen gastric irritation.
- Monitor weight.

**CV** Hypotension and bradycardia may develop, although the incidence is usually less than 3% of treated patients. As with other antiarrhythmic agents, tocainide may itself aggravate or induce arrhythmias in some patients.

- Monitor blood pressure and pulse before each dose.

**Skin** Rashes occur in up to 12% of treated patients.

- Forewarn patients that rashes may develop, and instruct them to notify physician if skin changes do appear.

**Patient and family education**
- See entry for drug class (p. 66).
- Review anticipated benefits and possible side effects of drug therapy with patients.

---

# verapamil hydrochloride (ver-AP-a-mill) class IV antiarrhythmic*

- verapamil hydrochloride: Calan, ♣Isoptin

**MECHANISM OF ACTION** Verapamil blocks calcium channels in various cells. Blockade of calcium channels in the SA and AV nodes slows conduction and may cause bradycardia. Verapamil has a greater effect on the AV node than other calcium channel blocking agents, making it more useful as an antiarrhythmic agent.

**INDICATIONS** **Paroxysmal supraventricular tachycardia** Verapamil often converts this arrhythmia to sinus rhythm. • The arrhythmia is often produced by AV nodal reentry, a process that can be stopped by the action of verapamil in slowing conduction through the AV node. **Ventricular tachycardia caused by atrial flutter or fibrillation** Verapamil slows conduction through the AV node and may therefore slow ventricular rates even though sinus rhythm is rarely restored.

**CONTRAINDICATIONS** See verapamil under Calcium channel blockers (p. 126).

**DOSAGE** IV: **ADULTS:** For arrhythmias, initial doses are 5 to 10 mg given as a bolus over 2 minutes (3 minutes for elderly patients). After 30 minutes an additional 10 mg (0.15 mg/kg) may be given if necessary. **CHILDREN:** For ages up to 1 year, initial doses should be 0.1 to 0.2 mg/kg body weight as a bolus over 2 minutes with constant ECG monitoring; the same dose may be repeated 30 minutes later, if necessary. For ages 1 to 15 years, initial doses should be 0.1 to 0.3 mg/kg as a bolus over 2 minutes, but the dose should not exceed 5 mg; the same dose may be repeated 30 minutes later, if necessary. *Special patient populations:* **ELDERLY:** IV doses in the elderly should be administered over 3 minutes to minimize adverse reactions. **PREGNANCY:** FDA pregnancy category B.

**PREPARATIONS** See verapamil under Calcium channel blockers (p. 126).

**DRUG INTERACTIONS** See verapamil under Calcium channel blockers (p. 126).

**FATE** See verapamil under Calcium channel blockers (p. 126).

**❦ NURSING CONSIDERATIONS**

**Side effects, toxicities, and associated nursing actions**
- See entry for drug class (p. 66).
- Verapamil may cause dangerous hypotension if overdosage occurs.
- AV blockade may occur with high doses of verapamil. For other information on verapamil, see Chapter 8 on calcium channel blocking agents.

*Also calcium channel blocker.

# Chapter Seven
# Antihypertensive drugs

**Centrally acting drugs**
clonidine
guanabenz
methyldopa

**Centrally and peripherally acting agents**
rauwolfia alkaloids

**Ganglionic blocking drugs**
mecamylamine
trimethaphan

**Neuroeffector blockers**
debrisoquin
guanadrel
guanethidine

**Vasodilators**
diazoxide
hydralazine
minoxidil
sodium nitroprusside

**Angiotensin antagonists**
captopril
enalapril

**Miscellaneous**
metyrosine
pargyline

The following drugs are also widely used antihypertensive drugs:

**Beta-adrenergic blockers (see Chapter 5, p. 40)**
acebutolol
atenolol
metoprolol
nadolol
pindolol
propranolol
timolol

**Alpha adrenergic blockers (see Chapter 5, p. 48)**
labetolol
prazosin
phentolamine
phenoxybenzamine
terazosin

**Calcium channel blockers (see Chapter 8, p. 121)**
diltiazem
nifedipine
verapamil

**INTRODUCTION**  **Chronic hypertension** Hypertension is generally defined as a resting diastolic blood pressure greater than 90 mm Hg in an adult. About 15% of adults in North America are hypertensive. No primary cause of hypertension can be found in 90% of hypertensive individuals. Hypertension of unknown origin is called *essential hypertension*.

The effectiveness of treating moderate to severe hypertension (diastolic pressure greater than 105 mm Hg) is well established. Untreated, moderate to severe hypertension is associated with the development of congestive heart failure, renal failure, aneurysms, and strokes. Hypertension with diastolic pressures of 90 to 105 mm Hg is borderline to mild hypertension. Mild hypertension is associated with increased morbidity when atheroslerosis is also a factor, as in sudden death (usually from electrical dysfunction of the heart secondary to poor coronary circulation) or myocardial infarction. Many physicians reserve treatment of mild hypertension for those patients with significant risk factors for atherosclerosis: smoking, high cholesterol values, high lipid levels, abnormal glucose tolerance test, ECG abnormalities, and a family history of atherosclerosis.

Blood pressure is regulated by renal mechanisms that influence the circulating blood volume through adjustments of body salt and water and cardiovascular mechanisms that influence the activity of the heart and blood vessels. Antihypertensive drug therapy is designed to modify the renal and cardiovascular mechanisms controlling blood pressure. These mechanisms are described with each drug class.  **Stepped therapy for chronic hypertension** Therapy is changing as more is learned about hypertension and as new drugs become available. Current therapy is based on a modified stepped-care approach in which drugs are added by class until blood pressure is brought under control. This approach is summarized in Table 7-1.

Step 1 is usually the administration of an oral diuretic, commonly a thiazide or thiazidelike diuret-

| Table 7-1. | Stepped-care therapy in treating chronic hypertension |
|---|---|
| GOAL | The goal is to bring blood pressure into the normal range: systolic pressure under 140 mm and diastolic pressure below 90 mm. Drug therapy is individualized, and drugs are added in steps as necessary. |
| STEP 1 | Encourage weight loss and a reduction in sodium intake. Drugs: diuretic (usually a thiazide diuretic) or sympathetic depressant (usually a beta-blocker) |
| STEP 2 | ADD  Sympathetic depressant (if not added in step 1) or  diuretic (if not added in step 1)  Angiotensin-converting enzyme inhibitor (with a diuretic)  or calcium channel blocker (with a diuretic) |
| STEP 3 | ADD  Vasodilator or  angiotensin-converting enzyme inhibitor  or  calcium channel blocker |
| STEP 4 | Substitute guanethidine for the step 2 drug |

ic. Diuretics inhibit renal tubular reabsorption, which causes diuresis that in turn reduces body salt and water (extracellular fluid). The loss of extracellular fluid is associated with reduced arterial blood pressure, but the mechanism of this hypotensive action remains obscure. This hypotensive effect is not seen in normotensive patients. The volume depletion also reduces plasma volume, although it is not clear that this reduction in plasma volume persists after the first month of therapy. In addition, many antihypertensive drugs cause fluid retention, an action that limits their antihypertensive effect. Diuretics (Chapter 9) are therefore commonly given with other antihypertensive drugs.

Instead of a diuretic, a beta-blocker may be given as the first drug. A beta-blocker is indicated for a patient who has coronary artery disease. Beta-blockers have been shown to have a protective effect against sudden death in individuals who have had a heart attack, however, diuretics may, by lowering potassium levels, increase the vulnerability of the compromised heart to sudden failure.

Step 2 in antihypertensive therapy is the addition of a sympathetic depressant drug to diuretic therapy. The sympathetic drug is commonly a beta-blocker. Other sympathetic depressants that might be used include methyldopa, clonidine, prazosin, reserpine, or the new sympathetic depressants, quanabenz or guanadrel. In addition, calcium channel-blockers and angiotensin-converting enzyme inhibitors are proving effective as drugs for step 2.

Step 3 is the addition of a vasodilator to the antihypertensive therapy. Hydralazine, minoxidil, and prazosin are the vasodilators most frequently used. Angiotensin-converting enzyme (ACE) inhibitor or a calcium channel blocker may alternatively be added as a step 3 drug.

Step 4 is normally used only to control severe hypertension. Guanethidine, a potent sympathetic depressant, is substituted for the step 2 depressant.

As can be seen in stepped therapy, drugs that inhibit the sympathetic tone of blood vessels by a variety of mechanisms have played a key role with diuretics in controlling hypertension. Two new drugs classes have been rapidly incorporated into antihypertensive therapy. The first new drug class, the angiotensin-converting enzyme (ACE) inhibitors, block the formation of the endogenous vasoconstrictor, angiontensin II. Angiotensin II is the end product following the release of renin by the kidney in response to high blood pressure. One major action of beta-blockers is to inhibit renin production by the kidney, so the actions of beta-blockers and ACE inhibitors are not additive.

The second new drug class is the calcium channel blockers. Calcium channel blockers decrease cardiac activity and reduce arterial tone, and each of these actions is characteristic of the particular drug. Nifedipine is a potent vasodilator and was the first calcium channel blocker approved for use in hypertensive patients. Verapamil is a potent cardiac depressant and may find use as a substitute for beta-blockers in selected cases.

Patients with essential hypertension must take drugs for the rest of their lives to control the hypertension. Drug therapy can rarely be discontinued after the blood pressure is brought into a normal range. Frequently the drug dosage can be reduced with time. This is important, since antihypertensive drugs can produce uncomfortable side effects, whereas the hypertension itself may not produce uncomfortable symptoms, a situation that can make patient compliance with drug therapy difficult. Obesity and high salt intake are factors that aggravate hypertension. If a patient reduces weight and salt intake, drug requirements frequently may also be reduced. Sympathetic depressants include the following drug classes: alpha-blockers, beta-blockers, centrally acting drugs, ganglionic blockers, and neuroeffector blockers. New drugs are being released as antihypertensive agents that blur the distinctions among the steps. For instance, quanadrel, a drug with a mechanism like guanethidine, is a step 2 drug. Some sympathetic depressant drugs, the beta-blockers and quanfacine, are sometimes used without a diuretic.

## ❦ NURSING CONSIDERATIONS

**Side effects, toxicities, and associated nursing actions**   The toxicities and side effects for different groups of antihypertensive drugs vary widely. They share the potential to cause:

**CV:** *Severe hypotension:*
- Monitor the blood pressure and pulse before initiating therapy, at the start of therapy, and whenever dosage is changed.
- Monitor blood pressure with the patient in lying, sitting, and standing positions.
- The blood pressure in some patients varies significantly between arms. Occasionally check the pressure in both arms. If one arm differs from the other, note which arm is used for each blood pressure determination.
- If hypotension is severe, instruct the patient to sit or lie down.
- Monitor fluid intake and output and weight.
- Supervise ambulation of hospitalized patients to guard against injury if the patient becomes dizzy.
- Use nightlights and bed siderails.
- Monitor the elderly closely; they are often more sensitive to hypotensive effects of drugs.

**Nursing interventions related to drug administration**
- In some acute situations, it is necessary to administer antihypertensive drugs by constant intravenous infusion. Use microdrip tubing and a volume control device or electronic infusion monitor.
- With intravenous administration, monitor the blood pressure and pulse every 3 to 5 minutes until stable, then every 15 minutes. The dose of medication is usually ordered to be titrated to the patient's response.
- After intravenous administration, keep the patient recumbent for at least 1 hour following drug administration. Keep the side rails up.
- Depending on the patient's condition, cardiac monitoring may be indicated during parenteral administration.

**Patient and family education**
- Inform patients of the desired effects of each drug prescribed, common side effects, and possible toxic effects. Ask the patient to report the appearance of any new sign or symptom.
- Hypotension is a common side effect, especially when the patient moves rapidly from a recumbent to a sitting or standing position (postural hypotension). Symptoms include dizziness, lightheadedness, weakness, and syncope. If symptoms occur, instruct the patient to sit or lie down until symptoms pass, then to rise slowly. Postural hypotension is often worse in the mornings and may be aggravated by long periods of standing, hot weather, hot showers or baths, ingestion of alcohol, and exercise, especially if the exercise is followed by immobility. Hypotension is also worse when patients are beginning therapy and during periods of dosage adjustment.
- Losing weight, adhering to a low-sodium diet, avoiding smoking and excessive caffeine, and adhering to a regular exercise program may decrease the need for antihypertensives.
- If indicated, refer the patient to a dietitian for instruction about sodium restriction. The need for

sodium restriction depends on the patient's general medical condition, other medications, and usual dietary habits; consult the physician. Instruction should be directed to the patient and to others in the household who regularly cook.

- Selected patients may be instructed to record and monitor their weight at regular intervals at home. Weight gain in excess of 2 lb/day or 5 lb/week should be reported to the health care provider.
- If a drug is associated with fluid retention, instruct patients to report signs of fluid retention such as tight rings, shoes, or clothing.
- Patients taking antihypertensives should avoid the concomitant use of other medications causing hypotension (e.g., alcohol, barbiturates, central nervous system depressants) or causing hypertension (e.g., sympathomimetics commonly found in cold remedies). Caution the patient to avoid taking any over-the-counter medications without prior clearance from the physician, and to keep all health care providers informed of all medications being taken.
- Review with patients appropriate actions for missed doses. If the missed dose is remembered soon after it was due, it may be taken and the usual schedule resumed. If the missed dose is remembered close to the time of the next dose, the patient should NOT double up, or take two doses close together in time. Advise patients to seek clarification from the physician or nurse when in doubt about medication schedules.
- Remind patients to keep all medications out of the reach of children.

# Centrally acting and centrally acting–peripherally acting antihypertensive drugs

**Centrally acting drugs (alpha-2 adrenergic agonists)** clonidine ~ guanabenz ~ methyldopa ~ **Centrally and peripherally acting drugs** rauwolfia alkaloids ~ reserpine ~ whole root rauwolfia ~ alseroxylon ~ deserpidine ~ rescinnamine

**DRUG COMBINATIONS**   clonidine and chlorthalidone: Combipress • methyldopa and chlorothiazide: Aldochlor • methyldopa and hydrochlorothiazide: Aldoril • reserpine and hydralazine HC1: Serpasil-Apresoline HC1 • reserpine and hydralazine HC1 and Hydrochlorothiazide: Ser-Ap-Es and others • resperpine and chlorothiazide: Diupres and others • resperpine and chlorthalidone: Regroton • reserpine and hydrochlorothiazide: Serpasil-Esidrix, Hydropres, others • reserpine and hydroflumethiazide: Hydro-Fluserpin and others • reserpine and methclothiazide: Diutensin • reserpine and polythiazide: Renese • reserpine and quinethazone: Hydromox • reserpine and trichlormethiazide: Metatensin • rauwolfia serpentina and bendroflumethiazide: Rauzide • rauwolfia serpentina and bendroflumethiazide and potassium chloride: Rautrax-N • rauwolfia serpentina and flumethiazide and potassium chloride: Rautrax • deserpidine and hydrochlorothiazide: Oreticyl • desperidine and methyclothiazide: Enduronyl, Eseridine, Meth-Desperidine

**OVERVIEW OF THE DRUG CLASS**   Blood pressure is in part controlled through the central nervous system. Baroreceptors in the aorta and carotid sinus monitor the blood pressure and send the information to the brain. The brain integrates this information and adjusts the heart rate and resistance of the blood vessels, largely through the sympathetic nervous system, to fine-tune the blood pressure. The centrally acting sympathetic depressants are drugs that act at this CNS center to lower heart rate and blood pressure.

**MECHANISM OF ACTION**   The centrally acting antihypertensives are sympathetic depressants. The vasomotor center in the medulla is a major center in the brain that controls blood pressure. In the CNS, norepineprine is the neurotransmitter for nerve tracts that ultimately decrease blood pressure. Centrally acting antihypertensive agents are alpha-2 adrenergic agonists that prevent the reuptake of norepinephrine. The resulting increase in CNS norepinephrine leads to a decrease in sympathetic tone in the periphery. This is in contrast to the peripheral nervous system, where norepinephrine increases blood pressure through a direct stimulation of alpha-1 adrenergic receptor, constricting blood vessels.

**INDICATIONS**   **Hypertension** Centrally acting antihypertensive drugs are used as step 2 drugs in the control of mild to moderate hypertension.

**CONTRAINDICATIONS**  See individual drugs.
**DRUG INTERACTIONS**  See individual drugs.

## clonidine  (KLOE-ni-deen)                              centrally acting antihypertensive

- clonidine (clonidine hydrochloride): Catapres, ✤Dixarit

**MECHANISM OF ACTION**   Clonidine is an alpha-2 adrenergic agonist. The antihypertensive effect is through the central nervous system, where clonidine inhibits peripheral sympathetic tone by stimulating alpha-2 adrenergic receptors in the vasomotor center of the medulla. The decrease in peripheral sympathetic tone is seen as a decrease in heart rate and in peripheral vascular resistance.

**INDICATIONS**   **Hypertension** Clonidine is used with a diuretic.  **Opiate withdrawal** Clonidine controls the sympathetic hyperactivity characteristic of opiate withdrawal.  **Migraine** Clonidine can reduce the severity and frequency of migraine attacks.  **Menopause** Clonidine decreases the severity and frequency of menopausal flushing.

**CONTRAINDICATIONS**   **Compromised cardiovascular status** Clonidine should be used with caution with patients having coronary insufficiency, cerebral vascular disease, recent myocardial infarction, or chronic renal failure.

**DOSAGE**   **Adults:**  PO: Initially, 0.1 mg twice daily, this dose is increased 0.1 or 0.2 mg/day until the desired response is achieved. Maintenance doses are usually in the range of 0.2-0.3 mg/day. Daily doses should not exceed 2.4 mg/day.  *Special patient populations:*  ELDERLY: The dose is individually titered and, in general, elderly patients require smaller doses.  PREGNANCY: FDA pregnancy category C.

**PREPARATIONS**   **Clonidine** *Transdermal:* 0.1 mg/24 hours (2.5 mg/3.5 cm$^2$), 0.2 mg/24 hours (5 mg/7 cm$^2$), 0.3 mg/24 hours (7.5 mg/10.5 cm$^2$).  **Clonidine hydrochloride** *Tablets:* 0.1, 0.2, 0.3 mg. *Combinations:* Clonidine hydrochloride, 0.1, 0.2, 0.3 mg with chlorthalidone 15 mg.

**DRUG INTERACTIONS**   **Alcohol and barbiturates** have CNS depressant effects that are enhanced by clonidine. **Tolazoline and tricyclic antidepressants** can block the antihypertensive effects of clonidine.

**FATE**   The *onset* of action is 30 to 60 minutes, and the *duration* of action is 12 to 24 hours. Clonidine and its metabolites are excreted in the urine. The duration of action doubles in patients with impaired renal function.

### ❦ NURSING CONSIDERATIONS
#### Side effects, toxicities, and associated nursing actions
- See Overview: Antihypertensive Drugs.

**CNS** Drowsiness occurs in about one third of patients. Dizziness, headache, and fatigue are occasionally noted. Rare side effects include depression or hallucinations.
- Caution patients to avoid driving or operating hazardous equipment until the effects of the medication can be evaluated.
- Assess the patient for signs of depression: anorexia, insomnia, neglect of personal appearance, withdrawal, changes in mood or affect.
- Assess patients for the appearance of other signs and symptoms.

**CV** Overdose usually produces hypotension and a slow heart rate. Occasionally, a paradoxical increase in blood pressure is seen. Clonidine therapy should never be abruptly discontinued; a rebound hypertension commonly accompanies abrupt withdrawal. Doses should be reduced over a period of 2 to 4 days.
- Impress on patients that suddenly stopping the drug can be dangerous. Instruct patients to have prescriptions refilled before the supply on hand runs out. Unreliable patients should not take this drug.

**GI** Constipation occurs in about one third of patients. This decreases in severity with time.
- If constipation occurs, instruct patients to increase fluid intake to 2500 to 3000 ml/day, increase dietary intake of fruit, fruit juices, and fiber, and increase daily exercise.

**Ophthalmic** Because retinal changes were noted in animal studies, periodic ophthalmic examinations are advisable for patients taking clonidine.
- Encourage patients to see an ophthalmologist early in therapy and at least yearly for continued monitoring.

**Allergic** Rashes.
- Instruct patients to report the development of skin changes.

**Other** Dry mouth, like constipation, is a common anticholinergic side effect. Sexual dysfunction is occasionally experienced.
- Instruct the patient to suck on sugarless candy or chew sugarless gum; others find relief sucking on ice chips. Some patients may wish to try commercially available saliva substitutes.
- Assess tactfully for sexual dysfunction, which may cause some patients to stop taking prescribed medications. Encourage patients to take medications as ordered for best effect, and caution them to consult with physician before stopping medication. Provide emotional support as needed.

**Patient and family education**    See Overview: Antihypertensive Drugs.

---

## guanabenz acetate    (GWAN-a-benz)    centrally acting antihypertensive

- guanabenz acetate: Wytensin

**MECHANISM OF ACTION**    Like clonidine, guanabenz is an alpha-2 adrenergic agonist. The antihypertensive effect is through the central nervous system, where guanabenz inhibits peripheral sympathetic tone by stimulating alpha-2 adrenergic receptors in the vasomotor center of the medulla. The decrease in peripheral sympathetic tone is seen as a decrease in heart rate and in peripheral vascular resistance.

**INDICATIONS**    **Hypertension** Guanabenz is administered with a diuretic to control mild to moderate hypertension.

**CONTRAINDICATIONS**    Severe coronary insufficiency. • Recent myocardial infarction. • Severe vascular disease. • Severe hepatic or renal failure.

**DOSAGE**    **Adults:**    **PO:** Initially, 4 mg twice daily. Dose may be increased in 4 to 8 mg daily increments every 1 to 2 weeks until the desired response is seen. Maximum dose: 32 mg twice daily.    *Special patient populations:*    **ELDERLY:** Geriatric patients are often more sensitive to sympathetic inhibition and are more susceptible to hypotension as a side effect. The dose is individually titered and, in general, elderly patients require smaller doses.    **PREGNANCY:** FDA pregnancy category C.

**PREPARATIONS**    *Tablets:* 4, 8, 16 mg.

**DRUG INTERACTIONS**    **Alcohol and other CNS depressants** diminish tolerance to guanabenz.

**FATE**    Guanabenz is about 75% absorbed from the gastrointestinal tract. *Onset* is in 1 hour, with a *peak* effect in 2 to 4 hours. Duration of action is about 8 hours.

### 🐝 NURSING CONSIDERATIONS

#### Side effects, toxicities, and associated nursing actions

**CNS** Sedation is a common side effect, particularly at higher doses. Overdose produces hypotension, drowsiness, lethargy, irritability, miosis, and a slow heart rate.
- Caution patients to avoid driving or operating hazardous equipment until the effects of the medication can be evaluated.
- Assess patients for the appearance of other signs and symptoms.

**CV** Dizziness, weakness, and headache are other common side effects.
- See Overview: Antihypertensive Drugs (p. 89).
- Monitor weight, intake, and output.

**GI** Dry mouth is experienced by about one third of patients taking guanabenz. Nausea, vomiting, and diarrhea are occasionally reported.
- Keep a record of bowel movements.
- If constipation develops, instruct the patient to maintain a fluid intake of 2500 to 3000 ml/day (if not contraindicated by the medical condition), increase the intake of fruits and fiber, maintain a regular

exercise program, and judiciously use foods known to stimulate defecation. In some patients it may be necessary to use a stool softener.

• Instruct the patient to suck on sugarless candy or chew sugarless gum; others find relief sucking on ice chips. Some patients may wish to try commercially available saliva substitutes.

• If GI symptoms are severe or persistent, notify physician.

**Respiratory** Nasal congestion.

• Advise patients of this annoying side effect. Caution patients to avoid over-the-counter treatments without first clearing them with the physician.

**Other** Like clonidine, guanabenz should not be abruptly discontinued. Dosage should be reduced over a few days to avoid a rebound hypertension.

• Reinforce to patients the need to take this drug as ordered and to avoid stopping the drug before discussing it with the physician. Patients should learn to have prescriptions refilled before the supply on hand runs out. Unreliable patients should not take this drug.

**Patient and family education** See Overview: Antihypertensive Drugs (p. 89).

---

## methyldopa (meth-ill-DOE-pa) centrally acting antihypertensive

• methyldopa: Aldomet, ✚Dopamet, ✚Medimet-250, ✚Novomedopa

**MECHANISM OF ACTION** Methyldopa depresses sympathetic nervous system activity through an action in the central nervous system. Methyldopa, like clonidine, enhances alpha-2 adrenergic activity in the vasomotor center of the medulla and thereby depresses sympathetic outflow. Methyldopa is metabolized to alpha-methylnorepinephrine, and this metabolite (a false neurotransmitter) is an alpha-2 agonist. As an antihypertensive, methyldopa decreases peripheral resistance but produces little change in heart rate or cardiac output. Blood flow through the kidneys, brain, and heart is maintained.

**INDICATIONS** **Hypertension** Methyldopa is used with a diuretic to control all degrees of hypertension.

**CONTRAINDICATIONS** **Hypersensitivity** A few patients develop allergic reactions to methyldopa. **Active liver disease** Methyldopa causes abnormal liver function test results, so the course of liver disease cannot be accurately monitered. **Blood dyscrasias** Methyldopa can cause a positive Coomb's test.

**DOSAGE** **PO:** **ADULT:** First week, 250 mg at bedtime; a second 250 mg dose may be added and then increased gradually to control blood pressure. Maximum dose, 2 g daily. **CHILDREN:** First week, 10 mg/kg daily divided into 2 to 4 doses. The dose is then adjusted every 2 days or more to control blood pressure. Maximum dose, 65 mg/kg daily. **IV:** **ADULTS:** 250 to 500 mg every 6 to 8 hours as needed. **CHILDREN:** 20 to 40 mg/kg daily in divided into four doses. *Special patient populations:* **ELDERLY:** The dose is individually titered and, in general, elderly patients require smaller doses. **PREGNANCY:** Methyldopa has been used without adverse fetal effects.

**PREPARATIONS** **Methyldopa** *Tablets:* 125, 250, 500 mg; *suspension:* 250 mg/5 ml. **Methyldopate hydrochloride** *Parenteral:* 50 mg/ml in 5 ml containers. *Combinations:* methyldopa, 250 mg, and chlorothiazide, 150 to 250 mg; or hydrochlorthiazide, 15, 25, 30, or 50 mg.

**DRUG INTERACTIONS** **Anesthetic** doses are reduced in patients treated with methyldopa. Vasopressors are used to control the hypotension during anesthesia. **Tolbutamide** metabolism is impaired by methyldopa, enhancing the hypoglycemic effect of the usual dose. **Phenoxybenzamine** combined with methyldopa can produce total urinary incontinence, which is reversible when the drugs are discontinued. **Lithium** combined with methyldopa may produce symptoms of lithium toxicity, although lithium levels are not increased. **Haloperidol** combined with methyldopa can produce psychiatric symptoms: irritability, aggressiveness, or dementia.

**DIAGNOSTIC TEST INTERFERENCE** Methyldopa interferes with several standard laboratory tests: Urinary uric acid by the phosphotungstate method. Serum creatinine by the alkaline picrate method. AST (SGOT) by colorimetric methods. Urinary catecholamines by fluorescent methods. A positive Coomb's test may occur with methyldopa therapy.

**FATE** Methyldopa is not well absorbed from the gastrointestinal tract. The *peak* antihypertensive effect is 4 to 6 hours after administration, and the *duration* of antihypertensive effect persists for up to 24 hours.

Methyldopa and its metabolites are eliminated by renal excretion, and patients with renal insufficiency can accumulate the drug.

## ❦ NURSING CONSIDERATIONS

### Side effects, toxicities, and associated nursing actions

**CNS** Drowsiness is a common side effect. Some patients experience a reduced mental acuity. Mental depression may occur.

- Caution patients to avoid hazardous activities (driving, operating machinery) until the effects of the medication can be evaluated.
- Scheduling the dose at bedtime may reduce the drowsiness during the day.
- Observe the patient for changes in mood or affect. Be alert to signs and symptoms frequently encountered in depression: insomnia, anorexia, withdrawal, neglect of personal appearance.

**CV** Sodium and water retention are common if a diuretic is not also administered. Orthostatic hypotension may occur.

- Monitor weight and serum electrolytes.
- See Overview: Antihypertensive Drugs (p. 89).

**GI** Dry mouth, nausea, vomiting, and diarrhea are occasionally reported.

- If dry mouth occurs, instruct patients to suck on ice chips, chew sugarless gum, or suck on sugarless hard candy. Some patients may wish to try a commercially available saliva substitute.
- If nausea, vomiting, or diarrhea are severe or persistent, notify the physician, and monitor intake, output, and weight.
- Monitor serum electrolytes.

**Respiratory** Nasal congestion.

- Assess patients for this annoying side effect.
- Caution patients to avoid over-the-counter medications for this problem without first consulting the physician. Nasal decongestants should be used only as directed.

**Metabolic** Alterations of liver function test results and increased AST and alkaline phosphatase levels may be seen in the first 3 months of therapy. Since these tests may reflect drug-induced hepatitis, liver function should be monitored during the first 4 months of therapy. The hepatitis is usually reversible.

- Monitor liver function studies.
- Instruct the patient to report the appearance of jaundice, right upper quadrant abdominal pain, or change in the color or consistency of stools.

**Renal** Methyldopa is eliminated by the kidneys; patients with renal insufficiency may accumulate the drug.

- Monitor the intake and output.
- Monitor the BUN and creatinine levels.
- Patients receiving dialysis may need an extra dose at the completion of dialysis; monitor the blood pressure.

**Other** Sexual dysfunction is occasionally reported.

- Assess tactfully for this problem. Sexual problems may result in poor patient compliance.
- Remind patients to take drugs as ordered for best result, and to consult with physician before discontinuing medication.
- Provide emotional support as needed.

**Hematologic** A positive Coomb's test appears for about 20% of patients receiving methyldopa; however, the actual occurrence of hemolytic anemia with methyldopa is rare and usually reversible when the drug is discontinued.

- Monitor blood counts before initiating therapy and at regular intervals during therapy.

### Patient and family education   See Overview: Antihypertensive Drugs (p. 89).

- If sedation is a problem, instruct the patient to add any increases in dosage in the evening rather than the morning, as this may reduce sedation interfering with work.
- Urine may darken when left exposed to the air.

# rauwolfia alkaloids  (rah-WOOL-fee-a)  centrally acting antihypertensives

See Table 7-2 for a listing of the rauwolfia alkaloids and their trade names.

**MECHANISM OF ACTION**  Rauwolfia alkaloids deplete stores of catecholamines. Since norepinephrine is the major catecholamine, this depletion reduces sympathetic tone and decreases peripheral resistance. However, the major antihypertensive effect is due to reduced cardiac output. Reserpine also depletes catecholamine and serotonin stores in the central nervous system, causing sedation and indifference. Serious mental depression is sometimes experienced.

**INDICATIONS**  **Hypertension** Reserpine is used to control mild hypertension. The other rauwolfia alkaloids may also be used.  **Hypertensive crisis** Reserpine can be administered intramuscularly. Antihypertensive action is seen in about 2 hours and persists for about 10 hours.  **Psychotic episodes** Reserpine can be used intramuscularly or orally to control psychotic episodes acutely or chronically. The antipsychotic drugs have essentially replaced reserpine for this use, however.

**CONTRAINDICATIONS**  • Hypersensitivity to rauwolfia derivatives. • Depression: Reserpine can itself cause serious depression. • Peptic ulcer, ulcerative colitis, gallstones: Depression of sympathetic tone allows a relative increase in cholinergic tone. The increase in stomach acid secretion and gastrointestinal secretions and motility are harmful in these conditions. • Pregnancy: Infants born to mothers taking reserpine show increased respiratory secretions, nasal congestion, cyanosis, and anorexia.

**DRUG INTERACTIONS**  **Digitalis and quinidine** may precipitate cardiac arrhythmias in patients taking reserpine.  **Antihypertensive drugs** Doses must be adjusted carefully if given with reserpine.  **Beta blocking agents** may have an additive effect with reserpine, producing hypotension and excessive slowing of the heart.  **MAO inhibitors** should not be given with reserpine.

**FATE**  Although the *onset* of antihypertensive effect may be seen within hours of initial administration, *peak* antihypertensive effect may take a week or more, depending on the time it takes to deplete norepinephrine stores. Similarly, the *duration* of antihypertensive effect may persist for several weeks after discontinuing reserpine. Reserpine is highly lipid soluble and is metabolized by the liver for excretion. The *half-life* is 50 to 100 hours.

## ❦ NURSING CONSIDERATIONS

### Side effects, toxicities, and associated nursing actions

**CNS** Effects include drowsiness, depression, dizziness, and headaches. Nightmares are common. Nervousness and anxiety may be noted. Parkinsonlike symptoms are infrequently seen. Serious depression, with suicidal intentions, is associated with higher doses of reserpine. Overdose causes extreme drowsiness or even coma; hypotension, hypothermia, respiratory depression, bradycardia, and miosis are further symptoms of overdose.
- Assess the patient for signs of depression: anorexia, insomnia, neglect of personal appearance, withdrawal, changes in mood or affect. It may be necessary to ask family members about these changes also.
- Caution patients to avoid driving or operating hazardous equipment until the effects of the medication can be evaluated.
- Assess patients for the appearance of other signs and symptoms.
- Be alert to signs of overdose, particularly if there is a recent history of depression.
- In an overdose serious enough to require vasopressor therapy, phenylephrine, levarterenol, or metaraminol should be used.

**CV** Effects include arrhythmias, slow heart rate, hypotension, and angina-like symptoms.
- See Overview: Antihypertensive Drugs (p. 89).

**GI** Problems include dry mouth, hypersecretion, nausea and vomiting, diarrhea, anorexia and bleeding.
- For dry mouth, instruct the patient to suck on sugarless candy or chew sugarless gum; others find relief sucking on ice chips. Some patients may wish to try commercially available saliva substitutes.
- If GI symptoms are severe or persistent, notify the physician.

**Respiratory** Nasal congestion is frequent.
- Advise patients of this annoying side effect. Caution patients to avoid over-the-counter treatments without first clearing them with physician.

Table
7-2.

## Rauwolfia alkaloids: trade names, dosage, and preparations

| Generic name | Trade names | Initial daily dose (mg) | Maintenance daily dose (mg) | Preparations |
|---|---|---|---|---|
| Alseroxylon | Rauwiloid | 1 | 2 | Tablets, 2 mg |
| Deserpidine | Harmonyl | 0.25 | 0.25 | Tablets, 0.25 mg |
| Rauwolfia Serpentina | Hiwolfia, Raudixin Rauserpa, Rauval Rauverid, Ru-Hy-T. Serfolia, Wolfina | 50 | 100 | Tablets, 50, 100 mg |
| Rescinnamine | ♣Moderil | 0.25 | 2 | Tablets, 0.25, 0.5 mg |
| Reserpine* | ♣Novareserpine, Rau-Sed ♣Reserfia, Reserpoid Sandril, Serpalan Serpasil, Serpate | 0.1 | 0.25 | Tablets, 0.1, 0.25, 1 mg |

Drug combinations:

Rauwolfia serpentina, 50 mg, with bendroflumethizide, 4 mg; with bendroflumethiazide, 4 mg, and potassium chloride, 400 mg; with Flumethiazide, 400 mg, and potassium chloride, 400 mg.

Deserpidine, 0.125 mg, with hydrochlorothiazide, 25, 50 mg; 0.25 mg with hydrochlorthiazide, 25 mg; 0.25, 0.5 mg with methyclothiazide, 5 mg.

Reserpine, 0.1 mg, with 25 mg hydralazine hydrochloride, with 25 mg hydralazine hydrochloride and 15 mg hydrochlorothiazide, with 25, 50 mg hydrochlorothiazide, with 2.5 mg methyclothiazide, with 2 mg trichlormethiazide; reserpine, 0.125 mg with 250, 500 mg chlorothiazide, with 25 mg chlorthalidone, with 25, 50 mg hydrochlorothiazide, with 25, 50 mg hydroflumethiazide, with 50 mg quinethazone; reserpine 0.2 mg with 50 mg hydralazine hydrochloride; reserpine, 0.25 mg, with 50 mg chlorthalidone, with 2 mg polythiazide.

*Reserpine may also be used in hypertensive emergencies: IM: Adults, Initial dose is 0.5 to 1 mg, followed by 2 and 4 mg doses at 3 hour intervals if necessary to control the hypertensive crisis, parenteral: 2.5 mg/ml in 10 ml vials or 2 ml ampules.

**Other** Sexual dysfunction, weight gain, and breast engorgement are sometimes reported.
- Assess tactfully for sexual dysfunction; many patients are uncomfortable relating sexual problems. Sexual dysfunction may prompt patient to discontinue medication without notifying physician. Provide emotional support as needed. Consult physician about possible drug or dosage change. Reinforce to patients the need to take medications as ordered for best effects.
- Assess for breast engorgement.
- Monitor weight.

**Patient and family education**   See Overview: Antihypertensive Drugs (p. 89).
- Patients may find this group of drugs convenient to take because once-a-day therapy is usually sufficient.
- Instruct the patient that reserpine and related compounds have a delayed onset of action and may require as long as 4 to 6 weeks of therapy before the full effect can be seen. When the drug is discontinued, effects may persist for several weeks.
- Taking this and related drugs with meals or a snack may reduce the gastric irritation that often accompanies the use of these drugs.
- Caution patients and family members to report the appearance of any unexpected sign or symptom.

• Many of the rauwolfia alkaloids, in single-drug or combination products, contain FD & C yellow dye #5 (tartrazine), which may cause an allergic reaction in susceptible individuals. While rare, this reaction is seen more commonly in persons with aspirin hypersensitivity. The following trade name products contain tartrazine (if in doubt, consult the pharmacist): Rauwiloid; Raudixin 50 mg and 100 mg; Rauzide; Rautrax-N; Rautrax; Serpasil-Apresoline Hydrochloride #1 and #2; Serpasil-Esidrix #1 and #2; Metatensin #2; Naquival.

# Antihypertensive blocking agents

**Ganglionic blocking drugs**     mecamylamine  ~  trimethaphan
**Neuroeffector blocking agents**      guanadrel  ~  guanethidine

**DRUG COMBINATIONS**   Guanethidine and hydrochlorothiazide: Esimil

**OVERVIEW OF THE DRUG CLASS**   Several drug classes are represented in antihypertensive therapy that block the action of norepinephrine on blood vessels by various mechanisms. Since norepinephrine is the sympathetic neurotransmitter that increases the tone of blood vessels and maintains blood pressure, blocking the action of norepinephrine lowers blood pressure. In this section two drug classes are presented, the ganglionic blockers and the neuroeffector blocking agents. Drugs that specifically block alpha-adrenergic receptors in the vasculature are covered in Chapter Five. All of these drug classes are sympathetic depressants because they block the action of norepinephrine to constrict blood vessels.

**MECHANISM OF ACTION**   Ganglionic blockers are actually antagonists of acetylcholine that act selectively at the ganglia of the autonomic nervous system. Ganglionic blockers inhibit the activation of the sympathetic and parasympathetic postganglionic neurons. In general, these drugs produce severe side effects in addition to lowering blood pressure. Neuroeffector blocking agents act at the postganglionic sympathetic nerve terminal to inhibit the release of norepinephrine and, over time, to deplete norepinephrine stores. Alpha-adrenergic blocking drugs are antagonists of norepinephrine, acting at the alpha-adrenergic receptors on the blood vessels to prevent the action of norepinephrine. This drug class is presented in Chapter Five.

**INDICATIONS**   • Moderate hypertension: guanadrel. • Severe hypertension: mecamylamine, guanethidine. • Hypertensive emergency: trimethaphan.

**CONTRAINDICATIONS**   See individual drugs.

**DRUG INTERACTIONS**   See individual drugs.

## mecamylamine hydrochloride
(mek-a-MILL'a-meen)                                                     ganglionic blocker antihypertensive

● mecamylamine hydrochloride: Inversine

**MECHANISM OF ACTION**   Mecamylamine is a potent ganglionic blocker. As such, it blocks receptor sites for acetylcholine in the autonomic ganglia and inhibits neurotransmission to both the sympathetic and parasympathetic branches of the autonomic nervous system.

**INDICATIONS**   In severe or malignant hypertension oral mecamylamine is effective.

**CONTRAINDICATIONS**   **Coronary insufficiency or recent myocardial infarction** Mecamylamine may further compromise cardiac function.   **Renal insufficiency (especially with uremia)** Mecamylamine may cause urinary retention.   **Chronic pyelonephritis** Mecamylamine may cause urinary retention, interfering with the antibiotics and sulfonamides used to treat chronic pyelonephritis.   **Glaucoma** Mecamylamine may aggravate glaucoma.

**DOSAGE**   **Adults:**   **PO:** Initially, 2.5 mg twice daily. Dose is adjusted in 2.5 mg increments every 2 days or so to achieve the desired response. For severe cases, four or more daily doses may be necessary. *Special patient populations:*   **PREGNANCY:** Safe use has not been established.

**PREPARATIONS**   *Tablets:* 2.5 mg.

**DRUG INTERACTIONS**    **Diuretics** will decrease the required dose of mecamylamine by about 50%.    **Anesthetics, alcohol, and other antihypertensive drugs** will potentiate the action of mecamylamine.

**FATE**    Mecamylamine is well absorbed from the gastrointestinal tract. *Onset of action* is 30 to 120 minutes; *duration* is 6 to 12 hours.

### ☙ NURSING CONSIDERATIONS

#### Side effects, toxicities, and associated nursing actions

**CNS** Effects include sedation, weakness, and fatigue.

• Caution patients to avoid driving or operating hazardous equipment until the effects of the medication can be evaluated.

**CV** Orthostatic hypotension is a common side effect. The dosage may need to be decreased.

• See Overview: Antihypertensive Drugs (p. 89).

**GI** Effects include anorexia, dry mouth, glossitis, nausea, vomiting, and constipation.

• Keep a record of bowel movements and monitor weight.

• If constipation develops, instruct patients to maintain a fluid intake of 2500 to 3000 ml/day (if not contraindicated by the medical condition); increase the intake of fruits, fruit juices, and fiber; maintain a regular exercise program, and judiciously use food known to stimulate defecation. In some patients it may be necessary to use a stool softener.

• If constipation is severe, auscultate for bowel sounds; paralytic ileus has been reported rarely.

• For dry mouth, instruct the patient to suck on sugarless candy or chew sugarless gum; others find relief sucking on ice chips. Some patients may wish to try commercially available saliva substitutes.

• If GI symptoms are severe or persistent, notify the physician.

**Ophthalmic** Dilated pupils and blurred vision are anticholinergic effects.

• Caution patients to avoid driving or operating hazardous equipment if visual problems occur; notify the physician.

**GU** Sexual dysfunction; urinary retention.

• Assess tactfully for sexual dysfunction; many patients are uncomfortable discussing sexual problems. Sexual dysfunction may prompt patient to discontinue medication without notifying the physician. Provide emotional support as needed. Consult the physician about possible drug or dosage change. Reinforce to patients the need to take medications as ordered for best effects.

• Instruct patients to report difficulty in urination, feeling that the bladder has not emptied, or pain in the bladder area.

#### Patient and family education

• Review with patients the anticipated benefits and possible side effects of drug therapy. Instruct patients to report the appearance of any new sign or symptom.

• Instruct patients to take this medication in a consistent way, either with or without food. Taking the drug after meals is the preferred time for dosing.

• Impress on patients that stopping the drug suddenly can be dangerous. Patients should learn to have prescriptions refilled before the supply on hand runs out. Unreliable patients should not take this drug.

• Sodium bicarbonate, found in some antacids, may contribute to toxicity from this drug. Instruct patients to obtain approval from the physician before using any medications, including home remedies.

---

## trimethaphan camsylate    (trye-METH-a-fan)    ganglionic blocker antihypertensive

• trimethaphan camsylate: Arfonad

**MECHANISM OF ACTION**    Trimethaphan is a short-acting ganglionic blocker. As such, trimethaphan blocks receptor sites for acetylcholine in the autonomic ganglia and inhibits neurotransmission to both the sympathetic and parasympathetic branches of the autonomic nervous system.

**INDICATIONS**    **Hypertensive emergency** Trimethaphan is used for short-term control of hypertension.    **Con-**

**trolled hypotension** Trimethaphan produces controlled hypotension during surgery. **Pulmonary hypertensive emergency** Trimethaphan is used to control pulmonary edema associated with pulmonary hypertension and systemic hypertension.

**CONTRAINDICATIONS**  Conditions in which hypotension is dangerous. These include shock, asphyxia, respiratory insufficiency, hypovolemia, and anemia.

**DOSAGE**  **Adults:**  IV: 3 to 4 mg/min, adjusted to maintain desired degree of hypotension. Rates required vary from 0.3 to 6 ml/min. *Dilution:* 10 ml (500 mg) of stock is diluted to 500 ml in 5% dextrose to give a solution 1 mg/ml. This solution should not be used as a vehicle to administer other drugs.  *Special patient populations:*  PREGNANCY: Safe use has not been established.

**PREPARATIONS**  *Parenteral:* 50 mg/ml in 10 ml ampule.

**DRUG INTERACTIONS**  **Antihypertensives and diuretics** An additive hypotensive effect may be seen with other antihypertensive drugs and diuretics.  **Anesthetics (especially spinal anesthetics)** These may cause severe hypotension with trimethaphan.

**FATE**  Trimethaphan has an immediate *onset of action* and a short *duration of action* on intravenous infusion.

☙ **NURSING CONSIDERATIONS**

### Side effects, toxicities, and associated nursing actions

**CV** Hypotension is especially a problem with elderly, debilitated, or very young patients. Hypotension may be reversed with phenylephrine HCl or mephentermine sulfate.

• See Overview: Antihypertensive Drugs (p. 89).
• Patients receiving this drug should be in the intensive care setting, where proper equipment for monitoring blood pressure and side effects is available.
• Raising the head of the bed may increase the hypotensive effects; cerebral anoxia is to be avoided.

**GI** Anorexia, nausea, vomiting, paralytic ileus (rare).

• Paralytic ileus is rare unless the drug is administered for longer than 48 hours.
• Monitor the frequency of bowel movements. Auscultate bowel sounds and assess for abdominal distention and pain.

**Allergic** Trimethaphan may liberate histamine stores to produce allergic symptoms.

• Assess patient for allergic type responses.
• It may be necessary to change drugs if response is severe.

**Ophthalmic** Cycloplegia and mydriasis.

• Since mydriasis (dilated pupils) is common, this sign should not be interpreted as anoxia or used to monitor depth of anesthesia.

**GU** Urinary retention.

• Monitor intake and output.
• If a urinary catheter is not in place, question the patient about difficulty voiding or bladder pain.
• Palpate the bladder for distention if indicated. Be especially alert to this problem in elderly male patients who may also have prostatic hypertrophy.

### Nursing interventions related to drug administration

• See Overview: Antihypertensive Drugs (p. 89).
• For proper dilution, see Dosage section.
• Consult with physician about guidelines for dosage titration.

### Patient and family education

• This drug is used in the intensive care setting and would not be used for self-medication.
• Keep the patient and family informed of changes in the treatment plan.

---

## guanadrel sulfate  (GWAN-a-drel)  neuroeffector blocker antihypertensive

• guanadrel sulfate: Hylorel

**MECHANISM OF ACTION**  Guanadrel is a neuron-blocking agent that acts like guanethidine.

**INDICATIONS**  **Moderate to severe hypertension** Guanadrel is usually administered with a thiazide.
**CONTRAINDICATIONS**  • Hypersensitivity to guanadrel. • Pheochromocytoma. • Congestive heart failure.
• Use of MAO inhibitors.
**DOSAGE**  **Adults:**  PO: Initially, 10 mg/day in two doses; dose is adjusted weekly or monthly as needed. Usual dosage range is 20 to 75 mg daily.  *Special patient populations:*  PREGNANCY: FDA pregnancy category B.
**PREPARATIONS**  *Tablets:* 10, 25 mg.
**DRUG INTERACTIONS**  **Rauwolfia alkaloids** in combination with guanadrel may lead to excessive hypotension, slowing of the heart, and mental depression.  **Digitalis** will further slow the heart rate. **Amphetaminelike compounds, tricyclic antidepressants, antipsychotics, and oral contraceptives** These drugs reduce the effectiveness of guanadrel.  **Exogenous catecholamines** When norepinephrine stores are depleted, effector cells become more sensitive to catecholamines. Vasopressor drugs may produce an exaggerated response in the patient treated with guanethidine.
**FATE**  Guanadrel is rapidly absorbed after oral administration. The *onset of action* is about 2 hours, with a *peak* response in 4 to 6 hours. The *half-life* of guanadrel is 10 hours, and about 85% of the drug is excreted in the urine in 24 hours. About 40% of the drug is unchanged.

## ❧ NURSING CONSIDERATIONS

### Side effects, toxicities, and associated nursing actions  Side effects for guanadrel are those characteristic of guanethidine, but less severe.

**CV** Sympathetic blockade causes dizziness, weakness, lassitude, and fainting. Unopposed parasympathetic activity causes a slow heart rate. Orthostatic hypotension is common and severe.
• See Overview: Antihypertensive Drugs (p. 89).
• Be especially alert to bradycardia if the patient is also receiving other drugs known to slow the pulse, such as cardiac glycosides.
• Caution patients to avoid driving or operating hazardous equipment if dizziness, weakness, or fainting occur.
• Assess for the presence of side effects. If severe, changing drugs may be necessary.
**GI** Severe diarrhea, secondary to unopposed parasympathetic activity, is common.
• Monitor intake and output if diarrhea is present. Monitor electrolytes and patient weight.
**GU** Inhibition of ejaculation is common. Assess male patients tactfully for this problem; many patients are reluctant to discuss sexual problems. Sexual problems may prompt patients to discontinue medications without notifying the physician. Consult with physician about possible changes in drug or dosage. Provide emotional support as needed. Reinforce to patients the importance of taking medications as ordered for best effect.
**Metabolic** Sodium retention is common, so guanadrel is usually administered with a thiazide diuretic.
• Monitor weight. Instruct patients to monitor and record weight at home. Instruct patients to notify physician of weight gain greater than 2 lb/day or 5 lb/week.
• Instruct patients to notify physician of tight rings, shoes, or clothing or of the development of edema (swelling).
• Monitor serum electrolytes, assess for development of edema, monitor intake and output.

### Patient and family education
• See Overview: Antihypertensive Drugs (p. 89).
• Instruct selected patients to monitor and record the pulse at regular intervals. Give the patients guidelines of what to do if the pulse rate is below the acceptable limit for that patient (usually 60 beats per minute in an adult, but individual patients may need other guidelines).
• Caution the patient to report the development of diarrhea. Severe diarrhea may need medical attention. Be alert to electrolyte imbalances in patients with severe chronic diarrhea.
• This drug may cause hypoglycemia. Caution patients with diabetes about this side effect. Diabetics may want to monitor blood and urine glucose levels more frequently until the effect can be evaluated and may need a dosage adjustment of antidiabetic medications.
• If dry mouth occurs, instruct the patient to suck on sugarless candy or chew sugarless gum; others find relief sucking on ice chips. Some patients may wish to try commercially available saliva substitutes.

- Nasal congestion may be a problem. Instruct patients about this possible side effect, but caution them to avoid the use of over-the-counter remedies to treat nasal congestion until approved by the physician.

## guanethidine sulfate (gwahn-ETH-i-deen) neuroeffector blocker antihypertensive

- guanethidine sulfate: ♣Apo-Guanethidine, Ismelin

**MECHANISM OF ACTION** Guanethidine is a peripherally acting neuroeffector blocker. Guanethidine acts at the postganglionic sympathetic nerve terminal, inhibiting norepinephrine release and depleting norepinephrine stores.

**INDICATIONS** • Moderate and severe hypertension. • Renal hypertension.

**CONTRAINDICATIONS** Hypersensitivity to guanethidine. • Pheochromocytoma. • Congestive heart failure. • Use of MAO inhibitors.

**DOSAGE** PO: ADULTS: *Ambulatory patients:* Initial dose is 10 mg daily in a single dose, increased gradually every 7 to 10 days if necessary. The average daily dose is 25 to 50 mg/day. *Hospitalized patients:* Initial dose is 25 to 50 mg, increased by 25 to 50 mg every other day if necessary. *Combination therapy:* Low doses are gradually added to a thiazide and/or hydralazine. MAO inhibitors should be withdrawn for at least 1 week before guanethidine. *Special patient populations:* PREGNANCY: Safe use has not been established.

**PREPARATIONS** *Tablets:* 10, 25 mg. The 10 mg tablets have tartrazine. *Combination:* 10 mg with 25 mg hydrochlorothiazide.

**DRUG INTERACTIONS** **Rauwolfia alkaloids** in combination with guanethidine may lead to excessive hypotension, slowing of the heart, and mental depression. **Cardiac glycosides** will further slow heart rate. **Amphetaminelike compounds, tricyclic antidepressants, antipsychotics, and oral contraceptives** reduce the effectiveness of guanethidine. **Exogenous catecholamines** When norepinephrine stores are depleted, effector cells become more sensitive to drugs with catecholamine effects. Vasopressor drugs may produce an exaggerated response in the patient treated with guanethidine.

**FATE** Guanethidine has an *onset of action* of about 8 hours. The *half-life* is about 8 days, and guanethidine accumulates in the body. The drug is partly metabolized and excreted in the urine. Reduced doses are necessary with impaired renal function.

### 🐾 NURSING CONSIDERATIONS

**Side effects, toxicities, and associated nursing actions** Guanethidine is a potent drug with serious possible side effects:

**CV** Sympathetic blockade causes dizziness, weakness, lassitude, and fainting. Unopposed parasympathetic activity causes a slow heart rate. Orthostatic hypotension is common and severe.
- See Overview: Antihypertensive Drugs (p. 89).
- Be especially alert to bradycardia if the patient is also receiving other drugs known to slow the pulse, such as cardiac glycosides.
- Caution patients to avoid driving or operating hazardous equipment if dizziness, weakness, or fainting occur.
- Assess for the presence of side effects. If severe, changing drugs may be necessary.

**GI** Severe diarrhea, secondary to unopposed parasympathetic activity, is common.
- Monitor intake and output if diarrhea is present. Monitor electrolytes and patient weight.

**GU** Inhibition of ejaculation is common.
- Assess male patients tactfully for this problem; many patients are reluctant to discuss sexual problems. Sexual problems may prompt patients to discontinue medications without notifying the physician. Consult with the physician about possible changes in drug or dosage. Provide emotional support as needed. Reinforce to patients the importance of taking medications as ordered for best effect.

**Metabolic** Sodium retention is common, so guanethidine is usually administered with a thiazide diuretic.

- Monitor weight. Instruct patients to monitor and record weight at home. Instruct patients to notify physician of weight gain greater than 2 lb/day or 5 lb/week.
- Instruct patients to notify physician of tight rings, shoes, or clothing or of the development of edema (swelling).
- Monitor serum electrolytes, assess for development of edema, and monitor intake and output.

**Patient and family education**

- See Overview: Antihypertensive Drugs (p. 89).
- Instruct selected patients to monitor and record the pulse at regular intervals. Give the patients guidelines of what to do if the pulse rate is below the acceptable limit for that patient (usually 60 beats per minute in an adult, but individual patients may need other guidelines).
- Caution the patient to report the development of diarrhea. Severe diarrhea may need medical attention. Be alert to electrolye imbalances in patients with severe chronic diarrhea.
- This drug may cause hypoglycemia. Caution patients with diabetes about this side effect. Diabetics may want to monitor blood and urine glucose more frequently until the effect can be evaluated and may need a dosage adjustment of antidiabetic medications.
- If dry mouth occurs, instruct the patient to suck on sugarless candy or chew sugarless gum: others find relief sucking on ice chips. Some patients may wish to try commercially available saliva substitutes.
- Nasal congestion may be a problem. Instruct patients about this possible side effect, but caution them to avoid the use of over-the-counter remedies to treat nasal congestion until approved by the physician.

# Antihypertensive vasodilators

diazoxide ~ hydralazine ~ minoxidil ~ sodium nitroprusside

**DRUG COMBINATIONS**    hydralazine HCl and hydrochlorothiazide: Apresazide, Aprozide, Apresodis, Apresoline-Esidrix and others • hydralazine HCl and reserpine: Serpasil-Apresoline HCl • hydralazine HCl and hydrochlorothiazide: Ser-Ap-Es and others

**OVERVIEW OF THE DRUG CLASS**    Vasodilators are used as emergency drugs (diazoxide and sodium nitroprusside) or as step 3 drugs (hydralazine and minoxidil) added to a diuretic and a sympathetic depressant.

**MECHANISM OF ACTION**    Vasodilators act directly on vascular smooth muscle to cause relaxation. The profound vasodilation lowers blood pressure, but in compensation there is an increase in heart rate, plasma renin, and fluid retention.

**INDICATIONS**    **Moderately severe to severe hypertension** Step 3 drugs—hydralazine and minoxidil.    **Hypertensive emergency** Diazoxide and sodium nitroprusside.

**CONTRAINDICATIONS**    See individual drugs.

**DRUG INTERACTIONS**    See individual drugs.

## diazoxide    (dye-az-OX-ide)    vasodilator

- diazoxide: Hyperstat

**MECHANISM OF ACTION**    Diazoxide relaxes arteriolar smooth muscle to reduce blood pressure. The prompt drop in blood pressure causes a reflex increase in heart rate and cardiac output.

**INDICATIONS**    **Hypertensive emergencies** Diazoxide is used in emergencies to promptly lower diastolic blood pressure.    **Insulinoma** Diazoxide counteracts hypoglycemia.

**CONTRAINDICATIONS**   **Cardiac conditions** that might be compromised by the action of diazoxide, which include aortic coarctation, arteriovenous shunt, coronary artery disease, and dissecting aortic aneurysm.   **Hypersensitivity** to diazoxide, thiazides, or other sulfonamide derivatives.

**DOSAGE**   **Hypertensive emergency:**   *Adults:*   IV: 1 to 3 mg/kg, up to 150 mg, undiluted, by IV push into a peripheral vein. May repeat after 5- to 15-minute intervals to achieve satisfactory decrease in blood pressure. Patient should be lying down. Further administration may be necessary at intervals of 4 to 24 hours to keep blood pressure down. Oral antihypertensive medication should be initiated as soon as possible. Diazoxide should not be given for more than 4 or 5 days.   **Insulinoma:**   *Adults:*   PO: 3 to 8 mg/kg daily in two or three divided doses.   *Special patient populations:*   PREGNANCY: Safe use has not been established. Teratogenic effects have been demonstrated in animals, including skeletal and cardiovacular abnormalities and fetal islet destruction.

**PREPARATIONS**   Parenteral: 15 mg/ml in 20 ml ampule; *capsule* 50 mg; *suspension: 50 mg/ml*. The suspension contains alcohol.

**DRUG INTERACTIONS**   **Coumarin anticoagulants and other protein-bound drugs such as phenytoin** may be displaced by diazoxide, which is highly protein bound.   **Insulin** doses of diabetic patients may have to be adjusted. Diazoxide has an hyperglycemic effect.   **Thiazides and other diuretics** may be potentiated by diazoxide.   **Antihypertensive drugs** The hypotensive effects of other antihypertensive drugs such as methyldopa and reserpine and other drugs causing peripheral dilation (hydralazine, nitrates, papaverinelike compounds) will be exaggerated by diazoxide. Serious hypotensive episodes may occur.

**FATE**   Diazoxide's *onset of action* occurs within 5 minutes. Because diazoxide is more than 90% bound to plasma protein, the *duration of action* is about 12 hours. The plasma *half-life* of diazoxide is about 28 hours. It is excreted unchanged in the urine.

## ❦ NURSING CONSIDERATIONS

### Side effects, toxicities, and associated nursing actions

**CV:** *Hypotension:* Diazoxide is a drug for emergency use for the hospitalized patient who can be carefully monitored. *Headache and/or flushing:* These symptoms may result from the arteriolar dilation. *Severe hypotension, anginal symptoms, cerebral ischemia, semiparalysis, and myocardial infarction:* These reactions are infrequent but serious complications of diazoxide therapy. *Reflex increase in heart rate and force of contraction:* See Overview: Antihypertensive Drugs (p. 89).

- Monitor blood pressure closely. Do not leave patient unattended during parenteral administration. Monitor electrocardiogram. Keep siderails up.

**Metabolic:** *Hyperglycemia:* This is usually transitory in healthy patients but may become serious in diabetic patients. *Sodium and water retention:* Although related chemically to the thiazide diuretics, diazoxide has no diuretic action itself. *Hyperuricemia:* This is usually transitory.

- Monitor blood and urine glucose levels, serum electrolytes, and serum uric acid.
- Monitor intake, output, and weight.
- Treatment of hyperuricemia often involves pushing fluids to ensure a good urinary output; this approach may be contraindicated in patients receiving diazoxide.

**GI** Nausea, vomiting, loss of appetite.

- Monitor intake, output, and weight.
- Be alert to gastrointestinal side effects. If pronounced or persistent, switching to another drug may be necessary.

### Nursing interventions related to drug administration

- See Overview: Antihypertensive Drugs (p. 89).
- Diazoxide may be administered undiluted, at a rapid rate (e.g., 150 mg over 30 seconds), or diluted and given as a slow infusion over a period of 20 to 30 minutes.
- The medication is highly alkaline and should not be given intramuscularly or subcutaneously. Inspect IV line for patency before administering, and monitor insertion site for signs of irritation or extravasation. Avoid extravasation, but should it occur, apply ice packs.
- Severe hypotension can be treated with a sympathomimetic such as norepinephrine.

### Patient and family education

- See Overview: Antihypertensive Drugs (p. 89).

- Parenteral forms of this drug are used only in the acute care setting. Keep patient and family informed of changes in the patient's condition and the treatment plan.
- Review with diabetic patients methods to monitor blood or urine glucose; a change in insulin or diet may be necessary.
- Teach selected patients to monitor and record weight or blood pressure in the home setting. Reinforce to patients the importance of returning for regular medical follow-up.

---

## hydralazine hydrochloride    (hye-DRAL-a-zeen)                    vasodilator

- hydralazine hydrochloride: Apresoline

**MECHANISM OF ACTION**    Hydralazine relaxes arterial smooth muscle to reduce blood pressure. A sympathetic depressant is commonly given with hydralazine to limit the reflex increase in heart rate and cardiac output. Blood flow to the kidneys and brain is maintained or increased.

**INDICATIONS**    **Moderate to severe hypertension** Hydralazine is usually given with a diuretic and a sympathetic depressant.    **Hypertensive crisis** Hydralazine may be given parenterally to control a hypertensive emergency; however, diazoxide or sodium nitroprusside is generally preferred.

**CONTRAINDICATIONS**    • Coronary artery disease. • Hypersensitivity to hydralazine. • Increased cranial pressure. Hydralazine may cause cerebral ischemia if given parenterally to patients with increased cranial pressure.

**DOSAGE**    **PO:**    **ADULTS:** Initially, 10 to 25 mg two or three times daily. If necessary, the dose is increased in 10 to 25 mg increments to achieve the desired reduction in blood pressure. The maximum total daily dose is 300 mg.    **CHILDREN:** Begin with 0.75 mg/kg divided into four daily doses. If necessary, increase over three to four weeks to a maximum of 7.5 mg/kg/day.    **IV or IM:**    **ADULTS:** 10 to 40 mg, repeated if necessary. Blood pressure should begin to fall in a few minutes and continue to fall for 10 to 80 minutes, depending on the dose.    *Special patient populations:*    **PREGNANCY:** Safe use has not been established.

**PREPARATIONS**    *Tablets:* 10, 25, 50, 100 mg; *Parenteral:* 20 mg/ml injection in 1 ml ampule.    **Combinations:** *Capsules:* Hydralazine hydrochloride 25 mg with hydrochlorothiazide, 25 mg; 50, 100 mg with 50 mg hydrochlorothiazide. *Tablets:* 25 mg with 15 mg hydrochlorothiazide and 0.1 mg reserpine; 50 mg with 0.2 mg reserpine.

**DRUG INTERACTIONS**    **Sympathomimetic drugs** may aggravate a fast heart rate or angina.    **Diazoxide** may cause profound hypotension in patients taking hydralazine.

**FATE**    When taken orally, hydralazine is extensively metabolized by the liver on absorption (first pass metabolism). Hydralazine is largely acetylated by the liver; some people are slow acetylators and therefore react longer to hydralazine. Hydralazine is also largely bound to plasma protein, and the plasma *half-life* is 2 to 8 hours. The *onset of action* is about 45 minutes after oral ingestion and the *duration of action* is about 6 hours.

☙ **NURSING CONSIDERATIONS**

### Side effects, toxicities, and associated nursing actions

**CV** Headache, palpitations, fast heart rate, and angina are common cardiovascular side effects of hydralazine. All drugs in this class may cause fluid retention and reflex increase in heart rate and force of contraction.
- See Overview: Antihypertensive Drugs (p. 89).
- Monitor weight. Inspect for development of edema. Monitor serum electrolytes and intake and output.
- Instruct patient to notify physician if these side effects develop.

**Allergic** *Hypersensitivity* is usually seen as a rash, fever, chills, or arthralgia. A few patients develop the symptoms of acute systemic *lupus erythematosus:* arthralgia, myalgia, dermatoses, fever, anemia, and splenomegaly. This is most common in patients receiving large doses who are slow acetylators. The symptoms usually disappear when hydralazine is discontinued.

- Monitor temperature, hematocrit, and hemoglobin.
- Assess the patient for joint or muscle pain.

**Other:** *Peripheral neuropathy* is an infrequent side effect and may be reversed with pyridoxine administration.
- Assess the patient for complaints of tingling or discomfort in the fingers, hands, or feet.

**GI** Anorexia, nausea, vomiting, diarrhea.
- Monitor intake and output and weight.
- Assess patients for these symptoms. If symptoms are persistent or severe, it may be necessary to switch drugs.

### Nursing interventions related to drug administration
- See Overview: Antihypertensive Drugs (p. 89).
- Parenteral administration is rarely used.

### Patient and family education
- See Overview: Antihypertensive Drugs (p. 89).
- Instruct patients to report the signs of peripheral neuritis should they occur: numbness, tingling, and paresthesias of the extremeties.
- Some brands of hydralazine contain FD & C coloring #5 (tartrazine), which may cause an allergic response in some individuals. Although rare, this response is more common in individuals with aspirin hypersensitivity. Patients who have this sensitivity should request a brand without this coloring (the pharmacist has access to this information) and should be instructed not to switch brands.
- Inform the patient of the desired effects of the drug, common side effects, and possible toxic effects. Ask the patient to report the appearance of any new sign or symptom.
- Taking the prescribed oral dose with meals or food may lessen gastric irritation.

---

## minoxidil (mi-NOX-i-dill) vasodilator

- minoxidil: Loniten

**MECHANISM OF ACTION** Minoxidil relaxes arteriolar smooth muscle to reduce blood pressure. The prompt drop in blood pressure causes a reflex increase in heart rate and cardiac output.

**INDICATIONS** **Severe hypertension** Minoxidil is used with a diuretic, usually furosemide, and sympathetic depressant drug in patients refractory to other antihypertensive drug combinations.

**CONTRAINDICATIONS** **Mild hypertension** Because minoxidil can produce serious side effects, it is used only for patients whose hypertension is not controlled with other drugs. **Pheochromocytoma** Minoxidil may stimulate catecholamine secretion from this tumor.

**DOSAGE** **PO:** **ADULTS AND CHILDREN OVER 12 YEARS:** Initially, 5 mg twice daily. The dosage may be increased at 3 day intervals to 10 mg, 20 mg and 40 mg daily if necessary. The usual dose is 10 to 40 mg daily; the maximum dose is 100 mg daily. The dose may be adjusted every 6 hours in hospitalized patients who are closely monitored. **CHILDREN UNDER 12 YEARS:** 0.2 mg/kg/day in two divided doses. Dosage may be increased gradually by 0.1 to 0.2 mg/kg/day to a maximum of 50 mg/kg/day if necessary. Usual doses are 0.25 to 1 mg/kg/day. *Special patient populations:* **PREGNANCY:** Safe use has not been established.

**PREPARATIONS** *Tablets:* 2.5, 10 mg.

**DRUG INTERACTIONS** **Guanethidine or quanadrel** Minoxidil will cause profound orthostatic hypotension in patients receiving guanethidine or guanadrel. These drugs should be discontinued before administration of minoxidil, or the patient should be hospitalized.

**FATE** Minoxidil is well absorbed from the gastrointestinal tract. The *onset of action* is about 30 minutes and the *peak effect* is seen in 2 to 3 hours. Although the plasma *half-life* of minoxidil is 4 hours, minoxidil accumulates in smooth muscle and is effective for about 3 days. Minoxidil is extensively metabolized to glucuronide and excreted in the urine.

## ❦ NURSING CONSIDERATIONS
### Side effects, toxicities, and associated nursing actions

**CV** *Fluid retention* can lead to congestive heart failure unless a diuretic, usually furosemide, is administered concurrently. *Tachycardia:* The reflex increase in heart rate can be prevented by concurrent administration of a sympathetic depressant, usually propranolol or another beta-blocker. *Cardiac lesions:* Animal studies have indicated that minoxidil may cause cardiac lesions; however, these lesions have not yet been found in autopsies of human patients receiving minoxidil. *Pericardial effusion:* If excessive fluid retention cannot be managed by diuretics or dialysis, minoxidil should be discontinued. About 3% of patients with impaired renal function have developed pericardial effusion while on minoxidil in spite of being dialyzed to reduce fluid retention. *ECG abnormalities:* Flattening of the T wave and increased QRS peaks are often seen in patients on minoxidil. These changes are usually asymptomatic and disappear when minoxidil is discontinued.
- See Overview: Antihypertensive Drugs (p. 89).
- Monitor the electrocardiogram on a regular basis.
- Monitor heart and lung sounds and assess for distended neck veins and edema. Monitor weight, intake and output, and serum electrolytes

**Allergic:** *Hypersensitivity:* Rashes are occasionally reported.
- Visually inspect patient for rashes. Instruct patients to report skin changes.

**Metabolic:** *Hypertrichosis:* Minoxidil causes an increased hair growth after 1 to 2 months of therapy in about 80% of patients. This hair growth begins on the face and later extends to the back, arms, legs, and scalp. Efforts are being made to develop topically effective minoxidil for treatment of baldness.
- Caution patients about this problem.
- Do a careful baseline assessment of hair distribution and quality before beginning therapy and at regular intervals thereafter.

### Patient and family education
- See Overview: Antihypertensive Drugs (p. 89).
- If hypertrichosis (see previous section) is bothersome, the hair may be bleached, shaved, or removed, depending on severity and location. Some patients prefer to change drugs. Caution patients not to discontinue the medication without contacting the physician.
- Instruct appropriate patients to monitor and record pulse and weight at home. Weight gain in excess of 2 lb/day or 5 lb/week should be reported. Pulse increases of 20 beats per minute or more should be reported.
- Caution all patients to report the development of swelling or tight rings, shoes, or clothing.

---

## sodium nitroprusside    (nye-troe-PRUH-side)    vasodilator

- sodium nitroprusside: Nipride, Nitropress

**MECHANISM OF ACTION**    Sodium nitroprusside is a potent vasodilator that relaxes both arteriolar and venous smooth muscle to reduce blood pressure. The prompt drop in blood pressure causes a reflex increase in heart rate, but cardiac output remains largely unchanged because venous tone and return decrease.

**INDICATIONS**    **Controlled hypotension during surgery.    Hypertensive emergency** Sodium nitroprusside is effective in reducing blood pressure immediately regardless of the cause of hypertension.

**CONTRAINDICATIONS**    • Patients with arteriovenous shunt or coarctation of the aorta. • Moribund patients or those with impaired cerebral circulation.

**DOSAGE**    **Continuous intravenous infusion:**    ADULTS AND CHILDREN: For patients not on antihypertensive drugs, the dose is adjusted from 0.5 to 10 µg/kg/min as required to lower the blood pressure 30% to 40% and stabilize it there. A device such as an infusion pump or microdrip regulator should be used. *Special patient populations:*    PREGNANCY: Safe use has not been established.

**PREPARATIONS**   Powder 50 mg.   **Preparation of the solution** The contents of a 50 mg vial are dissolved with about 3 ml of 5% dextrose and diluted into 250 ml (final, 0.2 mg/ml), 500 ml (final, 0.1 mg/ml) or 1 L (final 0.05 mg/ml) of 5% dextrose. The diluted solution is faint brown and must immediately be wrapped in aluminum foil or other opaque covering to protect it from light. Keep no more than 12 hours and discard earlier if the solution turns color (blue, green, dark red).

**DRUG INTERACTIONS**   **Ganglionic blockers and halogenated anesthetics** halothane or enflurane augment the hypotensive effect of sodium nitroprusside.   **Antihypertensive drugs** make patients more sensitive to sodium nitroprusside.

**FATE**   Sodium nitroprusside has an immediate *onset of action* and a *peak* effectiveness within 2 minutes. If discontinued, blood pressure returns to pretreatment levels within 10 minutes. Sodium nitroprusside is metabolized to cyanomethemoglobin and free cyanide. The free cyanide is quickly converted by the liver to thiocyanate, which has a plasma half-life of 4 days and is excreted in the urine.

## ☙ NURSING CONSIDERATIONS

### Side effects, toxicities, and associated nursing actions

**CNS** Disorientation, delirium, and psychotic behavior have been noted with sodium nitroprusside.
**Other** Muscle twitching.
- Obtain systematic neurologic and mental status exam at regular intervals.
- Reorient patients as needed. Do not leave unattended for long periods. Keep side rails up. Use night lights.

**CV** Rapid lowering of the blood pressure can cause nausea, vomiting, headache, palpitations, restlessness, and sweating.
- See Overview: Antihypertensive Drugs (p. 89).
- Titrate dosage carefully.

**Metabolic** Overdosage can lead to cyanide poisoning, particularly in patients with impaired liver function. Metabolic acidosis is one sign of cyanide poisoning.
- Calculate and administer doses carefully.
- Monitor liver function studies and blood gases.
- Thiocyanate levels should be determined daily if the drug is used longer than 72 hours. If serum thiocyanate levels do not exceed 10 mg/dl, it is probably safe to continue the drug.
- To treat overdose, discontinue the infusion. Administer amyl nitrite for 15 to 30 seconds each minute until a sodium nitrite solution for intravenous administration can be prepared. A 3% sodium nitrite solution should be administered intravenously at a rate of 2.5 to 5 ml/min up to a total dose of 10 to 15 ml. After this, inject sodium thiosulfate intravenously, 12.5 g in 50 ml of 5% dextrose in water over a 10 minute period. Monitor the patient carefully throughout. Signs of overdose can reappear for up to several hours, and sodium nitrite and sodium thiosulfate can be repeated at half the dose listed.

### Nursing interventions related to drug administration
- See Overview: Antihypertensive Drugs (p. 89).
- See section on metabolic side effects.

### Patient and family education
- See Overview: Antihypertensive Drugs (p. 89).
- Do not use this drug outside the intensive care setting.
- Keep patient and family informed of changes in the patient's condition and treatment plan.

---

# Angiotensin antagonists

captopril ～ enalapril

**DRUG COMBINATIONS**   captopril and hydrochlorothiazide: Capozide • enalapril and hydrochlorothiazide: Vaserectic

**OVERVIEW OF THE DRUG CLASS**   Angiotensin-converting enzyme inhibitor is a new class of antihypertensive agent in clinical use.

**MECHANISM OF ACTION**   Angiotensin II is a potent vasoconstrictor formed from angiotensin I by angiotensin converting enzyme (ACE). Inhibition of this enzyme decreases the amount of the potent vasoconstrictor and thereby contributes to a lowering of blood pressure.

**INDICATIONS**   See individual drugs.

**CONTRAINDICATIONS**   See individual drugs.

**DRUG INTERACTIONS**   See individual drugs.

---

## captopril   (KAP-toe-pril)                                    angiotensin-converting enzyme inhibitor

- captopril: Capoten

**MECHANISM OF ACTION**   Captopril is an inhibitor of angiotensin-converting enzyme (ACE), the enzyme responsible for converting angiotensin I to the potent vasoconstrictor, angiotensin II. Angiotensin II also promotes the secretion of aldosterone, the hormone promoting sodium and fluid retention. As an inhibitor of ACE, captopril blocks the formation of angiotensin II.

**INDICATIONS**   **Chronic hypertension** Captopril potentially has serious side effects so is used when other drug regimens have proven unacceptable. Captopril is usually used with a thiazide-type diuretic.   **Congestive heart failure** Captopril can be added to digitalis and diuretic therapy when these alone have proven inadequate.

**CONTRAINDICATIONS**   **Renal impairment** Use of captopril requires careful monitoring of kidney function.

**DOSAGE**   Hypertension:   *Adults:*   PO: Initial dose is 25 mg three times daily; at 1 to 2 week intervals, the dose may be increased by 50 mg increments; maximum dosage is 150 mg three times daily. A diuretic is usually given concurrently.   **Congestive heart failure:**   *Adults:*   PO: Initially, 25 mg three times daily. A lower dose of 6.35 or 12.5 mg three times daily is preferable in patients treated with diuretics who may be hypokalemic and hypovolemic. Dosage may be increased gradually. Most patients respond to 50 or 100 mg three times daily. The maximum daily dose is 450 mg.   *Special patient populations:*   PREGNANCY: Safe use has not been established.

**PREPARATIONS**   *Tablets:* 12.5, 25, 50, 100 mg; *combinations:* 25, 50 mg with 15, 25 mg hydrochlorothiazide.

**DRUG INTERACTIONS**   **Diuretics** potentiate the hypotensive action of captopril and are usually given concurrently to reduce the dose of captopril required.   **Nitroglycerin and other antianginal nitrates** may act synergistically with captopril.   **Sympathetic depressants** may compromise the support of blood pressure in patients on captopril and a diuretic. The use of sympathetic depressants and captopril is not recommended.   **Potassium-sparing diuretics or potassium supplements** Captopril will cause a slight increase in serum potassium levels. The use of potassium-sparing diuretics or potassium supplements may lead to hyperkalemia if given concurrently with captopril.

**DIAGNOSTIC TEST INTERFERENCE**   **Urine acetone** Captopril may cause a false-positive reaction for urine acetone.

**FATE**   Captopril is well and rapidly absorbed from the gastrointestinal tract but should be taken 1 hour before meals because food impairs absorption. The *peak* reduction in blood pressure is in 60 to 90 minutes. The *duration of action* is dose dependent. About half the drug is metabolized, and the metabolized and unchanged drug is eliminated in the urine.

### ☙ NURSING CONSIDERATIONS
#### Side effects, toxicities, and associated nursing actions

**CV** Captopril has few cardiovascular side effects, unlike many antihypertensive drugs. Cardiovascular symptoms such as hypotension, fast heart rate, or angina are not common.
- See Overview: Antihypertensive Drugs (p. 89).
- Hypotension is more common when hyponatremia is present. Monitor the electroytes.
- Overdose is controlled by administering normal saline.

**GI** Gastrointestinal irritation is occasionally experienced.
- If GI irritation is severe or persistent, notify physician.

**Metabolic** Some patients have elevated levels of liver enzymes, but this is rarely associated with liver damage. *Hyperkalemia:* Captopril tends to increase plasma potassium levels. *Proteinuria:* About 1% of patients receiving captopril develop proteinuria. Over half of the patients have had prior renal disease. Proteinuria usually develops at the eighth month of treatment. Current practice is to test for proteinuria before therapy and monthly thereafter for at least the first 9 months.

- Obtain urine protein before starting therapy and at regular intervals thereafter.
- Monitor serum electrolytes and liver function tests.

**Allergic** About 10% of patients will develop a rash in the first few weeks of therapy. This usually disappears with reduction of the dose.

**Neutropenia** Neutropenia develops in only a small (0.3%) percentage of patients. Those most at risk are those with impaired renal function, serious autoimmune disease, or taking other drugs known to affect white cells or the immune system.

- Monitor the white blood cell count and differential before starting therapy and at regular intervals thereafter.
- Caution patients to report any fever, sore throat, rash, or sign of infection.

### Patient and family education
- See Overview: Antihypertensive Drugs (p. 89).
- This drug should be taken 1 hour before meals because absorption is reduced when the drug is taken with food.
- Loss of taste, with associated weight loss, has been reported. Instruct patients to report the development of this side effect.

## enalapril maleate (en-AL-ah-pril) angiotensin-converting enzyme inhibitor

- enalapril maleate: Vasotec

**MECHANISM OF ACTION** Enalapril is administered in an inactive form (prodrug) that is activated in the body. Enalapril is de-esterified to the active drug, which is an inhibitor of angiotensin converting enzyme like captopril.

**INDICATIONS** **Chronic hypertension** Enalapril potentially has serious side effects so is used when other drug regimens have proven unacceptable. Enalapril is usually used with a thiazide-type diuretic. **Heart failure** Enalapril can be added to digitalis and diuretic therapy when these alone have proven inadequate.

**CONTRAINDICATIONS** **Renal impairment** Use of enalapril requires careful monitoring of kidney function.

**DOSAGE** **Adults:** PO: 10 to 20 mg daily. *Special patient populations:* PREGNANCY: Safe use has not been established.

**PREPARATIONS** *Tablets:* 5, 10, 20 mg; *combination:* 10 mg with 25 mg hydrochlorothiazide.

**DRUG INTERACTIONS** **Diuretics** potentiate the hypotensive action of enalapril and are usually given concurrently to reduce the dose of enalapril required. **Nitroglycerin and other antianginal nitrates** may act synergistically with enalapril. **Sympathetic depressants** may compromise the support of blood pressure in patients on enalapril and a diuretic. The use of sympathetic depressants and enalapril is not recommended. **Potassium-sparing diuretics or potassium supplements** Enalapril will cause a slight increase in serum potassium levels. The use of potassium-sparing diuretics or potassium supplements may lead to hyperkalemia if given concurrently with enalapril.

**FATE** Enalapril is well absorbed orally and converted to its active form. The *onset* of action is 1 to 2 hours; the *peak effect* is in 4 to 6 hours. The *duration* of action is 12 to 16 hours. The drug *half-life* is about 2 hours. The drug and metabolites are excreted in the urine.

### ☙ NURSING CONSIDERATIONS
#### Side effects, toxicities, and associated nursing actions
**CV** Enalapril has few cardiovascular side effects, unlike many antihypertensive drugs. Cardiovascular symptoms such as hypotension, fast heart rate, or angina are not common.

- See Overview: Antihypertensive Drugs (p. 89).
- Hypotension is more common when hyponatremia is present. Monitor electrolytes.

- Overdose is controlled by administering normal saline.

**GI** Gastrointestinal irritation is occasionally experienced.

- If GI irritation is severe or persistent, notify the physician.

**Metabolic** Some patients have elevated levels of liver enzymes, but this is rarely associated with liver damage. *Hyperkalemia:* Enalapril tends to increase plasma potassium levels. *Proteinuria:* About 1% of patients receiving enalapril develop proteinuria. Over half of the patients have had prior renal disease. Proteinuria usually develops at the eighth month of treatment. Current practice is to test for proteinuria before therapy and monthly thereafter for at least the first 9 months.

- Obtain urine protein before starting therapy and at regular intervals thereafter.
- Monitor serum electrolytes and liver function tests.

**Allergic** About 10% of patients will develop a rash in the first few weeks of therapy. This usually disappears with reduction of the dose.

**Neutropenia** Neutropenia develops in only a small (0.3%) percentage of patients. Those most at risk are those with impaired renal function, serious autoimmune disease, or taking other drugs known to affect white cells or the immune system.

- Monitor the white blood cell count and differential before starting therapy and at regular intervals thereafter.
- Caution patients to report any fever, sore throat, rash, or sign of infection.

### Patient and family education

- See Overview: Antihypertensive Drugs (p. 89).
- This drug should be taken 1 hour before meals because absorption is reduced when the drug is taken with food.
- Loss of taste, with associated weight loss, has been reported. Instruct patients to report the development of this side effect.

---

# Miscellaneous antihypertensive agents

metyrosine ~ pargyline

**OVERVIEW OF THE DRUG CLASS**   Miscellaneous antihypertensive agents include metyrosine and pargyline. Each drug has limited use in the treatment of hypertension.

**MECHANISM OF ACTION**   See individual drugs.

**INDICATIONS**   See individual drugs.

**CONTRAINDICATIONS**   See individual drugs.

**DRUG INTERACTIONS**   See individual drugs.

---

## metyrosine   (me-TIE-row-seen)                    miscellaneous antihypertensive

- metyrosine: Demser

**MECHANISM OF ACTION**   Metyrosine blocks the synthesis of catecholamines. It is an inhibitor of the enzyme tyrosine hydrolase, which catalyzes the first step in the synthesis of catecholamines from tyrosine.

**INDICATIONS**   **Pheochromocytoma** Metyrosine is used only preoperatively to control output from this catecholamine-secreting tumor.

**CONTRAINDICATIONS**   • Hypersensitivity to metyrosine.

**DOSAGE**   **Adults and children over 12:**   **PO:** Initially, 250 mg four times daily. To control catecholamine output, this dose may be increased daily by 250 to 500 mg to a maximum daily dose of 4 g. Metyrosine is administered during the week before surgery. The goal in normotensive patients is to decrease urinary catecholamine metabolites by 50%. In hypertensive patients, the goal is to normalize blood pressure and phenoxybenzamine is added if necessary. *Special patient populations:*   **PREGNANCY:** Safe use has not been established.

**PREPARATIONS**  *Capsules:* 250 mg.

**DRUG INTERACTIONS**  **Phenothiazines and haloperidol** Metyrosine may potentiate their extrapyramidal effects.  **Alcohol or other CNS depressants** Metyrosine may have additive CNS depressant effects.

**DIAGNOSTIC TEST INTERFERENCE**  **Urinary catecholamine measurements** Metabolites of metyrosine may give false increases in urinary catecholamine measurements.

**FATE**  Metyrosine is well absorbed from the gastrointestinal tract. Although 50% to 90% of the drug is echolamine determination.

## ☙ NURSING CONSIDERATIONS

### Side effects, toxicities, and associated nursing actions

**CNS** Moderate to severe sedation is common. *Extrapyramidal symptoms:* occur in about 10% of patients. *Anxiety and other mental disturbances* such as depression, hallucinations, disorientation, and confusion may be experienced, especially at high doses.

* Caution patients to avoid driving or operating hazardous equipment until the effects of the medication can be evaluated.
* Assess the patient for signs of depression: anorexia, insomnia, neglect of personal appearance, withdrawal, changes in mood or affect.
* Assess patients for other signs and symptoms. If side effects are severe or persistent, it may be necessary to change drugs.

**GI:** *Diarrhea:* Severe in about 10% of patients.

* Monitor intake and output and weight.
* Instruct patient to report the development of this side effect.

**Other** Symptoms of loss of sympathetic activity. These are infrequent but include nasal congestion, dry mouth, headache, nausea, vomiting, abdominal pain, and sexual dysfunction.

* See Overview: Antihypertensive Drugs (p. 89).
* If dry mouth occurs, instruct the patient to suck on sugarless candy or chew sugarless gum; others find relief sucking on ice chips. Some patients may wish to try commercially available saliva substitutes.
* Nasal congestion may occur. Instruct patients about this side effect, but caution them to avoid the use of over-the-counter decongestants unless drugs are first cleared by the physician.
* Assess tactfully for sexual dysfunction; many patients are unwilling to discuss sexual difficulties. Sexual dysfunction may prompt the patient to discontinue the medication without notifying the physician. Provide emotional support as needed. Reinforce to the patient the importance of taking the medication as ordered.
* Maintenance of fluid volume is important during and after surgery for removal of a pheochromocytoma. Force fluids to 3000 ml/day or as ordered.
* Monitor intake and output.

### Patient and family education

* See Overview: Antihypertensive Drugs (p. 89).
* Concomitant with the use of this drug, the patient may need to be collecting 24 hour urine specimens to monitor the urinary catecholamines. Stress the importance of taking the drugs as ordered and the relationship between the drug and the catecholamine output.

---

## pargyline hydrochloride  (PAR-gi-leen)  monoamine oxidase inhibitor

* pargyline hydrochloride: Eutonyl Filmtabs

**MECHANISM OF ACTION**  Pargyline is a monoamine oxidase inhibitor and therefore inhibits the degradation of catecholamines. The antihypertensive mechanism is not understood. MAO inhibitors have primary use as antidepressants.

**INDICATIONS**  **Moderate to severe hypertension** Usually administered with a diuretic.

**CONTRAINDICATIONS** • Pheochromocytoma. • Paranoid schizophrenia. • Hyperthyroidism. • Advanced renal failure. • Malignant hypertension. • Patients taking CNS stimulants. • Foods containing tyramine. • Tricyclic antidepressants and other MAO inhibitors.

**DOSAGE**   **Adults:**   PO: Initially, 25 mg once a day. The dosage may be increased weekly to obtain the desired response; maximum dose, 200 mg daily.   *Special patient populations:*   ELDERLY: Altered doses for the elderly have not been specifically established.   CHILDREN: Not recommended for children under 12 years old.   PREGNANCY: Safe use has not been established.

**PREPARATIONS**   *Tablets:* 10, 25, 50 mg; *combination:* 25 mg with 5 mg methyclothiazide.

**DRUG INTERACTIONS**   **Drugs with CNS action** should be used cautiously and at reduced dosage. Caffeine, alcohol, antihistamines, sedatives, hypnotics, tranquilizers, and narcotics are included in this category.   **CNS stimulants** are contradindicated.   **Tricyclic antidepressants and other MAO inhibitors** may act synergistically to cause vascular collapse and hyperthermia and are contraindicated.   **Methyldopa and dopamine** may cause hyperexcitability.   **Local anesthetics** may be ineffective for patients taking pargyline.   **Antiparkinsonian drugs** such as levodopa may have exaggerated hypertensive effects.

**FATE**   Pargyline is excreted primarily in the urine. Clinical response may take 2 to 3 weeks to appear after therapy begins and may persist that long after therapy ends.

### ☙ NURSING CONSIDERATIONS
#### Side effects, toxicities, and associated nursing actions

**CV** Orthostatic hypotension; fluid rentention. Patients with impaired renal function may accumulate pargyline.
• See Overview: Antihypertensive Drugs (p. 89).
• Monitor serum BUN and creatinine, weight, blood pressure.

**CNS** Insomnia, nightmares, muscle twitching, extrapyramidal symptoms. Overdose can cause agitation, hallucinations, hyperreflexia, high fever, convulsions, hypotensive and hypertensive episodes.
• Assess the patient for these side effects. If side effects are persistent or severe, the drug may need to be changed.
• Monitor the patient's temperature every 4 hours if overdose is suspected.
• Monitor the blood pressure and pulse.

**Metabolic** Can cause hypoglycemia and should be used cautiously in diabetic patients.
• Monitor serum glucose levels.
• Caution patients with diabetes to monitor blood glucose more frequently until the effects of the drug can be evaluated. An adjustment of antidiabetic medication may be needed.

**Renal** The drug may accumulate in the presence of renal impairment.
• Monitor BUN and creatinine levels.
• Monitor intake and output.
• Monitor weight.

**Other** Symptoms of lack of sympathetic activity: dry mouth, sweating, nausea, headache, blurred vision, difficulty in urination, sexual dysfunction.
• If dry mouth occurs, instruct the patient to suck on sugarless candy or chew sugarless gum; others find relief sucking on ice chips. Some patients may wish to try commercially available saliva substitutes.
• If constipation develops, instruct the patient to maintain a fluid intake of 2500 to 3000 ml/day (if not contraindicated by the medical condition), increase the intake of fruits and fiber, maintain a regular exercise program, and judiciously use foods known to stimulate defecation. In some patients it may be necessary to use a stool softener.
• Sexual dysfunction has been reported. Question patients carefully about this and other side effects. Caution patients to report the occurrence of any new sign or symptom.
• Instruct patients to avoid driving or operating hazardous equipment if blurred vision occurs; notify the physician.
• Caution patients to report any new sign or symptom. If the patient consumes foods containing tyramine while taking pargyline, hypertensive crisis may be precipitated.

- Instruct the patient and family about this hazard (see Patient and Family Education).
- Phentolamine is used to reduce the blood pressure in hypertensive crisis.

### Patient and family education

- See Overview: Antihypertensive Drugs (p. 89).
- Review the necessary dietary restriction with the patient and family. The following foods, which contain tyramine, should be avoided while the patient is receiving pargyline and for 14 days following the cessation of therapy with that drug: avocados, bananas, beer, bologna, canned figs, chocolate, cheese (except cottage cheese), cheese-containing foods such as pizza or macaroni and cheese, liver, meat extracts like Marmite, Bovril, Offal, papaya products (including meat tenderizers), pâté, pickled and kippered herring, pepperoni, pods of broad beans (fava beans), raisins, raw yeast or yeast extracts, salami, sausage, sour cream, soy sauce, wine, chianti, and yogurt. Excessive amounts of caffeine should be avoided, although caffeine in small amounts is acceptable.
- Symptoms of hypertensive crisis that might occur after ingestion of tyramine-rich foods include headache, palpitations, visual changes, neck stiffness or soreness, nausea, vomiting, sweating, photophobia, pupillary changes, and bradycardia or tachycardia. Hypertensive crisis is an emergency, and the patients should seek medical attention if these symptoms occur.
- Instruct the patient to report any jaundice, change in skin color, right upper quadrant abdominal pain, or change in the color or consistency of stools, as these symptoms may indicate liver dysfunction.

# Chapter Eight

# Agents to improve blood flow

**Antianginal nitrates and nitrites**
amyl nitrite
erythrityl tetranitrate
isosorbide dinitrate
nitroglycerin
pentaerythritol tetranitrate

**Calcium-channel blockers (drugs for angina, hypertension, arrhythmias)**
diltiazem
lidoflazine (investigational)
nifedipine
verapamil

**Agents to improve blood flow**
cyclandelate
isoxsuprine
niacin
nicotinyl alcohol
nylidrin
papaverine
tolazoline

**Drug to improve blood viscosity**
pentoxifylline

**INTRODUCTION**    Four classes of drugs are presented in this chapter. These drug classes are used to improve blood flow, mainly in clinical situations where blood flow is impeded, most commonly by atherosclerosis.

The *antianginal nitrates* are used as needed and prophylactically to relieve angina pectoris, the pain associated with insufficient blood flow to the heart. The *calcium channel blockers* are new drugs but are already in wide use not only as antianginal agents, but also as antihypertensive and antiarrhythmic drugs. The *peripheral vasodilators* are used to improve blood flow in peripheral and cerebrovascular disease. *Pentoxifylline* is a new drug, unique in its ability to improve blood viscosity by altering red blood cell deformability.

## Antianginal nitrates and nitrites

amyl nitrite  ~  erythrityl tetranitrate  ~  isosorbide dinitrate  ~  nitroglycerin ~  pentaerythritol tetranitrate

**OVERVIEW OF THE DRUG CLASS**    Angina is the pain that results when the heart does not have sufficient oxygen for its workload. Nitrates relieve this pain by reducing the work of the heart so that the heart requires less oxygen. Table 8-1 compares the nitrates and nitrites.

**MECHANISM OF ACTION**    Nitrates and nitrites relax vascular smooth muscle. The molecular basis of this action is not known; however, this relaxation reduces the cardiac workload in the following manner. The smooth muscle of the arterial and venous blood vessels is relaxed, but the effects on the venous blood vessels predominate. Dilation of the venous blood vessels promotes pooling of the blood in the periphery, which decreases the venous return of the blood to the heart. This decrease in the venous return of blood reduces the filling of the left ventricle. With the reduced filling of the left ventricle, the work of the heart to pump out that blood is also reduced. The heart requires less oxygen with a reduced workload so that angina is relieved. Technically, this overall effect of nitrates and nitrites on the venous system is a reduction in left ventricular end-diastolic pressure, which is termed a *preload reduction*.

Nitrates and nitrites also affect the arterial circulation, reducing the systemic blood pressure. The pressure against which the heart pumps out blood is reduced and so the workload of the heart is reduced. This is termed an *afterload reduction* in cardiac work.

**INDICATIONS**    **Acute angina** Inhaled amyl nitrite, sublingual nitroglycerin, and sublingual or chewable isosorbide dinitrate can quickly relieve an anginal attack or prevent an attack when taken before exertion, which can lead to an anginal attack.    **Prophylaxis for angina** Nitroglycerin in slow-release forms and oral forms of isosorbide dinitrate, erythrityl tetranitrate, and pentaerythritol tetranitrate are used for the long-term management of angina.    **Congestive heart failure, acute myocardial infarction** Nitrates are being evaluated in the management of congestive heart failure and acute myocardial infarction.

**CONTRAINDICATIONS**    **Hypersensitivity** Nitrates or nitrites should not be given to individuals allergic to these drugs.    **Head trauma or cerebral hemorrhage** Nitrates and nitrites increase intracranial pressure. **Hypertrophic cardiomyopathy** In this condition abnormal muscle tissue commonly obstructs outflow of the blood from the left ventricle. Nitrates and nitrites worsen the effects of this obstruction.

**DRUG INTERACTIONS**    **Alcohol** Enhances the hypotensive effects of nitrates and nitrites.

## ❦ NURSING CONSIDERATIONS

### Side effects, toxicities, and associated nursing actions

**CV** Headaches, flushing, and dizziness are common at the beginning of therapy. These can be minimized by starting with low doses.

- Caution the patient about these side effects (see Patient and Family Education). The patient should sit or lie down when anginal pain is experienced.
- Assessment of the patient with chest pain includes vital signs and blood pressure, auscultation of lung and heart sounds; assessment of intensity, duration, location, and quality of pain; response to medication; presence of diaphoresis; ECG changes; precipitating factors; patient history; and other subjective complaints. Chest pain in the patient with a history of angina pectoris may be due to other causes also.

**Other** Tolerance may develop during prolonged therapy. This tolerance is due to diminished vascular response and to increased drug metabolism.

- Evaluate with patients on a regular basis the continued effectiveness of the medication. It may be necessary to revise the drug regimen for individual patients.
- Maintain an ongoing record of use and effectiveness of nitrates for each patient.

**Dependence** Nitrate dependence is not common clinically, but high doses of nitrates should not be discontinued abruptly.

- Caution patients not to discontinue medications abruptly (see Patient and Family Education).

### Patient and family education

- At the first sign of an attack of angina, the patient should stop activities and sit or lie down.
- Hypotension is common following use of these drugs. Caution the patient to move slowly from lying to sitting or standing if the patient feels dizzy or lightheaded.
- Instruct patients to keep a record of anginal attacks and events associated with them.
- Instruct patients to avoid the use of alcohol, as it potentiates the hypotensive effects of the antianginal agents.
- In addition to using antianginal drugs, patients may find additional relief by losing weight, stopping smoking, limiting intake of caffeine, avoiding extremes in temperature, and becoming involved in a regular exercise program; consult the physician.
- With the help of the health care team, the patient may be able to identify situations that trigger anginal attacks, and then develop a plan to avoid these situations.
- Patients with angina should be instructed to wear a medical indentification tag or bracelet.
- Caution patients not to discontinue drugs for angina without consulting the physician.
- Remind patients to keep these and all drugs out of the reach of children.
- Review with the patient and family how to administer the prescribed antianginal medications, and ask for a return demonstration if appropriate. Typical instructions follow, but these instructions may be modified by the health care team based on the patient's response.

**Sublingual tablets** Instruct the patient to sit or lie down and remain calm while waiting for the tablets to work.

- Instruct the patient to place the tablet under the tongue and let it dissolve. The patient should not drink or eat while the tablet is dissolving.
- If pain is not relieved, sublingual tablets may be taken at 5-minute intervals until three tablets are used. If pain has not subsided after three tablets, patient should contact physician.
- Headache frequently occurs after taking sublingual tablets. If it persists, the patient should contact physician.
- In some instances, patients may be instructed to take a sublingual tablet 5 to 10 minutes before engaging in activities that have previously triggered an anginal attack; consult the physician and instruct the patient.

**Table 8-1.**

## Comparison of antianginal nitrates and nitrites

| Drug | Dosage form | Onset | Duration |
|------|-------------|-------|----------|
| Amyl nitrite | Inhalant | 30 sec | 3 to 5 min |
| Nitroglycerin | Intravenous | Immediate | Transient |
| | Sublingual | 3 min | 10 to 30 min |
| | Transmucosal | 3 min | 6 hr |
| | Oral, sustained release | Slow | 8 to 12 hr |
| | Topical ointment | 30 to 60 min | 4 to 6 hr |
| | Transdermal | 30 to 60 min | 224 hr |
| Isosorbide dinitrate | Sublingual or chewable | 2 to 5 min | 1 to 3 hr |
| | Oral | 15 to 30 min | 4 to 6 hr |
| | Oral, sustained release | slow | 12 hr |
| Erythrityl tetranitrate | Sublingual or chewable | 5 min | 2 hr |
| | Oral | 30 min | Variable |
| Pentaerythritol tetra-nitrate | Oral, sustained release | Slow | 12 hr |

- Sublingual tablets decompose quickly when exposed to light and moisture. Instruct the patient to keep tablets in the original container and to check and abide by expiration dates. Many patients will keep a stock supply of tablets at home and carry a smaller number with them. Tablets carried with the patient should be carried in amber glass bottles with metal caps (consult the pharmacist for aid in obtaining small bottles). The patient should be instructed to replenish the personal supply frequently, even weekly. No other medications should be kept in the container with the nitrates. Tablets are generally not effective after 6 months and should be discarded. Fresh, potent tablets often cause a burning or stinging sensation when placed under the tongue, although some patients cannot detect this.
- Instruct patients to remove and discard the cotton stopper when a new bottle of tablets is opened. Also instruct the patient to avoid handling the tablets unnecessarily and to carry the tablets in purse or jacket pockets, but not close to body heat.
- The sublingual form is the only form effective for self-medication for relieving an acute attack; other forms are for prevention of anginal attacks.

**Extended release tablets** Instruct the patient that sustained-release formulations are used on a regular basis, not on an ''as needed'' basis for acute attacks of angina.

- Doses should be taken on an empty stomach, 1 hour before or 2 hours after meals. Tablets are swallowed, not chewed or allowed to dissolve in the mouth.

**Buccal extended release tablets** The tablet should be placed between the cheek and gum or between the upper lip and gum and allowed to dissolve. It usually requires 3 to 5 hours to dissolve the tablet.

- This dosage form is not affected by eating or drinking, but the patient must try not to swallow the tablet. Instruct the patient to place it between upper lip and gum when eating or drinking.
- If the patient is to use these throughout the day, each new tablet should be placed in the mouth within 1 hour of the dissolution of the previous tablet.

**Antianginal ointments** These doses are ordered in inches. Small sheets of paper marked in half-inch increments are supplied by the manufacturer and are used to apply the medication. The ordered dose is measured onto the paper, then the patient uses the paper as an applicator to spread the ointment over an area of the skin.

- The individual applying the medication should avoid contacting the ointment with the fingertips, as the drug can be absorbed through the fingers.
- Instruct the patient to rotate the sites of application. Rate of absorption varies slightly by site, but using the same site repeatedly may lead to irritation. The chest, back, thighs, and upper arms are

usually used. Avoid markedly hairy areas or clip the hair; avoid shaving the skin as it may lead to skin irritation.

- These ointments may stain clothing, so the site is often wrapped with plastic wrap after the ointment is applied.
- Although the ointment would cover a large surface area (several inches by several inches), the goal is not to massage the site or rub in the ointment, Spreading the measured dose on the plastic wrap before applying it to the skin will help avoid this.
- Skin irritation or contact dermatitis should be reported to the physician.

**Transdermal adhesive dosage forms** There are several unit dose adhesive formulations available. Patients should be instructed not to interchange products without consulting the physician. The transdermal unit should not be cut or trimmed in any way.

- Instruct the patient to rotate sites to avoid skin irritation. If the patch falls off or becomes loose before the next dose is due, it should be replaced with a fresh patch.
- The dose should be applied at the same time each day. The previous day's dose patch is removed when a new one is applied. Markedly hairy areas should be avoided or the hair clipped; shaving the skin may predispose to skin irritation.

**Chewable tablets** These tablets are designed to be chewed thoroughly (for several minutes), then held in the mouth for 2 to 3 minutes until all of the drug has been absorbed. The chewed tablet is then swallowed.

**Aerosol spray** One or two doses (sprays) are sprayed into the mouth. Doses may be repeated at 3 to 5 minute intervals, but no more than three doses in 15 minutes should be used.

---

## amyl nitrite  (AM-il)  antianginal

- amyl nitrite: Amyl Nitrite Aspirols, Amyl Nitrite Vaporoles

**MECHANISM OF ACTION**  Amyl nitrite relaxes vascular smooth muscle to cause dilation of arterial and venous blood vessels. This relieves angina by reducing the left ventricular preload and afterload work. See entry for drug class (p. 114).

**INDICATIONS**  **Acute angina** Amyl nitrate provides immediate relief from acute angina.  **Renal and gallbladder colic** Amyl nitrite provides prompt, symptomatic relief.  **Cyanide poisoning** Amyl nitrite converts hemoglobin to methemoglobin, which forms a nontoxic complex with cyanide.

**CONTRAINDICATIONS**  See those for the drug class (p. 115).

**DOSAGE**  **Inhalation:**  ADULTS: 0.18 or 0.3 ml as required.  ADULTS AND CHILDREN: For cyanide poisoning: 0.3 ml ampule is crushed and inhaled for about 20 seconds every minute while sodium nitrite infusion is being prepared. *Special patient populations:*  PREGNANCY: Safe use has not been established.

**PREPARATIONS**  Liquid packaged in ampules to be crushed and inhaled: 0.18, 0.3 ml ampules.

**DRUG INTERACTIONS**  **Alcohol** Severe hypotension and cardiovascular collapse may occur when amyl nitrite is inhaled after drinking.

**FATE**  Amyl nitrite is effective within seconds after being inhaled. The *duration of action* is 3 to 5 minutes. Amyl nitrite is a highly volatile liquid and is excreted by the kidneys.

### ❦ NURSING CONSIDERATIONS

#### Side effects, toxicities, and associated nursing actions

CNS Headache, flushing, and dizziness are common.

CV Orthostatic hypotension is common if the patient does not sit or lie down when using the drug.

- See entry for drug class (p. 115).

#### Patient and family education

- See entry for drug class (p. 115).
- Instruct patient and family to wrap glass ampule in a handkerchief or other cloth to prevent glass slivers from cutting the hand when breaking the ampule.

• Warn patient that even though drug has a strong odor, several deep breaths must be taken to achieve benefit from the drug.

## erythrityl tetranitrate    (e-RI-thri-till)                                     antianginal

• erythrityl tetranitrate: Cardilate

**MECHANISM OF ACTION**    Erythrityl tetranitrate relaxes vascular smooth muscle, causing dilation of arterial and venous blood vessels. This reduces the cardiac workload by decreasing both the preload and afterload work of the left ventricle. See entry for drug class (p. 114).

**INDICATIONS**    **Prophylaxis for angina** Erythrityl tetranitrate is a long-acting nitrate used to prevent attacks of angina.

**CONTRAINDICATIONS**    See those of the drug class (p. 115).

**DOSAGE**    **Adults:**    SUBLINGUAL: 10 mg before physical or emotional stress.    PO: 10 mg three times daily initially; may be increased up to 100 mg daily; bedtime doses for patients with nocturnal angina. *Special patient populations:*    PREGNANCY: Safe use has not been established.

**PREPARATIONS**    *Oral or sublingual tablets:* 5, 10, 15 mg.

**DRUG INTERACTIONS**    **Alcohol** is a vasodilator, and the hypotensive effects of erythrityl tetranitrate may be increased by alcohol.    **Nitroglycerin** Erythrityl tetranitrate may induce tolerance to the acute effects of nitroglycerin.

**FATE**    Erythrityl tetranitrate is degraded by the liver, and degradation products are excreted in the urine.

## ✿ NURSING CONSIDERATIONS

### Side effects, toxicities, and associated nursing actions

**CNS** Headache and dizziness are common.

**CV** Flushing is usual, and orthostatic hypotension is common if the patient does not sit or lie down after taking the drug.

**GI** Gastrointestinal disturbances are common with large doses.

• If GI side effects are severe or persistent, notify the physician, as a change in drug or dosage may be necessary.

**Allergic** A few patients develop a hypersensitivity to nitrate.

**Other** Tolerance may develop with extended use.

• See entry for drug class (p. 115).

### Patient and family education

• See entry for drug class (p. 115).

## isosorbide dinitrate    (eye-soe-SOR-bide)                                     antianginal

• isosorbide dinitrate: ♣ Cornex, Isogard, Isordil, ♣ Novosorbide, Sorate, Sorbitrate

**MECHANISM OF ACTION**    Isosorbide dinitrate, like the other nitrates and nitrites, relaxes vascular smooth muscle to cause dilation of arterial and venous blood vessels. This reduces the cardiac workload by decreasing the preload and afterload work of the left ventricle. See the entry for the drug class (p. 114).

**INDICATIONS**    **Acute angina** Sublinguinal or chewable isosorbide relieves acute angina or prevents acute angina if taken just before an exertion that usually precipitates angina.    **Prophylaxis for angina** Oral or sustained release isosorbide can prevent or lessen anginal attacks.

**CONTRAINDICATIONS**    See those of the drug class (p. 115).

**DOSAGE**    **Adults:**    SUBLINGUAL: 2.5 to 10 mg.    CHEWABLE: 5 mg initially, up to 10 mg if a severe hypotensive response is not experienced.    PO: *Tablets:* 5 to 30 mg four times daily, *sustained-release:* 40 mg every 6 to 12 hours.    *Special patient populations:*    PREGNANCY: Safe use has not been established.

**PREPARATIONS**   *Sublingual tablets:* 2.5, 5 mg., *chewable tablets:* 5, 10 mg., *tablets:* 5, 10, 20, 30, 40 mg.

**DRUG INTERACTIONS**   **Alcohol** is a vasodilator which may increase the hypotensive effects of isosorbide dinitrate.   **Nitroglycerin** Isosorbide dinitrate may induce tolerance to the acute effects.

**FATE**   *Onset of action* depends on the route used: sublingual or chewable, 2 to 5 minutes; oral, 15 to 30 minutes; sustained release, slow. *Duration of action* is also dependent on the route used: sublingual or chewable, 1 to 2 hours; oral, 4 to 6 hours; sustained release, 12 hours. Isosorbide dinitrate is rapidly degraded by the liver but is longer acting than nitroglycerin. Degradation products are excreted in the urine.

## 🌿 NURSING CONSIDERATIONS

### Side effects, toxicities, and associated nursing actions

**CNS** Headache and dizziness are common.

**CV** Flushing is usual, and orthostatic hypotension is common if the patient does not sit or lie down after taking the drug.

• See entry for drug class (p. 115).

**GI** Nausea and vomiting are sometimes experienced.

• If GI side effects are severe or persistent, notify the physician, as a change in drug or dosage may be necessary.

**Allergic** A few patients develop a hypersensitivity to nitrate.

### Patient and family education

• See entry for drug class (p. 115).

---

## nitroglycerin   (nye-troe-GLI-ser-in)                                                antianginal

• nitroglycerin: Ango-O-Span, Cardabid, klavidordal, N-G-C, Niong, Nitro-Bid, Nitrocap, Nitro-Dur, ♣ Nitrogard, Nitroglyn, Nitrol, Nitrolin, Nitro-long, Nitronet, Nitrong, Nitrospan, Nitrolingual Spray, ♣ Nitrostabilin, Nitrostat, Transderm-Nitro, Trates Granucaps, ♣ Tridil

**MECHANISM OF ACTION**   Nitroglycerin relaxes vascular smooth muscle to dilate arterial and venous blood vessels. This reduces the cardiac workload by decreasing the preload and afterload work of the left ventricle. See entry for drug class (p. 114).

**INDICATIONS**   **Acute angina** Sublinguinal nitroglycerin relieves acute angina or prevents acute angina if taken just before an exertion that usually precipitates angina.   **Prophylaxis for angina** Sustained-release oral or transmucosal nitroglycerin, topical or transdermal nitroglycerin can prevent or lessen anginal attacks.   **Congestive heart failure** Intravenous or topical nitroglycerin can aid in relieving severe congestive heart failure (investigational).   **Acute myocardial infarction** Intravenous or topical nitroglycerin can reduce the extent of infarction during a myocardial infarction (investigational).

**CONTRAINDICATIONS**   See those for the drug class (p. 115).

**DOSAGE**   **Adult:**   **SUBLINGUAL:** 0.15 to 0.6 mg. If no relief in 5 minutes, may repeat dose but no more than three tablets in 15 minutes.   **ORAL, TIMED RELEASE TABLETS OR CAPSULES:** 2.6 to 13 mg four times a day.   **LINGUAL:** one or two sprays (0.4 to 0.8 mg) is sprayed on the oral mucosa. The can should not be shaken and the spray should not be inhaled or swallowed.   **TRANSMUCOSAL (BUCCAL):** 1 to 2 mg three times daily. This is a tablet kept in the cheek pouch. The nitroglycerin is embedded in a polymer that releases the drug over several hours.   **TOPICAL:** The 2% ointment contains 15 mg nitroglycerin per inch. One-half inch is the initial dose, spread over a 6 by 6 inch area on the chest, back, abdomen, or anterior thighs. The usual dosage is 1 to 2 inches every 8 hours; maximum, 5 inches every 4 hours.   **TRANSDERMAL:** A nitroglycerin-impregnated polymer is bonded to an adhesive bandage. When applied to the body, drug is released over 24 hours, at which time the unit is replaced.   **IV:** 5 $\mu$g/min is infused initially. The dose is increased by 5 $\mu$g/min every 3 to 5 minutes until a response is noted. If no response is noted at 20 $\mu$g/min, further doses are increased by 10 to 20 $\mu$g/min. The responses desired are reduced chest pain and reduced pulmonary artery wedge pressure with a near-normal arterial perfusion pressure. Dilution of stock nitroglycerin should be with 5% dextrose or 0.9 sodium chloride. Manufacturers differ in the concentration of stock nitroglycerin solutions, so particular care must be exercised in making the final dilution. *Special patient populations:* PREGNANCY: Safe use has not been established.

**PREPARATIONS** *Sublingual tablets:* 0.15, 0.3, 0.4, 0.6 mg; *oral: sustained release tablets*—1.3, 2.6, 6.5, 9 mg; *sustained release capsules*—2.5, 6.5, 9 mg; *transmucosal (buccal) tablets:* 1, 2, and 3 mg; *lingual aerosol:* 0.4 mg/metered spray; *topical ointment:* 2% (15 mg/inch); *transdermal patch:* 2.5, 5, 7.5, 10, 15 mg/24 hours; *intravenous solution:* 0.8, 5 mg/ml.

**DRUG INTERACTIONS** **Alcohol** is a vasodilator which may increase the hypotensive effect of nitroglycerin. **Long-acting nitrates** increase liver metabolism and may induce tolerance to nitroglycerin.

**FATE** Nitroglycerin is rapidly metabolized by the liver, which accounts for the need to administer nitroglycerin sublingually, transdermally, topically, or in a sustained release transmucosal form. If swallowed, nitroglycerin is absorbed from the gastrointestinal tract into the portal vein and is metabolized by the liver without ever reaching systemic circulation. (This rapid degradation by the liver is called "the first-pass effect.") The nitrate degradation products are excreted in the urine.

## 🐦 NURSING CONSIDERATIONS

### Side effects, toxicities, and associated nursing actions

**CNS** Headache and dizziness are common.

**CV** Flushing is usual. Orthostatic hypotension is common if the patient does not sit or lie down after taking sublingual nitroglycerin.

• See entry for drug class (p. 115).

**GI** Nausea and vomiting are sometimes experienced.

• If GI side effects are severe or persistent, notify the physician, as a change in drug or dosage may be necessary.

**Other** A burning sensation is common with the sublingual tablets.

• Warn patients about this side effect, which may confirm that tablets are potent. If sensation is intolerable to the patient, notify the physician.

### Nursing interventions related to drug administration

• As noted under Dosage, preparation of intravenous dilution and final dosage must be done carefully. Nitroglycerin is not for direct intravenous infusion; it must be diluted.

• Use a microdrip infusion set and a volume control or rate controlling device to prevent overdosage and to more accurately titrate the dose.

• Nitroglycerin migrates into plastic tubing. Dilutions should be prepared and kept in glass bottles. If standard polyvinyl chloride (PVC) intravenous tubing must be used, as much as 80% of the drug is lost into the tubing. Use tubing supplied by the manufacturer. If a switch is made to different tubing, the dose for a patient must be adjusted.

• Monitor the blood pressure, heart rate, electrocardiogram, and pulmonary capillary wedge pressure. Use this drug only in settings where drugs and experienced personnel to treat cardiovascular emergencies are available.

### Patient and family education

• See entry for drug class (p. 115).

---

## pentaerythritol tetranitrate   (pen-ta-er-ITH-ri-tole)   antianginal

• pentaerythritol tetranitrate: Duotrate, Peritrate Plateau Caps

**MECHANISM OF ACTION** Pentaerythritol tetranitrate, like the other nitrates and nitrites, relaxes vascular smooth muscle, thus dilating arterial and venous blood vessels. This reduces the cardiac workload by decreasing the preload and afterload work of the left ventricle. See entry for drug class (p. 114).

**INDICATIONS** **Prophylaxis for angina** Pentaerythritol tetranitrate is a long-acting nitrate used to prevent attacks of angina.

**CONTRAINDICATIONS** See those of the drug class (p. 115).

**DOSAGE**  **Adults:**  PO: 10 or 20 mg three or four times daily initially; may be increased up to 40 mg four times daily. Should be taken on an empty stomach. Onset is 30 minutes, and duration of action is 4 to 5 hours. Sustained release forms: 30 to 80 mg every 12 hours. Onset is slow.  *Special patient populations:*  PREGNANCY: Safe use has not been established.

**PREPARATIONS**  *Tablets:* 10, 20, 40 mg; *sustained release capsules:* 30, 45, 60, 80 mg: *sustained release tablets:* 80 mg.

**DRUG INTERACTIONS**  **Alcohol** is a vasodilator which may increase the hypotensive effects of pentaerythritol tetranitrate.  **Nitroglycerin** Pentaerythritol tetranitrate may induce tolerance to the acute effects of nitroglycerin.

**FATE**  Pentaerythritol tetranitrate is degraded by the liver, and degradation products are excreted in the urine.

## ☙ NURSING CONSIDERATIONS

### Side effects, toxicities, and associated nursing actions

**CNS** Headache and dizziness are common.

**CV** Flushing is usual, and orthostatic hypotension is common if the patient does not sit or lie down after taking the drug.

• See entry for drug class (p. 115).

**GI** Nausea and vomiting are sometimes experienced.

• If GI side effects are severe or persistent, notify the physician, as a change in drug or dosage may be necessary.

**Allergic** A few patients develop a hypersensitivity to nitrate.

**Other** Tolerance may develop with extended use.

• See entry for drug class (p. 115).

### Patient and family education

• See entry for drug class (p. 115).

---

# Calcium channel blockers

diltiazem ~ lidoflazine (investigational) ~ nifedipine ~ verapamil

**OVERVIEW OF THE DRUG CLASS**  Calcium channel blockers, also called calcium antagonists or calcium entry blockers, are a new class of drugs used in the treatment of angina, certain arrhythmias, and hypertension.

**MECHANISM OF ACTION**  Skeletal muscle has extensive stores of calcium in the sarcoplasmic reticulum, but both cardiac muscle and vascular smooth muscle lack these stores and must depend on the influx of extracellular calcium for the maintenance of contraction or tone. The calcium activates the contractile mechanisms and must be removed for relaxation. The calcium channel blockers interfere with the initial influx of calcium through specific calcium channels on the cell surface. These drugs therefore cause relaxation by preventing the entrance of calcium needed for contraction.

The calcium channel blockers decrease the oxygen requirements of the heart through several actions that make them effective antianginal drugs. They reduce peripheral vascular resistance by a systemic vasodilation. This means that the workload of the heart is decreased. These agents dilate the coronary vessels by inhibiting contractility of coronary smooth muscle. This action is especially important for relief from variant angina, in which coronary spasm prevents blood flow. The calcium channel blockers also reduce cardiac contractility (negative inotropy), which decreases the oxygen requirement of the heart.

Calcium channel blockers increase coronary blood flow through coronary vasodilation more selectively than they inhibit cardiac contractility. Without this selective preference, the calcium channel blockers would not be clinically useful because they would overly compromise cardiac function. The various drugs of this class differ in the degree of selectivity in coronary vasodilation versus decreased cardiac contractility.

AV nodal function may also be affected by calcium channel blockers because cells in the node depend primarily on calcium rather than sodium flow to generate an action potential. If calcium channels are blocked, these cells take longer to depolarize than normal. Therefore AV conduction is delayed and can be blocked. Ectopic pacemakers arising within ischemic areas of the heart muscle also often depend on calcium flow to generate impulses. These cells can be prevented from depolarizing or generating ectopic beats by the calcium channel blockers.

**INDICATIONS**  • Angina pectoris caused by coronary artery spasm. • Angina of exertion. • Paroxysmal supraventricular tachycardia; verapamil is useful.

**CONTRAINDICATIONS**  • Severe hypotension. • Hypersensivity. • Sick sinus syndrome. • Severe congestive heart failure. • Pre-existing AV blockade.

**DRUG INTERACTIONS**  **Beta-blockers and digitalis** combined with a calcium channel blocker may have additive effects in prolonging AV conduction.  **Cimetidine** may block metabolism of some calcium channel blockers and cause accumulation of the drug, increasing the risk of toxicity.

---

## ☙ NURSING CONSIDERATIONS

### Side effects, toxicities, and associated nursing actions

**CNS** Dizziness or lightheadedness.
• Caution patients to avoid driving or operating hazardous equipment if CNS side effects occur.
• Monitor blood pressure.
• If symptoms persist, it may be necessary to adjust dose or change drugs; notify the physician.

**CV** Hypotension, bradycardia, or asystole may result from therapeutic doses but are more common when excessive accumulation of calcium channel blocking agents occurs.
• Monitor the pulse. Be alert for bradycardia, especially if the patient is receiving a cardiac glycoside concurrently.
• Monitor the blood pressure and electrocardiogram (if available).
• Assessment of the patient with chest pain includes vital signs and blood pressure; auscultation of lung and heart sounds; assessment of intensity, duration, location, and quality of pain; response to medications; presence of diaphoresis; electrocardiogram changes; precipitating factors; patient history; and other subjective complaints. Chest pain in the patient with a history of angina pectoris may be due to other causes also.

**CV** Edema secondary to peripheral vasodilation, hypotension.
• Monitor the blood pressure, intake and output, and weight.
• Observe for signs of fluid retention: peripheral edema, subjective complaints of tight shoes and rings, weight gain. Also observe for congestive heart failure: dyspnea on exertion, distended jugular veins, orthopnea. Auscultate the lungs for pulmonary rales.

**GI** Gastrointestinal disturbances.
• If severe or persistent, notify the physician.
• Instruct the patient to try taking doses with meals. If taking doses with meals is effective, instruct patients to be consistent in this regime—varying how doses are taken may produce variable results.

**Liver** Calcium channel blocking agents may cause liver damage, which may cause the drug to accumulate (see individual drugs).
• Be alert to development of side effects not previously troublesome to patient that indicate drug accumulation.
• Assess for right upper quadrant abdominal pain, jaundice, change in color or consistency of stools, malaise.
• Monitor liver function studies.

### Patient and family education

• Review with patients the expected benefits and possible side effects of drug therapy. Encourage the patient to report the appearance of any new sign or symptom.
• Selected patients may be appropriate candidates for instruction on taking and recording the pulse daily at home. Such patients may be those on multiple-drug regimens or those in whom control of side effects has been difficult. Instruct patients to report a change of 10 beats per minute at rest.
• If postural hypotension occurs, instruct the patient to move slowly from lying to sitting or standing. Postural hypotension may be aggravated by long periods of standing, excessive heat, hot showers or

baths, and the ingestion of alcohol. Some patients may find the use of waist-high elastic stockings helpful if the problem persists; consult the physician.

- Selected patients may be appropriate condidates for instruction to monitor and record their weight on a regular basis at home. Instruct patients to report a weight gain of greater than 2 lb/day or 5 lb/week. Instruct the patient to report the development of tight rings, shoes, or clothing or signs of peripheral edema.

- If constipation develops, instruct the patient to maintain fluid intake to 2500 to 3000 ml/day (if not contraindicated by the medical condition), increase the intake of fruits and fiber, maintain a regular exercise program, and judiciously use foods known to stimulate defecation. In some patients it may be necessary to use a stool softener.

- Because of the serious drug interactions encountered with these medications, caution patients to keep all health care providers informed of all drugs being taken. Caution patients to avoid the use of any over-the-counter preparations unless first cleared by the physician.

- It is best to take these drugs 1 hour before meals or 2 hours after. If gastric irritation does occur, it may be reduced by taking doses with meals; consult the physician first.

- In addition to using calcium channel blocking agents as prescribed, patients may find additional relief by losing weight, stopping smoking, limiting intake of caffeine, avoiding extremes in temperature, and becoming involved in a regular exercise program; consult the physician.

- The importance of taking these drugs as prescribed should be emphasized. The patient should not change dosage or discontinue these drugs without first consulting with the health care provider.

- If a dose is missed, patients should take the dose as soon as it is remembered, but not within 2 hours of the next scheduled dose. Patients should not "double up" on subsequent doses.

---

## diltiazem hydrochloride    (dil-TYE-a-zem)    calcium blocker

- diltiazem hydrochloride: Cardizem

**MECHANISM OF ACTION**    Diltiazem is a calcium channel blocker that is especially effective in dilating coronary vessels.

**INDICATIONS**    Angina pectoris caused by coronary artery spasm. • Angina of exertion.

**CONTRAINDICATIONS**    **Hypotension** Patients with systolic blood pressures less than 90 mm Hg may be unable to tolerate the hypotensive effects of diltiazem.    **Second or third-degree AV blockage** The AV nodal blocking effects of diltiazem may trigger asystole (no heart beat), unless an active ventricular (ectopic) pacemaker exists.    **Sick sinus syndrome** Diltiazem slows the heart and may produce dangerous bradycardia, especially in patients with sick sinus syndrome.    **Congestive heart failure** Diltiazem may lower contractility of the heart muscle (negative inotropic effect), which may be dangerous for patients with compromised cardiac function.

**DOSAGE**    **Adults:**    **PO:** Doses of 30 to 60 mg every 6 to 8 hours may be used initially. The dosage should be gradually increased every 24 to 48 hours until the optimal clinical response is achieved. The optimal dosage for many patients is between 180 to 240 mg daily, divided into three or four equal doses. *Special patient populations:*    **PREGNANCY:** FDA pregnancy category C.

**PREPARATIONS**    *Tablets:* 30, 60 mg.

**DRUG INTERACTIONS**    **Beta-adrenergic blockers** act synergistically with calcium channel blockers to depress AV conduction and depress cardiac contractility. Should not be used together.    **Digitalis glycosides** act additively with the calcium channel blockers to depress AV conduction. Diltiazem also causes the accumulation of digitalis glycosides.

**FATE**    Diltiazem is well absorbed orally but is sensitive to first-pass metabolism in the liver, therefore bioavailability of the tablets is about 40%. Ultimately, most of the dose is metabolized by the liver, with only 2% to 4% of the unchanged drug being excreted in the urine. Diltiazem is highly bound to plasma proteins and has an elimination *half-life* of 3.5 hours. Data are not yet available on the effect of hepatic or renal dysfunction on the pharmacokinetics of diltiazem.

## NURSING CONSIDERATIONS

### Side effects, toxicities, and associated nursing actions
**CNS** Headache and dizziness.
- See entry for drug class (p. 122).

**CV** Peripheral edema has been noted in 2% to 3% of patients. Bradycardia may arise from the excessive action of diltiazem on the SA and AV nodes. AV blockade increases with the dose of diltiazem. Hypotension may arise from excessive relaxation of peripheral arteries by diltiazem. Congestive failure may arise from the negative inotropic effect (reduced contractility) of diltiazem.
- See entry for drug class (p. 122).

**Metabolic** Rarely, hepatic damage has occurred, signaled by significant elevations of liver enzymes. The changes are apparently reversible.
- See entry for drug class (p. 122).

### Patient and family education
- See entry for drug class (p. 122).

---

## lidoflazine    (lye-doe-FLAE-zeen)                                    calcium blocker

- lidoflazine (investigational in U.S.): ♣ Angex

**MECHANISM OF ACTION**    Lidoflazine blocks calcium channels.

**INDICATIONS**    **Angina pectoris caused by exertion** May improve coronary oxygenation by dilating coronary arteries and may lessen the work load of the heart by dilating peripheral arteries and reducing blood pressure.    **Myocardial infarction** May reduce the incidence of a second heart attack but does not measurably improve the mortality rate.

**CONTRAINDICATIONS**    Not yet fully evaluated but expected to be like other calcium channel blockers.

**DOSAGE**    **Adult:**    **PO:** Initial dosage is 60 mg daily for 1 week, increased to 120 mg daily the second week and 180 mg daily the third week. Dosage is maintained at this level for 2 months to assess clinical response. If necessary, the dosage may gradually be increased up to 360 mg daily.    *Special patient populations:* **PREGNANCY:** Safe use has not been established.

**PREPARATIONS**    *Tablets:* 60 mg.

**DRUG INTERACTIONS**    Not fully evaluated but expected to be like other calcium channel blockers.

**FATE**    Lidoflazine is slowly absorbed from the GI tract, producing peak levels in the blood within 4 to 8 hours. The drug is extensively metabolized, Lidoflazine metabolites are excreted in the urine and feces. The elimination *half-life* of lidoflazine is 16 to 24 hours. The full therapeutic effects of lidoflazine may take months to develop.

## ❦ NURSING CONSIDERATIONS

### Side effects, toxicities, and associated nursing actions    See entry for drug class (p. 122).
**CNS** Headache, dizziness, ringing in the ears, depression.
- Assess for ringing in the ears.
- Be alert to changes in affect. Assess for signs of depression: weight loss, loss of appetite, lack of interest in personal appearance, insomnia, withdrawal. Instruct families to report the possible development of depression.

**CV** Ventricular arrhythmias.

**Allergic** Skin rashes.
- Visually inspect patient for skin changes. Instruct patient to report development of rashes.

**GI** Gastrointestinal disturbances.

### Patient and family education
- See entry for drug class (p. 122).

## nifedipine    (nye-FED-i-peen)                                   calcium blocker

- nifedipine: ✿ Adalat, Procardia

**MECHANISM OF ACTION**    Nifedipine blocks calcium channels. It is somewhat selective for vascular smooth muscle and has little or no clinically important effects on the SA or AV nodes. The primary action of nifedipine is vasodilation.

**INDICATIONS**    **Angina pectoris caused by coronary artery spasm** Nifedipine reduces the incidence of spasm by promoting relaxation of coronary arterial smooth muscle.    **Angina of exertion.**

**CONTRAINDICATIONS**    Hypersensitivity.

**DOSAGE**    **Adults:**    PO: Initial dosage is 10 mg three times daily. Decrease in angina should be monitored, as well as the development of hypotension. If needed and tolerated, the dose may be increased over 1 to 2 weeks up to 20 or 30 mg three times daily. Doses exceeding 30 mg at one time or daily doses exceeding 180 mg are not recommended.    *Special patient populations:*    ELDERLY: Doses are individualized. Begin with low doses and add small increments as needed.    PREGNANCY: Embryotoxic in animals, including monkeys. FDA pregnancy category C.

**PREPARATIONS**    *Capsules:* 10 mg. Store in original container and protect from light.

**DRUG INTERACTIONS**    **Beta-blockers** when combined with nifedipine can worsen existing congestive heart failure. If nifedipine therapy begins too soon after withdrawal of beta-blocker therapy, angina can worsen.    **Digitalis** accumulates in patients taking nifedipine.    **Coumarins** Nifedipine increases the prothrombin time in patients receiving a coumarin.    **Cimetidine** causes the accumulation of nifedipine, apparently by blocking the metabolism of nifedipine.

**DIAGNOSTIC TEST INTERFERENCE**    **Liver enzymes** Tests show transient elevations.

**FATE**    Nifedipine is rapidly absorbed from the stomach, with peak blood levels appearing 30 minutes after the oral dose. Protein binding is high, and the elimination *half-life* has been reported to range from 2 to 6 hours. Nifedipine is extensively metabolized, with most of the metabolites being excreted by the kidney (80%) and the remainder being excreted in the feces.

### ❦ NURSING CONSIDERATIONS

**Side effects, toxicities, and associated nursing actions**    See entry for drug class (p. 122).
  **CNS** Dizziness, lightheadedness.
  **CV** Slight hypotension; peripheral vasodilation that may lead to edema. Rarely, angina is worsened, apparently because of reflex sympathetic activity increasing heart rate and cardiac work load.
  **Metabolic** Liver function may be impaired, with an increase in liver enzymes.
  **GI** Nausea and vomiting.
  • See entry for drug class (p. 122).

**Patient and family education**
  • See entry for drug class (p. 122).

## verapamil hydrochloride    (ver-AP-a-mill)                         calcium blocker

- verapamil hydrochloride: Calan, Isoptin

**MECHANISM OF ACTION**    Verapamil blocks calcium channels in various cells and is effective as a coronary and peripheral vasodilator. Verapamil is especially effective in blocking calcium channels in the SA and AV nodes, making it effective in treating some arrhythmias.

**INDICATIONS**    **Angina pectoris** caused by coronary artery spasm.    **Angina of exertion.**    **Paroxysmal supraventricular tachycardia** Verapamil often converts this arrhythmia to sinus rhythm. The arrhythmia is often produced by AV nodal reentry, a process that can be stopped by the action of verapamil in slowing conduction through the AV node.    **Ventricular tachycardia** caused by atrial flutter or fibrillation: Verapamil slows conduction through the AV node and may therefore slow ventricular rates even though sinus rhythm is rarely restored.

**CONTRAINDICATIONS**   **Severe hypotension** Verapamil may lower blood pressure rapidly to dangerously low levels, especially in patients whose starting blood pressure is below 90 mm Hg.   **Second- or third-degree AV blockade** Verapamil also slows conduction through the AV node and may cause complete block.   **Sick sinus syndrome** Verapamil can cause severe bradycardia or even asystole (no heart beat) when the SA node is inadequate.   **Severe congestive heart failure** Verapamil may worsen this condition by decreasing contractility of the heart muscle.   **Hypersensitivity** to the drug.

**DOSAGE**

**Angina:   PO:   ADULTS:** Initial doses are 80 mg every 6 to 8 hours, increased as needed on a daily or weekly basis until desired clinical effects are achieved. Usual dosages range from 240 to 320 mg daily in divided doses.

**Arrhythmias:   IV:   ADULTS:** Initial dose is 5 to 10 mg given as a bolus over 2 minutes (3 minutes for elderly patients). After 30 minutes an additional 10 mg (0.15 mg/kg) may be given if necessary. **CHILDREN—NEONATE TO 1 YEAR:** Initial dose 0.1 to 0.2 mg/kg as a bolus over 2 minutes with constant ECG monitoring; repeat in 30 minutes if necessary.   **CHILDREN—1 TO 15 YEARS:** Initial dose 0.1 to 0.3 mg/kg as a bolus over 2 minutes. Dose should not exceed 5 mg. Repeat in 30 minutes if necessary. *Special patient populations:* **ELDERLY:** Doses are individualized. Altered doses for the elderly have not been specifically established, but IV doses are administered more slowly.   **PREGNANCY:** Verapamil is embryotoxic in animals. FDA pregnancy category C.

**PREPARATIONS**   *Ampules:* 5 mg in 2 ml, 10 mg in 4 ml; *vials:* 5 mg in 2 ml or 10 mg in 4 ml; *syringes:* 5 mg in 2 ml, 10 mg in 4 ml (store solutions between 59° and 86° F and protect from light); *tablets:* 80, 120 mg.

**DRUG INTERACTIONS**   **Beta-blockers** when given IV with IV verapamil may cause serious depression of contractility and AV nodal conduction.   **Disopyramide** should not be administered within 48 hours of starting verapamil or within 24 hours after verapamil.   **Digitalis** has additive effects with verapamil on AV conduction. Watch patients on both drugs closely for AV block or excessive bradycardia (slowing of the heart).

**FATE**   Verapamil is rapidly and almost completely absorbed orally, but extremely rapid metabolism destroys much of the drug on the first pass through the liver. As a result, bioavailability of oral verapamil is only about 20% to 35%. Metabolism in the liver is ultimately responsible for eliminating most of an oral or IV dose. Seventy percent of a dose is excreted as metabolites in the urine, 16% in feces, and less than 10% as unchanged in the urine. The elimination *half-life* of verapamil increases from around 2 hours initially to as much as 16 hours after several doses have been given. Hepatic damage can cause accumulation of verapamil.

### ❧ NURSING CONSIDERATIONS

#### Side effects, toxicities, and associated nursing actions   See entry for drug class (p. 122).

**CNS** Dizziness, headache in about 4% of patients.

**CV** Hypotension in about 3% of patients taking the drug orally, 10% for IV. Peripheral edema in about 2% of patients.

**Metabolic** Impaired liver function with elevated liver enzymes and bilirubin.

**GI** Nausea, constipation.

#### Nursing interventions related to drug administration

- For intravenous administration, review Dosage.
- The patient should be connected to a cardiac monitor, and resuscitation equipment should be readily available.
- The patient should remain recumbent for at least 1 hour following intravenous administration. Monitor the blood pressure before allowing the patient to get up. Keep the side rails up.

#### Patient and family education

- See entry for drug class (p. 122).

# Agents to improve blood flow

**Peripheral vasodilators** ~ cyclandelate ~ isoxsuprine hydrochloride ~ niacin ~ nicotinyl alcohol ~ nylidrin ~ papaverine ~ tolazoline hydrochloride **Drug to improve viscosity** ~ pentoxifylline

**OVERVIEW OF THE DRUG CLASS**   Blood flow to the arms and legs, particularly the hands and feet, can be limited by arteriosclerosis or by spasm of the vessels. If the vessel narrowing is a result of arteriosclerosis, vasodilator drugs will be of little value. Vasodilator drugs may worsen the condition because vessels narrowed by arteriosclerosis will not dilate; adjacent vessels will dilate and shunt blood away from the occluded area, further reducing blood flow to the occluded area. Vasodilators are more rational in treating vasospastic diseases, but they have proved of limited value. In general, vasodilator therapy for peripheral vasular disease is of limited clinical value. Vasodilator drugs are also used to treat impaired cerebral blood flow. The effectiveness of this therapy is doubtful. Short-term improvement of symptoms is sometimes noted.

**MECHANISM OF ACTION**   The peripheral vasodilators act directly on vascular smooth muscle to cause vasodilation. This vasodilation seems independent of alpha- and beta-adrenergic receptors or of histamine receptors. Pentoxifylline is a new drug that is not a vasodilator; pentoxifylline acts on red blood cells to make them less stiff so that the red blood cells can more easily pass through narrowed vessels.

**INDICATIONS**   **Vasospastic disorders** Most common is Raynaud's phenomenon. Primarily involved are the hands, particularly the digits. Vasospasm is precipitated by cold or by stress and involves an increase of sympathetic tone, which further decreases blood flow. Raynaud's phenomenon can also be secondary to collagen diseases, occlusive arterial disease, or some drugs, especially beta-adrenergic blocking drugs. Pentoxifylline is used only for intermittent claudication.

**CONTRAINDICATIONS**   **Occlusive peripheral vascular disease** Vasodilators are not indicated for poor peripheral circulation due to atherosclerosis. Atherosclerotic vessels cannot dilate, and vasodilators may worsen circulation. This is because only the neighboring vessels will dilate, further reducing blood flow in the affected area. However, pentoxifylline, by acting on the red blood cells rather than the blood vessels, can improve blood flow in atherosclerotic vessels.

**DRUG INTERACTIONS**   **Tobacco** smoking leads to significant reduction of peripheral blood flow.

## ❦ NURSING CONSIDERATIONS

### Side effects, toxicities, and associated nursing actions

**CV** Hypotension, flushing, headache, dizziness, fast heart rate.
- Monitor the blood pressure and pulse when beginning therapy or when changing doses.
- Assess for the presence of other symptoms. Warn patients about the flushing, which may be startling.
- Caution patients to avoid driving or operating hazardous equipment if dizziness occurs.

**GI** Gastrointestinal disturbances, nausea, and vomiting.
- May be alleviated by taking doses with meals or antacids (see Patient and Family Education).
- If symptoms persist, consult the physician.

**Allergic:** *Hypersensitivity reactions:* A skin rash is the most common hypersensitivity reaction.
- Visually inspect the patient for development of rash. Instruct patients to report skin changes.

### Patient and family education

- Instruct patients about the expected outcomes of therapy, and possible side effects and toxic effects. Ask patients to report the development of any sign or symptom.
- Symptoms of hypotension include vertigo, dizziness, lightheadedness, syncope, and increased heart rate. If postural hypotension occurs, instruct patients to move slowly from sitting to standing.
- Hypotension may be potentiated in patients receiving vasodilators who are also receiving other drugs that can cause hypotension, such as diuretics, antihypertensives, central nervous system depressants, narcotics, and sedatives. Instruct patients to keep all health care providers informed of all medications being taken.
- If a dose of medication is missed, caution patients not to ''double up'' on the next dose to catch up.
- Caution patients to avoid the use of alcohol as it potentiates the hypotensive effects of vasodilators.
- Instruct patient to avoid smoking as it reduces peripheral blood flow.

- Instruct patient to avoid smoking as it reduces peripheral blood flow.
- Instruct patients to lose weight to ideal body weight to help decrease symptoms from peripheral vascular disease.
- Instruct patients to take oral preparations with meals or a snack to decrease gastric irritation.
- Instruct patients that timed-release formulations must be swallowed whole and not crushed or chewed.

## cyclandelate   (sye-KLAN-de-late)                                     peripheral vasodilator

- cyclandelate: Cyclospasmol

**MECHANISM OF ACTION**   Cyclandelate directly dilates vascular smooth muscle to cause vasodilation.

**INDICATIONS**   **Vasospastic and obstructive vascular disease** Possibly effective as an adjunct in the treatment of intermittent claudication, atherosclerosis, thrombophelebitis, nocturnal leg cramps, Raynaud's phenomenon, cerebral vascular disease.

**CONTRAINDICATIONS**   • Hypersensitivity to cyclandelate.

**DOSAGE**   **Adults:**   **PO:** Initially, 1200 to 1600 mg/day divided into four doses. When a clinical response is established, the dose is gradually lowered in 200 mg increments. The usual maintenance dosage is 400 to 800 mg daily in two to four doses.   *Special patient populations:*   **PREGNANCY:** Safe use has not been established.

**PREPARATIONS**   *Tablets:* 100 mg; *capsules:* 200, 400 mg.

**DRUG INTERACTIONS**   No drug interactions described.

**FATE**   Not well characterized. Therapeutic improvement is usually noted rapidly, but improvement requires continued therapy.

### ☙ NURSING CONSIDERATIONS

#### Side effects, toxicities, and associated nursing actions

**CV** Flushing, headache, dizziness, fast heart rate may be experienced, particularly early in therapy.
**GI** May be best tolerated by taking with meals and using antacids.
- See entry for drug class (p. 127).

#### Patient and family education

- See entry for drug class (p. 127 ).
- Reinforce to patients that ongoing use of the drug, as prescribed, is necessary for continued benefit.

## isoxsuprine hydrochloride   (eye-SOX-syoo-preen)                     peripheral vasodilator

- isoxsuprine hydrochloride: Vasodilan

**MECHANISM OF ACTION**   The mechanism of action is not clear. In addition to being a direct-acting vasodilator, isoxsuprine may be a beta-2 adrenergic receptor agonist since it primarily improves blood flow in skeletal muscle.

**INDICATIONS**   **Vasospastic and obstructive vascular disease** Possibly effective as an adjunct in the treatment of intermittent claudication, atherosclerosis, thrombophlebitis, nocturnal leg cramps, Raynaud's phenomenon, cerebral vascular disease.

**CONTRAINDICATIONS**   **Hypersensitivity** Discontinue if a severe rash develops.

**DOSAGE**   **Adults:**   **PO:** 10 to 20 mg three or four times a day.   **IM:** 5 to 10 mg two or three times a day.   *Special patient populations:*   **PREGNANCY:** Safe use has not been established. Isoxsuprine has been tested as an agent to control premature labor.

**PREPARATIONS**   *Tablets:* 10, 20 mg: *parenteral:* 5 mg/ml in 2 ml ampule.

**DRUG INTERACTIONS**   **Beta-Blockers** should diminish the response.

**FATE**  Not well characterized. Isoxsuprine does cross the placenta and can cause hypotension, tachycardia, hypoglycemia, and hypocalcemia in the newborn.

## 🐛 NURSING CONSIDERATIONS

### Side effects, toxicities, and associated nursing actions

**CV:** *Hypotension and fast heart rate:* These may be noted after IM administration of 10 mg doses, but only rarely otherwise.
- See entry for drug class (p. 127).

**GI** Nausea, vomiting, abdominal distress, and dizziness are infrequently experienced.

### Nursing interventions related to drug administration

- If used to control premature labor, monitor intensity, frequency, and duration of uterine contractions. Monitor fetal heart rate at regular intervals.

### Patient and family education

- See entry for drug class (p. 127).
- Reinforce to patients that ongoing use of the drug, as prescribed, is necessary for continued benefit.

---

## niacin   (NYE-a-sin)                                          peripheral vasodilator

- niacin (nicotinic acid): Nicobid

See nicotinyl alcohol tartrate below.

---

## nicotinyl alcohol tartrate   (nik-oh-TIN-ill)                peripheral vasodilator

- nicotinyl alcohol tartrate: Roniacol

**MECHANISM OF ACTION**  Nicotinyl alcohol is metabolized to niacin (nicotinic acid), which is a directly acting vasodilator, particularly in the blush area of the skin. There is little effect on blood vessels in the lower extremities.

**INDICATIONS**  **Deficient circulation** Possibly effective as adjunctive therapy in treating peripheral vascular disease, vascular spasm, varicose ulcers, bed sores, Meniere's syndrome, and vertigo.

**CONTRAINDICATIONS**  • Hepatic dysfunction. • Active peptic ulcer. • Severe hypotension. • Hemorrhaging or arterial bleeding.

**DOSAGE**  **Niacin:**  *Adults:*  **PO:** 100 to 150 mg three to five times daily or, for the extended release form, 300 to 400 mg every 12 hours.  **Nicotinyl alcohol:**  *Adults:*  **PO:** 50 to 100 mg three times daily. *Special patient populations:*  **PREGNANCY:** Safe use has not been established.

**PREPARATIONS**  **Niacin** *Capsules (timed release):* 125, 250, 400, 500 mg; *tablets:* 25, 50, 100, 500 mg. **Nicotinyl alcohol tartrate** Tablets: 50 mg; timed release tablets: 150 mg (as tartrate salt); elixir: 50 mg/5 ml.

**DRUG INTERACTIONS**  **Antihypertensive drugs with sympathetic depressant activity** Nicotinyl alcohol may have additive vasodilator activity and cause postural hypotension.

**FATE**  Nicotinyl alcohol is metabolized to niacin (nicotinic acid), which is vitamin $B_3$.

## 🐛 NURSING CONSIDERATIONS

### Side effects, toxicities, and associated nursing actions

**CV:** *Flushing,* particularly in the blush area. Tingling of the extremities, faintness, dizziness, and hypotension are occassionally experienced.

**GI** Gastrointestinal distress.
- See entry for drug class (p. 127).

### Patient and family education
- See entry for drug class (p. 127).
- Reinforce to patients that ongoing use of the drug, as prescribed, is necessary for continued benefit.
- Caution patients to avoid using medications containing niacin (e.g., vitamin preparations) without first checking with physician.

## nylidrin hydrochloride    (NYE-li-drin)    peripheral vasodilator

- nylidrin hydrochloride: Adrin, Arlidin, ✤PMSNylidrin

**MECHANISM OF ACTION**    Nylidrin is a beta-2 adrenergic agonist. It dilates arterioles in skeletal muscle, increases cerebral blood flow, and diminishes vascular resistance.

**INDICATIONS**    **Peripheral vascular disease** Possibly effective as an adjunctive aid in the treatment of atherosclerosis, Buerger's disease, diabetic vascular disease, nocturnal leg cramps, Raynaud's phenomenon, frostbite, and thrombophlebitis.

**CONTRAINDICATIONS**    **Myocardial infarction, paroxysmal tachycardia, angina, and thyrotoxicosis** Conditions in which beta-adrenergic stimulation would be harmful.

**DOSAGE**    **Adults:**    PO: 3 to 12 mg, three or four times daily.    *Special patient populations:*    PREGNANCY: Safe use has not been established.

**PREPARATIONS**    *Tablets*: 6, 12 mg.

**DRUG INTERACTIONS**    **Beta-blocking drugs** do not eliminate the action of nylidrin, suggesting a direct mechanism of action for nylidrin in addition to beta-adrenergic stimulation.

**FATE**    Not well characterized.

### ☙ NURSING CONSIDERATIONS

#### Side effects, toxicities, and associated nursing actions
**CNS** Nervousness, trembling, weakness, dizziness.
- Caution patients to avoid driving or operating hazardous equipment if weakness or dizziness occur.
- If CNS effects are severe or persistent, notify the physician.

**CV** Palpitations; postural hypotension. Overdose may stimulate the heart rate. This is dangerous in patients with congestive heart failure.
- See entry for drug class (p. 127).

**GI** Nausea and vomiting.

#### Patient and family education
- See entry for drug class (p. 127).
- Reinforce to patients that ongoing use of the drug, as prescribed, is necessary for continued benefit.

## papaverine hydrochloride    (pa-PAV-er-een)    peripheral vasodilator

- papaverine hydrochloride: Cerespan, Dilart, Genabid, Myodbid, Papacon Concaps, Pavabid Plateau Caps, Pavacap Unicelles, Pavacen Cenules, Pavadur, Pavagen, Pavased, Pavasule, Pavatine, Pavatym, Paverine Spancaps, Paverolan Lanacaps, Vasocap-150 and -300, Vasospan

**MECHANISM OF ACTION**    Papaverine directly relaxes smooth muscle, especially spasmodically contracted muscle. This action is seen in the vascular system, in the bronchial smooth muscle, and in the gastrointestinal, biliary, and urinary tracts. Papaverine also stimulates respiration by acting on the carotid and aortic body chemoreceptors. Blood flow is increased through the cerebral blood vessels, and these vessels are dilated, effects which may benefit some cases of cerebral vascular insufficiency. Papaverine also has a cardiac action, depressing conductivity and irritability and prolonging the refractory period. These actions limit premature systoles and ventricular arrhythmias.

**INDICATIONS**    The therapeutic value of papaverine has not been demonstrated; however, papaverine is widely used as a therapeutic aid in treating peripheral vascular diseases.

**CONTRAINDICATIONS**    **Atrial-ventricular (AV) block** Papaverine further depresses AV conduction.

**DOSAGE**    **Adults:**    PO: 60 to 300 mg, one to five times daily.    PO, TIMED-RELEASE: 150 mg every 12 hours; if required, increase dose to 300 mg or increase frequency to every 8 hours.    IV, IM: 30 to 120 mg every 3 hours. The IV dose should be injected slowly over 1 to 2 minutes. If cardiac extrasystoles are being treated, two doses should be given 10 minutes apart. Do not add to lactated Ringer's; papaverine will precipitate out.    *Special patient populations:*    ELDERLY: Doses are individualized. Altered doses for the elderly have not been specifically established.    CHILDREN: 6 mg/kg daily in four IM or IV doses.    PREGNANCY: Safe use has not been established.

**PREPARATIONS**    *Tablets:* 30, 60, 100, 200, 300 mg; *timed-release capsules:* 150, 300 mg; *timed release tablets:* 200 mg; *parenteral:* 30 mg/ml.

**DRUG INTERACTIONS**    None described.

**FATE**    Although papaverine is well absorbed, it binds to albumin and also accumulates in fat, factors that limit its distribution. Papaverine is metabolized by the liver, and metabolites are excreted in the urine.

## NURSING CONSIDERATIONS

### Side effects, toxicities, and associated nursing actions

**CNS** Drowsiness, sedation, malaise, vertigo. Symptoms of an overdose include drowsiness, weakness, nystagmus, double vision, incoordination; coma, cyanosis, and respiratory depression can develop.
- Caution patients to avoid driving or operating hazardous equipment if drowsiness, sedation, double vision, incoordination, or other CNS side effects occur; notify the physician.
- If CNS effects are severe or persistent, notify the physician.

**CV** Sweating, flushing, headache. Increased heart rate and depth of respiration; slight increase in blood pressure.
- See entry for drug class (p. 127).

**GI** Nausea, abdominal distress, loss of appetite, constipation, or diarrhea.
- Monitor weight; keep a record of stools.

**Allergic** Skin rash. Hepatic hypersensitivity has been reported, causing jaundice, eosinophilia, and altered liver function tests.
- Visually inspect patient for skin changes.
- Assess patient for malaise, fever, right upper quadrant abdominal pain, change in color or consistency of stools, jaundice.
- Monitor complete blood count, white blood cell differential, liver function tests.

**Chronic poisoning** Symptoms include depression, drowsiness, weakness, anxiety, incoordination, headache, blurred vision, upset stomach, and a skin rash. Blood counts may be low. The dose of papaverine is reduced or the drug is discontinued, depending on the severity.
- Assess for these signs of chronic poisoning.
- Review with patients at regular intervals the dose and dosing schedule the patient is following.

### Nursing interventions related to drug administration    Administer IV doses undiluted at a rate of 30 mg or less over 1 minute.
- If possible, monitor the electrocardiogram during IV administration.
- Monitor pulse, respirations, and blood pressure during IV administration and for 1 hour afterward.

### Patient and family education
- See entry for drug class (p. 127).
- Reinforce to patients that ongoing use of the drug, as prescribed, is necessary for continued benefit.

## tolazoline hydrochloride    (toe-LAZ-a-leen)    peripheral vasodilator

- tolazoline hydrochloride: Priscoline

**MECHANISM OF ACTION**    Tolazoline relaxes vascular smooth muscle directly. Tolazoline also has alpha-adrenergic blocking and histamine mimicking actions that cause vasodilation.

**INDICATIONS**    **Vasospastic vascular disease** Possibly effective as an adjunct in the treatment of intermittent claudication, atherosclerosis, thrombophlebitis, Buerger's disease., Raynaud's phenomenon, frostbite, gangrene, scleroderma, endocarditis, acrocyanosis, acroparesthesia.

**CONTRAINDICATIONS**    • Coronary artery disease. • Stroke. • Hypersensitivity.

**DOSAGE**    **Adults:**  SC, IM, IV: 10 to 50 mg four times daily.    **INTRA-ARTERIAL:** This route is used only in selected cases when parenteral administration has not yielded maximum benefit. A test dose of 25 mg (1 ml) is given slowly and the response determined. Further doses may be 50 to 75 mg. Initial doses are one or two injections daily; maintenance doses are two or three injections weekly.

**PREPARATIONS**    *Parenteral:* 25 mg/ml in 10 ml vials.

**DRUG INTERACTIONS**    **Alcohol** Tolazoline gives a disulframlike reaction and alcohol should not be ingested. **Epinephrine, norepinephrine** Tolazoline may reduce blood pressure, followed by an exaggerated rebound, if epinephrine or norepinephrine is injected.

**FATE**    Tolazoline is slowly absorbed parenterally. It is excreted primarily unchanged in the urine.

### ❦ NURSING CONSIDERATIONS

#### Side effects, toxicities, and associated nursing actions

**CNS** Apprehension; flushing, tingling.
- If CNS effects are severe or persistent, notify the physician.

**CV** Angina, arrhythmias, fast heart rate; change in blood pressure, including a marked hypertensive or hypotensive response. May precipitate a myocardial infarction. Symptoms of an overdose include goose-bumps, peripheral vasodilation, flushing of the skin, and occasionally, hypotension. The patient should be kept lying down with the head low; administer IV fluids. If the blood pressure must be raised, ephedrine is preferred because of its central and peripheral effects. Epinephrine or norepinephrine may be dangerous (see drug interactions).
- Observe carefully during parenteral administration. Monitor vital signs and blood pressure.
- See entry for drug class (p. 127).

**GI** Nausea, vomiting, diarrhea, GI upset; an existing peptic ulcer may be aggravated.

#### Nursing interventions related to drug administration    Administer IV doses undiluted at a rate of 10 mg or less over 1 minute.

#### Patient and family education    See entry for drug class (p. 127).
- Reinforce to patients that ongoing use of the drug, as prescribed, is necessary for continued benefit.

## pentoxifylline    (pen-tox-EYE-fi-leen)    hemorrheologic

- pentoxifylline: Trental

**MECHANISM OF ACTION**    Pentoxifylline is not a vasodilator but a hemorrheologic agent and represents a new type of drug. Pentoxifylline improves blood flow by decreasing blood viscosity and improving red blood cell flexibility.

**INDICATIONS**    **Chronic occlusive arterial disease of the limbs** Pentoxifylline significantly increases tissue oxygen levels in patients with peripheral arterial disease and intermittent claudication.

**CONTRAINDICATIONS**    **Hypersensitivity or intolerance to methylxanthines** Such compounds include caffeine and theophylline and theobromine, which are the active ingredients in coffee, tea, and chocolate.

**DOSAGE**    **Adults:**    PO: 400 mg three times daily with meals. An effect is usually apparent in 2 to 4 weeks. The drug should be tried for at least 8 weeks. *Special patient populations:*    ELDERLY: Doses are individualized. Altered doses for the elderly have not been specifically established.    CHILDREN: Pediatric doses have not been established.    PREGNANCY: Safe use has not been established.

**PREPARATIONS**    *Timed-release tablet:* 400 mg.

**DRUG INTERACTIONS**    **Anticoagulant or antiplatelet drugs** Since pentoxifylline decreases blood viscosity and prevents platelet aggregation, patients taking anticoagulant or antiplatelet medications should be monitored.

**FATE**    Pentoxifylline is well absorbed and reaches peak concentrations 2 or 3 hours after administration. Pentoxifyllin is metabolized by the liver, and the metabolite is excreted in the urine.

## 🦌 NURSING CONSIDERATIONS

### Side effects, toxicities, and associated nursing actions

**CNS** Dizziness, flushing, and headache are reduced by the timed-release formulation.
- Monitor the blood pressure and pulse when beginning therapy or when changing doses.
- Assess for the presence of other symptoms. Warn patients about the flushing, which may be startling.
- Caution patients to avoid driving or operating hazardous equipment if dizziness occurs.

**GI:** Intolerance to pentoxifylline has been reduced by the timed-release formulation. Nausea and an upset stomach are the most common reactions.
- May be alleviated by taking doses with meals or antacids.
- If symptoms persist, consult the physician.

### Patient and family education

- Instruct patients about the expected outcomes of therapy and possible side effects and toxic effects. Ask patients to report the development of any sign or symptom.
- Note Contraindications; obtain history of drug or food allergy before administering this drug.
- If a dose of medication is missed, caution patients not to ''double up'' on the next dose to catch up.
- Caution patients to avoid the use of aspirin or aspirin-containing products while taking pentoxifylline. Caution patients to keep all health care providers informed of all drugs being used.
- Instruct patients to avoid smoking, as it reduces peripheral blood flow.
- Instruct patients to lose weight to ideal body weight to help decrease symptoms from peripheral vascular disease.
- Instruct patients to take oral preparations with meals or a snack to decrease gastric irritation.
- Instruct patients that timed-release formulations must be swallowed whole and not crushed or chewed.
- Reinforce to patients to the need to take drug as ordered; several weeks of therapy may be necessary before improvement is noted.

# DIURETICS, FLUIDS, ELECTROLYTES, AND PARENTERAL NUTRITION PRODUCTS

**III**

**INTRODUCTION**  Fluid and electrolyte balance may be disturbed by many medical conditions, and it is often necessary to intervene to restore balance. Diuretics mobilize fluid for excretion from the body, along with a variety of solutes. Fluids and specific electrolytes may be returned to a patient by use of appropriate IV solutions. These solutions may contain calories in various forms for short-term or long-term use. Successful use of diuretics or IV solutions depends on careful monitoring of the patient so that as existing problems are corrected, new ones are not created.

# Chapter Nine
# Diuretic drugs

**Carbonic anhydrase inhibitors**
acetazolamide
dichlorphenamide
methazolamide

**Loop diuretics**
bumetanide
ethacrynic acid
furosemide

**Osmotic diuretics**
mannitol
urea

**Potassium-sparing diuretics**
amiloride
spironolactone
triamterene

**Thiazides and thiazidelike diuretics**
bendroflumethiazide
benzthiazide
chlorothiazide
chlorthalidone*
cyclothiazide
hydrochlorothiazide
hydroflumethiazide
indapamide*
methyclothiazide
metolazone*
polythiazide
quinethazone*
trichlormethiazide

**INTRODUCTION**  Diuretic drugs increase the elimination of water and electrolytes through the kidneys. Such an effect can occur by several mechanisms. *Carbonic anhydrase inhibitors* increase sodium ion excretion by increasing elimination of bicarbonate ion. *Loop diuretics* block reabsorption of chloride and associated sodium ions, increasing salt excretion. *Thiazide* and *thiazidelike* diuretics also block reabsorption of chloride and sodium but in a different part of the nephron than the loop diuretics. *Potassium-sparing diuretics* block the pump that exchanges sodium for potassium in a portion of nephron, leading to increased sodium excretion. For all these drugs, water accompanies the sodium excreted. *Osmotic diuretics* produce a urine with high osmotic strength so that water is excreted as it enters the tubule to dilute the urine.

Although the actions of the diuretics are similar, the clinical uses of these compounds vary (Table 9-1). Diuretics are often included in combination products (Table 9-2). The use of a single preparation containing two diuretics with differing mechanisms of action for treating hypertension reduces the number of tablets that must be taken daily. Combining a potassium-sparing diuretic with a thiazide often limits the potassium depletion that can complicate long-term therapy with thiazides alone. Combinations have the disadvantage of often being more expensive and making individualization of doses more difficult.

# Carbonic anhydrase inhibitors

acetazolamide  ~  dichlorphenamide  ~  methazolamide

**OVERVIEW OF THE DRUG CLASS**  Although carbonic anhydrase inhibitors have well-documented diuretic action, these drugs are most often used clinically for their actions in organs other than the kidneys (see Table 9-1). Members of this class of drugs are effective in controlling glaucoma and relieving the symptoms of acute mountain sickness and, when combined with other therapy, can aid in controlling seizures.

**MECHANISM OF ACTION**  Carbonic anhydrase inhibitors block secretion of hydrogen ion into the renal tubule, thereby increasing the excretion of bicarbonate. Sodium ion is excreted along with bicarbonate. Potassium ions are also lost, along with water. The diuretic action of these drugs is self-limiting because they produce metabolic acidosis, which blocks their renal effects.

**INDICATIONS**  Open-angle glaucoma Carbonic anhydrase inhibitors block secretion of aqueous humor and may reduce intraocular pressure in simple, noncongestive open-angle glaucoma. This action is inde-

*Nonthiazides with similar mechanisms.

| Table 9-1. | Summary of clinical uses of diuretic drugs | | | | | |
|---|---|---|---|---|---|---|
| Conditions responding to diuretics | Loop diuretics | Thiazides and related compounds | Potassium-sparing diuretics | Carbonic anhydrase inhibitors | Osmotic diuretics |
| Essential hypertension | + | + | + | | |
| Edema caused by congestive heart failure, renal disease, cirrhosis of liver | + | + | + | | |
| Pulmonary edema | + | | | | |
| Diabetes insipidus | | + | | | |
| Acute mountain sickness | | | | + | |
| Open-angle glaucoma | | | | + | |
| Excessive intraocular pressure | | | | + | + |
| Brain edema | | | | | + |

pendent of diuretic activity.    **Acute mountain sickness** The metabolic acidosis produced by carbonic anhydrase inhibitors lessens sleep hypoxia and the symptoms of acute mountain sickness.    **Convulsive disorders** Carbonic anhydrase inhibitors may have direct actions in the central nervous system or may reduce seizure activity indirectly by producing metabolic acidosis.    **Congestive heart failure** Carbonic anhydrase inhibitors can be used in congestive heart failure for diuretic action, but therapy should be on alternate days to avoid producing metabolic acidosis that terminates the drug effect.

**CONTRAINDICATIONS    Electrolyte imbalance** Excessive potassium loss is a special danger with carbonic anhydrase inhibitors.    **Severe pulmonary obstruction** These patients cannot compensate for the metabolic acidosis produced by carbonic anhydrase inhibitors because they cannot increase alveolar ventilation.    **Chronic noncongestive angle-closure glaucoma** This form of glaucoma may progress during use of the drugs.

**DRUG INTERACTIONS    ACTH and glucocorticoids** induce potassium loss, which when combined with the loss caused by carbonic anhydrase inhibitors may become severe.    **Amphotericin B** increases potassium loss, which may become severe when combined with the loss induced by carbonic anhydrase inhibitors.    **Thiazide and loop diuretics** increase potassium loss, which may become severe when combined with the loss induced by carbonic anhydrase inhibitors.    **Digitalis** toxicity may be increased because carbonic anhydrase inhibitors deplete potassium; low potassium levels increase sensitivity to digitalis.    **Quinidine** excretion may be impaired when carbonic anhydrase inhibitors are used because these agents alkalize the urine. • See individual drugs for other specific interactions.

**DIAGNOSTIC TEST INTERFERENCE    Blood ammonia, blood glucose, urinary glucose, plasma chloride levels, serum bilirubin, serum uric acid, urinary calcium, and urinary urobilinogen** may be increased by carbonic anhydrase inhibitors.    **Plasma bicarbonate, serum potassium, and urinary citrate levels** may be reduced by carbonic anhydrase inhibitors.    **Iodide uptake** may be decreased by carbonic anhydrase inhibitors.

## ☙ NURSING CONSIDERATIONS
### Side effects, toxicities, and associated nursing actions
**CNS** Nervous system effects may include paresthesias, sedation, depression, weakness, fatigue and other signs.
- Obtain baseline history and physical assessment before starting therapy.
- Monitor blood pressure regularly under standard conditions.
- Note that sedation, depression, weakness, and fatigue may be inadvertently attributed to aging or the effects of chronic illness, instead of drug side effects.

**Table 9-2.**

## Combination products containing diuretics

| Trade name | Diuretic component | Other ingredients | Use |
|---|---|---|---|
| Alazide | Hydrochlorothiazide (thiazide), spironolactone (potassium-sparing) | — | Antihypertensive, diuretic |
| Aldactazide | Hydrochlorothiazide (thiazide), spironolactone (potassium-sparing) | — | Antihypertensive, diuretic |
| Aldochlor | Chlorothiazide (thiazide) | Methyldopa (antihypertensive) | Antihypertensive |
| Aldoril | Hydrochlorothiazide (thiazide) | Methyldopa (antihypertensive) | Antihypertensive |
| Apresazide | Hydrochlorothiazide (thiazide) | Hydralazine (vasodilator) | Antihypertensive |
| Apresodex | Hydrochlorothiazide (thiazide) | Hydralazine (vasodilator) | Antihypertensive |
| Apresoline-Esidrix | Hydrochlorothiazide (thiazide) | Hydralazine (vasodilator) | Antihypertensive |
| Aquapres | Hydrochlorothiazide (thiazide) | Reserpine (rauwolfia) | Antihypertensive |
| Aquaserp | Hydrochlorothiazide (thiazide) | Reserpine (rauwolfia) | Antihypertensive |
| Capozide | Hydrochlorothiazide (thiazide) | Captopril (ACE-inhibitor) | Antihypertensive |
| Cherapas | Hydrochlorothiazide (thiazide) | Hydralazine (vasodilator), reserpine (rauwolfia) | Antihypertensive |
| Chloroserp | Chlorothiazide (thiazide) | Reserpine (rauwolfia) | Antihypertensive |
| Chloroserpine | Chlorothiazide (thiazide) | Reserpine (rauwolfia) | Antihypertensive |
| Combipres | Chlorthalidone (thiazide-like) | Clonidine (antihypertensive) | Antihypertensive |
| Corzide | Bendroflumethiazide (thiazide) | Nadolol (beta-blocker) | Antihypertensive |
| Diupres | Chlorothiazide (thiazide) | Reserpine (rauwolfia) | Antihypertensive |
| Diurese-R | Trichlormethiazide (thiazide) | Reserpine (rauwolfia | Antihypertensive |
| Diutensin | Methyclothiazide (thiazide) | Cryptenamine (veratrum alkaloid) | Antihypertensive |
| Diutensin-R | Methylclothiazide (thiazide) | Reserpine (rauwolfia) | Antihypertensive |
| Dyazide | Hydrochlorothiazide (thiazide), triamterene (potassium-sparing) | — | Antihypertensive |
| Enduronyl | Methyclothiazide (thiazide) | Deserpidine (rauwolfia) | Antihypertensive |
| Esimil | Hydrochlorothiazide (thiazide) | Guanethidine (antihypertensive) | Antihypertensive |
| Eutron | Methyclothiazide (thiazide) | Pargyline (MAO inhibitor) | Antihypertensive |
| Exna-R | Benzthiazide (thiazide) | Reserpine (rauwolfia) | Antihypertensive |
| H-H | Hydrochlorothiazide (thiazide) | Hydralazine (vasodilator) | Antihypertensive |
| HHR | Hydrochlorothiazide (thiazide) | Reserpine (rauwolfia), hydralazine (vasodilator) | Antihypertensive |
| Hydro-Fluserpine | Hydroflumethiazide (thiazide) | Reserpine (rauwolfia) | Antihypertensive |
| Hydromox R | Quinethazone (thiazide) | Reserpine (rauwolfia) | Antihypertensive |
| Hydropine | Hydroflumethiazide (thiazide) | Reserpine (rauwolfia) | Antihypertensive |
| Hydropres | Hydrochlorothiazide (thiazide) | Reserpine (rauwolfia) | Antihypertensive |
| Hydro-reserpine | Hydrochlorothiazide (thiazide) | Reserpine (rauwolfia) | Antihypertensive |
| Hydrosine | Hydrochlorothiazide (thiazide) | Reserpine (rauwolfia) | Antihypertensive |
| Hydrotensin | Hydrochlorothiazide (thiazide) | Reserpine (rauwolfia) | Antihypertensive |
| Hyserp | Hydrochlorothiazide (thiazide) | Reserpine (rauwolfia) | Antihypertensive |
| Inderide | Hydrochlorothiazide (thiazide) | Propranolol (beta-blocker) | Antihypertensive |
| Lopressor HCT | Hydrochlorothiazide (thiazide) | Metoprolol (beta-blocker) | Antihypertensive |
| Mallopress | Hydrochlorothiazide (thiazide) | Reserpine (rauwolfia) | Antihypertensive |
| Maxzide | Hydrochlorothiazide (thiazide), triamterene (potassium-sparing) | — | Antihypertensive |
| Metatensin | Trichlormethiazide (thiazide) | Reserpine (rauwolfia) | Antihypertensive |

**Table 9-2.**

## Combination products containing diuretics—cont'd

| Trade name | Diuretic component | Other ingredients | Use |
|---|---|---|---|
| Methy-deserpidine | Methyclothiazide (thiazide) | Deserpidine (rauwolfia) | Antihypertensive |
| Minizide | Polythiazide (thiazide) | Prazosin (alpha-blocker) | Antihypertensive |
| Moduretic | Hydrochlorothiazide (thiazide), amiloride HCl (potassium-sparing) | — | Antihypertensive |
| Naquival | Trichlormethiazide (thiazide) | Reserpine (rauwolfia) | Antihypertensive |
| Naturetin | Bendroflumethiazide (thiazide) | Potassium chloride | Antihypertensive |
| Oreticyl | Hydrochlorothiazide (thiazide) | Deserpidine (rauwolfia) | Antihypertensive |
| Rautrax | Bendroflumethiazide (thiazide) | Rauwolfia serpentina, potassium chloride | Antihypertensive |
| Rauzide | Bendroflumethiazide (thiazide | Rauwolfia serpentina | Antihypertensive |
| Regroton | Chlorthalidone (thiazide-like) | Reserpine (rauwolfia) | Antihypertensive |
| Renese-R | Polythiazide (thiazide) | Reserpine (rauwolfia) | Antihypertensive |
| R-HCTZ-H | Hydrochlorothiazide (thiazide) | Reserpine (rauwolfia), hydralazine (vasodilator) | Antihypertensive |
| Salazide | Hydroflumethiazide | Reserpine (rauwolfia) | Antihypertensive |
| Salutensin | Hydroflumethiazide (thiazide) | Reserpine (rauwolfia) | Antihypertensive |
| Ser-A-Gen | Hydrochlorothiazide (thiazide) | Reserpine (rauwolfia), hydralazine (vasodilator) | Antihypertensive |
| Seralazide | Hydrochlorothiazide (thiazide) | Reserpine (rauwolfia), hydralazine (vasodilator) | Antihypertensive |
| Ser-Ap-Es | Hydrochlorothiazide (thiazide) | Reserpine (rauwolfia), hydralazine (vasodilator) | Antihypertensive |
| Serathide | Hydrochlorothiazide (thiazide) | Reserpine (rauwolfia), hydralazine (vasodilator) | Antihypertensive |
| Ser Hydra Zine | Hydrochlorothiazide (thiazide) | Reserpine (rauwolfia), hydralazine (vasodilator) | Antihypertensive |
| Serpaside-Esidrix Serpazide | Hydrochlorothiazide (thiazide) | Reserpine (rauwolfia) | Antihypertensive |
| Spiractazide | Hydrochlorothiazide (thiazide), spironolactone (potassium-sparing) | — | Antihypertensive, diuretic |
| Spironazide | Hydrochlorothiazide (thiazide), spironolactone (potassium-sparing) | — | Antihypertensive, diuretic |
| Spirozide | Hydrochlorothiazide (thiazide), spironolactone (potassium-sparing) | — | Antihypertensive, diuretic |
| Tenoretic | Chlorthalidone (thiazide-like) | Atenolol (beta-blocker) | Antihypertensive |
| Timolide | Hydrochlorothiazide (thiazide) | Timolol (beta-blocker) | Antihypertensive |
| Thianal | Hydrochlorothiazide (thiazide) | Reserpine (rauwolfia) | Antihypertensive |
| Thiaserp | Chlorothiazide (thiazide) | Reserpine (rauwolfia) | Antihypertensive |
| Tri-Hydroserpine | Hydrochlorothiazide (thiazide) | Reserpine (rauwolfia), hydralazine (vasodilator) | Antihypertensive |
| Unipres | Hydrochlorothiazide (thiazide) | Reserpine (rauwolfia), hydralazine (vasodilator) | Antihypertensive |
| Vaseretic | Hydrochlorthiazide (thiazide), enalapril maleate (ACE inhibitor) | — | Antihypertensive |

**Allergic** Fever, rash, and signs of drug fever may occur.
- Monitor unexplained fever carefully.
- Assess for history of allergy to sulfonamide antibacterials, thiazide diuretics, or other sulfonamide-derivative diuretics before therapy, as cross-sensitivity to carbonic anhydrase inhibitors may occur.

**Blood** Blood dyscrasias such as thrombocytopenia, pancytopenia, and agranulocytosis have been reported.
- Monitor complete blood cell count and platelet count regularly.

**GI** Nausea, anorexia, or constipation may occur.
- Monitor intake and output.
- Keep record of bowel movements. If constipation occurs, instruct the patient to increase fluid intake to 2500 to 3000 ml/day (if not contraindicated by the medical condition), increase intake of fruit, fruit juices, and fiber, and increase level of exercise.

**Renal** Urinary frequency, renal colic, or stone formation may occur.
- Urinary frequency may occur due to the diuretic effect; it should lessen with continued use of the drug. Teach patients to take the last dose of the day before 6 PM to reduce the frequency of voiding at night. Instruct patients taking a single daily dose to take it in the morning for the same reason.
- Some patients may be instructed to increase daily fluid intake to 3000 ml or more to reduce the incidence of stone formation; consult with the physician.

**Metabolic** Weight loss and flaccid paralysis are observed rarely.
- Weigh patient regularly.
- Dehydration may occur with any diuretic. Monitor for thirst, decreased skin turgor, nausea, light-headedness, weakness, increased pulse, oliguria, decreased blood pressure, elevated hemoglobin level, hematocrit, and blood urea nitrogen (BUN).
- Monitor serum electrolytes. Assess for signs of hypokalemia: muscle weakness, apathy, abdominal distention, and paralytic ileus; ECG changes include flattened or inverted T waves, prolonged QT segment, and a prominent U wave.

**Patient and family education** Review with patients expected effects and possible side effects. Instruct patients to report the appearance of any unexpected sign or symptom.
- Instruct patient to report the appearance of any unexpected bruising or bleeding (signs of thrombocytopenia) or fever, rash, or sore throat (signs of agranulocytosis).
- Instruct patient to avoid the use of alcohol, which may potentiate hypotension.
- If postural hypotension occurs, caution patient to move slowly from lying to sitting or standing. Hypotension occurs more frequently in the elderly.
- If a potassium supplement is prescribed, teach the patient the importance of taking it as ordered. Dietary sources of potassium include citrus fruits and juices; grape, cranberry, apple, pear, and apricot juices; bananas; meat, fish, and fowl; cereals; and tea and cola beverages. Some patients with borderline low potassium levels can maintain potassium levels by increasing their daily intake of potassium-rich foods. Note that some potassium-rich foods are also high in sodium and may be contraindicated on that basis. Remind patients not to make dietary adjustments unless directed to do so; not all patients need to increase potassium intake, and for some it may be harmful.
- Remind patients to keep all health care providers informed of all medications being used.
- Remind patients to keep these and all medications out of the reach of children.

## acetazolamide   (a-seat-a-ZOLE-a-mide)   anticonvulsant, antiglaucoma, diuretic

- acetazolamide (acetazolamide sodium): Acetazolam, AK-Zol, Apo-acetazolamide Dazamide, Diamox

**MECHANISM OF ACTION** Acetazolamide, like other carbonic anhydrase inhibitors, blocks secretion of hydrogen ion into the renal tubule, thereby increasing excretion of bicarbonate, sodium, potassium ions, and water. The diuretic action of acetazolamide is self-limiting, because acetazolamide causes metabolic acidosis, which blocks renal effects of the drug. In some therapeutic applications, the desired action of acetazolamide is the production of mild metabolic acidosis.

**INDICATIONS**   **Open-angle glaucoma** Acetazolamide blocks secretion of aqueous humor and may reduce intraocular pressure. This action is independent of diuretic activity.   **Acute altitude sickness** Acetazolamide produces metabolic acidosis that lessens sleep hypoxia and alleviates the symptoms of acute mountain sickness.   **Convulsive disorders** Acetazolamide may act directly in the central nervous system or may reduce seizure activity indirectly by producing metabolic acidosis.   **Diuretic** Acetazolamide may be used in conditions such as congestive heart failure when diuresis is required. The drug should be given intermittently so that metabolic acidosis is not produced; metabolic acidosis terminates the diuretic action of acetazolamide.   **Periodic paralysis** Acetazolamide alters potassium utilization by muscle cells, thereby relieving paralysis.

**CONTRAINDICATIONS**   **Electrolyte imbalance** Excessive potassium loss is a special danger with acetazolamide.   **Severe pulmonary obstruction** These patients cannot compensate for the metabolic acidosis produced by acetazolamide because they cannot increase alveolar ventilation.   **Chronic noncongestive angle-closure glaucoma** This form of glaucoma may progress during use of acetazolamide.   **Severe respiratory acidosis** Acetazolamide produces acidosis, which may worsen the pre-existing acidotic state.   **Hepatic disease** Acetazolamide may precipitate hepatic coma in patients with severe cirrhosis or hepatic impairment.

**DOSAGE**   **For open-angle glaucoma:**   PO:   *Adult:* 250 mg one to four times daily for open-angle glaucoma, titrated to patient response; secondary glaucoma or preoperative treatment, 250 mg every 4 hours.   *Children:* 8 to 30 mg/kg body weight, or 300 to 900 mg/$M^2$ body surface area, in divided doses.   IV:   *Adult:* 500 mg to immediately reduce intraocular pressure in acute glaucoma; otherwise, dosage is as for oral forms.   *Children:* 5 to 10 mg/kg body weight every 6 hours.   **For acute mountain sickness:**   PO:   *Adult:* 500 mg daily for 24 to 48 hours before and during rapid ascent and for 48 hours after arrival.   **For convulsive disorders:**   PO:   *Adults or children:* 8 to 30 mg/kg body weight daily in two to four divided doses; range usually 375 mg to 1 g daily.   **As diuretic:**   PO:   *Adults or children:* 5 mg/kg body weight daily as single dose in the morning for 2 days, followed by 1 day without drug. The dose may be repeated, but acetazolamide is not ideal for prolonged diuretic therapy.   IV:   *Children:* 5 mg/kg body weight or 150 mg/$M^2$ for 1 or 2 days, alternating with days when no drug is given.   **For periodic paralysis:**   PO:   *Adults:* 250 mg to 1.5 g daily in divided doses.   *Special patient populations:*   PREGNANCY: Acetazolamide should not be administered to pregnant patients or those who may become pregnant during therapy unless the benefit clearly exceeds the risk of exposure. Carbonic anhydrase inhibitors are teratogenic and embryocidal at high doses in animals, although these effects are not documented in humans at therapeutic doses.

**PREPARATIONS**   *Tablets:* 125 or 250 mg; *capsules for sustained release:* 500 mg; *solution for parenteral administration:* A vial containing 500 mg of acetazolamide as the sodium salt is reconstituted with 5 ml sterile water for injection before use. The solution contains no preservative and should be refrigerated and used within 24 hours.

**DRUG INTERACTIONS**   Acetazolamide is subject to the same interactions as other members of the class (see p. 137). In addition, the following interactions may be important.   **Carbamazepine, phenobarbital, phenytoin, or primidone** may induce osteopenia (loss of bone mass), an action that is often enhanced by acetazolamide.   **Insulin or oral hypoglycemic agents** may require dosage adjustments when acetazolamide is also given, because acetazolamide can induce hyperglycemia and glycosuria.

**DIAGNOSTIC TEST INTERFERENCE**   See entry for drug class (p. 137).

**FATE**   Acetazolamide is well absorbed orally, with *peak* plasma concentrations occurring 2 to 4 hours after dosage with regular tablets. When used for treating glaucoma, the *onset* of action is about 1 hour and the *duration* of action is from 8 to 12 hours. Sustained release capsules produce an *onset* at 2 hours, *peak* action at 8 to 12 hours, and *duration* of action from 18 to 24 hours. Intravenous administration produces a *peak* effect at 15 minutes and a *duration* of action of 4 to 5 hours. Effects of acetazolamide when used to treat conditions other than glaucoma may take longer to be measured. Nearly all of administered acetazolamide is excreted by the kidneys as unchanged drug. The *half-life* for elimination is 2.4 to 5.8 hours.

## ❦ NURSING CONSIDERATIONS

### Side effects, toxicities, and associated nursing actions    See entry for drug class (p. 137).

**Metabolic** Metabolic acidosis is expected with continuous administration of acetazolamide.

- Monitor arterial pH. Metabolic acidosis is a pH below 7.35. Assess for signs and symptoms of headache, mental dullness, rapid and deep respirations, stupor, or coma. Death can occur.
- If acidosis is severe or persists, intermittent therapy (every other day) may be an acceptable alternative for treatment of edema; consult with the physician.
- Monitor carefully patients with other medical conditions predisposing to acidosis, such as patients with obstructive pulmonary disease.

**Renal** Acetazolamide may cause discomfort or pain on urination, signaling nephrotoxicity resembling that produced by sulfonamides.

- Monitor intake and output.
- Assess for renal colic (severe flank pain), hematuria (blood in urine), oliguria, and signs and symptoms of renal calculus formation.

**Blood** Tiredness or weakness is common and may signal blood dyscrasia or electrolyte imbalance.

- Monitor electrolytes.
- Monitor for hypokalemia (serum potassium level less than 3.5 mEq/L). Signs and symptoms include vomiting, leg cramps, muscle weakness, apathy, abdominal distention, paralytic ileus, and electrocardiogram (ECG) changes such as sagging S-T segments, depressed T waves, and elevated U waves.
- Monitor ECG at regular intervals.
- Monitor CBC and platelet count at regular intervals.

**GI** Loss of appetite, nausea, vomiting, diarrhea, and weight loss have been reported.

- Weigh patient regularly under standard conditions.
- Assess for dehydration. Symptoms include thirst, decreased skin turgor, nausea, lightheadedness, weakness, increased pulse, oliguria, decreased blood pressure, elevated hemoglobin level, hematocrit, and blood urea nitrogen (BUN).
- Assess for thirst, a frequent patient complaint. Before permitting patient to drink fluids as desired, consult with physician. Ingestion of too much fluid may compound possible electrolyte imbalances and defeat purpose of diuretics.
- Monitor intake and output. Persistent vomiting or diarrhea may contribute to electrolyte imbalances.

**Peripheral nervous system** Tingling or numbness in extremities or mouth may occur.

- Perform thorough physical assessment on regular basis to confirm deviations from baseline.

### Nursing interventions related to drug administration

- Read orders for oral preparations carefully; both tablets and extended-release capsules are available.
- If an oral liquid form is needed, tablets may be crushed and suspended in any highly flavored carbohydrate syrup. Elixirs, fruit juices, or vehicles containing alcohol or glycerin are not recommended. Tablets may also be softened in hot water and added to honey; prepare this form just before administration. For additional guidance about oral liquids, consult a pharmacist.
- Parenteral acetazolamide may be given direct IV push, added to standard IV solutions, or given IM (see Preparations). IM administration is painful.
- Administer direct IV push at a rate of 500 mg over at least 1 minute.

### Patient and family education

- See entry for drug class (p. 140).
- Review with patients expected effects and possible side effects. Instruct patients to report appearance of any unexpected sign or symptom.
- Instruct patients that diuretics work best when taken as ordered. Patients should not double up if a dose is missed. If a patient remembers a missed dose within a couple of hours of when it should have been taken, patient should take the missed dose. If the patient remembers the missed dose close to the time when the next dose is ordered, the patient should skip the missed dose, and begin with the next dose as prescribed.
- Instruct the patient to avoid driving or operating hazardous equipment if drowsiness, dizziness, lightheadedness, or visual changes occur. Notify the physician.

- Metallic taste in the mouth may occur. Sucking on sugarless hard candy, chewing sugarless gum, and frequent oral hygiene may help.
- Photosensitivity may occur. Instruct patients to avoid prolonged exposure to the sun, to wear a hat and long-sleeved clothing if sensitivity occurs, and to use maximum protection sunscreens.
- Instruct patient not to switch brands unless approved by physician. Different brands may not be bioequivalent.
- Diabetic patients may require an adjustment of insulin or oral hypoglycemic agent because acetazolamide can induce hyperglycemia and glycosuria. Instruct diabetic patients about this effect.
- Teach patients taking this drug as an anticonvulsant not to discontinue the medication suddenly; reinforce to the patient the need to work with the physician for drug and dosage adjustment.

## dichlorphenamide (dye-klor-FEN-a-mide) antiglaucoma

- dichlorphenamide: Daranide

**MECHANISM OF ACTION** As for other carbonic anhydrase inhibitors. See entry for drug class (p. 136).

**INDICATIONS** **Open-angle glaucoma** Dichlorphenamide blocks secretion of aqueous humor and may reduce intraocular pressure.

**CONTRAINDICATIONS** As for other carbonic anhydrase inhibitors. See entry for drug class (p. 137).

**DOSAGE** **PO:** **ADULTS:** 100 to 200 mg initially, then 100 mg twice daily until response is satisfactory; maintenance is with 25 to 50 mg one to three times daily. *Special patient populations:* **CHILDREN:** Doses not established. **PREGNANCY:** Carbonic anhydrase inhibitors are teratogenic and embryocidal at high doses in animals, although such effects have not been observed at therapeutic doses in humans. Nevertheless, dichlorphenamide is not usually given to pregnant patients or those likely to become pregnant during therapy.

**PREPARATIONS** *Tablets:* scored, 50 mg.

**DRUG INTERACTIONS** As for other carbonic anhydrase inhibitors. See entry for drug class (p. 137).

**DIAGNOSTIC TEST INTERFERENCE** • See entry for drug class (p. 137).

**FATE** Dichlorphenamide is effectively absorbed orally, with reduction of intraocular pressure occurring within 30 to 60 minutes. *Peak* activity is observed at 2 to 4 hours and *duration* is from 6 to 12 hours—similar to the values observed with acetazolamide. The route of excretion of dichlorphenamide is unknown.

### 🌸 NURSING CONSIDERATIONS

**Side effects, toxicities, and associated nursing actions** See entry for drug class (p. 137).

**Metabolic** Metabolic acidosis is less likely with dichlorphenamide than with other carbonic anhydrase inhibitors.

- Monitor arterial pH. Metabolic acidosis is a pH below 7.35. Assess for signs and symptoms of headache, mental dullness, rapid and deep respirations, stupor, coma, and eventually death.
- If acidosis is severe or persists, intermittent therapy (every other day) may be an acceptable alternative for treatment of edema; consult with the physician.
- Monitor carefully patients with other medical conditions predisposing to acidosis, such as patients with obstructive pulmonary disease.

**Renal** Dichlorphenamide may cause discomfort or pain on urination, signaling nephrotoxicity resembling that produced by sulfonamides.

- Monitor intake and output.
- Assess for renal colic (severe flank pain), hematuria (blood in urine), and oliguria, signs and symptoms of renal calculus formation.

**Blood** Tiredness or weakness is common and may signal blood dyscrasia or electrolyte imbalance.

- Monitor electrolytes.
- Monitor for hypokalemia (serum potassium level less than 3.5 mEq/L). Signs and symptoms include vomiting, leg cramps, muscle weakness, apathy, abdominal distention, paralytic ileus, and electrocardiogram (ECG) changes such as sagging S-T segments, depressed T waves, and elevated U waves.

- Monitor ECG at regular intervals.
- Monitor CBC and platelet count at regular intervals.

**GI** Loss of appetite, nausea, vomiting, diarrhea, and weight loss have been reported.

- Weigh patient regularly under standard conditions.
- Assess for dehydration. Symptoms include thirst, decreased skin turgor, nausea, lightheadedness, weakness, increased pulse, oliguria, decreased blood pressure, elevated hemoglobin level, hematocrit, and blood urea nitrogen (BUN).
- Assess for thirst, a frequent patient complaint. Before permitting the patient to drink fluids as desired, consult with the physician. Ingestion of too much fluid may compound possible electrolyte imbalances and defeat the purpose of diuretics.
- Monitor intake and output. Persistent vomiting or diarrhea may contribute to electrolyte imbalances.

**Peripheral nervous system** Tingling or numbness in extremities or mouth may occur.

- Perform thorough physical assessment on regular basis to confirm deviations from baseline.

**Patient and family education**   See entry for drug class (p. 140).

- Review with patients expected effects and possible side effects. Instruct patients to report appearance of any unexpected sign or symptom.
- Instruct patients that diuretics work best when taken as ordered. Patients should not double up if a dose is missed. If a patient remembers a missed dose within a couple of hours of when it should have been taken, patient should take missed dose. If the patient remembers the missed dose close to the time when the next dose is ordered, the patient should skip the missed dose, and begin with the next dose as prescribed.
- Instruct the patient to avoid driving or operating hazardous equipment if drowsiness, dizziness, lightheadedness, or visual changes occur. Notify the physician.
- A metallic taste in the mouth may occur. Sucking on sugarless hard candy, chewing sugarless gum, and frequent oral hygiene may help.
- Photosensitivity may occur. Instruct patients to avoid prolonged exposure to the sun, to wear a hat and long-sleeved clothing if sensitivity occurs, and to use maximum protection sunscreens.
- Diabetic patients may require an adjustment of insulin or oral hypoglycemic agent because dichlorphenamide can induce hyperglycemia and glycosuria. Instruct diabetic patients about this effect.

---

## methazolamide   (meth-a-ZOLE-a-mide)                                    antiglaucoma

- methazolamide: Neptazane

**MECHANISM OF ACTION**   As for other carbonic anhydrase inhibitors. See entry for drug class (p. 136).

**INDICATIONS**   **Open-angle glaucoma** Methazolamide blocks secretion of aqueous humor and may reduce intraocular pressure.

**CONTRAINDICATIONS**   As for other carbonic anhydrase inhibitors. See entry for drug class (p. 137).

**DOSAGE**   **Adult:**   **PO:** 25 to 100 mg two or three times daily.   *Special patient populations:*   **CHILDREN:** Doses not established.   **PREGNANCY:** Carbonic anhydrase inhibitors are teratogenic and embryocidal at high doses in animals, although such effects have not been seen at therapeutic doses in humans. Nevertheless, methazolamide is not usually administered to pregnant patients or those likely to become pregnant during therapy.

**PREPARATIONS**   *Tablets:* 50 mg scored.

**DRUG INTERACTIONS**   As for other carbonic anhydrase inhibitors. See entry for drug class (p. 137).

**DIAGNOSTIC TEST INTERFERENCE**   • See entry for drug class (p. 137).

**FATE**   Absorption of methazolamide is slower than with acetazolamide or dichlorphenamide. The *onset* of action in reducing intraocular pressure is 2 to 4 hours, and *peak* effects are not seen until 6 to 8 hours after administration. The *duration* of action is 10 to 18 hours. Renal excretion of methazolamide accounts for about 15% to 30% of administered drug, which appears unchanged in the urine. The fate of the remainder of the drug is unknown. The *half-life* for elimination of methazolamide is 14 hours.

## ❧ NURSING CONSIDERATIONS

### Side effects, toxicities, and associated nursing actions

- See entry for drug class (p. 137).

**Metabolic** Metabolic acidosis is expected with continuous administration of methazolamide.

- Monitor arterial pH. Metabolic acidosis is a pH below 7.35. Assess for signs and symptoms of headache, mental dullness, rapid and deep respirations, stupor, or coma. Death may occur.
- If acidosis is severe or persists, intermittent therapy (every other day) may be an acceptable alternative for treatment of edema; consult with the physician.
- Monitor carefully patients with other medical conditions predisposing to acidosis, such as patients with obstructive pulmonary disease.

**Renal** Methazolamide may cause discomfort or pain on urination, signaling nephrotoxicity resembling that produced by sulfonamides.

- Monitor intake and output.
- Assess for renal colic (severe flank pain), hematuria (blood in urine), oliguria, and signs and symptoms of renal calculus formation.

**Blood** Tiredness or weakness is common and may signal blood dyscrasia or electrolyte imbalance.

- Monitor electrolytes.
- Monitor for hypokalemia (serum potassium level less than 3.5 mEq/L). Signs and symptoms include vomiting, leg cramps, muscle weakness, apathy, abdominal distention, paralytic ileus, and electrocardiogram (ECG) changes such as sagging S-T segments, depressed T waves, and elevated V waves.
- Monitor ECG at regular intervals.
- Monitor CBC and platelet count at regular intervals.

**GI** Loss of appetite, nausea, vomiting, diarrhea, and weight loss have been reported.

- Weigh patient regularly, under standard conditions.
- Assess for dehydration. Symptoms include thirst, decreased skin turgor, nausea, lightheadedness, weakness, increased pulse, oliguria, decreased blood pressure, elevated hemoglobin level, hematocrit, and blood urea nitrogen (BUN).
- Assess for thirst, a frequent patient complaint. Before permitting patient to drink fluids as desired, consult with the physician. Ingestion of too much fluid may compound possible electrolyte imbalances and defeat the purpose of diuretics.
- Monitor intake and output. Persistent vomiting or diarrhea may contribute to electrolyte imbalances.

**Peripheral nervous system** Tingling or numbness in extremities or mouth may occur.

- Perform thorough physical assessment on regular basis to confirm deviations from baseline.

### Patient and family education

- See entry for drug class (p. 140).
- Review with patients expected effects and possible side effects. Instruct patients to report appearance of any unexpected sign or symptom.
- Instruct patients that diuretics work best when taken as ordered. Patients should not double up if a dose is missed. If a patient remembers a missed dose within a couple of hours of when it should have been taken, patient should take the missed dose. If the patient remembers the missed dose close to the time when the next dose is ordered, the patient should skip the missed dose, and begin with the next dose as prescribed.
- Instruct the patient to avoid driving or operating hazardous equipment if drowsiness, dizziness, lightheadedness, or visual changes occur. Notify the physician.
- A metallic taste in the mouth may occur. Sucking on sugarless hard candy, chewing sugarless gum, and frequent oral hygiene may help.
- Photosensitivity may occur. Instruct patients to avoid prolonged exposure to the sun, to wear a hat and long-sleeved clothing if sensitivity occurs, and to use maximum protection sunscreens.
- The diabetic patient may require an adjustment of insulin or oral hypoglycemic agent because

methazolamide can induce hyperglycemia and glycosuria. Instruct diabetic patients about this effect.

# Loop diuretics

bumetanide ~ ethacrynic acid ~ furosemide

**OVERVIEW OF THE DRUG CLASS**   Loop diuretics are the most powerful diuretics in clinical use. The high potency of these agents is helpful in controlling a variety of serious edematous states. The high potency of these agents also increases the risks of using them; many of the side effects noted with loop diuretics arise from excessive diuretic action. Patients must be carefully monitored to avoid profound dehydration and salt depletion.

**MECHANISM OF ACTION**   Bumetanide, ethacrynic acid, and furosemide inhibit active reabsorption of chloride ion in the ascending limb of Henle's loop in the kidney. Because chloride ion reabsorption is prevented, the passive reabsorption of sodium ion is also blocked. As a result, sodium chloride is retained in the tubule and excreted in the urine, carrying body water along with it. Potassium ion is also excreted in higher than normal amounts in response to loop diuretics.

**INDICATIONS**   **Edematous states** Edema caused by congestive heart failure, hepatic disease, renal disease, nephrotic syndrome, and malignancies may be controlled with loop diuretics.   **Hypertension** Loop diuretics may be used in step 1 care of hypertensive patients or in combination with other antihypertensive agents. The loop diuretics are especially helpful in treating hypertensives with a degree of renal insufficiency, a condition limiting the use of thiazide diuretics.

**CONTRAINDICATIONS**   **Anuria** Loop diuretics are effective during renal insufficiency but should not be administered when renal function has virtually ceased.   **Severe hepatic disease** Loop diuretics can be used to control edema in patients with hepatic disease, but if hepatic function is too severely impaired, the profound dehydration and electrolyte disturbances produced by these drugs may induce hepatic coma.

**DRUG INTERACTIONS**   **ACTH and glucocorticoids** induce potassium loss, which when combined with the loss caused by loop diuretics may become severe.   **Alcohol, barbiturates, or narcotics** may increase orthostatic hypotension induced by loop diuretics.   **Aminoglycoside antibiotics** are ototoxic (produce hearing loss or the loss of equilibrium). Concomitant therapy with loop diuretics, which are themselves ototoxic, greatly increases this risk. The combination is avoided except in life-threatening situations.   **Amphotericin B** causes potassium loss, which when combined with the loss caused by loop diuretics, may become severe.   **Antihypertensive agents** (peripheral adrenergic blocking agents or ganglionic blocking drugs) are potentiated by the action of loop diuretics. This interaction is often exploited when furosemide is used therapeutically in combination with other drugs for increased control of hypertension.   **Digitalis toxicity** may be increased because loop diuretics deplete potassium; low potassium levels increase sensitivity to digitalis.   **Indomethacin** may block the diuretic action of loop diuretics by an unknown mechanism.   **Lithium** toxicity may be enhanced by loop diuretics because they block the excretion of lithium and cause accumulation of toxic levels of the element.   **Nondepolarizing neuromuscular blocking agents (e.g., tubocurarine)** may have prolonged actions in the presence of loop diuretics because these diuretic agents tend to deplete potassium. **Probenecid** may block the diuretic action of loop diuretics by blocking the entry of the diuretics into the tubule where they exert their effects.   **Salicylate toxicity** may increase when loop diuretics are also given, as these agents interfere with salicylate excretion.   **Warfarin anticoagulant activity** may be enhanced by loop diuretics because these drugs can displace warfarin from plasma protein binding sites and increase the concentration of free, active anticoagulant.

## ❦ NURSING CONSIDERATIONS

**Side effects, toxicities, and associated nursing actions**

**Renal** Excessive diuresis may lead to dehydration and electrolyte imbalance.

**GI** Nausea, vomiting, and diarrhea may occur. Excessive diarrhea may signal a dangerous effect that requires discontinuing the diuretic.

- Monitor serum electrolytes and arterial blood gases, intake and output, and weight. Weigh patients under standard conditions.
- Monitor for hypokalemia (serum potassium less than 3.5 mEq/L). Signs and symptoms include vomiting, leg cramps, muscle weakness, apathy, abdominal distention, paralytic ileus, and electrocardiogram (ECG) changes such as sagging S-T segments, depressed T waves, and elevated V waves.
- Monitor for hyponatremia (serum sodium level below 135 mEq/L). Signs and symptoms include muscle weakness, leg cramps, irritability or confusion, lethargy, headache, hypotension, nausea, vomiting, and abdominal discomfort.
- Monitor for hypocalcemia (serum calcium level below 4.3 mEq/L). Signs and symptoms include tingling of the fingers, toes, nose, and ears, muscle spasms (tetany), and convulsions.
- Monitor for metabolic acidosis (arterial pH below 7.35). Signs and symptoms include headache, mental dullness, rapid and deep respirations, stupor, coma, and eventually death.
- Monitor for metabolic alkalosis (arterial pH above 7.45). Signs and symptoms include mental confusion, dizziness, tetany, and convulsions. When a result of diuretic therapy it is often related to potassium loss, and the symptoms are similar to hypokalemia.
- Monitor for hypochloremic alkalosis (serum chloride below 95 mEq/L with an associated arterial pH above 7.45) caused by prolonged vomiting, excessive nasogastric suctioning or drainage, or diuretic therapy. Symptoms are those of metabolic alkalosis.
- Monitor blood pressure.
- Assess for dehydration. Symptoms include thirst, decreased skin turgor, nausea, lightheadedness, weakness, increased pulse, oliguria, decreased blood pressure, elevated hemoglobin level, hematocrit, and blood urea nitrogen (BUN).
- Dehydration and hypovolemia can contribute to thromboembolic disorders. Observe for chest pain, shortness of breath, and pain in the calves or pelvis, which might indicate thromboembolism.

**Blood** Various blood dyscrasias have been reported.
- Monitor CBC and platelet count.
- Obtain physical assessment and history before starting therapy.
- Assess for petechiae, bruising, unexplained bleeding, fever, and sore throat.

**Ototoxicity** Ringing in the ears (tinnitus) or a sensation of fullness in the ears may signal the onset of permanent damage with hearing loss.
- Obtain a baseline assessment of hearing before starting therapy.
- Assess for tinnitus (ringing in the ears), reduced hearing acuity, and vertigo.

**CNS** Headaches, dizziness, blurred vision, and paresthesias may occur.
- Assess for the development of side effects.
- Instruct patients to avoid driving or operating hazardous equipment if dizziness or blurred vision develop; notify the physician.

**Allergic** Rashes and other allergic signs may develop, especially in patients with reported allergies to sulfonamides, drugs that are chemically related to the loop diuretics.
- Question the patient about a history of allergy to other medications before starting therapy.
- Observe for the development of allergic response.

**Metabolic** Alteration in glucose metabolism may occur with loop diuretics.
- Monitor blood glucose. Be especially vigilant with diabetic patients.
- Instruct diabetic patients to monitor blood glucose levels frequently, especially during periods of drug dosage adjustment, as a change in diet or dose of hypoglycemic agent may be necessary.

### Patient and family education
- Review with the patients the expected effects and possible side effects of the medication. Instruct patients to report the appearance of any unexpected sign or symptom.
- Instruct patients to report the appearance of any unexpected bruising or bleeding (signs of thrombocytopenia) or fever, rash, or sore throat (signs of agranulocytosis).
- Instruct patients to avoid the use of alcohol, which may potentiate hypotension.
- If postural hypotension occurs, caution patients to move slowly from lying to sitting or standing. Hypotension is more common in the elderly.

- If a potassium supplement is prescribed, teach the patient the importance of taking it as ordered. Dietary sources of potassium include citrus fruits and juices; grape, cranberry, apple, pear, and apricot juices; bananas; meat, fish, and fowl; cereals; and tea and cola beverages. Some patients with borderline low potassium levels can maintain potassium levels by increasing their daily intake of potassium-rich foods. Note that some potassium-rich foods are also high in sodium and may be contraindicated on that basis. Teach patients not to make dietary adjustments unless directed to do so; for some patients too much potassium could be harmful.
- Poor patient compliance is sometimes a result of annoyance with frequent and excessive urination. If a diuretic is ordered once a day, it should be taken in the morning to prevent interruption of sleep for urination. A twice-daily dose could be taken at 8 AM and 2 PM for the same reason; consult with physician.
- Instruct patients that diuretics work best when taken as ordered. Patients should not double up if a dose is missed.
- Note the drug interactions previously described. Instruct patients to keep all health care providers informed of all medications being taken. Other drugs may also cause hypotension, electrolyte imbalance, or other side effects and may contribute to the development of severe side effects in the patient.
- Photosensitivity may occur. Instruct patients to avoid prolonged exposure to the sun, to wear a hat and long-sleeved clothing if sensitivity occurs, and to use maximum protection sunscreens.
- Instruct diabetic patients to monitor blood glucose levels carefully, especially at the initiation or cessation of therapy or during periods of dosage adjustment. An adjustment of insulin or oral hypoglycemic agent may be necessary.
- Losing weight to reach ideal body weight, stopping smoking, engaging in regular exercise, and modifying the diet may be appropriate in individualized treatment of heart disease, hypertension, liver disease, or renal disease. After developing an individualized plan of care for the patient, refer the patient to the dietitian, visiting nurse, or other members of the health care team as needed.
- Instruct patients to notify physician if they develop vomiting or diarrhea that lasts longer than a day, as electrolyte imbalances may develop that may be compounded by diuretic use.
- Remind patients to keep these and all medications out of the reach of children.
- Teach patients to store medications away from heat and direct light and to avoid storing them in the bathroom, where heat and moisture may cause drugs to break down.
- Nurses need to be aware that these drugs may be abused by persons seeking rapid weight loss.

## bumetanide  (byoo-MET-a-nide)                    diuretic antihypertensive

- bumetanide: Bumex

**MECHANISM OF ACTION**    Bumetanide inhibits reabsorption of chloride and sodium ion in the ascending limb of Henle's loop, causing the increased excretion of salt with associated body water. Excretion of potassium ion is also increased, but excretion of lithium and uric acid is blocked.

**INDICATIONS**    **Edema caused by congestive heart failure** Bumetanide not only reduces the edema but also relieves some of the associated symptoms such as pulmonary distress, enlarged liver (hepatomegaly), high blood pressure, and rapid heart rate.    **Edema caused by hepatic disease** Bumetanide is useful in controlling edema and ascites associated with cirrhosis, but care must be taken to prevent hypokalemia (low blood potassium).    **Edema caused by renal disease** Bumetanide reduces fluid accumulation in renal insufficiency and may be used in nephrotic syndrome.    **Hypertension** Bumetanide may be used alone or in combination with other antihypertensive medications but is most useful in patients with a degree of renal insufficiency.

**CONTRAINDICATIONS**    **Anuria** Bumetanide is effective during renal insufficiency but should not be administered when renal function has virtually ceased.    **Severe hepatic disease** If hepatic function is too severely impaired, the profound dehydration and electrolyte disturbances produced by bumetanide may induce hepatic coma. **Allergy to sulfonamides** Bumetanide is chemically related to sulfonamide antibacterial agents and may be cross-allergenic.

**DOSAGE**    **Adult:**    **PO:** 0.5 to 2 mg daily as a single dose or divided into two equal doses administered morning and evening.    **IV, IM:** 0.5 to 1 mg initially, followed by repeated doses as necessary each 2 to 3 hours. Maximum daily dose is 10 mg.    *Special patient populations:*    **CHILDREN:** Doses not established.    **PREGNANCY:** FDA pregnancy category C.

**PREPARATIONS**    *Tablets:* 0.5 and 1 mg, scored; *solution for injection:* 0.25 mg/ml with 1% benzyl alcohol as a preservative.

**DRUG INTERACTIONS**    • See entry for drug class (p. 146).

**DIAGNOSTIC TEST INTERFERENCE**    Serum bilirubin, LDH, SGOT (AST), SGPT (ALT), and alkaline phosphatase may be elevated by bumetanide.

**FATE**    The *bioavailability* of bumetanide is high, with rapid and almost complete absorption following oral administration. The *onset* of action occurs within 0.5 to 1 hour following oral doses, 40 minutes following IM doses, and almost immediately following IV doses. The *peak* plasma concentration of the drug occurs within 0.5 to 2 hours following oral administration and *peak* effect is observed between 1 and 2 hours. With IM administration, peak effect also occurs between 1 and 2 hours. With IV doses, *peak* effects occur within 1 hour. The *duration* of action is about 4 hours with oral or IM administration of 1 to 2 mg of bumetanide. Diuresis persists longer with higher doses. IV administration results in a duration of about 2 to 3 hours. Bumetanide is partially metabolized in the liver. Metabolites of bumetanide are excreted in the feces via the bile, but most of the unchanged drug and metabolites are excreted in urine. The *half-life* for elimination in healthy adults is 1 to 1.5 hours.

## 🐾 NURSING CONSIDERATIONS

### Side effects, toxicities, and associated nursing actions    See entry for drug class (p. 146).

**Renal** Excessive diuresis may lead to dehydration and electrolyte imbalance.

**GI** Nausea, vomiting, stomach and intestinal discomfort, and diarrhea are possible but are reported by only about 1% of treated patients.

**CV** Bumetanide may cause orthostatic hypotension if combined with other hypotensive agents. Occasional patients show ECG changes and chest pain.
- Monitor arterial blood gases and renal function studies, including BUN and creatinine.
- Monitor intake and output and weight. Weigh patients under standard conditions.
- Monitor ECG.
- Monitor for electrolyte imbalances: see entry for drug class (p. 147).
- Monitor blood pressure and pulse every 4 hours. It may be necessary to monitor blood pressure with patient in lying, sitting, and standing positions and in both arms.

**Blood** Bumetanide is associated with blood dyscrasias such as alterations in hemoglobin concentration, prothrombin time, hematocrit, and leukocyte numbers or differential counts. Although these effects are rare (less than 1%) and usually transient, a few serious reactions and one fatality have been reported.
- Monitor CBC and platelet count, hematocrit and hemoglobin, and prothrombin time.
- See entry for drug class (p. 147).

**Ototoxicity** Bumetanide seems less likely to cause this reaction than other loop diuretics because of the high diuretic potency of bumetanide. At the lower doses used in oral therapy the incidence is about 1%; higher doses cause ototoxicity in up to 6.4% of patients.
- Assess hearing before starting therapy.
- Assess for tinnitus (ringing in the ears), reduced hearing acuity, and vertigo.

**CNS** Headaches, dizziness, weakness, and fatigue have been reported in 1% of treated patients.
- Assess for the development of side effects.

**Allergic** Urticaria and rash are rarely reported. One patient suffered a Stevens-Johnson reaction.
- Question patients about history of allergy to other medications before starting therapy.
- Observe for the development of allergic response: rash or fever. Symptoms of Stevens-Johnson syndrome include stomatitis with ulcerations of the oral mucosa, high fever, and erythematous skin eruptions.

**Metabolic** Hyperglycemia occurs in about 7% of treated patients. Glycosuria, proteinuria, and decreased glucose tolerance are more rare.
• Monitor blood glucose. Be especially vigilant with diabetic patients.
**Liver** Bumetanide alters liver function tests and may cause encephalopathy in patients with pre-existing liver disease.
• Monitor liver function studies (see Diagnostic Test Interference).
• Obtain mental status examination before beginning therapy, and monitor regularly if liver disease is present.
**Muscle** Musculoskeletal pain is reported by a few patients receiving bumetanide. The pain begins about 4 hours after an oral dose and may persist 6 to 12 hours.
• Forewarn patients about this side effect.

### Nursing interventions related to drug administration
• Parenteral bumetanide may be administered intravenously or intramuscularly.
• Visually inspect solution before administering. If it is discolored or contains particulate matter, discard.
• For IV injection, administer dose over 1 to 2 minutes.
• For IV infusion, dilute drug in 5% dextrose, 0.9% sodium chloride, or lactated Ringer's solution. Administer within 24 hours.
• Following intravenous administration, monitor blood pressure every 15 to 30 minutes until stable. Keep side rails up, and supervise ambulation.

### Patient and family education
• See entry for drug class (p. 147).
• Review with the patients the expected effects and possible side effects of the medication. Instruct patients to report the appearance of any unexpected sign or symptom.

---

## ethacrynic acid    (eth-a-KRI-nik)                                        diuretic

• ethacrynic acid (ethacrynate sodium): Edecrin

**MECHANISM OF ACTION**    Ethacrynic acid inhibits reabsorption of chloride and sodium in the ascending limb of Henle's loop, causing the increased excretion of salt with associated body water. Excretion of potassium ion is also increased, but excretion of lithium and uric acid is blocked.

**INDICATIONS**    **Edema caused by congestive heart failure** Ethacrynic acid relieves peripheral and pulmonary edema and thereby improves cardiac function.    **Edema caused by hepatic disease** This condition is relatively refractory to therapy with ethacrynic acid.    **Edema caused by renal disease** Ethacrynic acid reduces fluid accumulation in renal insufficiency and may be used in nephrotic syndrome. Low protein concentrations in these patients may impair the action of ethacrynic acid.    **Edema caused by malignancies** Ascites may be temporarily and partially controlled with ethacrynic acid.    **Hypertensive crises** Intravenous ethacrynic acid may be used in conjunction with other drugs to control acute hypertensive attacks.

**CONTRAINDICATIONS**    **Anuria** Ethacrynic acid should not be used in patients with anuria. If patients receiving the drug develop azotemia, oliguria, or electrolyte imbalances, therapy should be discontinued.    **Electrolyte imbalances** Ethacrynic acid will contribute to dangerous progression of imbalances in patients with metabolic alkalosis and hypokalemia or in dehydrated patients with low serum sodium concentrations.    **Hypotension** The hypotensive effects of ethacrynic acid will add to the existing problem and may dangerously lower blood pressure.    **Severe hepatic disease** Ethacrynic acid may control edema in patients with hepatic disease, but in advanced disease the drug may dangerously depress hepatic function. The result may be hepatic coma and death.    **Lupus erythematosus** This autoimmune disease may be activated by ethacrynic acid.

**DOSAGE**    **PO:**    **ADULT:** Initial dosage is 50 mg once a day following a meal. Dosage is increased in increments of 25 to 50 mg daily to achieve desired clinical effects. Maintenance dosages range from 50 to 200 mg daily, usually administered twice daily after meals. Daily doses should not exceed 400 mg.    **CHILDREN:** Initial doses of 25 mg may be used cautiously and increased in 25 mg increments to achieve desired clinical effects.   **IV:**   **ADULT ONLY:** 50 mg, or 0.5 to 1 mg/kg, is the usual dose. Up to 100 mg may be administered if required. The dose may be repeated if necessary in 2 to 4 hours, but a new site may be required to prevent thrombophlebitis.   *Special patient populations:*   **ELDERLY:** Elderly patients are more sensitive to ethacrynic acid than younger adults; dangerous dehydration may result. Geriatric patients require smaller doses and more gradual adjustment of dose.   **CHILDREN:** IV doses are not recommended for children, although PO use of the drug is possible (see under PO). Infants should not receive ethacrynic acid.   **PREGNANCY AND LACTATION:** Ethacrynic acid causes fetal abnormalities in animals and is not recommended for use in pregnant patients or nursing mothers.

**PREPARATIONS**   **Ethacrynic acid** *Tablets:* 25 and 50 mg, scored.   **Ethacrynate sodium** *Solution for injection:* 50 mg equivalent of ethacrynic acid with mannitol and thimerosal. Solutions that are not clear should not be used; reconstituted solutions should be discarded after 24 hours at room temperature.

**DRUG INTERACTIONS**   Ethacrynic acid is subject to the same interactions as other members of the class (see entry for drug class, p. 146). In addition, the following interaction may be important. **Hypoglycemic drugs** such as insulin and the oral agents may be less effective when patients are hypokalemic. Because ethacrynic acid tends to deplete potassium, the diuretic may interfere with the hypoglycemic action of these drugs.

**FATE**   The *bioavailability* of ethacrynic acid is high; doses are rapidly absorbed from the GI tract. The *peak* effect of an oral dose occurs at about 2 hours, with a *duration* of about 6 to 8 hours. IV administration gives a *peak* effect in 15 to 30 minutes and a *duration* of action of about 2 hours. Ethacrynic acid is partially metabolized by the liver, and 40% of a dose is excreted in bile. Up to 60% is secreted in the proximal tubule in the kidney.

## ☙ NURSING CONSIDERATIONS

### Side effects, toxicities, and associated nursing actions   See entry for loop diuretics (p. 146).

**Renal** Excessive diuresis may lead to dehydration and electrolyte imbalance.

**GI** Anorexia, nausea, vomiting, and GI discomfort may occur, especially with large doses or when doses must be continued over long periods of time. Severe watery diarrhea is cause to permanently discontinue the drug. GI bleeding has also occurred.

**CV** Ethacrynic acid may cause orthostatic hypotension or acute hypotensive episodes.
- Monitor arterial blood gases and renal function studies including BUN and creatinine.
- Monitor intake and output and weight. Weigh patients under standard conditions.
- Monitor ECG.
- Monitor serum electrolytes: see entry for drug class (p. 147).
- Monitor blood pressure and pulse every 4 hours. It may be necessary to monitor blood pressure with patient in lying, sitting, and standing positions and in both arms.

**Blood** Ethacrynic acid may cause blood dyscrasias, especially in severely ill patients. Hematuria is sometimes observed. When given by IV, ethacrynic acid may cause thrombophlebitis.
- Monitor CBC and platelet count, hematocrit, and hemoglobin, and perform urinalysis.
- Inspect IV sites for signs of thrombophlebitis: redness, pain, or increased warmth.

**Ototoxicity** Vertigo, tinnitus, a feeling of fullness in the ears, and hearing loss may occur. Ototoxicity is most likely with sodium ethacrynate administered IV to severely ill patients.
- Obtain baseline assessment of hearing before starting therapy.
- Assess for tinnitus (ringing in the ears), reduced hearing acuity, and vertigo.

**CNS** Confusion, apprehension, and headache may signal CNS effects.
- Assess for the development of side effects.
- Instruct patients to avoid driving or operating hazardous equipment if confusion develops.

**Allergic** Rash, fever, and chills are sometimes reported.
- Question patients about history of allergy to other medications before starting therapy.
- Observe for the development of an allergic response.

**Metabolic** Glucose metabolism may be altered by ethacrynic acid, especially at high doses. Glycosuria and hyperglycemia can result.
- Monitor blood glucose. Be especially vigilant with diabetic patients.

**Liver** Ethacrynic acid may precipitate hepatic coma and death in severely ill patients with pre-existing liver disease.

- Monitor liver function studies.
- Obtain mental status examination before beginning therapy, and monitor regularly if liver disease is present.

### Nursing interventions related to drug administration

- Ethacrynate sodium should not be given intramuscularly or subcutaneously.
- Visually inspect solution before administering. If it is discolored or contains particulate matter, discard.
- The usual dilution is 50 mg of ethacrynate sodium in 50 ml of 5% dextrose in water or sodium chloride injection.
- A single dose should not exceed 100 mg (100 ml).
- The drug may be administered by direct intravenous injection or by continuous infusion. Do not mix with other medications, do not add to intravenous solutions, and do not mix with blood or its derivatives.
- The rate of administration should not exceed 10 mg (10 ml) per minute.
- Check the infusion site carefully; thrombophlebitis is common, and extravasation causes pain and tissue irritation.
- Following intravenous administration, monitor blood pressure every 15 to 30 minutes until stable. Keep side rails up, and supervise ambulation.

### Patient and family education

- See entry for drug class (p. 147).
- Review with the patients the expected effects and possible side effects of the medication. Instruct patients to report the appearance of any unexpected sign or symptom.

---

## furosemide   (fyoo-ROH-se-mide)                                    diuretic antihypertensive

- furosemide: ✤Furoside, Lasix, Neo-Renal, ✤Novosemide, ✤Uritol

**MECHANISM OF ACTION**   Furosemide inhibits reabsorption of chloride and sodium in the ascending limb of Henle's loop, causing the increased excretion of salt with associated body water. Excretion of potassium ion is also increased, but excretion of lithium and uric acid is blocked.

**INDICATIONS**   **Edema caused by congestive heart failure** Furosemide relieves peripheral and pulmonary edema and thereby improves cardiac function.   **Edema caused by hepatic disease** This condition is relatively refractory to therapy with furosemide.   **Edema caused by renal disease** Furosemide reduces fluid accumulation in renal insufficiency and may be used in nephrotic syndrome.   **Hypertension** Intravenous furosemide may be used in conjunction with other drugs to control acute hypertensive attacks. In stepped care of chronic hypertension, furosemide is occasionally added along with other agents for a short time or substituted for a thiazide in patients with renal insufficiency.

**CONTRAINDICATIONS**   **Anuria** Furosemide should not be used in patients with anuria. If patients receiving the drug develop azotemia, oliguria or electrolyte imbalances, therapy should be discontinued. **Electrolyte imbalances** Furosemide will contribute to dangerous progression of imbalances.   **Hypotension** The hypotensive effects of furosemide will add to the existing problem and may dangerously lower blood pressure.   **Lupus erythematosus** This autoimmune disease may be activated by furosemide.

**DOSAGE**   **PO:**   **ADULTS:** For edema, initial dosage is 20 to 80 mg, once in the morning. Dosage is increased in increments of 20 to 40 mg at 6 to 8 hour intervals to achieve desired clinical effects. Maintenance dosages up to 600 mg daily may be required. As an antihypertensive, dosage is 40 mg twice daily. Higher doses are usually avoided.   **CHILDREN:** For edema, initial doses of 2 mg/kg as a single dose may be used. If required, doses may be increased in increments of 1 to 2 mg/kg every 6 to 8 hours to achieve desired clinical effects. The maximum daily dose for children is 6 mg/kg.   **IM, IV:**   **ADULT:** For edema, 20 to 40 mg as a single injection is the usual dose. The dose may be repeated if necessary in 2 hours with increases of 20 mg until desired effects are achieved. After dosage adjustment, doses are usually given once or twice daily. For acute pulmonary edema, IV doses of 40 mg initially may be followed with 80 mg 1 hour later if required. For acute hypertensive crises, doses of 100 to 200 mg IV have been used. **CHILDREN:** For acute pulmonary edema, doses are 1 mg/kg; subsequent doses may be increased by 1 mg/kg at 2 hour intervals. Daily doses should not exceed 6 mg/kg. *Special patient populations:* **ELDERLY:** Elderly patients are more sensitive to furosemide than younger adults; dangerous dehydration may result. Geriatric patients require smaller doses and more gradual adjustment of dose. **PREGNANCY AND LACTATION:** FDA pregnancy category C. Furosemide is not recommended for use in nursing mothers.

**PREPARATIONS** *Tablets:* 20, 40 (scored) and 80 mg; *solution for oral use:* 10 mg/ml, containing 11.5% alcohol and sorbitol; *solution for injection:* 10 mg/ml. The solution for oral use should be refrigerated, but not frozen, and protected from light. The solution for parenteral use may be stored at room temperature but should be protected from light. Discard the solution if it is yellow. Solutions should be used within 24 hours of preparation.

**DRUG INTERACTIONS** Furosemide is subject to the same interactions as other members of the class. See entry for drug class (p. 146). In addition, the following interactions may be important. **Antihypertensive agents (peripheral adrenergic blocking agents or ganglionic blocking drugs)** are potentiated by the action of furosemide. This interaction can be exploited therapeutically when furosemide is used in combinations with other drugs for increased control of hypertension. **Hypoglycemic drugs such as insulin and the oral agents** may be less effective when patients are hypokalemic. Because furosemide tends to deplete potassium, the diuretic may interfere with the hypoglycemic action of these drugs. **Chloral hydrate followed by IV furosemide** can cause hot flashes, diaphoresis, and acute blood pressure changes. **Clofibrate** may increase the likelihood of muscular pain and stiffness with furosemide.

**FATE** Furosemide is rapidly absorbed from the GI tract, but only about 60% of an oral dose reaches the blood. The *onset* of action after oral doses is 30 minutes with *peak* effects at 1 to 2 hours. The *duration* of action is about 2 hours. IM doses show similar onset, peak, and duration as oral doses; IV doses have a slightly more rapid onset. Furosemide is partially metabolized by the liver. About 50% of a dose is excreted in the kidney, with the rest being eliminated in the feces or by liver mechanisms.

## ☙ NURSING CONSIDERATIONS

### Side effects, toxicities, and associated nursing actions  See entry for drug class (p. 146).

**Renal** Excessive diuresis may lead to dehydration and electrolyte imbalance.

**GI** Anorexia, nausea, vomiting, and GI discomfort may occur. The sorbitol content of solutions for oral use may contribute to diarrhea, especially in children receiving large doses.

**CV** Furosemide may cause orthostatic hypotension or acute hypotensive episodes.

- Monitor arterial blood gases and renal function studies, including BUN and creatinine.
- Monitor intake and output and weight. Weigh patients under standard conditions.
- Monitor ECG.
- Monitor serum electrolytes: see entry for drug class (p. 147).
- Monitor blood pressure and pulse every 4 hours. It may be necessary to monitor blood pressure with patient in lying, sitting, and standing positions and in both arms.

**Blood** Various blood dyscrasias may occur. Thrombophlebitis can occur after IV administration.

- Monitor CBC and platelet count, hematocrit, and hemoglobin.
- Inspect IV site for signs of thrombophlebitis: redness, pain, increased warmth.

**Ototoxicity** Vertigo, tinnitus, a feeling of fullness in the ears, and hearing loss may occur. Ototoxicity is most likely with rapid administration of large parenteral doses.

- Obtain a baseline assessment of hearing before starting therapy.
- Assess for tinnitus (ringing in the ears), reduced hearing acuity, and vertigo.

**CNS** Confusion, apprehension, blurred vision, vertigo, and headache may signal CNS effects.

- Assess for the development of side effects.
- Instruct patients to avoid driving or operating hazardous equipment if blurred vision or vertigo develop; notify the physician.

**Allergic** Rash, photosensitivity, pruritis, and erythema multiforme have occurred. Patients allergic to sulfonamides are also likely to react to furosemide.

- Question patients about a history of allergy to other medications before starting therapy.

- Observe for the development of allergic response.

**Metabolic** Glucose metabolism may be altered by furosemide, especially at high doses. Glycosuria and hyperglycemia can result.

- Monitor blood glucose. Be especially vigilant with diabetic patients.

**Liver** Hepatic impairment can occur.

- Monitor liver function studies.
- Obtain mental status examination before beginning therapy, and monitor regularly if liver disease is present.

### Nursing interventions related to drug administration

- Furosemide is incompatible with acidic solutions, but it will mix with isotonic solutions, 5% dextrose in water, and lactated Ringer's solution. If in doubt, consult the pharmacy; flush tubing before administering intravenously.
- Visually inspect solution before administering; if it is discolored, discard.
- For IV injection, administer undiluted at a rate not to exceed 20 mg over a 2-minute period.
- Do not mix with other medications in a syringe.
- Following intravenous administration, monitor blood pressure every 15 to 30 minutes until stable. Keep side rails up, and supervise ambulation.
- Intramuscular injection may produce transient pain at the injection site.

### Patient and family education

- See entry for drug class (p. 147).
- Review with the patients the expected effects and possible side effects of the medication. Instruct patients to report the appearance of any unexpected sign or symptom.
- Instruct patients receiving oral solution to store solution in refrigerator.

---

# Osmotic diuretics

mannitol ~ urea

**OVERVIEW OF THE DRUG CLASS**  Osmotic diuretics are used to manipulate fluid distribution in various ways in the body. They are used to maintain urine volume and protect the kidneys from permanent damage during acute renal failure. These agents are also used to increase the osmolality of plasma, which reduces osmotic pressure inside the eye and central nervous system.

**MECHANISM OF ACTION**  Osmotic diuretics are nonelectrolytes that are filtered by the glomerulus in the kidney but are not significantly reabsorbed or metabolized; therefore the osmotic diuretics are highly concentrated in renal tubular fluid. In the tubule the high osmolality, which is determined by the concentration of solutes, reduces the reabsorption of water, causing urine production to increase. Sodium excretion is usually not increased. Secondly, by increasing the osmolality of plasma, water is forced to move from spaces inaccessible to the osmotic diuretics into the plasma. As a result, osmotic pressure is reduced in the eye and central nervous system as water moves into the blood compartment.

**INDICATIONS**  **Oliguric acute renal failure** Extensive trauma with hemorrhage and shock can cause acute renal failure. Burns and transfusion reactions can also cause the kidneys to acutely fail. Osmotic diuretics maintain urine flow and prevent renal tubular necrosis under these conditions.  **Cerebral edema** Swelling of the brain occurs following trauma or neurosurgery, as well as during diabetic coma or ketoacidosis. The resulting increase in intracranial pressure can be damaging or even fatal. Osmotic diuretics remove water from the brain compartment and move it to the plasma compartment, relieving the pressure inside the skull.  **Increased intraocular pressure** Osmotic diuretics lower pressure inside the eye by moving water to the plasma compartment from the eye. This action is helpful as preparation for eye surgery or in controlling acute episodes of glaucoma, a disease that elevates intraocular pressure.

**CONTRAINDICATIONS**  **Anuria** Osmotic diuretics can produce circulatory overload if renal failure has progressed to tubular necrosis and anuria.  **Dehydration** Osmotic diuretics can facilitate water loss and tissue dehydration. Patients should be adequately hydrated before these agents are administered.

**Severe pulmonary congestion or edema** Osmotic diuretics can worsen the condition of patients suffering from pulmonary congestion or edema caused by congestive heart failure. These diuretics expand the extracellular fluid volume and may increase the workload of the heart.    **Intracranial bleeding** Active bleeding may be intensified by osmotic diuretics.

**DRUG INTERACTIONS**    Few drug interactions have been reported with osmotic diuretics.

## ❦ NURSING CONSIDERATIONS

### Side effects, toxicities, and associated nursing actions

**CV** Osmotic diuretics can cause overexpansion of extracellular fluid volume, producing circulatory overload. Pulmonary congestion, chest pain, and rapid heart beat may indicate congestive heart failure.

* Monitor vital signs and blood pressure, intake and output, and daily weight.
* Assess breath and heart sounds on a regular basis.
* Assess for signs of pulmonary congestion and/or congestive heart failure: dyspnea, labored respirations, tachypnea and tachycardia, distended neck veins, rales, agitation, fluid retention, and weight gain.
* Determine with physician desired daily fluid balance. Infusion rate may be titrated to output. Oral fluids may or may not be permitted. Occasional ice chips may be permitted to help patient relieve thirst.

**Renal** Electrolyte imbalances can occur, as can dehydration. A few patients suffer direct renal damage.

**CNS** Acidosis and possible acute renal failure may alter the permeability of the blood-brain barrier so that osmotic diuretics can enter the brain and cause excessive dehydration. Brain damage and death have resulted.

* Monitor intake and output every 2 hours and weight daily. If urine output is less than 30 to 50 ml/hour or weight gain in excess of 3 lb/day occurs, notify the physician.
* Monitor serum and urine electrolytes, blood urea nitrogen (BUN), serum creatinine, arterial blood gases, and central venous pressure.
* Assess for hyponatremia (serum sodium level below 135 mEq/L). Signs and symptoms include muscle weakness, leg cramps, irritability or confusion, lethargy, headache, hypotension, nausea, vomiting, and abdominal discomfort.
* Assess for hypernatremia (serum sodium level above 145 mEq/L). Signs and symptoms include restlessness; thirst; flushed, dry skin and mucous membranes; tachycardia; fluid retention and weight gain.
* Assess for hypokalemia (serum potassium below 3.5 mEq/L). Signs and symptoms include vomiting, leg cramps, muscle weakness, apathy, abdominal distention, paralytic ileus, and electrocardiogram (ECG) changes such as sagging S-T segments, depressed T waves, and elevated U waves.
* Assess for hyperkalemia (serum potassium above 5.0 mEq/L). Signs and symptoms include weakness, spasticity, flaccid paralysis (late signs), nausea, colic, diarrhea, oliguria, and ECG changes such as tall, tent-shaped T waves, and later, atrial asystole, widening of the QRS, and irregular ventricular rhythms.
* Assess for metabolic acidosis (arterial pH below 7.35). Signs and symptoms include headache, mental dullness, rapid and deep respirations, stupor, coma, and eventually death.
* Monitor neurologic status regularly.

**Skin** If allowed to extravasate, osmotic diuretics cause local skin and tissue damage.

* Before instituting infusion, ascertain that IV infusion is secure and patent, with no signs of redness or infiltration, and that rate of flow is not sluggish.
* Inspect infusion site regularly.
* If infiltration is suspected, discontinue infusion and restart in another site.

### Patient and family education

* Review expected effects and possible side effects with patient and family.
* Keep the patient and family informed of changes in the patient's condition.

## mannitol  (MAN-i-tole)                                     osmotic diuretic

- mannitol: Mannitol, Osmitrol, Resectisol

**MECHANISM OF ACTION**   Mannitol, like other osmotic diuretics, increases water excretion. Sodium excretion is usually not increased, although sodium and lithium excretion can increase under certain conditions. See entry for drug class (p. 154).

**INDICATIONS**   **Oliguric acute renal failure** Mannitol can be used to maintain urine flow and prevent renal tubular necrosis following extensive trauma, hemorrhage, shock, burns, or transfusion reactions. **Cerebral edema** Mannitol osmotically removes water from the brain compartment and moves it to the plasma compartment, relieving dangerous increases of pressure inside the skull during cerebral edema. Swelling of the brain occurs following trauma or neurosurgery, as well as during diabetic coma or ketoacidosis.   **Increased intraocular pressure** Mannitol lowers intraocular pressure by moving water from the eye to the plasma compartment. This action is helpful as preparation for eye surgery or in controlling acute episodes of glaucoma, which elevates intraocular pressure.   **Detoxification following poisoning with renally excreted drugs** Mannitol is often combined with other diuretics to assist urinary elimination of salicylates (e.g., aspirin), imipramine, bromides, or some barbiturates. Alone, mannitol increases excretion of lithium, an action unlike other diuretics.   **Irrigation during transurethral prostatic resection** Mannitol solutions prevent hemolysis, which can occur when water is used for irrigation during this surgical procedure.   **Diagnostic aid to determine glomerular filtration rate (GFR)** Mannitol is freely filtered by the glomerulus but is not significantly reabsorbed; the excretion rate of mannitol therefore gives an estimate of GFR.

**CONTRAINDICATIONS**   • See entry for drug class (p. 154).

**DOSAGE**   **For oliguric renal failure:**   IV:   *Adults:* Before therapy is started, patients with suspected renal failure should receive a test dose of 12.5 g (0.2 g/kg) given as an infusion with a 15% or 20% solution over 3 to 4 minutes. If the patient produces at least 30 to 50 ml of urine each hour over the next 2 or 3 hours, mannitol therapy can be started. To prevent oliguria or acute renal failure, 50 to 100 g as a 5% to 25% solution is administered at a rate sufficient to cause production of 30 to 50 ml of urine hourly. Maximum daily doses should not exceed 6 g/kg.   *Children:* 2 g/kg or 60 g/$M^2$ of body surface as a 15% to 20% solution, given over 2 to 6 hours.   **For cerebral edema or glaucoma (systemic osmotic agent):**   IV:   *Adults:* 1 to 2 g/kg body weight as a 15% to 25% solution, administered over 30 to 60 minutes. Small or debilitated patients may require only 500 mg/kg. Maximum daily doses should not exceed 6 mg/kg.   *Children:* 1 to 2 g/kg body weight or 30 to 60 g/$M^2$ body surface as a 15% to 20% solution administered over 30 to 60 minutes. Small or debilitated patients may require only 500 mg/kg.   **For detoxification of renally excreted drugs:**   IV:   *Adults:* 50 to 200 g as a 5% to 25% solution, administered at a rate that will produce 100 to 500 ml of urine per hour.   *Children:* Up to 2 g/kg body weight or 60 g/$M^2$ body surface as a 5% to 10% solution.   **For irrigation in transurethral resection:**   ADULTS: 3.5% to 5% mannitol solutions are used for irrigating.   **For determination of GFR:**   ADULTS: 100 ml of a 20% solution (equivalent to 20 g) is diluted with 180 ml of sodium chloride injection; the resulting 7.2% mannitol solution is infused at 20 ml/min.   *Special patient populations:*   ELDERLY: Altered doses for the elderly have not been specifically established, but small or debilitated patients require lowered dosage.   PREGNANCY: Problems during pregnancy or breast-feeding have not been documented.

**PREPARATIONS**   *Solutions for injection:* 5%, 10%, 15%, 20%, or 25% solutions as mannitol injection or Osmitrol; *solution for irrigation:* 5% solution (Resectisol).

**DRUG INTERACTIONS**   **Lithium** excretion can be hastened by mannitol, possibly impairing therapeutic effects of lithium.

**FATE**   Mannitol is eliminated primarily by renal excretion; there is little metabolism of the drug. The *half-life* for elimination is about 100 minutes. Following IV administration, cerebrospinal and intraocular fluid pressure begins to fall within 15 minutes, whereas the onset of diuresis may be 1 to 3 hours. *Peak* reduction of intraocular pressure occurs within 30 to 60 minutes. The *duration* of fluid pressure reduction in the CNS and eye is up to 8 hours. Rebound increases in intracranial and intraocular pressure can occur 12 hours after therapy.

## ☙ NURSING CONSIDERATIONS
### Side effects, toxicities, and associated nursing actions
**CV** Mannitol can cause overexpansion of extracellular fluid volume, producing circulatory overload. Pulmonary congestion, chest pain, and rapid heartbeat may indicate congestive heart failure. Thrombophlebitis with redness, swelling, and pain at the injection site can occur.
- See entry for drug class (p. 155).
- Assess infusion site for redness and development of thrombophlebitis on regular basis (see Skin).

**Renal** Electrolyte imbalances can occur, as can dehydration. Signs include muscle cramps or pain, unusual tiredness, weakness, and heaviness of the legs. A few patients suffer direct renal damage.
**CNS** Acidosis and possible acute renal failure may alter permeability of the blood-brain barrier so that mannitol can enter the brain and cause excessive dehydration. Brain damage and death have resulted.
- See entry for drug class (p. 155).

**Skin** If allowed to extravasate, osmotic diuretics cause local skin and tissue damage.
- Before instituting infusion, ascertain that IV infusion is secure and patent, with no signs of redness or infiltration, and that rate of flow is not sluggish.
- Inspect infusion site regularly.
- If infiltration is suspected, discontinue infusion and restart in another site.

### Nursing interventions related to drug administration
- Before administering, check ampule or bottle for crystallization, a frequent problem. If crystals are present, warm the container under running water until crystals dissolve. Let cool to body temperature before administering.
- Dilution of mannitol before IV administration is not necessary. Mannitol should not be added to other intravenous solutions or medications or mixed with blood.
- The rate of intravenous administration is usually 1 to 2 g/kg over 30 to 90 minutes, but up to 3 g/kg has been given. See Dosage for other uses and dosages.
- An in-line filter should be used for intravenous administration.
- Read the order carefully. Mannitol comes in several concentrations. If in doubt, consult the physician.
- Do not confuse mannitol with mannitol hexanitrate, an antianginal drug.
- If blood must be administered concomitantly, 20 mEq of sodium chloride must be added to each liter of mannitol to prevent pseudoagglutination.

### Patient and family education
- Review expected effects and possible side effects with patient and family.
- Keep patient and family informed of changes in the patient's condition.
- Instruct patients to report the development of any unusual subjective complaint or feeling.

---

## urea   (yoo-REE-ah; KAR-ba-mide) osmotic diuretic

- urea (carbamide in Canada): Uremol, Urisec, Ureaphil, Velvelan

**MECHANISM OF ACTION**   Urea at high doses elevates the osmolality of plasma, causing shifts of water from tissues into extracellular fluid. This action is used to reduce intracranial and intraocular pressure. Urea is also concentrated in renal tubular fluid, causing water to be retained in the tubule and excreted as excess urine. Sodium, potassium, chloride, and lithium excretion is also increased by urea.

**INDICATIONS**   **Reduction of intracranial pressure** Urea osmotically removes water from the brain compartment, relieving dangerous increases in pressure from cerebral edema caused by surgery, trauma, disease, or drug intoxication.   **Reduction of intraocular pressure** Urea may reduce intraocular pressure when other means have failed. When indicated, urea can be useful in controlling pressure from acute glaucoma attacks or surgical trauma. Unlike mannitol, urea does penetrate the eye, which complicates the use of urea.   **Dermatologic conditions requiring a keratolytic agent** Creams and lotions containing urea are active and useful keratolytic preparations (Table 9-3).   **Abortifacient** Transabdominal intra-amniotic injection may be used to terminate a second-trimester pregnancy.

| Table 9-3. | Preparations of urea for topical use | | | |
|---|---|---|---|---|
| **Trade name** | **Form** | **Urea concentration (%)** | | **Other ingredients** |
| Alphaderm | Cream | 10 | | 1% hydrocortisone |
| Aquacare | Cream or lotion | 2, 10 | | — |
| Carmol 10 | Lotion | 10 | | — |
| Carmol 20 | Cream | 20 | | — |
| Carmol HC | Cream | 10 | | 1% hydrocortisone acetate |
| Nutraplus | Cream or lotion | 10 | | — |
| Rea-Lo | Cream | 30 | | — |
| | Lotion | 15 | | — |
| Ultra-Mide 25 | Lotion | 25 | | — |
| Ureacin | Cream | 20, 40 | | — |

**CONTRAINDICATIONS**   **Severe renal failure** Unless the kidneys can eliminate urea, the drug may accumulate and cause circulatory overload.   **Dehydration** Urea facilitates water loss and tissue dehydration. Patients should be hydrated before administering urea.   **Hepatic disease** Urea can be broken down into ammonia, which normally would be eliminated by the liver. When liver function is drastically impaired, ammonia may accumulate to dangerous levels in the blood.   **Intracranial bleeding** Active bleeding may be intensified by urea and is not used except in craniotomies.   **Cardiovascular impairment** Urea may expand the extracellular fluid volume and increase the work load of the heart. This action may precipitate or worsen congestive heart failure.   **Fructose intolerance caused by aldolase deficiency** These patients should not receive urea solutions that contain fructose.   **Ruptured amniotic membranes** Urea should not be used to induce abortion in these patients.   **Diabetes mellitus** Urea may increase risk of thrombosis.   **Sickle cell disease** Urea may increase the risk of hemolysis or thrombosis.

**DOSAGE**   **IV:**   **ADULTS:** Using a 30% solution, 0.5 to 1.5 g/kg is infused over 1 to 2.5 hours (4 to 6 ml/min). No more than 120 g should be given in 24 hours.   **CHILDREN OVER 2 YEARS:** 0.5 to 1.5 gm/kg body weight or 35 g/$M^2$ body surface area in 24 hours.   **CHILDREN YOUNGER THAN 2 YEARS:** 0.1 g/kg may suffice.   **Intra-amniotic:**   **ADULTS:** Remove up to 250 m amniotic fluid and replace with same amount of 40% to 60% urea solution (in 5% dextrose), all by transabdominal tap.   *Special patient populations:*   **PREGNANCY:** FDA pregnancy category C.

**PREPARATIONS**   *Crystals:* 40 g of crystals for reconstitution with appropriate diluent before use. Diluents commonly used are 5% or 10% dextrose or 10% invert sugar (fructose and dextrose) solutions. Because manufacturers differ, check the package insert for specific instructions for dilution. Solutions should be discarded after 24 hours and should not be used at all unless they are clear and colorless.

**DRUG INTERACTIONS**   **Lithium** excretion may be hastened by urea, reducing the therapeutic effects of lithium.

**FATE**   Urea is distributed into extracellular and intracellular fluids, entering blood, lymph, bile, CSF, aqueous humor, and amniotic fluid. The *onset* of pressure-lowering and diuretic effects occurs within 10 minutes, and the *peak* effects occur in 1 to 2 hours. The *duration* of these effects is usually 3 to 10 hours, although intraocular pressure may return to pretreatment values in 5 hours. Urea is excreted by the kidneys and hydrolyzed by bacterial enzymes in the gut. The *half-life* for elimination is 1.2 hours.

## ☙ NURSING CONSIDERATIONS
### Side effects, toxicities, and associated nursing actions
- See entry for drug class (p. 155).

**CV** Thrombophlebitis with redness, swelling, and pain at the injection site can occur. Thrombosis can occur in the legs, especially in the elderly. Occasionally irregular heart beats can arise.
* Assess infusion site for redness and development of thrombophlebitis on regular basis (see Skin).

**Renal** Urea can cause electrolyte imbalances such as hyponatremia and hypokalemia, as well as dehydration. Signs include muscle cramps or pain, unusual tiredness, weakness and heaviness of the legs.

**CNS** Nervousness and confusion have resulted from too rapid IV administration.

**Skin** If allowed to extravasate, urea causes local skin and tissue damage.

**Blood** Urea can cause hemolysis if administered too rapidly. Capillary bleeding can be increased.
* Before instituting infusion, ascertain that IV infusion is secure and patent, with no signs of redness or infiltration, and that rate of flow is not sluggish.
* Inspect infusion site regularly, and check infusion rate carefully.
* If infiltration is suspected, discontinue infusion and restart in another site.

**GI** Nausea and vomiting can occur.
* Warn patient of this possible side effect.
* If GI symptoms are severe or persist, notify the physician. It may be necessary to discontinue medication.

**Nursing interventions related to drug administration**
* Urea must be diluted to make a 30% solution (30% solution equals 30 g of urea per 100 ml or 300 mg/1 ml). Dilution may be done with 5% or 10% dextrose in water or with 10% invert sugar in water; some manufacturers supply the diluent. Patients with hereditary fructose intolerance (aldolase deficiency) may have a severe reaction to the invert sugar solution if it is used as a diluent. Symptoms include hypoglycemia, nausea, vomiting, tremors, coma, or convulsions.
* Rate of infusion should not exceed 4 ml/min (1200 mg/min).
* Only fresh solutions should be used; discard any unused portions.
* Do not mix urea with blood or other drugs in the same syringe.
* Check intravenous insertion site frequently and avoid extravasation. Venous irritation is more common with urea than mannitol. The use of hypothermia while urea is being administered increases the risk of venous thrombosis and hemoglobinuria (hemoglobin in the urine).

**Patient and family education**
* Review expected effects and possible side effects with patient and family.
* Keep patient and family informed of changes in the patient's condition.

# Potassium-sparing diurectics

amiloride ~ spironolactone ~ triamterene

**OVERVIEW OF THE DRUG CLASS**   Potassium-sparing diuretics are unique among diuretics in causing the retention of potassium, rather than its loss. When combined with other diuretics, the net effect is often potassium balance. The diuretic action of these drugs is weak but is additive with other agents because the mechanism of action is different from other diuretic classes.

**MECHANISM OF ACTION**   Potassium-sparing diuretics prevent the exchange of sodium for potassium in the late distal tubule. Normally at this site, a small fraction of the total sodium in the tubular fluid is exchanged for potassium, causing potassium to be excreted and some sodium to be retained. By blocking this exchange, this class of diuretics causes a small increase in sodium excretion leading to mild diuresis. The more important effect of the drugs is in preventing loss of potassium; it is for this action that they are normally employed.

**INDICATIONS**   **Hypokalemia induced by potassium depleting diuretics** Potassium-sparing diuretics are frequently combined with thiazide or loop diuretics to prevent or treat potassium depletion caused by these agents.   **Edema** Potassium-sparing diuretics have additive diuretic effects with other classes of diuretics and may be combined with them to prevent potassium depletion.   **Hypertension** Potassium-sparing diuretics may have weak hypotensive effects but are useful in combinations to prevent potassium depletion.

**CONTRAINDICATIONS** **Hyperkalemia** Elevated levels of potassium in the blood may be dangerously elevated further by potassium-sparing diuretics. **Serious renal impairment** Potassium-sparing diuretics may worsen electrolyte imbalances. **Diabetes** Diabetics with renal disease may be more likely to develop electrolyte disturbances.

**DRUG INTERACTIONS** **Antihypertensive drugs** have additive hypotensive effects with potassium-sparing diuretics. **Lithium** excretion is blocked by potassium-sparing diuretics, which may cause lithium toxicity. **Potassium** in food or other drugs may cause dangerously high blood potassium levels. Food sources of concentrated potassium include salt substitutes, potassium supplements, and low-salt milk. Drugs that contain high potassium include parenteral penicillin G and oral penicillin V preparations, as well as others. Blood from blood banks contains high potassium, especially after long storage. **Potassium-sparing diuretics** should never be combined with each other; dangerous hyperkalemia results, and deaths have been reported. **Thiazides, loop diuretics, and other diuretic classes** have additive diuretic effects with potassium-sparing diuretics.

## NURSING CONSIDERATIONS

### Side effects, toxicities, and associated nursing actions

**Renal** Hyperkalemia (high blood potassium) is possible with potassium-sparing diuretics. Metabolic acidosis may also occur. BUN values may be increased.

- Monitor serum electrolytes, BUN, and arterial blood gases.
- Assess for metabolic acidosis: deep rapid respirations, weakness, disorientation.
- Assess for hyperkalemia: nausea, colic, diarrhea, skeletal muscle spasms.
- Monitor intake, output, blood pressure, pulse, and weight.

**CNS** Confusion, dizziness, headache, and weakness occur in less than 10% of patients.

- Monitor patients carefully when initiating drug therapy.
- If confusion or dizziness occur, caution patient to avoid driving or operating hazardous equipment until the effects of medication wear off. Notify the physician.

### Patient and family education

- Review with patients the anticipated benefits and possible side effects of therapy. Instruct patients to report the development of any unexpected sign or symptom.
- If postural hypotension occurs, caution patient to move slowly from lying to sitting or standing. Hypotension is more common in the elderly.
- If patients have been switched to a potassium-sparing diuretic, or a potassium-sparing diuretic is prescribed in addition to a potassium-losing diuretic, impress on patients the need to *omit* previous potassium supplements that may have been ordered; consult the physician.
- Instruct patients to avoid salt substitutes, which contain potassium, while taking potassium-sparing diuretics.
- Instruct patients that diuretics work best when taken as ordered. Patients should not double up if a dose is missed.
- Instruct patients to keep all health care providers informed of all medication being taken. Other drugs may cause hypotension, electrolyte imbalance, or other side effects and may contribute to the development of severe side effects in the patient.
- Caution patients to avoid the use of alcohol, which may contribute to hypotension.
- Losing weight to reach ideal body weight, stopping smoking, engaging in regular exercise, and modifying the diet may be appropriate in the individualized treatment of heart disease or hypertension. After developing an individualized plan of care for the patient, refer the patient to the dietitian, visiting nurse, or other members of the health care team as needed.
- Poor patient compliance is sometimes a result of annoyance with frequent and excessive urination. A diuretic ordered once a day should be taken in the morning to prevent interruption of sleep for urination. A twice-daily dose could be taken at 8 AM and 2 PM for the same reason; consult with physician.
- Teach patients to notify the physician if vomiting or diarrhea occurs that lasts longer than 1 day, as electrolyte imbalances may be aggravated.
- Remind patients to keep these and all medications out of the reach of children.

# amiloride hydrochloride  (a-MILL-oh-ride)  potassium-sparing diuretic

- amiloride hydrochloride: Midamor

**MECHANISM OF ACTION**   Amiloride, like other potassium-sparing diuretics, prevents the exchange of sodium for potassium in the late distal tubule, causing potassium to be retained and some additional sodium to be excreted. Mild diuresis results.

**INDICATIONS**   **Edema** In combination with other diuretics, amiloride can improve fluid excretion in patients with congestive heart failure, cirrhosis of the liver, and other conditions. The most important role of amiloride is often to reverse the potassium loss of the more powerful diuretics with which it is combined.   **Hypertension** Amiloride may be used alone in or combination with other antihypertensive agents to control mild to moderate hypertension.   **Hypokalemia caused by potassium-wasting diuretics** Amiloride reverses or prevents potassium loss induced by thiazide or loop diuretics. This action of amiloride is important for patients receiving long-term diuretic therapy for conditions such as congestive heart failure and hypertension. Amiloride can also reverse metabolic alkalosis associated with long-term use of thiazide diuretics.

**CONTRAINDICATIONS**   **Hyperkalemia** Amiloride should not be given to patients having serum potassium concentrations above 5.5 mEq/L because amiloride may dangerously increase the serum potassium concentrations even further.   **Anuria, renal insufficiency, diabetic nephropathy** Amiloride is dangerous in these patients because they are particularly prone to rapid development of hyperkalemia and other electrolyte imbalances.

**DOSAGE**   **Adult:**   PO: Initially, 5 mg daily added to the established dosage of the potassium-wasting antihypertensive or diuretic drugs being administered. Doses increases in 5 mg increments at appropriate intervals, if necessary. Doses above 10 mg daily are rare. Dosage should be periodically evaluated and reduced if possible. *Special patient populations:* CHILDREN: Doses not established. PREGNANCY: FDA pregnancy category B. Amiloride appears in the milk of lactating animals; for this reason, patients and physicians may choose to avoid the drug if possible during lactation or discontinue breast-feeding when receiving the drug.

**PREPARATIONS**   *Tablets:* 5 mg; *tablets, combination:* 5 mg amiloride with 50 mg hydrochlorothiazide. The trade name of the combination is Moduretic.

**DRUG INTERACTIONS**   Amiloride is subject to the same interactions as other members of the class (See Overview, p. 160). In addition, the following interactions may be important.   **Antibiotics** may be administered as potassium salts (e.g., potassium penicillin V), which can contribute to potassium accumulation with amiloride.   **Digoxin** clearance may be altered by amiloride, presumably because amiloride decreases clearance of digoxin by the liver.   **Salt substitutes, low-salt milk, or dietetic foods** may contain high amounts of potassium, which would increase the risk of potassium accumulation with amiloride.

**DIAGNOSTIC TEST INTERFERENCE**   **Glucose tolerance tests** should not be done on patients receiving amiloride; dangerously high serum potassium concentrations have resulted. The drug should be discontinued at least 3 days before testing glucose tolerance.   **BUN, uric acid, and urinary calcium** may be increased.   **Blood glucose** may be increased in diabetics.

**FATE**   Oral absorption of amiloride is incomplete and further diminished by food in the stomach. The *onset* of diuretic action following oral doses is about 2 hours with *peak* concentrations appearing in blood at 3 to 4 hours. The *duration* of action is about 24 hours. Amiloride is eliminated primarily by renal excretion of unchanged drug; small amounts may be metabolized by the liver. The elimination *half-life* determined with multiple doses of amiloride may be 21 hours or longer.

## ❦ NURSING CONSIDERATIONS

### Side effects, toxicities, and associated nursing actions

**Metabolic** Metabolic acidosis may occur, which can increase the risk of hyperkalemia.
- See entry for drug class (p. 160).

- Monitor serum electrolytes and arterial blood gases.
- Assess for signs of metabolic acidosis: headache, mental dullness, rapid and deep-respirations, stupor, coma, and eventually death.

**Renal** Hyperkalemia (high potassium concentration in blood) may arise. BUN and serum creatinine concentrations may rise temporarily. Proteinuria and glycosuria are rare. Polyuria, dysuria, urinary frequency, or bladder spasms occur in up to 3% of patients.

- Monitor serum electrolytes, BUN, serum creatinine, and serum glucose levels. Monitor urinalysis.
- Hyperkalemia is more common in the elderly and in patients with renal disease or diabetes.
- Assess for urinary symptoms. If urinary frequency, dysuria, or spasm occur, check for urinary tract infection (monitor temperature, urinalysis, urine for culture and sensitivity). If urinary symptoms are not due to infection, it may be necessary to stop the drug.

**GI** Up to 8% of treated patients report nausea, vomiting, anorexia, or diarrhea. Abdominal pain, flatulence, bloating, heartburn, or GI bleeding occur less frequently.

- Monitor intake and output and weight.
- Assess for GI symptoms. Severe or persistent GI symptoms may require reducing the dosage or changing the drug.

**CNS** Up to 8% of patients report headache. Weakness, dizziness, encephalopathy, tremors, confusion, depression, paresthesia, or nervousness occur less frequently.

- If dizziness, confusion, or encephalopathy develop, caution patients to avoid driving or operating hazardous equipment until the effects of the medication can be evaluated.
- Assess for changes in mental status. Observe for signs of depression: sad affect, neglect of personal appearance, anorexia.

**CV** Up to 1% of patients suffer angina pectoris, palpitations, orthostatic hypotension, or cardiac arrhythmias.

- Monitor blood pressure and pulse.
- Be alert to cardiac side effects in patients with a history of cardiac disease.

**Liver** Jaundice is rare, but if liver disease already exists, patients may develop hepatic encephalopathy with tremors, confusion, coma, and increasingly severe jaundice.

- Assess for jaundice. Monitor liver function tests.
- Monitor mental status and level of consciousness.

**Blood** Various blood dyscrasias, including positive Coombs' test may occur.

- Monitor hematocrit, hemoglobin, white blood cell differential.

**Eye** Intraocular pressure may increase in up to 1% of patients.

- Be alert in giving this drug to patients with a history of glaucoma.
- Patients on long-term therapy should have periodic assessment of intraocular pressure.

**Other** Up to 3% of patients report muscle cramps.

- Assess for muscle cramps. If severe or persistent, notify the physician.

### Nursing interventions related to drug administration
- Taking the ordered dose with meals or a snack will help decrease gastric irritation.

### Patient and family education
- See entry for drug class (p. 160).
- Review with patients the potential dangers associated with salt substitutes, low-salt milk, or dietetic foods (see Drug Interactions).

## spironolactone   (spy-roe-noh-LAK-tone)                    potassium-sparing diuretic

- spironolactone: Aldactone, ✢Novospiroton, ✢Sincomen

**MECHANISM OF ACTION**   Spironolactone blocks the action of aldosterone in the kidney. Because aldosterone promotes sodium and water retention, the blockade of this action by spironolactone increases salt and water excretion. The diuretic effect of spironolactone is seen only in the presence of aldosterone. Spironolactone also reduces potassium excretion by actions in the distal tubule.

**INDICATIONS** Edema Spironolactone may reduce idiopathic edema or edema associated with congestive heart failure, cirrhosis of the liver, or nephrotic syndrome, conditions in which aldosterone actions are increased. **Hypertension** Spironolactone may substitute for thiazide diuretics in patients with gout or diabetes mellitus who cannot tolerate thiazides. Spironolactone is rarely used alone for hypertension and is most commonly used in combination with a thiazide diuretic. **Primary aldosteronism** Spironolactone can be used to treat the symptoms of excessive aldosterone and is occasionally useful in diagnosis of aldosteronism. **Hypokalemia** Spironolactone, like other potassium-sparing diuretics, can be used to prevent potassium depletion.

**CONTRAINDICATIONS** **Severe renal impairment or anuria** Spironolactone should not be used when renal function is severely impaired because of the risk of dangerous imbalances in potassium and other electrolytes. **Hyperkalemia** Patients with high serum potassium concentrations can rapidly develop dangerous potassium accumulation when spironolactone is added.

**DOSAGE** PO: **ADULT**: Daily dosages range from 25 to 200 mg in one to four doses. Initially 100 mg is given for 5 days, after which dosage may be adjusted. If needed, other diuretics may be added at this stage to maximize therapeutic response. In treating hypertension, the initial dose may need to be evaluated for as long as 2 weeks before other agents are added. **CHILDREN**: 3.3 mg/kg or 60 mg/M$^2$ daily as single or divided doses. *Special patient populations:* **ELDERLY**: Elderly patients are often overly sensitive to the hypotensive effects of spironolactone. Doses may need careful adjustment. **PREGNANCY**: Safe use during pregnancy has not been established. A metabolite of spironolactone appears in breast milk; nursing women should not use the drug.

**PREPARATIONS** *Tablets:* 25 mg; *tablets, film-coated:* 25, 50 (scored) and 100 mg (scored). Spironolactone is also included in the following combinations: *tablets:* 25 mg with 25 mg hydrochlorothiazide available as regular tablets (Spirozide), scored tablets (Spironazide), and film-coated tablets (Aldactazide 25/25); 50 mg spironolactone with 50 mg hydrochlorothiazide available as a film-coated tablet (Aldactazide 50/50).

**DRUG INTERACTIONS** Spironolactone is subject to the same interactions as other members of the class (see entry for drug class, p. 160). In addition, the following interactions may be important. **Potassium supplements, salt substitutes, low-salt milk, or dietetic foods** may contribute to dangerously high potassium accumulation when spironolactone is also administered. **Regional or general anesthesia** may be dangerous in patients receiving spironolactone because the diuretic may reduce vascular responses to norepinephrine, thereby impairing maintenance of normal blood pressure.

**DIAGNOSTIC TEST INTERFERENCE** **Assay of 17-hydroxycorticosteroids (cortisol)** in plasma and urine is interfered with by spironolactone. **BUN, uric acid and urinary calcium** may be increased. **Blood glucose** may be increased in diabetics.

**FATE** Spironolactone has a *bioavailability* exceeding 90% in the currently marketed formulations. Spironolactone is rapidly metabolized in the liver to form the active metabolite canrenone, as well as other minor metabolites. *Peak* serum concentrations of canrenone appear 2 to 4 hours after an oral dose of spironolactone. The *onset* of diuretic action is slow, taking 2 or 3 days to develop fully. The elimination *half-life* of canrenone ranges from 13 to 24 hours. Spironolactone and its metabolite canrenone are distributed into breast milk and cross the placenta.

## 🐦 NURSING CONSIDERATIONS

### Side effects, toxicities, and associated nursing actions

- See entry for drug class (p. 160).

**CNS** Headache, drowsiness, confusion, and ataxia may be signs of hyperkalemia.

- Monitor serum electrolytes.
- Assess ambulation for signs of ataxia.
- If drowsiness or confusion occur, caution patient to avoid driving or operating hazardous equipment until the effects of the medication can be evaluated. Notify the physician.

**GI** Anorexia, nausea, vomiting, diarrhea, and cramping.

- Monitor intake, output, blood pressure, pulse, weight.
- Monitor skin turgor, and assess mucous membranes.
- Notify physician for severe or persistent GI symptoms.

**Renal** Hyperkalemia is the most serious side effect of spironolactone and is more likely to occur in patients with pre-existing renal disease or patients taking potassium supplements. Dehydration and

low serum sodium concentrations can lead to dry mouth, thirst, drowsiness, and lethargy; these complications are especially dangerous in patients with hepatic damage.
* Monitor intake, output, blood pressure, pulse, weight.
* Monitor skin turgor, and assess mucous membranes.
* Ascertain that patients are not taking potassium supplements, which may have been prescribed before therapy with spironolactone.

**Metabolic** Hyperchloremic metabolic acidosis is a reversible alteration usually associated with hyperkalemia.
* Monitor blood gases and serum electrolytes.

**Allergic** Rashes are rare.
* Inspect patient for development of rashes; notify physician if rash appears.

**Endocrine** In males, spironolactone may cause gynecomastia, decreased libido, and relative impotence. In females, breast soreness, altered menstrual periods, amenorrhea, or postmenopausal bleeding can occur.
* Obtain a baseline physical appraisal before starting drug therapy.
* Assess carefully, through visual inspection and careful history taking, for development of endocrine abnormalities. The development of these side effects often contributes to the patient ceasing therapy. If side effects occur, notify the physician. Provide emotional support as needed. Remind patients not to stop therapy without first consulting the physician.
* In rare instances, breast cancer has been reported in men and women receiving spironolactone and other drugs, but cause and effect has not been established.

### Nursing interventions related to drug administration
* Taking ordered doses with meals or snacks may decrease gastric irritation.
* Tablets may be crushed and mixed in syrup or in fluid of patient's choice.

### Patient and family education
* See entry for drug class (p. 160).

---

## triamterene  (try-AM-ter-een)                               potassium-sparing diuretic

* triamterene: Dyrenium

**MECHANISM OF ACTION**   Triamterene is similar to amiloride, having no effect on aldosterone but blocking sodium reabsorption and potassium excretion in the distal tubule of the kidney. The result is mild diuresis with relative retention of potassium.

**INDICATIONS**   **Edema** Because triamterene takes effect slowly, the drug should not be used alone in conditions requiring rapid reduction of edema, e.g., congestive heart failure. Triamterene is often combined with more potent and rapid-acting diuretics to prevent excessive loss of potassium during therapy. **Hypertension** Triamterene may be combined with more potent diuretics to improve control of hypertension without excessive potassium loss.

**CONTRAINDICATIONS**   **Severe renal impairment** Triamterene should not be used when renal function is severely impaired because of the risk of dangerous imbalances in potassium and other electrolytes. **Hyperkalemia** Patients with high serum potassium concentrations can rapidly develop dangerous potassium accumulation when triamterene is added.   **Severe hepatic disease** Triamterene should not be used when hepatic function is severely impaired because dangerous imbalances in potassium and other electrolytes may precipitate hepatic coma.

**DOSAGE**   **PO:**   **ADULT:** Initial dose is 100 mg twice daily after meals; maintenance may require as little as 100 mg daily or every other day. Dosage should be individualized based on response, but daily dosage should not exceed 300 mg.   **CHILDREN:** Initial dose of 4 mg/kg or 115 mg/M$^2$ twice daily after meals; pediatric dosage should not exceed 300 mg daily.   *Special patient populations:*   **PREGNANCY:** Safe use not established. The drug passes into milk in lactating animals; nursing mothers should avoid triamterene.

**PREPARATIONS**    *Capsules:* 50, 100 mg; *capsule, combination:* 50 mg triamterene with 25 mg hydrochlorothiazide (trade name: Dyazide); *tablet, combination:* 75 mg triamterene with 50 mg hydrochlorothiazide (trade name: Maxide).

**DRUG INTERACTIONS**    Triamterene is subject to the same interactions as other members of the class (see entry
for drug class, p. 160). In addition, the following interactions may be important.    **Potassium supplements** may contribute to dangerously high potassium accumulation when triamterene is also
administered.    **Indomethacin or other nonsteroidal anti-inflammatory agents** may impair renal
function when given with triamterene, increasing the risk of dangerous electrolyte imbalances or
causing anuria.

**DIAGNOSTIC TEST INTERFERENCE**    **Quinidine assays** based on fluorescence are unreliable because both
quinidine and triamterene fluoresce at similar wavelengths.    **Urinary enzyme assays (e.g., lactic
dehydrogenase)** that depend on fluorescence measurements may be unreliable because triamterene
fluoresces.    **BUN, uric acid, and urinary calcium** may be increased.    **Blood glucose** may be
increased in diabetics.

**FATE**    Triamterene absorption following oral dosage is rapid but variable and incomplete. The *onset* of
diuresis is 2 to 4 hours, and the *duration* of action is up to 24 hours. Triamterene is metabolized,
probably in the liver. Excretion of triamterene and its metabolites is through the kidneys. The elimination *half-life* is 100 to 150 minutes.

### ☙ NURSING CONSIDERATIONS

**Side effects, toxicities, and associated nursing actions**    See entry for drug class (p. 160).

**CNS** Mental confusion, anxiety, weakness, and numbness in hands or feet may be signs of hyper-
kalemia.
- Monitor serum electrolytes.
- Assess for changes in neurologic function.

**CV** Cardiac arrhythmias may arise from hyperkalemia.
- Obtain ECG or cardiac rhythm strip at regular intervals.
- Be alert to arrhythmias in patients with a history of heart disease.

**Blood** Granulocytopenia and eosinophilia have been reported. Megaloblastic anemia can arise in
patients with alcoholic cirrhosis of the liver.
- Monitor complete blood count and white blood cell differential.
- Monitor for signs of granulocytopenia: fever, malaise, altered level of consciousness, cough, sore
  throat, symptoms of urinary tract infection.

**GI** Nausea, vomiting, and diarrhea may be direct actions of triamterene or indirectly related to elec-
trolyte imbalances.
- Monitor intake, output, blood pressure, weight.
- Assess skin turgor and mucous membranes.
- Monitor serum electrolytes.

**Renal** Hyperkalemia is the most serious reaction to triamterene; this imbalance may trigger a variety of
signs and symptoms. Hyponatremia (low sodium concentration in blood) may cause drowsiness,
thirst, and dry mouth. Increased BUN and uric acid concentrations may occur. Some patients have
increased risk of forming renal stones.
- Monitor serum electrolytes, BUN, uric acid.
- If drowsiness occurs, caution patients to avoid driving or operating hazardous equipment until the
  effects of the medication wear off. Notify the physician.

**Metabolic** Metabolic acidosis may arise because triamterene decreases serum concentrations of bicarbonate.
- Monitor arterial blood gases.

**Allergic** Skin rash or itching may signal an allergic reaction.
- Visually inspect patients for development of rash.
- If allergic-type response occurs, notify the physician.

**Other** Photosensitivity is possible with triamterene.
- If photosensitivity occurs, instruct the patient to avoid prolonged exposure to sun, to wear a wide-
  brimmed hat and long-sleeved clothing, and to use maximum protection sunscreens.

| Table 9-4. | **Pharmacokinetics of selected orally administered diuretics*** | | |

| | Diuretic effect | | |
|---|---|---|---|
| Generic name | Onset | Peak | Duration |
| Acetazolamide | 1-2 hr | 2-4 hr | 8-12 hr |
| Amiloride | 2 hr | 3-4 hr | 24 hr |
| Bendroflumethiazide | 1-2 hr | 6-12 hr | 18-24 hr |
| Benzthiazide | 2 hr | 4-6 hr | 12-18 hr |
| Bumetanide | 0.5-1 hr | 1-2 hr | 4 hr |
| Chlorothiazide | 2 hr | 4 hr | 6-12 hr |
| Chlorothiazide sodium (intravenous) | 15 min | 30 min | 6-12 hr |
| Chlorthalidone† | <2 hr | 2 hr | 48-72 hr |
| Cyclothiazide | 6 hr | 7-12 hr | 18-24 hr |
| Ethacrynic acid | 0.5 hr | 2 hr | 6-8 hr |
| Furosemide | 0.5-1 hr | 1-2 hr | 6-8 hr |
| Hydrochlorothiazide | 2 hr | 4 hr | 6-12 hr |
| Hydroflumethiazide | 1-2 hr | 3-4 hr | 18-24 hr |
| Indapamide† | 1-2 hr | 2.3-3.5 hr | 24-72 hr |
| Methyclothiazide | 2 hr | 6 hr | 24 hr |
| Metolazone† | 1 hr | 2 hr | 12-24 hr |
| Polythiazide | 2 hr | 6 hr | 36 hr |
| Quinethazone† | 2 hr | 6 hr | 18-24 hr |
| Spironolactone | Days | 2-3 days‡ | 2-3 days |
| Triamterene | 2-4 hr | Days‡ | 7-9 hr |
| Trichlormethiazide | 2 hr | 6 hr | 24 hr |

*All drugs were used orally, except for chlorothiazide sodium, which was used intravenously. Acetazolamide is a carbonic anhydrase inhibitor (p. 136); Amiloride, spironolactone, and triamterene are potassium-sparing diuretics (p. 159); bumetanide, ethacrynic acid, and furosemide are loop diuretics (p. 146); the remainder are thiazide or thiazidelike diuretics.
†Thiazidelike diuretics.
‡Peak effect requires multiple doses over several days.

### Nursing interventions related to drug administration
- Taking ordered doses with meals or a snack will lessen gastric irritation.
- Contents of capsule may be opened and mixed with food or fluid to aid patients who have difficulty swallowing capsules.

### Patient and family education
- See entry for drug class (p. 160).

# Thiazide and thiazidelike diuretics

bendroflumethiazide ~ benzthiazide ~ chlorothiazide ~ chlorthalidone*
~ cyclothiazide ~ hydrochlorothiazide ~ hydroflumethiazide ~ indapamide*
~ methyclothiazide ~ metolazone* ~ polythiazide ~ quinethazone*
~ trichlormethiazide

**OVERVIEW OF DRUG CLASS**    Thiazide and thiazidelike diuretics promote loss of sodium and water, reduce blood pressure, and alter metabolism by a variety of mechanisms. The potency of the thiazides and thiazidelike diuretics is less than that of loop diuretics but greater than other classes of diuretics.

*Nonthiazides with similar mechanisms.

Thiazides are widely used for treating hypertension, often increasing the response to additional antihypertensive drugs when combinations are required for control. Several thiazide and thiazidelike diuretics are available, differing primarily in the duration of diuretic action (Table 9-4).

**MECHANISM OF ACTION** Thiazides and related drugs block reabsorption of chloride and sodium in the distal tubule of the nephron. This action increases excretion of sodium chloride and body water, establishing a new balance with less salt and water retained in the body. This action is sought when these drugs are used as diuretics. Thiazides also inhibit carbonic anhydrase in the kidney, but the effect is temporary and not related to long-term diuretic action of these compounds. Thiazides and related drugs enhance potassium excretion by the kidney, but this action is not required for diuresis and is one of the most troublesome side effects of these agents.

**INDICATIONS** **Edema** Thiazides and related drugs may control edema arising from many causes, such as congestive heart failure, cirrhosis of the liver, and nephrotic syndrome. Metolazone is the most effective drug of the class for use in moderate renal failure. **Hypertension** Thiazide and related drugs are the most widely used agents for hypertension. In stepped-care management, the initial treatment is often with thiazides alone. When necessary, a beta-blocking drug may be added to a thiazide as step 2; the effects of these classes of drugs are additive. If control is not achieved with the combination of a thiazide and a beta-blocking drug, then a third drug with a different mechanism of action is added (step 3).

**CONTRAINDICATIONS** **Severe renal disease or anuria** Thiazides and related drugs lower glomerular filtration rates, reducing renal function. Renal failure may be precipitated. **Allergy to sulfonamide derivatives** Thiazides are chemically related to sulfonamide antibacterial agents and to sulfonylurea hypoglycemic agents. Allergies to these drugs may increase the risk of allergic reactions toward thiazide diuretics. **Hypokalemia** Thiazides and related drugs lower potassium levels in the body and may precipitate dangerous electrolyte imbalances. **Liver failure and hepatic coma** Thiazides and related drugs may alter electrolyte balance and precipitate hepatic coma in patients with pre-existing hepatic disease. **Pregnancy** Risks of fetal or neonatal jaundice or thrombocytopenia are increased.

**DRUG INTERACTIONS** **Amphotericin B** causes potassium loss, which when combined with the loss caused by thiazides can become dangerous. **Antihypertensive agents** have additive effects with thiazide and related diuretics. This interaction is therapeutically beneficial in the control of hypertension. **Corticosteroids and ACTH** cause potassium loss, which when combined with the loss caused by thiazides can become dangerous. **Digitalis glycosides** can cause a variety of dangerous toxic reactions, including fatal arrhythmias. The risk of these complications is increased by potassium depletion, which may be caused by thiazide diuretics. **Hypoglycemic agents** may appear less effective when thiazides and related drugs are used because these diuretics tend to elevate blood glucose. Dosage adjustment may be necessary. **Lithium** excretion is blocked by thiazides and related drugs. Lithium accumulation and toxicity are expected unless the dose of lithium is reduced.

**DIAGNOSTIC TEST INTERFERENCE** **Tests for pheochromocytoma** may be falsely negative when thiazides are taken. Tests affected include the tyramine test, phentolamine test, and the histamine test. **Total urinary estrogen and the estriol assay** may be falsely lowered by hydrochlorothiazide. Other thiazides may not show the reaction. **Urinary 17-hydroxycorticosteroid assays** may be falsely lowered by thiazides and related drugs.

**FATE** Thiazides and related drugs are well absorbed orally and distribute throughout the body, including across the placenta and into breast milk. Only chlorothiazide is administered parenterally. When given orally, the *onset* of diuretic action for thiazides is usually within 2 hours; the *onset* for antihypertensive effects is 3 or 4 days. The *peak* effect for diuresis is around 6 hours for most thiazides; the *duration* of action ranges from 6 to 24 hours. Thiazides are eliminated primarily as unchanged drug through the kidneys. Thiazide and related diuretics differ from one another primarily in pharmacokinetics; these differences are summarized in Table 9-4.

## 🌿 NURSING CONSIDERATIONS

### Side effects, toxicities, and associated nursing actions

**CNS** Headache, dizziness, vertigo, and paresthesias can occur.
- Assess for the development of these side effects.
- If dizziness or vertigo occur, caution patients to avoid driving or operating hazardous equipment

until the effects of the medication can be evaluated. Notify the physician.

**CV** Potassium depletion caused by thiazide and related diuretics can cause dangerous arrhythmias, especially in patients receiving cardiac glycosides (digitalis). Orthostatic hypotension may occur, and a few patients have suffered hypotension during surgery.

- Monitor serum electrolytes, especially potassium. Monitor blood pressure and pulse.
- Assess for signs of hypokalemia: vomiting, leg cramps, muscle weakness, apathy, abdominal distention, paralytic ileus, and ECG changes such as sagging S-T segments, depressed T waves, and elevated U waves.
- If orthostatic hypotension is a problem, instruct patients to move slowly from lying to sitting or standing positions. Hypotension is aggravated by prolonged periods of standing and hot showers. In some patients, support stockings may be beneficial.

**GI** Nausea, vomiting, anorexia, irritation of the stomach and intestinal tract, cholestatic jaundice, and pancreatitis have occurred. Monitor intake, output, weight.

- Assess for development of jaundice, right upper quadrant abdominal pain, change in color or consistency of stools.
- Assess for development of upper left quadrant abdominal pain, nausea, vomiting, fever.
- Monitor SGPT (ALT), SGOT (AST), LDH, and serum amylase.

**Renal** Potassium depletion occurs in almost every patient receiving thiazides and related diuretics, but the imbalance can be controlled by dietary management or potassium supplementation in most patients. Intervention with potassium-sparing diuretics is required in some patients. Hypochloremic alkalosis, dilutional hyponatremia, hypercalcemia, hypomagnesemia, and hyperuricemia can occur but are often triggered by other risk factors adding to the effects of the diuretics.

- Monitor serum electrolytes, uric acid, magnesium, and arterial blood gases.
- Assess for hyponatremia: muscle weakness, leg cramps, irritability or confusion, lethargy, headache, nausea, vomiting, and abdominal discomfort.
- Assess for hypercalcemia: thirst, polyuria, anorexia, nausea, vomiting, constipation, and altered level of consciousness.
- Assess for hypochloremic alkalosis: same as for metabolic alkalosis: mental confusion, dizziness, tetany, and convulsion.
- Assess for hypomagnesemia: confusion, hallucinations, tremors, muscle spasms, paresthesia, convulsion, and hyperactive reflexes.

**Metabolic** Hyperglycemia and glycosuria occur in predisposed or diabetic patients. Serum cholesterol, triglycerides, and very-low-density lipoprotein (VLDL) cholesterol are elevated by thiazides. Calcium metabolism may be affected, not only by changes in renal function but also by direct action on the parathyroid gland; hypercalcemia may result.

- Obtain baseline values of serum glucose, serum cholesterol, triglycerides, and lipoprotein levels before starting therapy and at regular intervals after therapy has begun.
- Assess for hypercalcemia (see preceding section).
- Instruct diabetic patients to monitor blood glucose levels more frequently after beginning thiazide therapy or changing doses. It may be necessary to change dose of insulin or oral hypoglycemic agent.

**Allergic** Skin reactions can occur, but allergic reactions may also include pneumonitis and interstitial nephritis.

- Inspect patient for skin changes.
- Maintain a high degree of suspicion for allergic reactions when unusual signs and symptoms develop.

**Other** Photosensitivity has been reported.

- If photosensitivity occurs, caution patient to avoid prolonged exposure to the sun, to wear a wide-brimmed hat and long-sleeve clothing, and to use a maximum protection sunscreen on exposed skin when in the sun.

### Nursing interventions related to drug administration

- Administer oral doses with meals or snack to lessen gastric irritation.

### Patient and family education

- Review with patients the anticipated benefits and possible side effects of drug therapy. Instruct

patients to report the development of any unexpected sign or symptom.
- Instruct patients to avoid the use of alcohol, which may potentiate hypotension.
- If a potassium supplement is prescribed, teach the patient the importance of taking it as ordered. Dietary sources of potassium include citrus fruits and juices; grape, cranberry, apple, pear, and apricot juices; bananas; meat, fish, and fowl; cereals; and tea and cola beverages. Some patients with borderline low potassium levels can maintain potassium levels by increasing their daily intake of potassium-rich foods. Note that some potassium-rich foods are also high in sodium and may be contraindicated on that basis.
- Poor compliance is sometimes a result of annoyance with frequent and excessive urination. If a diuretic is ordered once a day, it should be taken in the morning to prevent interruption of sleep for urination. A twice-daily dose could be taken at 8 AM and 2 PM and no later than 6 PM for the same reason; consult with the physician. For patients taking a thiazide diuretic for treatment of diabetes insipidus, the drug will help the patient *retain* fluid, not lose fluid, and concerns about excessive urination will not apply.
- Instruct patients that diuretics work best when taken as ordered. Patients should not double up if a dose is missed.
- Instruct patients to keep all health care providers informed of all medications being taken. Other drugs may also cause hypotension, electrolyte imbalance, or other side effects and may contribute to the development of severe side effects in the patient.
- Losing weight to reach ideal body weight, stopping smoking, engaging in regular exercise, and modifying the diet may be appropriate in individualized treatment of heart disease, hypertension, liver disease, or renal disease. After developing an individualized plan of care for the patient, refer the patient to the dietitian, visiting nurse, or other members of the health care team.
- Point out to patients that fatigue, lethargy, and other side effects may diminish with time.
- Some patients are eventually able to be controlled on alternate-day therapy. If prescribed, review with patients a way to remember the days to medicate and the days to omit the medication.
- Teach patients to notify the physician if vomiting or diarrhea occur for longer than 1 day and that electrolyte imbalances may be precipitated in patients who are also taking diuretics.
- Remind patients to keep these and all medications out of the reach of children.

## bendroflumethiazide (ben-droe-floo-meth-EYE-a-zide) thiazide diuretic

- bendroflumethiazide (bendrofluazide or benzydroflumethiazide in Canada): Naturetin

**MECHANISM OF ACTION** See entry for drug class (p. 167).

**INDICATIONS** See entry for drug class (p. 167).

**CONTRAINDICATIONS** See entry for drug class (p. 167).

**DOSAGE** PO: ADULT: Doses range from 2.5 to 20 mg daily, usually as a single dose given in the morning. Doses must be adjusted according to the response of the patient. CHILDREN: Initial doses are 0.1 to 0.4 mg/kg or 3 to 12 mg/M$^2$ daily. Maintenance doses for diuresis range from 0.05 to 0.1 mg/kg or 1.5 to 3 mg/M$^2$. *Special patient populations:* ELDERLY: The elderly may be at increased risk of orthostatic hypotension with this and other thiazides. PREGNANCY: Thiazides should be avoided in pregnancy because they cross the placenta and may cause blood dyscrasia or jaundice. The drugs also appear in milk of lactating mothers and may trigger allergic reactions in nursing infants.

**PREPARATIONS** *Tablets:* 2.5, 5 (scored), or 10 (scored) mg; all contain tartrazine. *Tablets, combinations:* 4 mg with 50 mg rauwolfia serpentina (Rauzide) contains tartrazine; 4 mg with 50 mg rauwolfia serpentina and 400 mg potassium chloride (Rautrax-N) (contains tartrazine); 5 mg with 40 mg nadolol (Corzide 40/5) or with 80 mg nadolol (Corzide 80/5), scored; 5 mg with 500 mg potassium chloride (Naturetin with K) (contains tartrazine).

**DRUG INTERACTIONS** • See entry for drug class (p. 167).

**DIAGNOSTIC TEST INTERFERENCE** • See entry for drug class (p. 167).

**FATE** • See entry for drug class (p. 167).

### ❦ NURSING CONSIDERATIONS

#### Side effects, toxicities, and associated nursing actions
- See entry for drug class (p. 167).

#### Nursing interventions related to drug administration
- See Preparations. Note that many contain FD & C yellow dye #5 (tartrazine), which may cause an allergic response in susceptible individuals. While rare, this side effect is seen more commonly in persons with aspirin hypersensitivity.

#### Patient and family education
- See entry for drug class (p. 168).

## benzthiazide    (benz-THYE-a-zide)                          thiazide diuretic

- benzthiazide: ✽Aquatag, Exna, Marazide

**MECHANISM OF ACTION**   See entry for drug class (p. 167).

**INDICATIONS**   See entry for drug class (p. 167).

**CONTRAINDICATIONS**   See entry for drug class (p. 167).

**DOSAGE**   PO:   **ADULT:** Doses range from 50 to 200 mg daily, with maintenance dosage often being reduced to 25 to 150 mg daily. Doses must be adjusted according to the response of the patient.   **CHILDREN:** Initial doses are 1 to 4 mg/kg or 30 to 120 mg/M$^2$ daily in three divided doses.   *Special patient populations:*   **ELDERLY:** The elderly may be at increased risk of orthostatic hypotension with this and other thiazides.   **PREGNANCY:** Thiazides should be avoided in pregnancy because they cross the placenta and may cause blood dyscrasias or jaundice. The drugs also appear in milk of lactating mothers and may trigger allergic reactions in nursing infants.

**PREPARATIONS**   *Tablets:* 25 to 50 mg. The 50 mg tablets sold under the trade names of Exna and Aquatag contain tartrazine.

**DRUG INTERACTIONS**   • See entry for drug class (p. 167).

**DIAGNOSTIC TEST INTERFERENCE**   • See entry for drug class (p. 167).

**FATE**   • See entry for drug class (p. 167).

### ❦ NURSING CONSIDERATIONS

#### Side effects, toxicities, and associated nursing actions
- See entry for drug class (p. 167).

#### Nursing interventions related to drug administration
- See Preparations. Note that some contain FD & C yellow dye #5 (tartrazine), which may cause an allergic response in susceptible individuals. While rare, this side effect is seen more commonly in persons with aspirin hypersensitivity.

#### Patient and family education
- See entry for drug class (p. 168).

## chlorothiazide    (klor-oh-THYE-a-zide)                          thiazide diuretic

- chlorothiazide (chlorothiazide sodium): Diuril, SK-Chlorothiazide

**MECHANISM OF ACTION**   See entry for drug class (p. 167).

**INDICATIONS**   See entry for drug class (p. 167).

**CONTRAINDICATIONS**   See entry for drug class (p. 167).

**DOSAGE**   Adult:   **PO, IV:** Doses range from 500 mg to 2 g daily in one or two doses. Doses must be adjusted according to the response of the patient and maintenance doses may be smaller than initial doses.   **Children 6 months to 12 years:**   **PO:** Usual daily doses are 20 to 22 mg/kg or 600 mg/M$^2$ in two divided doses.   **Infants up to 6 months:**   **PO:** Doses up to 33 mg/kg in two divided doses have been used.    *Special patient populations:*    ELDERLY: The elderly may be at increased risk of orthostatic hypotension with this and other thiazides.    PREGNANCY: Thiazides should be avoided in pregnancy because they cross the placenta and may cause blood dyscrasias or jaundice. The drugs also appear in milk of lactating mothers and may trigger allergic reactions in nursing infants.

**PREPARATIONS**    Chlorothiazide *Tablets:* 250 or 500 mg. Most tablets are scored. • *Oral suspension:* 250 mg/5 ml, includes 0.5% alcohol, benzoic acid, and parabens. • *Tablets, combinations:* 250 or 500 mg with 0.125 mg reserpine (Chloroserp, Chloroserpine, or Diupres [scored]). • *Tablets film-coated, combinations:* 150 or 250 mg with 250 mg methyldopa (Aldoclor).    **Sodium chlorothiazide,** *Solution for injection:* 500 mg (equivalent of chlorothiazide) with 250 mg mannitol, 0.4 mg thimerosal, and sodium hydroxide. Reconstitute with 18 ml of sterile water and discard after 24 hours. Solution is 25 mg/ml when reconstituted in this way.

**DRUG INTERACTIONS**    • See entry for drug class (p. 167)

**LABORATORY TEST INTERFERENCE**    • See entry for drug class (p. 167).

**FATE**    Chlorothiazide is incompletely absorbed. Food may increase the amount of drug absorbed. See entry for drug class (p. 167).

**NURSING CONSIDERATIONS**

### Side effects, toxicities, and associated nursing actions
• See entry for drug class (p. 167).

### Nursing interventions related to drug administration    This is the only thiazide diuretic available for IV administration. Dilute each 500 mg in at least 18 ml of compatible IV solution. Administer at a rate of 500 mg or less over 5 minutes. May be further diluted and administered via intermittent infusion. • Do not administer IM.

### Patient and family education
• See entry for drug class (p. 168).

---

# chlorthalidone    (klor-THAL-i-done)                    thiazidelike diuretic

• chlorthalidone, also chlorphthalidone or chlortalidone: Hygroton, Hylidone, ✽Novothalidone, Thalitone, ✽Uridon

**MECHANISM OF ACTION**    See entry for drug class (p. 167).

**INDICATIONS**    See entry for drug class (p. 167).

**CONTRAINDICATIONS**    See entry for drug class (p. 167).

**DOSAGE    PO:**    ADULT: Doses range from 25 to 200 mg daily, but usual doses are 25 to 100 mg daily as a single dose after breakfast. Doses must be adjusted according to the response of the patient. Daily doses should not exceed 200 mg, because no additional effect is produced above this dose. Doses may be given on alternate days for control of edema.    CHILDREN: Initial doses are 2 mg/kg or 60 mg/$M^2$ three times a week.    *Special patient populations:*    ELDERLY: The elderly may be at increased risk of orthostatic hypotension with this and other thiazides.    PREGNANCY: The safety of chlorthalidone in pregnancy and lactation has not been established.

**PREPARATIONS**    *Tablets:* 25, 50 or 100 mg; *tablets, combinations:* 15 mg with 0.1, 0.2, or 0.3 mg clonidine hydrochloride (Combipres), scored; 25 mg with 50 or 100 mg atenolol (Tenoretic); 25 mg with 0.125 or 0.25 mg reserpine (Regroton).

**DRUG INTERACTIONS**    • See entry for drug class (p. 167).

**DIAGNOSTIC TEST INTERFERENCE**    • See entry for drug class (p. 167).

**FATE**    • See entry for drug class (p. 167).

**NURSING CONSIDERATIONS**

### Side effects, toxicities, and associated nursing actions
• See entry for drug class (p. 167).

## cyclothiazide    (sye-kloe-THYE-a-zide)                         thiazide diuretic

- cyclothiazide: Anhydron

**MECHANISM OF ACTION**  • See entry for drug class (p. 167).
**INDICATIONS**  • See entry for drug class (p. 167).
**CONTRAINDICATIONS**  • See entry for drug class (p. 167).
**DOSAGE**  PO: ADULT: Doses range from 1 to 2 mg daily, with maintenance dosage often being reduced by administering 1 or 2 mg on alternate days or two to three times weekly. Doses must be adjusted according to the response of the patient.  CHILDREN: Initial doses are 0.02 to 0.04 mg/kg or 0.6 to 1.2 mg/M$^2$ daily in a single morning dose. These doses are reduced, if possible, for maintenance. *Special patient populations:*  ELDERLY: The elderly may be at increased risk of orthostatic hypotension with this and other thiazides.  PREGNANCY: Thiazides should be avoided in pregnancy because they cross the placenta and may cause blood dyscrasias or jaundice. The drugs also appear in milk of lactating mothers and may trigger allergic reactions in nursing infants.
**PREPARATIONS**  *Tablets:* 2 mg, scored.
**DRUG INTERACTIONS**  • See entry for drug class (p. 167).
**DIAGNOSTIC TEST INTERFERENCE**  • See entry for drug class (p. 167).
   **FATE**  • See entry for drug class (p. 167).
**🐦 NURSING CONSIDERATIONS**

**Side effects, toxicities, and associated nursing actions**
- See entry for drug class (p. 167).

**Nursing interventions related to drug administration**
- See entry for drug class (p. 167).

**Patient and family education**
- See entry for drug class (p. 168).

## hydrochlorothiazide    (hye-droe-klor-oh-THYE-a-zide)                  thiazide diuretic

- hydrochlorothiazide: ♣Apo-Hydro, Aquazide, Diaqua, ♣Diuchlor H, Esidrix, HydroDiuril, Mictrin, ♣Natrimax, ♣Nefrol, ♣Neo-Codema, Oretic, SK-Hydrochlorothiazide, Thiuretic, ♣Urozide

**MECHANISM OF ACTION**  • See entry for drug class (p. 167).
**INDICATIONS**  • See entry for drug class (p. 167).
**CONTRAINDICATIONS**  • See entry for drug class (p. 167).
**DOSAGE**  PO:  ADULT: Doses range from 25 to 200 mg daily divided into one to three doses. Maintenance doses may be lower. Doses must be adjusted according to the response of the patient.  CHILDREN 6 MONTHS TO 12 YEARS: Usual doses are 2 to 2.2 mg/kg or 60 mg/M$^2$ daily divided in two doses, not to exceed 100 mg daily.  CHILDREN UNDER 6 MONTHS: Doses may be as high as 3.3 mg/kg daily divided in two doses, not to exceed 37.5 mg daily.  *Special patient populations:*  ELDERLY: The elderly may be at increased risk of orthostatic hypotension with this and other thiazides.  PREGNANCY: Thiazides should be avoided in pregnancy because they cross the placenta and may cause blood dyscrasias or jaundice. The drugs also appear in milk of lactating mothers and may trigger allergic reactions in nursing infants.

**PREPARATIONS**   *Tablets:* 25, 50, or 100 mg. Some tablets are scored. *Solution,* for oral use: 50 mg/5 ml or 100 mg/ml. *Tablets, combinations:* See Table 9-2 (p. 138).

**DRUG INTERACTIONS**   • See entry for drug class (p. 167).

**DIAGNOSTIC TEST INTERFERENCE**   • See entry for drug class (p. 167).

**FATE**   • See entry for drug class (p. 167).

☙ **NURSING CONSIDERATIONS**

**Side effects, toxicities, and associated nursing actions**
   • See entry for drug class (p. 167).

**Nursing interventions related to drug administration**
   • See Preparations. Note that Serpasil-Esidrex brand combination product Nos. 1 and 2 contain FD & C yellow dye #5 (tartrazine), which may cause an allergic response in susceptible individuals. While rare, this side effect is seen more commonly in persons with aspirin hypersensitivity.

**Patient and family education**
   • See entry for drug class (p. 168).

---

## hydroflumethiazide   (hye-droe-floo-meth-EYE-a-zide)   thiazide diuretic

   • hydroflumethiazide: Diucardin, Saluron, Sonazide

**MECHANISM OF ACTION**   • See entry for drug class (p. 167).

**INDICATIONS**   • See entry for drug class (p. 167).

**CONTRAINDICATIONS**   • See entry for drug class (p. 167).

**DOSAGE**   **PO:**   **ADULT:** Doses range from 25 to 200 mg daily. Doses must be adjusted according to the response of the patient but should not exceed 200 mg daily. Doses above 100 mg daily should be given in divided doses.   **CHILDREN:** Initial doses are 1 mg/kg or 30 mg/M$^2$ daily in a single dose. *Special patient populations:*   **ELDERLY:** The elderly may be at increased risk of orthostatic hypotension with this and other thiazides.   **PREGNANCY:** Thiazides should be avoided in pregnancy because they cross the placenta and may cause blood dyscrasias or jaundice. The drugs also appear in milk of lactating mothers and may trigger allergic reactions in nursing infants.

**PREPARATIONS**   *Tablets:* 50 mg, scored; *tablets, combinations:* 25 or 50 mg with 0.125 mg reserpine (Hydro-Fluserpine, Hydropine, Salazide, Salutensin).

**DRUG INTERACTIONS**   • See entry for drug class (p. 167).

**DIAGNOSTIC TEST INTERFERENCE**   • See entry for drug class (p. 167).

**FATE**   • See entry for drug class (p. 167).

☙ **NURSING CONSIDERATIONS**

**Side effects, toxicities, and associated nursing actions**
   • See entry for drug class (p. 167).

**Nursing interventions related to drug administration**
   • See entry for drug class (p. 167).

**Patient and family education**
   • See entry for drug class (p. 168).

---

## indapamide   (in-DAP-a-mide)   thiazidelike diuretic

   • indapamide: ✿Lozide, Lozol

**MECHANISM OF ACTION**   • See entry for drug class (p. 167).

**INDICATIONS**   • See entry for drug class (p. 167).

**CONTRAINDICATIONS**   • See entry for drug class (p. 167).

**DOSAGE**    PO:   **ADULT:** Doses range from 2.5 to 5 mg daily as a single dose in the morning. Doses must be adjusted according to the response of the patient.   *Special patient populations:*   **ELDERLY:** The elderly may be at increased risk of orthostatic hypotension.   **CHILDREN:** Doses not established.   **PREGNANCY:** Indapamide, like the thiazides, should be avoided in pregnancy because the drug may cause blood dyscrasias or jaundice. Indapamide should be avoided during lactation until safety is established.

**PREPARATIONS**    *Tablets, film-coated:* 2.5 mg.

**DRUG INTERACTIONS**    • See entry for drug class (p. 167).

**DIAGNOSTIC TEST INTERFERENCE**    • See entry for drug class (p. 167).

**FATE**    Unlike the thiazides, indapamide is extensively metabolized in the liver, and little active drug is excreted in urine. The elimination *half-life* of indapamide is 14 to 18 hours, which allows the drug to be used as single daily doses.

### ☙ NURSING CONSIDERATIONS

**Side effects, toxicities, and associated nursing actions**
• See Overview of Drug Class (p. 167).

**Nursing interventions related to drug administration**
• See Overview of Drug Class (p. 168).

**Patient and family education**
• See Overview of Drug Class (p. 168).

---

## methyclothiazide    (meth-i-kloe-THYE-a-zide)    thiazide diuretic

• methyclothiazide: Aquatensen, ✿Duretic, Enduron, Ethon

**MECHANISM OF ACTION**    • See entry for drug class (p. 167).

**INDICATIONS**    • See entry for drug class (p. 167).

**CONTRAINDICATIONS**    • See entry for drug class (p. 167).

**DOSAGE**    PO:   **ADULT:** Doses range from 2.5 to 10 mg daily, usually as a single dose in the morning. Doses must be adjusted according to the response of the patient. The maximum daily dose is 10 mg; higher doses are ineffective and may increase toxicity.   **CHILDREN:** Initial doses are 0.05 to 0.2 mg/kg or 1.5 to 6 mg/M$^2$ daily in a single dose.   *Special patient populations:*   **ELDERLY:** The elderly may be at increased risk of orthostatic hypotension with this and other thiazides.   **PREGNANCY:** Thiazides should be avoided in pregnancy because they cross the placenta and may cause blood dyscrasias or jaundice. The drugs also appear in milk of lactating mothers and may trigger allergic reactions in nursing infants.

**PREPARATIONS**    *Tablets:* 2.5 or 5 mg, scored; *tablets, combinations:* 2.5 mg with 2 mg cryptenamine (Diutensen). 2.5 mg with 0.1 mg reserpine (Diutensen-R); 5 mg with 0.25 or 0.5 mg deserpidine (Enduronyl, Eserdine, Methy-Deserpidine). *Tablets film-coated, combinations:* 5 mg with 25 mg pargyline hydrochloride (Eutron Filmtab).

**DRUG INTERACTIONS**    • See entry for drug class (p. 167).

**DIAGNOSTIC TEST INTERFERENCE**    • See entry for drug class (p. 167).

**FATE**    • See entry for drug class (p. 167).

### ☙ NURSING CONSIDERATIONS

**Side effects, toxicities, and associated nursing actions**
• See entry for drug class (p. 167).

**Nursing interventions related to drug administration**
• See entry for drug class (p. 168).

**Patient and family education**
• See entry for drug class (p. 168).

## metolazone  (me-TOLE-a-zone)                thiazidelike diuretic

- metolazone: Diulo, Zaroxolyn

**MECHANISM OF ACTION**  • See entry for drug class (p. 167).

**INDICATIONS**  Some studies suggest that metolazone is more effective than other thiazide and thiazidelike drugs in patients with renal disease. See entry for drug class (p. 167).

**CONTRAINDICATIONS**  • See entry for drug class (p. 167).

**DOSAGE**  **PO:**  **ADULT:** Doses range from 2.5 to 20 mg daily as a single dose in the morning. Doses must be adjusted according to the response of the patient.  *Special patient populations:*  **ELDERLY:** The elderly may be at increased risk of orthostatic hypotension with this and other thiazides.  **CHILDREN:** Doses not established.  **PREGNANCY:** Safety in pregnancy and lactation not established.

**PREPARATIONS**  *Tablets:* 2.5, 5, or 10 mg.

**DRUG INTERACTIONS**  • See entry for drug class (p. 167).

**DIAGNOSTIC TEST INTERFERENCE**  • See entry for drug class (p. 167).

**FATE**  Absorption of metolazone is reduced in cardiac patients. Otherwise the drug is similar to thiazides. See entry for drug class (p. 167).

### 🐦 NURSING CONSIDERATIONS

#### Side effects, toxicities, and associated nursing actions
- See entry for drug class (p. 167).

#### Nursing interventions related to drug administration
- See entry for drug class (p. 168).

#### Patient and family education
- See entry for drug class (p.168).


## polythiazide  (poll-i-THYE-a-zide)                thiazide diuretic

- polythiazide: Renese

**MECHANISM OF ACTION**  • See entry for drug class (p. 167).

**INDICATIONS**  • See entry for drug class (p. 167).

**CONTRAINDICATIONS**  • See entry for drug class (p. 167).

**DOSAGE**  **PO:**  **ADULT:** Doses range from 1 to 4 mg daily as a single dose in the morning. Doses must be adjusted according to the response of the patient.  **CHILDREN:** Initial doses are 0.02 to 0.08 mg/kg or 2 mg/$M^2$ daily in a single dose.  *Special patient populations:*  **ELDERLY:** The elderly may be at increased risk of orthostatic hypotension with this and othr thiazides.  **PREGNANCY:** Thiazides should be avoided in pregnancy because they cross the placenta and may cause blood dyscrasias or jaundice. The drugs also appear in milk of lactating mothers and may trigger allergic reactions in nursing infants.

**PREPARATIONS**  *Tablets:* 1, 2, or 4 mg, scored; *tablets, combinations:* 2 mg with 0.25 mg reserpine (Renese-R), scored; *capsules, combinations:* 0.5 mg with 1, 2, or 5 mg of prazosin (Minizide).

**DRUG INTERACTIONS**  • See entry for drug class (p. 167).

**DIAGNOSTIC TEST INTERFERENCE**  • See entry for drug class (p. 167).

**FATE**  • See entry for drug class (p. 167).

### 🐦 NURSING CONSIDERATIONS

#### Side effects, toxicities, and associated nursing actions
- See entry for drug class (p. 167).

#### Nursing interventions related to drug administration
- See entry for drug class (p. 168).

#### Patient and family education
- See entry for drug class (p. 168).

## quinethazone    (kwin-ETH-a-zone)    thiazidelike diuretic

• quinethazone: ✤Aquamox, Hydromox

**MECHANISM OF ACTION**    • See entry for drug class (p. 167).
**INDICATIONS**    • See entry for drug class (p. 167).
**CONTRAINDICATIONS**    • See entry for drug class (p. 167).
**DOSAGE**    PO:    ADULT: Doses range from 50 to 200 mg daily as single or divided doses. Doses must be adjusted according to the response of the patient, but doses above 100 mg daily are seldom appropriate.    *Special patient populations:*    ELDERLY: The elderly may be at increased risk of orthostatic hypotension with this and other thiazides.    CHILDREN: Doses not established.    PREGNANCY: Safety in pregnancy and lactation not established.
**PREPARATIONS**    *Tablets:* 50 mg; *tablets, combinations:* 50 mg with 0.125 mg reserpine (Hydromox R).
**DRUG INTERACTIONS**    • See entry for drug class (p. 167).
**DIAGNOSTIC TEST INTERFERENCE**    • See entry for drug class (p. 167).
**FATE**    • See entry for drug class (p. 167).
### ❧ NURSING CONSIDERATIONS
#### Side effects, toxicities, and associated nursing actions
• See entry for drug class (p. 167).
#### Nursing interventions related to drug administration
• See entry for drug class (p. 168).
#### Patient and family education
• See entry for drug class (p. 168).

## trichlormethiazide    (try-klor-meth-EYE-a-zide)    thiazide diuretic

• trichlormethiazide: Aquazide, Diurese, Metahydrin, Naqua, Niazide, Triazide, Trichlorex

**MECHANISM OF ACTION**    • See entry for drug class (p. 167).
**INDICATIONS**    • See entry for drug class (p. 167).
**CONTRAINDICATIONS**    • See entry for drug class (p. 167).
**DOSAGE**    PO:    ADULT: Doses range from 1 to 4 mg daily as a single dose in the morning or in divided doses. Doses must be adjusted according to the response of the patient.    CHILDREN: Initial doses are 0.07 mg/kg or 2 mg/M$^2$ daily in single or divided doses.    *Special patient populations:*    ELDERLY: The elderly may be at increased risk of orthostatic hypotension with this and other thiazides.    PREGNANCY: Thiazides should be avoided in pregnancy because they cross the placenta and may cause blood dyscrasias or jaundice. The drugs also appear in milk of lactating mothers and may trigger allergic reactions in nursing infants.
**PREPARATIONS**    *Tablets:* 2 or 4 mg. The tablets sold under the trade names of Metahydrin and Trichlorex contain tartrazine. *Tablets, combinations:* 2 or 4 mg with 0.1 mg reserpine (Diurese -R, Metatensin, Naquival). Tablets sold under the trade names of Metatensin and Naquival contain tartrazine.
**DRUG INTERACTIONS**    • See entry for drug class (p. 167).
**DIAGNOSTIC TEST INTERFERENCE**    • See entry for drug class (p. 167).
**FATE**    • See entry for drug class (p. 167).
### ❧ NURSING CONSIDERATIONS
#### Side effects, toxicities, and associated nursing actions
• See entry for drug class (p. 167).
#### Nursing interventions related to drug administration
• See Preparations. Note that some contain FD & C yellow dye #5 (tartrazine), which may cause an allergic response in susceptible individuals. While rare, this side effect is seen more commonly in persons with aspirin hypersensitivity.
#### Patient and family education
• See entry for drug class (p. 168).

# Chapter Ten

# Intravenous fluids and solutions

amino acids
ammonium chloride
calcium carbonate (oral only)
calcium chloride
calcium glubionate (oral only)
calcium gluceptate
calcium gluconate
calcium glycerophosphate
calcium lactate
calcium phosphates, dibasic and tribasic (oral only)
dextran
dextrose
fat emulsions
fructose

hetastarch
invert sugar
magnesium sulfate
potassium acetate
potassium bicarbonate (oral only)
potassium chloride
potassium citrate (oral only)
potassium gluconate (oral only)
potassium phosphates, monobasic and dibasic
Ringer's solution
sodium bicarbonate
sodium chloride
sodium lactate

**OVERVIEW OF THE DRUG CLASS**   A variety of fluids and solutions are administered intravenously to control many imbalances that can arise from disease or trauma. The reasons for employing these agents are to replace fluid loss, to alter fluid distribution, to correct an electrolyte imbalance, to supply a required vitamin or nutrient, or to supply calories. This chapter also covers a few preparations used orally for chronic control of imbalances (e.g., potassium preparations and calcium products).

**MECHANISM OF ACTION**   Agents that replace fluid loss include blood, plasma, solutions of blood proteins, and isotonic solutions of sodium chloride or dextrose. The primary action of these agents is to increase extracellular fluid volume without greatly altering the composition of body fluids. Hypertonic or hypotonic solutions might be administered to cause fluid to move between plasma and interstitial spaces. Solutions of salts, vitamins, dextrose or other sugars, or amino acids may be used to correct specific deficiencies. Calories may be supplied in dextrose solutions, amino acid solutions, or suspensions of lipids.

**INDICATIONS**   **Fluid loss** Fluid depletion caused by dehydration, blood loss, or excessive vomiting and diarrhea can be treated with isotonic solutions of saline or dextrose or with blood or blood replacements. • Exact therapy depends on the specific condition and its cause.   **Electrolyte imbalances** Specific therapy to replace sodium, potassium, bicarbonate, calcium, magnesium, and other ions may be required for particular patients. • Signs of electrolyte imbalance are summarized in Table 10-1. **Nutritional support** Patients may require vitamins to treat a specific deficiency. • Patients unable to take sufficient nutrition by mouth require calories that may be supplied by dextrose for short-term support. • Long-term support of such patients requires more complex nutritional mixtures.

**CONTRAINDICATIONS**   **Congestive heart failure or hypertension** In general these patients do not tolerate extra fluid or sodium loads. When IV fluids must be used, care should be taken to prevent excessive fluid retention.   **Renal disease** Patients with renal disease may be unable to eliminate potassium, magnesium, or other ions efficiently. • Solutions or supplements containing electrolytes may cause these patients to accumulate dangerous concentrations of the ion. • See drug monographs for specific contraindications on individual preparations.

**DRUG INTERACTIONS**   See drug monographs for specific interactions.

---

## ❦ NURSING CONSIDERATIONS

### Nursing interventions related to drug administration

- Follow institutional or agency guidelines for IV insertion and management of IV fluids. Some general guidelines are listed below.
- Whenever possible, use stainless steel needles for infusions (to reduce the incidence of phlebitis). Perform venipuncture using aseptic conditions into a large, straight vein located in a place where the needle/cannula can be securely fastened.
- Using aseptic technique, change IV tubing every 48 to 72 hours.

| Table 10-1. | Common electrolyte imbalances | | | |
|---|---|---|---|---|
| **Solute ion** | **Normal plasma concentration** | **Signs of deficiency** | **Signs of excess** | |
| Sodium | 136-145 mEq/L 135-145 mmole/L | Anorexia, nausea, vomiting; increased intracranial pressure; oliguria leading to anuria | Dry, sticky membranes; fever; weakness and disorientation; oliguria | |
| Potassium | 3.5-5.0 mEq/L 3.5-5.0 mmol/L | Muscle weakness, diminished tendon reflexes, paralytic ileus, cardiac arrhythmia | Nausea and vomiting, muscle weakness, changes on ECG | |
| Bicarbonate | 24-31 mEq/L 21-28 mmol/L (pH 7.35-7.45) | Metabolic acidosis (pH<7.35); weakness; deep, rapid breathing (Kussmaul); stupor or unconsciousness | Metabolic alkalosis (pH>7.45), hypertonicity of muscles, depressed respirations, tetany | |
| Calcium | 4.7-5.6 mEq/L 2.12-2.62 mmol/L* | Tetany, prolonged QT interval on ECG | Weakness, fatigue, thirst; nausea, anorexia; muscle cramping | |
| Magnesium | 1.3-2.3 mEq/L 0.8-1.0 mmol/L | Flushing, hypertension, neuromuscular irritability | Nausea, vomiting, diarrhea, colic | |

*Serum concentration.

- Use inline filters and change as directed by agency policy (controversy continues about the necessity of filters for all IV solutions).
- Inspect IV bottles or bags carefully before using. If the container seems punctured or contaminated, the fluid is discolored, or particulate matter is present, the container should be discarded and a new bag or bottle obtained. Most IV solutions are clear. Exceptions include fat emulsion, blood, and blood products. If there is a question, consult the pharmacist.
- Calculate infusion rates carefully and monitor IV infusions hourly. If IV infusion rate falls markedly behind, investigate cause. Speeding up the infusion to ''catch up'' is potentially dangerous, as the patient may experience fluid overload or toxicity from too rapid infusion of a medication.
- Assess for signs of fluid overload: distended neck veins, edema, and noisy or rapid respirations. Monitor intake and output, weight, blood pressure, heart and breath sounds, central venous pressure or pulmonary capillary wedge pressure (if available), and urine specific gravity. Monitor skin turgor.
- Monitor the patient for the following problems: *infiltration* or *extravasation* occurs when the needle or cannula punctures the vein wall, and infusing fluid leaks into surrounding tissues. Extravasation of some fluids may lead to tissue necrosis. Assess insertion site for edema, burning, pain, coolness to touch, and usually slowing of IV rate. Change IV insertion site, and apply warm compresses to area of infiltration unless there are specific guidelines for treatment of extravasation of certain medications (e.g., some cancer chemotherapy drugs). *Phlebitis,* inflammation or irritation of the vein, may result from bacterial contamination, mechanical irritation (as when the cannula is not fastened securely), or chemical irritation, as from inadequately diluted drugs or too rapid infusion of medications. Assess for patient complaints of discomfort, swelling, red streak up extremity, warmth to touch, and usually a slowing of IV rate. Change IV insertion site and apply warm compresses to the area. *Generalized septicemia:* assess for fever, chills, hypotension, and symptoms of shock. There may be nothing amiss at the IV insertion site. *Occluded infusion:* assess for decreased infusion rate and backup of blood in tubing. There may be no discomfort. Occluded infusion may be caused by needle or cannula against vein wall, occlusion of needle or tubing by particulate matter or kinking of tubing, poor immobilization of the needle or cannula, or poor positioning of the extremity. Inspect the insertion site, reposition patient or extremity, check infusion rate, and check for kinks in tubing. Infusion should not be irrigated as there is risk of dislodging a clot or particulate matter into the vascular system. It may be necessary to change the insertion site.

- Use microdrip or minidrip infusion sets with infants and small children, when the dose of medication must be carefully titrated, or when there are factors predisposing to fluid overload, as in patients with severe cardiac or renal disease.
- When available, use electronic infusion monitors. These do not replace careful observation but may assist the nurse in delivering prescribed fluids and drugs at a steady rate.
- Use volume control devices (e.g., Volutrol) to help prevent administration of excessive volume by accident. Use in infants and small children, when the dose of drug must be carefully titrated, or when medications requiring additional dilution are being administered.

### Patient and family education
- If the patient's condition permits, patient should be informed of all medications being administered. Review with patient expected benefits and possible side effects of therapy.
- If patient's condition permits, involve patient and family in efforts to maintain well-functioning infusion. Instruct patient to call if infusion stops or slows markedly, when fluid container is nearly empty, or if pain, edema, redness, or change in color develops.

## amino acid injections   (a-MEE-noe)                      parenteral nutrition

- amino acid injections: Aminess, Aminosyn, BranchAmin, FreAmine, HepatAmine, Nephr-Amine, Novamine, ✿Nutrimix, ProcalAmine, RenAmin, Travasol, TrophAmine, ✿Vamin

**MECHANISM OF ACTION**   Amino acid solutions replace dietary protein. Solutions normally contain eight essential amino acids and additional amino acids, electrolytes, or carbohydrates. These preparations prevent or treat negative nitrogen balance.

**INDICATIONS**   **Parenteral nutrition** Patients unable to receive adequate nutrition by mouth may receive amino acid solutions to prevent negative nitrogen balance. • For long-term support, these solutions may be used along with lipid and carbohydrate preparations to achieve adequate caloric intake along with proper nutritional balance.   **Hypermetabolic states** Patients with extensive burns, severe sepsis, or severe trauma may not be able to take sufficient protein in the diet to supply metabolic needs. • Parenteral solutions of amino acids may be used to supplement dietary intake.

**CONTRAINDICATIONS**   **Renal failure** Amino acids increase the concentration of blood urea nitrogen, which may be difficult to eliminate if renal function is inadequate. • To minimize this problem, some preparations are formulated to supply only the essential amino acids plus histidine and arginine (Table 10-2) (e.g., Nephramine, Aminosyn-RF, Aminess).   **Hepatic failure** Nitrogenous wastes accumulate in hepatic failure and may precipitate hepatic coma. • Amino acid solutions may increase the accumulation of these nitrogenous materials. • Some preparations of amino acids are formulated to include large amounts of branched-chain amino acids (HepatAmine, BranchAmine) (Table 10-2), based on the theory that use of these amino acids controls hepatic encephalopathy.   **Patients intolerant of potassium or sodium** Patients with renal or cardiovascular disease frequently must restrict potassium and/or sodium intake. • If these patients must receive amino acid solutions, care should be taken to select one with the appropriate electrolyte content.

**DOSAGE**   IV:   **ADULTS, CHILDREN:** Individualized to accommodate nutritional requirements and fluid tolerance of the patient. *Special patient populations:* **PREGNANCY:** Altered doses not established. **RENAL OR HEPATIC FAILURE:** See Contraindications above.

**PREPARATIONS**   *Solutions, IV:* the composition of available solutions is shown in Table 10-2.

**DRUG INTERACTIONS**   None reported.

**FATE**   Amino acids are metabolized as the natural breakdown products of protein digestion. Amino acids may be incorporated into newly synthesized protein by the body, metabolized and stored, or used for energy.

**Table 10-2.**

## Amino acid solutions for parenteral use

| Trade name | Other components present | Nitrogen, g/100 ml |
|---|---|---|
| Aminess 5.2%* | Only essential amino acids with histidine and acetate | 0.66 |
| Aminosyn 3% | Acetate, sodium | 0.55 |
| Aminosyn 3% with dextrose | Acetate, dextrose (5% or 25%), potassium | 0.55 |
| Aminosyn 3.5% M | Acetate, chloride, magnesium, phosphate, potassium, sodium | 0.55 |
| Aminosyn 4.5% with dextrose | Acetate, chloride, dextrose (25%), potassium | 0.67 |
| Aminosyn 5% | Acetate, potassium | 0.786 |
| Aminosyn 7% | Acetate, potassium | 1.1 |
| Aminosyn 7% & electrolytes | Acetate, chloride, magnesium, phosphate, potassium, sodium | 1.1 |
| Aminosyn 8.5% | Acetate, chloride, potassium | 1.34 |
| Aminosyn 8.5% & electrolytes | Acetate, chloride, magnesium, phosphate, potassium, sodium | 1.34 |
| Aminosyn 10% | Acetate, potassium | 1.57 |
| Animosyn RF 5.2% | Only essential amino acids with arginine, histidine, acetate, potassium | 0.787 |
| BranchAmin 4% | Contains only isoleucine, leucine, valine with phosphate | 0.443 |
| FreAmine III 3% & electrolytes | Acetate, chloride, magnesium, phosphate, potassium, sodium | 0.46 |
| FreAmine 6.9% HBC | Acetate, chloride, sodium | 0.97 |
| FreAmine III 8.5% | Acetate, chloride, potassium, sodium | 1.3 |
| FreAmine III 10% | Acetate, chloride, potassium, sodium | 1.53 |
| HepatAmine 8% | Acetate, chloride, sodium | 1.2 |
| NephrAmine 5.4% | Only essential amino acids with histidine, cysteine, acetate, chloride, sodium | 0.65 |
| Novamine 8.5% | Acetate | 1.35 |
| Novamine 11% | Acetate | 1.8 |
| ProcalAmine 3% with 3% glycerin | Acetate, calcium, chloride, magnesium, phosphate, potassium, sodium | 0.46 |
| RenAmin 6.5% | Acetate, chloride | 1.0 |
| Travasol M & Electrolyte No. 45 | Acetate, chloride, magnesium, phosphate, potassium, sodium | 0.59 |
| Travasol 5.5% | Acetate, chloride | 0.926 |
| Travasol 5.5% & electrolytes | Acetate, chloride, magnesium, phosphate, potassium, sodium | 0.926 |
| Travasol 8.5% | Acetate, chloride | 1.42 |
| Travasol 8.5% & electrolytes | Acetate, chloride, magnesium, phosphate, potassium, sodium | 1.42 |
| Travasol 10% | Acetate, chloride | 1.65 |
| TrophAmine 6% | Acetate, chloride, sodium | 0.93 |

*Percentages following the name of the preparation indicate the concentration of protein.

### ❦ NURSING CONSIDERATIONS

#### Side effects, toxicities, and associated nursing actions

**CNS** CNS disorders and coma can arise when large quantities of NephrAmine or Aminess are administered because these preparations lack arginine.
- Perform neurologic assessment at regular intervals.

**CV** Fluid and electrolyte imbalances may occur.
- Monitor intake and output, weight, blood pressure, and pulse. Assess heart and breath sounds at regular intervals.
- Monitor serum electrolyte, magnesium, blood ammonia, phosphate, serum protein, BUN, pH, arterial blood gases, cholesterol, and serum glucose levels. Monitor ketones.

**Blood** Thrombophlebitis can occur during infusion.
- When possible, amino acids should be administered through a large central vein. If administered peripherally, amino acids should be diluted with 5% or 10% dextrose.
- **GI** Nausea can occur during infusion.
- Slowing the infusion rate or changing brands of amino acids may help if nausea is severe. If nausea is severe or persistent, notify physician.

**Other** Fever and flushing have been reported rarely.
- Monitor temperature at least every 4 hours.

#### Nursing interventions related to drug administration
- See entry for drug class (p. 177).
- Amino acids should be administered at a steady rate. An electronic infusion monitor should be used if possible.
- The use of an IV filter is recommended.
- Infusion rate should not exceed 4 mg of nitrogen/kg/hr.
- Once opened, a bottle should be used within 24 hours.
- Usually, infusions of amino acids are started slowly and gradually increased. When amino acid infusions are discontinued, the rate is usually slowed over several days.
- Medications, other than insulin, are rarely mixed with parenteral nutrition fluids. Consult the pharmacist if in doubt.

#### Patient and family education
- See entry for drug class (p. 179).

## ammonium chloride (a-MO-nee-um) acidifying agent

- ammonium chloride: Sold under generic name

**MECHANISM OF ACTION**  Ammonium chloride dissociates to form an ammonium ion, which is converted to urea by the normal liver. This reaction releases a hydrogen ion that neutralizes one bicarbonate ion. The chloride ion released from dissociation of ammonium chloride associates with other bases in the body and reduces alkaline reserves. The overall result of all these effects is a shift toward more acidic pH. The increase in chloride ion concentration increases the excretion of chloride in the kidney and promotes mild, temporary diuresis.

**INDICATIONS**  **Metabolic acidosis** may follow excessive chloride loss through excessive vomiting, gastric lavage, pyloric stenosis, or gastric drainage. • Hypochloremia can also arise from prolonged use of certain diuretics.  **Edematous conditions associated with hypochloremia** Ammonium chloride is useful for periods of less than about 3 days because the diuretic effect is only temporary.  **Urinary tract infections** Lowering the pH of urine increases the effectiveness of some antibacterial preparations. • Ammonium chloride may be prescribed along with an antibacterial agent.

**CONTRAINDICATIONS**  **Hepatic insufficiency** These patients cannot convert all the ammonium ion to urea and may suffer ammonia toxicity.  **Renal insufficiency** Patients of this type who also lack sodium must have both sodium and chloride supplied; ammonium chloride alone will not meet their needs.  **Primary respiratory acidosis** Patients with high total carbon dioxide and buffer base should not receive ammonium chloride.  **Pulmonary insufficiency or cardiac edema** Patients with these conditions should be carefully monitored for acid/base balance and respiratory function if ammonium chloride is given.

**DOSAGE**    **PO:**    **ADULTS:** 4 to 12 g daily in divided doses every 4 to 6 hours, after meals when possible. **CHILDREN:** 75 mg/kg daily in 4 doses after meals when possible.    **IV:**    **ADULTS, CHILDREN:** To treat metabolic alkalosis, ammonium chloride is administered by infusion, with dosage guided by the carbon dioxide combining power measured for the particular patient.    *Special patient populations:* **PREGNANCY:** Safe use has not been established.    **RENAL OR HEPATIC FAILURE:** See Contraindications above.

**PREPARATIONS**    *Tablets, enteric-coated:* 486 or 500 mg. *Concentrate for injection:* 26.75% (5 mEq, or 5 mmol, of ammonium and chloride ion per milliliter). Before use, this solution is diluted; 20 ml of concentrate is added to 500 ml of 0.9% sodium chloride or 40 ml of concentrate is added to 1000 ml of 0.9% sodium chloride. The resulting solution is 200 mEq (or 200 mmol) of ammonium ion per liter and 354 mEq (or 354 mmol) of chloride ions per liter. Infusion in adults should not exceed 5 ml/min.

**DRUG INTERACTIONS**    **Basic drugs such as amphetamines, mecamylamine, and quinidine** are more rapidly excreted in acidic urine. Elimination of these drugs is therefore enhanced by ammonium chloride. **Acidic drugs such as salicylates and barbiturates** are more readily reabsorbed from acidic urine. Elimination of these drugs is therefore lowered by ammonium chloride.

**FATE**    Ammonium chloride dissociates to ammonium and chloride ions. The liver converts ammonium ions to urea, which is then eliminated by the kidneys. Chloride ions also are excreted by the kidneys.

## ❦ NURSING CONSIDERATIONS

### Side effects, toxicities, and associated nursing actions

**CNS** Local or generalized twitching, asterixis, tonic seizures, and coma can arise from ammonia toxicity, which can occur when the liver is unable to metabolize all the ammonium ion being administered.

• Assess for twitching and asterixis (hand-flapping tremor). Monitor level of consciousness.
• Monitor serum ammonia levels.

**CV** Pallor, bradycardia, and other cardiac arrhythmias are all possible signs of ammonia toxicity.

• Monitor pulse and, if available, ECG rhythm strip.

**GI** Vomiting may be a sign of ammonia toxicity.

• Monitor intake and output, serum electrolyte level, and, if available, arterial blood gases.
• Note that excessive vomiting may have contributed to the alkalosis that is being treated by the ammonium chloride. After therapy with ammonium chloride is begun, assess carefully the continued or new development of vomiting.

**Other** Sweating and irregular breathing may be signs of ammonia toxicity.

• Monitor respiratory rate (increased rate may signal acidosis).

### Nursing interventions related to drug administration

• See Preparations above.
• See entry for drug class (p. 177).
• If crystallization of the concentrate for injection has occurred, warm the bottle under running water until crystals disappear.
• To avoid venous irritation and thrombophlebitis, administer IV doses slowly.
• Oral doses may be very irritating. Taking doses with meals or food may help lessen gastric irritation.

### Patient and family education

• See entry for drug class (p. 179).

---

## calcium    (KAL-see-um)                                                    mineral

• calcium carbonate
• calcium chloride
• calcium glubionate
• calcium gluceptate
• calcium gluconate

- calcium glycerophosphate
- calcium lactate
- calcium phosphate dibasic
- calcium phosphate tribasic: See Preparations for trade names

**MECHANISM OF ACTION**  Calcium is vital to proper functioning of cells and tissues. For this reason, calcium concentrations in blood and cells are closely regulated by the body. Short-term derangements in calcium concentrations cause severe symptoms, including tetany, and can cause death. Calcium in bones and teeth gives structural support. Long-term depletion of calcium weakens these structures.

**INDICATIONS**  **Calcium deficiency** Relative calcium deficiency can occur in normal conditions such as pregnancy and lactation and in healthy women during menopause. • Calcium deficiency can also be associated with diseases such as hypoparathyroidism, achlorhydria, chronic diarrhea, steatorrhea, sprue, pancreatitis, and renal failure. • Vitamin D deficiency, alkalosis, and hyperphosphatemia can also induce calcium deficiency. • The use of citrated blood can induce hypocalcemia because of the ability of citrate to bind to calcium.

**CONTRAINDICATIONS**  **Hypercalcemia** Patients with high concentrations of calcium in the blood should not receive additional calcium.   **Ventricular fibrillation** Calcium infusions may further compromise cardiac function.   **Cor pulmonale, respiratory acidosis, renal disease, or respiratory failure** Calcium chloride should not be used in patients with these conditions because this form of calcium is acidifying and therefore dangerous in these conditions.

**DOSAGE**  **PO:**  **ADULTS:** 1 to 2 g daily in 3 or 4 doses to prevent or treat calcium depletion.  **CHILDREN:** 45 to 65 mg/kg daily; neonatal hypocalcemia may require 50 to 150 mg/kg but should not exceed 1 g daily.  **IV:**  **ADULTS:** Actual doses depend upon the status of the patient. Average doses range from 7 to 14 mEq*/kg initially.  **CHILDREN:** Doses are individualized based on the status of the patient. Average doses range from 0.45 to 0.7 mEq/kg initially. Neonates being treated for tetany may receive a total daily dose of up to 2.4 mEq/kg administered in divided doses.  **IM:**  **ADULTS:** 2 to 5 mEq may be administered when IV administration is impossible. *Special patient populations:*  **PREGNANCY:** Pregnant and lactating women require more calcium than other women; dietary adjustments and supplementation may be necessary.

**PREPARATIONS**  **Calcium carbonate,** *pieces, chewable:* 1.2 g, equivalent to 600 mg or 30 mEq of calcium (Suplical). *Powder: generic. Suspension:* 1 g, equivalent to 400 mg or 20 mEq or calcium in 5 ml (Titralac); 1.25 g, equivalent to 500 mg or 25 mEq of calcium in 5 ml (calcium carbonate suspension). *Tablets:* 625 mg, equivalent to 260 mg or 13 mEq of calcium (generic); 1.25 g, equivalent to 500 mg or 25 mEq of calcium (BioCal, Os-Cal); 1.5 g, equivalent to 600 mg or 30 mEq of calcium (Caltrate). *Tablets, chewable:* 350 mg, equivalent to 140 mg or 7 mEq of calcium (Amitone); 420 mg, equivalent to 168 mg or 8.4 mEq of calcium, with glycine (Calcilac, Calglycine, Mallamint, Titralac); 500 mg, equivalent to 200 mg or 10 mEq of calcium (Chooz, Dicarbosil, Tums); 625 mg, equivalent to 250 mg or 12.5 mEq of calcium (BioCal); 750 mg, equivalent to 300 mg or 15 mEq of calcium (Cal-Sup with glycine, Tums E-X); 850 mg, equivalent to 340 mg or 17 mEq of calcium (AlkaMints).   **Calcium chloride,** *powder: generic. Solution, injection:* 10% (1.36 mEq of calcium and chloride in 1 ml). **Calcium glubionate,** *solution, oral:* 1.8 g, equivalent to 115 mg or 5.75 mEq in 5 ml (Dorcol Children's Liquid Calcium Supplement, Neo-Calglucon).   **Calcium gluceptate,** *powder: generic. Solution, injection:* 22% (0.9 mEq of calcium in 1 ml).   **Calcium gluconate,** *powder: generic. Tablets:* 500 mg, equivalent to 45 mg calcium; 650 mg, equivalent to 58.5 calcium; 1 g, equivalent to 90 mg, calcium. All generic. *Solution, injection:* 10%, equivalent to 0.45 to 0.48 mEq in 1 ml (Kalcinate).   **Calcium glycerophosphate,** *powder: generic.*   **Calcium glycerophosphate and calcium lactate,** *solution, injection:* 0.094 mEq of calcium in 1 ml (Calphosan).   **Calcium lactate,** *powder: generic. Tablets:* 325 mg, equivalent to 42.25 mg calcium; 650 mg, equivalent to 84.5 mg calcium. Both generic.   **Calcium phosphate dibasic,** *powder: generic. Tablets:* 500 mg of dihydrate, equivalent to 115 mg or 5.75 mEq calcium. Generic.   **Calcium phosphate tribasic,** *powder: generic. Tablets, film-coated:* 1604 mg, equivalent to 600 mg or 30 mEq of calcium (Posture). *Tablets, film-coated, combinations:* 650 mg, equivalent to 300 mg or 15 mEq of calcium, with 62.5 IU of

*1 mEq = 0.5 mmol of calcium.

vitamin D (Posture-D); 1300 mg, equivalent to 600 mg or 30 mEq of calcium, with 125 IU of vitamin D (Posture-D, scored).

**DRUG INTERACTIONS**   **Cardiac glycosides** have increased inotropic and toxic effects when given with calcium. The combination should be avoided if possible. If calcium must be given to such a patient, the dose must be small and administered slowly; the patient should be carefully observed for arrhythmias. **Tetracycline antibiotics** are irreversibly bound (chelated) by calcium. Oral or parenteral forms of the two agents should never be combined.

**DIAGNOSTIC TEST INTERFERENCE**   **Serum and urinary magnesium values** measured by the Titan yellow method may be falsely lowered by IV calcium salts.

**FATE**   Calcium is incompletely absorbed following oral administration in a process that is regulated by vitamin D. Calcium absorption and excretion by the kidneys is regulated by interactions between vitamin D, parathyroid hormone, and possibly calcitonin. These agents also regulate the release of calcium from stores in bone and the deposition of calcium in new or remodeled bone.

## ☙ NURSING CONSIDERATIONS

### Side effects, toxicities, and associated nursing actions

**CNS** A sense of oppression or other mood changes is occasionally reported with IV calcium.
- Assess for changes in mood. Remain with patient if mood changes are severe or frightening to patient.

**CV** Cardiac arrhythmias, vasodilation, decreased blood pressure, syncope, and even cardiac arrest have followed too rapid IV injection of calcium salts. Calcium injected directly into the heart rather than into the ventricular space may lacerate coronary arteries, with dangerous results.
- Monitor blood pressure and vital signs. Monitor ECG during IV administration.
- Monitor serum calcium levels.
- Be especially alert for the development of arrhythmias when administering a calcium preparation to a patient receiving a cardiac glycoside. The calcium preparation increases toxicity from the cardiac glycoside.

**GI** Oral calcium preparations may irritate or cause constipation. Calcium chloride, via any route of administration, is most often linked with this complication.
- Assess patients for GI side effects. If the patient is taking a calcium preparation for its antacid effects, it may be possible to switch antacids or alternate two antacid combination products to avoid diarrhea or constipation. See Chapter 60.
- If constipation occurs, instruct patient to increase fluid intake to 2500 to 3000 ml per day (if not contraindicated by medical condition); increase dietary intake of fruit, fruit juices, or fiber; and increase level of exercise. Use of a stool softener may be necessary.

### Nursing interventions related to drug administration

- See Preparations above.
- The following preparations may be given intravenously: calcium chloride, calcium gluceptate, and calcium gluconate. Read order and labels carefully. When possible, the drug should be warmed to body temperature before administering. Administer at a rate not exceeding 0.7 to 1.5 mEq/min. The IV route of administration is preferred in infants, but avoid using a scalp vein, as extravasation may cause tissue necrosis. Monitor ECG during IV administration (see CV side effects above). The patient should remain recumbent for 30 minutes following IV administration; monitor the blood pressure.
- The following preparations may be administered intramuscularly if IV administration is not possible: calcium gluceptate, calcium gluconate, or a combination of calcium glycerophosphate and calcium lactate. *Calcium chloride* may only be administered intravenously or intracardially. Use a large muscle mass such as the dorsogluteal site or rectus femoris muscle in adults. In children, the IV route is preferred; however, if the IM route must be used, use the vastus lateralis muscle.
- If 5 ml or more is to be administered intramuscularly to an adult, divide the dose and administer via two injections.
- The following preparations may be administered orally: the carbonate, glubionate, gluconate, lactate, and phosphate salts.

- Severe hypocalcemia may manifest as tetany. Chvostek's sign and Trousseau's sign may be positive (see a physical assessment book for illustration of these signs). Pad the side rails. Have resuscitation equipment readily available.

**Patient and family education**
- See entry for drug class (p. 179).
- Instruct patients to take oral calcium preparations 1 to 1 1/2 hours after eating and/or to take the dose with milk.
- Review with patients dietary sources of calcium: milk products, cheese, yogurt; dark green leafy vegetables such as spinach, kale, and greens; and sardines, clams, and oysters.

---

## dextran  (DEX-tran)                                                            blood substitute

- dextran 40: Gientran, LMD, Rheomacrodex
- dextran 70: Macrodex
- dextran 75

**MECHANISM OF ACTION**    Dextrans given intravenously have a colloidal osmotic effect that draws fluid from the interstitial spaces into the blood compartment. The result is an expansion of plasma volume. The large molecular weights of the dextrans cause them to be retained in the blood much like albumin. Dextran 40 decreases erythrocyte aggregation and lowers blood viscosity, actions not shared by the other forms of dextran.

**INDICATIONS**    **Shock** Dextran increases plasma volume and improves circulation in these patients. • Dextran is a substitute for blood or blood products when action must be taken before blood can be cross-matched. • Other fluids and electrolytes, as well as other drugs, may be required.    **Prophylaxis of venous thrombosis or pulmonary emboli** Hip replacement and certain other surgical procedures carry a high risk of embolitic complications. • Dextran 40 can be used prophylactically because of its effect on microcirculation, preventing blood sludging.

**CONTRAINDICATIONS**    **Thrombocytopenia or clotting disorders** At high doses dextrans may interfere with platelet function or promote bleeding by hemodynamic effects.    **Impaired renal function, pulmonary edema, or congestive heart failure** Dextrans may cause vascular overload in these compromised patients, with increased venous pressures, worsened pulmonary edema, and other signs.    **Dehydration** Dextran 40 may be dangerous to such patients, precipitating renal failure. • Anuria or oliguria may be a sign of impending renal failure; dextran 40 should be discontinued and an osmotic diuretic administered to restore urine flow.

**DOSAGE**    **IV:**    **ADULTS:** For shock, doses should not exceed 2 g/kg for the first day and 1 g/kg daily thereafter. Therapy should not continue beyond 5 days. For prophylaxis of venous thrombosis and pulmonary embolism, doses of 1 g/kg may be given for 3 days, followed by a 2-week period in which the same dose is given every 2 to 3 days.    *Special patient populations:*    **CHILDREN:** Doses have not been established.    **PREGNANCY:** Safe use has not been established.

**PREPARATIONS**    *Dextran 40, solution, injection:* 10% dextran 40 in 5% dextrose or 10% dextran 40 in 0.9% sodium chloride injection. *Dextran 70, solution injection:* 6% dextran 70 in 5% dextrose or 6% dextran 70 in 0.9% sodium chloride injection. *Dextran 75, solution, injection:* 6% dextran 75 in 5% dextrose or 6% dextran 75 in 0.9% sodium chloride injection.

**DRUG INTERACTIONS**    **Heparin** may cause unexpectedly profound depression of clotting in patients also receiving dextran 70 or dextran 75 because these dextrans can alter erythrocyte agglutination and platelet function. Data on dextran 40 are less complete, but some interaction with heparin might be expected.

**DIAGNOSTIC TEST INTERFERENCE**    **Blood glucose determinations** may yield falsely high values if the method used includes hydrolysis with sulfuric or acetic acid.    **Cross-matching of blood by proteolytic enzyme techniques** is not accurate because of interference from dextrans.    **Total protein assays using Biuret reagent** cannot be performed because dextrans cause turbidity in the sample.    **Bilirubin assays using alcohol** cannot be performed because dextrans cause turbidity in the sample.

**FATE**    Dextrans are normally eliminated by the kidneys, with the smaller molecular weight material being eliminated more rapidly than the larger. Dextran with molecular weight greater than 50,000 is not excreted at significant rates by the kidneys but is slowly metabolized to glucose and thence to carbon dioxide and water.

### ❦ NURSING CONSIDERATIONS

#### Side effects, toxicities, and associated nursing actions

**CV** Overloading of the vascular system may occur, with symptoms of fluid retention.
- Monitor weight, blood pressure and pulse, and intake and output; inspect for development of edema, especially in dependent areas (sacral area, feet, and legs). See entry for drug class (p. 177) for additional discussion of potential fluid overload.

**Blood** The hematocrit may be reduced but should not be allowed to fall below 30%. Protein concentration may also fall.
- Monitor hematocrit and hemoglobin, serum protein, and serum protein electrophoresis.
- Monitor for development of bleeding. Visually inspect patient for bruising, petechiae, or overt bleeding. Check stool for occult blood.

**GI** Nausea, vomiting, and involuntary defecation have occurred.
- Assess for development of GI symptoms. If severe or persistent, notify physician.
- Monitor intake and output.

**Renal** The urinary viscosity and specific gravity may greatly increase, especially with dextran 40. Hydration must be adequate to maintain urine flow.
- Monitor intake and output. If urine output falls below 30 to 50 ml/hr, notify physician.
- Monitor serum electrolyte level and urinary specific gravity.

**Allergic** Anaphylactoid reactions are possible within minutes of injection, even with small amounts of dextran. Symptoms include generalized urticaria, wheezing, a feeling of tightness in the chest, hypotension, nausea, and vomiting.
- Anticipate the possibility of allergic reaction by having readily available drugs, equipment, and personnel for treatment of an acute reaction.
- After beginning the infusion, remain at the beside of the patient for 15 to 30 minutes to assess the development of an allergic response.
- Monitor the vital signs. At the first sign of an allergic reaction, stop the infusion and notify the physician.

#### Nursing interventions related to drug administration
- See entry for drug class (p. 177).
- Monitor pulse, blood pressure, and central venous pressure (CVP) if available every 5 minutes initially, then every 15 minutes for an hour. Continue measurements at least hourly. For significant increases in CVP, slow or stop infusion and notify physician.
- If blood is to be administered, change tubing or flush tubing well with normal saline solution between infusions of dextran and blood. Dextran causes blood to coagulate in tubing.
- If crystallization has occurred, heat bottle in warm water bath until crystals dissolve before administering.
- Use only clear solutions. After opening a bottle, unused portions should be discarded.
- If blood is drawn for laboratory tests while patient is receiving dextran, note on the lab request that dextran is being infused. Dextran causes false high serum glucose levels and alterations in other blood tests.

#### Patient and family education
- See entry for drug class (p. 179).

---

## dextrose   (DEX-trose)                                    sugar

- dextrose (D-glucose): Sold under the generic name

**MECHANISM OF ACTION**   Dextrose is a naturally-occurring sugar in food and is a product of metabolism of more complex carbohydrates. Dextrose is further metabolized to carbon dioxide and water, supplying energy to cells.

**INDICATIONS**   **Hypoglycemia** Dextrose may be administered orally to conscious diabetic patients to reverse hypoglycemia. • IV dextrose may be required in unconscious diabetics.   **Fluid loss or dehydration** Both water and calories may be supplied by dextrose solutions.   **Parenteral nutrition** Patients unable to receive adequate nutrition by mouth may receive dextrose solutions to supply needed calories. • If long-term support is required, hypertonic solutions of dextrose may be used along with amino acids or suspensions of lipids to achieve adequate caloric intake along with proper nutritional balance.

**CONTRAINDICATIONS**   **Anuria** Hypertonic dextrose (concentrations exceeding 5%) may worsen renal damage.   **Hemorrhage in the central nervous system** Hypertonic dextrose (concentrations exceeding 5%) may increase the damage.   **Delirium tremens** If dehydrated, these patients cannot tolerate hypertonic dextrose (concentrations exceeding 5%).   **Diabetic coma** These patients already suffer from dangerously elevated blood glucose concentrations and cannot metabolize any additional sugar.   **Allergy to corn products** Because most dextrose is produced commercially from corn starch, the possibility of allergic reactions exists.

**DOSAGE**   **PO:**   **ADULTS:** In diabetics suffering from hypoglycemic reactions, 10 to 20 g, followed by self-monitoring of blood glucose with a repeat dose in 10 to 20 minutes if necessary.   **IV:**   **ADULTS OR CHILDREN:** For hypoglycemia, 20 to 50 ml of a 50% dextrose solution may be administered at rates not exceeding 3 ml/min. When administered for rehydration and/or calories, the dosage depends on the status of the patient, but rates should not exceed 0.8 g/kg in an hour.   **NEONATES AND INFANTS:** For hypoglycemia, doses are usually 2 ml/kg of 10% to 25% dextrose solution. When administered for rehydration and/or calories, the dosage depends on the status of the patient, but rates should not exceed 0.8 g/kg in an hour.   *Special patient populations:*   **PREGNANCY:** Special doses have not been established.

**PREPARATIONS**   *Tablets:* 500 mg. *Tablets, chewable:* 5 g. *Gel, oral:* 40% (2 g in 5 ml). *Solution, injection:* dextrose is available alone or in various combinations as hypotonic (2.5%), isotonic (5%), or hypertonic solutions (7.7% to 70%). See Table 10-3.

**DRUG INTERACTIONS**   **Hypoglycemic agents** (insulins, sulfonylureas) have less effect in lowering blood glucose when additional glucose is added to the system by administering oral or IV dextrose (glucose).

**FATE**   Dextrose is readily metabolized to carbon dioxide and water. When administered orally, the sugar is readily absorbed, with *peak* increases in blood glucose concentrations at 40 minutes after the dose.

## ❦ NURSING CONSIDERATIONS

### Side effects, toxicities, and associated nursing actions

**CNS** Mental confusion and loss of consciousness may signal hyperglycemia and impending hyperosmolar syndrome.
- Monitor level of consciousness.
- Monitor serum glucose level.

**CV** Water intoxication can arise if infusions of dextrose are continued for prolonged periods.

**Metabolic** Hyperglycemia can occur, especially with infusion rates greater than 0.5 g/kg in an hour. Hypokalemia, hypophosphatemia, and hypomagnesemia can occur.
- See entry for drug class (p. 177) for discussion of fluid overload.
- Monitor serum electrolyte, phosphorus, and magnesium levels, intake and output, and weight.

**Other** Rebound hypoglycemia can occur when infusions of dextrose are discontinued, especially if infusion of a concentrated solution is halted abruptly.
- Slowly discontinue infusing concentrations of 10% or greater by decreasing the rate over several hours or days. If hyperalimentation or total parenteral nutrition is discontinued suddenly, many institutions have standing orders to start a peripheral infusion of 10% dextrose immediately to avoid hypoglycemia.

### Nursing interventions related to drug administration
- See entry for drug class (p. 177).
- See Dosage above.
- Dextrose concentrations greater than 10% are usually administered through a large central line. Infusions of 10% or less can be safely administered via peripheral infusion. The exception to this is treatment of an acute hypoglycemic reaction, when concentrations of up to 50% may be given slowly by direct IV push.

- Tablets and gel preparations are used primarily by alert diabetics experiencing a hypoglycemic reaction. After a dose is taken, the blood glucose must be monitored, as it may be necessary to repeat the dose.

**Patient and family education**
- See entry for drug class (p. 179).

---

# fat emulsion
parenteral nutrition

- fat emulsion: Intralipid, Liposyn, Travamulsion

**MECHANISM OF ACTION**   Lipid mixtures are a concentrated source of calories for patients requiring all nutrition by parenteral routes.

**INDICATIONS**   **Long-term parenteral nutrition** For long-term support, patients must receive a balance of calories from carbohydrate, protein, and lipids.

**CONTRAINDICATIONS**   **Intolerance or allergy to components of the mixtures** The mixtures contain lipids from soybeans, egg yolk, and safflower.

**DOSAGE**   **IV:**   **ADULTS:** Administered by peripheral veins, 10% solutions at 1 ml/min and 20% solutions at 0.5 ml/min. The solutions are essentially isotonic because of added glycerol. The total amount of solution added is determined by the nutritional needs of the patient, but no more than 60% of the required calories should be supplied by fat emulsions. The daily limit ranges from 2.5 to 4 g/kg daily. **CHILDREN:** Infusion rates should be lower than adult rates, with initial test infusions at 0.05 ml/min for 20% emulsions and 0.1 ml/min for 10% emulsions. Rates for maintenance should not exceed about 1 g/kg in 4 hours.   *Special patient populations:*   **PREGNANCY:** Safe use has not been established.

**PREPARATIONS**   *Emulsions for administration:* 10% or 20%.

**DRUG INTERACTIONS**   **IV drugs and solutions** should not be combined with fat emulsions to avoid breaking down the structure of the emulsion.

**FATE**   Oils, fatty acids, and phospholipids in these mixtures are metabolized by the liver and other tissues to supply energy and intermediates for maintenance of cell structure.

## ☙ NURSING CONSIDERATIONS
### Side effects, toxicities, and associated nursing actions
**CV** Pain in the chest has rarely been reported.
- Monitor vital signs. If pain in the chest occurs, slow the infusion and assess the patient.

**Blood** Thrombophlebitis, thrombocytopenia, and anemia.
- Monitor platelet count. Observe for signs of thrombocytopenia: bleeding gums, nosebleeds, petechiae, change in the color of urine (which may indicate bleeding), and bleeding in the stool.
- Monitor hematocrit and hemoglobin levels.

**Liver** Liver function tests should be monitored.

**Metabolic** Transient elevations of triglycerides are common. Lipemia should clear between infusions of the fat emulsion.
- Monitor liver function tests and triglycerides.

### Nursing interventions related to drug administration
- See entry for drug class (p. 177).
- Fat emulsions may be administered via central or peripheral infusion.
- Inspect bottle carefully. Fat emulsions are milky in color. If the emulsion has "cracked" (the oil and other products have separated), it should not be used. Do not shake fat emulsions.
- Product manufacturers supply excellent instructions with the various products. Review these carefully before administering fat emulsions.
- Fat emulsions should not be filtered. If administering "piggyback," the fat emulsion must be attached to the primary line below any inline filters (that is, between the filter and the patient).
- Begin infusions slowly. Monitor vital signs. If the patient experiences no apparent difficulty, increase infusion rate to desired rate after 30 minutes. Consult manufacturer's literature.

**Patient and family education**
- See entry for drug class (p. 179).

---

## fructose   (FRUK-tose)                                    sugar

- fructose (D-frutose, fruit sugar, laevulose, levulose): Sold under generic name; Travert (combination product)*

**MECHANISM OF ACTION**   Fructose is a readily metabolized sugar that can supply energy to cells. Unlike dextrose, fructose can be taken into cells and metabolized even in the absence of insulin. Fructose is more readily converted to glycogen than is dextrose.

**INDICATIONS**   **Fluid depletion** Fructose solutions are used to supply calories and water for hydration.

**CONTRAINDICATIONS**   **Deficiency in aldolase B** Patients with the genetically determined lack of aldolase B activity cannot completely metabolize fructose. • These patients show signs of impaired renal function (Franconi's syndrome), which resolves when fructose is discontinued.

**DOSAGE**   IV:   ADULTS: Usual doses are 1 to 3 L of 10% solution daily.   *Special patient populations:* CHILDREN: Doses have not been established.   PREGNANCY: Safe use has not been established.

**PREPARATIONS**   *Solution, injection:* 10%. *Solution injection, combinations:* Invert sugar (equimolar concentrations of dextrose and fructose), 10% solution for injection. Invert sugar (equimolar concentrations of dextrose and fructose), 10% solution with electrolytes (Ionosol, Multiple Electrolyte, Electrolyte No. 1, Electrolyte No. 2).

**DRUG INTERACTIONS**   None reported.

**FATE**   Fructose is rapidly converted by fructokinase activity in the liver to fructose-1-phosphate, which is further metabolized by the action of aldolase B. The products of these sequential reactions may be used in several metabolic pathways. Lactic acid production is increased by fructose metabolism. Uric acid production often increases as well. Fructose is available to most tissues of the body but is not used by the CNS. For this reason fructose cannot reverse the CNS effect of acute hypoglycemia.

### ❧ NURSING CONSIDERATIONS

#### Side effects, toxicities, and associated nursing actions
**Renal** Fanconi's syndrome can be precipitated by fructose when patients lack aldolase B, an enzyme involved in metabolizing the sugar.
- Question patient about aldolase B deficiency before administering the infusion.
- Fanconi's syndrome is a disturbance of proximal renal tubular function. Findings include aminoaciduria, glycosuria, hyperphosphaturia, and renal loss of potassium, bicarbonate, and water.
- Monitor intake and output and weight.
- Monitor urinalysis. Abnormalities of glucose and protein should be further investigated, as should indications of renal disease. Fanconi's syndrome will resolve when fructose is discontinued.

**Metabolic** Lactic acidosis can occur, especially with high doses. Uric acid production may also be stimulated, resulting in hyperuricemia.
- Monitor arterial blood gases if available.
- Monitor serum uric acid level.

#### Nursing interventions related to drug administration
- See entry for drug class (p. 177).
- Infusion rate should not exceed 1 g/kg/hr.

#### Patient and family education
- See entry for drug class (p. 179).

---

## hetastarch   (HET-a-starch)                              blood substitute

- hetastarch (HES, hydroxyethyl starch): Hespan

---

*Equimolar mixture of dextrose and fructose; also called invert sugar.

**Table 10-3.**

## Dextrose solutions for parenteral use

| Dextrose concentration | Other components present | Calories/L* | Clinical use |
|---|---|---|---|
| 2.5% | — | 85 | To provide calories and water IV by peripheral veins |
| 2.5% | 0.45% Sodium chloride | 85 | To provide calories, salt, and water IV by peripheral veins |
| 2.5% | 1/2 Strength lactated Ringer's injection | 85 | To provide calories, water, and electrolytes IV by peripheral veins |
| 4% | Modified lactated Ringer's injection | 135 | To provide calories, water, and electrolytes IV by peripheral veins |
| 5% | — | 170 | To provide calories and water IV by peripheral veins |
| 5% | 0.11%, 0.2%, 0.225%, 0.3%, 0.45%, or 0.9% Sodium chloride | 170 | To provide calories, salt, and water IV by peripheral veins |
| 5% | 0.075%, 0.15%, 0.224%, or 0.3% Potassium chloride | 170 | To provide calories, potassium, and water IV by peripheral veins |
| 5% | 0.2% Sodium chloride and 0.075%, 0.15%, 0.22%, 0.224%, or 0.3% potassium chloride | 170 | To provide calories, water, and electrolytes IV by peripheral veins |
| 5% | 0.225% Sodium chloride and 0.075%, 0.15%, 0.224%, or 0.3% potassium chloride | 170 | To provide calories, water, and salt IV by peripheral veins |
| 5% | 0.33% Sodium chloride and 0.15% potassium chloride | 170 | To provide calories, salt, and water IV by peripheral veins |
| 5% | 0.45% Sodium chloride and 0.075%, 0.15%, 0.22%, 0.224%, 0.3% potassium chloride | 170 | To provide calories, salt, and water IV by peripheral veins |
| 5% | Acetated Ringer's injection | 170 | To provide calories, water, and electrolytes IV by peripheral veins |
| 5% | Lactated Ringer's injection | 170 | To provide calories, water, and electrolytes IV by peripheral veins |
| 5% | Ringer's injection | 170 | To provide calories, water, and electrolytes IV by peripheral veins |
| 5% | Electrolyte mixtures (Electrolyte No. 48, Electrolyte No. 75, Ionosol, Isolyte, Normosol, Plasma-Lyte) | 170–190 | To provide calories, water, and electrolytes IV by peripheral veins |

**Table 10-3.**

## Dextrose solutions for parenteral use—cont'd

| Dextrose concentration | Other components present | Calories/L* | Clinical use |
|---|---|---|---|
| 5% | 5% Alcohol (ethanol) | 450 | To provide calories IV by peripheral veins |
| 5% | 10% Alcohol (ethanol) | 720 | To provide calories IV by peripheral veins |
| 5% | 10% Dextran 40 | 170 | Rehydration; see drug monograph |
| 5% | 6% Dextran 70 or dextran 75 | 170 | Rehydration; see drug monograph |
| 7.7% | — | 260 | To provide calories and water IV by large veins |
| 10% | — | 340 | To provide calories and water IV by large veins |
| 10% | 0.45% or 0.9% sodium chloride | 340 | To provide calories, salt, and water IV by large veins |
| 10% | 0.2% Sodium chloride and 0.15% potassium chloride | 340 | To provide calories, water, and electrolytes IV by large veins |
| 10% | Electrolyte mixtures (Ionosol, Isolyte) | 340 | To provide calories, water, and electrolytes IV by large veins |
| 11.5% | — | 390 | To provide calories and water IV by large veins |
| 20% | — | 680 | To provide calories and water IV by central veins |
| 25% | — | 850 | To provide calories IV by central veins after dilution |
| 30% | — | 1020 | To provide calories IV by central veins after dilution |
| 38% | — | 1290 | To provide calories IV by central veins after dilution |
| 38% | Electrolyte pattern T | 1290 | To provide calories and electrolytes IV by central veins after dilution |
| 38.5% | — | 1310 | To provide calories IV by central veins after dilution |
| 40% | — | 1360 | To provide calories IV by central veins after dilution |
| 50% | — | 1700 | To provide calories IV by central veins after dilution |
| 50% | Electrolytes (pattern A, pattern B, pattern N, or with acetate) | 1700 | To provide calories and electrolytes IV by central veins after dilution |
| 60% | — | 2040 | To provide calories IV by central veins after dilution |
| 70% | — | 2380 | To provide calories IV by central veins after dilution |

*Each gram of glucose supplies 3.4 calories (Kcalories) or 11.3 kilojoule.

**MECHANISM OF ACTION**    Hetastarch has colloidal properties similar to albumin. Because of these properties hetastarch draws water from the interstitial space into the vascular compartment. Solutions of hetastarch are therefore useful to increase plasma volume.

**INDICATIONS**    **Shock** Shock induced by many causes is accompanied by reduced circulating plasma volume. • Solutions of hetastarch may be used to expand plasma volume. • Other fluids and electrolytes, as well as other drugs, may be required. • Hetastarch is a substitute for blood or blood products when fluids must be administered before blood can be cross-matched.

**CONTRAINDICATIONS**    **Severe bleeding disorders** Hetastarch can interfere with platelet function.    **Severe congestive heart failure** These patients may be unable to tolerate the volume expansion and may suffer signs of fluid overload or pulmonary edema. • Arterial and venous pressures may increase, as well as work load on the heart.    **Renal failure** Anuria or oliguria may signal renal failure. • These patients are more sensitive to fluid overload.

**DOSAGE**    IV:    ADULTS: Usual doses of a 6% solution are 500 to 1000 ml (30 to 60 g), not to exceed 1500 ml (90 g) or 20 ml/kg each hour (1.2 g/kg). Doses are adjusted to the degree of volume depletion of the patient and other clinical signs.    *Special patient populations:*    ELDERLY: Aged patients are more sensitive to fluid overload and should receive hetastarch under carefully controlled conditions to avoid this danger.    CHILDREN: Older children may receive hetastarch as adults, but the very young may be more sensitive to fluid overlaod and should receive hetastarch under carefully controlled conditions to avoid this danger.    PREGNANCY: Safe use has not been established.

**PREPARATIONS**    *Solution, injection:* 6% in 0.9% sodium chloride.

**DRUG INTERACTIONS**    None reported.

**FATE**    Hetastarch exists as a mixture of polymers with molecular weights ranging from 10,000 to 1,000,000. Those molecules with molecular weights under 50,000 are cleared from the body within 24 hours by the kidneys. Larger molecules are slowly degraded, releasing smaller polymers, glucose, and hydroxyethyl-glucose. Glucose is metabolized; the smaller polymers and hydroxyethyl-glucose are eliminated by the kidney. Elimination of 99% of the drug may take 2 weeks or longer.

## NURSING CONSIDERATIONS

### Side effects, toxicities, and associated nursing actions
**CV** Volume expansion may be accompanied by increased arterial and venous pressure, increased stroke volume, and increased work load on the heart.
• Monitor heart rate, blood pressure, and ECG strip if available.
**Blood** Hematocrit, hemoglobin, plasma proteins, and platelets may decrease, especially with large doses of hetastarch. Hetastarch also increases erythrocyte sedimentation rates and prolongs clotting times.
• Monitor hematocrit and hemoglobin, platelet count, erythrocyte sedimentation rate, and clotting times.
• Assess for signs of bleeding: unexplained bruising, bleeding from gums or nose, blood in urine or stool, and petechiae.
**Allergic** Allergic reactions include fever, chills, itching, vomiting, headache, flulike symptoms, and anaphylaxis.
• Monitor vital signs.
• Remain with patient for 15 to 30 minutes after beginning infusion. If signs of an allergic reaction appear, discontinue infusion.
• Have available drugs, equipment, and personnel to treat an acute allergic response.

### Nursing interventions related to drug administration
• See Dosage above for infusion rate.
• See entry for drug class (p. 177).
• Unused portions should be discarded.

### Patient and family education
• See entry for drug class (p. 179).

## magnesium sulfate  (mag-NEE-zi-um)  electrolyte*

- magnesium sulfate (epsom salt): Sold under generic name

**MECHANISM OF ACTION**  Magnesium is an important cofactor in many enzyme reactions and is required for maintenance of normal membrane function. Magnesium is in general a CNS depressant, but the exact mechanism of anticonvulsant action is unknown. Administered orally, magnesium salts are cathartics.

**INDICATIONS**  **Seizures in eclampsia or preeclampsia** The mechanism of the magnesium effect is not known. • In other types of seizures magnesium may be effective because it replaces depleted magnesium pools in the body.  **Magnesium deficiency** Total parenteral nutrition, prolonged IV therapy with magnesium-free fluids, malabsorption syndrome, alcoholism, cirrhosis of the liver, and acute pancreatitis may all be associated with magnesium depletion. • Parenteral magnesium can be administered to correct acute deficiencies.  **Barium poisoning** Parenteral magnesium sulfate controls muscle stimulation caused by barium poisoning. • Orally administered magnesium can precipitate the barium and cause catharsis.

**CONTRAINDICATIONS**  **Heart block or myocardial damage** Magnesium may worsen heart block.  **Renal impairment** Patients with renal disease may be unable to eliminate magnesium rapidly enough to prevent toxic accumulations of magnesium.

**DOSAGE**  **PO:**  **ADULT:** 10 to 30 g (81 to 243 mEq† of magnesium) as a laxative.  **CHILDREN 6 TO 12 YEARS:** 5 to 10 g as a laxative.  **CHILDREN 2 TO 5 YEARS:** 2.5 to 5 g as a laxative.  **IV:**  **ADULTS:** Doses should be guided by monitoring clinical response and magnesium concentrations in serum. For eclampsia, initial doses include 4 g in 250 ml of 5% dextrose given by IV infusion, with additional doses given intramuscularly. Total daily doses should not exceed 30 to 40 g. The concentration of magnesium in IV fluids should not exceed 20% (200 mg/ml); the rate of infusion should not exceed 150 mg/min (1.5 ml of a 10% solution). For barium poisoning, 1 to 2 g is usual. For parenteral nutrition, 0.5 to 3 g daily is sufficient to prevent magnesium depletion.  **CHILDREN:** 0.25 to 1.25 g of magnesium in infants is sufficient for supplementation in parenteral nutrition.  **IM:**  **ADULTS:** 1 to 5 g may be given in the buttock at 4- to 6-hour intervals; the lower doses are adequate for magnesium repletion, but the higher doses may be required in treating eclampsia. The concentration of solution administered is usually 25% (250 mg/ml) or 50% (500 mg/ml).  **CHILDREN:** Doses up to 100 mg/kg may be administered at 4- to 6-hour intervals. The concentration of drug administered should not exceed 20%.  *Special patient populations:*  **PREGNANCY:** Magnesium does pass to the fetus when magnesium is used to treat eclampsia. Because of the danger of neuromuscular and respiratory depression, magnesium should not be administered within 2 hours of delivery of the infant.  **RENAL FAILURE:** See Contraindications above.

**PREPARATIONS**  *Crystals, powder:* for preparation of oral solutions. *Solution, injection:* 10%, 12.5%, or 50%.

**DRUG INTERACTIONS**  **Opiates, barbiturates, general anesthetics,** and other CNS depressants may cause additive CNS depression with magnesium sulfate.  **Neuromuscular blocking agents** have additive effects with magnesium and may cause excessive blockade in patients receiving magnesium.  **Digitalis-treated** patients may be more prone to heart block if they must receive calcium after treatment with magnesium.

**FATE**  Magnesium administered intravenously takes action immediately and persists for about 30 minutes. The *onset* of action following IM administration is about 1 hour, with a *duration* of 3 to 4 hours. Elimination of magnesium is through the kidneys.

## ☙ NURSING CONSIDERATIONS

### Side effects, toxicities, and associated nursing actions

**CNS** Depression of reflexes (patellar reflex), flaccid paralysis, hypothermia, and CNS depression are signs of magnesium intoxication.
- Monitor patellar reflex, temperature, and level of consciousness.
- Monitor serum magnesium levels.

**CV** Flushing, hypotension, circulatory collapse, and depression of cardiac function are signs of magnesium intoxication.

*Also cathartic, anticonvulsant.

†1 mEq = 1 mmol of potassium.

- Monitor blood pressure and pulse. In pregnant women, monitor fetal heart sounds. In severe eclampsia or preeclampsia, it may be appropriate to monitor ECG tracing of the mother and attach fetal monitor to assess infant status.
- Monitor intake and output. If urinary output falls below 30 to 100 ml per hour, it may indicate magnesium toxicity.

  **Other** Respiratory failure may be the cause of death in magnesium intoxication.

- Monitor respiratory rate. Respiratory rate should be at least 16 per minute before administration of a parenteral dose.
- Newborn infants of mothers who received parenteral magnesium sulfate should be monitored carefully during the first several hours after birth for signs of magnesium toxicity (see Table 10-1).

### Nursing interventions related to drug administration

- See Dosage above for information about rate of parenteral administration.
- See entry for drug class (p. 177).
- Treatment of overdosage is with parenteral calcium gluconate or calcium gluceptate.
- IM magnesium sulfate is painful. To reduce discomfort, 1 ml of 2% lidocaine may be added to the drug dose (with physician approval). Administer the injection slowly.

### Patient and family education

- See entry for drug class (p. 179).

---

## potassium    (poe-TASS-ee-um)                                          electrolyte

- potassium acetate
- potassium bicarbonate
- potassium chloride
- potassium citrate
- potassium gluconate
- potassium phosphate, monobasic or dibasic: Parenteral products sold under generic name

Oral products, see Table 10-4.

**MECHANISM OF ACTION**   Potassium is present in highest concentrations within cells, where the ion maintains isotonicity. Potassium is required for proper electrical activity of cells in nerves, heart, and muscles. The ion is also required by a variety of metabolic processes.

**INDICATIONS**   **Potassium depletion (hypokalemia)** Potassium depletion can arise from many causes including chronic diseases (renal diseases, familial periodic paralysis, hyperadrenalism), gastrointestinal or nutritional disorders (prolonged vomiting, diarrhea, malnutrition, malabsorption syndrome, negative nitrogen balance), metabolic derangements (metabolic alkalosis, metabolic acidosis, diabetic acidosis), medical procedures (prolonged drainage of GI fluids, dialysis, prolonged parenteral nutrition without added potassium), or drug therapy (thiazide diuretics, loop diuretics, carbonic anhydrase inhibitors, ACTH, natural corticosteroids, aminosalicylic acid, amphotericin B).

**CONTRAINDICATIONS**   **Renal impairment** Oliguria, anuria, or azotemia may signal insufficient renal function that will lead to dangerous accumulation of potassium if the ion is administered.   **Addison's disease (chronic adrenocortical insufficiency)** Potassium tends to accumulate in this condition if it is untreated; additional potassium may cause dangerously high concentrations.   **Dehydration** Potassium levels are already elevated in these patients.   **Severe burns or extensive tissue destruction** Destroyed cells release potassium, which can significantly elevate potassium levels in the blood.
- Additional potassium may be dangerous.   **Hyperkalemia** Excessive potassium in the blood from any cause is a contraindication for potassium administration.

**DOSAGE**   **PO:**   **ADULTS:** To prevent hypokalemia, 20 mEq* of potassium daily. To treat potassium depletion, 40 to 100 mEq of potassium daily. Doses must be individualized based on laboratory and clinical data

*1 mEq = 0.5 mmol of magnesium.

for each patient. Supplementation should begin gradually (3 to 7 days), and the daily dosage should be divided into 2 to 4 doses. Daily dosage should not exceed 150 mEq. **CHILDREN:** To replace potassium deficits, 2 to 3 mEq/kg or 40 mEq/M$^2$. Daily dosage should not exceed 3 mEq/kg. Doses should be divided. **IV:** **ADULTS:** Doses are adjusted for patient needs. The concentration of potassium in the IV fluid should not exceed 40 mEq/L, and the solutions should not be administered any faster than 20 mEq/hr. **CHILDREN:** As oral doses. *Special patient populations:* **ELDERLY:** Dehydration is not uncommon in elderly patients. If severe, potassium levels may already be elevated. **PREGNANCY:** Altered doses have not been established. **RENAL FAILURE:** See Contraindications, page 194.

**PREPARATIONS** Potassium bicarbonate, potassium chloride, potassium gluconate, potassium acetate, and potassium citrate are available in a variety of formulations for oral administration: *tablets for solution, capsules, powder for solution, solutions, and elixirs* (Table 10-4). Potassium acetate, potassium chloride, and potassium phosphates are available as solutions for parenteral use. In addition to the solutions listed below, potassium is included in Ringer's solution (see drug monograph) and in electrolyte mixtures that are frequently combined with dextrose, fructose, or invert sugar (see drug monographs). *Potassium chloride, solution, injection:* 2 or 4 mEq* in each milliliter. *Potassium chloride, solution, injection:* 1.5, 2.0, 2.4, 3.0, and 3.2 mEq in each milliliter. *Solution combinations, injection:* 5% dextrose with 0.075% (10 mEq/L), 0.15% (20 mEq/L), 0.224% (30 mEq/L), or 0.3% (40 mEq/L) potassium chloride. 0.9% Sodium chloride with 0.15% (20 mEq/L) or 0.3% (40 mEq/L) potassium chloride. 5% Dextrose and 0.2% sodium chloride with 0.075% (10 mEq/L), 0.15% (20 mEq/L), 0.22% (30 mEq/L), 0.224% (30 mEq/L), or 0.3% (40 mEq/L) potassium chloride. 5% Dextrose and 0.225% sodium chloride with 0.075% (10 mEq/L), 0.15% (20 mEq/L), 0.224% (30 mEq/L), or 0.3% (40 mEq/L) potassium chloride. 5% Dextrose and 0.33% sodium chloride with 0.15% potassium chloride. 5% Dextrose and 0.45% sodium chloride with 0.075% (10 mEq/L), 0.15% (20 mEq/L), 0.22% (30 mEq/L), 0.224% (30 mEq/L), or 0.3% (40 mEq/L) potassium chloride. 10% Dextrose and 0.2% sodium chloride with 0.15% (20 mEq/L) potassium chloride. *Potassium phosphates (monobasic and dibasic), solution, injection:* 4.4 mEq potassium and 3 mm phosphate per milliliter or 4.5 mEq potassium and 3 mm phosphate per milliliter.

**DRUG INTERACTIONS** **Potassium-sparing diuretics** should not be used with potassium supplements because of the danger of potassium accumulation and toxicity. **Salt substitutes and low-salt milk** contain significant potassium and may lead to dangerous accumulations when used along with potassium supplements. **Penicillins, blood, and blood plasma** may contain significant potassium that should be taken into account when administering potassium orally or parenterally.

**FATE** Potassium salts are rapidly absorbed following oral administration. Enteric-coated tablets release potassium chloride primarily in the small intestine, where high local concentrations can irritate or ulcerate the intestinal lining. Potassium is removed from the blood and concentrated in cells by the action of Na$^+$, K$^+$-ATPase. Elimination of potassium is primarily by the kidneys.

## ❦ NURSING CONSIDERATIONS

### Side effects, toxicities, and associated nursing actions

**CNS** Paresthesias, confusion, listlessness, and flaccid paralysis may be signs of hyperkalemia.
- Monitor level of consciousness. Question patient about development of paresthesias.
- Monitor serum electrolyte level.

**CV** ECG abnormalities may reflect hyperkalemia.

**Blood** Hyperkalemia is the most likely and most dangerous side effect of potassium administration. Death can be caused by cardiovascular collapse.
- Monitor ECG. ECG changes that may indicate hyperkalemia include peaking of T waves, flattening of P waves, prolonged P-R interval, and widening of the QRS. Ultimately, hyperkalemia may lead to ventricular fibrillation and cardiac standstill.

**GI** Potassium salts are irritating and may cause nausea, vomiting, diarrhea, and abdominal pain. Enteric-coated forms may cause perforation of the small bowel.

*1mEq = 1 mmol of potassium.

**Table 10-4.**

| Potassium for use as oral supplementation | | | | |
|---|---|---|---|---|
| Trade name | Potassium form | Dosage form | Potassium content | Other components |
| Bayon | Gluconate | Elixir | 6.7 mEq/5 ml | 5% alcohol; sugar-free |
| Bi-K | Citrate | Solution | 6.7 mEq/5 ml | Sorbitol |
| Cena-K | Chloride | Solution | 6.7 or 13.3 mEq/5 ml | Sugar-free |
| Duo-K | Chloride, gluconate | Solution | 6.7 mEq/5 ml | — |
| K-G | Gluconate | Elixir | 6.7 mEq/5 ml | 5% alcohol |
| K-Lor | Chloride | Powder dissolve | 15 mEq/packet | — |
| K-Lor | Chloride | Powder dissolve | 20 mEq/packet | Sugar-free |
| K-Lyte | Bicarbonate | Tablet dissolve | 25 mEq | 2.1 g citric acid |
| K-Lyte/CL | Chloride | Powder dissolve | 25 mEq/dose | — |
| K-Lyte/CL | Bicarbonate, chloride | Tablets dissolve | 25 mEq | 0.91 g lysine, 0.55 g citric acid |
| K-Lyte/CL 50 | Bicarbonate, chloride | Tablets dissolve | 50 mEq | 3.65 g lysine, 1 g citric acid |
| K-Lyte DS effervescent tablets | Bicarbonate, citrate | Tablets dissovle | 50 mEq | 2.1 g citric acid |
| K-Tab | Chloride | Tablets extended-release | 10 mEq | — |
| Kaochlor 10% | Chloride | Solution | 6.7 mEq/5 ml | 5% Alcohol, tartrazine |
| Kaochlor-Eff | Bicarbonate, chloride, citrate | Tablets dissolve | 20 mEq | Tartrazine, 1.84 g betaine HCl, sugar-free |
| Kaochlor 10% SF | Chloride | Solution | 6.7 mEq/5 ml | 5% Alcohol, sugar-free |
| Kaon | Gluconate | Tablets | 2 or 5 mEq | — |
| Kaon Elixir | Gluconate | Elixir | 6.7 mEq/5 ml | 5% Alcohol, sugar-free |
| Kaon-Cl 10% | Chloride | Tablets extended-release | 10 mEq | — |
| Kaon-Cl 20% | Chloride | Solution | 13.3 mEq/5 ml | 5% Alcohol, sugar-free |
| Kaon-Cl | Chloride | Tablets extended-release | 6.7 mEq | Tartrazine |
| Kato | Chloride | Powder dissolve | 20 mEq/packet | 0.5 mEq sodium |
| Kay Ciel | Chloride | Powder dissolve | 20 mEq/packet | Sugar-free |
| Kay Ciel Elixir | Chloride | Elixir | 6.7 mEq/5 ml | 4% Alcohol, sugar-free |
| Kaylixir | Gluconate | Elixir | 6.7 mEq/5 ml | 5% Alcohol |
| Klor-10% | Chloride | Solution | 6.7 mEq/5 ml | — |
| Klor-Con | Chloride | Powder dissolve | 20 mEq/packet | Sugar-free |
| Klor-Con | Chloride | Powder dissolve | 25 mEq/dose | — |
| Klor-Con | Chloride | Solution | 13.3 mEq/5 ml | Tartrazine |
| Klor-Con/EF | Bicarbonate | Tablets dissolve | 25 mEq | 2.1 g citric acid |
| Klorvess | Bicarbonate, chloride | Tablets dissolve | 20 mEq | 0.913 g lysine, sugar-free |

**Table 10-4.**

## Potassium for use as oral supplementation—cont'd

| Trade name | Potassium form | Dosage form | Potassium content | Other components |
|---|---|---|---|---|
| Klorvess 10% | Chloride | Solution | 6.7 mEq/5 ml | 0.7% Alcohol |
| Klorvess Effervescent Granules | Bicarbonate, chloride | Granules dissolve | 20 mEq/packet | 0.913 g lysine, sugar-free |
| Klotrix | Chloride | Tablets extended-release | 10 mEq | — |
| Kolyum | Chloride, gluconate | Powder | 20 mEq/5 g | Sorbitol, sugar-free |
| Kolyum | Chloride, gluconate | Solution | 6.7 mEq/5 ml | Sorbitol, sugar-free |
| Micro-K Extencaps | Chloride — | Capsules — | 8 mEq — | — — |
| Micro-K Extencaps | Chloride | Capsules | 10 mEq | — |
| Pota-Chlor 10% | Chloride | Solution | 6.7 mEq/5 ml | 5% Alcohol |
| Pota-Chlor 20% | Chloride | Solution | 13.3 mEq/5 ml | — |
| Potage | Chloride | Powder dissolve | 20 mEq/packet | Sugar-free |
| Potasalan | Chloride | Solution | 6.7 mEq/5 ml | 4% Alcohol |
| Potassine | Chloride | Solution | 5 mEq/5 ml | — |
| Potassium Chloride Enseals | Chloride | Tablets enteric-coated | 4 mEq | — |
| Potassium Chloride Enseals | Chloride | Tablets enteric-coated | 13.4 mEq | — |
| Quic-K | Bicarbonate | Tablet | 6.5 mEq | — |
| Rum-K | Chloride | Solution | 10 mEq/5 ml | Sugar-free |
| SK-Potassium Chloride 10% | Chloride | Solution | 6.7 mEq/5 ml | — |
| SK-Potassium Chloride 20% | Chloride | Solution | 13.3 mEq/5 ml | — |
| Slow-K | Chloride | Tablets extended-release | 8 mEq | — |
| Tri-K | Acetate, bicarbonate, citrate | Solution | 2.5 mEq/5 ml | — |
| Trikates | Acetate, bicarbonate, citrate | Solution | 15 mEq/5 ml | — |
| Twin-K | Citrate, gluconate | Solution | 6.7 mEq/5 ml | Sorbitol |
| Twin-K-CL | Citrate, gluconate | Solution | 5 mEq/5 ml | Ammonium chloride, 1.3 mEq/5 ml; sorbitol |

• Work with the patient to find an oral form of potassium that the patient is willing to take. Taking oral preparations with a snack or meals may lessen irritation. Effervescent preparations may be unpalatable to the patient, but some patients are willing to use this form. Diluting liquid preparations in milk or juice may diminish gastric irritation. Powder for solution should be completely dissolved before taking. Enteric-coated forms should be avoided if possible.

### Nursing interventions related to drug administration

• *Dilute* parenteral potassium preparations before administering and give via slow IV infusion. See Dosage above.
• See entry for drug class (p. 177).
• Do not administer wax matrix formulations to patients with esophageal compression from an enlarged left atrium; use liquid preparations for these patients.
• Do not administer potassium in patients with minimum or absent kidney function.

### Patient and family education

• See entry for drug class (p. 179).
• Instruct the patient about dietary sources of potassium: citrus fruits and juices; grape, cranberry, apple, pear, and apricot juices; bananas; whole grain cereals; tea and cola beverages; peanut butter; and nuts. Note that many of these food items are also high in sodium and so may be contraindicated on that basis for some patients.
• Licorice can cause potassium excretion. Caution patients with hypokalemia to avoid licorice.
• Some oral preparations contain FD & C coloring #5 (tartrazine), which may cause an allergic response in some individuals. Although rare, this response is more common in individuals with aspirin hypersensitivity. Caution patients who have this allergy to avoid switching brands of potassium preparation.
• Oral potassium is available plain, in sugar-free formulations, and in formulations containing one or more of the following: sorbitol, alcohol, citric acid, or sodium. If the patient has a history of allergy or prescribed dietary restrictions that would limit the preparations that should be used, the patient, pharmacist, physician, and nurse should work together to find a formulation that is satisfactory for the patient (see Table 10–4).

## Ringer's injection    (RING-ers)                                    electrolyte solution

• Ringer's injection: Sold under generic name

**MECHANISM OF ACTION**    Ringer's injection is a multiple electrolyte solution that is intended to supply the proper balance of electrolytes, as well as water when used for hydration. The solution contains 147 mEq/L sodium, 4 mEq/L potassium, 4.5 mEq/L calcium, and 156 mEq/L chloride. Modifications of the solution include adding dextrose or other sugars to supply calories. Added acetate and lactate act as precursors of bicarbonate and are therefore alkalinizing agents.

**INDICATIONS**    **Dehydration** Fluid loss or reduced plasma volume can be treated with administration of Ringer's injection.    **Mild acidosis** Ringer's injection with acetate or lactate can be used to replace fluids and electrolytes when mild acidosis is also present.

**CONTRAINDICATIONS**    **Congestive heart failure or pulmonary edema** Patients with these conditions cannot tolerate excess fluid.    **Hyperkalemia, hypercalcemia,** or other conditions in which any of the components of the mixture should be avoided: patients must be able to eliminate the sodium, potassium, calcium, and chloride ions supplied by the Ringer's solution.

**DOSAGE**    IV:    ADULTS: Dosage is adjusted to the patient's condition and needs; 90 to 125 ml/hr is commonly employed.    *Special patient populations:*    CHILDREN: Special pediatric doses have not been established.    PREGNANCY: Safe use has not been established.

**PREPARATIONS**    *Solution, injection:* Ringer's injection (pH 5.5 to 6.1, 309 mOsm/L) contains in mEq/L the following ions: 147 sodium, 4 potassium, 4.5 calcium and 156 chloride.

Ringer's injection with 5% dextrose (pH 4 to 4.6, 561 mOsm/L) supplies 170 calories/L (565 kilojoules/L), in addition to the electrolytes listed above for Ringer's injection.

Acetated Ringer's injection (pH 6.7, 275 mOsm/L) contains in mEq/L the following ions: 131 sodium, 4 potassium, 3 calcium, 109 chloride, and 28 acetate.

Acetated Ringer's injection with 5% dextrose (pH 4.7, 540 mOsm/L) supplies 170 calories/L (565 kilojoules/L), in addition to the electrolytes listed above for acetated Ringer's injection.

Lactated Ringer's injection (pH 6.2 to 6.7, 273 mOsm/L) contains in mEq/L the following ions: 130 sodium, 4 potassium, 3 calcium, 109 chloride, and 28 lactate.

Lactated Ringer's injection with 5% dextrose (pH 4.7 to 5.1, 525 to 530 mOsm/L) supplies 170 to 180 calories/L (565 to 598 kilojoules/L), in addition to the electrolytes listed above for lactated Ringer's injection.

Lactated Ringer's injection 1/2 strength with 2.5% dextrose (pH 5, 263 mOsm/L) supplies 85 to 89 calories/L (283 to 296 kilojoules/L) and the following ions, in mEq/L: 65 sodium, 2 potassium, 1 to 1.5 calcium, 55 chloride, and 14 lactate.

Modified lactated Ringer's injection with 4% dextrose (pH 5, 255 mOsm/L) supplies 135 calories/L (449 kilojoules/L) and the following ions, in mEq/L: 26 sodium, <1 potassium, <1 calcium, 22 chloride, and 6 lactate.

**DRUG INTERACTIONS**   See specific interactions for sodium, potassium, and calcium.

**FATE**   Sodium, potassium, calcium, and chloride ions are eliminated by the kidneys. Acetate and lactate are metabolized, contributing bicarbonate to alkalinize the system.

## 👻 NURSING CONSIDERATIONS

### Side effects, toxicities, and associated nursing actions

**CV** Signs of fluid overload may occur.

**Blood** Specific electrolyte imbalances may occur, including alkalosis if acetate or lactate have been administered.

• Monitor serum electrolyte level and arterial blood gases.

### Nursing interventions related to drug administration

• See entry for drug class (p. 177).

### Patient and family education

• See entry for drug class (p. 179).

---

## sodium bicarbonate   (SODE-ee-um)                    alkalinizing agent

• sodium bicarbonate (sodium acid carbonate, sodium hydrogen carbonate): Arm & Hammer Baking Soda, Neut, Soda Mint

**MECHANISM OF ACTION**   Sodium bicarbonate dissociates in the body to release sodium and bicarbonate ions. Sodium is eliminated by the kidneys. The bicarbonate ion contributes to the buffering system composed of bicarbonate, carbon dioxide, and carbonic acid. This buffering system is the primary one regulating extracellular pH. The bicarbonate ion is the base in this system. Addition of bicarbonate raises extracellular pH.

**INDICATIONS**   **Metabolic acidosis** can be caused by many diseases, as well as by drugs or chemicals (carbonic anhydrase inhibitors, ammonium chloride, methyl alcohol).   **Phenobarbiturate or salicylate intoxication** The elimination of these drugs is enhanced in the alkaline urine produced by sodium bicarbonate.   **Bicarbonate depletion** Extensive diarrhea can deplete bicarbonate.   **Hyperkalemia** Bicarbonate may be required in addition to other therapy to promote the reuptake of potassium into cells.

**CONTRAINDICATIONS**   **Metabolic or respiratory alkalosis** Bicarbonate worsens the alkalosis.   **Hypocalcemia** Alkalosis in these patients may cause tetany.   **Hypochloremia** Excessive loss of stomach fluids or treatment with certain diuretics depletes chloride ion and may cause alkalosis, which is worsened by bicarbonate.   **Edema and congestive heart failure** The sodium content of sodium bicarbonate may not be tolerated by patients with relative fluid overload.

**DOSAGE    PO:    ADULTS:** To treat metabolic acidosis, 20 to 36 mEq* of sodium bicarbonate is given daily in divided doses. The dose is adjusted to create plasma bicarbonate concentrations of 18 to 20 mEq/L. To alkalinize the urine, 48 mEq (4 g) is given initially, then 1 to 2 g every 4 hours, not to exceed 16 g daily.    **CHILDREN:** To alkalinize the urine, 1 to 2 mEq/kg may be used, with adjustments as necessary to maintain pH at the desired level.    **IV:    ADULTS:** To treat metabolic acidosis, 2 to 5 mEq/kg as a 4- or 8-hour infusion. Subsequent doses depend on patient response.    **CHILDREN:** Older children receive adult doses. Neonates and infants up to 2 years should receive hypertonic sodium bicarbonate by slow infusion of a 4.2% solution. The maximum daily dose is 8 mEq/kg.    ***Special patient populations:*    CHILDREN:** Rapid injection is dangerous in small children, leading in some cases to intracranial hemorrhage.    **PREGNANCY:** Safe use has not been established.

**PREPARATIONS**    *Tablets:* 300, 325, 600, and 650 mg. *Powder, oral:* sold as baking soda. *Solution, for nebulization:* 4.2% (2.5 mEq/5 ml) for inhalation. *Solution, injection:* 4.2% (2.5 mEq/5 ml), 5% (3 mEq/5 ml), 7.5% (4.46 mEq/5 ml), and 8.6% (5 mEq/5 ml). *Solution, to adjust pH of injections:* 4% (2.4 mEq/5 ml), 4.2% (2.5 mEq/5 ml).

**DRUG INTERACTIONS:    Amphetamines, methadone, quinidine, and quinine** are reabsorbed more readily from alkaline urine and are therefore excreted more slowly when sodium bicarbonate is given. **Aspirin, salicylates,** and other acidic drugs are excreted more rapidly when urine is alkaline.    **Lithium** excretion may be enhanced by the excess sodium supplied as sodium bicarbonate.    **Methenamine** is a urinary antiseptic that requires acidic pH to be effective. Sodium bicarbonate counteracts the antiseptic effect by raising urinary pH.

**FATE**    Sodium bicarbonate is readily absorbed following oral administration. Sodium and bicarbonate ions are eliminated in the urine in processes carefully regulated by the kidneys so that electrolyte and acid/base balances are preserved.

### ❦ NURSING CONSIDERATIONS

#### Side effects, toxicities, and associated nursing actions

**CNS** Cerebral dysfunction, altered consciousness, seizures, and tetany can result from alkalosis induced by sodium bicarbonate.

**Metabolic** Alkalosis.
- Monitor level of consciousness.
- Monitor arterial blood gases.
- If alkalosis is present, pad siderails. Have resuscitation equipment available. Have available calcium gluconate and 2.14% ammonium chloride solution to treat overdose.

**CV** Fluid retention can arise from the sodium content of sodium bicarbonate. Congestive heart failure may be worsened.
- Monitor intake and output, weight, and blood pressure. Assess breath sounds.

**GI** Oral doses of sodium bicarbonate cause gastric distension and flatulence. Mixing sodium bicarbonate with acid results in the release of carbon dioxide gas.
- Instruct patient to chew oral forms thoroughly and to drink a full glass of liquid.
- Dissolve powder forms completely in water before drinking.

#### Nursing interventions related to drug administration
- See entry for drug class (p. 177).
- Except during resuscitation, dilute sodium bicarbonate before IV administration. Prepackaged syringes for emergency use are found on most crash carts or in the emergency drug box.
- When used to alkalinize the urine, monitor urine pH.

#### Patient and family education
- See entry for drug class (p. 179).

---

## sodium chloride                                                                electrolyte

- sodium chloride: Sold under generic name

*1 mEq = 1 mmol of sodium bicarbonate.

**MECHANISM OF ACTION** Sodium chloride dissociates in water to sodium and chloride ions. Sodium is the most abundant positively charged ion in extracellular fluid and is the primary determinant of osmotic pressure of that fluid. Normal saline solution (0.9% sodium chloride) is isotonic; it has an osmolarity of 308 mOsm/L, similar to body fluids. Chloride and sodium, along with bicarbonate and other ions, also contribute to acid-base balance in the body.

**INDICATIONS** **Dehydration** Isotonic or hypotonic solutions of sodium chloride can be used to replace water and sodium chloride in patients who have suffered excessive fluid loss. • These solutions essentially restore extracellular fluid volume. **Metabolic alkalosis with sodium depletion** Mild imbalances of this sort often respond to replacement of sodium chloride. **Hyponatremia** Severe sodium depletion may require rapid replacement with hypertonic solutions of sodium chloride.

**CONTRAINDICATIONS** **Congestive heart failure, edema, or other sodium-retaining conditions** Patients with these conditions may accumulate sodium and associated fluid to dangerous degrees. **Hypernatremia or hyperchloremia** Additional sodium or chloride should not be added in patients with these conditions.

**DOSAGE** **PO:** ADULTS: 1 to 2 g three times daily. **IV:** ADULTS: Dosage is guided by clinical status of the patient. Usual doses are 1 L of 0.9% sodium chloride daily or 1 to 2 L of 0.45% sodium chloride. Hypertonic solutions (3% or 5%) may be given through a large vein, 100 ml/hr; additional doses should be withheld until electrolyte and acid-base status can be evaluated. *Special patient populations:* ELDERLY: Altered doses for the elderly have not been specifically established, but the elderly require special care to avoid electrolyte imbalances or fluid overloads. CHILDREN: Benzyl alcohol used as a bacteriostatic agent in sodium chloride solutions has caused death in neonates. Solutions of sodium chloride containing benzyl alcohol should not be used to dilute drugs or to flush IV lines in neonates. PREGNANCY: The risk in pregnancy is primarily from electrolyte, acid-base, or osmotic imbalances.

**PREPARATIONS** *Tablets:* 250 and 650 mg. Sold as salt tablets. *Tablets, enteric-coated:* 1 g. *Solution, injection:* 0.45%, 0.9%, 3%, or 5%. 0.9% Solutions marked ''bacteriostatic'' also contain benzyl alcohol or parabens. *Solution, for preparation of IV admixtures:* 2.5 or 4 mEq/ml. *Solution, combinations:* 0.11%, 0.2%, 0.225%, 0.3%, 0.45%, or 0.9% sodium chloride with dextrose (2.5%, 5%, or 10%). 0.2%, 0.225%, 0.33%, 0.45%, or 0.9% sodium chloride with dextrose (5% or 10%) and potassium chloride (0.075%, 0.15%, 0.22%, 0.224%, 0.3%). 0.9% Sodium chloride with 6% dexran 70 or dextran 75. 0.9% Sodium chloride with 6% hetastarch.

**DRUG INTERACTIONS** **Lithium** excretion may be enhanced by the excess sodium supplied as sodium chloride. **Corticotropin** or **corticosteroids** may promote salt and water retention.

**FATE** Sodium and chloride are excreted by the kidneys. Excretion is regulated by the kidneys to maintain salt and water balance.

## ❧ NURSING CONSIDERATIONS

### Side effects, toxicities, and associated nursing actions
**CNS** Weakness and disorientation may be signs of sodium excess.
**Blood:** Dilution of electrolytes other than sodium and chloride can occur. Other imbalances such as hypokalemia are possible.
• Monitor level of consciousness.
• Monitor serum electrolyte level.
**CV** Fluid retention may lead to signs of congestive heart failure in patients with preexisting cardiac impairment.
• Monitor intake and output and weight. Assess heart and breath sounds.

### Nursing interventions related to drug administration
• See Dosage above. Preparations containing benzyl alcohol should not be used to dilute drugs or flush IV lines in neonates.
• See entry for drug class (p. 177).
• Oral tablets should be taken with a full glass of water.

**Patient and family education**
- See entry for drug class (p. 179).

---

# sodium lactate                                          alkalinizing agent

- sodium lactate: Sold under generic name

**MECHANISM OF ACTION**    Sodium lactate acts as an alkalinizing agent because the lactate ion is converted to bicarbonate by the liver.

**INDICATIONS**    **Mild to moderate metabolic acidosis** The bicarbonate derived from lactate corrects the acidosis.

**CONTRAINDICATIONS**    **Edema, congestive heart failure,** or **sodium retention** Patients with these conditions may not be able to tolerate the sodium content of sodium lactate and may suffer fluid overload. **Metabolic or respiratory alkalosis** The alkalosis produced by sodium lactate may cause dangerous symptoms.    **Hepatic insufficiency, shock, congestive heart failure, hypoxia, or beriberi** Lactate utilization is reduced in patients with these conditions. • The lactate supplied in sodium lactate may therefore not be metabolized and may accumulate to dangerous levels.    **Lactic acidosis** Sodium lactate may worsen this condition.

**DOSAGE**    **PO:**    **ADULTS:** 30 ml/kg daily of 1/6 molar solution to alkalinize the urine.    **IV:**    **ADULTS:** Dosage is determined by the condition of the patient and the degree of acidosis. The dosage should not exceed 300 ml/hr of a 1/6 molar solution. *Special patient populations:* **CHILDREN:** Special pediatric doses have not been established.    **PREGNANCY:** Safe use has not been established.

**PREPARATIONS**    *Solution, injection:* 1/6 molar. This solution is also occasionally used orally. *Solution, injection for preparation of IV admixtures:* 2.5 mEq/ml.

**DRUG INTERACTIONS**    None reported.

**FATE**    Sodium lactate dissociates to sodium and lactate ions. The sodium ion can be excreted by the kidneys. The lactate ion can be metabolized to bicarbonate in the liver, but the process takes 1 to 2 hours.

**❦ NURSING CONSIDERATIONS**

**Side effects, toxicities, and associated nursing actions**

**CV** Fluid retention and edema.
- Monitor intake and output, weight, and vital signs.

**Renal** Hypernatremia and electrolyte imbalances.

**Metabolic** Metabolic alkalosis.
- Monitor serum electrolyte level and arterial blood gases.

**Nursing interventions related to drug administration**
- See Dosage above for rate of IV administration.
- See entry for drug class (p. 177).
- If used to alkalinize the urine, monitor the urine pH.

**Patient and family education**
- See entry for drug class (p. 179).

# AGENTS TO MODIFY BLOOD

**IV**

**INTRODUCTION**   Blood is liquid tissue that performs many functions. The coagulation system provides mechanisms for repairing leaks or dislodging or preventing deposits in the vasculature. A variety of drugs are available to alter blood coagulation. Antiplatelet drugs may have prophylactic value in preventing strokes and heart attacks. Heparin is a direct-acting anticoagulant drug that is widely used in the hospital to prevent blood coagulation in a variety of situations. The oral anticoagulants, often called ''blood thinners'' by the lay community, are indirect-acting anticoagulants. They have a multitude of interactions with other drugs. Thrombolytic drugs are used to dissolve a clot that has already formed. Recent use has expanded their use to treating acute myocardial infarctions. Systemic hemostatic agents are used to promote blood coagulation.

Lipids transported in the blood are bound to complex proteins. Abnormally high concentrations of blood lipids are associated with atherosclerosis. Drugs are effective in reducing abnormally high plasma lipid values. These drugs help to slow atherosclerosis, a leading cause of strokes and heart attacks.

Iron, vitamin $B_{12}$, and folic acid are all nutritional agents necessary for the production of mature red blood cells, the transport system for oxygen. Deficiencies of any one of these can lead to anemia, and so these agents are used therapeutically to overcome the specific nutritional anemias arising in their absence.

# Chapter Eleven

# Drugs altering blood coagulation

**Antiplatelet drugs**
aspirin (see Chapter 47)
dipyridamole
sulfinpyrazone (see Chapter 50)

**Direct-acting anticoagulant**
heparin

**Indirect-acting (oral) anticoagulants**
anisindione
dicumarol
phenprocoumon
warfarin

**Thrombolytic agents**
streptokinase
urokinase

**Systemic hemostatic agents**
aminocaproic acid
antihemophilic factor
factor IX complex
menadione/menadiol
phytonadione

**INTRODUCTION**   The process of blood coagulation is diagrammed in Fig. 11-1. The initial step can be an event in the intrinsic pathway, the activation of the blood component factor XII (the Hageman factor) by contact with exposed collagen, or an event in the extrinsic pathway, that is, the release of tissue factor by damaged tissue. All pathways activate factor X. Factor Xa (activated factor X) forms a complex with platelet phospholipids, calcium, and factor V. This complex, which is sometimes called throm-

**Figure 11-1.** The stages of blood coagulation are diagrammed. Actions of drug classes discussed in this chapter include four stages.
*Stage I:*
   a. Antiplatelet drugs inhibit platelet aggregation in the intrinsic pathway.
   b. Citrate and EDTA, which chelate calcium, prevent the formation of factor Xa.
   c. Heparin, by activating antithrombin III, neutralizes factor Xa and stops coagulation at stage 1.
   d. Oral acticoagulants prevent the synthesis of factors VII, IX, and X, which are necessary for stage 1.
   e. Local hemostatic agents provide a contact to activate the intrinsic pathway.
*Stage II:* Oral anticoagulants prevent the synthesis of prothrombin.
*Stage III:* Heparin activates antithrombin III to prevent thrombin
*Stage IV:*
   a. Aminocaproic acid inhibits the activation of profibrinolysin and so inhibits clot degradation.
   b. Streptokinase and urokinase activate profibrinolysin to aid clot digestion.

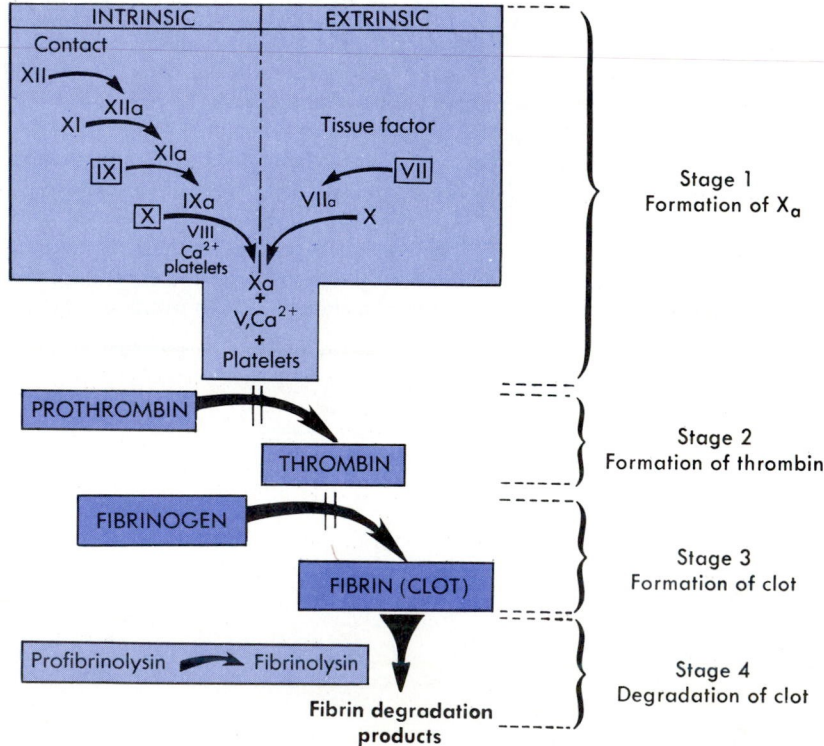

Ⅱ  Indicates the step is blocked by heparin

☐  Indicates a clotting factor that is not synthesized when oral anticoagulants are present

boplastin, catalyzes the conversion of prothrombin (factor II) to thrombin. Thrombin then catalyzes the conversion of fibrinogen to fibrin. After cross-linking of fibrin by factor XIIIa, fibrin becomes insoluble, forming a mesh that is the blood clot.

Blood clots in the arterial system are initially composed largely of platelets with a fibrin mesh (white thrombus). Blood clots in the venous sytem have only a few platelet aggregates and are composed largely of fibrin with trapped red blood cells (red thrombus). A thrombus in either the arterial or venous system may dislodge, becoming an embolus. Venous emboli often lodge in the small arteries of the pulmonary circulation, thereby markedly blocking the oxygenation capacity of the lungs and increasing the blood pressure in the pulmonary system, a life-threatening situation. Thrombi tend to form in veins when blood flow is low, favoring the accumulation of activated clotting factors. Patients at risk for venous thrombosis include anyone immobilized as a result of trauma or surgery or anyone with a history of thromboembolism.

*Antiplatelet* drugs are those drugs that interfere with the aggregation of platelets, the first step in intrinsic coagulation. Clinical trials are in progress to see if prophylactic therapy with these agents decreases the incidence of stroke or myocardial infarction.

*Anticoagulant* drugs, direct or indirect acting, are those drugs that interfere with any of the steps leading to the formation of fibrin. Blood coagulation is often referred to as a cascade phenomenon, since the process becomes magnified at every step. Each activated factor is a catalyst leading to the formation of many molecules of the next activated factor. The earlier in the process that a step can be blocked, the more efficient will be the inhibition of blood coagulation.

*Thromolytic* drugs are those that aid in the process to dissolve clots.

*Systemic hemostatic* drugs are those agents that aid in clot formation.

# Antiplatelet drugs

aspirin (see Chapter 47)  ~  dipyridamole  ~  sulfinpyrazone (see Chapter 50)

**OVERVIEW OF THE DRUG CLASS**  The role of platelet aggregation as the initial step leading to blood coagulation is well established. In particular, the blood clots forming in the arterial system, as opposed to the venous system, are highly linked to conditions promoting platelet aggregation. Patients readily identified as at risk for arterial clots are those who have already suffered a myocardial infarction or a stroke. Clinical trials are in progress to test whether aspirin, dipyridamole, or sulfinpyrazone will decrease the incidence of recurrent strokes or heart attacks when taken prophylactically by patients who have already experienced a heart attack or stroke. Antiplatelet drugs are used prophylactically in patients with heart valve prostheses, heart valve disorders, and shunts.

**MECHANISM OF ACTION**  Antiplatelet drugs interfere with the aggregation of platelets. When there is a break in the endothelial lining exposing collagen, platelets readily attach to the collagen in the exposed tissue. This attachment starts reactions that promote the attachment of platelets to each other. Blood clots in the arterial system begin with platelet aggregation. A clot beginning in a cardiac vessel can cause a myocardial infarction. A clot beginning in a cranial vessel can lead to a stroke.

**INDICATIONS**  **Transient ischemic attack** Aspirin has proved effective for preventing further attacks in men. **Stroke** Clinical trials are examining whether prophylactic treatment with aspirin, dipyridamole, or sulfinpyrazone decreases the recurrence of strokes.  **Myocardial infarction** Clinical trials are examining whether prophylactic treatment with aspirin, dipyridamole, or sulfinpyrazone decreases the recurrence of heart attacks.

**CONTRAINDICATIONS**  • See individual drugs.

**DRUG INTERACTIONS**  • See individual drugs.

## dipyridamole  (dye-peer-ID-a-mole)                                    antiplatelet

• dipyridamole: Persantine

**MECHANISM OF ACTION**   Dipyridamole inhibits at least two enzymes, which allows the accumulation of adenosine, a coronary vasodilator, and of cyclic AMP, which can also lead to vasodilation and inhibition of platelet aggregation.

**INDICATIONS**   **Angina** Coronary vasodilation is one action of dipyridamole; however, studies have not demonstrated the efficiency of long-term therapy with dipyridamole in decreasing the frequency or severity of anginal attacks. It is not effective for acute relief of angina.   **Antiplatelet function** Investigational use of dipyridamole as an antiplatelet drug has been effective in preventing thromboembolic complications only when dipyridamole is used in combination with other drugs.

**CONTRAINDICATIONS**   • None.

**DOSAGE**   **PO:**   **ADULTS:** For chronic angina: 50 mg three times daily at least 1 hour before meals. For prevention of thromboembolic disorders: 150 to 400 mg daily, in combination with aspirin or an anticoagulant.   *Special patient populations:*   **PREGNANCY:** Safe use has not been established.

**PREPARATIONS**   *Tablets:* 25, 50, 75 mg; *tablets (film-coated):* 25, 50, 75 mg.

**DRUG INTERACTIONS**   **Aspirin** and dipyridamole have an additive inhibition on platelet aggregation.   **Oral anticoagulants** can be safely combined with dipyridamole, since dipridamole alone does not affect prothrombin time.

**FATE**   Dipyridamole is metabolized in the liver, and products are excreted in the bile.

### ☙ NURSING CONSIDERATIONS

#### Side effects, toxicities, and associated nursing actions

**CNS** Headache, dizziness.
- Caution patients to avoid driving or operating hazardous equipment if dizziness develops.
- Instruct patients to notify the physician if CNS symptoms are severe or persistent, as a change in dose may be indicated.

**CV** Peripheral vasodilation, fainting.
- Warn the patient about the possibility of fainting. If fainting occurs regularly, instruct the patient to notify the physician, as dosage may need adjustment.

**GI** Nausea, vomiting.
- Instruct patients to take the drug with a full glass of water to lessen gastric irritation. The drug should be taken on an empty stomach, 1 hour before or 2 hours after meals.
- Although the drug works best on an empty stomach, taking the drug with meals or snack may lessen gastric irritation.
- Instruct patients to notify the physician if GI symptoms are severe or persistent.

**Allergic** Rash.
- Instruct patients to report the development of rash or any new sign or symptom.

#### Nursing interventions related to drug administration
- Persantine brand 25 mg tablets contain FD & C yellow dye #5 (tartrazine), which may cause an allergic reaction in susceptible individuals. Although rare, this side effect is seen more often in persons with aspirin hypersensitivity.

#### Patient and family education
- Review anticipated benefits and possible side effects of drug therapy with patients.
- Forewarn patients that several months of therapy may be needed before desired effects are seen; provide positive reinforcement and support
- Caution patients not to switch brands unless directed to do so by the physician, as brands vary in bioavailability.
- Instruct patients to space doses throughout the day. If a dose is missed, instruct the patient to take the dose as soon as remembered, unless within 4 hours of the next dose, in which case the forgotten dose should be omitted and the usual dosing schedule resumed with the next dose. Instruct patients not to double up to make up for missed doses.
- Dipyridamole may be prescribed with aspirin. Caution patients not to take more aspirin than prescribed. Consult the physician about appropriate treatment of headache, fever, or other problems for which aspirin might be used.
- Remind patients to keep these and all medications out of the reach of children.

# Direct-acting anticoagulant
heparin

## heparin calcium    (HEP-a-rin)                                    anticoagulant

- heparin calcium: ✣Calcilen, Calciparine
- heparin sodium: ✣Hepalean, Liquaemin, ✣Minihep, Monoparin

**OVERVIEW**   Heparin is a direct-acting anticoagulant that can be administered to the patient to slow coagulation (in vivo use) or can be added to a storage container to prevent the coagulation of blood (in vitro use).

Other direct-acting agents that can be added to a storage container to prevent the coagulation of blood are citrate and ethylenediamine tetra-acetic acid (EDTA). These compounds bind to calcium, forming a complex that makes calcium unavailable for blood coagulation. Since calcium is essential for many biochemical events, anticoagulants that complex calcium can only be used in storage containers (in vitro), not in a patient (in vivo).

**MECHANISM OF ACTION**   Heparin activates a plasma protein, antithrombin III. As the name indicates, antithrombin III neutralizes thrombin; however, antithrombin III also neutralizes factor Xa, the step before the activation of prothrombin to thrombin. This inhibition of factor Xa, rather than the inhibition of thrombin, appears to be primarily responsible for the effective anticoagulant action of heparin in low doses. Heparin may also serve as an antiplatelet drug. In vitro, heparin actually stimulates platelet aggregation. In vivo, however, heparin appears to coat the endothelial lining of the vessels. Since heparin is a very negatively charged polymer, heparin adds a negative charge to the endothelium that keeps platelets from attaching and forming a thrombus.

**INDICATIONS**   **In vitro anticoagulation** Heparin prevents the coagulation of blood that is stored or taken for laboratory samples. A heparin sodium lock flush solution maintains the patency of indwelling arterial and venous catheters.   **Prophylaxis for postoperative thromboembolism** Low doses of heparin prevent thromboembolisms in the patient population at risk: those over 40 years of age undergoing thoracoabdominal surgery.   **In vivo anticoagulation** Heparin in high doses prevents the further growth of venous thrombi, accelerates the resolution of fresh pulmonary emboli, and may reduce the incidence of arterial and pulmonary embolism in patients with mitral valve disease or chronic atrial fibrillation.   **Disseminated intravascular coagulation** The use of heparin therapy to treat this condition is controversial. **Extracorporal circulation and dialysis** Heparin controls clot formation.

**CONTRAINDICATIONS**   • Hypersensitivity to heparin. • Uncontrolled bleeding. • Pregnancy: During the last trimester and the immediate postpartum period, maternal hemorrhage is a risk of heparin therapy.

**DOSAGE**   **IV:**   **ADULTS:** Continuous infusion: an initial loading dose is 5000 units followed by 20,000 to 40,000 units in 1 L of 0.9% saline over 24 hours.   **CHILDREN:** The initial loading dose is 50 units/kg followed by 100 units/kg infused over each 4 hour period or 20,000 units/$M^2$/kg per 24 hours. **Intermittent IV infusion:**   **ADULTS:** The initial dose is 10,000 units followed by 5,000 to 10,000 units every 4 to 6 hours.   **CHILDREN:** The initial dose is 100 units/kg followed by 50 to 100 units/kg every 4 hours. These high dosages are adjusted according to coagulation test results, determined just before each injection. The whole blood clotting time should be approximately 2.5 to 3 times control value, or the partial thromboplastin time (PTT), which is 1.5 to 2.5 times control value. Coagulation tests are performed frequently during continuous intravaneous infusion.   **SC:**   **ADULTS:** In low-dose heparin therapy for postoperative prophylaxis, 5000 units is administered 2 hours before surgery and every 8 to 12 hours after surgery for 5 to 7 days or until the patient is ambulatory, whichever is longer. **CHILDREN:** Low-dose therapy is not commonly used in children.   **OTHER:** Not effective orally. Intramuscular injections are avoided because they create painful hematomas.   *Special patient populations:*   **PREGNANCY:** Safe use has not been established. Heparin does not cross the blood-brain barrier. Use in the last trimester may increase the risk of maternal hemorrhage.

**PREPARATIONS**    *Parenteral:* 25,000 units/ml (heparin calcium); 1000, 2500, 5000, 7500, 10,000, 15,000, 20,000, 40,000 units/ml (heparin sodium); *lock flush solution:* 10, 100 units/ml.

**DRUG INTERACTIONS**    **Aspirin, dextran, phenylbutazone, ibuprofen, indomethacin, dypridamole, and hydroxychloroquine** interfere with coagulation and accentuate the anticoagulation effect of heparin. **Streptokinase, urokinase** Use of heparin with these thrombolytic drugs will increase the risk of hemorrhage.

**DIAGNOSTIC TEST INTERFERENCE**    Heparinized blood should not be used for isoagglutin, complement, erhthrocyte fragility tests, or platelet counts. Heparinized plasma cannot be used for lipid or fatty acid determinations because heparin activates the enzyme lipoprotein lipase, which degrades plasma triglycerides to fatty acids and glycerol. Tests that may have falsely low values include cholesterol, direct Coombs' test, and levels of sodium calcium and the enzyme acid phosphatase.

**FATE**    Heparin is a normal body constituent found in mast cells, although the physiologic role of heparin has not been established. Although some heparin may appear in the urine when large doses are administered, low doses of heparin are apparently taken up by mast cells. The plasma *half-life* of heparin is 1 to 2 hours in healthy adults.

## ☙ NURSING CONSIDERATIONS

### Side effects, toxicities, and associated nursing actions

**Hematologic hemorrhage** Bleeding complications occur in up to 20% of patients receiving heparin, especially with high-dose therapy.
- Visually inspect the patient at least twice a day for the appearance of bruising and petechiae.
- Check stool for guaiac/blood at least twice per week.
- Instruct patients to report the appearance of any bleeding: bloody nose, blood in urine, stool, or vomitus, coughing up blood, bleeding gums, prolonged menses.
- Monitor vital signs at regular intervals. Be alert to signs of hemorrhage: hypotension, rapid pulse, or other signs of shock. In pregnant women, hemorrhage most likely occurs in the third trimester or immediate postpartum period.
- Monitor ordered blood work, especially when high-dose heparin (>15,000 units per 24 hours) is prescribed for anticoagulation. Monitor partial thromboplastin time (PTT): the goal of anticoagulation therapy is 1.5 to 2 times normal. Monitor activated PTT (aPTT): the goal of anticoagulation therapy is 1.5 to 3 times normal. Little change is these tests should be noted when low-dose therapy is prescribed. Blood specimens for these tests are usually obtained ½ hour before an ordered dose for intermittent therapy.
- Monitor platelet counts. Thrombocytopenia increases the risk of hemorrhage.
- Check most current laboratory work before administering each dose of heparin. Omit the dose and notify the physician if blood work indicates excessive anticoagulation.
- Keep protamine sulfate, the antidote for heparin, available. Unless frank hemorrhage is present, the usual treatment for excessive anticoagulation is temporary discontinuation of heparin.

**Allergic** Hypersensitivity reactions associated with heparin include chills, fever, and urticaria. If these appear, they usually begin about a week after therapy is initiated. Less common are asthma, rhinitis, lacrimation, and anaphylaxis.
- Before administering heparin, question patients about previous allergic responses to heparin.
- Have emergency drugs, equipment, and personnel available in settings where heparin is used.
- An unusual immune response called white clot syndrome is occasionally seen. In this syndrome, the presence of heparin stimulates a reaction that causes platelets to aggregate and form clots. Monitor platelet counts. Be alert to signs and symptoms of clot development: chest pain, neurologic deficits, diminished or absent pulses in extremities.
- Transient alopecia has been reported up to several months after therapy. Reassure patients that this is temporary.

### Nursing interventions related to drug administration
- Read the label on heparin carefully because there are many strengths available.
- Note above each patient's bed (or as is customary in the institution) when the patient is on heparin therapy so that personnel from the laboratory will use the appropriate technique to avoid bleeding after venipuncture.

### Subcutaneous administration
- Any commonly used subcutaneous site may be chosen, but the abdomen is preferred because there are few muscles there, and bruising is less of a cosmetic problem. Avoid the arms.
- Rotate sites, even if the abdomen is used exclusively.
- Avoid areas within 2 inches of the umbilicus. Avoid abdominal scars.
- Try to avoid bruising, which will sometimes occur even with the best technique. Avoid using areas that are bruised.
- Do not inject the skin with the same needle used to draw up the medication.
- Inject at a 45 to 90 degree angle with a ⅝ to ½ inch, 25 or 26 gauge needle after careful assessment of the patient to avoid injection into muscle.
- There is disagreement about pinching the skin as would be done in administering insulin. Pinching may contribute to more bruising.
- Do not aspirate before injecting the medication.
- Do not rub the site after administration. Apply gentle pressure over the site for 15 seconds after administration.
- Keep an accurate record of all injections sites.

**Continuous intravenous administration of heparin** Microdrip tubing and an electronic infusion monitoring device should be used. The infusion rate should be checked regularly to ascertain that the patient is receiving the prescribed dose.
- Heparin is incompatible with many other medications. If other intravenous medications must be administered, establish a second infusion line for these other medications, or flush the tubing containing heparin with normal saline before and after administration of the other medication.

**Establishing and using the heparin well (heparin lock):**  **INTERMITTENT INTRAVENOUS HEPARIN VIA HEPARIN WELL:**
- Insert heparin well into vein using accepted sterile venipuncture technique.
- Secure device in place with tape, and "prime" the well with a small amount (1 to 2 ml) of heparin of the same dosage strength as will be used for anticoagulation.
- Inject each prescribed dose of heparin into the heparin well. The injected dose displaces the heparin remaining in the well each time a dose is given, so flushing the well after the dose is administered is not necessary. Individual institutional policy should be followed if it differs from that described.

**OTHER INTRAVENOUS MEDICATIONS VIA HEPARIN WELL:** One method for administering other medications via heparin well is to insert and secure as described, then prime with 1 ml of a solution of normal saline containing 10 or 100 units of heparin per milliliter. These solutions are available in prepackaged syringes, multiple-dose vials, or can be prepared by the nurse or the pharmacy. Each time a drug is administered, the procedure is:
- Flush the heparin well with 1 to 2 ml of normal saline.
- Administer the prescribed medication via push or infusion.
- Flush the well again with 1 to 2 ml of normal saline.
- Finally, administer 1 ml of the dilute heparin solution. The exact procedure of the agency should be followed.

**AVOIDING INFILTRATION:** When administering any solution of drug via heparin well, infiltration should be avoided. It may be difficult to ascertain whether the needle is in place; procedures for checking this vary. It should be possible to aspirate blood from the heparin well if it is in the vein. In addition, drugs being injected should go in smoothly, with no patient discomfort and little resistance to the infusion. Finally, there should be no swelling, discoloration, redness, or tenderness around the insertion site. If there is doubt that the heparin well is in the correct place, it should be removed and a new one inserted.
- If possible, avoid the intramuscular route of administration for medications for patients receiving heparin because of the danger of intramuscular bleeding. If absolutely unavoidable, intramuscular injections should be scheduled for times when the coagulation time is the shortest, such as ½ to 1 hour before the next dose of heparin. This is of little concern for patients on low-dose heparin therapy.
- Many hospitals require that each dose of heparin be checked by two professionals before the drug is administered.

**Patient and family education**   Heparin is rarely used outside of the hospital setting. If prescribed for use at home, the patient or family must be taught correct injection technique, the need for regular follow-up with the physician, the need to keep all health care providers, especially dentists, informed of all medications being used, and the need to wear a medical identification tag or bracelet stating that heparin is being used.

- Review with patients the goal of heparin therapy and side effects associated with its use.
- Instruct patients and families that individuals on heparin therapy should avoid the use of products containing aspirin or salicylates. Patients should avoid the use of any over-the-counter medications without first clearing their use with the physician.
- Caution patients to use electric razors while taking high-dose heparin to avoid cutting themselves.
- Caution patients and families to report any signs of bleeding from any site: nosebleeds, hematuria, bloody or tarry stools, bleeding gums, change in menstrual flow, excessive bruising, or excessive bleeding from any cut or scratch.
- Patients should brush their teeth gently, with a soft-bristle brush, and floss gently. Patients may find it necessary to forego flossing while on anticoagulant therapy, and some may even have to give up toothbrushing because of excessive bleeding from gums. If patients cannot brush their teeth, assist them to find other acceptable ways to provide oral hygiene, such as a water-spray device, swabbing the mouth, or using mouthwashes. Note that excessive bleeding may indicate overmedication and should be reported.

# Indirect-acting (oral) anticoagulants

anisindione ~ dicumarol ~ phenprocoumon ~ warfarin

**OVERVIEW OF THE DRUG CLASS**   Four clotting factors, II (prothrombin), VII, IX, and X, are synthesized in the liver, with vitamin K as a necessary cofactor. If vitamin K is deficient, these clotting factors will be synthesized in a functionally inactive state, which impairs blood coagulation.

Two classes of drugs, the coumarins and the indandiones, interfere with the regeneration of active vitamin K in the liver and thereby produce an effective vitamin K deficiency. These drugs are active only when administered to the patient. These drugs are inactive in preventing the coagulation of blood collected for storage.

**MECHANISM OF ACTION**   Oral anticoagulants prevent the action of vitamin K in the liver. The normal action of vitamin K in the liver is to promote the synthesis of the active form of four of the clotting factors: factors II (prothrombin), VII (proconvertin), IX (Christmas factor or plasma thromboplastin component), and X (Stuart-Prower factor). The activation of these clotting factors requires the oxidation and reduction of vitamin K. The oral anticoagulants prevent the reduction of oxidized vitamin K, thereby interrupting the activation cycle. As a result, these clotting factors do not have the carboxylated glutamic acid residues needed to bind calcium and thereby orient the clotting factors on the membrane surface phospholipid. This membrane binding is required to generate thrombin.

The oral anticoagulants have no effect on clotting factors II, VII, IX, and X that have already been activated. The action of the oral anticoagulants is therefore not evident until existing activated clotting factors have been largely eliminated from circulation. The half-life of clotting factors ranges from 5 to 6 hours for factor VII to 60 hours for factor II.

**INDICATIONS**   **Venous thrombosis and pulmonary embolism** Generally, coumarin is given to follow up large-dose heparin therapy for the prophylaxis or treatment of these conditions.   **Thromboembolism or embolism** Prophylaxis or treatment of these conditions associated with mitral valve disease, atrial fibrillation, or prosthetic heart valves.   **Prophylaxis for thrombosis** This use is not well documented for immobilized geriatric orthopedic patients, for patients after coronary artery bypass surgery, or following myocardial infarction.

**CONTRAINDICATIONS**   **Pregnancy and lactation** Fetal malformation and hemorrhage have been documented. **Patients at hemorrhagic risk** These include patients with hemorrhagic tendencies; patients with bleeding lesions or other problems in which hemorrhaging might present a life-threatening risk, such as severe hypertension or an aneurysm; and patients with recent or contemplated surgery of the eye or CNS. Procedures such as spinal puncture or insertion of an IUD are contraindicated in anticoagulated patients.

**DRUG INTERACTIONS**    Oral anticoagulants have more clinically significant drug interactions than other drug classes. Careful monitoring is required when oral anticoagulants are used with other drugs.    **Drugs enhancing the anticoagulant effects**    • Oral antibiotics decrease the availability of vitamin K. • Chloral hydrate, chlofibrate, phenylbutazone, salicylates, sulfonamides, sulfonylureas, and triclofos displace anticoagulants from albumin. • Alcohol, allopurinol, chloramphenicol, cimetidine, co-tri-maxoazole, disulfiram, metronidazole, phenylbutazone, sulfinpyrazone, and sulfonamides inhibit the metabolism of oral anticoagulants. • Anabolic steroids, danazol, glucagon, quinidine, sulindac, and thyroid increase the anticoagulant effect by unknown mechanisms.    **Drugs increasing the bleeding tendency** • Dipyridamole, indomethacin, oxyphenbutazone, phenylbutazone, salicylates, and sulfin-pyrazone inhibit platelet aggregation. • Alkylating agents, antimetabolites, quinidine, quinine, and salicylates inhibit the synthesis of coagulant factors. • Glucocorticoids, indomethacin, oxyphenbuta-zone, phenylbutazone, potassium salts, salicylates, and sulfinpyrazone tend to cause ulcers.    **Drugs decreasing the anticoagulant effect** • Barbiturates, carbamazepine, chlorinated insecticides, ethchlr-vynol, glutethimide, griseofulvin, phenytoin, and rifampin induce drug-metabolizing enzymes. • Es-trogens, oral contraceptives, and vitamin K promote the synthesis of clotting factors. • Cholestyram-ine and colestipol inhibit the absorbtion of oral anticoagulants.    **Drugs whose actions are altered by oral anticoagulants** • Sulfonylurea oral hypoglycemic agents (chlorpropamide and tolbutamide) and phenytoin: oral anticoagulants inhibit the metabolism of these drugs. These drugs become more active and toxic.

**FATE**    Oral anticoagulants are tightly bound to plasma albumin. This tight binding creates a reservoir or depot of drug in the body that is released as the free drug is metabolized and eliminated. This tight binding contributes to the long duration of action of the oral anticoagulants, which ranges from a few days (anisindione and warfarin) to a week or more (dicumerol and phenprocoumon). Some of the drug interactions previously detailed arise from a second drug displacing or being displaced by an oral anticoagulant. The concentration of free drug so displaced may be great enough to cause toxic effects.

Oral anticoagulants are metabolized by the liver microsomal enzymes. Drugs that induce these metabolizing enzymes increase the elimination of oral anticoagulants; drugs that inhibit these enzymes decrease the elimination of the oral anticoagulants.

## ❧ NURSING CONSIDERATIONS

**Side effects, toxicities, and associated nursing actions**    Indandiones have a greater incidence of adverse effects on the liver, skin, and blood than do the coumarins.

**CV:    HEMORRHAGE:** Long-term hematopoietic damage may include aplastic anemia, leukopenia, red cell aplasia, atypical mononuclear cells, thrombocytopenia, agranulocytosis, and the presence of leukocyte agglutinins.

• Visually inspect the patient at regular intervals for the appearance of bruising or petechiae.
• Check stool for guaiac/blood at regular intervals.
• Monitor vital signs at regular intervals. Be alert to signs of hemorrhage: hypotension, rapid pulse, or other signs of shock.
• Monitor ordered blood work and prothrombin time (PT): goal of anticoagulation therapy is 2 to 2.5 times the control in seconds or 20% to 30% (or as prescribed by physician).
• Check most current laboratory work before administering each dose. Omit the dose and notify the physician if blood work indicates excessive anticoagulation.
• Monitor complete blood count, white blood cell differential, and platelet count.
• Oral anticoagulant therapy is frequently initiated while patients are still receiving heparin.
• Monitor complete work appropriate to both drugs if patient is receiving both. Since heparin can alter PT levels, specimens for PT determination should be drawn just before the next ordered dose of heparin.
• Keep vitamin $K_1$ or phytonadione available to treat overdose with coumarins and indandiones.

Unless frank hemorrhage is present, the usual treatment for excessive anticoagulation is temporary discontinuation of the anticoagulant. If immediate and/or partial reversal of hemorrhage is necessary, fresh-frozen plasma is transfused.

**Allergic** A rash is the common skin reaction.
- Visually inspect the patient at regular intervals for the appearance of a rash.
- Potentially fatal skin lesions characterized by infarction, vasculitis, and thrombosis have occurred. Any subjective or objective changes in the skin should be reported to the physician.

**Metabolic** Liver damage may be evidenced as jaundice or hepatitis.
- Monitor liver function studies if available.
- Assess patients for the presence of jaundice, right upper quadrant abdominal pain, anorexia, intermittent nausea and vomiting, enlarged, tender liver, change in the color of urine or stool.

## Nursing interventions related to drug administration
- Note above each patient's bed (or as is customary in the institution) when the patient is on anticoagulant therapy so personnel from the laboratory will use appropriate techniques to prevent patient from bleeding after venipuncture.
- Read the physician's order carefully to prepare the correct dose. Do not confuse Liquaemin (heparin trade name) with Liquamar (phenprocoumon trade name).
- Intramuscular injections should be avoided if possible in patients receiving anticoagulants.

### Parenteral administration of warfarin
- Warfarin is available for intravenous or intramuscular use, although these routes of administration are less common than the oral route.
- Diluent is supplied by the manufacturer and makes a solution of 25 mg/ml.
- For intravenous use, give via intravenous injection and do not mix with intravenous fluids. Flush tubing before and after administration.
- Warfarin is compatible with heparin in a syringe but incompatible with many other medications; consult the pharmacy.
- Rate of administration should not exceed 25 mg (1 ml) per minute.

## Patient and family education
- Teach patients receiving anticoagulants (''blood thinners'') about why they are taking the medication, the importance of taking the correct dose as directed, and precautions to observe to avoid bleeding.
- Caution patients to avoid contact sports and activities associated with a high chance of injury such as construction work, carpentry, or foundry work. Obviously, patients are not usually able to change occupations, but they should be cautioned to avoid injury if at all possible.
- Caution patients to use electric razors while taking anticoagulants because there is less risk of cutting themselves.
- Teach patients to report any signs of bleeding from any site: nosebleeds, hematuria, bloody or tarry stools, bleeding gums, change in menstrual flow, excessive bruising, or excessive bleeding from any cut or scratch.
- Patients should not go barefoot.
- Patients should brush their teeth gently, with a soft-bristle brush, and floss gently. Patients may find it necessary to forego flossing while on anticoagulant therapy, and some may even have to give up toothbrushing because of excessive bleeding from gums. If patients cannot brush their teeth, assist them to find other acceptable ways to provide oral hygiene, such as a WaterPik, swabbing the mouth, or using mouthwashes. Note that excessive bleeding may indicate overmedication and should be reported.
- Remind patients to keep all health care providers informed of any medications they are taking. Specifically point out that dentists need to know if patients are receiving anticoagulants.
- Patients should wear a medical alert bracelet or tag stating their anticoagulant medication.
- Women of child-bearing age should be informed of the risks associated with the use of anticoagulants and should consider the use of birth control measures while on therapy. If in the first trimester when beginning therapy, some women may elect to terminate the pregnancy. Advise women to discuss the question of pregnancy with their physicians.

- Note the large number of drug interactions with oral anticoagulants. Caution patients to avoid the use of any medications without clearance from their physicians. Point out to the patient that this includes even over-the-counter preparations such as aspirin, vitamins, cold remedies, and cough medicines. Aspirin is particularly dangerous because of its potent antiplatelet effects.
- Instruct the patient to report unexplained fever, unusual fatigue, sore throat, or chills (signs of agranulocytosis), rash, jaundice, abdominal pain, skin changes, or any other unusual symptoms that might indicate a drug side effect.
- Patients should be instructed not to "double up" if a dose is missed. It may be necessary to help the patient devise a way to remember to take the daily dose of anticoagulant, for example, a calendar that the patient marks each day the medication is taken.
- Instruct patients to take the prescribed dose at the same time each day.
- Caution patients to limit the use of alcohol while on oral anticoagulants.
- Vitamin K deficiency or excess in the diet may alter the anticoagulation effects of the oral anticoagulants. Dietary sources of vitamin K include green leafy vegetables such as cabbage, spinach, kale, and lettuce, cauliflower, tomatoes, wheat bran, cheese, egg yolk, and liver. Encourage patients to include these foods as part of their daily intake.
- Because of alterations in bioavailability, caution patients not to switch brands of anticoagulant prescribed.
- Instruct patients to keep these and all medications out of the reach of children.
- Panwarfin brand 7.5 mg tablets may contain FD & C yellow #5 (tartrazine) and may cause allergic type reactions in some individuals. This allergic reaction is seen more often in individuals with aspirin hypersensitivity.

---

## anisindione   (an-iss-in-DYE-one)   oral anticoagulant

- anisindione: Miradon

**MECHANISM OF ACTION**   Anisindione is the only anticoagulant of the indandione chemical class used in the United States. See entry for drug class (p. 210).

**INDICATIONS**   • See entry for drug class (p. 210).

**CONTRAINDICATIONS**   • See entry for drug class (p. 210).

**DOSAGE**   **PO:**   **ADULT:** First day, 300 mg; second day, 200 mg; third day, 100 mg; maintenance doses range from 25 to 250 mg, as required, based on prothrombin time determinations.   *Special patient populations:*   **PREGNANCY AND LACTATION:** Fetal malformation and hemorrhage have been documented.

**PREPARATIONS**   *Tablets:* 50 mg.

**DRUG INTERACTIONS**   • See entry for drug class (p. 211).

**DIAGNOSTIC TEST INTERFERENCE**   Indandione metabolites may color alkaline urine red-orange, which may interfere with some laboratory spectrophotometric tests.

**FATE**   Peak *action* is 1 to 3 days. The plasma *half-life* is 3 to 5 days, and *duration of action* is 1 to 6 days, making anisindione a long-acting drug.

### 🐦 NURSING CONSIDERATIONS

**Side effects, toxicities, and associated nursing actions**
See entry for drug class (p. 211).

**Nursing interventions related to drug administration**
See entry for drug class (p. 212)

**Patient and family education**
See entry for drug class (p. 212).

---

## dicumarol, bishydroxycoumarin   (dye-KOO-ma-role)   anticoagulant

- Sold under generic name

**MECHANISM OF ACTION**    Dicumarol is chemically a coumarin. See entry for drug class (p. 210).
**INDICATIONS**    • See entry for drug class (p. 210).
**CONTRAINDICATIONS**    • See entry for drug class (p. 210).
**DOSAGE**    PO:    ADULT: First day, 200 to 300 mg; maintenance doses range from 25 to 250 mg daily and must be individualized based on prothrombin times for each patient.    *Special patient populations:* PREGNANCY AND LACTATION: Fetal malformation and hemorrhage have been documented.
**PREPARATIONS**    *Tablets:* 25, 50, 100 mg.
**DRUG INTERACTIONS**    • See entry for drug class (p. 211).
**FATE**    See entry for drug class (p. 211). Dicumarol is irregularly absorbed, making dosage highly individual. *Peak action* is seen in 1 to 3 days. The plasma *half-life* is 1 to 2 days, and the *duration of action* is 2 to 10 days.

## ❦ NURSING CONSIDERATIONS
### Side effects, toxicities, and associated nursing actions
• See entry for drug class (p. 211).
### Nursing interventions related to drug administration
• See entry for drug class (p. 212).
### Patient and family education
• See entry for drug class (p. 212).

---

## phenprocoumon    (fen-proe-KOO-mon)                    oral anticoagulant

---

• phenprocoumon: Liquamar

**MECHANISM OF ACTION**    Warfarin is chemically a coumarin. • See entry for drug class (p. 210).
**INDICATIONS**    • See entry for drug class (p. 210).
**CONTRAINDICATIONS**    • See entry for drug class (p. 210).
**DOSAGE**    PO:    ADULT: First day, 24 mg. Maintenance doses range from 0.75 to 6 mg daily.    *Special patient populations:*    PREGNANCY AND LACTATION: Fetal malformation and hemorrhage have been documented.
**PREPARATIONS**    *Tablets:* 3 mg.
**DRUG INTERACTIONS**    • See entry for drug class (p. 211).
**FATE**    Phenprocoumon has its *peak action* in 1½ to 3 days. The *duration of action* is 7 to 14 days, and the plasma *half-life* is very long, 6 to 7 days.

## ❦ NURSING CONSIDERATIONS
### Side effects, toxicities, and associated nursing actions
• See entry for drug class (p. 211).
### Nursing interventions related to drug administration
• See entry for drug class (p. 212).
### Patient and family education
• See entry for drug class (p. 212).

---

## warfarin potassium                                    oral anticoagulant

---

• warfarin potassium: Arthrombin-K
• warfarin sodium: Coufarin, Coumadin, Panwarfin

**MECHANISM OF ACTION**    Warfarin is chemically a coumarin. • See entry for drug class (p. 210).
**INDICATIONS**    • See entry for drug class (p. 210).
**CONTRAINDICATIONS**    • See entry for drug class (p. 210).

**DOSAGE   PO:   ADULT:** 10 to 15 mg daily for 2 to 5 days or until the desired prothombin time is reached. The initial dose may be 40 to 60 mg for adults and 20 to 30 mg for elderly patients. Maintenance doses range from 2 to 10 mg daily. Parenteral doses are the same as oral doses.   *Special patient populations:*   **PREGNANCY AND LACTATION:** Fetal malformation and hemorrhage have been documented.

**PREPARATIONS**   *Tablets:* 2, 2.5, 5, 7.5, 10 mg; *parenteral:* 50 mg.

**DRUG INTERACTIONS**   • See entry for drug class (p. 211).

**FATE**   Warfarin is better absorbed than other oral anticoagulants; however, brands differ in bioavailability. *Peak action* is in ½ to 3 days. The plasma *half-life* is ½ to 3 days, and the *duration of action* is 2 to 5 days.

**☙ NURSING CONSIDERATIONS**

**Side effects, toxicities, and associated nursing actions**
   • See entry for drug class (p. 211).

**Nursing interventions related to drug administration**
   • See entry for drug class (p. 212).

**Patient and family education**
   • See entry for drug class (p. 212).

## Thrombolytic agents

alteplase ~ streptokinase ~ urokinase

**OVERVIEW OF THE DRUG CLASS**   The protein, fibrin, provides the network for a blood clot (thrombus). Normally, fibrin is degraded slowly by the proteolytic enzyme, plasmin. In some clinical situations where tissue damage is threatened by ischemia, it is desirable to degrade the clot much more quickly. Thrombolytic drugs are used to rapidly degrade blood clots. Streptokinase and urokinase have been used for a few years, but researchers are seeking new agents. The thrombolytic agents under active clinical investigation include tissue-type plasminogen activator (tPA) and anisoylated-plasminogen-streptokinase activator complex (APSAC).

**MECHANISM OF ACTION**   Plasminogen is part of the natural system that degrades blood clots. Plasminogen is a proenzyme, the inactive precursor of plasmin. The activation of plasminogen is carefully regulated by tissue activators and natural inhibitors. Thrombolytic drugs activate plasminogen to its active form, plasmin, thereby aiding clot digestion.

**INDICATIONS**   • Pulmonary embolism. • Deep vein thrombosis. • Coronary artery thrombosis and myocardial infarction.

**CONTRAINDICATIONS**   • Active internal bleeding. • Invasive procedures within 10 days, including a major surgery and organ biopsy. • Stroke within the previous 2 months. • Pregnancy or recent childbirth. • Gastrointestinal bleeding. • Prior allergic reaction to the drug. • Thrombi present for more than 7 days. • Brain tumor.

**DRUG INTERACTIONS**   **Heparin or oral anticoagulants** These anticoagulants increase the risk of hemorrhage. **Aspirin, dipyridamole, indomethacin, phenylbutazone, and sulfinpyrazone** These drugs decrease platelet adhesiveness and increase the risk of hemorrhage if given with a thrombolytic drug.

## alteplase recombinant   (AL-teh-place)                                     thrombolytic

   • alteplase recombinant: Activase, ✦Activase rt-PA

**MECHANISM OF ACTION**   Alteplase is a tissue plasminogen activator, produced by recombinant DNA technology. Alteplase is an enzyme that binds to fibrin and becomes very active in catalyzing the conversion of plasminogen to plasmin. Plasmin is the enzyme that degrades fibrin, dissolving a thrombus (clot). Because alteplase has little activity unless it is bound to fibrin, alteplase may be infused into the bloodstream, but it will localize at a clot. Alteplase is also known as TPA.

**INDICATIONS**   **Acute myocardial infarction** Best results are when administered within the first 6 hours.

**CONTRAINDICATIONS**   • Active bleeding. • History of strokes. • Recent (2 months) intracranial or intraspinal surgery. • Brain tumor. • Aneurysm. • Severe hypertension.

**DOSAGE**   **IV infusion:**   ADULTS: 100 mg total. Sixty mg is infused over the first hour with, 6 to 10 mg administered as an initial bolus over 1 to 2 minutes. During the second and third hours 20 mg/hr is administered. Doses higher than 150 mg are associated with an increased incidence of intracranial bleeding.   *Special patient populations:*   PREGNANCY: Pregnancy category C.

**PREPARATIONS**   *Lyophilized powder:* 20 and 50 mg/vial. Reconstitute with sterile water to 1 mg/ml. May be further diluted 1:1 with 0.9% sodium chloride or 5% dextrose to 0.5 mg/ml for infusion.

**DRUG INTERACTIONS**   **Heparin** increases incidence of bleeding.   **Aspirin, dipyridamole** increase incidence of bleeding.

**FATE**   Alteplase is rapidly cleared by the liver. The plasma *half-life* is 5 minutes. The decrease in thrombus size can be demonstrated in 1.5 to 2 hours.

❦ **NURSING CONSIDERATIONS**

### Side effects, toxicities, and associated nursing actions

**CNS** Intracranial bleeding, especially at doses greater than 150 mg.

**CV** Bleeding and hypotension.

• Monitor the vital signs at regular intervals. Be alert to signs of hemorrhage: hypotension, rapid pulse, or other signs of shock. Monitor pupil size and reactivity and level of consciousness.

• Monitor ordered blood work, including hemoglobin, hematocrit, thrombin time, activated partial thromboplastin time, prothrombin time, and platelet counts.

• Inspect patients for the appearance of bruising, petechiae, or any signs of bleeding.

• Check stools for guaiac/blood daily.

• Use caution in handling and moving patient to avoid excessive bruising.

• If arterial puncture is necessary, apply pressure to the puncture site for 30 minutes following the procedure. Check the site regularly for signs of bleeding.

**GI** Nausea and vomiting.

• Monitor for GI side effects; if severe, notify physician.

• Monitor intake and output and weight.

### Nursing interventions related to drug administration

• The use of this agent should be restricted to the acute care setting, where personnel and equipment for continuous patient monitoring are present.

• Continuous ECG monitoring should be done during therapy with this drug.

• For continuous infusion, use microdrip tubing and an electronic infusion monitoring device.

• IM injections of any medication are contraindicated during therapy with this drug.

• Venipuncture should be minimized, and pressure must be applied to the site for a minimum of 15 minutes.

• Note above each patient's bed (or as is customary in the institution) when patient is receiving alteplase therapy so that personnel from the laboratory will use appropriate technique to avoid patient bleeding after venipuncture.

### Patient and family education

• This drug is not used for self-management. Keep patient and family informed of anticipated benefits of drug therapy and any changes in the patient's condition.

---

## streptokinase   (strep-toe-KYE-nase)                                           thrombolytic

• streptokinase: Kabikinase, Streptase

**MECHANISM OF ACTION**   Streptokinase interacts with plasminogen to form plasmin, the active enzyme that degrades fibrin.

**INDICATIONS**   • Pulmonary embolism. • Deep-vein thrombosis. • Arterial thrombosis and embolism. • Coronary artery thrombosis and myocardial infarction: recent studies demonstrate a reduced amount of cardiac damage following streptokinase administered during an ongoing myocardial infarction. • Occluded arteriovenous cannulae.

**CONTRAINDICATIONS** • Active internal bleeding. • Invasive procedures within 10 days, including major surgery and organ biopsy. • Stroke within the previous 2 months. • Pregnancy or recent childbirth. • Gastrointestinal bleeding. • Prior allergic reaction to the drug. • Thrombi present for more than 7 days. • Brain tumor.

**DOSAGE** **Adults:** IV: The initial loading dose is 250,000 IU infused over 30 minutes. Thereafter, the solution is infused at 100,000 IU/hr. Usual durations of infusion are 24 hours for pulmonary embolism or acute myocardial infarction, 24 to 72 hours for arterial thromboses or embolism, and 72 hours for deep vein thrombosis. **INTRA-ARTERIAL CANNULA:** 250,000 IU in 2 ml are instilled over 30 minutes, after which the cannula is clamped for 2 hours. The contents are then aspirated, and the cannula is flushed with saline. **INTRACORONARY:** For angiography, the patient is heparinized with 5000 to 10,000 units of heparin administered intra-arterially. After the obstructed coronary vessel is identified, 2000 IU/min streptokinase is administered through the catheter to the occluded site. Clot lysis is monitored every 15 minutes. The total dose is 150,000 to 250,000 IU. *Special patient populations:* **PREGNANCY:** Safe use has not been established. To prevent premature separation of the placenta, streptokinase should not be administered during the first 18 weeks of pregnancy (pregnancy category A).

**PREPARATIONS** *Powder (lyophilized):* 250,000, 600,000, and 750,000 IU. The powder is reconstituted with normal saline or 5% dextrose, usually to 45 ml. Foaming and flocculation are minimized by gentle agitation rather than shaking and dissolving the powder. The reconstituted solution should be stored at 2° to 4° C.

**DRUG INTERACTIONS** **Heparin or oral anticoagulants** increase the risk of hemorrhage. **Aspirin, dipyridamole, indomethacin, phenylbutazone, and sulfinpyrazone** decrease platelet adhesiveness and increase the risk of hemorrhage if given with a thrombolytic drug. **Aminocaproic acid** inhibits the activation of plasminogen by streptokinase.

**DIAGNOSTIC TEST INTERFERENCE** **Blood coagulation tests** are altered, with increase in thromboplastin time (TT), activated partial thromboplastin time (aPTT), and prothrombin time (PT).

**FATE** Streptokinase is bound by antibodies and rapidly cleared from circulation.

## NURSING CONSIDERATIONS

### Side effects, toxicities, and associated nursing actions

**Hematologic** Bleeding is frequent and may be hard to control.
- Monitor vital signs at regular intervals. Be alert to signs of hemorrhage: hypotension, rapid pulse, or other signs of shock. Temporary increases in systolic blood pressure have been reported. If systolic blood pressure increases more than 25 mm Hg, notify the physician.
- Monitor ordered blood work. A drop in hematocrit will be experienced by 20% to 30% of patients even if clinical bleeding has not occurred. Other blood work includes thrombin time (TT), activated partial thromboplastin time (aPTT), prothrombin time (PT), and platelet counts. If patient has been on heparin, streptokinase is withheld until TT is less than two times normal control. If heparin is to be started after streptokinase therapy, heparin is withheld until TT is less than two times normal control.
- Visually inspect the patient at least twice a day for the appearance of bruising, petechiae, or any signs of bleeding.
- Check stool for guaiac/blood daily.
- The hemostatic status of the patient may be altered more with this drug than with heparin or oral anticoagulants. If any sign of bleeding occurs, notify the physician.
- Instruct the patient to report the appearance of any bleeding: bloody nose, blood in urine, stool, or vomitus, coughing up blood, bleeding gums, prolonged menses, oozing from previous injection sites.
- Use caution in handling and moving the patient to avoid excessive bruising.
- If arterial puncture is necessary, it should be done by a physician in the radial or brachial artery rather than the femoral. Pressure to the puncture site should be applied for 30 minutes following the procedure, and the site should be checked at regular intervals for signs of bleeding.

- If hemorrhage occurs, discontinue streptokinase infusion and notify the physician. Treatment may be with one or more of the following: plasma volume expanders other than dextran, cryoprecipitate, fresh-frozen plasma, packed red blood cells, and aminocaproic acid.

**Allergic** Streptokinase is a product of beta-hemolytic streptococci and is highly antigenic. About 30% of patients have a febrile reaction. Anaphylaxis is reported to occur in about 2.5% of patients. Milder allergic reactions, including urticaria, itching, flushing, nausea, headache, and musculoskeletal pain, are reported by about 12% of patients.

- Observe the patient for the signs and symptoms of allergic response.
- Have drugs, equipment, and personnel readily available to treat possible anaphylactic shock.
- Antihistamines and/or corticosteroids may be used to diminish allergic response. Do *not* use aspirin to reduce fever (see Drug Interactions).

**Other** Phlebitis may occur at the injection site.

- Observe IV insertion site and extremity for signs of phlebitis: redness, irritation, patient complaints of pain. If phlebitis appears, change IV sites.
- Decreasing the rate of infusion or increasing the dilution of drug may lessen the phlebitis.

### Nursing interventions related to drug administration

- Restrict the use of this agent to the acute care setting, where personnel and equipment for continuous patient monitoring are present.
- Continuous ECG monitoring should be done during direct IV push therapy, during investigational use, for coronary catheter procedures, or whenever assessment of the patient indicates that monitoring is indicated.

### Continuous IV infusion

- Use microdrip tubing and an electronic infusion monitoring device. The infusion rate should be checked regularly to ascertain that the patient is receiving the prescribed dose.

### Intra-arterial cannula

- See Dosage. Before using streptokinase, attempt to clear occluded cannulae with heparinized saline. Follow institutional guidelines.
- Streptokinase should not be mixed with any other medications in a syringe or infusion.

**Intramuscular injections** of any medication are absolutely contraindicated because of the possibility of intramuscular bleeding.

**Venipunctures** should be minimized, and pressure must be applied to the site for a minimum of 15 minutes.

- Note above each patient's bed (or as is customary in the institution) when the patient is on streptokinase therapy so personnel from the laboratory will use appropriate technique to avoid causing patient bleeding after venipuncture.

### Patient and family education
This drug is not used for self-management. Keep patient and family informed of anticipated benefits of drug therapy and changes in patient's condition.

---

## urokinase   (yoor-oh-KIE-nase)                                              thrombolytic

- urokinase: Abbokinase

**MECHANISM OF ACTION**   Urokinase is a direct activator of plasminogen, resulting in the formation of the thrombolytic enzyme, plasmin. Plasmin degrades fibrin clots.

**INDICATIONS**   • Pulmonary embolism. • Deep vein thrombosis. • Coronary artery thrombosis and myocardial infarction. • Occluded IV catheters: Urokinase clears catheters occluded by blood clots or fibrin.

**CONTRAINDICATIONS**   • Active internal bleeding. • Invasive procedures within 10 days, including major surgery and organ biopsy. • Stroke within the previous 2 months. • Pregnancy or recent childbirth. • Gastrointestinal bleeding. • Prior allergic reaction to the drug. • Thrombi present for more than 7 days. • Brain tumor.

**DOSAGE**   IV:   **ADULTS:** 4400 IU/kg is infused over 10 minutes, followed by the continuous infusion of 4400 IU/kg/hr for 12 to 24 hours.   **OCCLUDED IV CATHETER:** 5000 IU/ml is gently instilled into the catheter in a volume equivalent to the internal volume of the catheter. After 5 to 10 minutes, the contents of the catheter are aspirated. The procedure may be repeated if necessary.   *Special patient populations:*   PREGNANCY: Safe use has not been established (pregnancy category B).

**PREPARATIONS**   *Powder (lyophilized):* 5000 IU, 250,000 IU. The powder is dissolved in sterile water and used immediately. Unused portions should be discarded. The powder is stored at 2° to 4° C.

**DRUG INTERACTIONS**   **Heparin or oral anticoagulants** These anticoagulants increase the risk of hemorrhage. **Aspirin, dipyridamole, indomethacin, phenylbutazone, or sulfinpyrazone** These drugs decrease platelet adhesiveness and increase the risk of hemorrhage if given with a thrombolytic drug.

**FATE**   Urokinase is rapidly cleared from the blood. The plasma *half-life* is 10 to 20 minutes.

## 🐦 NURSING CONSIDERATIONS

### Side effects, toxicities, and associated nursing actions

**Hematologic** Hemorrhage is the most frequent side effect of urokinase.

- Monitor vital signs at regular intervals. Be alert to signs of hemorrhage: hypotension, rapid pulse, or other signs of shock.
- Monitor ordered blood work. A drop in hematocrit will be experienced by 20% to 30% of patients even if clinical bleeding has not occurred. Other blood work includes thrombin time (TT), activated partial thromboplastin time (aPTT), prothrombin time (PT), and platelet counts. If the patient has been on heparin, urokinase is withheld until TT is less than two times normal control. If heparin is to be started after urokinase therapy, heparin is withheld until TT is less than two times normal control.
- Visually inspect the patient at least twice a day for the appearance of bruising, petechiae, or any signs of bleeding.
- Check stool for guaiac/blood daily.
- The hemostatic status of the patient may be altered more with this drug than with heparin or oral anticoagulants. If any sign of bleeding occurs, notify the physician.
- Instruct the patient to report the appearance of any bleeding: bloody nose, blood in urine, stool, or vomitus, coughing up blood, bleeding gums, prolonged menses, oozing from previous injection sites.
- Use caution in handling and moving patient to avoid excessive bruising.
- If arterial puncture is necessary, it should be done by a physician in the radial or brachial artery rather than the femoral. Pressure to the puncture site should be applied for 30 minutes following the procedure, and the site checked at regular intervals for signs of bleeding.
- If hemorrhage occurs, discontinue urokinase infusion and notify the physician. Treatment may be with one or more of the following: plasma volume expanders other than dextran, cryoprecipitate, fresh-frozen plasma, packed red blood cells, and aminocaproic acid.

**Lung** Bronchospasm is reported, but rarely.

- Assess lung sounds and respiratory function at regular intervals.

**Allergic** Unlike streptokinase, urokinase is not highly antigenic, and allergic reactions are not common.

- Observe the patient for the signs and symptoms of allergic response.
- Have drugs, equipment, and personnel readily available to treat possible anaphylactic shock.
- Antihistamines and/or corticosteroids may be used to diminish allergic response. Do *not* use aspirin to reduce fever (see Drug Interactions).

### Nursing interventions related to drug administration

- Restrict the use of this agent to the acute care setting, where personnel and equipment for continuous patient monitoring are present.
- Continuous ECG monitoring should be done during direct IV push therapy, during investigational use, for coronary catheter procedures, or whenever assessment of the patient indicates that monitoring is indicated.

**Continuous IV infusion** Use microdrip tubing and an electronic infusion monitoring device. The infusion rate should be checked regularly to ascertain that the patient is receiving the prescribed dose.

**Intra-arterial cannula**

- See Dosage. Before using urokinase, attempt to clear the occluded cannulae with heparinized saline. Follow institutional guidelines.
- Urokinase should not be mixed with any other medications in a syringe or infusion.

- Intramuscular injections of any medication are absolutely contraindicated because of the possibility of intramuscular bleeding.
- Venipunctures should be minimized, and pressure must be applied to the site for a minimum of 15 minutes.
- Note above each patient's bed (or as is customary in the institution) when patient is on urokinase therapy so that personnel from the laboratory will use appropriate technique to avoid bleeding after venipuncture.

**Patient and family education**   This drug is not used for self-management. Keep the patient and family informed of anticipated benefits of drug therapy and changes in patient's condition.

# Systemic hemostatic agents

aminocaproic acid ~ antihemophilic factor ~ factor IX complex ~ menadione/menadiol ~ phytonadione

**OVERVIEW OF THE DRUG CLASS**   Drugs used as systemic hemostatic agents are a varied group not only chemically, but also with respect to their mechanism of action.

**MECHANISM OF ACTION**   Systemic hemostatic agents have varied mechanisms of action. Aminocaproic acid interferes with the activation of the fibrinolytic process. Antihemophilic factor and factor IX complex are blood products needed by individuals genetically lacking them. Menadione and phytonadione are forms of vitamin K that promote the synthesis of certain clotting factors.

**INDICATIONS**   • Hemorrhage.

**CONTRAINDICATIONS**   • See individual drugs.

**DRUG INTERACTIONS**   • See individual drugs.

## aminocaproic acid   (a-mee-noe-ka-PROE-ik)                    systemic hemostatic agent

- aminocaproic acid: Amicar

**MECHANISM OF ACTION**   Aminocaproic acid inhibits fibrinolysis and is useful in treating excessive bleeding resulting from overactivity of the fibrinolytic system.

**INDICATIONS**   **Excessive bleeding** when resulting from systemic hyperfibrinolysis and urinary fibrinolysis or associated with surgical complications following heart surgery and portacaval shunt; in hyperfibrinolysis associated with carcinoma of the lung, prostate, cervix, or stomach; or in hematologic disorders such as aplastic anemia.   **Hematuria,** whether surgical or nonsurgical, arising from the bladder, prostate, or urethra.   **Prophylaxis for patients with hemophilia** before dental surgical procedures. **Antidote for thrombolytic drug (streptokinase, urokinase) toxicity.**

**CONTRAINDICATIONS**   **Disseminated intravascular coagulation** Serious or fatal thrombus formation may result.   **Hemorrhage secondary to the loss of vascular integrity** Aminocaproic acid is ineffective in controlling bleeding not due to excessive fibrinolysis.

**DOSAGE**   **IV, PO:**   **ADULTS:** 5 to 6 g is given initially, followed by 1 g at hourly intervals or 6 g every 6 hours. Maximum dose: 30 g in 24 hours. A dose of 6 g/24 hr is effective in prostate surgery because the drug is concentrated in the urine.   **CHILDREN:** 100 mg/kg every 6 hours for 6 days.   *Special patient populations:*   **PREGNANCY:** Safe use has not been established. Aminocaproic acid is teratogenic in rat studies.

**PREPARATIONS**   *Tablets:* 500 mg; *solution* (syrup): 1.25 g/5 ml; *parenteral:* 250 mg/ml.

**DRUG INTERACTIONS**   • None described.

**FATE**   Aminocaproic acid is well absorbed and widely distributed in the body. It is excreted in the urine, largely unchanged. About 50% is excreted in 24 hours. The kidney concentrates aminocaproic acid by filtration and reabsorption, and therapeutic levels can be readily achieved in the urinary tract.

## ☙ NURSING CONSIDERATIONS

### Side effects, toxicities, and associated nursing actions

**CNS** Dizziness, tinnitus, malaise, and headache are reported. High doses are associated with anorexia.

• Assess for the presence of these side effects. Since therapy is usually for a short period, reassure the patient that these effects are temporary.
• If dizziness occurs, caution the hospitalized patient to call for assistance before attempting to ambulate. Keep side rails up. Patients at home should avoid driving or engaging in hazardous activities until dizziness wears off.

**CV** Bradycardia and arrhythmia have been reported after IV injection.

• Monitor vital signs before administration and at regular intervals during infusions. If possible, continuous cardiac monitoring should be done during infusions.

**Eye** Conjunctival suffusion.

• Assess the conjunctiva for irritation. If eyes become painful or irritation continues, notify the physician, or instruct the outpatient department to call the patient's personal physician.

**GI** Nausea, cramping, diarrhea.

• Assess for these side effects. Monitor intake and output if severe.
• If symptoms persist, the outpatient department should notify the physician.

**Metabolic** Weakness, fatigue, elevated serum concentrations of creatine kinase (CK), creatinine phosphokinase (CPK), aldolase, and AST (SGOT).

• Assess for these signs and symptoms. Monitor blood work if available. If symptoms persist, outpatient should notify physician.

**Allergic** Rash.

• Visually inspect skin at least daily in hospitalized patients. Instruct the outpatient department to notify physician if rash persists.

**Other** Some patients with hemophilia report dry ejaculation for a short period following use of aminocaproic acid.

• Inform patients about this possible side effect. Assess for this problem. Reassure patients that this effect is only temporary.

### Nursing interventions related to drug administration

• This drug should be administered orally or by infusion. Avoid direct IV push of this drug as it is associated with hypotension, bradycardia, and arrhythmias.
• Since the drug may cause clot formation, be alert to signs of possible thrombosis: pain in extremities, one extremity colder than others, loss of pulse in an extremity, shortness of breath, chest pain, Homan's sign.

### Patient and family education

• Review with patients possible side effects. Instruct patient to call a physician if any unexpected sign or symptom appears.

---

## antihemophilic factor   (an-tee-hee-moe-FILL-ik)        systemic hemostatic

• antihemophilic factor (AHF, AHG, factor VIII): Factorate, Generation II, Hemofil

**MECHANISM OF ACTION**   Factor VIII is a blood coagulation factor that is missing in classic hemophilia (hemophilia A).

**INDICATIONS**  • Hemophilia A (classic hemophilia).

**CONTRAINDICATIONS**  • Not effective for treating von Willebrand's disease.

**DOSAGE**   IV:   **ADULTS AND CHILDREN:** Dosage must be individualized according to the situation. For prophylaxis, patients weighing less than 50 kg are given 250 units daily in the morning; patients weighing more than 50 kg are given 500 units daily in the morning. For overt bleeding, an initial dose is 15 to 25 units/kg, followed by 8 to 15 units every 8 to 12 hours for 3 to 4 days. In general, the plasma level of antihemophilic factor need only be 10% of normal to prevent bleeding but 30% of normal to stop a hemorrhage. Levels approaching normal are required before surgery.   *Special patient populations:* **PREGNANCY:** Antihemophilic factor is used in pregnancy only when clearly needed. Because hemophilia is a sex-linked disease, its incidence is low in females.

**PREPARATIONS**   Antihemophilic factor (AHF) is a sterile, lyophilized powder prepared by cold-precipitation from pooled human venous plasma. The activity is not less than 100 antihemophilic factor unit (AFU) per milligram of protein. The powder is stable for about 2 years when refrigerated but may be stored at room temperature for up to 6 months. The diluent should not be frozen. AHF is reconstituted with sterile water for injection and should be used within 3 hours.

**DRUG INTERACTIONS**   • None reported.

**FATE**   The *half-life* of antihemophilic factor is 4 to 24 hours.

## ☙ NURSING CONSIDERATIONS

### Side effects, toxicities, and associated nursing actions

**CNS** Headaches, somnolence, lethargy, clouding, or loss of consciousness.

**CV** Tachycardia, hypotension.

**Eye** Disturbance of vision.

**GI** Nausea, vomiting.

• Most side effects clear spontaneously within 15 to 20 minutes and may be related to rate of infusion.

• Monitor pulse and blood pressure before starting infusion and at regular intervals during infusion.

• Keep side rails up on hospitalized patients.

• If these or any other side effects persist or are severe, notify the physician.

**Allergic** Fever, chills, urticaria.

• Question patients about a history of allergy to this product before administering.

• Patients with a history of allergic response to this product may have an antihistamine prescribed before the AHF.

• Monitor vital signs.

• Have drugs, equipment, and personnel available to treat an acute response.

**Other** Because antihemophilic factor is derived from pooled blood, there is a risk of hepatitis and acquired immune deficiency syndrome (AIDS). The incidence of these serious diseases from use of AHF has been decreased by new screening methods. Some preparations of AHF are heat treated. This inactivates the hepatitis virus.

• Hepatitis B vaccine may be ordered as a prophylactic measure.

• Both hepatitis and AIDS may require months to develop. Assess patients for the development of signs and symptoms (listed in Patient and Family Education). Encourage patients to return for regular follow-ups with the health care team.

### Nursing interventions related to drug administration

• Antihemophilic factor may be administered via direct IV push or via IV infusion. If given via direct IV push, only plastic syringes should be used, as AHF solution adheres to glass syringes.

• Observe expiration date.

• Powder and diluent should be at room temperature before reconstitution. Follow manufacturer's instructions to reconstitute. Gently rotate vial to dissolve concentrate; do not shake vigorously. It may require 5 to 10 minutes to completely dissolve concentrate.

• Reconstituted preparations should be administered within 3 hours of reconstitution. Reconstituted preparations should not be refrigerated. The solution should be at room temperature during infusion.

• AHF should be filtered before administration.

• The rate of administration is based on patient response and concentration of specific brand used (number of units per milliliter will be indicated on label). Monitor the pulse during administration; if the pulse rate increases significantly, slow the infusion or stop it if necessary. Solutions containing greater than 34 AHF units per milliliter (e.g., Hemofil or Hemofil T brands) must be administered at a rate not exceeding 2 ml/min. AHF solutions containing less than 34 AHF units per milliliter may be administered at a rate of 10 to 20 ml per 3 minute period. Profilate brand should be administered at a rate not exceeding 10 ml/min.

- Cryoprecipitated factor VIII is prepared differently than AHF. It is made from the freezing and thawing of fresh plasma from individual donors. Because it is not made from pooled plasma, the risk of hepatitis and AIDS is less, however, the amount of factor VIII per bag varies, so the response is less predictable. Cryoprecipitated factor VIII is kept frozen until ready to use, then thawed to room temperature in a 37° C (98.6° F) water bath. It is administered in the same way as blood. It must be administered within 3 hours of thawing. A typical dose may be 10 to 15 bags.
- Monitor available blood work, including factor VIII levels, hemoglobin, and hematocrit.

### Patient and family education

- Review with patients possible side effects and anticipated benefits of therapy.
- Patients with hemophilia may be quite knowledgeable about their own body's response to injury. These patients are often able to accurately indicate that bleeding has begun in a joint or other location prior to objective signs being clearly present. Encourage patients to report the subjective appearance of any sign or symptom.
- Instruct patients to report the appearance of signs or symptoms which may indicate the development of hepatitis or AIDS: malaise, fatigue, right upper quadrant abdominal pain, change in the color or consistency of stools, anorexia, jaundice.
- Instruct patients to wear a medical identification tag or bracelet indicating factor VIII deficiency.
- Remind patients to keep all health care providers informed of their medical condition.

# factor IX complex
systemic hemostatic

- factor IX complex: Konyne, Profilnine, Proplex

**MECHANISM OF ACTION**   Factor IX (Christmas factor or plasma thromboplastin component) is a blood coagulation factor required to convert prothrombin to thrombin.

**INDICATIONS**   **Hemophilia B or Christmas disease** A hereditary, sex-linked disorder characterized by a deficiency of factor IX.   **Hemorrhage** Secondary to an overdose of oral anticoagulant when rapid reversal is required.

**CONTRAINDICATIONS**   • Of value only for a deficiency of factor IX.

**DOSAGE**   IV:   ADULTS AND CHILDREN: Doses are highly individualized. To stop nonthreatening bleeding, 75 units/kg are administered, repeated after 8 to 12 hours if necessary. *Special patient populations:* PREGNANCY: Antihemophilic factor is used in pregnancy only when clearly needed. Because hemophilia is a sex-linked disease, its incidence is low in females.

**PREPARATIONS**   Factor IX complex is a sterile, lyophilized concentrate of blood coagulation factors II, VII, IX, and X derived from fresh venous plasma. One unit of factor IX complex is defined as the average of factor II, VII, IX, and X activity present in 1 ml of normal fresh pooled plasma less than 1 hour old. The powder is reconstituted with sterile water and should be used within 12 hours. While the powder is stored refrigerated, the reconstituted solution should not be refrigerated.

**DRUG INTERACTIONS**   • None reported.

**FATE**   The *half-life* of factor IX is 12 to 24 hours.

## ❦ NURSING CONSIDERATIONS

### Side effects, toxicities, and associated nursing actions

**Allergic** Transient fever, chills, headache, flushing, tingling, and changes in pulse rate and blood pressure may be experienced on administration.

- Monitor vital signs and blood pressure before starting therapy and at regular intervals.
- Have adequate drugs, equipment, and personnel available for rapid response.
- These side effects may be lessened by slowing the rate of infusion.

**Other** Because factor IX complex is derived from pooled blood, there is a risk of hepatitis and acquired immune deficiency syndrome (AIDS). The incidence of these serious diseases from use of factor IX complex has been decreased by new screening methods. Some preparations of factor IX complex are heat treated, which inactivates the hepatitis virus.

- Hepatitis B vaccine may be ordered as a prophylactic measure.

- Both hepatitis and AIDS may require months to develop. Assess patients for the development of signs and symptoms (listed in Patient and Family Education). Encourage patients to return for regular follow-ups with the health care team.

### Nursing interventions related to drug administration

- Factor IX complex may be administered via direct IV push or via IV infusion.
- Observe the expiration date.
- Powder and diluent should be at room temperature before reconstitution. Follow the manufacturer's instructions to reconstitute. Gently rotate the vial to dissolve concentrate; do not shake vigorously. It may require 5 to 10 minutes to completely dissolve the concentrate.
- Reconstituted preparations should be administered within 3 hours of reconstitution. Reconstituted preparations should not be refrigerated. The solution should be at room temperature during infusion.
- Factor IX complex should be filtered before administration.
- The rate of administration is based on patient response, although approximately 100 units per minute is usually well tolerated. The rate should not exceed 10 ml/min. Monitor the pulse during administration; if the pulse rate increases significantly, slow the infusion, or stop it if necessary.
- Disseminated intravascular coagulation (DIC) has been reported in patients receiving factor IX complex postoperatively and in patients with liver disease. Assess for petechiae or purpura, mild oozing from puncture sites, peripheral thrombosis, tachycardia, tachypnea, bone or joint pain, abdominal tenderness, palpitations. Monitor coagulation studies.

### Patient and family education

- Review with patients possible side effects and anticipated benefits of therapy.
- Patients with hemophilia may be quite knowledgeable about their own body's response to injury. These patients are often able to accurately indicate that bleeding has begun in a joint or other location before objective signs are clearly present. Encourage patients to report the subjective appearance of any sign or symptom.
- Instruct patients to report the appearance of signs or symptoms that may indicate the development of hepatitis or AIDS: malaise, fatigue, right upper quadrant abdominal pain, change in the color or consistency of stools, anorexia, jaundice.
- Instruct patients to wear a medical identification tag or bracelet indicating factor IX deficiency.
- Remind patients to keep all health care providers informed of their medical condition.

---

## menadione  (men-a-DYE-one)                    systemic hematostatic agent

- menadione (menaphthone, vitamin $K_3$): generically available
- menadione sodium diphosphate: Synkayvite, ✤Synkavite

**MECHANISM OF ACTION**  Vitamin K is required for the synthesis of blood coagulation factors II (prothrombin), VII (proconvertin), IX (Christmas factor or plasma throboplastin component), and X (Stuart-Prower factor). These factors are synthesized in the liver. Their activation requires vitamin K for the carboxylation step. The gamma-carboxyglutamyl forms of the factors are required for the calcium-dependent phospholipid binding required for blood clotting.

**INDICATIONS**  **Vitamin K deficiency** Chiefly secondary to malabsorption syndromes from such causes as regional enteritis, prolonged diarrhea, and bowel resection.

**CONTRAINDICATIONS**  • Hypersensitivity.

**DOSAGE**  **PO:**  **ADULTS:** 2 to 10 mg daily.  **CHILDREN:** 50 to 100 μg daily.  **SC, IM:**  **ADULTS:** 5 to 15 mg one to two times daily.  **CHILDREN:** 5 to 10 mg one or two times daily.  *Special patient populations:*  **PREGNANCY:** Menadione or menadiol sodium diphosphate administered to women in the last weeks of pregnancy can cause toxic reactions in the neonate.

**PREPARATIONS**  **Menadione** *Powder.*  **Menadiol sodium diphosphate** *Tablets:* 5 mg; *injection:* 5, 10, 37.5 mg/ml.

**DRUG INTERACTIONS**    Oral anticoagulants response is decreased by vitamin K3.

**DIAGNOSTIC TEST INTERFERENCE**    Urinary 17-hydroxycorticosteroids Values as determined by the modified Reddy, Jenkin, Thorn procedure are falsely high in patients treated with menadione.

**FATE**    Menadione, but not menadiol sodium diphosphate, requires bile salts for absorption from the gastrointestinal tract. Menadiol is converted to menadione in the liver. When given to control bleeding, a response may be seen in about 2 hours. IM or SC administration provides a long *duration of action*.

## 🐦 NURSING CONSIDERATIONS

### Side effects, toxicities, and associated nursing actions

**GI** Gastric upset may occur after oral administration.
* Suggest that patients take medication with meals.

**Hematologic** Individuals who have glucose-6-phosphate deficiency can suffer hemolysis if menadione or menadiol sodium diphosphate is administered.
* Assess for history of glucose-6-phosphate deficiency prior to administration.

**Allergic** Rashes and urticaria are occasionally reported.
* Assess for history of allergy prior to administration.
* Assess for development of allergic response.

### Nursing interventions related to drug administration    Patients with bile deficiency who are receiving oral menadione need concomitant administration of bile salts for drug absorption.
* Monitor prothrombin time (PT) to evaluate effectiveness of therapy.
* For treatment and prevention of hemorrhagic disease in the newborn, phytonadione is preferred.
* Menadiol sodium diphosphate may be given IM, SC, or IV. The IM or SC routes may be contraindicated in hypoprothrombinemia because of the risk of hemorrhage or hematoma at the injection site.

**Systemic hemostatic agents**
* Intramuscular injections may cause pain at the injection site, nodule formation, and bleeding from the injection site. In older children and adults, the dorsogluteal or ventrogluteal injection sites are preferred. In infants and small children, the vastus lateralis injection site is preferred.
* Menadiol sodium diphosphate may be given intravenously undiluted or added to most infusion solutions; it is incompatible with protein hydrolysate. The undiluted dose may be administered over 1 minute.

### Patient and family education
* Review with patients the side effects and anticipated benefits of therapy.
* The dietary requirement for vitamin K has not been established but has been estimated at 0.03 μg/kg for adults and 1 to 5 μg/kg for children. Although it is not stored in the body for long periods, vitamin K deficiency is rare in adults on the basis of dietary deficiency alone. Dietary sources include tomatoes, green leafy vegetables, meats, dairy products, cereals, and fruits.

---

## phytonadione    (fye-toe-na-DYE-one)    systemic hematostatic agent

* phytonadione (phylloquinone, phytomenadion, vitamin K₁): Mephyton, AquaMEPHYTON, Konakion

**MECHANISM OF ACTION**    Vitamin $K_1$ is required for the synthesis of blood coagulation factors II (prothrombin), VII (proconvertin), IX (Christmas factor or plasma thromboplastin component), and X (Stuart-Prower factor). These factors are synthesized in the liver. Their activation requires vitamin K for the carboxylation step. The gamma-carboxyglutamyl forms of the factors are required for the calcium-dependent phospholipid binding, an important step in blood clotting.

**INDICATIONS**    **Hemorrhage** Phytonadione is the drug of choice to treat hemorrhage resulting from overdosage of oral anticoagulants.    **Hypothrombinemia** Phytonadione is used to treat this vitamin K deficiency. **Hemorrhagic disease of the newborn** Many states require, and the American Academy of Pediatrics recommends, routine administration of vitamin K at birth.

**CONTRAINDICATIONS**    **Liver disease** Patients with liver disease should not be given large doses repeatedly.

**DOSAGE**    PO, SC, IM:    **ADULTS AND CHILDREN:** 2.5 to 25 mg for hypoprothrombinemic states.    IV, IM, SC:    **NEWBORNS:** 0.5 to 1 mg immediately after birth for prophylaxis.    IV:    **ADULTS:** 1 to 5 mg for mild overdose of oral anticogulants.    *Special patient populations:*    **PREGNANCY:** 1 to 5 mg may be given to the mother 12 to 24 hours before delivery as prophylaxis for the baby instead of directly to the baby after delivery. Vitamin K is also found in breast milk.

**PREPARATIONS**    *Tablets:* 5 mg; *solutions:* 1, 2, and 10 mg/ml.

**DRUG INTERACTIONS**    **Oral anticoagulants, salicylates, phenylbutazone, sulfonamides, quinine, quinidine, broad-spectrum antibiotics** Vitamin K reverses the anticoagulant effect of these drugs.    **Cholestyramine, mineral oil** decrease the absorption of vitamin K from the intestine.

**FATE**    Vitamin $K_1$ is well absorbed orally. Absorption is through the intestinal lymph and requires bile salts. The *onset of action* is in 6 to 12 hours after oral administration and 1 to 2 hours after parenteral administration.

## ❧ NURSING CONSIDERATIONS

### Side effects, toxicities, and associated nursing actions

**Allergic** Rarely, severe anaphylactic reactions are seen after IV administration: cramplike pains, cardiac irregularities, chest pain, cyanosis, dulled consciousness, flushing, circulatory collapse, difficulty in breathing, sweating.

- Assess for a history of allergy before administering.
- Monitor vital signs and blood pressure. Remain with the patient for 5 to 10 minutes following administration.
- Appropriate drugs, equipment, and personnel for treatment of an acute response should be readily available.

**Other** Pain, swelling, and tenderness may be noted at the injection site.

- Record and rotate injection sites systematically.
- In older children and adults, the dorsogluteal or ventrogluteal injection sites are preferred. In infants and small children, the vastus lateralis injection site is preferred.
- Some patients with severe local reactions may find that a switch to menadiol sodium diphosphate causes less irritation.

### Nursing interventions related to drug administration

- Monitor prothrombin time (PT) to evaluate the effectiveness of therapy.

**Systemic hemostatic agents**

- Read labels carefully. Konakion brand is for intramuscular injection only. AquaMEPHYTON brand may be given IM, IV, or subcutaneously.
- The IM or subcutaneous routes may be contraindicated in hypoprothrombinemia because of the risk of hemorrhage or hematoma at the injection site.
- Phytonadione (AquaMEPHYTON) should be diluted for intravenous administration with normal saline solution, 5% dextrose in water or 5% dextrose in normal saline solution. All of the diluents should be preservative free. No other diluents should be used. Administer slowly at a rate not exceeding 1 mg/min. Review possible allergic reactions (see Side Effects), and monitor the patient closely.
- Phytonadione is light sensitive. Administer dosage immediately after preparing. If administered via slow infusion, infusion solution should be protected from light.
- Patients with bile deficiency who are receiving oral menadione need concomitant administration of bile salts for drug absorption.

### Patient and family education

- Review with patients the side effects and anticipated benefits of therapy.
- The dietary requirement for vitamin K has not been established but has been estimated at 0.03 μg/kg for adults and 1 to 5 μg/kg for children. Although it is not stored in the body for long periods, vitamin K deficiency is rare in adults on the basis of dietary deficiency alone. Dietary sources include tomatoes, green leafy vegetables, meats, dairy products, cereals, and fruits.

Chapter Twelve
# Antilipemic drugs

cholestyramine resin
clofibrate
colestipol hydrochloride
dextrothyroxine

gemfibrozil
lovastatin
niacin
probucol

**OVERVIEW OF THE DRUG CLASS**    There are two main types of lipids in the blood: triglyceride and cholesterol. These lipids are bound to special proteins to form soluble lipoproteins. There are four major classes of lipoproteins: chylomicrons, very low density lipoproteins (VLDLs), low density lipoproteins (LDLs), and high density lipoproteins (HDLs). Chylomicrons and VLDLs are composed largely of triglycerides and transport triglycerides to tissues for metabolic use or storage. LDLs and HDLs transport cholesterol.

Hyperlipidemia is associated with an abnormal concentration of one or more of the four lipoproteins. Five major types of hyperlipidemia have been described, depending on which lipoproteins are present in abnormally high concentrations. The characteristics of the five types of hyperlipidemia are given in Table 12-1. All hyperlipidemias can be genetically determined but may also be secondary to diabetes, obesity, alcoholism, hypotyhyroidism, and liver and kidney disease. Only two kinds of hyperlipidemias are commonly encountered: type II and type IV. These two common types of hyperlipidemia are associated with a high production of triglycerides (type IV) or cholesterol (type II) by the liver. Type IV hyperlipidemia (high VLDL) is often well controlled by calorie restriction with emphasis on lowering weight and on reducing carbohydrates from which the liver synthesizes triglycerides. When diet alone does not reduce blood lipid levels to acceptable ranges, a few drugs have been found effective for lowering the concentration of blood lipids. The type of hyperlipidemia determines which drug may be effective.

**Table 12-1.**

### Types of hyperlipidemias

| | Type I | Type II | Type III | Type IV | Type V |
|---|---|---|---|---|---|
| Lipoprotein content of fasting plasma | | | | | |
| 1. Chylomicrons | Markedly increased | Absent | May be present | Absent | Increased |
| 2. VLDL | Normal or decreased | Normal or increased | Increased | Increased | Increased |
| 3. LDL | Normal or decreased | Increased | Increased | Normal | Normal or decreased |
| Lipids | | | | | |
| Cholesterol | Increased | Increased | Increased | Normal or Increased | Increased |
| Triglyceride | Increased | Normal or increased | Increased | Increased | Increased |
| Incidence | Rare | Common | Relatively uncommon | Common | Relatively uncommon |
| Usual age at detection | Early childhood | Early adulthood (can be detected in infancy or childhood) | Early adulthood | Adulthood (middle age) | Early adulthood |
| Risk of atherosclerosis | Normal | Greatly increased | Greatly increased | Probably increased | Unknown |

**Figure 12-1.** Diagram of origin and fate of lipids. Sites of action of drugs that can lower excessive plasma concentrations of lipids: (1) Drugs that lower cholesterol by increasing the excretion of bile acids—*cholestyramine* and *cholestipol*. (2) Drugs that lower triglycerides by inhibiting hepatic triglyceride synthesis-*gemfibrozil* and *niacin*. (3) Drug that lowers VLDL, inhibiting its release and activating lipoprotein lipase-*clofibrate*. (4) Drug that lowers cholesterol by stimulating LDL degradation-*dextrothyroxine*. (5) Drugs that lower cholesterol by inhibiting cholesterol synthesis—*lovastatin, probucol*. (6) Drug that lowers cholesterol by increasing cholesterol excretion into bile—*clofibrate*.

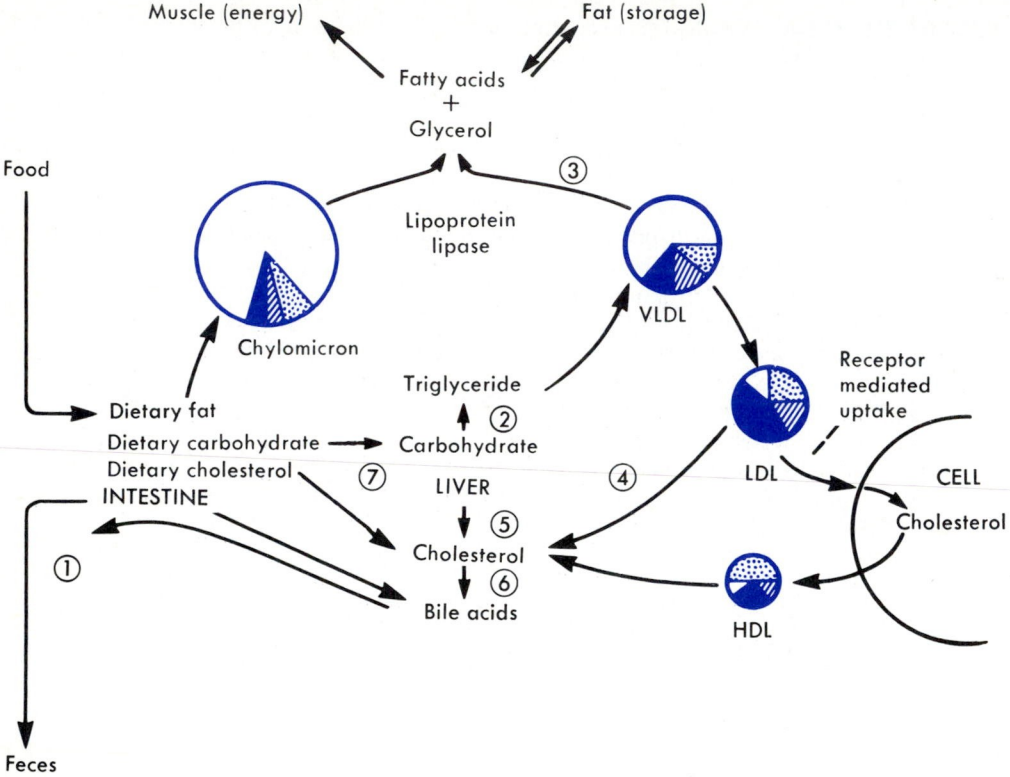

**MECHANISM OF ACTION**   Drugs that lower plasma triglycerides or cholesterol act by a variety of mechanisms that interfere with the synthesis, storage, or degradation of these lipids. The sites of action are diagrammed in Fig. 12-1.

**INDICATIONS**   **Hyperlipidemia** Normal levels of cholesterol and triglycerides depend on sex and age. Individuals with with values greatly elevated for their sex and age group should be treated with diet and drugs added if diet alone is not effective.

**CONTRAINDICATIONS**   • Hyperlipidemia controlled by diet.

**DRUG INTERACTIONS**   • See individual drugs.

## 🐦 NURSING CONSIDERATIONS
### Side effects, toxicities, and associated nursing actions

**GI** Most of these drugs can produce GI symptoms, including constipation, impaction, abdominal pain, distention, bloating, flatulence, nausea, vomiting, diarrhea, loss of appetite (see individual drugs).

• Forewarn patients about these side effects. GI symptoms may be severe enough to cause patients to discontinue the medications. Provide emotional support as needed. Reinforce to patients the importance of taking the drug as prescribed for best effect.

• Assess GI complaints. Keep a record of bowel movements. If constipation is severe, auscultate bowel sounds. Encourage a fluid intake of 2500 to 3000 ml/day, an increased intake of fruit, fruit juice, and fiber, and an increase in daily exercise. A stool softener may be indicated in some cases.

- For diarrhea, monitor weight, intake, and output.
- If GI symptoms are severe or persistent, consult the physician about a change in drug or dose.

**Patient and family education**

- Review the side effects and anticipated benefits of therapy with patients. Caution patients to report the appearance of any sign or symptom.
- Patients requiring diet modification will probably benefit from referral to a dietitian. Diet requirements can become very complicated if patients need to limit calories, carbohydrates, saturated fats, cholesterol, sodium, potassium, or other component parts of their diet based on other medical needs.
- Most antilipemics must be taken for 3 months or more before effects can be seen. These drugs should not be continued indefinitely if there is no positive response to them.
- If the drug produces the desired effect in lowering blood lipids, it is important for the patient to understand that it may be necessary to continue treatment for years.
- Remind patients to keep this and all medications out of the reach of children.

## cholestyramine resin    (koe-less-TIR-a-meen)    antilipemic

- cholestyramine: Questran

**MECHANISM OF ACTION**    Cholestyramine resin binds bile acids, decreasing their reabsorption through the enterohepatic circulation. Bile acids are the degradation products of cholesterol that are produced in the liver and excreted into the intestine through the biliary tract. The net effect of cholestyramine, when taken several times a days, is to increase the excretion of cholesterol.

**INDICATIONS**    **Type II hyperlipidemia** Cholestyramine resin is effective in lowering cholesterol levels in individuals with values above the ninetieth to ninety-fifty percentile who fail to respond adequately to dietary management. The effect takes about 1 month.    **Pruritus associated with partial cholestasis** Symptomatic relief is associated with removal of bile acids.    **Cardiac glycoside toxicity** Cholestyramine binds cardiac glycosides and can prevent absorption if given shortly after the glycoside is ingested. Since digitoxin enters the enterohepatic circulation, the concentration of this cardiac glycoside is lowered by cholestyramine even some time after ingestion of the cardiac glycoside.

**CONTRAINDICATIONS**    **Complete biliary obstruction.**

**DOSAGE**    **PO:**    **ADULTS:** 4 g three to four times daily, taken before meals and bedtime.    **CHILDREN OVER 12 YEARS OF AGE:** 8 to 16 g daily in two or three doses; 2 or 4 g twice daily before meals; 80 mg/kg three times daily.    *Special patient populations:*    **PREGNANCY:** Safe use has not been established. The drug is not absorbed and therefore will not produce direct fetal harm; however, cholestyramine can interfere with absorption of fat-soluble vitamins.

**PREPARATIONS**    *Powder.*

**DRUG INTERACTIONS**    **Other drugs** Cholestyramine is an anion-exchange resin that may bind other drugs to delay or reduce their absorption. In general, patients should take other drugs at least 1 hour before or 4 hours after cholestyramine. Specific drugs known to be bound by cholestyramine include oral anticoagulants, thyroid hormones, digitoxin and digoxin, vitamin K, chenodiol, iron salts, phenylbutazone, thiazide diuretics, phenobarbital, tetracycline, and loperamide.

**FATE**    Cholestyramine resin is not absorbed systemically and is excreted in the feces.

## ☙ NURSING CONSIDERATIONS

**Side effects, toxicities, and associated nursing actions**

**CNS** Headache, anxiety, vertigo, dizziness, fatigue, tinnitus, syncope, drowsiness, femoral nerve pain, paresthesias.

- Assess patients for these side effects.
- If dizziness, vertigo, syncope, or drowsiness develop, caution the patient to avoid activities such as driving or operating hazardous equipment until side effects wear off.

**CV** Claudication, arteritis, thrombophlebitis, myocardial ischemia, angina, myocardial infarction.

**Eye** Arcus juvenilis and uveitis.

**GU** Hematuria, dysuria, burnt odor to urine, diuresis.

**Allergic** Rash.

**Other** Xanthomas of hands and fingers, weight loss or gain, increased libido, swollen glands, edema, dental bleeding, fatigue, weakness, shortness of breath.

- Obtain a complete history and perform a thorough baseline assessment before starting therapy.
- Monitor intake, output, and weight. Monitor urinalysis.
- Warn patients about possible changes in the odor of urine.
- Visually inspect the patient for development of rash or xanthomas.
- Monitor vital signs.
- Instruct the patient to report the development of any new sign or symptom. Any problem that persists should be reported to the physician.

**Metabolic** Hyperchloremic acidosis may result from the absorption of chloride released from the resin and absorbed in place of bicarbonate. Urinary calcium excretion is increased.

- Monitor serum electrolytes and arterial blood gases in acutely ill patients.
- Assess for signs of acidosis: headache, mental dullness, Kussmaul's respirations, disorientation, coma.

**Hematologic** Decreased prothrombin time, ecchymosis, anemia.

- Monitor hematocrit, hemoglobin, and prothrombin time.
- Assess for pallor, fatigue, bruising.

**GI** Constipation occurs in 20% of patients. Constipation may include impaction and aggravation of hemorrhoids. Other effects include abdominal pain and distention, bloating, flatulence, nausea, vomiting, diarrhea, loss of appetite, heartburn, and biliary colic.

- See entry for drug class (p. 228).
- Review with patient the correct way to prepare the powder (see following section).

### Nursing interventions related to drug administration

- See Drug Interactions. If therapeutic dosage levels for a drug have been determined with the patient taking cholestyramine resin and the antilipemic is later discontinued, the dose of the other drug may then be too high. This has occurred with digitalis preparations and oral anticoagulants.
- Cholestyramine resin should not be taken in its dry form. Always mix with fluid or with food or fruit having a high fluid content. Fill a glass with 4 to 6 ounces of water, milk, or juice. Put the correct dose of medication on top of the fluid and let it stand, without stirring, for 1 to 2 minutes. This allows the medicine to absorb moisture and will help prevent lumps. Stir and drink the moisture while the drug is still suspended. Add a little more of the selected beverage to rinse the glass, and drink this also. The drug should be taken before meals.
- Applesauce, crushed pineapple, and soups with high fluid content may also be used.
- Carbonated beverages may be used, but the addition of the medication will cause excessive foaming initially, so a large glass should be used.
- Because this drug interferes with absorption of fat-soluble vitamins, supplemental vitamins may be necessary.

### Patient and family education

- See entry for drug class (p. 229).
- Ascertain that the patient can prepare the ordered dose correctly.
- Ascertain that the patient has worked out an appropriate schedule to take all prescribed medications while avoiding taking cholestyramine at the same time as other medications.
- Questran brand contains FD & C yellow dye #5 (tartrazine), which may cause an allergic response in some individuals. Although rare, it is seen more often in persons with aspirin hypersensitivity.

---

## clofibrate (kloe-FYE-brate)                                              antilipemic

- clofibrate: Atromid S

**MECHANISM OF ACTION** Clofibrate reduces the plasma concentration of triglycerides by two mechanisms. First, clofibrate activates the enzyme lipoprotein lipase, thereby accelerating the breakdown of

VLDLS. Second, clofibrate inhibits the release of VLDLS by the liver. Clofibrate also decreases plasma cholesterol concentrations by increasing the excretion of cholesterol into the bile.

**INDICATIONS** • Types II, III, IV, and V hyperlipidemias.

**CONTRAINDICATIONS** • Hepatic or renal dysfunction. • Primary biliary cirrhosis.

**DOSAGE** PO: ADULTS: 2 g daily in divided doses. *Special patient populations:* PREGNANCY: Clofibrate has been shown to accumulate in the fetuses of test animals and is therefore contraindicated during pregnancy. Clofibrate is excreted in breast milk and should not be taken by nursing mothers.

**PREPARATIONS** *Capsules:* 500 mg.

**DRUG INTERACTIONS** **Oral anticoagulants** The dose must be reduced by half since clofibrate displaces albumin-bound coumarins. **Phenytoin and tolbutamide** doses must be reduced, since the protein-bound drugs are displaced by clobifrate. **Furosemide** taken concurrently with clofibrate enhances the effects of both drugs.

**DIAGNOSTIC TEST INTERFERENCE** **Abnormal liver function test results** (increased SGOT [AST] and SGPT [ALT]); proteinuria, BSP retention, increased creatine phosphokinase. **Fasting blood glucose and serum insulin** levels may be decreased in diabetic patients.

**FATE** The free drug is rapidly hydrolyzed in the liver and the metabolite excreted in the urine. Clofibrate is active as the metabolite and is about 90% bound to albumin in the blood. The drug *half-life* is variable, from 6 to 25 hours, and is markedly increased by cirrhosis or renal impairment.

## ❦ NURSING CONSIDERATIONS

### Side effects, toxicities, and associated nursing actions

**CNS** Fatigue, weakness, drowsiness, dizziness, and headache.

**CV** Increased or decreased angina and arrhythmias.

**GU** Impotence and decreased libido; dysuria, hematuria, proteinuria, and decreased urine output.

**Skin** Rash, alopecia, pruritis, dry skin and hair.

**Other** Weight gain and polyphagia.

- Obtain a complete history and perform a thorough baseline assessment before starting therapy.
- Caution patient that if dizziness or drowsiness occurs, the patient should avoid driving or operating hazardous equipment until the effects of medication wear off.
- Monitor intake, output, and weight. Monitor urinalysis.
- Visually inspect the patient for development of rash or xanthomas.
- Monitor vital signs.
- Assess for sexual problems; patients may be reluctant to discuss sexual problems, but these problems may prompt the patient to discontinue the medication without notifying the physician. Provide emotional support as needed. Remind patients to continue the medication as ordered for best effect. Consult the physician about a change in drug or dosage.
- Instruct the patient to report the development of any new sign or symptom. Any problem that persists should be reported to the physician.
- Monitor urinalysis.

**GI** Nausea is the most common reaction. Other effects include diarrhea, bloating, flatulence, abdominal distress, gallstones, enlarged liver, vomiting.

- Taking doses with meals may decrease gastric irritation.
- See entry for drug class (p. 228).

**Hematologic** Leukopenia, potentiation of anticoagulant effect, anemia, eosinophilia.

- Monitor complete blood count and white blood cell differential.
- Assess for pallor, fatigue, fever, sore throat, bruising, bleeding.

### Patient and family education

- See entry for drug class (p. 229).
- Caution diabetic patients to monitor blood glucose carefully (see Diagnostic Test Interference), as an adjustment in insulin or diet may be necessary.

## colestipol hydrochloride (koe-LES-ti-pole) antilipemic

- colestipol hydrochloride: Colestid

**MECHANISM OF ACTION**   Colestipol, like cholestyramine, is a resin that binds bile acids, decreasing their reabsorption through the enterohepatic circulation. Bile acids are the degradation products of cholesterol that are produced in the liver and excreted into the intestine through the biliary tract. The net effect of colestipol, when taken several times a days, is to increase the excretion of cholesterol.

**INDICATIONS**   **Type II hyperlipidemia** Cholestipol is effective in lowering cholesterol levels in individuals with values above the ninetieth to ninety-fifth percentile who fail to respond adequately to dietary management. The effect takes about 1 month.   **Pruritus associated with partial cholestasis** Symptomatic relief is associated with removal of bile acids.   **Cardiac glycoside toxicity** Cholestipol binds cardiac glycosides and can prevent absorption if given shortly after the glycoside is ingested. Since digitoxin undergoes enterohepatic circulation, the concentration of this cardiac glycoside is lowered by colestipol even some time after ingestion of the cardiac glycoside.

**CONTRAINDICATIONS**   • Complete biliary obstruction.

**DOSAGE**   PO:   ADULTS: 15 to 30 g daily in divided doses taken before meals.   **CHILDREN OVER 12 YEARS OF AGE:** 10 to 20 g daily in two or three doses, or 500 mg/kg daily in two to four divided doses. *Special patient populations:* PREGNANCY: Safe use has not been established. The drug is not absorbed and therefore will not produce direct fetal harm; however, colestipol can interfere with the absorption of fat-soluble vitamins.

**PREPARATIONS**   *Beads*.

**DRUG INTERACTIONS**   **Other drugs** Colestipol is an anion-exchange resin that may bind other drugs to delay or reduce their absorption. In general, patients should take other drugs at least 1 hour before or 4 hours after colestipol. Specific drugs known to be bound by colestipol include oral anticoagulants, thyroid hormones, digitoxin and digoxin, vitamin K, chenodiol, iron salts, phenylbutazone, thiazide diuretics, phenobarbital, tetracycline, and loperamide.

**FATE**   Colestipol resin is not absorbed systemically and is excreted in the feces.

### ☙ NURSING CONSIDERATIONS

#### Side effects, toxicities, and associated nursing actions

**CNS** Headache, anxiety, vertigo, dizziness, fatigue, tinnitus, syncope, drowsiness, femoral nerve pain, paresthesias.
- Assess patients for these side effects.
- If dizziness, vertigo, syncope, or drowsiness develop, caution the patient to avoid activities such as driving or operating hazardous equipment until side effects wear off.

**CV** Claudication, arteritis, thrombophlebitis, myocardial ischemia, angina, myocardial infarction.

**Eye** Arcus juvenilis and uveitis.

**GU** Hematuria, dysuria, burnt odor to urine, diuresis.

**Allergic** Rash.

**Other** Xanthomas of hands and fingers, weight loss or gain, increased libido, swollen glands, edema, dental bleeding, fatigue, weakness, shortness of breath.
- Obtain a complete history and perform a thorough baseline assessment before starting therapy.
- Monitor intake, output, and weight. Monitor urinalysis.
- Warn patients about the possible change in the odor of urine.
- Visually inspect the patient for development of rash or xanthomas.
- Monitor vital signs.
- Instruct patients to report the development of any new sign or symptom. Any problem that persists should be reported to the physician.

**Metabolic** Hyperchloremic acidosis may result from the absorption of chloride released from the resin and absorbed in place of bicarbonate. Urinary calcium excretion is increased.
- Monitor serum electrolytes and arterial blood gases in acutely ill patients.
- Assess for signs of acidosis: headache, mental dullness, Kussmaul's respirations, disorientation, coma.

**Hematologic** Decreased prothrombin time, ecchymosis, anemia.
- Monitor hematocrit, hemoglobin, and prothrombin time.
- Assess for pallor, fatigue, bruising.

**GI** Constipation occurs in 20% of patients. Constipation may include impaction and aggravation of hemorrhoids. Other effects include abdominal pain and distention, bloating, flatulence, nausea, vomiting, diarrhea, loss of appetite, heartburn, and biliary colic.
- See entry for drug class (p. 228).
- Review with the patient the correct way to prepare the powder (see following section).

#### Nursing interventions related to drug administration
- See Drug Interactions. If therapeutic dosage levels for a drug have been determined with the patient taking colestipol and the antilipemic is later discontinued, the dose of the other drug may then be too high. This has occurred with digitalis preparations and oral anticoagulants.
- Colestipol should not be taken in its dry form. Always mix with fluid or with food or fruit having a high fluid content. Fill a glass with 4 to 6 ounces of water, milk, or juice. Put the correct dose of medication on top of the fluid and let it stand, without stirring, for 1 to 2 minutes. This allows the medicine to absorb moisture and will help prevent lumps. Stir and drink the mixture while the drug is still suspended. Add a little more of the selected beverage to rinse the glass, and drink this also. The drug should be taken before meals.
- Applesauce, crushed pineapple, and soups with high fluid content may also be used.
- Carbonated beverages may be used, but the addition of the medication will cause excessive foaming initially, so a large glass should be used.
- Because this drug interferes with absorption of fat-soluble vitamins, supplemental vitamins may be necessary.

#### Patient and family education
- See entry for drug class (p. 229).
- Ascertain that the patient can prepare the ordered dose correctly.
- Ascertain that the patient has worked out an appropriate schedule to take all prescribed medications while avoiding taking colestipol at the same time as other medications.

---

## dextrothyroxine sodium   (dex-troe-thye-ROX-in)                    antilipemic

- dextrothyroxine sodium (D-thyroxine): Choloxin

**MECHANISM OF ACTION**   Dextrothyroxine is the inactive stereoisomer of the hormone thyroxine. Dextrothyroxine enhances the degradation of LDLs and thereby lowers plasma cholesterol levels.

**INDICATIONS**   **Type II hyperlipidemia** A 20% to 30% decrease in elevated cholesterol levels may be seen in 1 month.

**CONTRAINDICATIONS**   **Heart disease,** including agina, arrhythmias, history of myocardial infarction, rheumatic heart disease, congestive heart failure, and hypertension.   **Liver or kidney disease.   Pregnancy; nursing mothers.**

**DOSAGE**   PO:   ADULTS: Initially, 1 to 2 mg daily, increased in 1 to 2 mg increments monthly to a maximum of 4 to 8 mg daily.   CHILDREN: Initially, 0.05 mg/kg, increased in up to 0.05 mg/kg increments monthly. Maximum dose is 4 mg daily.   *Special patient populations:*   PREGNANCY: Safe use has not been established.

**PREPARATIONS**   *Tablets:* 1, 2, 4, 6 mg.

**DRUG INTERACTIONS**   **Catecholamines** Dextrothyroxine will sensitize the heart to the action of catecholamines.   **Oral anticoagulants** will be potentiated by dextrothyroxine.   **Thyroid preparations** increase the sensitivity to dextrothyroxine.   **Insulin and oral hypoglycemic** doses may have to be increased for the diabetic patient.

**DIAGNOSTIC TEST INTERFERENCE**   **Thyroid tests** PBI (protein-bound iodide) increased: iodine 131 uptake decreased.   **Fasting blood sugar** Value may be increased in diabetic patients.

**FATE**   Only about 25% is absorbed orally. The drug is almost completely protein bound. The plasma *half-life* is about 18 hours.

## ❦ NURSING CONSIDERATIONS
### Side effects, toxicities, and associated nursing actions
**CNS** Insomnia, nervousness, headache, tinnitus, dizziness, malaise.
- Assesses for presence of these side effects.
- If dizziness occurs, caution patient to avoid driving or operating hazardous equipment until the effects of the medication wear off.

**CV** Palpitations, ECG changes, worsening of peripheral vascular disease, angina.
- Obtain a careful history and thorough patient assessment before starting therapy.
- If possible, a baseline ECG should be done before therapy.
- Monitor the pulse. If the pulse is greater than 120 beats per minute, withhold the dose and notify the physician.
- Monitor peripheral pulses on a regular basis.
- Patients taking this drug and a cardiac glycoside are especially susceptible to cardiac side effects. Assess cardiovascular status carefully in these patients.

**Eye** Visual disturbances, exophthalmos, retinopathy.
- Assess the patient for subjective changes in vision.
- Observe monthly for development of exophthalmos.

**GI** Dyspepsia, nausea and vomiting, constipation, diarrhea, decrease in appetite.
- Taking ordered doses with meals may decrease gastric irritation.
- See entry for drug class (p. 228).

**GU** Menstrual irregularities, changes in libido, diuresis.
- Monitor weight, intake, and output.
- Assess tactfully for changes in libido; some patients may be reluctant to discuss sexual problems. Sexual problems may prompt some patients to discontinue medications without notifying the physician. Provide emotional support as needed.
- Remind patients to take drugs as ordered for best effects.
- Consult with the physician about changes in drug or dosage.

**Metabolic** Increased metabolism, gallstones.
- Monitor pulse and weight.
- Assess for symptoms related to gallstones: right upper quadrant abdominal pain, anorexia, vomiting, fever, fat intolerance, flatulence, nausea.
- This drug may increase blood glucose concentrations in diabetic patients. Diabetics may need an adjustment of oral hypoglycemic agent or insulin. If dextrothyroxine is discontinued, diabetics who required adjustment (increase) in antidiabetic medication will again need adjustment in dosages.

**Allergic** Skin rash (may be due to iodism).
- Visually inspect patient at regular intervals for rash.
- Assess for signs of iodism: metallic taste in the mouth, sneezing, swollen and tender thyroid gland, vomiting, and bloody diarrhea.

### Patient and family education
- Review side effects and anticipated benefits of therapy with patient. While some side effects may occur quickly after the start of therapy, others may require weeks or months.
- Instruct patients to report the development of any new sign or symptom.
- Cholixin brand 2 mg and 6 mg tablets contain FD & C yellow dye #5 (tartrazine), which may cause allergic reactions in some individuals. Although rare, this allergic response is seen more often in individuals with aspirin hypersensitivity.
- Advise the patient to wear a medical identification tag or bracelet indicating that this medication is being used.
- Caution the patient to keep all health care providers informed of all medications being taken.

# gemfibrozil  (gem-FI-broe-zil)                                  antilipemic
- gemfibrozil: Lopid

**MECHANISM OF ACTION**   Gemfibrozil is chemically related to clofibrate. Like clofibrate, it lowers VLDL levels to lower total triglyceride levels. Gemfibrozil also interferes with the transfer of fatty acids from adipose tissue to the liver and with the hepatic production of VLDL. Gemfibrozil has variable effects on total cholestrol levels. LDL levels appear to fall, whereas HDL levels appear to rise.

**INDICATIONS**   • Type IV hyperlipidemia

**CONTRAINDICATIONS**   • Hepatic or severe renal dysfunction. • Primary biliary cirrhosis. • Gallbladder disease. • Hypersensitivity.

**DOSAGE**   PO:   ADULTS: 1200 mg daily (range: 900 to 1500 mg), divided in two doses 30 minutes before the morning and evening meals.   *Special patient populations:*   PREGNANCY: Safe use has not been established. Animal tests have shown gemfibrozil to be tumorigenic. Although it is not known whether gemfibrozil is excreted in breast milk, it should not be used by nursing mothers (FDA pregnancy category B).

**PREPARATIONS**   *Capsules:* 300 mg.

**DRUG INTERACTIONS**   **Oral anticoagulants** Like clofibrate, gemfibrozil may displace oral anticoagulants bound to protein, thereby potentiating these drugs.

**FATE**   Gemfibrozil is absorbed rapidly and completely. The drug is highly protein bound and enters the enterohepatic circulation.

### ☙ NURSING CONSIDERATIONS

#### Side effects, toxicities, and associated nursing actions

**CNS** Headache, dizziness.

**Eye** Blurred vision.

• Assess for the presence of these side effects.

• If dizziness or blurred vision occur, caution the patient to avoid driving or operating hazardous equipment until the effects of the medication have worn off. The patient should notify the physician.

**GI** Abdominal pain, epigastric pain, and/or diarrhea occur in about 5% of patients. These symptoms may occasionally be severe. Nausea, vomiting, and flatulence are reported less frequently.

**Biliary** Cholelithiasis may occur due to increased cholesterol excretion in the bile.

• Assess for symptoms related to cholelithiasis: right upper quadrant abdominal pain, anorexia, vomiting, fever, fat intolerance, flatulence, and nausea.

**Metabolic** Gemfibrozil may cause an increase in fasting glucose and a decrease in glucose tolerance in some individuals.

• This drug may increase blood glucose concentrations in diabetic patients. Diabetics may need an adjustment of oral hypoglycemia agent or insulin. If gemfibrozil is discontinued, diabetics who required adjustment (increase) in antidiabetic medication will again need adjustment in dosages.

**Hematologic** Blood coagulation may occasionally be affected. Slight decreases in the hematocrit and leukocyte count have been reported.

• Monitor the complete blood count (CBC), hematocrit, and hemoglobin.

• Assess for pallor, fatigue, sore throat, fever.

**Allergic** Rash, dermatitis, eczema, exanthema, pruritis, urticaria.

• Visually inspect the patient for skin changes on a regular basis.

• Caution patients to report the development of skin changes to the physician.

**Other** Flu-like muscle symptoms: back and neck pain, arthralgia, bursitis, cramps, swollen joints. These are seen mainly in patients with impaired renal function.

• Caution patients to report the development of these symptoms.

• Monitor renal function studies: serum creatinine and blood urea nitrogen (BUN).

#### Patient and family education

• See entry for drug class (p. 229).

---

## lovastatin   (low-vah-STAT-in)                                  antilipemic

• lovastatin: Mevacor

**MECHANISM OF ACTION**   This is a new drug that acts by inhibiting the enzyme HMG-CoA reductase. This is a key enzyme in the synthesis of cholesterol.

**INDICATIONS**  • Hyperlipemia.

**CONTRAINDICATIONS**  • Liver disease. • Hypersensitivity to the drug. • Pregnancy, breast feeding.

**DOSAGE**  PO:  ADULTS: 20 to 80 mg daily. Begin with 20 mg once a day. Adjust to higher doses if needed only at 4-week intervals. If 80 mg is required, that dose may be divided into two to four doses. *Special patient populations:* PREGNANCY: Safe use has not been established. Lovastatin does produce fetal malformations at high doses in rats (FDA pregnancy category X).

**PREPARATIONS**  *Tablets:* 20 mg.

**DRUG INTERATIONS**  None reported.

**FATE**  Lovastatin is poorly absorbed from the gastrointestinal tract. About 85% of the drug appears in the feces and about 10% in the urine. Lovastatin may require 4 weeks of administration to see cholesterol lowering effects.

☙ **NURSING CONSIDERATIONS**

**Side effects, toxicities, and associated nursing actions**

**Eye** An eye examination is recommended before and during therapy because slight changes in the lens have been noted.

• Encourage patients to have regular eye examinations.

**GI** Constipation or diarrhea; flatulence; cramps and nausea.

• See entry for drug class (p. 228).

**Other** A liver function study should be performed every 4 to 6 weeks over the first 15 months of therapy. About 2% of patients show a threefold or greater increase in the level of serum transaminases, an indication of abnormal liver function; therapy should be discontinued. Muscle pain is occasionally reported.

• Monitor liver function tests.

• Instruct patients to report the development of malaise, fever, right upper quadrant abdominal pain, or change in the color or consistency of stools.

• Encourage patients to return for regular follow-up.

• Assess patients for the development of any new sign or symptom.

**Patient and family education**

• Review anticipated benefits and possible side effects of drug therapy with patient and family.

• See entry for drug class (p. 229).

---

## niacin  (NYE-a-sin)                                                    antilipemic

• niacin (nicotinic acid): Nicotinex, Nicolar, ✦Novoniacin

**MECHANISM OF ACTION**  Niacin is a B vitamin for which the minimum daily requirement (MDR) is 20 mg. At doses 10 to 20 times this, niacin is a vasodilator. At doses 100 to 200 times the MDR, niacin depresses the synthesis of VLDLs by the liver. This reduces LDL levels as well.

**INDICATIONS**  • Types II, III, IV, and V hyperlipemias.

**CONTRAINDICATIONS**  • Gallbladder disease. • Liver disease. • Gout. • Peptic ulcer. • Hemorrhaging or arterial bleeding.

**DOSAGE**  PO:  ADULTS: Dosage is highly individualized. Range: 1.5 to 6 g daily in two to four divided doses. Initially, 100 mg three times daily may be given, then decreased 300 mg daily every 4 to 7 days. *Special patient populations:* PREGNANCY: Safe use has not been established. Niacin is excreted into breast milk.

**PREPARATIONS**  *Powder; solution:* 50 mg/5 ml; *tablets:* 100, 250, 500 mg.

**DRUG INTERACTIONS**  **Ganglionic blocking agents** Nicotinamide potentiates the hypotensive effect of these agents.

**DIAGNOSTIC TEST INTERFERENCE**  **Urinary catecholamines** Nicotinamide produces flourescent compounds in the urine that may interfere with this test.  **Benedict's reagent** Nicotinamide may give false-positive reactions with cupric sulfate solution, which is used for urine glucose determination.

**Serum bilirubin, uric acid, alkaline phosphatase, ALT (SGPT), AST (SGOT), LDH** These values may be increased.

**FATE**   Niacin is well absorbed and readily metabolized to nicotinamide. Nicotinamide is further metabolized by the liver but when given in large amounts is also excreted unchanged in the urine.

### ❦ NURSING CONSIDERATIONS

#### Side effects, toxicities, and associated nursing actions

**CV** Cutaneous flushing within the first 2 hours. Tolerance develops to this reaction. Headache, itching, and tingling are also common. Hypotension.
- Monitor the blood pressure.
- Flushing may be ameliorated by taking 300 mg of aspirin 30 minutes before the niacin.
- Taking the prescribed dose with meals or in a sustained release form may lessen side effects.

**GI** General gastrointestinal upset.
- Taking the prescribed dose with meals may lessen GI side effects. For some patients, the sustained release formula intensifies GI side effects. These patients may respond better to regular formulations.
- See entry for drug class (p. 228).

#### Patient and family education
- See entry for drug class (p. 229).
- Nicotinamide (niacinamide), the niacin component of many multivitamin preparations, does not produce the characteristic blushing seen with other niacin formulations. Nicotinamide does not lower plasma cholesterol levels, so this preparation is useful only in vitamin replacement or in treatment of pellagra, a disease caused specifically by niacin deficiency. For additional information about the role of dietary niacin, refer to a text on nutrition.
- Nicolar brand tablets contain FD & C yellow dye #5 (tartrazine), which may cause an allergic reaction in susceptible individuals. Although rare, this allergic reaction is seen more often in individuals with aspirin hypersensitivity.

## probucol   (PROE-byoo-kole)                                    antilipemic

- probucol: Lorelco

**MECHANISM OF ACTION**   Probucol inhibits cholesterol synthesis, leading to a decrease in plasma LDL (low density lipoprotein).

**INDICATIONS**   • Type II hyperlipemia.

**CONTRAINDICATIONS**   • Recent myocardial infarction.

**DOSAGE**   **PO:**   **ADULTS:** 500 mg twice daily with the morning and evening meals.   *Special patient populations:*   **PREGNANCY:** Safe use has not been established. Animal studies have not shown adverse reproductive effects, but probucol is distributed into the milk of lactating animals.

**PREPARATIONS**   *Tablets:* 250 mg.

**DRUG INTERACTIONS**   **Clofibrate** Although the reduction in total cholesterol or LDL cholesterol is not marked, a pronounced drop in HDL cholesterol may be noted.

**FATE**   Probucol is poorly absorbed. Being highly lipophilic, probucol accumulates in fat. Excretion is slow, principally by billiary excretion in the feces.

### ❦ NURSING CONSIDERATIONS

#### Side effects, toxicities, and associated nursing actions

**CNS** Insomnia, tinnitus, dizziness, headache.

**Eye** Conjunctivitis, lacrimation, blurred vision.
- Assess patients regularly for these side effects.
- Caution patients that if dizziness or blurred vision occurs, patients should avoid driving or operating hazardous equipment until the effects of the medication can be evaluated.

**CV** ECG changes were seen in animal studies.
- Obtain baseline ECG before starting therapy, and monitor ECG at least annually.
- Monitor the pulse at regular intervals.

**GI** Diarrhea or loose stools are experienced by 10% of patients. Flatulence, abdominal pain, nausea and vomiting, indigestion, or GI bleeding occasionally occurs transiently.
- See entry for drug class (p. 228).

**GU** Nocturia; impotence.
- Question patients carefully for presence of these side effects. Patients who experience impotence due to drug side effects will often cease taking the medication. A switch to a different drug may be necessary. Provide emotional support as needed. Remind patients to take drugs as prescribed for best effect.

**Hematologic** Eosinophilia, decreased hematocrit, thrombocytopenia.

**Metabolic** Increases in serum concentrations of AST (SGOT), ALT (SGPT), bilirubin, alkaline phosphatase, creatine kinase (CK), creatinine phosphokinase (CPK), and uric acid are sometimes seen.
- Obtain baseline complete blood count (CBC), hematocrit and hemoglobin, platelet count, and liver function studies before starting therapy, and monitor at regular intervals.
- Caution patient to report the development of unexplained bruising or bleeding.

**Skin** Rash, pruritis, ecchymoses, petechiae, hyperhidrosis, fetid sweat.
- Visually inspect patients regularly for the development of these side effects.
- Warn patients that skin changes may occur.

## Patient and family education
- See entry for drug class (p. 229).

Chapter Thirteen

# Drugs to treat nutritional anemias

iron salts
vitamin B$_{12}$

folic acid
leucovorin calcium

**OVERVIEW OF THE DRUG CLASS**    Iron, folic acid, and vitamin B$_{12}$ are all required to produce red blood cells. A deficiency in any one of these agents will result in anemia.

**MECHANISM OF ACTION**    Iron is required for the synthesis of the heme part of hemoglobin. Folic acid and vitamin B$_{12}$ are required for DNA synthesis. The constant production of the immature precursors of red blood cells requires active DNA synthesis.

**INDICATIONS**    • Nutritional deficiency specific for iron, folic acid, or vitamin B$_{12}$.

**CONTRAINDICATIONS**    • See individual agent.

**DRUG INTERACTIONS**    • See individual agent.

---

## iron salts                                                        iron-deficiency anemia

- iron salts: ferrous fumarate, ferrous gluconate, ferrous sulfate, polysaccharide–iron complex, soy protein–iron complex

**MECHANISM OF ACTION**    Iron is a component of several enzymes necessary for energy transfer in biochemical reactions. Iron is also the part of the heme complex in hemoglobin and myoglobin that is responsible for oxygen transport in the blood and tissues, respectively.

When the body's supply of iron is deficient, hemoglobin cannot be synthesized. The result is that the red blood cells formed are small (microcytic) and pale (hypochromic).

**INDICATIONS**    Iron deficiency anemia This is most common in menstruating or pregnant women due to their high requirements for hemoglobin synthesis.

**CONTRAINDICATIONS**    • Hemochromatosis, hemosiderosis, chronic hemolytic anemias. • Cirrhosis of the liver. • Peptic ulcer, regional enteritis, ulcerative colitis.

**DOSAGE**    PO—recommended dietary allowances (RDA):    ADULTS: 10 mg for males, 18 mg for menstruating females; 30 to 60 mg for pregnant and lactating females.    CHILDREN: 10 to 15 mg;    TEENAGERS: 18 mg.    **For iron deficiency:** 6 mg/kg/day of elemental iron. The elemental iron content varies according to the salt form: ferrous gluconate is 11.6% elemental iron; ferrous fumarate, 33%; ferrous sulfate, 20%. Replacement therapy, in the absence of bleeding, rarely requires more than 6 months. *Special patient populations:*    CHILDREN: Children have higher relative requirements for iron because of their rapid growth.    PREGNANCY: Iron is a common supplement for pregnant and lactating women.

**PREPARATIONS**    **Ferrous fumarate (33% elemental iron)** *Suspension:* 45 mg/0.6 ml, 100 mg/5 ml; *tablets:* 60, 195, 200, 300, 324, 325 mg; *tablets, chewable:* 100 mg; *tablets, extended-release:* 300, 324 mg.    **Ferrous gluconate (11.6% elemental iron)** *Capsules:* 325, 435 mg; *solution:* 300 mg/5 ml; *tablets:* 300, 320, 325 mg; *tablets, film-coated:* 300 mg.    **Ferrous sulfate (20% elemental iron)** *Capsules, extended-release:* 150, 225, 250, 390 mg; *solution:* 90 mg/5 ml, 125 mg/5 ml, 220 mg/5 ml, 75 mg/0.6 ml; *tablets:* 195, 300, 324, 325 mg: *tablets, enteric-coated:* 325 mg: *tablets, extended-release:* 525 mg; *tablets, film-coated:* 300 mg.    **Polysaccharide–iron complex** *Capsules:* 150 mg iron; *solution:* 100 mg iron per 5 ml; *tablets:* 50 mg iron.    **Soy protein–iron complex** *Tablets:* 50 mg iron.

**DRUG INTERACTIONS**    **Tetracycline** absorption from the GI tract is inhibited by iron.    **Chloramphenicol** delays the response to iron therapy.    **Vitamin C** increases the absorption of iron.    **Antacids** decrease iron absorption.    **Penicillamine** absorption is decreased by iron.

**FATE**    The absorption of iron is tightly regulated by the transport protein transferrin. Iron stores consist of iron bound to specific proteins: ferritin and hemosiderin. Iron is highly conserved by the body, and little is excreted.

## ☙ NURSING CONSIDERATIONS

### Side effects, toxicities, and associated nursing actions

**GI** Iron is highly irritating and can cause bleeding.

- Monitor color and consistency of stools. Feces will be dark green or black and more tarry in consistency. If there is doubt about whether the cause of a change in color or consistency in stools is due to blood or to ingestion of iron, the stool should be tested for blood.
- Monitor hematocrit, hemoglobin, and reticulocyte count at regular intervals.

### Patient and family education

- Review with patients the side effects and anticipated benefits of therapy. Caution patients to report the appearance of any sign or symptom.
- Inform patients about anticipated changes in color and consistency of stools (see preceding section).
- Instruct patients to take iron on an empty stomach, if tolerable. If the drug cannot be taken on an empty stomach, advise patients to take the drug with meals. Absorption is reduced in the presence of milk, antacids, tetracycline, many cereals, and eggs. Since the absorption is increased with the ingestion of ascorbic acid (vitamin C), some patients may wish to take the iron with orange or another citrus juice.
- Some patients find that regular use of iron preparations causes diarrhea, whereas others may complain that the iron causes constipation. If the latter occurs, instruct patients to increase their daily fluid intake to at least 3000 ml, to add fiber and bulk to the diet, and to add to the diet foods known by the patient to stimulate defecation, such as fresh fruits, coffee, prune juice, or other foods.
- Decreasing the dose of iron while increasing the frequency of taking the iron may decrease the incidence or severity of side effects.
- Liquid iron preparations may stain the teeth, so they should be taken through a straw. Dilute the preparation well with water or fruit juice, and rinse the mouth out well after taking the dose.
- Review with the patient the dietary history and instruct as appropriate about modifications that could be made to increase the intake of iron-rich foods. Good sources of dietary iron include fish and meat, especially organ meats (liver, kidney, heart). Beans, prune juice, and iron-enriched cereals and breads are also good sources of iron. If appropriate, refer the patient to a dietitian in the hospital or health department for additional instruction.
- Remind patients to keep iron preparations, and all drugs, out of the reach of children. Emphasize the importance of seeking prompt medical attention if overdose is suspected. Because iron preparations are available so readily in over-the-counter preparations, adults may not realize the severity of overdose in children.

---

## iron dextran injection                                             antianemic

- iron dextran injection: Feostat, Hematran, Hydextran, Imferon, Irodex, Proferdex, Rocyte

**MECHANISM OF ACTION**    Iron is a component of several enzymes necessary for energy transfer in biochemical reactions. Iron is also the part of the heme complex in hemoglobin and myoglobin that is responsible for oxygen transport in the blood and tissues, respectively,

When the body's supply of iron is deficient, hemoglobin cannot be synthesized. The result is that the red blood cells formed are small (microcytic) and pale (hypochromic).

**INDICATIONS**    **Iron deficiency anemia** For use with those patients requiring parenteral therapy: intolerance to oral iron, poor absorption, GI disease.

**CONTRAINDICATIONS**    **Hypersensitivity to iron-dextran** Fatal anaphylactoid reactions have occurred.

**DOSAGE**    **IM, IV:**    ADULTS AND CHILDREN: Doses are individualized, based on estimates of total iron requirements. This is necessary because the body cannot excrete excess iron. A test dose is always given first to monitor for a possible anaphylactoid reaction.    **IV:** An IV dose is injected, undiluted, at a rate not exceeding 50 mg of iron per minute. If there are no adverse reactions to the test dose, subsequent doses may be increased to 100 mg or iron in 2 or 3 days and iron given daily until the total calculated dose has been administered.    **IM:** An IM should initially be no larger than 25 mg. Subsequent daily doses are based on body size. Maximum daily doses are infants under 10 pounds (4.5 kg), 25 mg; 10 to 20 pounds (4.5 to 9 kg), 50 mg; children and adults 20 to 110 pounds (9 to 50 kg), 100 mg; over 110 pounds (50 kg), 250 mg.    *Special patient populations:*    **PREGNANCY:** Iron-dextran has been shown to cause fetal abnormalities in animals when given early in gestation. Iron-dextran does cross the placenta.

**PREPARATIONS**    *Injection:* 50 mg iron/ml. Some preparations are for IM use only.

**DRUG INTERACTIONS**    Drug interactions are reported only for the oral forms of iron at the level of absorption from the GI tract.

**LABORATORY TEST INTERFERENCES**    IV doses greater than 100 mg of iron may color the serum brown. Falsely high serum bilirubin values and falsely low values of serum calcium are measured. Serum iron and total iron-binding capacity measurements are not meaningful for 3 weeks.

**FATE**    Iron dextran is absorbed IM through the lymphatic system. About 60% is absorbed in 3 days, 90% in 3 weeks, and the remainder over months. The staining of the skin at the injection site may remain for up to 2 years.

Release of iron depends on the ingestion of the complex by macrophages. Iron is gradually released and transferred to the transport protein transferrin.

## 🐦 NURSING CONSIDERATIONS

### Side effects, toxicities, and associated nursing actions

**Allergic** The most serious response is an anaphylactoid reaction; however, large IV doses are often accompanied by delayed reactions such as arthralgia, myalgia, and fever. Local inflammatory reactions may occur at the IM injection site.

- Monitor the vital signs.
- To decrease the possibility of severe anaphylactic reaction, it is suggested that a small test dose of 25 mg (0.5 ml) be given, and the patient observed carefully for at least 1 hour before the remainder of the initial dose is given.
- Appropriate drugs (epinephrine, antihistamines, steroids) and resuscitation equipment should be readily available in any setting where parenteral iron is being administered.
- Discontinue oral preparations when parenteral forms are being used to decrease the incidence of toxic reactions.

### Nursing interventions related to drug administration

**Intramuscular iron injections**

- Adminster these preparations only in the large muscle mass of the buttocks to avoid possible staining of the skin in more frequently visible areas. The following method of administration is suggested to help reduce the possibility of staining.
- After drawing up the ordered dose, add 0.1 ml of air to the syringe. Discard the needle used to draw up the medication and obtain a new one. Using the Z-track method of intramuscular administration, inject all of the medication and the 0.1 ml of air, the desired effect of the air being to flush any remaining medication out of the needle, then withdraw the needle.
- After an initial test dose, intravenous iron should be administered slowly via direct intravenous push at a rate not to exceed 1 ml (50mg) per minute. This drug is incompatible with other drugs in a syringe or with infusing fluids. Flush the IV line with 0.9% sodium chloride before and after administering the ordered dose.
- Read drug labels carefully. Some preparations contain phenol and are suitable for intramuscular administration only.
- Following intravenous administration, monitor vital signs and blood pressure. The patient should remain lying down for 30 minutes following drug administration.
- Monitor hematocrit, hemoglobin, and reticulocyte count.

### Patient and family education

- Review with patients the side effects and anticipated benefits of therapy. Caution patients to report the appearance of any sign or symptom.

# vitamin B$_{12}$ antianemic

- vitamin B$_{12}$ (cyanocobalamin concentrate, cyanocobalamin, hydroxocobalamin, liver extract, vitamin B$_{12}$ with intrinsic factor): generic only

**MECHANISM OF ACTION** Vitamin B$_{12}$ is required for a key reaction in the synthesis of thymidylate, a component of deoxyribonucleic acid (DNA). The synthesis of new red blood cells in the numbers required demands an adequate supply of vitamin B$_{12}$. A deficiency of vitamin B$_{12}$ also leads to neurologic damage because vitamin B$_{12}$ is a cofactor for an enzymatic step necessary for producing the myelin sheath of nerves.

**INDICATIONS** **Pernicious anemia** This arises from a deficiency of *intrinsic factor*, the binding protein for vitamin B$_{12}$ produced in the stomach. Absorption of dietary vitamin B$_{12}$ requires intrinsic factor. The body has a 2 to 5 year supply of vitamin B$_{12}$, so it takes some time for pernicious anemia to appear. The anemia resulting is a *megalobastic* (immature red blood cell), *macrocytic* (large cell) anemia like that produced by folic acid deficiency. A tingling sensation in the extremities, due to early neurologic damage, is one symptom of vitamin B$_{12}$ deficiency. Folic acid will correct the anemia, but not the neurologic damage.

**CONTRAINDICATIONS** • None: Vitamin B$_{12}$ is often misused as a tonic or to treat mental conditions.

**DOSAGE** **PO:** **ADULTS AND CHILDREN:** The recommended daily dietary allowance (RDA) is 0.5 to 3μg in children and 3μg in adults. **IM, SC (for pernicious anemia):** **ADULTS:** 30 μg daily for 5 to 10 days. Once clinical symptoms have disappeared, monthly maintenance doses of 100 to 200 μg are given. **CHILDREN:** Total dose is 1 to 5 mg, given in single doses of 100 μg over 2 or more weeks. Maintenance doses are 60 μg per month. *Special patient populations:* **PREGNANCY:** Vitamin B$_{12}$ administration is considered safe during pregnancy.

**PREPARATIONS** **Cyanocobalamin concentrate** *Tablets:* 25, 50, 100, 250 μg. **Cyanocobalamin** *Tablets:* 25, 50, 100, 250, 500, 1000 μg; *injection:* 30, 100, 1000 μg/ml; *injection, repository:* 1000 μg/ml. **Hydroxocobalamin** *Injection:* 1000 μg/ml. **Liver extract** *Injection:* 10, 20 μg/ml. **Liver extract crude** *Injection:* 2 μg/ml. **Vitamin B$_{12}$ with intrinsic factor** *Tablets:* 0.5 units.

**DRUG INTERACTIONS** **Alcohol, aminoglycoside antibiotics, colchicine, extended-release potassium preparations, aminosalicylic acid, anticonvulsants, cobalt irradiation of the small bowel, or excessive alcohol intake** decrease the absorption of vitamin B$_{12}$ from the GI tract. **Vitamin C** destroys dietary vitamin B$_{12}$. **Chloramphenicol** antagonizes the hematopietic response to vitamin B$_{12}$.

**DIAGNOSTIC TEST INTERFERENCE** **IF antibodies** Vitamin B$_{12}$ may lead to false-positive results for intrinsic factor antibodies.

**FATE** Vitamin B$_{12}$ requires intrinsic factor, synthesized by the parietal cells of the stomach, for binding and transport across the small intestine. Vitamin B$_{12}$ is stored in the liver. In the healthy person, stores are large enough to meet requirements for 2 to 5 years.

## ☙ NURSING CONSIDERATIONS

### Side effects, toxicities, and associated nursing actions

**GI** Mild diarrhea.
- Monitor consistency and frequency of stools.
- If diarrhea persists or is severe, a change in drug dose may be necessary.

**Hematologic** Peripheral vascular thrombosis.
- Obtain careful baseline vascular assessment.
- Monitor peripheral pulses regularly.

**Allergic** Urticaria; rarely, anaphylaxis.
- Monitor vital signs and blood pressure.
- Keep available appropriate drugs (epinephrine, antihistamines, steroids) and resuscitation equipment in any setting where vitamin B$_{12}$ is administered.

### Nursing interventions related to drug administration
- Vitamin B$_{12}$ should not be administered intravenously. The intramuscular route is preferred, although cyanocobalamin may be administered by deep subcutaneous injection.

- Read orders and labels carefully. A depot form is available, which would be administered every 2 to 3 weeks.

### Patient and family education
- Review with patients the side effects and anticipated benefits of therapy. Caution patients to report the appearance of any sign or symptom.
- Teach patients with pernicious anemia about their disease. It may be difficult for patients to understand why the vitamin $B_{12}$ cannot be taken orally and why it must be continued for life.
- In those rare cases in which vitamin $B_{12}$ deficiency is due to dietary causes, review the diet with the patient and instruct the patient about possible dietary sources of the vitamin. Sources of vitamin $B_{12}$ include animal protein, eggs, and dairy products. If appropriate, refer the patient to the hospital or health department dietitian for additional instruction.
- Patients should avoid the use of alcohol while taking vitamin $B_{12}$.
- Vitamin $B_{12}$ should not be taken within 1 hour of ascorbic acid.

## folic acid   (FOE-lick)                                                antianemic

- folic acid: generic

**MECHANISM OF ACTION**   Folic acid is required for a key reaction in the synthesis of thymidylate, a component of deoxyribonucleic acid (DNA). Vitamin $B_{12}$ is necessary for the regeneration of the active metabolite of folic acid. The synthesis of new red blood cells in the numbers required demands an adequate supply of folic acid. The anemia resulting from a deficiency of vitamin $B_{12}$ can be corrected by large doses of folic acid, but the neurologic damage resulting from vitamin $B_{12}$ deficiency will not be corrected by folic acid.

**INDICATIONS**   **Megaloblastic, macrocytic anemia** This is most common during pregnancy, and folic acid is usually given as a supplement to pregnant women.

**CONTRAINDICATIONS**   **Pernicious anemia** It is important to determine that a patient with megaloblastic, marcocytic anemia does not have pernicious anemia secondary to a deficiency of vitamin $B_{12}$. Folic acid will correct the anemia but will not affect the neurologic damage, which can become irreversible if not treated with vitamin $B_{12}$.

**DOSAGE**   **PO:**   **ADULTS AND CHILDREN:** 0.25 to 1 mg daily. Maintenance doses are 0.1 mg for infants; 0.3 mg for children under 4 years; 0.4 mg for children over 4 years to adult.   *Special patient populations:*   **PREGNANCY:** Folic acid is commonly given during pregnancy.

**PREPARATIONS**   *Tablets:* 0.1, 0.4, 0.8, 1 mg; *injection:* 5 mg/ml.

**DRUG INTERACTIONS**   **Phenytoin** Folic acid may increase the metabolism of phenytoin and cause lower serum concentrations.   **Chloramphenicol** may inhibit the hematopoietic response to folic acid.

**FATE**   Folic acid is rapidly absorbed and widely distributed in the body. Excess amounts are excreted in the urine. Unlike vitamin $B_{12}$, body stores of folic acid are not large, and a deficiency state can develop rapidly.

## NURSING CONSIDERATIONS

### Nursing interventions related to drug administration
- Oral preparations are used most frequently. There is a parenteral form available. The drug may be given IM, direct IV push, or added to most infusion solutions. Administer IV push at a rate not to exceed 5 mg/min.
- Although rare, anaphylaxis from parenteral administration has occurred.
- Monitor vital signs.
- Have drugs, equipment, and personnel available for resuscitation when parenteral forms are used.

### Patient and family education
- Review with patients the side effects and anticipated benefits of therapy. Caution patients to report the appearance of any sign of symptom.

- Review with patients their usual dietary intake, and instruct as needed about sources of folic acid. Good sources of folic acid include meats, fresh vegetables, and fresh fruits.
- Teach patients with pernicious anemia about their disease. It may be difficult for patients to understand why the vitamin $B_{12}$ cannot be taken orally and why it must be continued for life.
- In those rare cases in which vitamin $B_{12}$ deficiency is due to dietary causes, review the diet with the patient and instruct the patient about possible dietary sources of the vitamin. Sources of vitamin $B_{12}$ include animal protein, eggs, and dairy products. If appropriate, refer the patient to the hospital or health department dietitian for additional instuction.

## leucovorin calcium    (loo-koe-VOR-in)                                              antianemic

- leucovorin calcium: Wellcovorin

**MECHANISM OF ACTION**    Leucovorin is the active metabolite of folic acid.

**INDICATIONS**    **Antidote for folic acid antagonists** Leucovorin rescue: To diminish the toxicity of folic acid antagonists such as methotrexate, trimethoprim, and pyrimethamine.    **Megaloblastic anemia** Used when oral folic acid therapy is not feasible.

**CONTRAINDICATIONS**    • Pernicious anemia.

**DOSAGE**

**For leucovorin rescue of methotrexate toxicity:**    PO, IM, IV:    ADULTS AND CHILDREN: Give in an amount equal to the weight of the antagonist given, preferably within an hour. In cancer therapy with high-dose methotrexate, 10 mg/M$^2$ is given as a beginning dose within 24 hours and thereafter at 6 hour intervals for 72 hours. If after 24 hours the serum creatinine is increased by 50%, the dose of leucovorin is increased to 100 mg/m$_2$ every 3 hours.

**Megaloblastic anemias:**    IM:    ADULTS: 1 mg daily.    *Special patient populations:*    PREGNANCY: Safe use has not been established.

**PREPARATIONS**    *Tablets:* 5, 25 mg; *injection:* 50 mg; 5 mg/ml.

**DRUG INTERACTIONS**    **Methotrexate, trimethoprim, pyrimethanmine** Leucovorin is the antidote for these folic acid antagonists.

**FATE**    Leucovorin is rapidly absorbed and converted to other tetrahydrofolic acid derivatives.

## ☙ NURSING CONSIDERATIONS

### Side effects, toxicities, and associated nursing actions

- Hypersensitivity.

### Nursing interventions related to drug administration

- Read labels and orders carefully. Do not confuse with folic acid.
- Reconstitute as directed on vial for parenteral administration. Administer immediately after preparing; if left standing, precipitation may occur.
- Monitor vital signs after parenteral administration. Since allergic reactions have occurred with folic acid, there is theoretic possibility they may occur with leucovorin also.

### Patient and family education

- Review with patients the side effects and anticipated benefits of therapy. Caution patients to report the appearance of any sign or symptom.

# ANTIBACTERIAL AGENTS

**V**

**INTRODUCTION**   Antibacterial agents are selective poisons designed to attack bacteria within the human host without directly damaging human tissues. These drugs inhibit or destroy the bacteria, allowing the patient's immune system to resolve the infection. This clinical goal is achieved by a variety of mechanisms. *Penicillins, cephalosporins,* and other *beta-lactam* antibiotics block cell wall synthesis in bacteria. Because this process does not occur in mammalian cells, the drugs are selective for bacteria. *Aminoglycosides, tetracyclines, chloramphenicol,* and *erythromycin* inhibit protein synthesis carried out by bacterial ribosomes. Because mammalian ribosomes do not readily bind these agents, the drugs are selective for bacteria. *Rifampin* inhibits the enzyme that forms RNA from DNA. Because only the bacterial form of the enzyme is inhibited, rifampin is selective for bacteria. *Nalidixic acid, norfloxacin,* and other quinolones inhibit enzymes that control DNA structure. Because these drugs inhibit only the bacterial form of these enzymes, only bacteria are affected. *Sulfonamides, trimethoprim,* and *sulfones* block folic acid metabolism, preferentially affecting bacterial cells because of the different enzymes and enzyme forms found in bacteria. *Urinary tract antiseptics* are effective because they are highly concentrated in the urinary tract, where they can directly attack bacteria causing disease.

# Chapter Fourteen

# Penicillins

amdinocillin
amoxicillin trihydrate
amoxicillin with clavulanate potassium
ampicillin, ampicillin sodium, ampicillin trihydrate
ampicillin sodium with sulbactam sodium
azlocillin sodium
bacampicillin hydrochloride
benzathine penicillin G
carbenicillin disodium
carbenicillin indanyl sodium
cloxacillin sodium
cyclacillin

dicloxacillin sodium
hetacillin, hetacillin potassium
methicillin sodium
mezlocillin sodium
nafcillin sodium
oxacillin sodium
penicillin G potassium, penicillin G sodium
penicillin V, penicillin V potassium
piperacillin sodium
procaine penicillin G
ticarcillin disodium
ticarcillin disodium with clavulanate potassium

**OVERVIEW OF THE DRUG CLASS**   Penicillins are the most widely used family of antibiotics. In use since the 1940s, these drugs have proved safe and effective in many types of infections. Early penicillins came from natural sources and were used primarily against infections caused by gram-positive bacteria. Semisynthetic penicillins introduced later created new properties such as resistance to penicillinase, an enzyme produced by *Staphylococcus aureus* that destroyed earlier penicillins. These penicillinase-resistant drugs, as well as the original natural penicillins, have narrow antibacterial spectra. Other semisynthetic penicillins had extended antibacterial spectra against gram-negative bacteria primarily because they penetrate the cell envelope of these organisms better than older penicillins. A few of these compounds also have activity against *Pseudomonas aeruginosa,* a pathogen that resists the action of most antibacterial agents. Table 14-1 lists the classes of penicillins.

**MECHANISM OF ACTION**   Penicillins inhibit bacterial enzymes that assemble peptidoglycan, the substance that gives rigidity to the bacterial cell wall. Without rigid support, the cell wall is unable to withstand osmotic forces from within the cell, and the bacteria can rupture. Penicillins also alter the composition of the cell wall so that bacterial enzymes called autolysins become more active. Autolysins dissolve linkages in the cell wall, further weakening the structure. Penicillins are considered bactericidal because the actions described are capable of directly killing bacteria. Because penicillin does not act on mammalian cells, these drugs are relatively free of toxicity.

Resistance to the action of penicillins occurs in bacteria that produce penicillinases or beta-lactamases. These enzymes destroy the penicillin molecule before the drug can fatally disrupt the bacterial cell wall. Less common mechanisms of resistance do not involve beta-lactamases or penicillinases but arise from intrinsic resistance of the targets of penicillin action in the bacteria.

**INDICATIONS**   **Infections caused by gram-positive bacteria** Narrow-spectrum penicillins are usually preferred for these infections when the organisms are susceptible. • When penicillinase-producing strains of *aureus* are suspected, one of the penicillinase-resistant penicillins must be used (Table 14-1).   **Infections caused by gram-negative bacteria** Narrow-spectrum penicillins may be effective against *Neisseria* and *Pasteurella* but against most other gram-negative organisms, the extended spectrum penicillins must be used (Table 14-1).   **Infections caused by anaerobic bacteria** Narrow-spectrum penicillins are effective against many of these pathogens.   **Infections caused by spirochetes** Syphilis, yaws, pinta, and bejel may be controlled with narrow-spectrum penicillins (Table 14-1).

**CONTRAINDICATIONS**   **Allergy to penicillin or cephalosporin drugs** Anaphylaxis and death are possible outcomes. • The risk is greatest in those who report previous allergic reactions to penicillin and less in those previously reacting to cephalosporins.

**DRUG INTERACTIONS**   **Aminoglycosides** have additive or synergistic antibacterial action with penicillins when used to treat relatively resistant organisms. They may be inactivated if mixed in a syringe or IV bottle with penicillin solutions.   **Clavulanic acid** inhibits beta-lactamases that may destroy penicillin. Clavulanic acid may therefore be synergistic with penicillins.   **Probenecid** inhibits renal secretion of penicillins and may prolong the elimination half-life. Probenecid is used to prolong antibacterial

**Table 14-1.**

| Classification of penicillins | | |
| --- | --- | --- |
| Class | Properties | Representatives |
| Narrow spectrum | Primarily effective against gram-positive bacteria but are destroyed by the penicillinase from *S. aureus* | Penicillin G, benzathine penicillin G, procaine penicillin G, and penicillin V |
| Penicillinase-resistant | Narrow spectrum but resist the action of penicillinase from *S. aureus* | Cloxacillin, dicloxacillin, methicillin, nafcillin, and oxacillin |
| Extended spectrum | Improved action against gram-negative bacteria but often destroyed by penicillinase from *S. aureus* | Amdinocillin, amoxycillin, ampicillin, bacampicillin, cyclacillin, and hetacillin |
| Antipseudomonas | Used only for gram-negative bacteria, including *P. aeruginosa* and related organisms | Azlocillin, carbenicillin, mezlocillin, piperacillin, ticarcillin |

action of penicillins with short half-lives. **Sulbactam** inhibits beta-lactamases that may destroy penicillins. Sulbactam may therefore be synergistic with penicillins.   **Tetracyclines, chloramphenicol, or erythromycin** may interfere with bactericidal action of penicillins. • For drug interactions specific to individual agents, see individual drugs.

## 🦫 NURSING CONSIDERATIONS
### Side effects, toxicities, and associated nursing actions

**CNS** Although rare, seizures, hallucinations, confusion, twitching, hyperreflexia, dysphasia, and encephalopathy may occur, especially with very high doses of penicillins.
- Obtain a baseline assessment of neurologic function and mental status.
- Assess neurologic function every 4 hours in patients receiving large doses of penicillins.

**Blood** Eosinophilia and hemolytic anemia may be allergic reactions. Other transient effects such as thrombocytopenia, leukopenia, and neutropenia are most often seen with high IV doses but are considered by some physicians to be allergic reactions.
- Monitor complete blood count (CBC) and differential and platelets.
- Assess for development of unexplained bruising or bleeding, pallor, malaise, fever.

**GI** Oral penicillins irritate the GI tract, leading to nausea, vomiting, diarrhea, and intestinal distress. Suprainfections may cause diarrhea or the more serious antibiotic-associated pseudomembranous colitis.
- Assess the patient for development of GI symptoms. Report the development of diarrhea to the physician.
- Monitor intake and output if vomiting and/or diarrhea are severe or persist.
- Monitor weight of infants and children.

**Renal** Acute interstitial nephritis (fever, hematuria, proteinuria) occurs rarely with some penicillins. The sodium or potassium content of some penicillin preparations is associated with renal dysfunction and electrolyte imbalance in certain patients.
- Monitor serum electrolytes and intake and output in patients with known renal or cardiovascular disease.
- Caution patients to report the appearance of hematuria; monitor urinalysis.
- Monitor temperature, and report development of fever to the physician.

**Allergic** Allergic reactions are the most common side effect associated with penicillins, occurring in 2% to 5% of patients. Reactions range from rashes to anaphylaxis, which occurs in 0.05% of patients. Up to 10% of anaphylactic reactions prove to be fatal. Other allergic signs include blood dyscrasias (see Blood), serum sickness, renal or hepatic damage.

- Before administering any antibacterial agents, assess the patient for a history of previous allergy to any drugs. Use penicillins cautiously in patients with previous allergic response to penicillin or cephalosporin preparations (cross-sensitivity).
- Have drugs, equipment, and personnel readily available to treat acute allergic response in any setting where antibacterial agents are administered.
- Note clearly and prominently any drug allergy on patient's chart, Kardex, or other records.
- Inspect patients for development of rashes. Assess for other signs or symptoms that may indicate allergic response.
- Monitor vital signs.
- Serum sickness resembles an allergic response and is characterized by rapid onset or rash, urticaria, fever, arthralgia, edema, and hepatosplenomegaly. It usually develops 7 to 15 days after the patient begins using the drug but may develop sooner. The incidence increases with age.

**Other** Suprainfection can occur as with any broad-spectrum antibiotic. Suprainfection may arise when broad-spectrum antibiotics disrupt normal bacterial flora, allowing a sudden overgrowth of an endogenous or exogenous organism, thus producing an active infection where none had existed before.

- Assess for development of suprainfection: anogenital itching, vaginal itching and/or discharge, diarrhea, fever, oral irritation, or ulceration. Instruct patients to report the development of any unexpected sign or symptom.

### Nursing interventions related to drug administration
- Check for expiration date before preparing and administering the prescribed dose.
- Shake liquid suspension preparations well, as drug may have settled to the bottom of the bottle. Instruct patients to do the same if patient is to self-treat at home.
- Nurses allergic to an antibacterial drug in a class or chemically related class should wear gloves while preparing ordered doses of drugs to avoid skin contamination.
- IM antibacterial preparations should be administered in a large muscle mass such as the dorsogluteal site or rectus femoris muscle in adults or the vastus lateralis muscle in infants and small children. Aspirate carefully before injecting medication to avoid inadvertent intravenous injection. If blood is aspirated, withdraw the needle and prepare a fresh dose of medication. Record the injection site and rotate sites.
- Observe patients carefully for the development of acute allergic reactions for 30 minutes following parenteral doses.

### Patient and family education
- Review with the patient and family the expected benefits and possible side effects of therapy.
- Caution patients to report to the physician the development of any unexplained symptom or side effect.
- Review with patients the need to take the medication as ordered for the specified period of time (usually 7 to 10 days). Unused medications should be discarded. Patients should not share medications with others.
- Encourage patients with a history of allergic response to a drug to wear a medical identification tag or bracelet noting their allergy.
- Most penicillins interfere with urine glucose testing when methods using cupric sulfate are used (e.g., Benedict's solution, Clinitest). These antibacterials to not interfere with glucose oxidase tests (e.g., Diastix, Tes-Tape). Caution diabetic patients about this drug effect. Encourage patients to monitor blood glucose.
- Many antibacterial agents are excreted through breast milk. Instruct lactating women to check with their physicians before breast feeding while taking antibacterials.
- Instruct patients to read the label to check for the expiration date. Teach patients to discard medications that have passed the expiration date, as they may not work as well as desired.

- Instruct patients to store the liquid form of most penicillins in the refrigerator but to avoid freezing the drug. Specific instructions should be provided by the pharmacist who fills the prescription.
- Caution patients to keep these and all medications out of the reach of children.

## amdinocillin  (am-DEEN-oh-sill-in)  antibiotic*

- amdinocillin (mecillinam): Coactin

**MECHANISM OF ACTION**  Although amdinocillin binds to different target proteins than other penicillins and alters the cell wall in a different way, bactericidal action still occurs as a result of disruption of the cell wall. See entry for drug class (p. 246).

**INDICATIONS**  **Serious urinary tract infections** Common organisms causing these infections are *Enterobacter*, *Escheriehia coli*, and *Klebsiella*. • Not all strains of these organisms are susceptible to amdinocillin.

**CONTRAINDICATIONS**  **Allergy to penicillins or cephalosporins** Although cross-reaction is not complete, amdinocillin should be avoided if at all possible in these patients.

**DOSAGE**  IV, IM:  **ADULT:** 10 mg/kg every 4 hours; doses are reduced to 10 mg/kg every 6 hours if amdinocillin is combined with other antibiotics. In renal impairment (creatinine clearance below 30 ml/min), doses are 10 mg/kg every 6 to 8 hours.  *Special patient populations:*  **ELDERLY:** Special geriatric doses have not been established, although the elimination half-life of the drug is prolonged in elderly patients (see Fate).  **RENAL IMPAIRMENT:** Normal doses are administered every 6 to 8 hours to avoid drug accumulation in patients with moderate to severe impairment.  **CHILDREN:** Safe use has not been established, although doses of 10 mg/kg every 6 hours have been used without evident harm. In neonates the elimination half-life is prolonged (see Fate).  **PREGNANCY:** FDA pregnancy category B.

**PREPARATIONS**  *Powder for reconstitution:* 500 mg, 1 g. Sterile water is added to reconstitute the solution: 4.6 ml to 500 mg vial, 9.6 ml to 1 g vial. After shaking to dissolve, the contents of the vial should be transferred aseptically to 50 ml of 5% dextrose injection. The resulting solutions are 10 mg/ml (500 mg vial) or 20 mg/ml (1 g vial).

**DRUG INTERACTIONS**  • See entry for drug class (p. 246).

**DIAGNOSTIC TEST INTERFERENCE**  **ALT, AST, and alkaline phosphatase** concentrations in serum may be increased.

**FATE**  Amdinocillin is not absorbed adequately from the GI tract and must be administered parenterally. Orally available derivatives are not yet approved in the United States. Absorption from IM sites is good with *peak* serum concentrations at 25 to 45 minutes. Amdinocillin is distributed to most body tissues but does not enter the CNS unless the meninges are inflamed by disease. Amdinocillin crosses the placenta. The elimination *half-life* of amdinocillin is 0.6 to 1.6 hours in healthy young adults but averages about 4 hours in patients over 65 years of age and from 1.5 to 5.4 hours in neonates. Amdinocillin is eliminated primarily by the kidneys, but some metabolism may occur.

## ☙ NURSING CONSIDERATIONS

### Side effects, toxicities, and associated nursing actions

**CNS** Dizziness occurs in about 1% of treated patients. Drowsiness or lethargy is less common.
- Monitor patient's level of consciousness.
- If dizziness occurs, caution patients to avoid driving or operating hazardous equipment until effects of the medication wear off. Notify the physician.

**CV** Elevated blood pressure is rare.
- Monitor blood pressure.

**Blood** Eosinophilia and thrombocytosis occur in 5% of treated patients; anemia, neutropenia, and leukopenia in 1%; thrombocytopenia is less common. Thrombophlebitis, tenderness, and pain at the injection site are reported in 1% of patients.
- Monitor CBC and differential count.

*Extended spectrum penicillin.

- Observe for the development of fatigue, unexplained bruising or bleeding, hematuria, blood in stools, pallor, fever.
- Check the IV insertion site regularly for development of thrombophlebitis.
- Rotate IM injection sites.

**GI** Nausea, vomiting, or diarrhea occurs in about 1% of patients receiving the drug parenterally.

- Monitor for development of GI symptoms. If symptoms are severe or persistent, notify the physician.
- Monitor intake and output.

**Renal** Hypokalemia is a rare side effect.

- Monitor serum electrolytes. Assess for signs of hypokalemia: muscle weakness, apathy, abdominal distention, and paralytic ileus; ECG changes include inverted T waves, prolonged QT segment, and prominent U wave.
- Be alert to hypokalemia in patients receiving other drugs that may affect electrolyte status, such as diuretics.

**Allergic** Rash, itching, and/or pruritis occur in about 1% of patients; anaphylaxis has not yet been reported but should be expected as with other penicillins.

- Have drugs, equipment, and personnel available to treat acute allergic response, as noted in entry for drug class (p. 248).

### Nursing interventions related to drug administration
- See entry for drug class (p. 248).
- After preparing IV doses as ordered (see Preparations), prepared dose should be infused over 15 to 30 minutes. The drug should not be mixed with other medications.

### Patient and family education
- See entry for drug class (p. 248).

---

## amoxicillin trihydrate    (a-MOX-i-sill-in)                                    antibiotic*

- amoxicillin trihydrate (amoxycillin):  Amoxil, Larotid, Novamox, Polymox, Sumox, Trimox, Utimox, Wymox

**MECHANISM OF ACTION**  • See entry for drug class (p. 246).

**INDICATIONS**   **Infections caused by gram-positive aerobic bacteria** Bronchitis, epiglottitis, otitis media, pharyngitis, skin infections, sinusitis, and tonsilitis are often caused by strains of *Streptococcus* or *Staphylococcus* susceptible to amoxicillin. Amoxicillin is not effective against penicillinase-producing *Staphylococcus* strains. Penicillin G or penicillin V is usually preferred for group A beta-hemolytic streptococci, *Streptococcus pneumoniae,* and groups B, C, or G streptococci.   **Infections caused by enterococci** Urinary tract infections caused by *Streptococcus faecalis, S. faecium,* and *S. durans* often respond to high urinary concentrations of amoxicillin. Endocarditis caused by these organisms is best treated simultaneously with an aminoglycoside and a penicillin such as amoxicillin.   **Infections caused by gram-negative aerobic bacteria** Susceptible bacteria may include *Escherichia coli, Hemophilus influenzae, Neisseria gonorrhoeae, Proteus mirabilis,* and *Salmonella.* These organisms commonly cause infections of the urinary tract. *Hemophilus* causes ear infections and meningitis.   **Prophylaxis** Amoxicillin is used to prevent bacterial endocarditis in patients with prosthetic heart valves who must undergo minor procedures likely to seed bacteria into the blood, such as instrumentation of the genitourinary tract.

**CONTRAINDICATIONS**   **Allergy to penicillins or cephalosporins** Anaphylaxis and death are possible outcomes. The risk is greatest in those who report previous allergic reactions to penicillin and less in those previously reacting to cephalosporins.   **Mononucleosis** Rashes occur in a high percentage of patients with mononucleosis who are given amoxicillin.   **Penicillinase-producing *Staphylococcus* strains** These organisms are resistant to amoxicillin.

**DOSAGE**   **PO:**  **ADULT:** 250 to 500 mg every 8 hours, according to severity of the infection and organism susceptibility; therapy should normally be continued for 7 to 10 days or 48 to 72 hours after all signs of

*Extended spectrum penicillin.

infection have cleared. Doses must be lowered in renal failure. Single doses of 3 g amoxicillin with 1 gm$^2$ of probenecid may be used for gonorrhea (Neisseria gonorrhoeae). Disseminated cases require additional therapy with 500 mg every 6 hours for 7 days.   **CHILDREN OLDER THAN 1 MONTH:** Children weighing more than 20 kg receive adult doses. Below 20 kg, doses are 20 to 40 mg/kg or 500 mg to 1 g/M$^2$ daily, given as divided doses every 8 hours. Doses must be lowered in renal failure. *Special patient populations:*   **ELDERLY:** Special geriatric doses have not been established, but the drug may be excreted slowly (see Fate).   **PREGNANCY:** Safe use in pregnancy has not been established, although the drug has been used without apparent harm in pregnant women. Amoxicillin passes into the milk of nursing mothers; nursing should be suspended during amoxicillin therapy.

**PREPARATIONS**   *Tablets, chewable:* 125, 250 mg; *capsules:* 250, 500 mg; *oral suspension:* 125 mg/5 ml, 250 mg/5 ml, 50 mg/ml.

**DRUG INTERACTIONS**   **Oral contraceptives** may be less effective when amoxicillin or related penicillins are used because the antibiotic increases hepatic inactivation of the steroids in contraceptive preparations. **Allopurinol** may be more likely to cause rashes when given with amoxicillin and related penicillins. In addition, see entry for drug class (p. 246).

**DIAGNOSTIC TEST INTERFERENCE**   **Glucose** determinations by the cupric sulfate method are unreliable when amoxicillin is given.   **Coomb's test** (direct antiglobulin test) gives false-positive results with amoxicillin.   **ALT and AST** concentrations in serum may be increased.

**FATE**   Amoxicillin is almost completely absorbed from the GI tract and therefore produces higher serum concentrations than oral doses of the related drug, ampicillin. *Peak* concentrations occur 1 to 2 hours after oral doses of amoxicillin. The drug is well distributed to most tissues and enters the CNS adequately when the meninges are inflamed. Elimination is primarily renal; active metabolites have not been identified. The elimination *half-life* is 1 to 2 hours in healthy young adults; renal impairment can extend these values up to 21 hours. The elderly also have longer elimination half-lives, leading to some accumulation of the drug.

## 🐦 NURSING CONSIDERATIONS

### Side effects, toxicities, and associated nursing actions

**GI** Up to 5% of adults receiving oral amoxicillin report diarrhea. Loose stools are much more frequent in children: up to 42% in infants younger than 8 months; 20% of 8 to 16 month old children, and 8.5% of 2 to 3 year olds. Nausea and vomiting occur in about 2% of treated adults. For other side effects, see entry for drug class (p. 247).

### Nursing interventions related to drug administration

• See entry for drug class (p. 248).

### Patient and family education

• Amoxicillin may be taken without regard to meals.
• Note that a chewable tablet is available. Instruct patients to chew this form briefly before swallowing. Caution patients to keep this form briefly before swallowing. Caution patients to keep this form (and all drugs) out of the reach of children.
• The oral suspension may be taken as reconstituted or may be further diluted in juice, formula, milk, ginger ale, or water. The dose should be consumed immediately after it is prepared.
• For further guidelines, see entry for drug class (p. 248).

---

# amoxicillin with clavulanate potassium
### (a-MOX-i-sill-in; klav-yoo-LAN-ate)                                              antibiotic*

• amoxicillin with clavulanate potassium: Augmentin, ✿Clavulin

**MECHANISM OF ACTION**   • See entry for drug class (p. 246) for mechanism of amoxicillin. Clavulanic acid is an inhibitor of beta-lactamases. It is combined with amoxicillin to extend the action of amoxicillin against organisms that would ordinarily be marginally susceptible because they produce beta-lactamases.

*Extended spectrum penicillin.

**INDICATIONS**    Oral therapy of infections caused by organisms producing beta-lactamases Susceptible organisms include *Branhamella catarrhalis, Escherichia coli, Hemophilus influenzae, Klebsiella,* and *Staphylococcus aureus.* Amoxicillin alone may be effective if the strains do not produce beta-lactamases. These organisms cause otitis media, sinusitis, and infections of the respiratory tract, urinary tract, skin, and soft tissues.

**CONTRAINDICATIONS**    • As for amoxicillin (p. 246).

**DOSAGE**    PO:    ADULTS AND CHILDREN OVER 40 KG: 250 or 500 mg amoxicillin with 125 mg clavulanic acid every 8 hours.    CHILDREN: 20 to 40 mg/kg amoxicillin daily in doses every 8 hours. Dosage is calculated based on amoxicillin content of the combination.    *Special patient populations:*    PREGNANCY: FDA pregnancy category B.

**PREPARATIONS**    *Tablets, chewable:* 125 mg amoxicillin with 31.25 mg clavulanic acid or 250 mg amoxicillin with 62.5 mg clavulanic acid; *tablets, film-coated:* 250 or 500 mg amoxicillin with 125 mg clavulanic acid. *oral suspension:* 125 mg/5 ml amoxicillin with 31.25 mg/5 ml clavulanic acid or 250 mg/5 ml amoxicillin with 62.5 mg/5 ml clavulanic acid.

**DRUG INTERACTIONS**    • As for amoxicillin (p. 246).

**DIAGNOSTIC TEST INTERFERENCE**    • As for amoxicillin (p. 251).

**FATE**    Clavulanic acid is well absorbed and distributed in the body. The drug is metabolized extensively before excretion. The elimination *half-life* is 0.8 to 1.2 hours. The fate of amoxicillin is unaffected by the presence of clavulanic acid. See amoxicillin (p. 251).

**🐾 NURSING CONSIDERATIONS**

### Side effects, toxicities, and associated nursing actions

GI Up to 9% of adults receiving the combination of amoxicillin and clavulanate potassium report diarrhea. Nausea, vomiting, and other signs of GI distress are reported in up to 5% of patients receiving 250 or 500 mg amoxicillin with 125 mg clavulanic acid. Patients who inadvertently double the dose of clavulanic acid by taking two tablets each containing 250 mg amoxicillin and 125 mg clavulanic acid have a much higher incidence of GI distress. At this dose, up to 40% report nausea and vomiting.
• For other side effects, see entry for drug class (p. 247).

### Nursing interventions related to drug administration

• See entry for drug class (p. 248).
• Oral preparations of this drug are available in three forms (see Preparations). Because the ratio of amoxicillin with clavulanic acid varies among the three dosage forms, they should not be substituted for each other. Only the form ordered should be administered. If another form is desired to improve compliance or ease of administration, a new order from the physician should be obtained.

### Patient and family education

• See entry for drug class (p. 248).
• Amoxicillin with clavulanate potassium may be taken without regard to meals. Taking the drug with meals may decrease the incidence of GI symptoms.
• Note that a chewable tablet is available. Instruct patients to chew this form briefly before swallowing. Caution patients to keep this form (and all drugs) out of the reach of children.
• Instruct patients not to double up if a dose is missed. Efforts should be made to take the drug as ordered.

---

## ampicillin    (am-peh-SILL-in)                                        antibiotic*

• ampicillin (aminobenzylpenicillin): Omnipen, ✿Penbritin
• ampicillin sodium: ✿Ampicin, ✿Ampilean, NaMPICIL, Omnipen, Polycillin-N, Totacillin-N
• ampicillin trihydrate: Amcil, Penamp, Polycillin, Principen, Probampacin, SK-Ampicillin, Totacillin

**MECHANISM OF ACTION**    • See entry for drug class (p. 246).

**INDICATIONS**    Infections caused by gram-positive aerobic bacteria Bronchitis, epiglottitis, otitis media, pharyngitis, skin infections, sinusitis, and tonsilitis are often caused by strains of *Streptococcus* or *Staph-*

*Extended spectrum penicillin.

*ylococcus* susceptible to ampicillin. Penicillin G or penicillin V is usually preferred for group A beta-hemolytic *streptococci, Streptococcus pneumoniae,* and groups B, C, or G streptococci • Ampicillin is not effective against penicillinase-producing *Staphylococcus* strains.  **Infections caused by enterococci** Urinary tract infections caused by *Streptococcus faecalis, S. faecium,* and *S. durans* often respond to high urinary concentrations of ampicillin. Endocarditis caused by these organisms is best treated simultaneously with an aminoglycoside and a penicillin such as ampicillin.  **Infections caused by gram-negative aerobic bacteria** Susceptible bacteria may include *Escherichia coli, Hemophilus influenzae, Neisseria gonorrhoeae, Proteus mirabilis,* and *Salmonella.* • These organisms commonly cause infections of the urinary tract. • *Hemophilus* causes ear infections and meningitis. **Prophylaxis** Used to prevent bacterial endocarditis in patients with prosthetic heart valves who must undergo procedures likely to seed bacteria into the blood, such as surgery or instrumentation of the genitourinary, biliary, or GI tracts.

**CONTRAINDICATIONS**  **Allergy to penicillins or cephalosporins** Anaphylaxis and death are possible outcomes; the risk is greatest in those who report previous allergic reactions to penicillin and less in those previously reacting to cephalosporins.  **Mononucleosis** Rashes occur in a high percentage of patients with mononucleosis who are given ampicillin.  **Penicillinase-producing Staphylococcus strains** These organisms are resistant to ampicillin.

**DOSAGE**  **PO:**  **ADULT:** 250 to 500 mg every 6 hours, according to the severity of the infection and organism susceptibility; therapy should normally be continued for 7 to 10 days or 48 to 72 hours after all signs of infection have cleared. Doses must be lowered in renal failure. Single doses of 3.5 g ampicillin with 1 g of probenecid may be used for gonorrhea (*Neisseria gonorrhoeae*). Disseminated cases require additional therapy with 500 mg every 6 hours for 7 days.  **CHILDREN OLDER THAN 1 MONTH:** Children weighing more than 20 kg receive adult doses. Below 20 kg, doses are 25 to 50 mg/kg daily, given as divided doses every 6 hours. Doses must be lowered in renal failure.  **IV, IM:**  **ADULT:** 8 to 14 g or 150 to 200 mg/kg daily in divided doses given every 3 to 4 hours. These doses are for serious infections such as septicemia and bacterial meningitis.  **CHILDREN BELOW 40 KG BODY WEIGHT:** For septicemia or bacterial meningitis, 100 to 400 mg/kg daily, given as divided doses every 3 to 4 hours. Milder infections may be treated with 50 to 100 mg/kg given as divided doses every 6 to 8 hours. Neonates receive the same dosage divided into two doses daily. Daily doses in children should not exceed 12 g.  *Special patient populations:*  **ELDERLY:** Special geriatric doses have not been established, but the drug is eliminated more slowly in older adults.  **PREGNANCY:** Safe use in pregnancy has not been established although the drug has been used without apparent harm in pregnant women. Ampicillin passes into the milk of nursing mothers; nursing should be suspended during ampicillin therapy.

**PREPARATIONS**  **Ampicillin** *Capsules:* 250, 500 mg; *oral suspension:* 125 mg/5 ml, 250 mg/5 ml, 500 mg/5 ml, and 100 mg/ml.  **Ampicillin sodium** *Powder to prepare solution for injection:* 125 mg, 250 mg, 500 mg, 1 g, 2 g, or 10 g (10 g is pharmacy bulk package). *Powder to prepare solution for IV infusion:* 500 mg, 1 g, or 2 g.  **Ampicillin trihydrate** *Capsules:* 250, 500 mg. *Capsules, combinations:* single-dose bottle of nine capsules, each capsule containing 389 mg ampicillin and 111 mg probenecid for a total dose of 3.5 g ampicillin and 1 g probenecid. For single-dose therapy of gonorrhea. *oral suspension:* 125 mg/5 ml, 250 mg/5 ml, 500 mg/5 ml, and 100 mg/ml. *oral suspension, combinations:* 3.5 g ampicillin with 1 g probenecid. For single-dose therapy of gonorrhea.

**DRUG INTERACTIONS**  • See entry for drug class (p. 246).

**DIAGNOSTIC TEST INTERFERENCE**  **Allopurinol** may be more likely to cause rashes when given with amoxicillin and related penicillins.  **ALT and AST** concentrations in serum may be increased.  **Aminoglycoside assays** may be falsely lowered by ampicillin, which inactivates aminoglycoside antibiotics.  **Coombs test (direct antiglobulin test)** gives false-positive results with ampicillin.  **Glucose** determinations by the cupric sulfate method are unreliable when ampicillin is given.  **Oral contraceptives** may be less effective when ampicillin or related penicillins are used because the antibiotic increases hepatic inactivation of the steroids in contraceptive preparations.  **Uric acid** determinations by the copper-chelate method are falsely elevated.

**FATE**  Ampicillin is incompletely absorbed from the GI tract and therefore produces lower serum concentrations than the related drug, amoxicillin. *Peak* concentrations occur 1 to 2 hours after oral doses of ampicillin. Food decreases absorption. Administration IM more rapidly produces higher peak serum values. The drug is well distributed to most tissues and enters the CNS adequately when the meninges are inflamed. Elimination is primarily renal; active metabolites have not been identified. The elimination *half-life* is 0.7 to 1.4 hours in healthy young adults; renal impairment can extend these values up to 21 hours. The elderly also have longer elimination half-lives, leading to some accumulation of the drug.

## ❦ NURSING CONSIDERATIONS

### Side effects, toxicities, and associated nursing actions

**GI** Up to 17% of adults receiving oral ampicillin report diarrhea. In children, diarrhea may cause discontinuance of therapy in 8.5% of those treated. Nausea and vomiting occur in 2% to 3% of treated adults. *Pseudomembranous colitis* is reported in 0.3% to 5% of patients; ampicillin is one of the most frequently reported causes of this condition.
• Assess for diarrhea, and notify the physician immediately if diarrhea develops.
**Rash** Ampicillin causes a maculopapular rash unrelated to the usual urticarial allergic reactions caused by most penicillins. The maculopapular rash appears late in therapy (3 to 14 days). The incidence is reported to be 5% to 10% in children and 3.7% to 13.4% in adults. This rash is much more likely to occur in viral diseases and occurs in almost all patients with mononucleousis. The origin of this reaction is unknown. For other side effects, see entry for drug class (p. 247).

### Nursing interventions related to drug administration
• When given by direct IV push, administer each 500 mg over at least a 5 minute period.
• For infusion, dilute ordered dose in at least 50 ml of infusion fluid. If 5% dextrose in water, 5% dextrose in 0.45 sodium chloride, 10% invert sugar in water, or one sixth sodium lactate solution is used, infuse dose within 4 hours. If 0.9% sodium chloride is used, dilution is stable over at least 8 hours. Rate of infusion should never exceed 500 mg over at least 5 minutes.
• For further guidelines, see entry for drug class (p. 248).

### Patient and family education
• Ampicillin may be taken with meals, but maximum absorption occurs if the oral dose is taken 1 hour before or 2 hours after meals. Take dose with a full glass (8 ounces) of water.
• For further guidelines, see entry for drug class (p. 248).

---

# ampicillin sodium with sulbactam sodium
(am-peh-SILL-in; sool-BAK-tam)                                                    antibiotic*

• ampicillin sodium with sulbactam sodium: Unasyn

**MECHANISM OF ACTION** • See entry for drug class (p. 246) for mechanism of ampicillin. Sulbactam is an inhibitor of beta-lactamases. It is combined with ampicillin to extend the action of ampicillin against organisms that would ordinarily be marginally susceptible because they produce beta-lactamases.

**INDICATIONS** **Infections of skin** Serious infections caused by beta-lactamase-producing strains of *Staphylococcus aureus* and other bacteria may respond. **Intra-abdominal infections** Serious infections caused by beta-lactamase-producing strains of *Escherichia coli, Klebsiella, Bacteroides,* and other bacteria may respond **Gynecologic infections** Serious infections caused by beta-lactamase-producing strains of gram-negative and anaerobic bacteria may respond.

**CONTRAINDICATIONS** **Allergy to penicillins or cephalosporins** Anaphylaxis and death are possible outcomes. The risk is greatest in those who report previous allergic reactions to penicillin and less in those previously reacting to cephalosporins. **Mononucleosis** Rashes occur in a high percentage of patients with mononucleosis who are given ampicillin.

**DOSAGE** **IM, IV:** **ADULT:** 1.5 g (1 g ampicillin with 0.5 g sulbactam) or 3 g (2 g ampicillin with 1 g sulbactam) every 6 hours. *Special patient populations:* **CHILDREN:** Doses are not established. **PREGNANCY:** FDA pregnancy category B.

*Extended spectrum penicillin.

**PREPARATIONS** *Powder for reconstitution:* 1.5 g (1 g ampicillin with 0.5 g sulbactam) or 3 g (2 g ampicillin with 1 g sulbactam).

**DRUG INTERACTIONS** • As for ampicillin (p. 251).

**DIAGNOSTIC TEST INTERFERENCE** • As for ampicillin (p. 251).

**FATE** The pharmacokinetics of sulbactam are similar to those of ampicillin (p. 251). Both drugs appear in low levels in breast milk.

## 🦋 NURSING CONSIDERATIONS

### Side effects, toxicities, and associated nursing actions

**Allergy** Rashes are seen in up to 2% of patients. Itching, edema, facial swelling, erythema, and tightness in the throat are less common.
• Have drugs, equipment, and personnel available to treat acute allergic reactions.
• Check the patient every 5 minutes during the first 15 minutes following drug administration.

**GI** Up to 3% of patients experience diarrhea. Nausea, vomiting, flatulence, abdominal distention, and pseudomembranous colitis are less common.
• Assess for GI side effects. Notify the physician if diarrhea develops.
• Monitor intake, output, and weight.

**Blood** Various dyscrasias have been reported, including changes in platelets and white blood cells.
• Assess for bruising, unexplained bleeding, fever, malaise, sore throat, pallor, fatigue.
• Monitor complete blood cell count, differential, and platelet count.

**Local** Up to 16% of patients experience pain on IM injection; 3% report pain or thrombophlebitis at IV sites.
• Forewarn patients about pain at IM injection sites.
• Use anatomic landmarks to choose injection sites. Record and rotate injection sites.
• Inspect IV site for signs of thrombophlebitis: pain, warmth, redness. Instruct patient to call if IV infusion begins to cause pain or is not infusing well.

### Nursing interventions related to drug administration
• See Local.
• See entry for drug class (p. 248).
• Check manufacturer's instructions for dilution and rate of infusion.

### Patient and family education
• See entry for drug class (p. 248).

---

# azlocillin sodium (AZ-loh-sill-in) antibiotic*

• azlocillin sodium: Azlin

**MECHANISM OF ACTION** • See entry for drug class (p. 246).

**INDICATIONS** **Infections caused by gram-negative aerobic bacteria** Susceptible organisms may include *Enterobacter, Escherichia coli, Morganella morganii, Proteus mirabilis, Proteus vulgaris, Providencia rettgeri* and *Pseudomonas aeruginosa*. These organisms may cause septicemia and infections of the respiratory tract, urinary tract, abdominal cavity, skin, bones, and joints.

**CONTRAINDICATIONS** **Allergy to penicillins or cephalosporins** • See entry for drug class (p. 246). **Penicillinase-producing strains of *Staphylcoccus aureus*** Azlocillin is destroyed by this penicillinase and is therefore ineffective for infections caused by these strains.

**DOSAGE** **IV:** **ADULT:** Dosage ranges from 100 to 300 mg/kg daily, given as divided doses every 4 to 6 hours, depending on the site and severity of infection. Total doses should not exceed 350 mg/kg or 24 g daily. **CHILDREN:** Pediatric dosages are not fully established, but the drug has been used in children with

*Extended spectrum penicillin.

cystic fibrosis at doses of 75 mg/g every 4 hours up to a total of 24 g daily. *Special patient populations:* **RENAL IMPAIRMENT:** Doses must be reduced, based upon degree of renal impairment. **PREGNANCY:** FDA pregnancy category B.

**PREPARATIONS** *Powder to prepare solution for injection:* 2, 3, or 4 g. *Powder to prepare solution for IV infusion:* 2, 3, or 4 g. The sterile powder should be reconstituted with sterile water for injection, 5% dextrose injection or 0.9% sodium chloride injection, 10 ml for each gram of azlocillin. The fully dissolved drug may be injected directly IV or may be diluted further into compatible fluids.

**DRUG INTERACTIONS** • See entry for drug class (p. 246).

**DIAGNOSTIC TEST INTERFERENCE** **ALT and AST** concentrations in serum may be increased **Aminoglycoside assays** may be unreliable because azlocillin can inactivate aminoglycoside antibiotics. **Protein assays** by turbidometric or biuret methods may be unreadable or give false-positive results in the presence of azlocillin.

**FATE** Azlocillin is not absorbed from the GI tract and is administered intravenously. Azlocillin is distributed into most tissues, including the CNS; the drug passes the placenta and enters the fetus. Renal excretion is the primary route of elimination, but some metabolism and elimination in the bile occur. The elimination *half-life* is 0.8 to 1.3 hours in healthy adults but is extended in patients with renal impairment and in neonates. Patients with cystic fibrosis may have shorter elimination times than healthy adults.

## ❦ NURSING CONSIDERATIONS

### Side effects, toxicities, and associated nursing actions

**CV** Transient chest pain is reported when azlocillin is administered IV too rapidly.
• Rate of administration for direct IV push doses should be at least 5 minutes.
• If chest pain occurs, assess patient and slow infusion rate.

**Blood** Abnormal platelet aggregation and prolonged bleeding time may occur with azlocillin. In addition, up to 7.4% of patients may show eosinophilia, an allergic reaction.
• Monitor platelets, white blood cell differential, and bleeding time.
• Monitor for unexplained bruising or bleeding.

**GI** Up to 3% of patients suffer diarrhea with parenteral azlocillin. Other GI effects are occasionally reported.

**Renal** Hypokalemia, hypernatremia, increased BUN and creatinine, and increased serum uric acid are rare.
• Monitor serum electrolytes, BUN, uric acid, and creatinine.
• Monitor intake, output, and weight.
• Assess for signs of hypokalemia: muscle weakness, apathy, abdominal distention, and paralytic ileus. ECG changes include inverted T waves, prolonged QT segment, and prominent U waves. Assess for signs of hypernatremia: dry, sticky mucous membranes, low urinary output, and firm, ''rubbery'' tissue turgor.
• Azlocillin also causes other side effects common to penicillins; see entry for drug class (p. 247).

### Nursing interventions related to drug administration
• See CV side effects.
• If azlocillin is refrigerated, precipitation may occur. Warm the vial in warm water, then shake to reconstitute.
• Slightly discolored azlocillin may still be used.
• May be diluted to administer as an intermittent infusion to a solution not exceeding 100 mg/ml. A solution that is too strong may cause venous irritation. See manufacturer's literature. Administer diluted dose over 30 minutes.
• For additional guidelines, see entry for drug class (p. 248).

### Patient and family education
• See entry for drug class (p. 248).

## bacampicillin hydrochloride   (bay-KAM-peh-sill-in)      antibiotic*

- bacampicillin hydrochloride (carampicillin hydrochloride): ✿Penglobe, Spectrobid

**MECHANISM OF ACTION**    Bacampicillin is a prodrug with no antibacterial activity until it is metabolized in the body to release ampicillin. For the mechanism of action of ampicillin, see entry for drug class (p. 246).

**INDICATIONS**    • Bacampicillin substitutes for oral ampicillin (p. 246).

**CONTRAINDICATIONS**    **Allergy to penicillin or cephalosporin** Anaphylaxis and death are possible outcomes; the risk is greatest in those who report previous allergic reactions to penicillin and less in those previously reacting to cephalosporins.    **Mononucleosis** Rashes occur in a high percentage of patients with mononucleosis who are given bacampicillin.

**DOSAGE**    **PO:**    **ADULT:** 400 to 800 mg bacampicillin every 12 hours (equivalent to 280 or 560 mg ampicillin). For serious respiratory infections, up to 1.6 g bacampicillin (equivalent to 1.12 g ampicillin) may be used. Therapy should continue 7 to 10 days or for 2 to 3 days after all signs of infection have disappeared. For gonorrhea, 1.6 g with 1 g probenecid as a single dose.    **CHILDREN:** Children weighing more than 25 kg receive adult doses, below 25 kg, 12.5 to 25 mg/kg bacampicillin (equivalent to 8.75 to 17.5 mg/kg ampicillin) every 12 hours. *Special patient populations:* **PREGNANCY:** FDA pregnancy category B.

**PREPARATIONS**    *Tablets, film-coated:* 400 mg (equivalent to 280 mg ampicillin); *oral, suspension:* 125 mg/5 ml (equivalent to 87.5 mg/5 ml ampicillin).

**DRUG INTERACTIONS**    **Disulfiram** should not be used in patients receiving bacampacillin because metabolism of the penicillin releases small amounts of ethanol, which can interact with disulfiram to produce the characteristic reaction.    **Oral contraceptives** may be less effective when bacampacillin or related penicillins are used because the antibiotic may increase hepatic inactivation of the steroids in contraceptive preparations. • For other interactions, see ampicillin (p. 246).

**DIAGNOSTIC TEST INTERFERENCE**    • See ampicillin (p. 246).

**FATE**    Absorption of bacampicillin is nearly complete after oral administration. Esterases in the intestine and plasma rapidly release acetaldehyde, ethanol, carbon dioxide, and the active metabolite ampicillin. *Peak* serum levels occur at 30 to 90 minutes and are usually higher than an equivalent dose of ampicillin would produce. Ampicillin released in this way is handled exactly as ampicillin administered directly. See ampicillin (p. 251).

### ❦ NURSING CONSIDERATIONS

#### Side effects, toxicities, and associated nursing actions
- See ampicillin (p. 251).

#### Nursing interventions related to drug administration
- See entry for drug class (p. 248).

#### Patient and family education
- Tablets may be administered without regard to meals. Suspension should be administered 1 hour before or 2 hours after meals. Take dose with a full glass (8 ounces) of water.
- Remind patients to keep these and all medications out of the reach of children.
- For further guidelines, see entry for drug class (p. 248).

---

## benzathine penicillin G   (BENZ-uh-thine pen-i-SILL-in)      antibiotics†

- benzathine penicillin G (benzathine benzylpenicillin): Bicillin

**MECHANISM OF ACTION**    Benzathine penicillin G is relatively insoluble and is therefore slowly absorbed from intramuscular injection sites. Penicillin G is released as the active drug. For the mechanism of penicillin G, see entry for drug class (p. 246).

*Extended spectrum penicillin.
†Narrow spectrum penicillin.

**INDICATIONS** **Prophylaxis of recurrent rheumatic fever** Benzathine penicillin G is an effective alternative to oral penicillins. **Infections caused by staphylococci, streptococci, and spirochetes** These organisms are often susceptible to low concentrations of penicillin G.

**CONTRAINDICATIONS** • See penicillin G (p. 246).

**DOSAGE** **PO:** **ADULTS:** 400,000 to 600,000 units every 4 to 6 hours for 10 days. **CHILDREN UNDER 12 YEARS:** 25,000 to 90,000 units/kg daily in three to six divided doses. **IV** IV administration is absolutely contraindicated. **IM:** **ADULT:** 1.2 million units as a single injection. Higher doses may be required for neurosyphilis or yaws. **CHILDREN UNDER 27 KG:** 600,000 units as a single injection. **NEONATES:** 50,000 units as a single injection. *Special patient populations:* **PREGNANCY:** Safety not established.

**PREPARATIONS:** *Tablets:* 200,000 units containing tartrazine. *Suspension for IM injection:* 300,000 or 600,000 units/ml containing parabens and povidone. *Suspension for IM injection, combinations:* • 150,000 units benzathine penicillin G with 150,000 units procaine penicillin G in each milliliter; also contains parabens and povidone. • 300,000 units benzathine penicillin G with 300,000 units procaine penicillin G in each milliliter; also contains parabens and povidone. • 450,000 units benzathine penicillin G with 150,000 units procaine penicillin G in each milliliter; also contains parabenz and povidone.

**DRUG INTERACTIONS** • See penicillin G (p. 269).

**LABORATORY TEST INTERFERENCE** • See penicillin G (p. 270).

**FATE** Benzathine penicillin G is slowly absorbed from intramuscular sites, releasing the active drug penicillin G. Because of slow absorption, peak serum concentrations of penicillin G are low but very prolonged. Single doses of 1.2 million units produce measurable serum concentrations for up to 4 weeks. Orally administered benzathine penicillin G is absorbed but offers few advantages to other acid-stable penicillins that are used orally. The active penicillin G that is released from benzathine penicillin G is distributed and excreted just as penicillin G directly administered. See Penicillin G (p. 270).

## 🐝 NURSING CONSIDERATIONS

### Side effects, toxicities, and associated nursing actions

**Local** Benzathine penicillin G may occlude vessels or cause emboli if injected directly into arteries or veins.
- Choose IM injection sites carefully, using anatomic landmarks as guides. Use large muscle masses such as the dorsogluteal or rectoris femoris muscle in adults or the vastus lateralis in infants and small children. Aspirate carefully before injecting medication. If blood appears in the syringe, the needle should be withdrawn, and a fresh dose of medication prepared and administered.
- Record and rotate injection sites.

**Peripheral nerves** If benzathine penicillin G is injected near large nerves, severe and permanent damage to the nerve may occur.
- See Local side effects.
- Benzathine penicillin G causes all side effects associated with penicillins (see entry for drug class, p. 247).

### Nursing interventions related to drug administration
- See Local side effects.
- Commercially available tablets contain FD & C dye #5, tartrazine, which may cause an allergic reaction in susceptible individuals. Although rare, this side effect is seen more often in persons with aspirin hypersensitivity.

### Patient and family education
- Oral doses of benzathine penicillin G should be taken 1 hour before or 2 hours after meals, with a full glass (8 ounces) of water.
- For additional guidelines, see entry for drug class (p. 248).

## carbenicillin disodium   (car-BEN-i-sill-in)   antibiotic*

- carbenicillin disodium: Geopen, Pyopen

**MECHANISM OF ACTION**   • See entry for drug class (p. 246).

**INDICATIONS**   **Infections caused by gram-negative aerobic bacteria** Susceptible organisms may include *Enterobacter, Escherichia coli, Morganella morganii, Proteus mirabilis, Proteus vulgaris, Providencia rettgeri,* and *Pseudomonas aeruginosa.* These organisms may cause septicemia and infections of the respiratory tract, urinary tract, abdominal cavity, skin, bones, and joints.

**CONTRAINDICATIONS**   **Allergy to penicillins or cephalosporins** • See entry for drug class (p 246).   **Penicillinase-producing strains of *Staphylcoccus aureus*** Carbenicillin is destroyed by this penicillinase and therefore is ineffective for infections caused by these strains.   **Sodium restriction** Patients who must restrict salt intake because of hypertension or heart or renal disease should not take carbenicillin because of its high salt content.

**DOSAGE**   **IV:**   ADULTS AND CHILDREN OLDER THAN 1 MONTH: Dosage ranges from 200 to 500 mg/kg daily, given as divided doses every 4 hours or by continuous infusion, depending on the site and severity of infection. Total doses should not exceed 40 g daily. Doses must be reduced in renal failure.   **CHILDREN:** Neonates, 100 mg/kg as an initial loading dose followed by 75 mg/kg every 8 hours. Dosage may increase to 100 mg/kg every 8 hours after the first week of life. Doses must be reduced in renal failure.   **IM:**   ADULT: 1 to 2 g every 6 hours.   **CHILDREN:** 50 to 400 mg/kg daily in divided doses, the dose and interval being determined by the severity and site of infection as well as the age of the child.   *Special patient populations:*   RENAL IMPAIRMENT: Doses may be reduced. Patients may be more prone to hemorrhagic complications.   PREGNANCY: Safe use not established.

**PREPARATIONS**   Powder to prepare solution for injection: 1, 2, 5, 10, 20, or 30 g. The 10, 20, and 30 g forms are pharmacy bulk packages. Powder to prepare solution for IV infusion: 2, 5, and 10 g. Each gram of carbenicillin contains 5.3 mEq of sodium. The sterile powder should be reconstituted with sterile water for injection. For IM injection, the powder may be reconstituted in 0.5% lidocaine without epinephrine or in bacteriostatic water containing 0.9% benzyl alcohol.

**DRUG INTERACTIONS**   **Lithium** excretion may be altered by the high sodium content of carbenicillin preparations; blood levels of lithium should be carefully monitored when both drugs are used. • For additional interactions, see entry for drug class (p. 246).

**DIAGNOSTIC TEST INTERFERENCE**   **ALT and AST** concentrations in serum may be increased.   **Aminoglycoside assays** may be unreliable because carbenicillin can inactivate aminoglycoside antibiotics.   **Coomb's test** (direct antiglobulin test) may be falsely positive in the presence of carbenicillin.   **Glucose assays** using cupric sulfate are unreliable when carbenicillin is present.   **Uric acid** determined by the copper-chelate method may be falsely elevated by carbenicillin.   **Urinary specific gravity** may be elevated by the high sodium content of carbenicillin, especially if urine output is low.

**FATE**   Carbenicillin is not absorbed from the GI tract. *Peak* serum concentrations are achieved within 1 to 2 hours following IM administration. Carbenicillin is distributed into most tissues and enters fetuses. Entry into the CNS is best when the meninges are inflamed by infection. Renal excretion is the primary route of elimination. The elimination *half-life* is 0.8 to 1.0 hours in healthy adults but is extended in patients with renal or hepatic impairment and in neonates.

### ❧ NURSING CONSIDERATIONS

#### Side effects, toxicities, and associated nursing actions

**Blood** Abnormal platelet aggregation and prolonged bleeding time may occur with carbenicillin.
- Monitor platelets and bleeding time.
- Observe for unexplained bruising or bleeding.

**Renal** Hypokalemia, hypernatremia, increased BUN and creatinine, and increased serum uric acid are rare.
- Monitor serum electrolytes, BUN, creatinine, and uric acid.

*Extended spectrum penicillin.

- Assess for signs of hypokalemia: muscle weakness, apathy, abdominal distention, and paralytic ileus. ECG changes include inverted T waves, prolonged QT segment, and prominent U waves. Assess for signs of hypernatremia: dry, sticky mucous membranes, low urinary output, and firm, "rubbery" tissue turgor.
- Monitor intake and output.
- Carbenicillin also causes other side effects common to penicillins. See entry for drug class (p. 247).

### Nursing interventions related to drug administration

- May be administered direct IV push or as an intermittent infusion. Dilute as ordered on the package. Administer at a rate not exceeding 1 g over 5 minutes when given direct IV push. Administer ordered dose over at least 15 minutes in the newborn.
- For IM injection, select muscle mass carefully. In infants and small children, the vastus lateralis should be used. Record injection site and rotate sites.
- See entry for drug class (p. 248).

### Patient and family education

- See entry for drug class (p. 248).

## carbenicillin indanyl sodium (car-BEN-i-sill-in IN-da-neel) antibiotic*

- carbenicillin indanyl sodium (carindacillin sodium): Geocillin, ✸Geopen Oral

**MECHANISM OF ACTION** The mechanism is the same as for carbenicillin disodium. See entry for drug class (p. 246).

**INDICATIONS** **Urinary tract or prostatic infections caused by gram-negative aerobic bacteria** Susceptible organisms may include *Enterobacter, Escherichia coli, Morganella morganii, Proteus mirabilis, Proteus vulgaris, Providencia rettgeri,* and *Pseudomonas aeruginosa.*

**CONTRAINDICATIONS** **Allergy to penicillins or cephalosporins** • See entry for drug class (p. 246). **Penicillinase-producing strains of Staphylcoccus aureus** Carbenicillin is destroyed by this penicillinase and is therefore ineffective for infections caused by these strains.

**DOSAGE** **PO:** **ADULT:** 382 to 764 mg four times daily for 10 days or until signs of infection resolve. *Special patient populations:* **CHILDREN:** Safe doses not established. **PREGNANCY:** Safe use not established.

**PREPARATIONS** *Tablets, film-coated*: 382 mg of carbenicillin.

**DRUG INTERACTIONS** See entry for drug class (p. 246).

**DIAGNOSTIC TEST INTERFERENCE** **ALT and AST** concentration in serum may be increased. **Aminoglycoside assays** may be unreliable because carbenicillin can inactivate aminoglycoside antibiotics. **Coomb's test** (direct antiglobulin test) may be falsely positive in the presence of carbenicillin. **Glucose assays** using cupric sulfate are unreliable when carbenicillin is present. **Uric acid** determined by the copper-chelate method may be falsely elevated by carbenicillin.

**FATE** Carbenicillin indanyl sodium is poorly absorbed from the GI tract, with only 30% to 40% of a dose entering the blood. After absorption, the indanyl ester is cleaved, releasing carbenicillin as the active component. *Peak* serum concentrations of carbenicillin are achieved within 0.5 to 2 hours. Distribution and elimination are the same as for carbenicillin disodium. The clinical effect is achieved because the carbenicillin released is concentrated in urine. See carbenicillin disodium (p. 259).

### ☙ NURSING CONSIDERATIONS

#### Side effects, toxicities, and associated nursing actions

**GI** Nausea, vomiting, diarrhea, abdominal distress, and flatulence are dose-related side effects. Unpleasant tastes and smells are also reported.

**Other side effects of carbenicillin indanyl sodium** are as for carbenicillin disodium. See carbenicillin disodium (p. 259).

*Extended spectrum penicillin.

- See entry for drug class (p. 247).
- Tell the patient that the drug may come with a packet of a drying agent in the bottle. This packet should be left in the bottle until all of the medication is used, as it keeps moisture from getting into the drug, but the packet should then be discarded and *not* swallowed.

## cloxacillin sodium   (KLOX-uh-sill-in)                     antibiotic*

- cloxacillin sodium (chlorophenylmethyl isoxazolyl penicllin): Cloxapen, Tegopen

**MECHANISM OF ACTION**   Cloxicillin resists the action of penicillinase produced by *Staphylcoccus aureus*. Against other pathogens, cloxicillin has the same mechanism of action but is less potent than penicillin G. See entry for drug class (p. 246).

**INDICATIONS**   **Infections caused by penicillinase-producing Staphylococcus strains** Cloxacillin sodium and related drugs are not destroyed by this penicillinase and are therefore effective against infections that will not respond to other classes of penicillins.

**CONTRAINDICATIONS**   **Allergy to penicillins or cephalosporins** • See entry for drug class (p. 246).

**DOSAGE**   **PO:**   **ADULT:** 250 to 500 mg every 6 hours.   **CHILDREN:** 50 to 100 mg/kg daily in divided doses every 6 hours, up to a maximum daily dose of 4 g.   *Special patient populations:*   **CHILDREN:** Neonates may accumulate the drug unless special care is taken to monitor serum concentrations and reduce dosage appropriately.   **PREGNANCY:** Safe use not established.

**PREPARATIONS**   *Capsules*: 250 or 500 mg. *Solution, oral*: 125 mg/5 ml.

**DRUG INTERACTIONS**   **Aminoglycosides** have additive or synergistic antibacterial action with penicillins when used to treat relatively resistant organisms.   **Probenecid** inhibits renal secretion of penicillins and may prolong the elimination half-life.

**DIAGNOSTIC TEST INTERFERENCE**   **Aminoglycoside assays** may be falsely lowered by penicillins, which inactivate aminoglycoside antibiotics.   **AST** concentrations in serum may be increased.   **Protein assays** by turbidometric methods give false-positive results in the presence of cloxacillin and related penicillins.

**FATE**   Oral absorption of cloxacillin is incomplete but adequate. *Peak* serum concentrations occur 0.5 to 2 hours after a dose. Food diminishes absorption. The drug is found in the milk of nursing mothers and in fetuses. Active and inactive forms are excreted by the kidneys. Some drug is excreted via the bile. The elimination *half-life* of cloxicillin is 0.4 to 0.8 hours in healthy adults but is prolonged in patients with renal failure or in neonates.

## 🐾 NURSING CONSIDERATIONS

### Side effects, toxicities, and associated nursing actions

**Liver** Alkaline phosphatase, AST (SGOT), and ALT (SGPT) levels may be elevated by cloxacillin. Fever, anorexia, nausea, hepatomegaly, and other signs may also occur. Intrahepatic cholestasis is possible.
- Monitor liver function tests.
- Assess for development of liver dysfunction: development of jaundice, right upper quadrant abdominal pain, change in the character or consistency of stools, fever, or malaise.

**Other** For other side effects of cloxacillin, see entry for drug class (p. 247).

### Patient and family education
- Oral cloxacillin should be taken 1 hour before or 2 hours after meals, with a full glass (8 ounces) of water.
- For additional guidelines, see entry for drug class (p. 248).

## cyclacillin   (sye-kluh-SILL-in)                     antibiotic†

- cyclacillin (aminocyclohexyl penicillin): Cyclapen

**MECHANISM OF ACTION**   • See entry for drug class (p. 246).

*Penicillinase-resistant penicillin
†Extended spectrum penicillin.

**INDICATIONS** • Cyclacillin substitutes for oral ampicillin (p. 252).

**CONTRAINDICATIONS** • See ampicillin (p. 253).

**DOSAGE**  PO:  ADULT: 250 to 500 mg every 6 hours (equivalent to 280 or 560 mg ampicillin). Doses should not exceed 2 g daily.  CHILDREN OVER 20 KG: 250 mg every 8 hours.  CHILDREN BELOW 20 KG: Above 2 months of age, 125 mg every 8 hours or 50 to 100 mg/kg daily in divided doses. *Special patient populations:*  RENAL IMPAIRMENT: Doses must be reduced, based on degree of renal impairment.  CHILDREN: Safety in neonates has not been established.  PREGNANCY: Safety not established.

**PREPARATIONS**  *Tablets*: 250 or 500 mg; *oral suspension*: 125 mg/5 ml or 250 mg/5 ml.

**DRUG INTERACTIONS** • See entry for drug class (p. 246).

**DIAGNOSTIC TEST INTERFERENCE**  AST concentrations in serum may be increased.

**FATE**  Absorption of cyclacillin is nearly complete following oral administration. *Peak* serum levels occur at 30 to 60 minutes. The elimination *half-life* of cyclacillin is 0.5 to 0.8 hours. Most of the drug is eliminated unchanged in urine. Renal impairment increases the half-life.

### ❦ NURSING CONSIDERATIONS

#### Side effects, toxicities, and associated nursing actions
• See ampicillin (p. 254).

#### Patient and family education   At least one study has indicated that this drug may be safely taken with milk or milk formula. This drug may probably be taken without regard to meals.
• For additional guidelines, see entry for drug class (p. 248).

---

## dicloxacillin sodium   (DYE-klox-uh-sill-in)   antibiotic*

• dicloxacillin sodium (dichlorophenylmethyl isoxazolyl penicllin): Dycill, Dynapen, Pathocil

**MECHANISM OF ACTION**  Dicloxacillin resists the action of penicillinase produced by *Staphylococcus aureus*. Against other pathogens, dicloxacillin has the same mechanism of action but is less potent than penicillin G. See entry for drug class (p. 246).

**INDICATIONS:**  **Infections caused by penicillinase-producing Staphylococcus strains** Dicloxacillin sodium and related drugs are not destroyed by this penicillinase and are therefore effective against infections that will not respond to other classes of penicillins.

**CONTRAINDICATIONS**  **Allergy to penicillins or cephalosporins** Anaphylaxis and death are possible outcomes. The risk is greatest in those who report previous allergic reactions to penicillin and less in those previously reacting to cephalosporins.

**DOSAGE**  PO:  ADULTS AND CHILDREN OVER 40 KG: 125 to 250 mg every 6 hours.  CHILDREN OVER 1 MONTH OF AGE: 12.5 to 50 mg/kg daily in divided doses every 6 hours; severe infections such as osteomyelitis may require 50 to 100 mg/kg daily in divided doses every 6 hours.  *Special patient populations:* CHILDREN: Neonates may accumulate the drug unless special care is taken to monitor serum concentrations and reduce dosage appropriately.  PREGNANCY: Safe use not established.

**PREPARATIONS**  *Capsules*: 125, 250, or 500 mg. *Solution, oral*: 62.5 mg/5 ml.

**DRUG INTERACTIONS**  As for cloxacillin sodium (p. 261).

**DIAGNOSTIC TEST INTERFERENCE**  As for cloxacillin sodium (p. 261).

**FATE**  As for cloxacillin sodium (p. 261).

### ❦ NURSING CONSIDERATIONS

#### Side effects, toxicities, and associated nursing actions   As for cloxacillin sodium (p. 261).

#### Patient and family education   This drug should be administered 1 hour before or 2 hours after meals with a full glass (8 ounces) of water.
• For additional guidelines, see entry for drug class (p. 248).

*Penicillinase-resistant penicillin.

## hetacillin   (het-uh-SILL-in)

- hetacillin (phenazacillin): Versapen
- hetacillin potassium: Versaper

**MECHANISM OF ACTION**   Hetacillin is a prodrug with no antibacterial activity until it is metabolized in the body to release ampicillin. For the mechanism of action of ampicillin, see entry for drug class (p. 246).

**INDICATIONS**   Hetacillin may substitute for oral ampicillin (p. 252).

**CONTRAINDICATIONS**   • See ampicillin (p. 252).

**DOSAGE   PO:   ADULTS AND CHILDREN OVER 40 KG:** Dosage equivalent to 225 to 450 mg of ampicillin every 6 hours.   **CHILDREN BELOW 40 KG:** Dosage equivalent to 22.5 to 45 mg/kg of ampicillin in divided doses every 6 hours.   *Special patient populations:*   **PREGNANCY:** Safety not established.

**PREPARATIONS   Hetacillin** *Oral, suspension*: 112.5 mg/5 ml equivalent of ampicillin.   **Hetacillin potassium** *Capsules*: 225 mg equivalent of ampicillin.

**DRUG INTERACTIONS**   • See entry for drug class (p. 246).

**DIAGNOSTIC TEST INTERFERENCE**   • See ampicillin (p. 253).

**FATE**   Hetacillin is rapidly absorbed from the GI tract and converted to ampicillin. *Peak* serum levels of ampicillin occur at 30 to 90 minutes and are usually similar to an equivalent dose of ampicillin. Ampicillin released in this way is handled by the body exactly as ampicillin administered directly. See ampicillin (p. 253).

### 🦌 NURSING CONSIDERATIONS

#### Side effects, toxicities, and associated nursing actions
- See ampicillin (p. 254).

#### Patient and family education
- This drug should be administered 1 hour before or 2 hours after meals with a full glass (8 ounces) of water.
- For additional guidelines, see entry for drug class (p. 248).

## methicillin sodium   (meth-i-SILL-in)

- methicillin sodium (dimethoxyphenyl penicillin): Staphcillin

**MECHANISM OF ACTION**   Methicillin resists the action of penicillinase produced by *Staphylococcus aureus*. Against other pathogens, methicillin has the same mechanism of action but is less potent than penicillin G. See entry for drug class (p. 246).

**INDICATIONS   Infections caused by penicillinase-producing Staphylococcus strains** Methicillin is not destroyed by this penicillinase and is therefore effective against infections that will not respond to other classes of penicillins. • Methicillin-resistant strains of *Staphylococcus aureus* are known. • Penicillinases or beta-lactamases are not involved in methicillin resistance; these resistant organisms are often resistant to other antibiotics as well.

**CONTRAINDICATIONS   Allergy to penicillins or cephalosporins** Anaphylaxis and death are possible outcomes. • The risk is greatest in those who report previous allergic reactions to penicillin and less in those previously reacting to cephalosporins.   **Renal impairment** Methicillin may be contraindicated in some patients because methicillin frequently causes acute interstitial nephritis.

**DOSAGE   IM:   ADULTS AND CHILDREN OVER 40 KG:** 1 g methicillin sodium (equivalent to 900 mg methicillin) every 4 to 6 hours by deep IM injection into a large muscle mass.   **CHILDREN OVER 1 MONTH OF AGE:** 25 to 100 mg/kg methicillin sodium (equivalent to 22.5 to 90 mg/kg methicillin) every 6 hours.   **NEONATES:** 50 to 200 mg/kg methicillin sodium (equivalent to 45 to 180 mg/kg

*Extended spectrum penicillin
†Penicillinase-resistant penicillin.

methicillin) total daily dose in divided doses every 6 to 12 hours. Dose and frequency depend on the age and weight of the neonate, as well as severity of infection.   **IV:   ADULTS AND CHILDREN OVER 40 KG:** 1 to 2 g methicillin sodium (900 mg to 1.8 g methicillin) every 4 to 6 hours.   **CHILDREN AND INFANTS:** Although children have received doses as listed for IM route, doses for IV administration are not completely established.   *Special patient populations:* **RENAL IMPAIRMENT:** Doses must be reduced based on degree of renal impairment.   **CHILDREN:** Neonates may accumulate the drug unless special care is taken to monitor serum concentrations and reduce dosage appropriately.   **PREGNANCY:** Safe use not established.

**PREPARATIONS**   *Powder to prepare solution for injection:* 1, 4, 6, or 10 g methicillin sodium, equivalent to 0.9, 3.6, 5.4, and 9 g methicillin, respectively. The 10 g preparation is a pharmacy bulk package. *Powder to prepare solution for IV infusion:* 1 g (0.9 g methicillin) or 4 g (3.6 g methicillin) methicillin sodium. Solutions should be reconstituted in sterile water or saline (0.45% or 0.9%). For IM injection, concentrations of 500 mg/ml methicillin sodium are used. For IV administration, the drug should be diluted to 100 mg/ml or less.

**DRUG INTERACTIONS**   **Aminoglycosides antibiotics** have additive or synergistic antibacterial action with penicillins when used to treat relatively resistant organisms.   **Aminoglycoside antibiotics** may be inactivated when combined with methicillin.   **Probenecid** inhibits renal secretion of penicillins and may prolong the elimination half-life.

**LABORATORY TEST INTERFERENCE**   **Aminoglycoside assays** may be falsely lowered by penicillins, which inactivate aminoglycoside antibiotics.   **Coomb's test (direct antiglobulin test)** may be falsely positive.   **Protein assays** by turbidometric methods give false-positive results in the presence of methicillin and related penicillins.   **Uric acid assays** using the copper-chelate method may be falsely elevated.   **Urinary 17-hydroxycorticosteroids** may be falsely increased.

**FATE**   Oral absorption is inadequate for methicillin. *Peak* serum concentrations following IM doses occur at 0.5 to 1 hour. The drug is found in the milk of nursing mothers and in fetuses. Methicillin is not metabolized, and the active drug is excreted by the kidneys. The elimination *half-life* is 0.4 to 0.5 hours in healthy adults but is prolonged in patients with renal failure or in neonates and may be slightly prolonged in children.

## ☙ NURSING CONSIDERATIONS

### Side effects, toxicities, and associated nursing actions

**Liver** Alkaline phosphatase, AST (SGOT), and ALT (SGPT) may be elevated by methicillin. Fever, anorexia, nausea, hepatomegaly, and other signs may also occur.
- Monitor liver function tests.
- Assess for development of liver dysfunction: development of jaundice, right upper quadrant abdominal pain, change in the character or consistency of stools, fever, malaise.

**Renal** Interstitial nephritis occurs in up to 17% of patients receiving IV methicillin. Methicillin is the penicillin most likely to cause this reaction.
- Monitor intake and output.
- Monitor urinalysis; be alert for white blood cells and tubular casts, microscopic hematuria, and proteinuria.
- Monitor BUN and serum creatinine.

**Blood** In addition to blood dyscrasias common to other penicillins, methicillin causes local irritation to blood vessels. Thrombophlebitis and pain at the injection site are common with methicillin. Thrombophlebitis is especially a risk with elderly patients.
- Assess the IV insertion site carefully before administering each dose to ascertain that the needle is in the vein and infusing properly.
- Instruct patients to report tenderness or irritation near the site of the IV insertion site.
- Monitor the rate of infusion carefully.

**Other** For other side effects of methicillin, see entry for drug class (p. 247).

### Nursing interventions related to drug administration
- For parenteral administration, see Preparations.
- For IM injection, dilute as directed on vial. Use large muscle masses, such as the dorsogluteal site or rectus femoris in adults or the vastus lateralis in infants and small children. Record the injection site and rotate sites.

- For direct IV push, dilute as for IM injection. Further dilute with 50 ml of 0.45% or 0.9% sodium chloride injection. Administer at a rate of 10 ml/min.
- For intermittent infusion, dilute as for IM injection, then further dilute to a concentration of 2 to 20 mg/ml. Doses for intermittent infusion are usually administered over 20 to 30 minutes.
- See Blood side effects.

**Patient and family education**
- See entry for drug class (p. 248).

---

## mezlocillin sodium    (mez-loh-SILL-in)                                           antibiotic*

- mezlocillin sodium: Mezlin

**MECHANISM OF ACTION** • See entry for drug class (p. 246).

**INDICATIONS** **Infections caused by gram-negative aerobic bacteria** Susceptible organisms may include *Enterobacter, Escherichia coli, Klebsiella, Morganella morganii, Proteus mirabilis, Proteus vulgaris, Providencia rettgeri, Pseudomonas aeruginosa,* and *Serratia.* • These organisms may cause septicemia and infections of the respiratory tract, urinary tract, abdominal cavity, skin, bones, and joints.

**CONTRAINDICATIONS** **Allergy to penicillins or cephalosporins** Anaphylaxis and death are possible outcomes. • The risk is greatest in those who report previous allergic reactions to penicillin and less in those previously reacting to cephalosporins. **Penicillinase-producing strains of *Staphylcoccus aureus*** Mezlocillin is destroyed by this penicillinase and is therefore ineffective for infections caused by these strains.

**DOSAGE** **IM:** **ADULT:** 1.5 to 2 g every 6 hours (100 to 125 mg/kg daily) by deep IM injection. **IV:** **ADULT:** Dosage ranges from 1.5 to 4 g every 6 hours (100 to 300 mg/kg daily). Total doses should not exceed 350 mg/kg or 24 g daily. Doses are reduced in renal failure. **CHILDREN:** From 1 month to 12 years of age, 50 to 75 mg/kg every 4 hours. Neonates, 75 mg/kg every 12 hours during the first week of life and every 8 or 6 hours from the second through fourth weeks of life. *Special patient populations:* **RENAL IMPAIRMENT:** Doses must be reduced based on degree of renal impairment. **PREGNANCY:** FDA pregnancy category B.

**PREPARATIONS** *Powder to prepare solution for injection:* 1, 2, 3, or 4 g. *Powder to prepare solution for IV infusion:* 2, 3, or 4 g. For IM injection, the sterile powder should be reconstituted with sterile water for injection or lidocaine solution without epinephrine (0.5% or 1%), 3 to 4 ml for each gram of azlocillin. For IV administration, the sterile powder is reconstituted with sterile water for injection, 5% dextrose injection, or 0.9% sodium chloride injection. For each gram of drug, 10 ml of fluid should be added. The fully dissolved drug may be injected directly IV or may be diluted further into compatible fluids. Solutions for IV use should not exceed concentrations of 100 mg/ml.

**DRUG INTERACTIONS** • See entry for drug class (p. 246).

**DIAGNOSTIC TEST INTERFERENCE** **ALT, AST and alkaline phosphatase** concentrations in serum may be increased. **Aminoglycoside assays** may be unreliable because mezlocillin can inactivate aminoglycoside antibiotics. **Coombs' test (direct antiglobulin test)** may be falsely positive in the presence of mezlocillin. **Protein assays** by turbidometric or biuret methods may be unreadable or give false-positive results in the presence of mezlocillin.

**FATE** Mezlocillin is not absorbed from the GI tract and must be administered IM or IV. *Peak* serum concentrations following IM administration are at 45 to 90 minutes. Mezlocillin distributes into most tissues, but concentrations in the CNS are low unless the meninges are inflamed. The drug passes the placenta and enters the fetuses. Renal excretion is the primary route of elimination, but some metabolism and elimination in the bile occurs. The elimination *half-life* is 0.7 to 1.3 hours in healthy adults but is extended in patients with renal or hepatic impairment and in neonates.

*Extended spectrum penicillin.

## ✾ NURSING CONSIDERATIONS
### Side effects, toxicities, and associated nursing actions

**Blood** Abnormal platelet aggregation and prolonged bleeding time may occur with mezlocillin. In addition, up to 7.4% of patients may show eosinophilia, an allergic reaction.
- Monitor platelets, white blood cell differential count, and bleeding time.
- Monitor for unexplained bruising or bleeding.

**GI** Up to 3% of patients suffer diarrhea with parenteral mezlocillin. Other GI effects are occasionally reported.
- Assess for development of GI symptoms.
- Monitor intake and output.

**Renal** Hypokalemia, hypernatremia, increased BUN and creatinine, and increased serum uric acid are rare.
- Monitor serum electrolytes, BUN, uric acid, and creatinine.
- Assess for signs of hypokalemia: muscle weakness, apathy, abdominal distention, paralytic ileus. ECG changes include inverted T waves, prolonged QT segment, and prominent U waves. Assess for hypernatremia: dry, sticky mucous membranes, low urinary output, and firm, ''rubbery'' tissue turgor.
- Monitor intake, output, and weight.

**Other** Mezlocillin also causes other side effects common to penicillins. See entry for drug class (p. 247).

### Nursing interventions related to drug administration
- See Preparations.
- For direct IV push administration, dose should be administered over 3 to 5 minutes.
- For intermittent IV infusion, prepare dilution as directed. Dose should be administered over a 30 minute period.
- Mezlocillin should not be mixed with other drugs in a syringe or IV tubing.
- For IM injections, select the muscle mass carefully. In infants and small children, the vastus lateralis should be used. To lessen discomfort associated with IM administration, the ordered dose should be administered over 12 to 15 seconds. No more than 2 g should be administered in a single injection. Record the injection site and rotate sites.

### Patient and family education
- See entry for drug class (p. 248).

---

## nafcillin sodium    (naf-SILL-in)                                   antibiotic*

- nafcillin sodium (ethoxynaphthamido penicillin sodium): Nafcil, Nallpen, Unipen

**MECHANISM OF ACTION**    Nafcillin resists the action of penicillinase produced by *Staphylococcus aureus*. Against other pathogens, nafcillin has the same mechanism of action but is less potent than penicillin G. See entry for drug class (p. 246).

**INDICATIONS**    **Infections caused by penicillinase-producing Staphylococcus strains** Nafcillin is not destroyed by this penicillinase and is therefore effective against infections that will not respond to other classes of penicillins.

**CONTRAINDICATIONS**    **Allergy to penicillins or cephalosporins** Anaphylaxis and death are possible outcomes. The risk is greatest in those who report previous allergic reactions to penicillin and less in those previously reacting to cephalosporins.

**DOSAGE**    **PO:    ADULT:** 250 mg to 1 g every 4 to 6 hours, depending on the severity of infection.    **CHILDREN:** 30 to 40 mg/kg daily in three or four doses for neonates and up to 50 to 100 mg/kg daily every 6 hours for older children.    **IM:    ADULT:** 500 mg every 4 to 6 hours by deep IM injection into a large muscle mass.    **CHILDREN OVER 1 MONTH OF AGE:** 50 to 200 mg/kg daily in two to four

---

*Penicillinase-resistant penicillin.

divided doses. **NEONATES:** 20 mg/kg daily in two divided doses up to 200 mg daily in three divided doses. Dose and frequency depend on the age and weight of the neonate, as well as severity of infection. **IV: ADULT:** 500 mg to 2 g every 4 hours, depending on the severity of infection. **CHILDREN OVER 1 MONTH IN AGE:** 50 to 200 mg/kg daily every 4 to 6 hours, depending on severity of infection. **NEONATES:** Although children have received nafcillin IV, doses by this route are not completely established. *Special patient populations:* **CHILDREN:** Neonates may accumulate the drug unless special care is taken to monitor serum concentrations and reduce dosage appropriately. **PREGNANCY:** Safe use not established.

**PREPARATIONS** *Capsules:* 250 mg. *Tablets, film-coated:* 500 mg. *Solution, oral:* 250 mg in 5 ml. *Powder to prepare solution for injection:* 500 mg, 1 g, 2 g, or 10 g. The 10 g preparation is a pharmacy bulk package. *Powder to prepare solution for IV infusion:* 1, 1.5, 2 or 4 g. Solutions should be reconstituted in sterile water, bacteriostatic water, or saline 0.9%. For IM injection, concentrations of 250 mg/ml are used. For IV administration, the drug should be diluted to 50 mg/ml or less.

**DRUG INTERACTIONS** As for cloxacillin sodium (p. 261).

**DIAGNOSTIC TEST INTERFERENCE** **Protein assays** by the biuret method give false-positive results in the presence of nafcillin. Other interferences are as for cloxacillin sodium (p. 261).

**FATE** Oral absorption of nafcillin is erratic and incomplete. *Peak* serum concentrations following oral doses occur at 0.5 to 2 hours. *Peak* serum concentrations following IM doses occur at 0.5 to 1 hour. The drug is found in the milk of nursing mothers and in fetuses. Nafcillin is extensively metabolized to inactive metabolites in the liver and excreted primarily in bile. Very little active drug is excreted by the kidneys. Nafcillin is the only penicillin eliminated in this fashion. The elimination *half-life* is 0.5 to 1.5 hours in healthy adults, but elimination is prolonged in patients with renal or hepatic failure or in neonates.

## 🕊 NURSING CONSIDERATIONS

### Side effects, toxicities, and associated nursing actions

**Liver** Alkaline phosphatase, AST (SGOT), and ALT (SGPT) may be elevated by nafcillin. Fever, anorexia, nausea, hepatomegaly, and other signs may also occur.
* Monitor liver function tests.
* Monitor vital signs.
* Assess for development of liver dysfunction: development of jaundice, right upper quadrant abdominal pain, change in the character or consistency of stools, fever, malaise.

**Blood** In addition to blood dyscrasias common to other penicillins, nafcillin causes local irritation to blood vessels. Thrombophlebitis and pain at the injection site are common with nafcillin. Thrombophlebitis is especially a risk with elderly patients.
* Assess IV insertion site carefully before administering each dose to ascertain that the needle is in the vein and the IV is infusing properly. Also assess for redness, tenderness, and complaints of irritation or pain.
* Monitor the rate of IV infusion carefully.

**Other** For other side effects of nafcillin, see entry for drug class (p. 247).

### Nursing interventions related to drug administration

* See Preparations.
* For IM injection, select the muscle mass carefully, and try to avoid nerve injury. In adults, use the dorsogluteal site or rectus femoris muscle. In infants and small children, the vastus lateralis should be used. Drug powder that has been reconstituted with bacteriostatic water containing 0.9% benzyl alcohol should not be used in neonates. Record the injection sites and rotate sites.
* For direct IV push, dilute as indicated, and administer the dose over 5 to 10 minutes.
* For intermittent IV infusion, dilute as indicated. Infuse dose over 30 to 60 minutes.

### Patient and family education
Oral nafcillin should be administered 1 hour before or 2 hours after meals with a full glass (8 ounces) of water.
* For additional guidelines, see entry for drug class (p. 248).

## oxacillin sodium    (ox-uh-SILL-in)                                     antibiotic*

- oxacillin sodium (methylphenyl isoxazolyl penicillin): Bactocill, Prostaphlin

**MECHANISM OF ACTION**    Oxacillin resists the action of penicillinase from *Staphylcoccus aureus*. Against other pathogens, oxacillin has the same mechanism of action but is less potent than penicillin G. See entry for drug class (p. 246).

**INDICATIONS    Infections caused by penicillinase-producing Staphylococcus strains** Oxacillin sodium is not destroyed by this penicillinase and is therefore effective against infections that will not respond to other classes of penicillins.

**CONTRAINDICATIONS    Allergy to penicillin or cephalosporins** Anaphylaxis and death are possible outcomes. The risk is greatest in those who report previous allergic reactions to penicillin and less in those previously reacting to cephalosporins.

**DOSAGE    PO:    ADULTS AND CHILDREN OVER 40 KG:** 500 mg to 1 g every 4 to 6 hours.    **CHILDREN OVER 1 MONTH IN AGE:** 50 to 100 mg/kg daily in divided doses every 4 to 6 hours.    **IM, IV:    ADULTS AND CHILDREN OVER 40 KG:** 250 mg to 2 g every 4 to 6 hours, depending on the severity of the infection.    **CHILDREN OVER 1 MONTH IN AGE:** 50 to 200 mg/kg daily total as divided doses every 4 to 6 hours.    **NEONATES:** 25 to 200 mg/kg daily in divided doses every 6 to 12 hours.    *Special patient populations:*    **CHILDREN:** Neonates may accumulate the drug unless special care is taken to monitor serum concentrations and reduce dosage appropriately.    **PREGNANCY:** Safe use not established.

**PREPARATIONS**    *Capsules:* 250 or 500 mg. *Solution, oral:* 250 mg/5 ml; powder to prepare solution for injection: 250 mg, 500 mg, 1 g, 2 g, 4 g, or 10 g (4 and 10 g are pharmacy bulk packages); powder to prepare solution for IV infusion: 1, 2, or 4 g. For IM administration, oxacillin is diluted to 167 mg/ml by the addition of appropriate amounts of sterile water or saline (0.45% or 0.9%). The drug should be administered deep into a muscle mass. For IV administration, oxacillin is diluted to 50 or 100 mg/ml for direct IV injection or further diluted to 0.5 to 40 mg/ml for IV infusion.

**DRUG INTERACTIONS**    As for cloxacillin sodium (p. 261).

**DIAGNOSTIC TEST INTERFERENCE**    As for cloxacillin sodium (p. 261).

**FATE**    Oral absorption is incomplete but adequate for oxacillin. *Peak* serum concentrations occur 0.5 to 2 hours after a dose. Food diminishes absorption. IM administration produces peak serum concentrations within 0.5 hour. The drug is found in the milk of nursing mothers and in fetuses. Active and inactive forms are excreted by the kidneys. The elimination *half-life* of oxacillin is 0.3 to 0.8 hours in healthy adults but is prolonged in patients with renal failure or in neonates.

### ☙ NURSING CONSIDERATIONS
#### Side effects, toxicities, and associated nursing actions

**Liver** Alkaline phosphatase, AST (SGOT), and ALT (SGPT) may be elevated by oxacillin. Fever, anorexia, nausea, hepatomegaly, and other signs may also occur. Intrahepatic cholestasis is possible.
- Monitor liver function tests.
- Monitor vital signs.
- Assess for development of liver dysfunction: development of jaundice, right upper quadrant abdominal pain, change in the character or consistency of stools, fever, malaise.

**Other** For other side effects of oxacillin, see entry for drug class (p. 247).

#### Nursing interventions related to drug administration
- See Preparations.
- For IM injection, select the muscle mass carefully, and try to avoid nerve injury. In adults, use the dorsogluteal site or rectus femoris muscle. In infants and small children, the vastus lateralis should be used. Record the injection sites and rotate sites.
- For direct IV push, dilute as indicated, and administer the dose over 10 minutes. To lessen irritation of the vein, administer the dose as slowly as possible. Be alert to thrombophlebitis, especially in the elderly.

*Penicillinase-resistant penicillin.

- For intermittent IV infusion, dilute as indicated. Infusion time varies with total volume. A single dose may be infused for up to 6 hours.

**Patient and family education**

- Oral oxacillin should be administered 1 hour before or 2 hours after meals with a full glass (8 ounces) of water.
- For additional guidelines, see entry for drug class (p. 248).

## penicillin G   (pen-i-SILL-in Gee)    antibiotic*

- penicillin G potassium: ✤Megacillin, ✤Novopen, Pentids, Pfizerpen G, Pharmapen
- penicillin G sodium: ✤Crystapen

**MECHANISM OF ACTION**   Penicillin G interferes with synthesis and maintenance of bacterial cell walls, leading to destruction of rapidly growing bacteria. (See entry for drug class, p. 246).

**INDICATIONS**   **Infections caused by gram-positive aerobic bacteria** Septicemia, endocarditis, meningitis, and infections of bones, joints, and soft tissues may be treated. Susceptible organisms may include *Streptococcus pneumoniae, S. pyrogenes,* and other Streptococci; *Staphylcoccus aureus* and *epidermidis.* nonpenicillinase-producing strains; *Bacillis anthracis* (anthrax); *Corynebacterium diphtheriae* (diphtheria); *Listeria monocytogenes; Erysipelothrix rhusiopathiae.*   **Infections caused by gram-negative aerobic bacteria** Susceptible bacteria may include *Neisseria gonorrhoeae, N. meningitidis; Branhamella catarrhalis; Pasteurella multocida.* These bacteria may cause meningitis, gonorrhea, and septicemia.   **Infections caused by anaerobic bacteria** *Actinomyces, Peptococcus,* and *Peptostrieptococcus* are usually susceptible. • Strains of the following organisms may be susceptible: *Bacteroides, Clostridium,* and *Fusobacterium.* • These bacteria may cause abcesses and infections of soft tissues, abdominal cavity, and mouth.   **Infections caused by spirochetes** *Treponema pallidum* (syphilis and bejel), *T. carateum (pinta), T. pertenue* (yaws).

**CONTRAINDICATIONS**   **Allergy to penicillin or cephalosporin drugs** Anaphylaxis and death are possible outcomes. The risk is greatest in those who report previous allergic reactions to penicillin and less in those previously reacting to cephalosporins.

**DOSAGE**   **PO:**   **ADULTS AND CHILDREN OVER 12 YEARS:** 200,000 to 500,000 units every 6 to 8 hours or 800,000 units every 12 hours.   **CHILDREN:** 25,000 to 90,000 units/kg daily in three to six doses.   **IV:**   **ADULTS AND CHILDREN OVER 12 YEARS:** 2 to 50 million units daily by infusion or divided doses every 4 hours. The dose depends on the severity of infection and degree of sensitivity of infecting bacteria.   **CHILDREN:** 25,000 to 400,000 units/kg daily divided in doses every 4 to 6 hours. Longer intervals between doses may be required for neonates.   **IM:**   **ADULTS AND CHILDREN OVER 12 YEARS:** Doses by this route should not exceed 100 million units daily.   **CHILDREN:** As for IV doses.   *Special patient populations:*   **PREGNANCY:** Safe use is not established, although the drug is used without apparent harm in treating syphilis and gonorrhea during pregnancy.

**PREPARATIONS**   **Penicillin G potassium** *Tablets:* 200,000, 250,000, 400,000, 500,000, and 800,000 units. Some preparations sold under the trade "Pentids" contain tartrazine. *Solution, oral:* 200,000, 250,000, and 400,000 units in 5 ml. Preparations sold under the trade name "Pentids" contain tartrazine. *Powder to prepare solution for injection:* 200,000, 500,000, 1 million, 5 million, 10 million, and 20 million units.   **Penicillin G sodium** *For solution, injection:* 5 million units.

**DRUG INTERACTIONS**   **Aminoglycoside antibiotics** have additive or synergistic antibacterial action with penicillins when used to treat relatively resistant organisms.   **Aminoglycoside antibiotics** may be inactivated if mixed in a syringe or IV bottle with penicillin solutions.   **Probenecid** inhibits renal secretion of penicillins and may prolong the elimination half-life. Probenecid may be used to prolong the antibacterial action of penicillin G.   **Tetracyclines, chloramphenicol, or erythromycin** may interfere with the bactericidal action of penicillins.

*Narrow spectrum penicillin.

**DIAGNOSTIC TEST INTERFERENCE** **Aminoglycoside assays** may be falsely lowered because penicillin G potassium can directly inactivate aminoglycoside antibiotics. **Coombs' test (direct antiglobulin test)** is falsely positive in up to 3% of patients receiving large doses of penicillin G. **Folic acid assays** using *Lactobacillus casei* as a test organism cannot be used in the presence of penicillin G. **Glucose assays** using cupric sulfate give false-positive results in the presence of penicillin G. **Guthrie test for phenylketonuria** is unreliable in the presence of penicillin G unless the penicillin is inactivated before exposing the sample to the Bacillus subtilis test organism. **HLA tissue typing** may be unreliable because penicillin G reacts with some antigens. **Assays of 17-ketosteroids** by the Norymberski or Zimmerman methods may be falsely elevated. **Test for lead intoxication** using urinary concentrations of ALA (gamma-aminolevulinic acid) as a diagnostic sign are unreliable in the presence of penicillin G. **Protein assays** using biuret, Folin-Ciocalteau, or turbidometric methods may be falsely elevated by penicillin G. **Tests of renal function** using PAH (aminohippurate sodium) or PSP (phenolsulfonphthalein) are unreliable because penicillin G competes with these compounds for secretion by the kidney. **Urinary specific gravity** may be falsely elevated by high IV doses of penicillin G potassium. **Uric acid assays** using the copper-chelate method are falsely elevated by penicillin G.

**FATE** Penicillin G is incompletely absorbed orally. *Peak* serum concentrations are reached within 0.5 to 1 hour but are only about 0.5 unit/ml when the drug is administered orally. Absorption from IM sites is rapid and virtually complete, producing *peak* serum concentrations of 6 to 20 units/ml within 15 to 30 minutes. Penicillin G is well distributed to most tissues. Entry into the CNS is poor unless infection causes inflamation of the meninges. The drug also enters breast milk and crosses the placenta. Penicillin G, primarily as active drug, is eliminated efficiently by the kidneys, but small amounts also appear in bile. The elimination *half-life* is 0.4 to 0.9 hours in healthy adults but is extended in renal failure and in neonates.

### ☙ NURSING CONSIDERATIONS

#### Side effects, toxicities, and associated nursing actions
- See entry for drug class (p. 247).

#### Nursing interventions related to drug administration
- Read labels carefully in order to prepare correct dose and for correct preparation and correct route of administration.
- Prepare as directed on the vial for intermittent infusion. These drugs are not administered direct IV push.
- Do not mix penicillin G for infusion with other medications.
- See Preparations. Some strengths of Pentids brand tablets and solution contain FD & C dye #5, tartrazine, which may cause allergic reactions in some individuals. Although rare, it may be seen more often in persons with aspirin hypersensitivity.

#### Patient and family education
- Penicillin G potassium oral preparations should be administered 1 hour before or 2 hours after meals with a full glass (8 ounces) of water.
- Teach patients not to take acidic fruit juices such as orange or grapefruit juice or other acidic beverages within 1 hour of taking an oral dose of penicillin G, as the beverage may prevent the medication from working as well as desired.
- For additional guidelines, see entry for drug class (p. 248).

---

## penicillin V   (pen-i-SILL-in Vee)                                    antibiotic*

- penicillin V (phenoxymethyl penicillin) potassium: Beepen-VK, Betapen-VK, Ledercillin VK, Nadopen-V, Novopen-VK, Penapar VK, Pen-Vee K, Robicillin VK, SK-Penicillin VK, Suspen, Uticillin VK, V-Cillin K, Veetids

**MECHANISM OF ACTION**   • See entry for drug class (p. 246).

**INDICATIONS** **Infections caused by streptococci** Group A beta-hemolytic streptococci and *Streptococcus pneumoniae* are usually highly susceptible to penicillin V. • Infections caused by these organisms

*Narrow spectrum penicillin.

include otitis media, scarlet fever, erysipelas, tonsillitis, pharyngitis, and infections of the respiratory tract.    **Infections caused by nonpenicillinase-producing staphylococci** *Staphylococci* often cause infections of skin or other soft tissues. • Strains that produce penicillinase are resistant to penicillin V. **Prophylaxis of bacterial endocarditis** Penicillin V may be used during and immediately after procedures likely to introduce bacteria into the bloodstream (dental procedures, respiratory tract instrumentation). • Prophylaxis is necessary only for patients at risk because of previous surgery or disease. **Prophylaxis of recurrent rheumatic fever** Penicillin V can be used for long-term prophylaxis to prevent streptococcal infections from reestablishing disease.    **Necrotizing ulcerative gingivitis** Penicillin V is often effective against the anaerobic organisms causing this infection.

**CONTRAINDICATIONS**    **Allergy to penicillins or cephalosporins** Anaphylaxis and death are possible outcomes. • The risk is greatest in those who report previous allergic reactions to penicillin and less in those previously reacting to cephalosporins.

**DOSAGE**    **PO:**    **ADULTS AND CHILDREN OVER AGE 12:** 125 to 500 mg every 6 to 12 hours, depending on the severity of infection. For long-term prophylaxis, 125 to 250 mg every 12 hours is sufficient. For short-term prophylaxis of bacterial endocarditis, up to 2 g may be given at the time of the procedure with 1 g following 1 hour later.    **CHILDREN OLDER THAN 1 MONTH:** 15 to 62.5 mg/kg daily in three to six doses or 0.5 to 1 g/M$^2$ in divided doses.    *Special patient populations:* **PREGNANCY:** Safe use not established.

**PREPARATIONS**    **Penicillin V** *Tablets:* 250 and 500 mg; *solution, oral:* 125 or 250 mg in 5 ml.    **Penicillin V potassium** *Tablets:* 125, 250, or 500 mg; *tablets, film-coated:* 250 or 500 mg; *solution, oral:* 125 or 250 mg in 5 ml. Preparation sold under trade name of Veetids contains tartrazine. Penicillin V activity is also sometimes expressed in terms of penicillin units. By convention, 250 mg is considered equivalent to 400,000 units.

**DRUG INTERACTIONS**    **Oral contraceptives** may be less effective when penicillin V is used because the antibiotic increases hepatic inactivation of the steroids in contraceptive preparations. • For other possible interactions see entry for drug class (p. 246).

**DIAGNOSTIC TEST INTERFERENCE**    Expected to be similar to penicillin G (p. 270), except that penicillin V concentrations are lower, and therefore the frequency of interferences is lower.

**FATE**    Penicillin V is better absorbed orally than the related drug, penicillin G. This property offsets the lower potency of penicillin V, but the drug is appropriate only for oral administration. Other properties of the drug are similar to penicillin G (p. 270).

### ☙ NURSING CONSIDERATIONS

#### Side effects, toxicities, and associated nursing actions
• See entry for drug class (p. 247).

#### Nursing interventions related to drug administration
• Veetids brand 125 mg/5 ml oral solution contains FD & C dye #5, tartrazine, which may cause an allergic reaction in susceptible individuals. Although rare, this side effect is encountered more frequently in persons with aspirin hypersensitivity.

#### Patient and family education
• Penicillin V and penicillin V potassium may be given without regard to meals, but absorption is improved if doses are administered 1 hour before or 2 hours after meals.
• For additional guidelines, see entry for drug class (p. 248).

---

## piperacillin sodium    (pip-er-uh-SILL-in)                                                antibiotic*

• piperacillin sodium: Pipracil

**MECHANISM OF ACTION**    • See entry for drug class (p. 246).

**INDICATIONS**    **Infections caused by gram-negative aerobic bacteria** Susceptible organisms may include *Enterobacter, Escherichia coli, Klebsiella, Morganella morganii, Proteus mirabilis, Proteus vul-*

---

*Extended spectrum penicillin.

*garis, Providencia rettgeri, Pseudomonas aeruginosa,* and *Serratia.* • These organisms may cause septicemia and infections of the respiratory tract, urinary tract, abdominal cavity, skin, bones, and joints.   **Perioperative prophylaxis** Patients undergoing vaginal hysterectomy, abdominal hysterectomy, caesarian section, or other intra-abdominal procedures may receive piperacillin ½ to 1 hour before surgery and for up to 24 hours post surgery.

**CONTRAINDICATIONS**   **Allergy to penicillins or cephalosporins** Anaphylaxis and death are possible outcomes. The risk is greatest in those who report previous allergic reactions to penicillin and less in those previously reacting to cephalosporins.   **Penicillinase-producing strains of *Staphylcoccus aureus*** Piperacillin is destroyed by this penicillinase and is therefore ineffective for infections caused by these strains.

**DOSAGE**   **IM:**   **ADULT:** 6 to 8 g daily (100 to 125 mg/kg) in divided doses every 6 to 12 hours by deep IM injection.   **IV:**   **ADULT:** Dosage ranges from 100 to 300 mg/kg daily given as divided doses every 4 to 6 hours, depending on the site and severity of infection. Usual doses are from 8 to 18 g daily; total doses should not exceed 350 mg/kg or 24 g daily.   **CHILDREN:** Pediatric dosages are not fully established, but the drug has been used in children at doses of 50 mg/kg or 1.5 g/M$^2$ every 4 hours. *Special patient populations:*   **RENAL IMPAIRMENT:** Doses must be reduced, based on degree of renal impairment.   **PREGNANCY:** FDA pregnancy category B.

**PREPARATIONS**   *Powder to prepare solution for injection:* 2, 3, or 4 g; 40 g bulk pharmacy package. *Powder to prepare solution for IV infusion:* 2, 3, or 4 g. For IM injection, the sterile powder should be reconstituted with sterile or bacteriostatic water for injection, sterile or bacteriostatic 0.9% sodium chloride injection, or lidocaine without epinephrine (0.5% or 1%). Use 2 ml for each gram of piperacillin. For IV administration, the sterile powder should be dissolved in sterile or bacteriostatic water for injection or in 0.9% sodium chloride injection. Use 5 ml for each gram of piperacillin and inject directly or dilute with an additional 50 ml of solution for infusion.

**DRUG INTERACTIONS**   • See entry for drug class (p. 246).

**DIAGNOSTIC TEST INTERFERENCE**   **ALT and AST** concentrations in serum may be increased.   **Aminoglycoside antibiotic** assays may be unreliable because mezlocillin can inactivate aminoglycosides.   **Aminoglycoside antibiotics** may have additive or synergistic antibacterial action with piperacillin when used to treat relatively resistant organisms.   **Coombs' test (direct antiglobulin test)** may be falsely positive in the presence of piperacillin.   **Probenecid** inhibits renal secretion of piperacillin and may prolong the elimination half-life.   **Protein assays** by turbidometric or biuret methods may be unreadable or give false-positive results in the presence of piperacillin.

**FATE**   Piperacillin is not absorbed from the GI tract and must be administered IM or IV. *Peak* serum concentrations following IM administration are at 30 to 50 minutes. Piperacillin is distributed into most tissues. Concentrations in the CNS are low unless the meninges are inflamed. The drug passes the placenta and enters fetuses. Renal excretion is the primary route of elimination, but some elimination in the bile occurs. The elimination *half-life* is 0.6 to 1.3 hours in healthy adults but is extended in patients with renal or hepatic impairment and in neonates.

## ☙ NURSING CONSIDERATIONS
### Side effects, toxicities, and associated nursing actions

**Blood** Abnormal platelet aggregation and prolonged bleeding time may occur with piperacillin. In addition, up to 7.4% of patients may show eosinophilia, an allergic reaction.
• Monitor platelets, white blood cell differential count, and bleeding time.
• Monitor for unexplained bruising or bleeding.

**GI** Up to 3% of patients suffer diarrhea with parenteral piperacillin. Other GI effects are occasionally reported.
• Assess for development of GI symptoms.
• Monitor intake and output.

**Renal** Hypokalemia, hypernatremia, increased BUN and creatinine, and increased serum uric acid are rare.
• Monitor serum electrolytes, BUN, uric acid, and creatinine.
• Assess for signs of hypokalemia: muscle weakness, apathy, abdominal distention, paralytic ileus. ECG changes include inverted T waves, prolonged QT segment, and prominent U waves. Assess for

hypernatremia: dry, sticky mucous membranes, low urinary output, and firm, "rubbery" tissue turgor.

- Monitor intake, output, and weight.

**Other** Piperacillin also causes other side effects common to penicillins. See entry for drug class (p. 247).

## Nursing interventions related to drug administration

- See Preparations.
- For direct IV push, dilute as directed. Administer dose over 3 to 5 minutes.
- For intermittent infusion, dilute reconstituted drug with at least 50 ml of appropriate solution. Administer dose over at least 30 minutes.
- For IM injection, select muscle mass carefully, and try to avoid nerve injury. In adults, use the dorsogluteal site or rectus femoris muscle. In infants and small children, the vastus lateralis should be used. IM doses should not exceed 2 g at a single injection site. Record injection sites and rotate sites.

## Patient and family education

- For additional guidelines, see entry for drug class (p. 248).

---

## procaine penicillin G   (pro-kane pen-i-SILL-in gee)   antibiotic*

- procaine penicillin G (procaine benzylpenicillin): Crysticillin, Duracillin, Wycillin

**MECHANISM OF ACTION**   Procaine penicillin G is relatively insoluble and is therefore slowly absorbed from IM injection sites. Penicillin G is released as the active drug. For the mechanism of penicillin G, see entry for drug class (p. 246).

**INDICATIONS**   **Mild to moderate infections caused by staphylococci, streptococci, and spirochetes** These organisms are often susceptible to low concentrations of penicillin G.   **Follow-up therapy for infections initially treated with penicillin G** Procaine penicillin G can substitute for the shorter-acting penicillin G preparations after the need for high serum concentrations has passed.

**CONTRAINDICATIONS**   **Allergy to procaine** Patients who are allergic to procaine or related local anesthetics should not receive procaine penicillin G. • As for penicillin G (p. 269).

**DOSAGE**   IV: IV administration is absolutely contraindicated.   **IM: ADULT:** 600,000 to 1.2 million units daily in one or two doses. For eradication of the diphtheria carrier state, 300,000 units daily. For treatment of endocarditis, 4.8 million units daily in two to four doses. For gonorrhea or pelvic inflammatory disease, 4.8 million units with 1 g probenecid as a single injection. No more than 2.4 million units should be given at any one site. Injections are at deep IM sites.   **CHILDREN FROM 1 MONTH TO 12 YEARS:** 25,000 to 50,000 units/kg daily or 500,000 to 1 million units/$M^2$ as a single injection.   **NEONATES:** 50,000 units/kg daily as a single injection.   *Special patient populations:* **PREGNANCY:** Safety not established.

**PREPARATIONS**   *Suspension for IM injection:* 300,000, 500,000, or 600,000 units/ml containing parabens, phenol, and/or povidone. Suspension for IM injection, combinations: • 150,000 units benzathine penicillin G with 150,000 units procaine penicillin G in each milliter; also contains parabens and povidone. • 300,000 units benzathine penicillin G with 300,000 units procaine penicillin G in each milliliter; also contains parabens and povidone. • 450,000 units benzathine penicillin G with 150,000 units procaine penicillin G in each milliliter; also contains parabenz and povidone.

**DRUG INTERACTIONS**   • See penicillin G (p. 269).

**DIAGNOSTIC TEST INTERFERENCE**   • See penicillin G (p. 270).

**FATE**   Procaine penicillin G is slowly absorbed from IM sites, releasing the active drug penicillin G. Because of the slow absorption, *peak* serum concentrations of penicillin G at 1 to 4 hours are low, but measurable serum concentrations are maintained for 1 to 5 days. The active penicillin G that is released from procaine penicillin G is distributed and excreted just as penicillin G directly administered. See penicillin G (p. 270).

*Narrow spectrum penicillin.

## ☙ NURSING CONSIDERATIONS

### Side effects, toxicities, and associated nursing actions

**Local** Procaine penicillin G may occlude vessels or cause emboli if injected directly into arteries or veins.

**Peripheral nerves** If injected near large nerves, penicillin G may cause severe and permanent damage to the nerve.

- For IM injection, select the muscle mass carefully, using anatomic landmarks and trying to avoid nerve injury. In adults, use the dorsogluteal site or rectus femoris muscle. In infants and small children, the vastus lateralis should be used.
- Record the injection sites and rotate sites.
- Aspirate carefully before administering drug. If blood appears in the syringe, withdraw the needle and prepare a fresh dose.
- If the volume of drug is large, it may be divided and administered in two separate injections.

**Other** Procaine penicillin G causes all side effects associated with penicillins (p. 247).

### Nursing interventions related to drug administration

- Occasionally, patients are allergic to procaine. Assess for procaine allergy. Signs and symptoms include anxiety, confusion, agitation, fear of impending death, and convulsions. Treat as for all acute allergic responses.

### Patient and family education

- For additional guidelines, see entry for drug class (p. 248).

---

## ticarcillin disodium    (tye-kar-SILL-in)                                    antibiotic*

- ticarcillin disodium: Ticar

**MECHANISM OF ACTION**   • See entry for drug class (p. 246).

**INDICATIONS**   • As for carbenicillin disodium (p. 259).

**CONTRAINDICATIONS**   • As for carbenicillin disodium (p. 259).

**DOSAGE**   **IM:**   **ADULT:** 1 g every 6 hours.   **CHILDREN:** 50 to 300 mg/kg daily, in two to four doses, depending on the age of the child and severity of infection.   **IV:**   **ADULT:** Dosage ranges from 150 to 300 mg/kg daily given as divided doses every 3, 4, or 6 hours, depending on the site and severity of infection. Total doses should not exceed 24 g daily.   **CHILDREN:** As for IM administration.   *Special patient populations:*   **RENAL IMPAIRMENT:** Doses must be reduced, based on degree of renal impairment.   **PREGNANCY:** Safe use not established.

**PREPARATIONS**   *Solution, injection:* 1, 3, 6, and 20 g. The 20 g form is a pharmacy bulk package. *Solution for IV infusion:* 3 g. The sterile powder should be reconstituted with sterile water for IV injection using at least 4 ml for each gram of drug. Further dilute the drug to 50 mg/ml or less to minimize vein irritation. For IM injection, the powder may also be reconstituted in 1% lidocaine without epinephrine or in bacteriostatic water containing 0.9% benzyl alcohol. Use 2 ml for each gram of drug to produce solutions of 385 mg/ml.

**DRUG INTERACTIONS**   • See Carbenicillin disodium (p. 259).

**DIAGNOSTIC TEST INTERFERENCE**   Expected to be similar to carbenicillin. See Carbenicillin disodium (p. 259).

**FATE**   *Peak* serum concentrations are achieved within 0.5 to 1.25 hours. The elimination *half-life* is 0.9 to 1.3 hours in healthy adults. Other properties of ticarcillin are similar to carbenicillin. See Carbenicillin disodium (p. 259).

## ☙ NURSING CONSIDERATIONS

### Side effects, toxicities, and associated nursing actions   As for carbenicillin disodium (p. 259).

- Assess for signs of hypokalemia: muscle weakness, apathy, abdominal distention, paralytic ileus. ECG changes include inverted T waves, prolonged QT segment, and prominent U waves. Assess for

*Extended spectrum penicillin.

hypernatremia: dry, sticky mucous membranes, low urinary output, and firm, "rubbery" tissue turgor.
- Monitor intake, output, and weight.

**Nursing interventions related to drug administration**
- See Preparations.
- For IM injection, select the muscle mass carefully and try to avoid nerve injury. In adults, use the dorsogluteal site or rectus femoris muscle. In infants and small children, the vastus lateralis should be used. Drug powder that has been reconstituted with bacteriostatic water containing 0.9% benzyl alcohol should not be used in neonates. Do not exceed 2 g for one dose at a single injection site. Record the injection sites and rotate sites.
- For direct IV push, dilute as indicated, and administer the dose as slowly as possible to lessen venous irritation.
- For intermittent IV infusion, dilute as indicated. Infuse dose over 30 minutes to 2 hours in adults or over 10 to 20 minutes in neonates.
- See entry for drug class (p. 248).

**Patient and family education**
- For additional guidelines, see entry for drug class (p. 248).

---

# ticarcillin disodium with clavulanate potassium
(tye-kar-SILL-in; klav-yoo-LAN-ate)                                                    antibiotic*

- ticarcillin disodium with clavulanate potassium: Timentin
- clavulanate potassium

**MECHANISM OF ACTION**    Clavulanic acid is an inhibitor of beta-lactamases. It is combined with ticarcillin to extend the action of ticarcillin against organisms that would ordinarily be marginally susceptible because they produce beta-lactamase. For mechanism of action of ticarcillin, see entry for drug class (p. 246).

**INDICATIONS**    Infections caused by Staphylococcus *S. aureus* or *S. epidermidis*, including penicillinase-producing strains, are usually susceptible.    Infections caused by gram-negative aerobic bacteria Susceptible organisms may include beta-lactamase-producing strains of the following organisms: *Citrobacter, Enterobacter, Escherichia coli, Hemophilus influenzae, Klebsiella,* and *Serratia.* • These organisms may cause septicemia and infections of the respiratory tract, urinary tract, abdominal cavity, skin, bones, and joints.

**CONTRAINDICATIONS**    Allergy to penicillins or cephalosporins Anaphylaxis and death are possible outcomes. The risk is greatest in those who report previous allergic reactions to penicillin and less in those previously reacting to cephalosporins.

**DOSAGE**    IV:    ADULT AND CHILDREN OVER 12 YEARS: 3 g equivalent of ticarcillin with 100 mg equivalent of clavulanic acid every 4 to 8 hours. For patients under 60 kg, 200 to 300 mg/kg equivalent of ticarcillin with associated clavulanate every 4 to 6 hours. *Special patient populations:*    CHILDREN: Although clavulanate potassium has been used in children when combined with amoxycillin, the safety of clavulanate potassium combined with ticarcillin disodium has not been tested adequately in children.    RENAL IMPAIRMENT: Doses must be reduced, based on degree of renal impairment.    PREGNANCY: FDA pregnancy category B.

**PREPARATIONS**    *Solution, injection:* 3 g ticarcillin equivalent with 100 mg equivalent of clavulanic acid. The sterile powder should be reconstituted with 13 ml sterile water or sodium chloride for injection and used directly or further diluted.

**DRUG INTERACTIONS**    • As for carbenicillin disodium (p. 259).

**DIAGNOSTIC TEST INTERFERENCE**    • As for carbenicillin disodium (p. 259).

**FATE**    The elimination *half-life* of clavulanic acid is 1.1 to 1.5 hours in healthy adults. The drug is metabolized to some extent and excreted by the kidneys. See also Ticarcillin disodium (p. 274).

*Extended spectrum penicillin.

## ☙ NURSING CONSIDERATIONS

### Side effects, toxicities, and associated nursing actions

**Blood** Eosinophilia occurs in 5.5% of patients and is probably an allergic reaction. Thrombocytosis, leukopenia, neutropenia, lowered hemoglobin, lowered hematocrit, and prolonged bleeding time are less common.

• Monitor hematocrit and hemoglobin, WBC differential count, platelets, and bleeding time.

• Assess for bruising and unexplained bleeding, pallor, fatigue, malaise.

• Monitor vital signs.

**GI** Diarrhea or loose stools occur in about 1% of patients. Nausea, vomiting, flatulence, and other GI distress occur less frequently.

• Assess for development of GI signs and symptoms.

• Monitor intake and output.

• If diarrhea or vomiting are severe or persistent, notify the physician.

**Renal** Hypernatremia, increased serum creatinine or BUN, and altered serum potassium concentrations are not common.

• Monitor serum electrolytes, BUN, creatinine.

• Assess for signs of hypokalemia: muscle weakness, apathy, abdominal distention, paralytic ileus. ECG changes include inverted T waves, prolonged QT segment, and prominent U waves. Assess for hypernatremia: dry, sticky mucous membranes, low urinary output, and firm, ''rubbery'' tissue turgor.

• Monitor intake, output, and weight.

**Liver** Transient increases in serum concentrations of AST (SGOT), ALT (SGPT), alkaline phosphatase, LDH, and bilirubin may occur.

• Monitor liver function tests.

**Allergic** Rash and urticaria occur in about 1.6% of patients. Pruritis, fever, wheezing, arthralgia, myalgia, and anaphylactic reactions are less common.

• Assess patients for development of rash, urticaria, pruritis, and other allergic responses.

• Monitor vital signs.

• Have drugs, personnel, and equipment available to treat an acute allergic response.

**Other** 3.8% of patients suffer reactions at the injection site, including phlebitis. Signs include pain, swelling, burning, and induration at the site.

• Assess IV insertion site and extremity for signs of irritaion and phlebitis before administering each dose.

• Instruct patients to report pain, irritation, or redness.

### Nursing interventions related to drug administration

• See Preparations.

• See other side effects.

• Visually inspect solutions before administering. Do not administer solutions that are discolored or that contain particulate matter.

• For intermittent infusion, dilute as directed, then infuse dose over 30 minutes.

### Patient and family education

• See entry for drug class (p. 248).

# Chapter Fifteen

# Cephalosporins and related beta-lactam antibiotics

| | |
|---|---|
| aztreonam (a monobactam) | cefsulodin sodium |
| cefaclor | ceftazidime |
| cefadroxil | ceftizoxime sodium |
| cefamandole nafate | ceftriaxone sodium |
| cefazolin sodium | cefuroxime sodium |
| cefmenoxime (investigational) | cephalexin |
| cefonicid sodium | cephalothin sodium |
| cefoperazone sodium | cephapirin sodium |
| ceforanide | cephradine |
| cefotaxime sodium | imipenem (a carbapenem) |
| cefotetan disodium (a cephamycin) | moxalactam (an oxacephem) |
| cefoxitin sodium (a cephamycin) | |

**OVERVIEW OF THE DRUG CLASS**   Penicillins, cephalosporins, and the other drugs listed above are all beta-lactam antibiotics. Cephalosporins were introduced in the 1960s, in part to meet the challenge of increasing resistance to penicillins. Unlike the natural and extended-spectrum penicillins, cephalosporins are not destroyed by the penicillinase of *Staphylococcus aureus*. The cephalosporins that are referred to as first-generation drugs are otherwise generally similar to extended-spectrum penicillins. Second-generation cephalosporins may be less effective against gram-positive bacteria but more effective against certain gram-negative bacteria than are the first-generation drugs. Third-generation drugs are useful almost exclusively against gram-negative bacteria.

In the 1970s new classes of beta-lactams began to be developed. Cephamycins currently in use are similar to second-generation cephalosporins but are more resistant to beta-lactamases. Oxa-cephems such as moxalactam resemble third-generation cephalosporins but resist beta-lactamases like cephamycins. Monobactams such as aztreonam are unusual among beta-lactams because they are effective only against gram-negative bacteria. Carbapenems such as imipenem have the widest antimicrobial spectrum and highest potency of any beta-lactam antibiotic.

The properties of these beta-lactam antibiotics are summarized in Table 15-1.

**MECHANISM OF ACTION**   All beta-lactam antibiotics, including penicillins and cephalosporins, have the same mechanism of action. The cell wall is weakened because these drugs interfere with the synthesis of peptidoglycan, the rigid structural support of the wall. The action may be bactericidal because affected bacteria can rupture. Cephalosporins differ from penicillins in better penetration of cell walls of gram-negative bacteria and in better resistance to beta-lactamases. Some bacteria become resistant to cephalosporins by increasing beta-lactamase activity, lowering permeability of the cell wall, altering sensitivity of target enzymes, or by combinations of these mechanisms.

**INDICATIONS**   **Infections caused by gram-positive bacteria** First-generation cephalosporins may be effective against *Streptococcus pneumoniae,* group A and B streptococci, and *Staphylococcus*. • Penicillinase-producing *Staphylococcus* strains may be susceptible but methicillin-resistant strains are likely to be resistant. • Infections caused by susceptible bacteria include septicemia and infections of the upper respiratory tract, urinary tract, bones, joints, skin, and soft tissues.   **Infections caused by gram-negative bacteria** Cephalosporins and related beta-lactam antibiotics can be effective against most gram-negative bacteria. • First-generation drugs are least likely and third-generation drugs are most likely to be effective. • Against *Serratia* and *Pseudomonas aeruginosa,* only third-generation cephalosporins, aztreonam, moxalactam, and imipenem, are effective. • Infections caused by susceptible bacteria include septicemia and infections of the urinary tract, respiratory tract, bones, joints, skin, and soft tissues.   **Infections caused by anaerobic bacteria** Selected second- and third-generation drugs may be effective, as well as imipenem, moxalactam, and the cephamycins. • Infections caused by susceptible bacteria include abscesses and infections of bones, soft tissues, and the abdominal cavity.   **Infections caused by Neisseria gonorrhea** Second- or third-generation cephalosporins are

| Table 15-1. | Classification of cephalosporins and other beta-lactam antibiotics | | |
|---|---|---|---|
| **Class** | **Properties** | | **Representatives** |
| Cephalosporin, first-generation | Effective against gram-positive bacteria, including penicillinase-producing *Staphylococcus;* gram-negative bacteria, including *Escherichia coli* and *Klebsiella* | | Cefadroxil, cefazolin, cephalexin, cephalothin, cephapirin, cephradine |
| Cephalosporin, second-generation | Less active against gram-positive bacteria but better activity against gram-negative bacteria than first-generation drugs | | Cefaclor, cefamandole, cefonicid, ceforanide, cefuroxime |
| Cephalosporin, third-generation | Weak activity against gram-positive bacteria but broad activity against gram-negative bacteria, often including *Pseudomonas* and *Serratia* | | Cefoperazone, cefotaxime, cefsulodin, ceftazidime, ceftizoxime, ceftriaxone |
| Cephamycin | Highly resistant to beta-lactamases and active against anaerobic bacteria; spectrum resembles second-generation cephalosporins | | Cefotetan, cefoxitin |
| Oxa-cephem | Highly resistant to beta-lactamases, active against anaerobic bacteria, and resembles third-generation cephalosporins | | Moxalactam |
| Carbapenem | Extremely potent, broad-spectrum drug | | Imipenem |
| Monobactam | Highly resistant to beta-lactamases but effective only against aerobic gram-negative bacteria | | Aztreonam |

especially useful for infections caused by penicillinase-producing strains.　**Perioperative prophylaxis** Cephalosporins may be used immediately before and for a short time after surgery to lower risk of infection following cesarean section, cholecystectomy, vaginal hysterectomy, or other procedures.

**CONTRAINDICATIONS**　**Allergy to cephalosporin, penicillin, or other beta-lactam antibiotics** Anaphylaxis and death are possible. • Although cross-allergenicity is not complete, the risk of allergic reactions is increased by a history of reactions to related drugs.

**DRUG INTERACTIONS**　**Aminoglycosides** have additive or synergistic antibacterial action with some cephalosporins when used to treat relatively resistant organisms such as *Pseudomonas aeruginosa*. **Nephrotoxic drugs** such as the antibiotics vancomycin, colistin, polymyxin B, and aminoglycosides may increase the risk of renal damage with cephalosporins.　**Probenecid** slows excretion of most cephalosporins by blocking secretion sites in renal tubules.

**DIAGNOSTIC TEST INTERFERENCE**　**Coombs' test** (antiglobulin test) is falsely positive in about 3% of patients receiving cephalosporins.　**Creatinine** measured by the Jaffe reaction may be falsely elevated by cephalosporins.　**Glucose assays** using the cupric sulfate method may be falsely elevated by cephalosporins.

## ❦ NURSING CONSIDERATIONS
### Side effects, toxicities, and associated nursing actions
**CNS** Fatigue, dizziness, vertigo, malaise, and headache can occur. Toxic accumulation can cause paranoid reactions.

- Be alert for development of neurologic changes. Fatigue and malaise may be difficult to diagnose in seriously ill patients.
- If dizziness occurs, caution patients to avoid driving or operating hazardous equipment until the effects of the medication wear off.

**Blood** Cephalosporins cause a positive Coombs' test (direct antiglobulin test) in at least 3% of treated patients. Neutropenia, thrombocytopenia, thrombocythemia, and leukopenia are rare, mild, and usually reversible effects. Certain cephalosporins are more frequently associated with blood dyscrasias (see monographs for moxalactam, cefoperazone, and cefamandole).

- Monitor complete blood count, WBC differential count, and platelet count.
- Assess for bruising, unexplained bleeding, pallor, fatigue, malaise, fever, and sore throat.

**GI** Nausea, vomiting, diarrhea and other signs of GI distress are most common with oral cephalosporins. Pseudomembranous colitis may be induced by antibiotics of the cephalosporin class.

- Assess the patient for development of GI symptoms. Report the development of diarrhea to the physician.
- Monitor intake and output.
- Monitor weight of infants, children, and elderly patients.

**Renal** Transient increases in BUN and serum creatinine levels have been observed. Renal toxicity is increased in old age or by preexisting renal impairment.

- Monitor serum creatinine and BUN levels.
- Monitor intake and output and weight, especially in elderly or those with preexisting renal disease.
- Monitor serum electrolyte levels, especially in patients with known renal or cardiovascular disease.

**Liver** Transient increases in SGOT (AST), SGPT (ALT), or alkaline phosphatase have occurred. Other mild, reversible effects are rarely observed.

- Monitor liver function tests.
- Assess for development of liver dysfunction: jaundice, right upper quadrant abdominal pain, change in color or consistency of stools, fever, and malaise.

**Allergic** Allergic reactions are the most common side effects for most cephalosporins, occurring in up to 5% of patients. Reactions include rashes, urticaria, pruritis, fever, chills, eosinophilia, joint pain, edema, erythema, exfoliative dermatitis, serum sickness, and anaphylaxis.

- Before administering any antibacterial agents, assess patient for history of allergy to any drugs. Use cephalosporins cautiously in patients with previous allergic response to cephalosporins or penicillins (cross-sensitivity).
- Have readily available drugs, equipment, and personnel to treat acute allergic response in any setting where antibacterial agents are administered.
- Note clearly and prominently any drug allergy on patient's chart, kardex, or other records.
- Visually inspect patient regularly for development of rashes or skin changes. Assess for other signs or symptoms (see above) that may indicate allergic response.
- Monitor vital signs.
- Serum sickness resembles an allergic response, characterized by rapid onset of rash, urticaria, fever, arthralgia, edema, and hepatosplenomegaly. It usually develops 7 to 15 days after the drug is started but may develop sooner. The incidence increases with age.

**Other** Suprainfection can occur as with any extended-spectrum antibiotic. Suprainfection may arise when broad-spectrum antibiotics disrupt normal bacterial flora, allowing a sudden overgrowth of an endogenous or exogenous organism, thus producing an active infection where one had not before existed.

- Assess for development of suprainfection: anogenital itching, vaginal itching and/or discharge, diarrhea or fever, or oral irritation or ulceration. Instruct patient to report the development of any unexpected sign or symptom.

### Nursing interventions related to drug administration

- Check for expiration date before preparing and administering prescribed dose.
- Shake liquid suspension preparations well as drug may have settled to the bottom of the bottle.

Instruct patient to do the same if patient is to self-treat at home.

- Nurses allergic to an antibacterial drug in a class or chemically related class should wear gloves while preparing ordered doses of drugs to avoid skin contamination.
- IM antibacterial preparations should be administered in a large muscle mass, such as the dorsogluteal site or rectus femoris muscle in adults or the vastus lateralis muscle in infants and small children. Use anatomical landmarks to carefully identify site. Aspirate carefully before injecting medication to avoid inadvertent IV injection. If blood is aspirated, withdraw needle and prepare fresh dose of medication. Record injection site and rotate sites.
- Many of the IV cephalosporins are associated with phlebitis, thrombophlebitis, pain, and induration. Change IV insertion sites frequently, using small scalp vein needles when possible; monitor IV infusion rate carefully; inspect insertion site and extremity regularly for redness, swelling, and irritation; and ascertain that IV is infusing well and appears to be patent before administering IV doses. Instruct patient to report pain or signs of irritation.
- Observe patients carefully for the development of acute allergic reactions during the first 30 minutes following parenteral doses, especially the first dose.

**Patient and family education**

- Review with patient and/or family the expected benefits and possible side effects of therapy.
- Instruct patient to report the development of any unexplained symptom or side effect.
- Review with patients the need to take the medication as ordered, for the specified period of time (usually 7 to 10 days). Unused medications should be discarded. Patients should not share medications with others.
- Encourage patients with a history of an allergic response to a drug to wear a medical identification tag or bracelet noting their allergy.
- Cephalosporins interfere with urine glucose testing when methods using cupric sulfate are used (e.g., Benedict's solution, Clinitest). Cephalosporins do not interfere with glucose oxidase tests (e.g., Diastix, Tes-Tape). Inform diabetic patients about this drug effect and encourage them to monitor blood glucose while taking these drugs.
- Teach patients to read labels carefully and to discard drugs that have passed their expiration date, as they may not work as desired.
- Instruct patients to store liquid forms in the refrigerator unless directed otherwise on the bottle label. Store tablet or capsule forms in a cool, dry place. Avoid storing drugs in the bathroom where moisture and heat may cause the drugs to break down. Avoid freezing medications.
- Review with patients that cephalosporins can be taken on a full or empty stomach. If the medicine causes GI distress, it should be taken with meals or a snack. When taken on an empty stomach, the drug should be taken with a full glass (8 oz) of water or other liquid.
- Many antibacterial agents are excreted through breastmilk. Instruct lactating women to check with their physicians before breastfeeding while taking antibacterials.
- Instruct patients to keep these and all medications out of the reach of children.

## aztreonam   (az-TREE-oh-nam)         antibiotic*

- aztreonam: Azactam

**MECHANISM OF ACTION**   Monobactams are highly resistant to beta-lactamases and are chemically different from other beta-lactam antibiotics. Monobactams are also unusual by being effective only against gram-negative aerobic bacteria. The mechanism of action is apparently the same as for other beta-lactam antibiotics, as bacterial cell wall is disrupted. Bacterial growth is inhibited or the bacteria are killed.

**INDICATIONS**   **Infections caused by aerobic gram-negative bacteria** Susceptible bacteria include *E. coli, Haemophilus influenzae, Klebsiella, Neisseria gonorrhoeae, Proteus, Providencia, P. aeruginosa,* and *Serratia.* • Infections to be treated may include infections of the respiratory or genitourinary tract.

*Monobactam.

**CONTRAINDICATIONS**  **Allergy to cephalosporin, penicillin, or other beta-lactam antibiotics** Anaphylaxis and death are possible. • Although cross-allergenicity is not complete, the risk of allergic reactions is increased by a history of reactions to related drugs.

**DOSAGE**  **IM, IV:**  **ADULTS:** Doses of 0.5 to 2 g every 8 hours have been used in trials. Doses are reduced in renal failure.  *Special patient populations:*  **RENAL IMPAIRMENT:** Doses are reduced, based on the degree of renal failure.  **CHILDREN:** Doses have not been established.  **PREGNANCY:** FDA pregnancy category B.

**PREPARATIONS**  *Powder to prepare solution for injection:* 1 or 2 g.

**DRUG INTERACTIONS**  See entry for drug class (p. 278).

**DIAGNOSTIC TEST INTERFERENCE**  See entry for drug class (p. 278).

**FATE**  Aztreonam is poorly absorbed from the GI tract and must be administered parenterally. Absorption from IM sites is rapid and complete, with *peak* serum concentrations achieved within 1 hour. Distribution of the drug appears good, producing adequate concentrations in the CNS when the meninges are inflamed. Excretion is primarily renal as the unchanged drug. The elimination *half-life* is 1.7 hours but is extended in renal failure.

## ❦ NURSING CONSIDERATIONS

### Side effects, toxicities, and associated nursing actions

**Liver** AST and ALT are elevated in 5% of patients.

**Other** Fatigue and a strange taste during infusion are reported in 5% to 7% of treated patients.

• Assess for development of fatigue. Monitor liver function tests.

• Reassure patient that unusual taste occasionally occurs.

• Other reactions to aztreonam are similar to other beta-lactam antibiotics. See entry for drug class (p. 278).

### Nursing interventions related to drug administration

• See entry for drug class (p. 279).

### Patient and family education

• See entry for drug class (p. 280).

---

## cefaclor  (SEF-a-klor)  antibiotic*

• cefaclor: Ceclor

**MECHANISM OF ACTION**  See entry for drug class (p. 277).

**INDICATIONS**  **Infections caused by gram-positive bacteria** Susceptible bacteria include *Streptococcus pneumoniae*, group A beta-hemolytic streptococci, and staphylococci. • Infections caused by these organisms include otitis media, pneumonia, and upper respiratory tract infections.  **Infections caused by H. influenzae** Otitis media and pneumonia caused by this organism may respond to cefaclor.  **Urinary tract infections** Susceptible organisms may include *E. coli*, *Proteus mirabilis*, *Klebsiella*, or *Staphylococcus*.

**CONTRAINDICATIONS**  **Allergy to cephalosporin, penicillin, or other beta-lactam antibiotics** Anaphylaxis and death are possible. • Although cross-allergenicity is not complete, the risk of allergic reactions is increased by a history of reactions to related drugs.

**DOSAGE**  **PO:**  **ADULTS:** 250 to 500 mg every 8 hours not to exceed a total daily dose of 4 g.  **CHILDREN OLDER THAN 1 MONTH:** 20 to 40 mg/kg daily in divided doses every 8 hours, not to exceed a total daily dose of 1 g. *Special patient populations:*  **PREGNANCY:** FDA pregnancy category B.

**PREPARATIONS**  *Capsules:* 250 or 500 mg. *Suspension, oral:* 125 or 250 mg in each 5 ml. Reconstituted suspensions are stable 14 days at 2° to 8° C.

**DRUG INTERACTIONS**  See entry for drug class (p. 278).

**DIAGNOSTIC TEST INTERFERENCES**  See entry for drug class (p. 278).

**FATE**  Oral absorption is complete but may be impeded by food. *Peak* serum concentrations occur at 0.5 to 1 hour. Elimination is primarily renal as unchanged drug, with *half-life* of 0.6 to 0.9 hours.

*Second-generation cephalosporin.

## 🦋 NURSING CONSIDERATIONS

### Side effects, toxicities, and associated nursing actions

**Blood** Infants and children occasionally show transient lymphocytosis.

• Monitor WBC differential count.

**Allergic** Serum sickness is more common with cefaclor than with most other cephalosporins. This increased incidence is probably caused by the repeated use of the drug to treat episodes of otitis media.

• See entry for of drug class (p. 279) for a description of serum sickness. Discontinuing the medication and treating with corticosteroids and antihistamines may help.

• For other reactions, see entry for drug class (p. 278).

### Patient and family education

• This drug may be taken without regard to meals.

• For other guidelines, see entry for drug class (p. 280).

---

## cefadroxil    (sef-uh-DROX-ill)                                          antibiotic*

• cefadroxil: Duricef, Ultracef

**MECHANISM OF ACTION**    See entry for drug class (p. 277).

**INDICATIONS**    **Infections caused by gram-positive bacteria** Susceptible bacteria include group A beta-hemolytic streptococci and staphylococci. • Infections caused by these organisms include pharyngitis, tonsilitis, and skin and soft tissue infections.    **Urinary tract infections** Susceptible organisms may include *E. coli, P. mirabilis,* or *Klebsiella.*

**CONTRAINDICATIONS**    **Allergy to cephalosporin, penicillin, or other beta-lactam antibiotics** Anaphylaxis and death are possible. • Although cross-allergenicity is not complete, the risk of allergic reactions is increased by a history of reactions to related drugs.

**DOSAGE**    **PO:**    **ADULTS:** 1 to 2 g daily in 1 or 2 doses.    **CHILDREN:** 15 mg/kg twice daily.    *Special patient populations:*    **RENAL IMPAIRMENT:** Doses are reduced, based on the degree of renal failure.    **PREGNANCY:** FDA pregnancy category B.

**PREPARATIONS**    *Tablets:* 1 g. *Capsules:* 500 mg. *Suspension, oral:* 125, 250, or 500 mg in each 5 ml. Suspensions are stable 14 days at 2° to 8° C.

**DRUG INTERACTIONS**    See entry for drug class (p. 278).

**DIAGNOSTIC TEST INTERFERENCES**    See entry for drug class (p. 278).

**FATE**    Oral absorption is complete and, unlike cephalexin, not impeded by food. *Peak* serum concentrations occur at about 1 hour, which is similar to cephalexin. Elimination of both drugs is primarily renal. Cefadroxil has a slightly longer elimination *half-life* than cephalexin, accounting for the twice daily dosing of cefadroxil.

## 🦋 NURSING CONSIDERATIONS

### Side effects, toxicities, and associated nursing actions

• See entry for drug class (p. 278).

### Patient and family education

• This drug may be administered without regard to meals.

• For other guidelines, see entry for drug class (p. 280).

---

## cefamandole nafate    (sef-uh-MAN-dole)                                  antibiotic†

• cefamandole nafate: Mandol

**MECHANISM OF ACTION**    See entry for drug class (p. 277).

*First-generation cephalosporin.
†Second-generation cephalosporin.

**INDICATIONS**    **Infections caused by gram-positive bacteria** Susceptible bacteria include *S. pneumoniae*, group A beta-hemolytic streptococci, group D streptococci, and staphylococci. • Infections caused by these organisms include pneumonia, peritonitis, septicemia, and infections of the urinary tract, skin, and skin structures.    **Infections caused by Enterobacter** Urinary tract infections, peritonitis, and infections of skin or skin structures may respond to cefamandole.    **Infections caused by gram-negative bacteria** Susceptible organisms may include *E. coli, H. influenzae, Klebsiella,* or *P. mirabilis.* • Infections caused by these organisms include pneumonia, urinary tract infections, peritonitis, septicemia, and infections of skin and skin structures.    **Infections caused by anaerobic bacteria** Cefamandole has been used to treat or, in prophylaxis, to prevent mixed infections at sites including the respiratory and reproductive tracts.

**CONTRAINDICATIONS**    **Allergy to cephalosporin, penicillin, or other beta-lactam antibiotics** Anaphylaxis and death are possible. • Although cross-allergenicity is not complete, the risk of allergic reactions is increased by a history of reactions to related drugs.

**DOSAGE**    **IM, IV:**    **ADULTS:** 500 mg to 1 g every 4 to 8 hours, not to exceed a total daily dose of 12 g. **CHILDREN OLDER THAN 1 MONTH:** 50 to 100 mg/kg daily in divided doses every 4 to 8 hours; in rare cases dosage up to 150 mg/kg daily may be used. *Special patient populations:* **RENAL IMPAIRMENT:** Doses are reduced, based on the degree of renal failure. **PREGNANCY:** FDA pregnancy category B.

**PREPARATIONS**    *Solution, injection:* 500 mg, 1, 2, and 10 g. All contain 63 mg sodium carbonate for each gram of cefamandole. The 10 g preparation is a pharmacy bulk package. *Solution, infusion:* 1 or 2 g. Both contain 63 mg sodium carbonate for each gram of cefamandole. For IM administration, each gram of cefamandole should be dissolved in 3 ml sterile or bacteriostatic water, 0.9% sodium chloride injection, or bacteriostatic 0.9% sodium chloride injection. The solution to be injected is 285 mg/ml. For IV administration, each gram should be dissolved in 10 to 20 ml sterile water for injection, 5% dextrose injection, or 0.9% sodium chloride injection. One gram of cefamandole in 22 ml of water forms an isotonic solution. Avoid solutions containing magnesium or calcium (e.g., Ringer's or lactated Ringer's injection).

**DRUG INTERACTIONS**    **Alcohol** may cause a disulfiram-like reaction, with facial flushing, sweating, tachycardia, hypotension, headache, nausea, or other symptoms. For other interactions, see overview of drug class (p. 278).

**DIAGNOSTIC TEST INTERFERENCES**    See entry for drug class (p. 278).

**FATE**    Cefamandole nafate is not adequately absorbed orally. Absorption from IM sites is good, producing *peak* serum concentrations within 30 to 120 minutes. Cefamandole nafate is rapidly and almost completely hydrolyzed to cefamandole, a more active antibiotic than cefamandole nafate. Elimination is almost all by renal mechanisms. The elimination *half-life* is 0.5 to 2.1 hours in healthy adults but is increased in renal failure.

## ❦ NURSING CONSIDERATIONS

### Side effects, toxicities, and associated nursing actions

**Blood** Hypoprothrombinemia and vitamin K deficiency have been reported. These reactions are most likely to occur in elderly or debilitated patients or in those with alcohol dependency or impaired renal function. Vitamin K may be administered prophylactically in these patients to prevent serious bleeding reactions.
- Monitor prothrombin time.
- Assess for signs of bruising or bleeding, hematuria, nosebleed, or blood in stool.
- Vitamin K may be ordered prophylactically or because of documented vitamin K deficiency. IM injections in the presence of a prolonged prothrombin time may cause hematomas at the injection sites. Inspect injection sites closely. Apply firm but gentle pressure over injection site after administering injection to prevent hematoma formation.
- For other side effects, see entry for drug class (p. 278).

### Nursing interventions related to drug administration
- See Preparations above.

- For direct IV push injection, dilute as directed and administer dose over 3 to 5 minutes.
- For intermittent IV infusion, dilute as directed. Rate of administration varies with final volume.
- If an aminoglycoside is being administered concomitantly with cefamandole nafate, two separate infusion sites should be used for the two drugs.
- See entry for drug class (p. 279).

### Patient and family education
- See entry for drug class (p. 280).
- Disulfiram-like reactions may occur if alcohol is ingested within 48 to 72 hours of a dose of cefamandole. This intense reaction is characterized by flushing of the face, palpitations, rapid heart rate, and low blood pressure. Instruct patients to avoid the use of alcohol for at least 3 days following the last dose of this antibacterial.

## cefazolin sodium  (sef-AZ-oh-lin)  antibiotic*

- cefazolin sodium: Ancef, Kefzol

**MECHANISM OF ACTION**  See entry for drug class (p. 277).

**INDICATIONS**  **Infections caused by gram-positive bacteria** Susceptible bacteria include *S. pneumoniae*, streptococci including group A beta-hemolytic strains, and *Staphylococcus aureus*. • Infections caused by these organisms include septicemia, endocarditis, and infections of the respiratory tract, skin and soft tissue, biliary tract, bone, and joints.  **Infections caused by gram-negative bacteria** Susceptible organisms may include *Enterobacter, enterococci, E. coli, H. influenzae, Klebsiella,* and *P. mirabilis*. • Infections caused by these organisms include septicemia and infections of the respiratory tract, genitourinary tract, and biliary tract.  **Perioperative prophylaxis** Cafezolin is indicated only for certain surgical procedures likely to produce infections (vaginal hysterectomy, cholecystectomy with obstructions) or for high-risk patients (those with artificial heart valves, artificial joints).

**CONTRAINDICATIONS**  **Allergy to cephalosporin, penicillin, or other beta-lactam antibiotics** Anaphylaxis and death are possible. • Although cross-allergenicity is not complete, the risk of allergic reactions is increased by a history of reactions to related drugs.

**DOSAGE**  IM, IV:  ADULTS: 250 mg to 1.5 g every 6 hours, up to 12 g daily.  CHILDREN OVER 1 MONTH OF AGE: 25 to 50 mg/kg daily in 3 or 4 equal doses; the maximum dose is 100 mg/kg daily.  *Special patient populations:*  RENAL IMPAIRMENT: Doses are reduced, based on the degree of renal failure.  PREGNANCY: FDA pregnancy category B.

**PREPARATIONS**  *Cefazolin sodium, powder to prepare solution for injection:* 250 or 500 mg. 1, 5, and 10 g bulk packages are available for pharmacy use. *Powder to prepare solution for infusion:* 500 mg or 1 g. Some preparations contain 0.04% polysorbate 80. *Cefazolin sodium in dextrose, powder to prepare solution for injection:* 500 mg or 1 g in 5% dextrose. Cefazolin and its solutions should be protected from light. The sterile powder should be stored at 15° to 30° C; frozen preparations should be maintained below −20° C.

**DRUG INTERACTIONS**  See entry for drug class (p. 278).

**DIAGNOSTIC TEST INTERFERENCES**  See entry for drug class (p. 278).

**FATE**  Cefazolin is not absorbed orally and must be given intramuscularly or intravenously. *Peak* serum concentrations are achieved 1 to 2 hours following IM injections. Cefazolin penetrates most tissues adequately but is not reliably distributed to obstructed bile ducts, prostatic tissues, human milk, or cerebrospinal fluid. Cefazolin is excreted exclusively as unchanged drug by the kidneys. The elimination *half-life* is 1.2 to 2.2 hours in normal healthy adults but is greatly prolonged in renal failure.

### ☙ NURSING CONSIDERATIONS
#### Side effects, toxicities, and associated nursing actions
- See entry for drug class (p. 278).

---

*First-generation cephalosporin.

### Nursing interventions related to drug administration
- See Preparations above.
- For direct IV push, reconstitute powder as directed on vial. Further dilute these solutions with at least 5 ml for Ancef brand or 10 ml for Kefzol brand. Infuse ordered dose at a rate of 1 g over 5 minutes or longer, based on volume of fluid and age and condition of patient.
- For intermittent infusion, dilute reconstituted solution with 50 to 100 ml of a compatible IV solution. Infuse over 30 minutes to 1 hour, depending on volume of fluid and age and condition of patient.
- Commercially available frozen preparations should be thawed at room temperature before being administered. These thawed preparations are for intermittent infusion only, not direct IV push infusion.
- IM injections should be made into large muscle masses, as described in the entry for drug class (p. 279).

### Patient and family education
- See entry for drug class (p. 280).
- Disulfiram-like reactions may occur if alcohol is ingested within 48 to 72 hours of a dose of cefazolin. This intense reaction is characterized by flushing of the face, palpitations, rapid heart rate, and low blood pressure. Instruct patients to avoid the use of alcohol for at least 3 days following the last dose of this antibacterial.

---

## cefmenoxime sodium   (sef-men-OX-eem)   antibiotic*

- cefmenoxime sodium (investigational): Cefmax

**MECHANISM OF ACTION**   See entry for drug class (p. 277).

**INDICATIONS**   **Infections caused by gram-negative bacteria** Susceptible organisms may include *E. coli, Enterobacter, Serratia, Klebsiella,* or *P. mirabilis.* • Infections caused by these organisms include pneumonia, urinary tract infections, and septicemia.

**CONTRAINDICATIONS**   See entry for drug class (p. 278).

**DOSAGE**   IM, IV:   **ADULTS:** Not fully established.   *Special patient populations:*   **CHILDREN:** Doses not established.   **RENAL IMPAIRMENT:** Reduce dose in renal failure.   **PREGNANCY:** FDA pregnancy category B.

**PREPARATIONS**   *Solution for injection:* currently investigational in the United States.

**DRUG INTERACTIONS**   See entry for drug class (p. 278).

**DIAGNOSTIC TEST INTERFERENCES**   See entry for drug class (p. 278).

**FATE**   Cefmenoxime sodium is not adequately absorbed orally. Absorption from IM sites is good, producing *peak* serum concentrations within 1 hour. Cefmenoxime is not metabolized and is excreted by the kidneys. The elimination *half-life* is 1 hour in healthy adults but is increased in renal failure.

## ❧ NURSING CONSIDERATIONS

### Side effects, toxicities, and associated nursing actions
- See entry for drug class (p. 278).

### Nursing interventions related to drug administration
- Consult manufacturer's literature for current guidelines for dilution and rate of administration.
- For IM injection, large muscle masses should be used as described in the entry for drug class (p. 279).
- Inspect drug powder or solution before use. Discolored preparations or solutions containing particulate matter should not be used.
- If an aminoglycoside is being administered concurrently with cefmenoxime, two separate infusion sites should be used.

*Third-generation cephalosporin.

**Patient and family education**
- See entry for drug class (p. 280).

---

## cefonicid sodium    (sef-oh-NIGH-sid)                     antibiotic*

- cefonicid sodium: Monicid

**MECHANISM OF ACTION**    See entry for drug class (p. 277).

**INDICATIONS**    **Infections caused by gram-positive bacteria** Susceptible bacteria include *S. pneumoniae,* group A beta-hemolytic streptococci, and staphylococci. • Infections caused by these organisms include pneumonia, septicemia, and infections of the urinary tract, skin, and skin structures. • First-generation cephalosporins are generally more effective for these infections. **Infections caused by gram-negative bacteria** Susceptible organisms may include *E. coli, H. influenzae, Klebsiella,* or *P. mirabilis.* • Infections caused by these organisms include pneumonia, urinary tract infections, and septicemia.

**CONTRAINDICATIONS**    **Allergy to cephalosporin, penicillin, or other beta-lactam antibiotics** Anaphylaxis and death are possible. • Although cross-allergenicity is not complete, the risk of allergic reactions is increased by a history of reactions to related drugs.

**DOSAGE**    **IM, IV:**    **ADULTS:** 1 g once daily, with rare cases requiring up to 2 g daily. Dosage reduced in renal failure.    *Special patient populations:*    **RENAL IMPAIRMENT:** Doses are reduced, based on the degree of renal failure.    **CHILDREN:** Doses not established.    **PREGNANCY:** FDA pregnancy category B.

**PREPARATIONS**    *Powder to prepare solution for injection:* 500 mg, 1, 2, and 10 g. The 10 g preparation is a pharmacy bulk package. *Powder to prepare solution for infusion:* 1 g. Before reconstitution, vials should be stored at 2° to 8° C and protected from light. Solutions may turn yellow without loss of potency, but solutions with extensive discoloration or precipitates should be discarded. For IM administration, 500 mg should be dissolved in 2 ml sterile water. The solution to be injected is 250 mg/ml. Alternatively, 1 g is dissolved in 2.5 ml sterile water to produce a 325 mg/ml solution. For IV administration, cefonicid may be dissolved as for IM administration and used directly or further diluted in 50 to 100 ml for infusion.

**DRUG INTERACTIONS**    See entry for drug class (p. 278).

**DIAGNOSTIC TEST INTERFERENCES**    See entry for drug class (p. 278).

**FATE**    Cefonicid sodium is not adequately absorbed orally. Absorption from IM sites is good, producing *peak* serum concentrations within 1 to 2 hours. Cefonicid is not metabolized and is excreted by the kidneys. The elimination *half-life* is 3.5 to 5.8 hours in healthy adults but is increased in renal failure.

## ❦ NURSING CONSIDERATIONS

### Side effects, toxicities, and associated nursing actions
**Local effects** About 6% of patients receiving IM injections of cefonicid report pain and discomfort.
- Rotate injection sites.
- If a 2 g or larger dose is to be administered intramuscularly, divide the dose and administer as two injections.
- Other reactions to cefonicid are similar to those of other cephalosporins.
- See entry for drug class (p. 278).

### Nursing interventions related to drug administration
- See Preparations above.
- For direct IV push, reconstitute as directed, then administer prescribed dose over 3 to 5 minutes.
- For intermittent IV infusion, further dilute reconstituted solution in 50 to 100 ml of compatible IV fluid and administer over 20 to 30 minutes.

*Second-generation cephalosporin.

- IM injections should be made into large muscle masses, as described in the entry for drug class (p. 279).

**Patient and family education**
- See entry for drug class (p. 280).
- Disulfiram-like reactions may occur if alcohol is ingested within 48 to 72 hours of a dose of cefonicid. This intense reaction is characterized by flushing of the face, palpitations, rapid heart rate, and low blood pressure. Instruct patients to avoid the use of alcohol for at least 3 days following the last dose of this antibacterial.
- Some patients experience a flulike syndrome. Instruct patients to notify physician if they have a fever.

---

## cefoperazone sodium   (sef-oh-PEAR-uh-zone)                                    antibiotic*

- cefoperazone sodium: Cefobid

**MECHANISM OF ACTION**   See entry for drug class (p. 277).

**INDICATIONS**   **Infections caused by gram-positive bacteria** Although *S. pneumoniae,* group A beta-hemolytic streptococci, and staphylococci may be susceptible, penicillins or first-generation cephalosporins are more likely to be effective.   **Infections caused by gram-negative bacteria** Susceptible bacteria may include *Enterobacter, Escherichia coli, Haemophilus influenzae, Klebsiella, Proteus,* or *P. aeruginosa.* • Infections caused by these organisms include pneumonia, septicemia, peritonitis, gynecologic infections, and infections of the urinary tract, skin, or skin structures. • Although cefoperazone may be effective, other third-generation cephalosporins have higher potency.   **Infections caused by mixed aerobic-anaerobic bacteria** Peritonitis, abdominal abscesses, gynecologic infections, endometritis, and pelvic inflammatory disease (PID) have responded to cefoperazone. • Susceptible organisms contributing to these infections include *Bacteroides, Bacteroides fragilis,* and *Clostridium.*

**CONTRAINDICATIONS**   **Allergy to cephalosporin, penicillin, or other beta-lactam antibiotics** Anaphylaxis and death are possible. Although cross-allergenicity is not complete, the risk of allergic reactions is increased by a history of reactions to related drugs.

**DOSAGE**   **IM, IV:**   **ADULTS:** 2 to 4 g daily in equal doses every 12 hours. Doses as high as 16 g daily have rarely been used without evident harm.   **CHILDREN:** Pediatric doses are not established, although a few neonates and children have received 25 to 100 mg/kg every 12 hours.   *Special patient populations:*   **PREGNANCY:** FDA pregnancy category B.

**PREPARATIONS**   *Powder to prepare solution for injection:* 1 or 2 g. *Powder to prepare solution for IV infusion:* 1 or 2 g. Before reconstitution, vials should be stored at 2° to 8° C and protected from light. Solutions may turn slightly yellow without loss of potency. Manufacturer's directions for reconstitution should be followed. IM solutions require two-step dilution in water and lidocaine.

**DRUG INTERACTIONS**   See entry for drug class (p. 278).

**DIAGNOSTIC TEST INTERFERENCE**   See entry for drug class (p. 278).

**FATE**   Cefoperazone is not absorbed from the GI tract and must be administered intramuscularly or intravenously. *Peak* serum concentrations are achieved 1 to 2 hours following IM doses. Concentrations in the CNs are low in healthy adults but increase when inflammation is present. Cefoperazone is unusual among cephalosporins because the drug is eliminated principally in bile. The elimination *half-life* is 1.6 to 2.6 hours in healthy adults and in unchanged by renal impairment. The elimination half-life is extended in patients with impaired hepatic function and in neonates.

**❦ NURSING CONSIDERATIONS**
### Side effects, toxicities, and associated nursing actions
**Blood** Hypoprothrombinemia, vitamin K deficiency, and bleeding have occurred with cefoperazone. Patients most at risk are elderly or debilitated patients or those suffering from renal failure. Vitamin K often alleviates the condition. Vitamin K deficiency is most likely in patients with malabsorption, alcohol dependence, or in those receiving prolonged hyperalimentation.

---

*Third-generation cephalosporin.

- Monitor prothrombin time.
- Assess for signs of bruising or bleeding, hematuria, nosebleed, or blood in stool.
- Vitamin K may be ordered prophylactically or because of documented vitamin K deficiency. IM injections in the presence of a prolonged prothrombin time may cause hematomas at the injection sites. Inspect injection sites closely. Apply firm but gentle pressure over injection site after administering injection to prevent hematoma formation.

**GI** Up to 7% of treated patients experience diarrhea. There have been a few reports of antibiotic-induced colitis.
- Monitor patient for development of diarrhea.
- Monitor intake and output.
- Report development of diarrhea to physician.
- For other reactions, see entry for drug class (p. 278).

### Nursing interventions related to drug administration
- See Preparations above.
- Although direct IV infusion of this drug has been done, the manufacturer does not recommend this route of administration. Administer doses direct IV push over a 3- to 5-minute period.
- For intermittent IV infusion, the reconstituted drug should be further diluted with 20 to 40 ml per gram of drug. The resulting infusion should be administered over 15 to 30 minutes.
- For continuous infusion, the diluted drug may be administered over 6 to 24 hours, depending on total volume and concentration of drug.
- IM injections should be made into large muscle masses as described in the overview of drug class (p. 280).
- See manufacturer's directions for preparation of IM dilutions (two-step process is described).
- IM injections diluted with bacteriostatic water containing benzyl alcohol should not be administered to neonates.
- Patients with allergy to lidocaine should not receive dilutions containing lidocaine.
- If an aminoglycoside is being administered concurrently to the patient, separate infusion sites should be used.

### Patient and family education
- See entry for drug class (p. 280).
- Disulfiram-like reactions may occur if alcohol is ingested within 48 to 72 hours of a dose of cefoperazone. This intense reaction is characterized by flushing of the face, palpitations, rapid heart rate, and low blood pressure. Instruct patients to avoid the use of alcohol for at least 3 days following the last dose of this antibacterial.

## ceforanide    (seh-FOR-uh-nide)                                              antibiotic*

- ceforanide: Precef

**MECHANISM OF ACTION**    See entry for drug class (p. 277).

**INDICATIONS**    **Infections caused by gram-positive bacteria** Susceptible bacteria include *S. pneumoniae*, group A beta-hemolytic streptococci, group B streptococci, and staphylococci. • Infections caused by these organisms include pneumonia, septicemia, and infections of the bones, skin, and skin structures. • First-generation cephalosporins are generally more effective for these infections.    **Infections caused by gram-negative bacteria** Susceptible organisms may include *E. coli, Klebsiella,* or *P. mirabilis.* • Infections caused by these organisms include pneumonia, urinary tract infections, septicemia, and infections of bones, skin, or skin structures.

**CONTRAINDICATIONS**    **Allergy to cephalosporin, penicillin, or other beta-lactam antibiotics** Anaphylaxis and death are possible. Although cross-allergenicity is not complete, the risk of allergic reactions is increased by a history of reactions to related drugs.

**DOSAGE**    **IM, IV**    **ADULTS:** 0.5 to 1 g every 12 hours, with rare cases requiring up to 4 g every 12 hours. Dosage reduced in renal failure.    **CHILDREN OVER 1 YEAR:** 20 to 40 mg/kg daily in equal doses

*Second-generation cephalosporin.

every 12 hours. *Special patient populations:* RENAL IMPAIRMENT: Doses are reduced, based on the degree of renal failure. PREGNANCY: FDA pregnancy category B.

**PREPARATIONS** *Powder to prepare solution for injection:* 500 mg, 1 g, and 10 g. The 10 g preparation is a pharmacy bulk package. All preparations contain lysine. *Powder to prepare solution for infusion:* 500 mg or 1 g. Both preparations contain lysine. Vials must be shaken while the drug is being dissolved to ensure that ceforanide lysine is formed. Solutions may turn yellow without loss of potency, but solutions with extensive discoloration or precipitates should be discarded. For IM administration, ceforanide solutions should be 250 mg/ml. For IV administration, ceforanide may be dissolved as for IM administration and used for infusion. For direct IV injection, concentrations should not exceed 100 mg/ml.

**DRUG INTERACTIONS** See entry for drug class (p. 278).

**DIAGNOSTIC TEST INTERFERENCES** See entry for drug class (p. 278).

**FATE** Ceforanide is not adequately absorbed orally. Absorption from IM sites is good, producing *peak* serum concentrations within 1 hour. Ceforanide is not metabolized and is excreted by the kidneys. The elimination *half-life* is 2.6 to 3.3 hours in healthy adults but is increased in renal failure.

**♥ NURSING CONSIDERATIONS**

### Side effects, toxicities, and associated nursing actions

**Liver** Mild, transient increases in AST (SGOT), ALT (SGPT), and alkaline phosphatase occur in up to 11% of patients.
* Monitor liver function tests.
* Assess for development of liver dysfunction: jaundice, right upper quadrant abdominal pain, and change in color or consistency of stools.

**Renal** Up to 11% of patients show transient increases in serum creatinine and BUN.
* Monitor serum creatinine and BUN.
* Monitor intake and ouptut and weight, especially in the elderly or those with known renal disease.
* Monitor serum electrolytes, especially in patients with known renal or cardiovascular disease.
* Other reactions to ceforanide are similar to those of other cephalosporins. See entry for drug class (p. 278).

### Nursing interventions related to drug administration
* See Preparations above.
* For direct IV push, dilute as directed to a concentration not exceeding 100 mg/ml. Administer prescribed dose over 3 to 5 minutes.
* For intermittent IV infusion, dilute as directed and infuse dose over 30 minutes.
* For IM injections, large muscle masses should be used as described in the Overview Of Drug Class (p. 279).

### Patient and family education
* See entry for drug class (p. 280).

---

## cefotaxime sodium  (sef-oh-TAX-eem)        antibiotic\*

* cefotaxime sodium: Claforan

**MECHANISM OF ACTION** See entry for drug class (p. 277).

**INDICATIONS** **Infections caused by gram-positive bacteria** Although *S. pneumoniae,* group A beta-hemolytic streptococci, and staphylococci may be susceptible, penicillins or first-generation cephalosporins are more likely to be effective. **Infections caused by gram-negative bacteria** Susceptible bacteria may include *Citrobacter, Enterobacter, E. coli, H. influenzae, Klebsiella, Morganella morganii, Neisseria gonorrhoeae, Proteus, Providencia rettgeri, P. aeruginosa,* or *Serratia marcescens.* • Infections caused by these organisms include pneumonia, septicemia, peritonitis, gynecologic infections,

*\*Third-generation cephalosporin.*

and infections of the urinary tract, skin, or skin structures. **Infections caused by mixed aerobic-anaerobic bacteria** Peritonitis, abdominal abscesses, gynecologic infections, and skin infections have responded to cefotaxime. • Susceptible organisms contributing to these infections include *Bacteroides, Bacteroides fragilis, Peptococcus, Peptostreptococcus,* and *Clostridium.* **Gonorrhea** Cefotaxime is the only cephalosporin currently recommended as first-line therapy for infections caused by penicillinase-producing *Neisseria gonorrhoea* or nonpenicillinase-producing strains. **Meningitis** Cefotaxime may be effective alone or combined with other drugs to treat CNS infections caused by *E. coli, H. influenzae, Klebsiella pneumoniae, Neisseria meningitidis,* or *S. pneumoniae.*

**CONTRAINDICATIONS** **Allergy to cephalosporin, penicillin, or other beta-lactam antibiotics** Anaphylaxis and death are possible. • Although cross-allergenicity is not complete, the risk of allergic reactions is increased by a history of reactions to related drugs.

**DOSAGE** **IM, IV:** ADULTS AND CHILDREN OVER 50 KG: 1 to 2 g every 6 to 8 hours. Daily doses should not exceed 12 g. For gonorrhea, 1 g IM as a single dose. CHILDREN: 25 to 50 mg/kg every 12 hours for neonates or every 8 hours for ages 1 to 4 weeks. Older children receive 50 to 180 mg/kg daily in 4 to 6 equal doses. ***Special patient populations:*** PREGNANCY: FDA pregnancy category B.

**PREPARATIONS** *Powder to prepare solution for injection:* 1, 2, or 10 g. The 10 g preparation is a bulk pharmacy package. *Solution for IV infusion:* 1 or 2 g. Available as lyophiled powder for reconstitution with compatible fluids or as frozen solutions in 5% dextrose. Frozen solutions should be stored below −20° C. The powder or solutions may darken; this change may indicate loss of potency. For IM injection, sterile or bacteriostatic water is added to vials (3 ml to 1 g; 5 ml to 2 g) to make solutions of 300 to 330 mg/ml. For direct IV injection, solutions are 95 or 180 mg/ml. For infusion, solutions are approximately 18 mg/ml. Isotonic solution of cefotaxime is 1 g in 14 ml sterile water.

**DRUG INTERACTIONS** See entry for drug class (p. 278).

**DIAGNOSTIC TEST INTERFERENCE** **Glucose** assay with cupric sulfate may not be affected by cefotaxime, unlike other cephalosporins. **Creatinine** assays using the Jaffe reaction may not be affected by cefotaxime, unlike other cephalosporins. See entry for drug class (p. 278).

**FATE** Cefotaxime is not absorbed from the GI tract and must be administered IM or IV. *Peak* serum concentrations are achieved within 30 minutes following IM doses. Concentrations in the CNS are low in healthy adults but increase when inflammation is present. Cefotaxime is converted in the body to desacetylcefotaxime, an active metabolite. The elimination *half-life* of both active forms ranges from 0.9 to 1.9 hours in healthy adults. Up to 60% of a dose appears in urine as unchanged cefotaxime; an additional 24% appears in urine as desacetylcefotaxime, the active metabolite.

## NURSING CONSIDERATIONS

### Side effects, toxicities, and associated nursing actions

**Local effects** Pain, induration, phlebitis, or thrombophlebitis occurs at injection sites in up to 5% of patients.

- For other reactions, see entry for drug class (p. 278).

### Nursing interventions related to drug administration

- See Preparations above.
- For IM injection, large muscle masses should be used as described in the overview of drug class (p. 280). If an IM dose is 2 g or larger, the dose should be divided and administered in two separate injections.
- For direct IV push, dilute as directed and administer dose over 3 to 5 minutes.
- For intermittent IV infusion, dilute as directed in 50 to 100 ml of compatible IV solution. Administer dose over 20 to 30 minutes.
- Thaw frozen solutions at room temperature. Thawed solutions should be used only for intermittent IV infusions.
- Inspect drug powder or solution before use. Discolored preparations or solutions containing particulate matter should not be used.

### Patient and family education

- See entry for drug class (p. 280).

# cefotetan disodium   (sef-oh-TEE-tan)    antibiotic*

- cefotetan disodium: Cefotan

**MECHANISM OF ACTION**   Cephamycins are highly resistant to destruction by beta-lactamases and have a high degree of activity against anaerobic organisms. Other properties of cephamycins are much like those of second-generation cephalosporins. Cephamycins share the same mechanism of action as other beta-lactam antibiotics. See entry for drug class (p. 277).

**INDICATIONS**   **Infections caused by gram-positive bacteria** Although *S. pneumoniae*, group A beta-hemolytic streptococci, and staphylococci may be susceptible, penicillins or first-generation cephalosporins are more likely to be effective.    **Infections caused by gram-negative bacteria** Susceptible bacteria may include *Citrobacter, Enterobacter, E. coli, H. influenzae, Klebsiella, M. morganii, N. gonorrhoeae, Proteus, P. rettgeri,* or *S. marcescens*. • Infections caused by these organisms include pneumonia, peritonitis, gynecologic infections, and infections of the urinary tract, skin, or skin structures. **Infections caused by mixed aerobic-anaerobic bacteria** Peritonitis, abdominal abscesses, gynecologic infections, and skin infections have responded to cefotetan. • *Bacteroides fragilis* and a few other species of *Bacteroides* are reliably susceptible.

**CONTRAINDICATIONS**   **Allergy to cephalosporin, penicillin, or other beta-lactam antibiotics** Anaphylaxis and death are possible. Although cross-allergenicity is not complete, the risk of allergic reactions is increased by a history of reactions to related drugs.

**DOSAGE**   IM, IV:   ADULTS: 1 to 2 g every 12 hours; the maximum dose is 6 g daily.   *Special patient populations:*   RENAL IMPAIRMENT: Doses are reduced, based on the degree of renal failure. CHILDREN: Doses not established.   PREGNANCY: FDA pregnancy category B.

**PREPARATIONS**   *Powder to prepare solution for injection:* 1 to 2 g. *Powder to prepare solution for IV infusion:* 1 or 2 g. Vials should be stored below 22° C and protected from light. Reconstituted solutions are stable for 24 hours at room temperature and for 96 hours refrigerated. Strongly discolored solutions or solutions containing particulate matter should be discarded. For IM injection, 2 ml of diluent is added to 1 g vials to produce a concentration of 375 mg/ml or 3 ml diluent is added to 2 g vials to produce 471.5 mg/ml. Compatible diluents are sterile or bacteriostatic water, 0.5% or 1% lidocaine HCl, or normal saline solution. For IV use, dilute with sterile water 10 ml to each gram (97 to 98 mg/ml) for direct injection or dilute with 5% dextrose or 0.9% sodium chloride, 50 ml to each gram for IV infusion.

**DRUG INTERACTIONS**   See entry for drug class (p. 278).

**DIAGNOSTIC TEST INTERFERENCE**   See entry for drug class (p. 278).

**FATE**   Cefotetan is not absorbed from the GI tract and must be given parenterally. Cefotetan is not metabolized and is excreted as unchanged drug primarily by the kidneys. The elimination *half-life* is 3 to 4.6 hours in healthy adults and is increased in renal impairment.

## ❦ NURSING CONSIDERATIONS

### Side effects, toxicities, and associated nursing actions
- See entry for drug class (p. 278).

### Nursing interventions related to drug administration
- See Preparations above.
- For IM injection, large muscle masses should be used, as described in the overview of drug class (p. 280).
- For direct IV push, dilute as directed and administer dose over 3 to 5 minutes.
- For intermittent IV infusion, dilute as directed in 50 to 100 ml of compatible IV solution. Administer dose over 20 to 30 minutes.
- IM solutions reconstituted with lidocaine should not be used for IV doses.
- Inspect drug powder or solution before use. Discolored preparations or solutions containing particulate matter should not be used.

### Patient and family education
- See entry for drug class (p. 280).

*Cephamycin.

## cefoxitin sodium    (sef-OX-i-tin)                                    antibiotic*

- cefoxitin sodium: Mefoxin

**MECHANISM OF ACTION**    Cephamycins are highly resistant to destruction by beta-lactamases and have a high degree of activity against anaerobic organisms. Other properties of cephamycins are much like second-generation cephalosporins. Cephamycins share the same mechanism of action as other beta-lactam antibiotics. See entry for drug class (p. 277).

**INDICATIONS**    **Infections caused by gram-positive bacteria** Although *S. pneumoniae* and *S. aureus* may be susceptible, penicillins or first-generation cephalosporins are more likely to be effective.    **Infections caused by gram-negative bacteria** Susceptible bacteria may include *E. coli, H. influenzae, Klebsiella, M. morganii, N. gonorrhoeae, Proteus,* or *P. rettgeri*. • Infections caused by these organisms include septicemia, pneumonia, peritonitis, gynecologic infections, and infections of the urinary tract, skin, or skin structures.    **Infections caused by mixed aerobic-anaerobic bacteria** Peritonitis, septicemia, abdominal abscesses, gynecologic infections, and skin infections have responded to cefoxitin, even when combined therapy with aminoglycosides and clindamycin failed. • Organisms contributing to these infections include *Bacteroides, B. fragilis, Clostridium, Peptococcus,* and *Peptostreptococcus*.

**CONTRAINDICATIONS**    See entry for drug class (p. 278).

**DOSAGE**    **IM, IV:**    **ADULTS:** 1 to 2 g every 6 to 8 hours; the maximum dose is 12 g daily.    **CHILDREN OVER 3 MONTHS:** 80 to 160 mg/kg daily in 4 to 6 equal doses.    *Special patient populations:*    **RENAL IMPAIRMENT:** Doses are reduced, based on the degree of renal failure.    **CHILDREN:** Safe doses for children younger than 3 months have not been established.    **PREGNANCY:** FDA pregnancy category B.

**PREPARATIONS**    *Powder to prepare solution for injection:* 1, 2, or 10 g. The 10 g preparation is a pharmacy bulk package. *Powder to prepare solution for IV infusion:* 1 or 2 g. Also available as a frozen solution in 5% dextrose. Frozen solutions should be stored below −20° C. Solutions may darken without loss of potency. For IM injection, solutions in water or lidocaine (0.5% or 1%) are used at approximately 400 mg/ml. For IV administration, 10 ml of diluent is added to each gram for direct injection or 50 ml of diluent is added to each gram for IV infusion. Compatible diluents include 5% or 10% dextrose or 0.9% sodium chloride.

**DRUG INTERACTIONS**    See entry for drug class (p. 278).

**DIAGNOSTIC TEST INTERFERENCE**    See entry for drug class (p. 278).

**FATE**    Cefoxitin is not absorbed from the GI tract and must be given parenterally. Peak serum concentrations are achieved 20 to 30 minutes following Im administration. Cefoxitin is primarily excreted as unchanged drug by the kidneys. The elimination *half-life* is 0.7 to 1.1 hours in healthy adults and is increased in renal impairment.

## ❦ NURSING CONSIDERATIONS

### Side effects, toxicities, and associated nursing actions

**Local effects** The most common reaction includes pain, induration, and phlebitis or other signs of irritation at the injection site.
- For other reactions, see entry for drug class (p. 278).

### Nursing interventions related to drug administration
- See Preparations above.
- For IM injection, large muscle masses should be used, as described in the overview of drug class (p. 280).
- For direct IV push, dilute as directed and administer dose over 3 to 5 minutes.
- For intermittent IV infusion, dilute as directed in 50 to 100 ml of compatible IV solution. Administer dose over 20 to 30 minutes or as prescribed by physician.
- Thaw frozen solutions at room temperature. Thawed solutions should be used only for intermittent IV infusions.

*Cephamycin.

- Inspect drug powder or solution before use. Discolored preparations or solutions containing particulate matter should not be used.
- IM doses reconstituted with lidocaine should not be used for IV doses.
- Temporarily discontinue infusing IV fluids while infusing cefoxitin.
- If an aminoglycoside is being administered concurrently, separate infusion sites should be used.

### Patient and family education
- See entry for drug class (p. 280).

---

## cefsulodin sodium    (sef-SOOL-oh-din)                         antibiotic*

- cefsulodin sodium: Cefomonil

**MECHANISM OF ACTION**    See entry for drug class (p. 277).

**INDICATIONS**    **Infections caused by P. aeruginosa** Urinary tract infections, otitis, sinusitis, abscesses, septicemia, and infections of skin, bones, joints, and burns have been successfully treated. • For serious infections, combination therapy with an aminoglycoside or other agent may be required.

**CONTRAINDICATIONS**    **Allergy to cephalosporin, penicillin, or other beta-lactam antibiotics** Anaphylaxis and death are possible. • Although cross-allergenicity is not complete, the risk of allergic reactions is increased by a history of reactions to related drugs.

**DOSAGE**    IV:    **ADULTS:** By infusion, 500 mg to 3 g every 6 hours, not to exceed 12 g daily.    *Special patient populations:*    **RENAL IMPAIRMENT:** Doses are reduced, based on the degree of renal failure. **CHILDREN:** Doses not established.    **PREGNANCY:** Safe use in pregnancy and lactation has not been established.

**PREPARATIONS**    *Powder to prepare solution for infusion:* 1 g. One gram in 8 ml sterile water is isotonic. Protect drug from light.

**DRUG INTERACTIONS**    See entry for drug class (p. 278).

**DIAGNOSTIC TEST INTERFERENCE**    See entry for drug class (p. 278).

**FATE**    Cefsulodin is absorbed from IM sites but is most often administered by IV infusion for serious infections. The drug is partially metabolized, but most is excreted unchanged by the kidneys. The elimination *half-life* is 1 to 2.7 hours but is extended in renal failure.

### ✿ NURSING CONSIDERATIONS

#### Side effects, toxicities, and associated nursing actions
**Local effect** About 9% of treated patients report pain on IM administration.
- Rotate injection sites and record sites.
- Choose large muscle masses carefully, as described in the overview of drug class.
- For other reactions, see entry for drug class (p. 278).

#### Nursing interventions related to drug administration
- See Preparations above.
- For IM injection, large muscle masses should be used, as described in the overview of drug class (p. 280).
- For direct IV push, dilute as directed and administer dose over 3 to 5 minutes.
- For intermittent IV infusion, dilute as directed in 50 to 100 ml of compatible IV solution. Administer dose over 20 to 30 minutes or as prescribed by physician.
- Inspect drug powder or solution before use. Discolored preparations or solutions containing particulate matter should not be used.

#### Patient and family education
- See entry for drug class (p. 280).

*Third-generation cephalosporin.

# ceftazidime pentahydrate   (sef-TAZ-i-deem)   antibiotic*

- ceftazidime pentahydrate: Fortaz, Magnacef, Tazidime, Tazicef

**MECHANISM OF ACTION**   See entry for drug class (p. 277).

**INDICATIONS**   **Infections caused by gram-positive bacteria** Although *S. pneumoniae* and staphylococci may be susceptible, penicillins or first-generation cephalosporins are more likely to be effective.   **Infections caused by gram-negative bacteria** Susceptible bacteria may include *Enterobacter, E. coli, H. influenzae, Klebsiella, Proteus, P. aeruginosa,* or *Serratia.* • Infections caused by these organisms include pneumonia, septicemia, peritonitis, and infections of the urinary tract, bone, and skin or skin structures.   **Infections caused by mixed aerobic-anaerobic bacteria** Peritonitis and other mixed infections have responded to ceftazidime. • Susceptible organisms contributing to these infections include *Bacteroides* and *Peptostreptococcus.*

**CONTRAINDICATIONS**   See entry for drug class (p. 278).

**DOSAGE**   IM, IV:   **ADULTS AND CHILDREN OVER 12 YEARS:** 0.5 to 2 g every 8 to 12 hours. Daily doses should not exceed 6 g.   **CHILDREN:** 25 to 50 mg/kg daily in 2 equal doses for infants 1 to 2 months old or 30 to 100 mg/kg daily in 3 equal doses for ages 2 months to 12 years.   *Special patient populations:* **RENAL IMPAIRMENT:** Doses are reduced, based on the degree of renal failure. **PREGNANCY:** FDA pregnancy category B.

**PREPARATIONS**   *Powder to prepare solution for injection:* 500 mg, 1, 2, or 6 g. The 6 g preparation is a bulk pharmacy package. *Powder to prepare solution for IV infusion:* 1 or 2 g. For IM injection, sterile or bacteriostatic water or 0.5% or 1% lidocaine is added to vials (3 ml to each gram) to make solutions of 280 mg/ml. For direct IV injection, solutions are 95 to 180 mg/ml. For infusion, solutions are further diluted into compatible fluids.

**DRUG INTERACTIONS**   See entry for drug class (p. 278).

**DIAGNOSTIC TEST INTERFERENCE**   See entry for drug class (p. 278).

**FATE**   Ceftazidime is not absorbed from the GI tract and must be administered IM or IV. *Peak* serum concentrations are achieved within 1 hour following IM doses. Concentrations in the CNS are low in healthy adults but increase when inflammation is present. Ceftazidime is excreted primarily as unchanged drug by the kidneys. The elimination *half-life* is about 1.8 hours in healthy adults but is extended in renal impairment and in neonates.

## ❦ NURSING CONSIDERATIONS

### Side effects, toxicities, and associated nursing actions

**Local effects** Pain, induration, phlebitis, or thrombophlebitis occurs, at injection sites in up to 3% of patients.

- For other reactions, see entry for drug class (p. 278).

### Nursing interventions related to drug administration

- See Preparations above.
- For IM injection, large muscle masses should be used, as described in the overview of drug class (p. 280).
- For direct IV push, dilute as directed and administer dose over 3 to 5 minutes.
- For intermittent IV infusion, dilute as directed in 50 to 100 ml of compatible IV solution. Administer dose over 20 to 30 minutes or as prescribed by the physician.
- Thaw frozen solutions at room temperature. Thawed solutions should be used only for intermittent IV infusions.
- Inspect drug powder or solution before use. Discolored preparations or solutions containing particulate matter should not be used.
- IM solutions reconstituted with lidocaine should not be used for IV doses.
- If an aminoglycoside is being administered concurrently, separate IV infusion sites should be used.

*Third-generation cephalosporin.

**Patient and family education**
- See entry for drug class (p. 280).

---

## ceftizoxime sodium    (sef-tiz-OX-eem)    antibiotic*

- ceftizoxime sodium: Cefizox

**MECHANISM OF ACTION**   See entry for drug class (p. 277).

**INDICATIONS**   **Infections caused by gram-positive bacteria** Although *Streptococcus pneumoniae*, group A beta-hemolytic streptococci, and staphylococci may be susceptible, penicillins or first-generation cephalosporins are more likely to be effective.   **Infections caused by gram-negative bacteria** Susceptible bacteria may include *Enterobacter, E. coli, H. influenzae, Klebsiella, M. morganii, N. gonorrhoeae, P. rettgeri, Proteus, P. aeruginosa*, or *Serratia*. • Infections caused by these organisms include pneumonia, septicemia, peritonitis, and infections of the urinary or reproductive tract, bone, and skin or skin structures.   **Infections caused by mixed aerobic-anaerobic bacteria** Infections of the lower respiratory tract, abdominal cavity, and skin or skin structures have responded to ceftizoxime. • Susceptible organisms contributing to these infections include *Bacteroides, B. fragilis, Peptococcus*, and *Peptostreptococcus*.   **Meningitis** Susceptible bacteria include *H. influenzae* and *S. pneumoniae*.

**CONTRAINDICATIONS**   **Allergy to cephalosporin, penicillin, or other beta-lactam antibiotics** Anaphylaxis and death are possible. • Although cross-allergenicity is not complete, the risk of allergic reactions is increased by a history of reactions to related drugs.

**DOSAGE**   **IM, IV:**   **ADULTS:** 0.5 to 2 g every 8 to 12 hours. Daily dosage should not exceed 12 g.   **CHILDREN OVER 6 MONTHS:** 50 mg/kg every 6 to 8 hours. Dosage should not exceed 12 g daily.   *Special patient populations:*   **RENAL IMPAIRMENT:** Doses are reduced, based on the degree of renal failure.   **PREGNANCY:** FDA pregnancy category B.

**PREPARATIONS**   *Powder to prepare solution for injection:* 1 or 2 g. *Powder to prepare solution for IV infusion:* 1 or 2 g. Also available as frozen solutions in 5% dextrose. Vials should be protected from light. Frozen solutions should be stored below −20° C. For IM injection, sterile water is added to vials (3 ml to each gram) to make solutions of 270 mg/ml. For direct IV injection, solutions are 95 mg/ml. For infusion, solutions are further diluted into compatible fluids.

**DRUG INTERACTIONS**   See entry for drug class (p. 278).

**DIAGNOSTIC TEST INTERFERENCE**   See entry for drug class (p. 278).

**FATE**   Ceftizoxime is not absorbed from the GI tract and must be administered IM or IV. *Peak* serum concentrations are achieved within 0.5 to 1.5 hours following IM doses. Concentrations in the CNS are low in healthy adults but increase when inflammation is present. Ceftizoxime is excreted primarily as unchanged drug by the kidneys. The elimination *half-life* is about 1.4 to 1.9 hours in healthy adults but is extended in renal impairment.

## 🐾 NURSING CONSIDERATIONS

### Side effects, toxicities, and associated nursing actions

**Local effects** Pain, induration, phlebitis, or thrombophlebitis occurs at injection sites in up to 5% of patients.
- For other reactions, see entry for drug class (p. 278).

### Nursing interventions related to drug administration

- See Preparations above.
- For IM injection, large muscle masses should be used, as described in the entry for drug class (p. 280). If an IM dose is 2 g or larger, the dose should be divided and administered in two separate injections.
- For direct IV push, dilute as directed and administer dose over 3 to 5 minutes.
- For intermittent IV infusion, dilute as directed in 50 to 100 ml of compatible IV solution. Administer dose over 20 to 30 minutes or at rate prescribed.

*Third-generation cephalosporin.

- Thaw frozen solutions at room temperature. Thawed solutions should be used only for intermittent IV infusions.
- Inspect drug powder or solution before use. Discolored preparations or solutions containing particulate matter should not be used.

### Patient and family education
- See entry for drug class (p. 280).

## ceftriaxone sodium   (sef-tri-AX-ohne)                                antibiotic*

- ceftriaxone sodium: Rocephin

**MECHANISM OF ACTION**   See entry for drug class (p. 277).

**INDICATIONS**   **Infections caused by gram-positive bacteria** Although *S. pneumoniae,* group A and B streptococci, and *S. aureus* may be susceptible, penicillins or first-generation cephalosporins are more likely to be effective.   **Infections caused by gram-negative bacteria** Susceptible bacteria may include *Enterobacter, E. coli, H. influenzae, Klebsiella, N. gonorrhoeae, Proteus, P. aeruginosa,* or *Serratia.* • Infections caused by these organisms include pneumonia, septicemia, peritonitis, and infections of the reproductive or urinary tract, bone, and skin or skin structures.   **Meningitis** Susceptible bacteria may include *H. influenzae, N. meningitidis,* and *S. pneumoniae.*

**CONTRAINDICATIONS**   **Allergy to cephalosporin, penicillin, or other beta-lactam antibiotics** Anaphylaxis and death are possible. • Although cross-allergenicity is not complete, the risk of allergic reactions is increased by a history of reactions to related drugs.

**DOSAGE**   IM, IV:   **ADULTS AND CHILDREN OVER 12 YEARS:** 1 to 2 g in one or two doses. Daily doses should not exceed 4 g.   **CHILDREN:** 50 to 100 mg/kg daily in 2 equal doses.   *Special patient populations:*   **PREGNANCY:** FDA pregnancy category B.

**PREPARATIONS**   *Powder to prepare solution for injection:* 250, 500 mg, 1, 2, or 10 g. The 10 g preparation is a bulk pharmacy package. *Powder to prepare solution for IV infusion:* 1 or 2 g. Protect vials from light. For IM injection, sterile or bacteriostatic water, 0.9% sodium chloride, 5% dextrose, or 1% lidocaine is added to vials (3.6 ml to each gram) to make solutions of 250 mg/ml. For intermittent IV infusion, solutions are approximately 100 mg/ml.

**DRUG INTERACTIONS**   See entry for drug class (p. 278).

**DIAGNOSTIC TEST INTERFERENCE**   See entry for drug class (p. 278).

**FATE**   Ceftriaxone is not absorbed from the GI tract and must be administered IM or IV. *Peak* serum concentrations are achieved 1.5 to 4 hours following IM doses. Concentrations in the CNS are low in healthy adults but increase when inflammation is present. Ceftriaxone is excreted as unchanged drug by the kidneys; some drug is excreted as inactive metabolites in the feces. The elimination *half-life* is about 5.4 to 10.9 hours in healthy adults but is extended in renal impairment and in neonates. Ceftriaxone has the longest half-life among the cephalosporins.

### ❦ NURSING CONSIDERATIONS
#### Side effects, toxicities, and associated nursing actions
**GI** Diarrhea in up to 44% of treated children and 28% of treated adults has been reported in three studies. The incidence is lower in other reports.
- Monitor patient for development of diarrhea. If diarrhea develops, notify physician.
- Monitor intake and output.
- Monitor weight of infants and small children.
- For other reactions, see entry for drug class (p. 278).

#### Nursing interventions related to drug administration
- See Preparations above.
- For IM injection, large muscle masses should be used as described in the Overview of Drug Class (p. 280).
- For direct IV push, dilute as directed and administer dose over 2 to 4 minutes.

*Third-generation cephalosporin.

- For intermittent IV infusion, dilute as directed in 50 to 100 ml of compatible IV solution. Administer dose over 20 to 30 minutes in adults, over 10 to 30 minutes in neonates or small children, or as prescribed by the physician.
- IM solutions prepared with bacteriostatic water containing benzyl alcohol should not be administered to neonates.
- Inspect drug powder or solution before use. Discolored preparations or solutions containing particulate matter should not be used.
- IM solutions reconstituted with lidocaine should not be used for IV doses.
- If an aminoglycoside is being administered concurrently, separate IV infusion sites should be used.

### Patient and family education
- See entry for drug class (p. 280).

---

## cefuroxime sodium  (sef-yoor-OX-eem)  antibiotic*

- cefuroxime sodium: Zinacef

**MECHANISM OF ACTION**    See entry for drug class (p. 277).

**INDICATIONS**    **Infections caused by gram-positive bacteria** Susceptible bacteria include *S. pneumoniae,* group A beta-hemolytic streptococci, and *S. aureus.* • Infections caused by these organisms include pneumonia, septicemia, and infections of the skin and skin structures. • First-generation cephalosporins or penicillins are generally more effective for these infections.    **Infections caused by gram-negative bacteria** Susceptible organisms may include *Enterobacter, E. coli, H. influenzae, Klebsiella,* or *N. gonorrhoeae.* • Infections caused by these organisms include pneumonia, urinary tract infections, gonorrhea, and infections of skin or skin structures.    **Meningitis** Susceptible organisms may include *S. pneumoniae, S. aureus, N. meningitidis,* and *H. influenzae* (including ampicillin-resistant strains).

**CONTRAINDICATIONS**    **Allergy to cephalosporin, penicillin, or other beta-lactam antibiotics** Anaphylaxis and death are possible. • Although cross-allergenicity is not complete, the risk of allergic reactions is increased by a history of reactions to related drugs.

**DOSAGE**    **IM, IV:**    **ADULTS:** 750 mg to 1.5 g every 8 hours, with rare cases requiring up to 3 g every 8 hours. Dosage is reduced in renal failure.    **CHILDREN:** Older than 3 months, 50 to 100 mg/kg daily in divided doses every 6 to 8 hours; meningitis may require initial doses of 200 to 240 mg/kg daily, in divided doses every 6 to 8 hours.    *Special patient populations:*    **RENAL IMPAIRMENT:** Doses are reduced, based on the degree of renal failure.    **PREGNANCY:** FDA pregnancy category B.

**PREPARATIONS**    *Powder to prepare solution for injection:* 750 mg and 1.5 g. *Powder to prepare solution for infusion:* 750 mg and 1.5 g. Before reconstitution, vials should be protected from light. Solutions may turn yellow without loss of potency, but solutions with extensive discoloration or precipitates should be discarded. For IM administration, 750 mg should be dissolved in 3.6 ml sterile water to produce a suspension for injection of 208 mg/ml. For IV administration, cefuroxime may be dissolved in sterile water to produce a solution of 90 to 94 mg/ml for direct injection or 7.5 to 15 mg/ml for infusion.

**DRUG INTERACTIONS**    See entry for drug class (p. 278).

**DIAGNOSTIC TEST INTERFERENCES**    **Creatinine** assays using the Jaffe reaction may not be affected by cefuroxime, unlike the case with other cephalosporins. For other interferences, see entry for drug class (p. 278).

**FATE**    Cefuroxime is not adequately absorbed orally. Absorption from IM sites is good, producing *peak* serum concentrations within 15 minutes to 1 hour. Cefuroxime penetrates the CNS adequately when the meninges are inflamed. Cefuroxime is excreted unchanged by the kidneys. The elimination *half-life* is 1 to 2 hours in healthy adults but is increased in renal failure and in neonates.

---

*Second-generation cephalosporin.

## ❦ NURSING CONSIDERATIONS
### Side effects, toxicities, and associated nursing actions
**Local effects** Up to 95% of patients receiving IM injections of cefuroxime report pain and discomfort lasting 5 minutes or less.
- Use anatomical landmarks to identify muscle masses, as described in the entry for drug class (p. 280).
- Rotate injection sites and record sites.

**Blood** Up to 10% of patients show reduced hemoglobin and hematocrit levels.
- Monitor hematocrit and hemoglobin levels.
- Assess for fatigue and pallor.
- Other reactions to cefuroxime are similar to those of other cephalosporins.
- See entry for drug class (p. 278).

### Nursing interventions related to drug administration
- See Preparations above.
- For IM injection, large muscle masses should be used, as described in the overview of drug class (p. 280).
- For direct IV push, dilute as directed and administer dose over 3 to 5 minutes.
- For intermittent IV infusion, dilute as directed in 50 to 100 ml or compatible IV solution. Administer dose over 15 to 60 minutes in adults or as prescribed by the physician.
- Inspect drug powder or solution before use. Discolored preparations or solutions containing particulate matter should not be used.

### Patient and family education
- See entry for drug class (p. 280).

---

# cephalexin   (sef-uh-LEX-in)                                    antibiotic*

- cephalexin: Ceporex, Keflex, Novolexin

**MECHANISM OF ACTION**   See entry for drug class (p. 277).

**INDICATIONS**   **Infections caused by gram-positive bacteria** Susceptible bacteria include *S. pneumoniae*, group A beta-hemolytic streptococci, group B streptococci, and *S. aureus*. • Infections caused by these organisms include pharyngitis, tonsilitis, and skin and soft tissue infections.   **Urinary tract infections** Susceptible organisms may include *E. coli*, *P. mirabilis*, or *Klebsiella*.

**CONTRAINDICATIONS**   **Allergy to cephalosporin, penicillin, or other beta-lactam antibiotics** Anaphylaxis and death are possible. • Although cross-allergenicity is not complete, the risk of allergic reactions is increased by a history of reactions to related drugs.

**DOSAGE**   **PO:**   **ADULTS:** 250 to 500 mg every 6 to 12 hours. Daily doses should not exceed 4 g.   **CHILDREN:** 25 to 100 mg/kg daily in 2 or 4 doses.   *Special patient populations:*   **PREGNANCY:** Safe use in pregnancy and lactation has not been established.

**PREPARATIONS**   *Tablets:* 1 g. *Capsules:* 250 or 500 mg. *Suspension, oral:* 125 or 250 mg in each 5 ml, or 100 mg/ml. Suspensions are stable 14 days at 2° to 8° C.

**DRUG INTERACTIONS**   See entry for drug class (p. 278).

**DIAGNOSTIC TEST INTERFERENCES**   See entry for drug class (p. 278).

**FATE**   Oral absorption is complete but may be impeded by food. *Peak* serum concentrations occur at about 1 hour. Elimination is primarily renal as the unchanged drug. The elimination *half-life* is 0.5 to 1.2 hours.

## ❦ NURSING CONSIDERATIONS
### Side effects, toxicities, and associated nursing actions
- See entry for drug class (p. 278).

### Patient and family education
- Cephalexin may be taken without regard to meals.
- See entry for drug class (p. 280).

## cephalothin sodium   (sef-uh-LOW-thin)                    antibiotic*

- cephalothin sodium: Ceporacin, Keflin, Seffin

**MECHANISM OF ACTION**   See entry for drug class (p. 277).

**INDICATIONS**   **Infections caused by gram-positive bacteria** Susceptible bacteria include *S. pneumoniae,* group A beta-hemolytic streptococci, and staphylococci. • Infections caused by these organisms include respiratory infections, septicemia, pharyngitis, tonsilitis, and skin and soft tissue infections.   **Urinary tract infections** Susceptible organisms may include *E. coli, P. mirabilis,* or *Klebsiella.*

**CONTRAINDICATIONS**   **Allergy to cephalosporin, penicillin, or other beta-lactam antibiotics** Anaphylaxis and death are possible. • Although cross-allergenicity is not complete, the risk of allergic reactions is increased by a history of reactions to related drugs.

**DOSAGE**   **IM, IV:**   **ADULTS:** 500 mg to 2 g every 4 to 6 hours. The maximum daily dose is 12 g.   **CHILDREN:** 80 to 160 mg/kg daily, as divided doses.   *Special patient populations:*   **RENAL IMPAIRMENT:** Doses are reduced, based on the degree of renal failure.   **PREGNANCY:** FDA pregnancy category B.

**PREPARATIONS**   *Powder to prepare solution for injection:* 1, 2, 4, 10, or 20 g. The 4, 10, and 20 g preparations are pharmacy bulk packages. *Solution for infusion:* 1 or 2 g. Available as powder for reconstitution or as frozen solutions in 5% dextrose or 0.9% sodium chloride. Frozen solutions should be stored below -20° C. All preparations contain 30 mg sodium bicarbonate for each gram of cephalothin.

**DRUG INTERACTIONS**   See entry for drug class (p. 278).

**DIAGNOSTIC TEST INTERFERENCES**   See entry for drug class (p. 278).

**FATE**   Cephalothin is not absorbed from the GI tract and must be given parenterally. *Peak* serum concentrations occur within 30 minutes of IM administration. Cephalothin is extensively metabolized, mostly to desacetylcephalothin, which is only one fourth as active as cephalothin. The elimination *half-life* of cephalothin is 30 to 60 minutes in healthy adults but is extended in renal impairment.

### ☙ NURSING CONSIDERATIONS

#### Side effects, toxicities, and associated nursing actions
- See entry for drug class (p. 278).

#### Nursing interventions related to drug administration
- See Preparations above.
- For IM injection, large muscle masses should be used, as described in the entry for drug class (p. 280). If powder does not dissolve into amount of diluent specified on vial, 0.2 to 0.4 ml additional diluent may be added and the vial warmed under running water.
- For direct IV push, dilute as directed and administer dose over 3 to 5 minutes.
- For intermittent IV infusion, dilute as directed in 50 to 100 ml of compatible IV solution. Administer dose over 15 to 30 minutes in adults or as prescribed by physician.
- Inspect drug powder or solution before use. Discolored preparations or solutions containing particulate matter should not be used.
- Thaw frozen solutions at room temperature. Thawed solutions should be used only for intermittent IV infusions.

#### Patient and family education
- See entry for drug class (p. 280).

## cephapirin sodium   (sef-uh-PYRE-in)                    antibiotic*

- cephapirin sodium: Cefadyl

**MECHANISM OF ACTION**   See entry for drug class (p. 277).

---

*First-generation cephalosporin.

**INDICATIONS**   As for cephalothin (p. 299).

**CONTRAINDICATIONS**   **Allergy to cephalosporin, penicillin, or other beta-lactam antibiotics** Anaphylaxis and death are possible. • Although cross-allergenicity is not complete, the risk of allergic reactions is increased by a history of reactions to related drugs.

**DOSAGE**   **IM, IV:**   **ADULTS:** 500 mg to 2 g every 4 to 6 hours. Dosage is reduced in renal failure.   **CHILDREN OVER 3 MONTHS:** 40 to 80 mg/kg daily in 4 equal doses.   *Special patient populations:*   **RENAL IMPAIRMENT:** Doses are reduced, based on the degree of renal failure.   **PREGNANCY:** FDA pregnancy category B.

**PREPARATIONS**   *Powder to prepare solution for injection:* 500 mg, 1, 2, or 20 g. The 20 g preparation is a pharmacy bulk package. *Powder to prepare solution for infusion:* 1, 2, or 4 g. Solutions may turn yellow without loss of potency.

**DRUG INTERACTIONS**   See entry for drug class (p. 278).

**DIAGNOSTIC TEST INTERFERENCES**   See entry for drug class (p. 278).

**FATE**   Cephapirin is not absorbed from the GI tract and must be given parenterally. *Peak* serum concentrations occur within 30 minutes of IM administration. Cephapirin is metabolized mostly to desacetylcephapirin, which is only one half as active as cephapirin. The elimination *half-life* of cephapirin is 20 to 50 minutes in healthy adults but is extended in renal impairment.

☙ **NURSING CONSIDERATIONS**

**Side effects, toxicities, and associated nursing actions**
- See entry for drug class (p. 278).

**Nursing interventions related to drug administration**
- See Preparations above.
- For IM injection, large muscle masses should be used, as described in the entry for drug class (p. 280).
- For direct IV push, dilute as directed and administer dose over 3 to 5 minutes.
- For intermittent IV infusion, dilute as directed in 50 to 100 ml of compatible IV solution. Administer dose over 15 to 30 minutes in adults or as prescribed by physician.
- Inspect drug powder or solution before use. Discolored preparations or solutions containing particulate matter should not be used.

**Patient and family education**
- See entry for drug class (p. 280).

---

## cephradine   (SEF-ra-deen)                                                    antibiotic*

- cephradine: Anspor, Velosef

**MECHANISM OF ACTION**   See entry for drug class (p. 277).

**INDICATIONS**   **Infections caused by gram-positive bacteria** Susceptible bacteria include group A beta-hemolytic streptococci and staphylococci. • Infections caused by these organisms include pneumonia, otitis media, pharyngitis, tonsilitis, and skin and soft tissue infections.   **Urinary tract infections** Susceptible organisms include *E. coli, P. mirabilis,* or *Klebsiella.*

**CONTRAINDICATIONS**   **Allergy to cephalosporin, penicillin, or other beta-lactam antibiotics** Anaphylaxis and death are possible. Although cross-allergenicity is not complete, the risk of allergic reactions is increased by a history of reactions to related drugs.

**DOSAGE**   **PO:**   **ADULTS:** 250 mg to 1 g every 6 to 12 hours. Maximum daily dosage is 4 g. Dosage is reduced in renal failure.   **CHILDREN OVER 9 MONTHS:** 25 to 100 mg/kg daily in 2 to 4 equal doses.   **IM, IV:**   **ADULTS:** 500 mg to 1 g four times daily. Maximum daily dose is 8 g.   **CHILDREN OVER 1 YEAR:** 50 to 100 mg/kg daily, in 4 equal doses.   *Special patient populations:*   **RENAL IMPAIRMENT:** Doses are reduced, based on the degree of renal failure.   **PREGNANCY:** FDA pregnancy category B.

*First-generation cephalosporin.

**PREPARATIONS** *Capsules:* 250 or 500 mg. *Suspension, oral:* 125 or 250 mg in each 5 ml. Suspensions are stable 14 days at 2° to 8° C. *Powder to prepare solution for injection:* 250, 500 mg, and 1 g. Contains sodium carbonate. *Powder to prepare solution for injection or infusion:* 4 g with solium carbonate. *Powder to prepare solution for infusion:* 2 g sodium-free.

**DRUG INTERACTIONS** See entry for drug class (p. 278).

**DIAGNOSTIC TEST INTERFERENCES** See entry for drug class (p. 278).

**FATE** Oral absorption is complete but is impeded by food. *Peak* serum concentrations occur at about 1 hour, which is similar to cephalexin. Unlike other cephalosporins, cephradine may be used both parenterally and orally. *Peak* serum concentrations are achieved within 1 to 2 hours following IM administration. Elimination is primarily renal. The elimination *half-life* is 0.7 to 2 hours in healthy adults but is extended in renal impairment.

## ☙ NURSING CONSIDERATIONS

### Toxicities, side effects, and associated nursing actions
- See entry for drug class (p. 278).

### Nursing interventions related to drug administration
- See Preparations above.
- For IM injection, large muscle masses should be used, as described in the entry for drug class (p. 280).
- For direct IV push, dilute as directed and administer dose over 3 to 5 minutes.
- For intermittent IV infusion, dilute as directed in 50 to 100 ml of compatible IV solution. Administer dose over 15 to 30 minutes in adults or as prescribed by physician.
- Inspect drug powder or solution before use. Discolored preparations or solutions containing particulate matter should not be used.

### Patient and family education
- Cephradine may be taken without regard to meals.
- See entry for drug class (p. 280).

---

## imipenem   (em-ee-PEN-em)                                                                                   antibiotic*

- imipenem with cilastatin sodium: Primaxin

**MECHANISM OF ACTION** Cilastatin is an inhibitor of renal dipeptidase, an enzyme that destroys the antibiotic imipenem in the body. Imipenem is the active antibacterial agent in the combination and shares the same mechanism of action as other beta-lactam antibiotics. See entry for drug class (p. 277).

**INDICATIONS** Seriously ill patients with mixed or nosocomial infections or infections of unknown etiology Imipenem has a remarkably high potency and broad spectrum. • The only organisms known to be resistant in significant numbers are *Pseudomonas maltophilia*, *Streptococcus faecium*, *Flavobacterium*, anaerobic corynebacteria, methicillin-resistant staphylococci, *Pseudomonas cepacia*, and chlamydiae.

**CONTRAINDICATIONS** Allergy to cephalosporin, penicillin, or other beta-lactam antibiotics Anaphylaxis and death are possible. • Although cross-allergenicity is not complete, the risk of allergic reactions is increased by a history of reactions to related drugs.

**DOSAGE** IV: ADULTS: 250 mg to 1 g every 6 to 8 hours, not to exceed 50 mg/kg or 4 g daily. *Special patient populations:* RENAL IMPAIRMENT: Doses may be reduced, based on the degree of renal failure. CHILDREN: Doses not established. PREGNANCY: FDA pregnancy category C.

**PREPARATIONS** *Solution, injection:* 250 or 500 mg each of imipenem anhydrous and cilastatin sodium.

**DRUG INTERACTIONS** See entry for drug class (p. 278).

**DIAGNOSTIC TEST INTERFERENCE** See entry for drug class (p. 278).

**FATE** Imipenem is not adequately absorbed from the GI tract and must be administered parenterally. In the absence of cilastatin, imipenem is extensively metabolized in the kidneys. Cilastatin inhibits the renal

*Carbapenem.

dipeptidase that destroys imipenem and maintains activity of the antibiotic in the body. The elimination *half-life* of imipenem is about 1 hour and is extended in renal failure.

## 🐦 NURSING CONSIDERATIONS

### Side effects, toxicities, and associated nursing actions
- See entry for drug class (p. 278).

### Nursing interventions related to drug administration
- See Preparations above.
- For direct IV push, dilute as directed and administer dose over 3 to 5 minutes.
- For intermittent IV infusion, dilute as directed in 50 to 100 ml of compatible IV solution. Administer dose over 15 to 30 minutes in adults or as prescribed by physician.
- Inspect drug powder or solution before use. Discolored preparations or solutions containing particulate matter should not be used.

### Patient and family education
- See entry for drug class (p. 280).

---

## moxalactam    (mox-uh-LAK-tam)                                      antibiotic*

- moxalactam: Moxam

**MECHANISM OF ACTION**    See entry for drug class (p. 277).

**INDICATIONS**    **Infections caused by gram-positive bacteria** Although *Streptococcus pneumoniae,* group A beta-hemolytic streptococci, and *Staphylococcus aureus* may be susceptible, penicillins or first-generation cephalosporins are more likely to be effective.    **Infections caused by gram-negative bacteria** Susceptible bacteria may include *Enterobacter, E. coli, H. influenzae, Klebsiella, Proteus, P. aeruginosa,* or *Serratia.* • Infections caused by these organisms include pneumonia, septicemia, peritonitis, and infections of the reproductive or urinary tract, bone, and skin or skin structures.    **Mixed infections of aerobic and anaerobic bacteria** Septicemia, intraabdominal infections, and infections of skin or skin structures may respond. • Organisms contributing to these infections include *Bacteroides, B. fragilis, Clostridium, Eubacterium, Fusobacterium, Peptococcus,* and *Streptopeptococcus.* **Meningitis** Susceptible bacteria may include *Haemophilus influenzae, E. coli,* and *Klebsiella.*

**CONTRAINDICATIONS**    **Allergy to cephalosporin, penicillin, or other beta-lactam antibiotics** Anaphylaxis and death are possible. • Although cross-allergenicity is not complete, the risk of allergic reactions is increased by a history of reactions to related drugs.

**DOSAGE**    IM, IV:    **ADULTS:** 1 to 4 g daily, in equally divided doses every 8 to 12 hours. The maximum daily dose is 4 g.    **CHILDREN:** 50 mg/kg every 12 hours in neonates, every 8 hours in infants 1 to 4 weeks of age, and every 6 to 8 hours in children over 1 month of age. Doses may approach 200 mg/kg daily in serious infections. *Special patient populations:* **RENAL IMPAIRMENT:** Doses are reduced, based on the degree of renal failure. **PREGNANCY:** FDA pregnancy category C.

**PREPARATIONS**    *Powder to prepare solution for injection:* 1, 2, or 10 g. The 10 g preparation is a pharmacy bulk package. *Powder to prepare solution for infusion:* 1 or 2 g.

**DRUG INTERACTIONS**    See entry for drug class (p. 278).

**DIAGNOSTIC TEST INTERFERENCE**    See entry for drug class (p. 278).

**FATE**    Moxalactam is not absorbed from the GI tract and must be administered parenterally. *Peak* serum concentrations are achieved within 0.5 to 1 hour following IM administration. The drug is well distributed to most tissues and the CNS. Excretion is primarily by the kidneys. The elimination *half-life* is about 2 to 3.5 hours in healthy adults but is decreased in children 1 to 24 months of age to about 1.6 hours. Renal failure extends the half-life.

## 🐦 NURSING CONSIDERATIONS

### Side effects, toxicities, and associated nursing actions
**Blood** Bleeding is the greatest risk with moxalactam. Moxalactam causes both platelet dysfunction and hypoprothrombinemia. Hypoprothrombinemia can be prevented or partially reversed by admin-

---

*Oxa-cephem.

istrations of vitamin K, which is often given prophylactically when moxalactam must be used. Platelet dysfunction is not reversed by vitamin K. Serious or even fatal bleeding episodes are possible, especially if the maximum daily dose is exceeded.

- Monitor vital signs, blood pressure, and intake and output.
- Monitor patient for signs of unexplained bruising or bleeding: bleeding gums, nosebleeds, hematuria, blood in stools, bruises, or petechiae.
- Monitor prothrombin time.
- Vitamin K may be ordered prophylactically. IM injections in the presence of a prolonged prothrombin time may cause hematomas at the injection sites. Inspect injection sites closely. Apply firm but gentle pressure over injection site after administering injection to prevent hematoma formation.
- For other reactions to moxalactam, see entry for drug class (p. 278).

### Nursing interventions related to drug administration
- See Preparations above.
- For IM injection, large muscle masses should be used, as described in the entry for drug class (p. 280).
- For direct IV push, dilute as directed and administer dose over 3 to 5 minutes.
- For intermittent IV infusion, dilute as directed in 50 to 100 ml of compatible IV solution. Administer dose over 15 to 30 minutes in adults or as prescribed by physician.
- Inspect drug powder or solution before use. Discolored preparations or solutions containing particulate matter should not be used.
- If an aminoglycoside is being administered concurrently with moxalactam, two separate infusion sites should be used.

### Patient and family education
- Disulfiram-like reactions may occur if alcohol is ingested within 48 to 72 hours of a dose of moxalactam. This intense reaction is characterized by flushing of the face, palpitations, rapid heart rate, and low blood pressure. Instruct patients to avoid the use of alcohol for at least 3 days following the last dose of this antibacterial.
- See entry for drug class (p. 280).

# Chapter Sixteen

# Aminoglycosides and aminocyclitols

**Aminoglycosides**
amikacin
gentamicin
kanamycin
neomycin
netilmicin

paromomycin
streptomycin
tobramycin

**Aminocyclitols**
spectinomycin

**OVERVIEW OF THE DRUG CLASS**   Aminoglycoside antibiotics are among the most active agents used to treat infections caused by *Pseudomonas aeruginosa* and *Serratia,* but not all members of the class share this activity (Table 16-1). All of these antibiotics are capable of bactericidal action directed toward a broad range of gram-negative bacteria. The limitations to the use of aminoglycosides include the requirement for parenteral administration and the high risk of toxic reactions. Spectinomycin is used only to treat gonorrhea in situations when penicillin or other drugs cannot be used.

**MECHANISM OF ACTION**   Aminoglycosides and aminocyclitols inhibit protein synthesis in bacteria by binding to the bacterial ribosomes. Once bound by drugs, these ribosomes are unable to synthesize protein normally. In many circumstances the action of aminoglycosides is bactericidal and may involve additional unknown mechanisms of bacterial cell killing. The ribosomes found in mammalian cells do not bind aminoglycosides; therefore, mammalian cells are resistant.

**INDICATIONS**   **Serious infections caused by gram-negative aerobic bacteria** Susceptible organisms include *Acinetobacter, Citrobacter, Enterobacter, Escherichia coli, Klebsiella, Proteus, Providencia, Pseudomonas, Salmonella, Serratia,* and *Shigella.* Amikacin, gentamicin, netilmicin, and tobramycin are the aminoglycosides most active against these bacteria.   **Serious infections caused by *Pseudomonas aeruginosa*** Amikacin, gentamicin, netilmicin, and tobramycin are most active against this organism. **Serious infections caused by *Mycobacteria*** Tuberculosis caused by various species of *Mycobacteria* can be controlled with streptomycin or, more rarely, with kanamycin.   **Parasitic infestations** Infections caused by the ameba *Entamoeba histolytica* and certain helminthic infestations can be controlled with paromomycin.   **Gonorrhoea** Infections caused by *Neisseria gonorrhoeae* may respond to spectinomycin. Spectinomycin may be most useful in treating penicillinase-producing strains of *N. gonorrhoeae* (PPNG).

**CONTRAINDICATIONS**   **Renal impairment** Because aminoglycosides can cause renal tubular necrosis, the drugs should be avoided if possible in patients with renal impairment. When aminoglycosides must be used, the dosage must be reduced to prevent serious drug accumulation and toxicity. Serum creatinine or other tests of renal function must be evaluated regularly. To estimate dosing intervals, the following

**Table 16-1.**   Clinical use of aminoglycosides and aminocyclitols

|  | \ | \ | Cause of infection | \ | \ |
|---|---|---|---|---|---|
|  | Enterobac-teriaceae | Pseudomonas | Neisseria | Mycobacteria | Protozoa |
| Amikacin | + | + | − | − | − |
| Gentamicin | + | + | − | − | − |
| Kanamycin | + | − | − | + | − |
| Neomycin | + | − | − | − | − |
| Netilmicin | + | + | − | − | − |
| Paromomycin | − | − | − | − | + |
| Streptomycin | − | − | − | + | − |
| Tobramycin | + | + | − | − | − |
| Spectinomycin | − | − | + | − | − |

formula may apply: patient's serum creatinine concentration (mg/100 ml) $\times$ 9 = dose interval in hours for usual adult milligrams per kilogram dose. Alternatively, maintenance doses may be given every 12 hours, adjusted according to the following formula: Patient's creatinine clearance [ml/min] divided by normal creatinine clearance [ml/min] $\times$ 7.5 mg/kg = Adjusted maintenance dose in mg/kg. Remember these formulas are only representative of the many ways aminoglycoside doses may be adjusted.

**Hearing loss** Because aminoglycosides can cause hearing loss, the drugs should be avoided if possible in patients with pre-existing hearing problems. When aminoglycosides must be used, concentrations of the drug in serum should be monitored and doses adjusted to avoid serious accumulation. Hearing acuity should also be monitored.

**DRUG INTERACTIONS**    **Nephrotoxic drugs** such as amphotericin B, capreomycin, cephalosporins, colistin, cisplatin, methoxyflurane, polymyxin B, or vancomycin may increase the risk of renal damage from aminoglycosides.    **Ototoxic drugs** such as ethacrynic acid or furosemide may increase the risk of hearing loss with aminoglycosides.    **Dimenhydrinate** may mask the signs of ototoxicity caused by aminoglycosides.    **Succinylcholine, tubocurarine,** and other neuromuscular blocking agents may have additive effects with aminoglycosides, causing unexpectedly profound or prolonged paralysis. Respiratory paralysis is the most frequent sign.    **Beta-lactam antibiotics** such as penicillins and cephalosporins often have synergistic antibacterial activity with aminoglycosides. Combinations of these two classes of drugs are often used to treat serious infections caused by relatively resistant organisms such as *Pseudomonas aeruginosa*.

## ❦ NURSING CONSIDERATIONS

### Side effects, toxicities, and associated nursing actions

**CNS** Headache, tremor, lethargy, paresthesias, arachnoiditis, encephalopathy, coma, and depression are rare and may accompany intrathecal injection.

- Monitor the patient's level of consciousness. When intrathecal injections are being administered, be alert to alterations in the neurologic assessment.

**Peripheral nerve** Neuromuscular blockade is possible with aminoglycosides, especially when the neuromuscular junction is already depressed by neuromuscular blocking agents, general anesthetics, or diseases such as myasthenia gravis. Rare patients suffer respiratory depression. Paralysis may or may not respond to neostigmine or calcium.

- Be alert to neuromuscular blockade in susceptible patients.
- Have neostigmine and calcium available in settings where aminoglycosides are used with high-risk patients, such as the operating room, recovery room, and intensive care units.

**Ototoxicity** Hearing loss is a dose-related side effect of aminoglycosides. For this reason, high doses or drug accumulation must be avoided. Hearing loss is most commonly associated with amikacin, kanamycin, neomycin, or paromomycin. Vestibular damage, leading to dizziness or loss of balance, is most commonly associated with gentamicin, streptomycin, or tobramycin.

- Be alert to diminished hearing in patients. Be especially alert in elderly patients and patients with pre-existing tinnitus, vertigo, hearing loss, or who have previously received ototoxic drugs. Question patients about perceived hearing loss.
- If hearing loss is suspected, a complete audiologic examination should be performed. Newborns of mothers who received aminoglycosides during pregnancy or labor may suffer ototoxicity.
- Be alert to loss of balance in ambulatory patients. Question the patient about perceived dizziness.
- Monitor serum drug levels (see Table 16-2).

**Blood** Anemia, granulocytopenia, leukopenia, thrombocytopenia, or changes in reticulocyte count may rarely be seen.

- Monitor hematocrit and hemoglobin, white blood cell differential count, platelet count, and red blood cell count and reticulocyte count.
- Monitor temperature. Assess for malaise, pallor, sore throat.
- Observe for signs of bleeding: unexplained bruising, bleeding such as nosebleeds or bleeding gums, petechiae, blood in urine or stool.

**GI** Nausea, vomiting, and diarrhea are common when aminoglycosides are administered orally. Malabsorption syndrome and electrolyte imbalances may occur. GI reactions are rare with parenterally administered aminoglycosides.

- Monitor intake and output, especially if vomiting and/or diarrhea are present. If GI symptoms are persistent or severe, notify the physician.
- Monitor weight.
- Monitor electrolytes.

**Renal** Nephrotoxicity is a dose-related side effect of aminoglycosides. For this reason, high doses or drug accumulation must be avoided. Signs of renal damage include proteinuria, cells or casts in urine, decreased urine specific gravity, decreased creatinine clearance, increased serum creatinine, and increased BUN.

- Monitor urinalysis, serum creatinine and creatinine clearance, and BUN.
- Monitor intake and output, weight, and blood pressure. If urinary output begins to fall, notify the physician.
- Patients must be kept adequately hydrated. Analyze daily intake and output to determine if the patient is adequately hydrated for age and size.
- Visually inspect urine on a regular basis to note development of proteinuria, cells, or casts in urine.

**Liver** Hepatomegaly, hepatic necrosis, or transient increases in AST (SGOT), ALT (SGPT), LDH, alkaline phosphatase, and bilirubin are reported rarely.

- Monitor the laboratory test noted.
- Assess the patient for signs of liver impairment: jaundice, hepatomegaly, right upper quadrant abdominal pain, change in the color of consistency of stools, fever, malaise.

**Allergic** A few patients suffer rash, urticaria, pruritis, fever, and eosinophilia. Less common is transient agranulocytosis and anaphylaxis

- Question the patient about a history of allergic response to aminoglycosides, or any antibacterial agent, before administering the prescribed dose.
- Assess for signs of agranulocytosis: fever, malaise, altered level of consciousness, or development of new signs and symptoms: sore throat, urinary frequency, or dysuria.
- Observe for signs of allergic response: rash, urticaria, pruritus.
- Have drugs, equipment, and personnel readily available to treat an acute allergic response.
- Note clearly and prominently any drug allergy on the patient's chart, Kardex, or other records.
- Monitor vital signs.

**Table 16-2.**

| Aminoglycoside concentrations: guidelines for monitoring therapy* | | | |
|---|---|---|---|
| | Desired peak serum concentration ($\mu$g/ml) | Maximal trough concentration ($\mu$g/ml) | Maximal peak concentration ($\mu$g/ml) |
| Amikacin | 15–30 | 5–10 | 30–35 |
| Gentamicin | 4–10 | 1–2 | 10–12 |
| Kanamycin | 15–30 | 5–10 | 30–35 |
| Netilmicin | 6–12 | 0.5–2 | 16 |
| Streptomycin | 5–25 | 5 | 40–50 |
| Tobramycin | 4–10 | 1–2 | 10–12 |

*Aminoglycoside values may be assayed directly in serum as a guide to therapy. Blood samples are drawn immediately before a dose to assess the minimal concentration reached during therapy (trough); samples for peak concentrations are drawn at appropriate times after injection. If measured concentrations fail to achieve the range shown in the first column, therapeutic failure is likely. If measured concentrations exceed the values in the second or third columns, drug accumulation and toxicity are likely.

**Nursing interventions related to drug administration**
- Check expiration date before preparing and administering the prescribed dose.
- Nurses allergic to an antibacterial drug in a class should wear gloves while preparing ordered doses of the drug to avoid skin contamination.
- IM antibacterial preparations should be administered in a large muscle mass such as the dorsogluteal site or rectus femoris muscle in adults or the vastus lateralis muscle in infants and small children. Use anatomic landmarks to carefully identify sites. Aspirate carefully before injecting medication to avoid inadvertent intravenous injection. If blood is aspirated, withdraw the needle and prepare a fresh dose of medication. Record the injection site and rotate sites.
- Pain at the injection site can accompany any IM aminoglycoside.
- Observe patients carefully for the development of acute allergic reactions during the first 30 minutes following parenteral doses, especially after the first dose. Aminoglycosides are incompatible with other medications in a syringe.
- Because accurate peak and trough levels depend on drawing the blood sample in relation to when a dose of drug is given, aminoglycoside should be given as closely as possible to the ordered time if drug levels are to be measured.
- With topical preparations, ototoxicity and nephrotoxicity are rare but may occur. Factors influencing the likelihood of toxicity include the frequency of application, the size of the area to which the preparation is being applied, whether the skin surface is intact, and the amount and kind of other ototoxic or nephrotoxic drugs the patient might be receiving concomitantly.

**Patient and family education**
- Review with the patient and/or family the expected benefits and possible side effects of therapy.
- Caution the patient to report the development of any unexplained symptom or side effect.
- Encourage patients with a history of allergic response to wear a medical identification tag or bracelet noting their allergy.
- Review with patients the need to take the medication ordered for the specified period of time. Unused medications should be discarded. Patients should not share medications with others.
- Instruct patients to read the label to check for the expiration date. Teach patients to discard medications that have passed the expiration date, as the drugs may not work as well as desired.
- Many antibacterial agents are excreted through breast milk. Instruct lactating women to check with their physicians before breast-feeding while taking antibacterials.
- Remind patients to keep these and all medications out of the reach of children.

## amikacin sulfate (am-i-KAY-sin) aminoglycoside antibiotic

- amikacin sulfate: Amikin

**MECHANISM OF ACTION** • See entry for drug class (p. 304).

**INDICATIONS** **Serious infections caused by gram-negative bacteria** Susceptible organisms may include *Acinetobacter, Citrobacter, Enterobacter, Escherichia coli, Klebsiella, Proteus,* and *Providencia.* Infections caused by these bacteria include septicemia, complicated or recurrent infections of the urinary tract, and infections of the respiratory tract, skin, bones, joints, or central nervous system. **Serious infections caused by Pseudomonas aeruginosa** Susceptibility of the strain causing the infection should be tested, but amikacin is often effective. **Staphylococci** Amikacin may be indicated when staphylococci are contributing to mixed infections or when staphylococci or gram-negative aerobic bacteria might the causing the infection.

**CONTRAINDICATIONS** • See entry for drug class (p. 304).

**DOSAGE** **IM, IV:** ADULTS, CHILDREN AND OLDER INFANTS: 15 mg/kg (ideal body weight) daily in equally divided doses every 8 or 12 hours for persons with normal renal function. Daily doses should not exceed 15 mg/kg or 1.5 g and should not be administered for longer than 10 days. *Special patient populations:* ELDERLY: Doses may need adjustment because of the less efficient renal function of elderly patients.   **RENAL IMPAIRMENT:** Dosage in patients with renal disease must be reduced according to the degree of renal impairment. Loading doses followed by lower maintenance doses are used (see Overview, p. 304).   **NEONATES:** Amikacin is not recommended for neonates.   **PREG-NANCY:** Aminoglycosides can harm fetuses when the drugs are administered to pregnant women (FDA pregnancy category D).

**PREPARATIONS**   *Solution, injection:* 50 or 250 mg/ml with sodium bisulfite and sodium citrate.

**DRUG INTERACTIONS**   • See entry for drug class (p. 305).

**FATE**   Like all aminoglycosides, amikacin is not absorbed from the GI tract and must be administered parenterally. *Peak* serum concentrations are achieved within 45 minutes to 2 hours following IM administration. Amikacin is generally well distributed to most tissues except for the eye or normal CNS. Amikacin can be used for CNS infections, although intrathecal injections may be necessary. The drug concentrates in renal tissues and in certain structures in the inner ear. Amikacin crosses the placenta and enters fetuses. The excretion of amikacin is almost exclusively by glomerular filtration in the kidney. For this reason, even mild renal impairment can cause significant drug accumulation. The elimination *half-life* in healthy adults is 2 to 3 hours but may be as high as 30 to 86 hours in patients with severe renal impairment.

## ☙ NURSING CONSIDERATIONS

### Side effects, toxicities, and associated nursing actions
• See entry for drug class (p. 305).

### Nursing interventions related to drug administration
• For adults, the prescribed IV dose is diluted in 100 to 200 ml of usual IV fluids. The dose should be administered over 30 to 60 minutes.
• For infants, the dose should be well diluted in a volume determined by the dose and size of the child. The infant's dose should be infused over 1 to 2 hours. The dose in the older child should be infused over 30 to 60 minutes.
• See entry for drug class (p. 307).

### Patient and family education
• See entry for drug class (p. 307).

---

## gentamicin sulfate   (jen-tuh-MY-sin)                    aminoglycoside antibiotic

• gentamicin sulfate: Apogen, Cidomycin, Garamycin, Jenamicin

**MECHANISMS OF ACTION**   • See entry for drug class (p. 304).

**INDICATIONS**   **Serious infections caused by gram-negative bacteria** Susceptible organisms may include *Citrobacter, Enterobacter, E. coli, Klebsiella, Proteus,* and *Serratia.* Infections caused by these bacteria include septicemia, complicated or recurrent infections of the urinary tract, and infections of the respiratory tract, skin, bones, joints, or central nervous system.   **Serious infections caused by P. aeruginosa** Susceptibility of the strain causing the infection should be tested, but gentamicin is often effective. Increased effectiveness can be achieved by combination therapy with carbenicillin or another antipseudomonas penicillin.   **Serious infections caused by gram-positive bacteria** Serious infections such as endocarditis caused by group D streptococci or neonatal sepsis caused by staphylococci may respond best to combinations of gentamicin and an appropriate penicillin.

**CONTRAINDICATIONS**   **Severe or refractory skin lesions** Treatment of these lesions with topical preparations should be supplemented with administration of a systemic antibacterial agent. Extensive use of topical antibiotics occasionally leads to systemic absorption with subsequent toxicity or to local overgrowth of resistant organisms such as fungi. • For other contraindications, see entry for drug class (p. 304).

**DOSAGE**   **IM, IV:**   **ADULT:** 3 to 5 mg/kg (ideal body weight) daily in three or four equal doses. For most patients the preferred route is IM.   **CHILDREN:** Children and infants, 6 to 7.5 mg/kg daily in equal doses every 8 hours. Neonates, 2.5 mg/kg every 12 hours (5 mg/kg daily).   **Topical:**   **ADULTS OR CHILDREN:** Ophthalmic, 1 drop of a 0.3% solution every 4 to 8 hours or a 1 cm strip of 0.3% ointment every 6 to 12 hours. Otic, 3 or 4 drops in the ear canal every 4 to 8 hours. To skin, apply 0.1% cream or ointment three or four times daily.   *Special patient populations:*   **ELDERLY:** Doses may need adjustment because of the less efficient renal function of elderly patients.    **RENAL IMPAIRMENT:** Dosage in patients with renal disease must be reduced according to the degree of renal impairment (see Overview, p. 304).    **PREGNANCY:** Aminoglycosides can harm fetuses when the drugs are administered to pregnant women (FDA pregnancy category D).

**PREPARATIONS**    *Solution, IM or IV injection:* 10 or 40 mg/ml, with edetate disodium, parabens, and sodium bisulfite. *Solution, intrathecal injection:* 2 mg/ml, preservative-free. *Solution in 5% dextrose for IV infusion:* 60, 80, or 100 mg total, all at 1 mg/ml in dextrose. *Solution in 0.9% sodium chloride for IV infusion:* 40 mg at 0.4 or 0.8 mg/ml; 60 mg at 0.6, 1.0, or 1.2 mg/ml; 70 mg at 0.7 or 1.4 mg/ml; 80 mg at 0.8, 1.0, or 1.6 mg/ml; 90 mg at 0.9 or 1.8 mg/ml; 100 mg at 1.0 or 2.0 mg/ml; 120 mg at 1.2 or 2.4 mg/ml. *Ophthalmic-otic:* 0.3% ointment or solution. *Topical:* 0.1% ointment or cream.

**DRUG INTERACTIONS**    • See entry for drug class (p. 305).

**FATE**    Like all aminoglycosides, gentamicin is not absorbed from the GI tract and must be administered parenterally. *Peak* serum concentrations are achieved within 30 to 90 minutes following IM administration. Gentamicin is generally well distributed to most tissues. The drug does not readily enter the eye or the normal CNS but does concentrate in the kidneys and in certain structures in the inner ear. Gentamicin crosses the placenta and enters fetuses. Excretion is almost exclusively by renal glomerular filtration. For this reason, even mild renal impairment can cause significant drug accumulation. The elimination *half-life* of gentamicin in healthy adults is 2 to 3 hours but may be as high as 24 to 60 hours in patients with severe renal impairment.

## ❦ NURSING CONSIDERATIONS

### Side effects, toxicities, and associated nursing actions
• See entry for drug class (p. 305).

### Nursing interventions related to drug administration
• Dilute adult dose in 50 to 200 ml of 0.9% sodium chloride or 5% dextrose injection. Final dilution should not exceed 1 mg/ml. Administer dose over 30 minutes to 2 hours.
• For infants and children, the total volume of dilution would be smaller, but concentration should not exceed 1 mg/ml. Administer the dose to infants and children over 30 minutes to 2 hours.
• For intrathecal use, a preservative-free form is available.
• With topical use, patients may experience a sensitivity reaction to the gentamicin or to other agents in the cream preparation. Teach patients to report the development of skin irritation.
• With gentamicin eye drops, some patients experience irritation and redness. Teach patients to report the development of new or increased eye irritation.

### Patient and family education
• See entry for drug class (p. 307).

---

## kanamycin sulfate    (kan-uh-MY-sin)                                    aminoglycoside antibiotic

• kanamycin sulfate: Anamid, Kantrex, Klebcil

**MECHANISM OF ACTION**    • See entry for drug class (p. 304).

**INDICATIONS**    **Serious infections caused by gram-negative aerobic bacteria** Susceptible bacteria include *Acinetobacter, Enterobacter, Escherichia coli, Klebsiella, Proteus,* and *Serratia.* Infections that respond to kanamycin may include septicemia, peritonitis, complicated infections of the urinary tract, and infections of skin, bones, joints, and respiratory tract.    **Serious infections caused by gram-positive bacteria** Serious infections caused by staphylococci may respond to combinations of kanamycin and an appropriate penicillin.    **Tuberculosis** Kanamycin can be used for short-term therapy for strains of *Mycobacterium* shown to be susceptible.

**CONTRAINDICATIONS**    • See entry for drug class (p. 304).

**DOSAGE**    **IM, IV:**    **ADULTS, CHILDREN, AND INFANTS:** 15 mg/kg daily in equally divided doses every 8 or 12 hours. Daily dosage must not exceed 1.5 g.    **PO:**    **ADULT:** 4 to 12 g daily for reducing bacterial count in the bowel. Not for treatment of systemic infections.    **IP:**    **ADULT:** 500 mg in 20 ml sterile water for instillation.    **Inhalation:**    **ADULT:** 250 mg in 3 ml of 0.9% sodium chloride. Administer by nebulizer.    *Special patient populations:*    **ELDERLY:** Doses may need adjustment because of the less efficient renal function of elderly patients.   **RENAL IMPAIRMENT:** Dosage in patients with renal disease must be reduced according to the degree of renal impairment (see Overview, p. 304). **PREGNANCY:** Aminoglycosides can harm fetuses when the drugs are administered to pregnant women (FDA pregnancy category D).

**PREPARATIONS**   *Capsules:* 500 mg; *solution, injection:* 36.5, 250, or 333 mg/ml.

**DRUG INTERACTIONS**   • See entry for drug class (p. 305).

**FATE**   Like all aminoglycosides, kanamycin is not absorbed from the GI tract and must be administered parenterally. *Peak* serum concentrations are achieved within 1 hour following IM administration. Kanamycin is generally well distributed to most tissues except for the eyes or normal CNS. Kanamycin crosses the placenta and enters fetuses. Excretion is almost exclusively by renal glomerular filtration. For this reason, even mild renal impairment can cause significant drug accumulation. The elimination *half-life* of kanamycin in healthy adults is 2 to 4 hours but may be as high as 27 to 80 hours in patients with severe renal impairment.

## ❦ NURSING CONSIDERATIONS

### Side effects, toxicities, and associated nursing actions
• See entry for drug class (p. 305).

### Nursing interventions related to drug administration
• See entry for drug class (p. 307).
• For IV administration, dilute each 500 mg of drug in 100 to 200 ml of usual IV fluid. Infuse dose over 30 to 60 minutes.
• For infants and small children, the total volume will be reduced, but the dose should be infused over 30 to 60 minutes.

### Patient and family education
• See entry for drug class (p. 307).

---

## neomycin sulfate   (nee-oh-MY-sin)                              aminoglycoside antibiotic

• neomycin sulfate: Mycifradin, Myciguent

**MECHANISM OF ACTION**   • See entry for drug class (p. 304).

**INDICATIONS**   **Hepatic encephalopathy** Neomycin given orally may reduce the number of ammonia-producing organisms in the intestine. This action may relieve accumulation of nitrogenous wastes when hepatic failure has impaired the body's ability to eliminate them normally.   **Intestinal antisepsis** Neomycin may be used before colorectal surgery to minimize the possibility of peritoneal infections.   **Diarrhea** Enteropathogenic strains of *Escherichia coli* may be susceptible to oral neomycin.

**CONTRAINDICATIONS**   • See entry for drug class (p. 304).

**DOSAGE**   PO:   **ADULT:** 3 to 12 g of neomycin sulfate daily in four equal doses. Not for systemic infections. **CHILDREN:** 625 mg to 1.75 g $M^2$ for hepatic encephalopathy; alternatively, 50 to 100 mg/kg may be used.   *Special patient populations:*   **ELDERLY:** Doses may need adjustment because of the less efficient renal function of elderly patients.   **RENAL IMPAIRMENT:** Patients with renal failures are more likely to accumulate the drug and suffer toxicity, even when the drug is administered orally or topically.   **PREGNANCY:** Aminoglycosides can harm fetuses when the drugs are administered to pregnant women (FDA pregnancy category D).

**PREPARATIONS**   *Tablets:* 500 mg neomycin sulfate (equivalent to 350 mg neomycin). *Solution, oral:* 125 mg neomycin sulfate in each 5 ml. *Topical:* 0.5% neomycin sulfate (equivalent to 0.35% neomycin) as cream or ointment. *Combinations with other antibacterial agents, ophthalmic or topical:* • Neomycin sulfate 5 mg (3.5 mg neomycin equivalent) with 5000 units polymyxin B and 500 units bacitracin in each gram of ointment. • Neomycin sulfate 5 mg (3.5 mg neomycin equivalent) with 5000 units polymyxin B and 400 units bacitracin zinc in each gram of ointment. • Neomycin sulfate 2.5 mg (1.75 mg neomycin equivalent) with 5000 units polymyxin B and 25 µg gramicidin in each milliliter of ophthalmic solution. • Neomycin sulfate 5 mg (3.5 mg neomycin equivalent) with 10,000 units polymyxin B and 10 mg hydrocortisone in each milliliter of ophthalmic or otic solution or suspension.

**DRUG INTERACTIONS** • See entry for drug class (p. 305).

**FATE** Neomycin has similar properties to other aminoglycosides except that neomycin is more toxic than other members of this family. For this reason, neomycin should not be administered systemically. Administered topically or orally, neomycin is not absorbed significantly, and toxicity is unlikely.

**☙ NURSING CONSIDERATIONS**

**Side effects, toxicities, and associated nursing actions**
• See entry for drug class (p. 305).

**Nursing interventions related to drug administration**
• See entry for drug class (p. 307).

**Patient and family education**
• See entry for drug class (p. 307).

---

## netilmicin sulfate   (neh-till-MY-sin)                aminoglycoside antibiotic

• netilmicin sulfate: Netromycin

**MECHANISM OF ACTION** • See entry for drug class (p. 304).

**INDICATIONS** • As for gentamicin (p. 308).

**CONTRAINDICATIONS** • See entry for drug class (p. 304).

**DOSAGE** **IM, IV:** **ADULT:** 3 to 6.5 mg/kg ideal body weight daily in equal doses every 8 to 12 hours. Netilmicin must be given by deep IM injection. **CHILDREN:** 6 weeks to 12 years of age, 5.5 to 8 mg/kg daily in equal doses every 8 to 12 hours. Premature to 6 weeks of age, 4 to 6.5 mg/kg daily in equal doses every 12 hours. *Special patient populations:* **ELDERLY:** Doses may need adjustment because of the less efficient renal function of elderly patients. **RENAL IMPAIRMENT:** Dosage in patients with renal disease must be reduced according to the degree of renal impairment (see Overview, p. 304). **PREGNANCY:** Aminoglycosides can harm fetuses when the drugs are administered to pregnant women (FDA pregnancy category D).

**PREPARATIONS** *Solution, injection:* 25 mg/ml pediatric preparation, with propylparaben 0.2 mg, methylparaben 1.3 mg, edetate disodium 0.1 mg, sodium sulfate 2.6 mg, sodium metabisulfite 2.1 mg, and sodium sulfite 1.2 mg in each milliliter or 100 mg/ml with benzyl alcohol 10 mg, edetate disodium 0.1 mg, sodium metabisulfite 2.4 mg, and sodium sulfite 0.8 mg in each milliliter.

**DRUG INTERACTIONS** • See entry for drug class (p. 305).

**FATE** As for gentamicin (p. 309).

**☙ NURSING CONSIDERATIONS**

**Side effects, toxicities, and associated nursing actions**
• See entry for drug class (p. 305).

**Nursing interventions related to drug administration**
• See entry for drug class (p. 307).
• For IV administration, dilute the dose with 50 to 200 ml of usual IV solutions. Infuse the dose over 30 minutes to 2 hours.
• For infants and small children, the volume of fluid will be less but should be sufficient to infuse the dose over 30 minutes to 2 hours.

**Patient and family education**
• See entry for drug class (p. 307).

---

## paromomycin sulfate   (pair-oh-moh-MY-sin)                aminoglycoside antibiotic

• paromomycin sulfate: Humatin

**MECHANISM OF ACTION** The antibacterial effect of paromomycin sulfate is the same as for other aminoglycosides (see entry for drug class, p. 304). In addition, paromomycin has direct amebicidal effects and is effective against certain cestodes.

**INDICATIONS**    **Amebiasis** Paromomycin is effective only against the intestinal forms of the disease, killing both trophozoite or cysts forms of the ameba.    **Cestodiasis** Paromomycin may be effective against various tapeworms.

**CONTRAINDICATIONS**    **Ulcerative intestinal lesions or intestinal blockage** These conditions may lead to absorption of the drug systemically, causing toxicity.    **Impaired renal function** Small amounts of drug absorbed from the intestinal tract may accumulate in patients unable to excrete the agent.

**DOSAGE**    **PO:**    **ADULT:** For intestinal amebiasis, 25 to 35 mg/kg daily in equal doses every 8 hours for 5 to 10 days. For cestodiasis, 1 g every 15 minutes for four doses.    **CHILDREN:** For intestinal amebiasis, 750 mg/M$^2$ daily in equal doses every 8 hours for 5 days. For cestodiasis, 11 mg/kg every 15 minutes for four doses. *Special patient populations:* **PREGNANCY:** FDA pregnancy category D. **RENAL IMPAIRMENT:** See Contraindications.

**PREPARATIONS**    *Capsules:* 250 mg.

**DRUG INTERACTIONS**    Drug interactions are limited because the drug is not appreciably absorbed when used orally.

**FATE**    When administered orally, paromomycin is not absorbed significantly and is excreted in the feces.

**☙ NURSING CONSIDERATIONS**

### Side effects, toxicities, and associated nursing actions

**CNS** Headache and vertigo occur rarely.
- Assess for headache and vertigo. If vertigo develops, supervise the ambulation of hospitalized patients. Teach patients that if vertigo develops, patients should avoid driving or operating hazardous equipment until the effects of the medication wear off.

**Blood** Eosinophilia occurs rarely.
- Monitor white blood cell differential count.

**GI** Nausea, anorexia, vomiting, epigastric pain, abdominal cramping, diarrhea, pruritis ani, and malabsorption of nutrients have occurred.
- Assess for the development of these problems.
- Monitor intake, output, and weight.

**Renal** Hematuria is a rare, unexplained reaction.
- Visually inspect urine output for apparent development of hematuria.
- Monitor urinalysis.

**Allergic** Rash, exanthema, and eosinophilia may occur.
- If paromomycin is absorbed systemically, all the toxicities associated with other aminoglycosides can be expected. See entry for drug class (p. 305).

### Nursing interventions related to drug administration
- See entry for drug class (p. 307).

### Patient and family education
- See entry for drug class (p. 307).

---

## streptomycin sulfate    (strep-toh-MY-sin)    aminoglycoside antibiotic

- Sold under generic name

**MECHANISM OF ACTION**    • See entry for drug class (p. 304).

**INDICATIONS**    **Tuberculosis** Streptomycin is used along with one, two, or three other agents for initial therapy of serious cases of active tuberculosis.    **Tularemia (rabbit fever)** Streptomycin is the drug of choice for this zoonosis (disease caused by contact with infected animal).    **Plague** Streptomycin is effective against *Yersinia pestis,* the causative organism transmitted to humans from infected rodents by the bite of a flea.    **Endocarditis** This infection, usually caused by various forms of streptococci, is usually best treated by a combination of penicillin G with streptomycin or gentamicin.

**CONTRAINDICATIONS**    • See entry for drug class (p. 304).

**DOSAGE**    **IM, IV:**    **ADULT:** 1 to 4 g daily in equal doses every 6 to 12 hours. Doses must be reduced in renal failure.    **CHILDREN:** 20 to 40 mg/kg or 1 g/m$^2$ daily in equal doses every 6 to 12 hours.    *Special* *patient populations:* **ELDERLY**: Patients over 60 years receive 1 g daily in two equal doses for streptococcal endocarditis. Doses for all elderly patients should be adjusted, taking into account renal function and status of the eighth cranial nerve function (hearing and balance). **RENAL IMPAIRMENT**: Dosage in patients with renal disease must be reduced according to the degree of renal impairment (see Overview, p. 304). **PREGNANCY**: Aminoglycosides can harm fetuses when the drugs are administered to pregnant women (FDA pregnancy category D).

**PREPARATIONS** *Solution for IM injection:* 400 or 500 mg/ml, with sodium bisulfite, sodium citrate and phenol; *powder to prepare solution:* 1 or 5 g powder. Freshly prepared solutions are required for intrathecal, subarachnoid, or intrapleural injection.

**DRUG INTERACTIONS** • See entry for drug class (p. 305).

**LABORATORY TEST INTERFERENCE** **Glucose** assays using cupric sulfate may yield false-positive results in the presence of streptomycin.

**FATE** Like all aminoglycosides, streptomycin is not absorbed from the GI tract and must be administered parenterally. *Peak* serum concentrations are achieved within 1 to 2 hours following IM administration. Like all aminoglycosides, streptomycin does not enter the normal CNS but does concentrate in the kidneys and in certain structures in the inner ear and may cross the placenta and enter fetuses. Excretion is almost exclusively by renal glomerular filtration. For this reason, even mild renal impairment can cause significant drug accumulation. The elimination *half-life* is 2 to 3 hours in healthy adults but may be as high as 10 hours in neonates or 110 hours in patients with severe renal failure.

## ❧ NURSING CONSIDERATIONS

### Side effects, toxicities, and associated nursing actions
• See entry for drug class (p. 305).

### Nursing interventions related to drug administration
• Streptomycin should be administered deep IM. Follow directions on the container for dilution. The prepared dose should not have a concentration greater than 500 mg/ml.
• IV streptomycin is not recommended.

### Patient and family education
• See entry for drug class (p. 307).

## tobramycin sulfate  (toe-bra-MYE-sin)  aminoglycoside antibiotic

• tobramycin sulfate: Nebcin, Tobrex

**MECHANISM OF ACTION** • See entry for drug class (p. 304).

**INDICATIONS** **Serious infections caused by gram-negative bacteria** As for gentamicin (p. 308). **Serious infections caused by Pseudomonas aeruginosa** As for gentamicin (p. 308), including some strains resistant to gentamicin. **Serious infections caused by gram-positive bacteria** When *Staphylcoccus aureus* contributes to serious infections, tobramycin may be effective alone or may require combination therapy with a penicillin.

**CONTRAINDICATIONS** • See entry for drug class (p. 304).

**DOSAGE** IM, IV: **ADULT**: 3 to 5 mg/kg ideal body weight daily in equal doses every 8 hours. **CHILDREN**: Below 1 week of age, 4 mg/kg or less daily in equal doses every 12 hours. Older infants and children receive adult doses. *Special patient populations:* **ELDERLY**: Doses may need adjustment because of the less efficient renal function of elderly patients. **RENAL IMPAIRMENT**: Dosage in patients with renal disease must be reduced according to the degree of renal impairment (see entry for drug class, p. 304). **PREGNANCY**: Aminoglycosides can harm fetuses when the drugs are administered to pregnant women (FDA pregnancy category D).

**PREPARATIONS** *Solution, injection:* 10 to 40 mg/ml with edetate disodium, phenol, and sodium bisulfite; 1.2 g to dissolve for injection.

**DRUG INTERACTIONS** • See entry for drug class (p. 305).

**FATE** • As for gentamicin (p. 309).

## ❧ NURSING CONSIDERATIONS

### Side effects, toxicities, and associated nursing actions
- See entry for drug class (p. 305).

### Nursing interventions related to drug administration
- For IV infusion, reconstitute powder as directed on vial. Dilute the ordered dose further in 50 to 100 ml of usual IV solutions. Administer the dose over 20 to 60 minutes.
- Dilute pediatric doses in sufficient fluid to allow an infusion over 20 to 60 minutes.

### Patient and family education
- See entry for drug class (p. 307).

---

## spectinomycin hydrochloride  (spek-tin-oh-MYE-sin)  aminocyclitol antibiotic

- spectinomycin hydrochloride: Trobicin

**MECHANISM OF ACTION**  • Similar to aminoglycosides. See entry for drug class (p. 304).

**INDICATIONS**  • **Penicillinase-producing strains of Neisseria gonorrhoeae** Gonorrhea caused by penicillinase-producing strains are resistant to the penicillins that would otherwise be the drugs of choice. Spectinomycin can be used as single-dose therapy in uncomplicated cases. Alternative therapy is with a second- or third-generation cephalosporin. Spectinomycin is not effective against syphilis, chlamydial infections, or mycoplasma.

**CONTRAINDICATIONS**  **Allergy to spectinomycin** Previous allergic reactions are reasons to avoid exposure.

**DOSAGE**  IM:  ADULT: 2 g as single dose by deep IM injection.  CHILDREN: 40 mg/kg as a single dose by deep IM injection.  *Special patient populations:*  PREGNANCY: Safe use in pregnancy and lactation has not been established.

**PREPARATIONS**  *Solution, injection:* 2 or 4 g.

**DRUG INTERACTIONS**  Drug interactions are unlikely because spectinomycin is used only as a single dose.

**FATE**  Spectinomycin is not absorbed from the GI tract but is rapidly absorbed from IM sites, achieving *peak* serum concentrations within 1 hour. The elimination *half-life* of the drug is 1.2 to 2.8 hours in adults. Within 48 hours, 70% to 100% of the drug is excreted by the kidneys.

## ❧ NURSING CONSIDERATIONS

### Side effects, toxicities, and associated nursing actions
**CNS** Dizziness, headache, nervousness, and insomnia have been reported occasionally following a single dose of spectinomycin.
**Allergic** Urticaria, rashes, fever, or chills can occur.
- Assess the patient for these side effects.
- Request that the patient remain at the treatment center for 30 minutes following injection to see if side effects develop.
- Teach the patient to avoid driving or operating hazardous equipment if dizziness develops. Dizziness should diminish in time.
- Instruct the patient to notify the physician if fever, chills, or rash develop.
**GI** Nausea or vomiting occur occasionally.
- Teach the patient about this side effect. Instruct the patient to notify the physician if GI symptoms are severe or persistent.
**Local reactions** Pain at the injection site is the most frequently reported side effect.
- Warn the patient that this side effect may occur.

### Nursing interventions related to drug administration
- See entry for drug class (p. 307).

### Patient and family education  See entry for drug class (p. 307).
- If this drug is administered for treatment of gonorrhea, teach the patient about the disease and its transmission. Usual local procedures should be followed for reporting venereal disease and attempting to follow up with patient's sexual contacts.

# Chapter Seventeen

# Tetracyclines and chloramphenicol

**Tetracyclines**
chlortetracycline
demeclocycline hydrochloride
doxycycline calcium
doxycycline hyclate
doxycycline monohydrate
methacycline hydrochloride
minocycline hydrochloride

oxytetracycline
oxytetracycline hydrochloride
tetracycline
tetracycline hydrochloride

**Chloramphenicols**
chloramphenicol
chloramphenicol palmitate
chloramphenicol sodium succinate

**OVERVIEW OF THE DRUG CLASS**  Tetracyclines and chloramphenicol are classified as broad-spectrum antibiotics because they are effective against a variety of gram-positive and gram-negative bacteria as well as rickettsia and spirochetes. Resistance has developed against tetracyclines, lessening their clinical utility. In addition, broad-spectrum penicillins and cephalosporins have replaced tetracyclines in some but not all situations. Rare but potentially fatal side effects have limited the use of chloramphenicol. Nevertheless, tetracyclines and chloramphenicol remain useful in specific infections where other agents are not indicated and as topical agents (Table 17-1).

**MECHANISM OF ACTION**  Tetracyclines and chloramphenicol inhibit protein synthesis in bacteria. Growth and reproduction of bacteria are thereby inhibited, but the bacteria are not necessarily killed. In most circumstances, these drugs are therefore bacteriostatic. Protein synthesis in mammalian cells is normally not affected by these drugs for two reasons. First, the ribosomes found in the cytoplasm of mammalian cells do not as readily bind to the drugs as do the ribosomes from bacteria. Second, tetracyclines are concentrated in bacterial cells. The bacterial ribosomes are therefore exposed to higher concentrations of tetracycline than are mammalian cells.

**INDICATIONS**  **Infections caused by Rickettsia** Brill-Zinsser disease, Q fever, rickettsialpox, Rocky Mountain spotted fever, and typhus may be treated with tetracyclines or chloramphenicol.  **Infections caused by Chlamydia or Mycoplasma** Psittacosis (parrot fever) and infections of the genitourinary tract caused by *Chlamydia* or *Mycoplasma* often respond to tetracyclines. Tetracyclines are also used in atypical pneumonias caused by *Mycoplasma*.  **N. gonorrhoeae** Tetracyclines may be used in patients

**Table 17-1.**

| Summary of clinical uses of tetracyclines and chloramphenicol | | | | | | |
|---|---|---|---|---|---|---|
| **Antibacterial agent** | **Oral** | **IM** | **IV** | **Topical\*** | **Eye** | **Ear** |
| Chloramphenicol | + | | | + | + | + |
| Chloramphenicol palmitate | + | | | | | |
| Chloramphenicol sodium succinate | | | + | | | |
| Chlortetracycline | | | | + | + | |
| Demeclocycline CHl | + | | | | | |
| Doxycycline calcium | + | | | | | |
| Doxycycline hyclate | + | | + | | | |
| Doxycycline monohydrate | + | | | | | |
| Meclocycline sulfosalicylate | | | | + | | |
| Methacycline HCl | + | | | | | |
| Minocycline HCl | + | | | + | | |
| Oxytetracycline | + | + | | | | |
| Oxytetracycline HCl | + | | + | | | |
| Tetracycline | + | | | | | |
| Tetracycline HCl | + | + | + | + | + | |

\*Topical preparations are often used for acne.

unable to take penicillins.    **Brucellosis** Tetracyclines are used alone or with streptomycin or rifampin.
**Plague** Tetracyclines may be used with streptomycin.    **Cholera** Tetracyclines reduce the symptoms
and the excretion of the causative organism, *Vibrio cholerae*.    **Glanders or melioidosis** Tetracyclines
with streptomycin may be used for glanders *(Pseudomonas mallei); tetracyclines alone or with chloramphenicol may be used for melioidosis (Pseudomonas pseudomallei).    **Campylobacter fetus**
Strains may be susceptible to chloramphenicol, but all isolates should be tested.    **Granuloma inguinale** Tetracyclines may be effective.    **Infections caused by spirochetes** Tetracyclines may be the
drugs of choice for relapsing fever (*Borrelia recurrentis*) or Lyme's disease but are alternative drugs
for syphilis or yaws.    **Acne** Tetracyclines may be used in low doses over long periods for inflammatory acne vulgaris.    **Infections caused by gram-positive bacteria** Treatment of streptococcal
infections should be extended to 10 days to prevent the development of rheumatic fever or acute
glomerulonephritis.

**CONTRAINDICATIONS**    **Children under 8 years of age** Tetracyclines bind to and discolor permanent teeth in
this age group.    **Pregnancy** Pregnant women are at risk of severe hepatotoxicity from tetracyclines;
fetuses may suffer retardation of bone growth and discoloration of teeth. For these reasons, tetracyclines are routinely avoided in pregnancy.    **Renal impairment** Because tetracyclines diminish renal
function, these drugs are usually avoided in patients with pre-existing renal impairment. The exceptions are minocycline and doxycycline, which are highly lipid-soluble tetracyclines that are eliminated
efficiently by nonrenal mechanisms.

**DRUG INTERACTIONS**    **Aluminum, calcium, iron, magnesium, manganese, or zinc salts** bind to tetracyclines
and may impede absorption from the GI tract. Laxatives, antacids, or vitamin preparations may
contain high concentrations of one or more of these salts. The high calcium content of milk products
also impedes absorption of some tetracyclines.    **Oral anticoagulants** are more potent than expected
when tetracyclines are used. The antibiotics may lower vitamin K production by intestinal bacteria,
contributing to the anticoagulant effect.    **Barbiturates, phenytoin, and carbamazepine** increase the
rate of elimination of doxycycline and lower the serum concentrations of the antibiotic. Other tetracyclines are unaffected.    **Kaolin, pectin, or bismuth subsalicylate** may interfere with the absorption
of tetracyclines. These substances are common ingredients in antidiarrheal medications.    **Methoxyflurane** is nephrotoxic and may cause additive toxicity with tetracyclines. Fatal renal damage has
resulted.    **Penicillins and other beta-lactam antibiotics** are less effective when tetracyclines are also
given because the beta-lactam antibiotics are most effective against rapidly growing bacteria. The
bacteriostatic effect of the tetracyclines protects organisms from the bactericidal effect of the beta-
lactams.

## 🐛 NURSING CONSIDERATIONS
### Side effects, toxicities, and associated nursing actions
**CNS** Vestibular symptoms occur in most patients receiving minocycline; women are more prone to
this reaction than are men. All tetracyclines may cause dizziness, lightheadedness, vertigo, drowsi-
ness, fatigue, and ataxia. In infants, bulging fontanels are a clear sign of increased intracranial
pressure.
* Teach patients about the possibility of vestibular side effects; their appearance can be frighten-
  ing.
* Teach patients to avoid driving or operating hazardous equipment if dizziness, lightheadedness,
  vertigo, or drowsiness occur, and to notify the physician.
* Supervise the ambulation of ataxic patients.
* Monitor infants by palpating fontanels every 4 hours.
* Monitor the patient's level of consciousness for general changes in CNS functioning.

**Blood** Altered numbers and functions of white blood cells may occur, especially with prolonged
therapy. Hemolytic anemia and thrombocytopenia have occurred.
* Monitor the red blood cell count and reticulocyte count, platelet count, hematocrit and hemoglobin,
  and white blood cell differential count.
* Assess for signs of hemolytic anemia: jaundice, fever, chills, back or abdominal pain, fatigue, or
  hepatosplenomegaly.

- Assess for signs of thrombocytopenia: bleeding gums, nosebleeds, change of color of urine indicating possible hematuria, change of color of stools, excessive bruising, or development of petechiae.

**GI** These dose-related effects are the most common reactions to tetracyclines. Anorexia, nausea, vomiting, diarrhea, flatulence, abdominal discomfort, and epigastric distress are commonly reported symptoms. Suprainfections with *Candida* may cause stomatitis, dysphagia, sore throat, black hairy tongue, and anal lesions. Antibiotic-associated pseudomembranous colitis is possible.

- Assess for development of these GI symptoms. If nausea, vomiting, diarrhea, or any symptom is severe or persistent, notify the physician.
- Review with patients the signs of suprainfection. Teach patients not to treat these symptoms by increasing the dose of antibiotic.

**Renal** BUN levels often increase during therapy with tetracyclines; serum creatinine levels may also increase. Outdated or degraded preparations of tetracyclines may cause Fanconi's syndrome, which includes polyuria and proteinuria. Demeclocycline causes reversible diabetes insipidus in which the kidneys fail to respond normally to vasopressin; as a result large amounts of dilute urine are produced.

- Monitor BUN, serum creatinine, and urinalysis.
- Assess for signs of diabetes insipidus: copious amounts of dilute urine in excess of intake. Monitor urine specific gravity and intake and output, especially if urine output seems excessive or patient complains of frequent urination.
- Remind patients to discard unused antibiotics. Check the expiration date before preparing an ordered dose of tetracyclines. Teach patients to observe expiration dates.

**Liver** Fatty liver degeneration is possible, especially with large doses or in patients with pre-existing liver diseases. Pregnant women are also subject to this reaction.

- Monitor liver function tests if available. Other signs of possible fatty liver include nausea, vomiting, and hepatomegaly.

**Skin** Photosensitivity can occur with any tetracycline but seems most common with demeclocycline. An exaggerated sunburn reaction is the common sign of photosensitivity. Minocycline causes a blue-gray discoloration at sites of inflammation in some patients.

- Teach patients about these two side effects.
- Teach patients at risk for photosensitivity to avoid exposure to the sun and to wear long pants, a wide-brimmed hat, and long-sleeved shirt if outside. A maximum-protection sunscreen should also be used.

**Local effects** IM injections are painful, and IV injections are commonly associated with thrombophlebitis.

- IM route of administration is rarely used.
- Dilute IV injection as indicated and administer slowly to minimize thrombophlebitis. See entry for cephalosporins class (p. 280) for general guidelines about assessing thrombophlebitis.

**Allergy** Patients may develop rashes of various kinds or more dangerous signs such as angioedema, asthma, anaphylaxis, or serum sickness.

- Before administering any antibacterial agent, assess the patient for a history of allergy to any drug.
- Have drugs, equipment, and personnel readily available to treat acute an allergic response in any setting where antibacterial agents are administered.
- Note clearly and prominently any drug allergy on patient's chart, Kardex, or other records.
- Inspect the patient regularly for rashes or skin changes. Assess for other signs or symptoms (see preceding) that may indicate allergic response.
- Monitor vital signs.
- Serum sickness resembles an allergic response and is characterized by rapid onset of rash, urticaria, fever, arthralgia, edema, and hepatosplenomegaly. It usually develops 7 to 15 days after the patient begins drug therapy but may develop sooner. The incidence increases with age.

**Nursing interventions related to drug administration**

- Shake the liquid suspension preparations well, as the drug may have settled to the bottom of the bottle. Instruct the patient to do the same if the patient is to self-treat at home.

- Nurses allergic to an antibacterial drug in a class should wear gloves while preparing ordered doses of any drugs in the class to avoid skin contamination.
- Instruct patients taking tablets or capsules to take the dose with a full glass (8 ounces) of water or fluid.
- IM antibacterial preparations should be administered in a large muscle mass such as the dorsogluteal site or rectus femoris muscle in adults or the vastus lateralis muscle in infants and small children. Use anatomic landmarks to carefully identify the site. Aspirate carefully before injecting medication to avoid inadvertent intravenous injection. If blood is aspirated, withdraw the needle and prepare a fresh dose of medication. Record the injection site and rotate sites.
- Observe patients carefully for acute allergic reactions during the first 30 minutes following parenteral doses, especially after the first dose.

**Patient and family education**
- Review with the patient and/or family the expected benefits and possible side effects of therapy.
- Teach the patient to report the development of any unexplained symptom or side effect.
- Review with patients the need to take the medication as ordered for the specified period of time (usually 7 to 10 days). Unused medications should be discarded. Patients should not share medications with others.
- Encourage patients with a history of allergic response to a drug to wear a medication identification tag or bracelet noting the allergy.
- Many antibacterial agents are excreted through breast milk. Instruct lactating women to check with the physicians before breast-feeding while taking antibacterials.
- Teach patients to keep these and all medications out of the reach of children.
- Review with patients taking tetracyclines the drug interactions previously described. Note that most tetracyclines should not be taken with milk, antacids, laxatives, vitamin preparations, and many antidiarrhea preparations. Tetracyclines are best taken on an empty stomach. Teach patients to keep all health care providers informed of all medications being taken.

## chlortetracycline    (klor-tet-rah-SYE-klin)                    tetracycline antibiotic

- chlortetracycline: Aureomycin

**MECHANISM OF ACTION** • See entry for drug class (p. 315).
**INDICATIONS**   Chlortetracycline is used only as a topical agent for acne or as an antibacterial for the eye.
**DOSAGE**   Topical:   ADULTS AND CHILDREN: Apply ointment once or twice daily.   Ophthalmic:   ADULTS AND CHILDREN: Apply a 1 cm strip of ointment every 2 to 4 hours or more frequently.
**PREPARATIONS**   *Ointment, ophthalmic:* 1%; *ointment, topical:* 1%.
**❦ NURSING CONSIDERATIONS**
   **Side effects, toxicities, and associated nursing actions**   Systemic side effects are rarely seen with topical or ophthalmic preparations. Instruct patients to report the development of any unexpected sign or symptom. See entry for drug class (p. 316).

## demeclocycline hydrochloride    (dee-mek-loh-SYE-klin)           tetracycline antibiotic

- demeclocycline hydrochloride (demethylchlortetracycline): Declomycin

**MECHANISM OF ACTION** • See entry for drug class (p. 315).
**INDICATIONS** • See entry for drug class (p. 315).
**CONTRAINDICATIONS** • See entry for drug class (p. 316).
**DOSAGE**   PO:   ADULTS AND CHILDREN OVER 8 YEARS: 600 mg daily in two or four equal doses administered 1 hour before or 2 hours after meals. Dosage for children may be calculated based on body weight (6.6 to 13.2 mg/kg) or surface area (300 mg/M$^2$). *Special patient populations:*   ELDERLY: Special geriatric doses have not been established, but tetracyclines should not be administered at

normal doses to patients with impaired renal or hepatic function. **CHILDREN:** Children under 8 years of age should not receive tetracyclines because the drugs discolor permanent teeth. **PREGNANCY:** Avoid if possible in pregnancy and lactation. Fetal bones and teeth absorb tetracyclines administered to the mother. Fatal liver toxicity is possible in pregnant women.

**PREPARATIONS** *Tablets, film-coated:* 150 or 300 mg; *capsules:* 150 mg.

**DRUG INTERACTIONS** See entry for drug class (p. 316).

**DIAGNOSTIC TEST INTERFERENCE** **Glucose determinations** may be altered by tetracyclines. Assays using cupric sulfate may give false-positive results in the presence of tetracyclines. Assays using glucose oxidase may give false-negative values. **Urinary catecholamine assays** may be falsely increased when fluorimetric methods are used.

**FATE** Demeclocycline hydrochloride is administered orally because parenteral administration causes pain and phlebitis. Absorption from the GI tract is incomplete, with only 60% to 80% of a dose entering the blood. Food lowers absorption and may prevent effective concentrations from reaching the blood. *Peak* serum concentrations are reached in 3 to 4 hours in fasting adults. Excretion of demeclocycline involves renal and hepatic mechanisms. The elimination *half-life* in healthy adults is 10 to 17 hours but is extended in renal failure to 48 to 68 hours.

## ❧ NURSING CONSIDERATIONS

### Side effects, toxicities, and associated nursing actions
• See entry for drug class (p. 316).

### Nursing interventions related to drug administration
• See entry for drug class (p. 317).

### Patient and family education
• See entry for drug class (p. 318).
• Demeclocycline should be taken 1 hour before or 2 hours after meals or milk.
• Review with diabetics the possibility that taking this drug may interfere with accurate results of urine glucose determinations (see Diagnostic Laboratory Test Interference). Instruct patients to monitor blood glucose levels.

## doxycycline calcium (doxy-SYE-klin) tetracycline antibiotic

• doxycycline calcium: Vibramycin
• doxycycline hyclate
• doxycycline monohydrate

**MECHANISM OF ACTION** • See entry for drug class (p. 315).

**INDICATIONS** • See entry for drug class (p. 315).

**CONTRAINDICATIONS** • See entry for drug class (p. 316).

**DOSAGE** **PO:** **ADULTS AND CHILDREN OVER 8 YEARS:** 100 mg every 12 hours for the first day, then 50 to 100 mg every 12 hours. For children weighing less than 45 kg, 2.2 mg/kg every 12 hours for the first day, then 1.1 or 2.2 mg/kg every 12 hours **IV:** **ADULTS AND CHILDREN OVER 8 YEARS:** Doses as for PO administration. Infusions should be over 1 to 4 hours and the concentration of drug used should be 0.1 to 1 mg/ml. *Special patient populations:* **CHILDREN:** Children under 8 years of age should not receive tetracyclines because the drugs discolor permament teeth. **PREGNANCY:** Avoid if possible in pregnancy and lactation. Fetal bones and teeth absorb tetracyclines administered to the mother. Fatal liver toxicity is possible in pregnant women.

**PREPARATIONS** **Doxycycline calcium** *Oral, suspension:* 50 mg to 5 ml. **Doxycycline hyclate** *Tablets, film-coated:* 50 or 100 mg; *capsules:* 50 or 100 mg; *solution, injection:* 100 or 200 mg doxycycline with ascorbic acid. **Doxycyline monohydrate** *Oral, suspension:* 25 mg in 5 ml.

**DRUG INTERACTIONS** • See entry for drug class (p. 316).

**DIAGNOSTIC TEST INTERFERENCE** **Glucose determinations** may be altered by tetracyclines. Assays using cupric sulfate may give false-positive results in the presence of tetracyclines. Assays using glucose oxidase may give false-negative values. **Urinary catecholamine assays** may be falsely increased when fluorimetric methods are used.

**FATE** Because doxycycline is much more lipid-soluble than other tetracyclines, doxycycline is handled in the body differently than the rest of the class. Oral absorption of doxycycline is almost complete and is usually not impeded by food. *Peak* serum concentrations following oral doses appear by 1.5 to 4 hours. Doxycycline is eliminated primarily in feces, with less than one quarter of a dose being eliminated by the kidneys. The elimination *half-life* of doxycycline is 14 to 24 hours in healthy adults and 18 to 30 hours in patients with severe renal failure. Doses need not be adjusted in patients with renal impairment.

## ❦ NURSING CONSIDERATIONS

### Side effects, toxicities, and associated nursing actions
- See entry for drug class (p. 316).

### Nursing interventions related to drug administration
- See entry for drug class (p. 317).
- For IV administration, dilute each 100 mg or less with 10 ml of normal saline or sterile water for injection. Further dilute with 100 to 1000 ml of compatible IV solution. The final solution should be 0.1 to 1.0 mg/ml. Administer over 1 to 4 hours, although it is preferable to administer slowly; 100 mg diluted to 100 ml to a concentration of 1 mg/ml should be administered over 2 hours.
- Take care to avoid inadvertent introduction into adjacent soft tissues. Inspect IV insertion site carefully before initiating the infusion. Tell the patient to notify the nurse if the infusion rate slows or the IV becomes painful.

### Patient and family education
- See entry for drug class (p. 318).
- Oral doxycycline preparations may be taken without regard to meal time or milk products.
- Review with diabetics the possibility that taking this drug may interfere with accurate results of urine glucose determinations (see Diagnostic Test Interference). Instruct patients to monitor blood glucose levels.

---

## meclocycline   (mek-loh-SYE-klin)                 tetracycline antibiotic

- meclocycline: Meclan

**MECHANISM OF ACTION**   • See entry for drug class (p. 315).
**INDICATIONS**   Meclocycline is used only as a topical agent for acne.
**DOSAGE**   Topical:   **ADULTS AND CHILDREN:** Apply morning and evening to affected skin.
**PREPARATIONS**   *Cream* 1%.

## ❦ NURSING CONSIDERATIONS

### Side effects, toxicities, and associated nursing actions   Systemic side effects are rarely seen with topical or ophthalmic preparations. Instruct patients to report the development of any unexpected sign or symptom.
- See entry for drug class (p. 316).

---

## methacycline hydrochloride   (meth-uh-SYE-klin)        tetracycline antibiotic

- methacycline hydrochloride: Rondomycin

**MECHANISM OF ACTION**   • See entry for drug class (p. 315).
**INDICATIONS**   • See entry for drug class (p. 315).
**CONTRAINDICATIONS**   • See entry for drug class (p. 316).
**DOSAGE**   PO:   **ADULTS AND CHILDREN OVER 8 YEARS:** 600 mg daily in two or four equal doses, with or without an initial loading dose of 300 mg. Treatment of atypical pneumonia may require 900 mg daily for 6 days. Doses should be given 1 hour before or 2 hours after meals. Doses for children may be calculated on a weight basis (6.6 to 13.2 mg/kg daily) or on surface area (350 mg/$M^2$ daily) and given in two or four equal doses. *Special patient populations:*   **ELDERLY:** Special geriatric doses have

not been established, but tetracyclines should not be administered at normal doses to patients with impaired renal or hepatic function. **CHILDREN:** Children under 8 years of age should not receive tetracyclines because the drugs discolor permanent teeth. **PREGNANCY:** Avoid if possible in pregnancy and lactation. Fetal bones and teeth absorb tetracyclines administered to the mother. Fatal liver toxicity is possible in pregnant women.

**PREPARATION** *Capsules:* 150 or 300 mg.

**DRUG INTERACTIONS** • See entry for drug class (p. 316).

**DIAGNOSTIC TEST INTERFERENCE** **Glucose determinations** may be altered by tetracyclines. Assays using cupric sulfate may give false-positive results in the presence of tetracyclines. Assays using glucose oxidase may give false-negative values. **Urinary catecholamine assays** may be falsely increased when fluorimetric methods are used.

**FATE** Methacycline is administered orally because parenteral administration causes pain and phlebitis. Absorption from the GI tract is incomplete, with only 60% of a dose entering the blood. Food lowers absorption and may prevent effective concentrations from reaching the blood. *Peak* serum concentrations are reached in 2 to 3 hours in fasting adults. Excretion of methacycline involves both renal and hepatic mechanisms. The elimination *half-life* in healthy adults is 7 to 15 hours but is extended in renal failure to 44 hours.

## NURSING CONSIDERATIONS

### Side effects, toxicities, and associated nursing actions
• See entry for drug class (p. 316).

### Nursing interventions related to drug administration
• See entry for drug class (p. 317).

### Patient and family education
• See entry for drug class (p. 318).
• Methacycline should be taken 1 hour before or 2 hours after meals or milk.
• Review with diabetics the possibility that taking this drug may interfere with accurate results of urine glucose determinations (see Diagnostic Test Interference). Instruct patients to monitor blood glucose levels.

## minocycline hydrochloride (min-oh-SYE-klin) tetracycline antibiotic

• minocycline hydrochloride: Minocin

**MECHANISM OF ACTION** • See entry for drug class (p. 315).

**INDICATIONS** • See entry for drug class (p. 315).

**CONTRAINDICATIONS** • See entry for drug class (p. 316).

**DOSAGE** **PO, IV:** **ADULTS AND CHILDREN OVER 8 YEARS:** 200 mg initially, followed by 100 mg every 12 hours or 100 to 200 mg initially, followed by 50 mg every 6 hours. Children receive initial doses of 4 mg/kg followed by 2 mg/kg every 12 hours. *Special patient populations:* **CHILDREN:** Children under 8 years of age should not receive tetracyclines because the drugs discolor permanent teeth. **PREGNANCY:** Avoid if possible in pregnancy and lactation. Fetal bones and teeth absorb tetracyclines administered to the mother. Fatal liver toxicity is possible in pregnant women.

**PREPARATIONS** *Tablets, film-coated:* 50 to 100 mg; *capsules:* 50 or 100 mg; *oral suspension:* 50 mg in 5 ml, with 5% alcohol and parabens. *solution, infusion* 100 mg.

**DRUG INTERACTIONS** • See entry for drug class (p. 316).

**DIAGNOSTIC TEST INTERFERENCE** **Glucose determinations** may be altered by tetracyclines. Assays using cupric sulfate may give false-positive results in the presence of tetracyclines. Assays using glucose oxidase may give false-negative values. **Urinary catecholamine assays** may be falsely increased when fluorimetric methods are used. Minocycline may not cause this interference, but the other tetracyclines interfere.

**FATE** Minocycline is a highly lipid-soluble drug that is handled in the body much like doxycycline. Minocycline may also be used in patients with renal impairment, but doxycycline is more often chosen in this circumstance. See Doxycycline (p. 320).

## ❦ NURSING CONSIDERATIONS

### Side effects, toxicities, and associated nursing actions
- See entry for drug class (p. 316). Note that most patients suffer CNS side effects related to vestibular effects.

### Nursing interventions related to drug administration
- See entry for drug class (p. 317).
- For IV use, reconstitute as directed on vial with 5 ml of sterile water for injection. Further dilute each 100 mg of drug with 500 to 1000 ml of compatible IV fluid to make a solution of 100 to 200 µg/ml. Administer this dilute solution immediately after preparing and infuse over 6 hours.

### Patient and family education
- See entry for drug class (p. 318).
- Minocycline may be taken without regard to meals or milk.
- Review with diabetics the possibility that taking this drug may interfere with accurate results of urine glucose determinations (see Diagnostic Test Interference). Instruct patients to monitor blood glucose levels.

---

## oxytetracycline    (oxy-tet-rah-SYE-klin)                    tetracycline antibiotic

- oxytetracycline: Oxymycin, Terramycin
- oxytetracycline hydrochloride: E.P. Mycin, Uri-Tet

**MECHANISM OF ACTION** • See entry for drug class (p. 315).

**INDICATIONS** • See entry for drug class (p. 315).

**CONTRAINDICATIONS** • See entry for drug class (p. 316).

**DOSAGE**    **PO:** **ADULTS AND CHILDREN OVER 8 YEARS:** 1 to 2 g daily in four equal doses. For film-coated tablets, 500 mg (two tablets) initially, followed by 250 mg every 6 hours. Up to 4 g daily may be used. Doses for children are calculated by weight (25 to 50 mg/kg daily) or by surface area (0.6 to 1.2 g/M$^2$ daily), given in four equal doses.    **IM:** **ADULTS AND CHILDREN OVER 8 YEARS:** 250 mg as a single dose or 300 mg daily in two or three equal doses. For children, 15 to 25 mg/kg daily in two or three equal doses up to a maximal daily dose of 250 mg.    **IV:** **ADULTS AND CHILDREN OVER 8 YEARS:** When PO doses are not practical, 0.5 to 1 g daily may be given in two equal infusions. The maximal daily dose is 500 mg every 6 hours. For children, 10 to 20 mg/kg daily in two equal infusions.    *Special patient populations:*    **ELDERLY:** Special geriatric doses have not been established, but tetracyclines should not be administered at normal doses to patients with impaired renal or hepatic function.    **CHILDREN:** Children under 8 years of age should not receive tetracyclines because the drugs discolor permanent teeth.    **PREGNANCY:** Avoid if possible in pregnancy and lactation. Fetal bones and teeth absorb tetracyclines administered to the mother. Fatal liver toxicity is possible in pregnant women.

**PREPARATIONS**    **Oxytetracycline** *Tablets, film-coated:* 250 mg; *solution, injection:* 50 mg/ml or 125 mg/ml oxytetracycline in 2% lidocaine. For IM use.    **Oxytetracycline hydrochloride** *Capsules:* 250 mg; *solution, injection:* 250 or 500 mg with ascorbic acid. For IV use.    **Oxytetracycline hydrochloride combinations** *Capsules:* 250 mg oxytetracycline with 50 mg phenazopyridine hydrochloride and 250 mg sulfamethizole.

**DRUG INTERACTIONS** • See entry for drug class (p. 316).

**DIAGNOSTIC TEST INTERFERENCE**    **Glucose determinations** may be altered by tetracyclines. Assays using cupric sulfate may give false-positive results in the presence of tetracyclines. Assays using glucose oxidase may give false-negative values.    **Urinary catecholamine assays** may be falsely increased when fluorimetric methods are used.

**FATE**    Absorption of oxytetracycline from the GI tract is incomplete, with only 60% of a dose entering the blood. Food lowers absorption and may prevent effective concentrations from reaching the blood. *Peak* serum concentrations are reached in 2 to 4 hours in fasting adults. Excretion of oxytetracycline involves both renal and hepatic mechanisms. The elimination *half-life* in healthy adults is 6 to 10 hours but is extended in renal failure to 47 to 66 hours.

## ❦ NURSING CONSIDERATIONS

### Side effects, toxicities, and associated nursing actions
- See entry for drug class (p. 316).

### Nursing interventions related to drug administration
- See entry for drug class (p. 317).
- For IV use, dilute as directed on the vial to make a solution of 25 or 50 mg of oxytetracycline per milliliter. Further dilute in at least 100 ml of 0.9% sodium chloride injection, 5% dextrose injection, or Ringer's injection. The rate of administration should not exceed 100 mg over 5 minutes. The infusion must be completed within 12 hours of dilution.

### Patient and family education
- See entry for drug class (p. 318).
- Oxytetracycline should be taken 1 hour before or 2 hours after meals or milk products.
- Review with diabetics the possibility that taking this drug may interfere with accurate results of urine glucose determinations (see Diagnostic Test Interference). Instruct patients to monitor blood glucose levels.

---

## tetracycline  (tet-rah-SYE-klin)                     tetracycline antibiotic

- **tetracycline hydrochloride:** Achromycin, Bristacycline, Cyclopar, Medicycline, Neo-tetrine, Novatetra, Panmycin, Retet, Robitet, Sumycin, Tetra-C, Tetracyn, Tetralean, Tetrex

**MECHANISM OF ACTION** • See entry for drug class (p. 315).

**INDICATIONS** • See entry for drug class (p. 315).

**CONTRAINDICATIONS** • See entry for drug class (p. 316).

**DOSAGE**  PO: **ADULTS AND CHILDREN OVER 8 YEARS:** 1 to 2 g daily in two to four equal doses. For children, 25 to 50 mg/kg or 0.6 to 1.2 g daily in two to four equal doses.  IV: **ADULTS AND CHILDREN OVER 8 YEARS:** When PO doses are not practical, 250 to 500 mg may be given every 12 hours up to a maximum of 500 mg every 6 hours. For children, 10 to 20 mg/kg daily in two equal infusions.  IM: **ADULTS AND CHILDREN OVER 8 YEARS:** 250 mg daily as a single dose or 300 mg daily in two or three equal doses. For children, 15 to 25 mg/kg daily in two or three doses up to a maximum of 250 mg at one time.  **Topical:** **ADULTS OR CHILDREN:** Apply ointment once or twice daily to affected areas; apply solution for acne morning and evening.  **Eye:** **ADULTS AND CHILDREN:** Apply a 1 cm strip of ointment every 2 to 4 hours or more frequently; apply suspension 1 drop every 6 to 12 hours or more frequently.  *Special patient populations:* **ELDERLY:** Special geriatric doses have not been established, but tetracyclines should not be administered at normal doses to patients with impaired renal or hepatic function.  **CHILDREN:** Children under 8 years of age should not receive tetracyclines because the drugs discolor permanent teeth.  **PREGNANCY:** Avoid if possible in pregnancy and lactation. Fetal bones and teeth absorb tetracyclines administered to the mother. Fatal liver toxicity is possible in pregnant women.

**PREPARATIONS**  Tetracycline *Suspension, oral:* 125 mg in 5 ml; *capsules, combinations:* 250 mg with 50 mg amphotericin B; *suspension, oral combination:* 125 mg in 5 ml, with 25 mg amphotericin B in each 5 ml.  **Tetracycline hydrochloride** *Tablets, film-coated:* 250 to 500 mg; *capsules:* 100, 250, or 500 mg; *powder to prepare solution for IV injection:* 250 or 500 mg; *powder to prepare solution, injection combination:* 100 or 250 mg with 40 mg procaine hydrochloride; *ointment or suspension, ophthalmic:* 1%; *ointment or solution, topical:* 3% ointment or 2.2 mg/ml solution.

**DRUG INTERACTIONS** • See entry for drug class (p. 316).

**DIAGNOSTIC TEST INTERFERENCE**  **Glucose determinations** may be altered by tetracyclines. Assays using cupric sulfate may give false-positive results in the presence of tetracyclines. Assays using glucose oxidase may give false-negative values.  **Urinary catecholamine assays** may be falsely increased when fluorimetric methods are used. Minocycline may not cause this interference, but the other tetracyclines interfere.

**FATE**    Absorption of tetracycline from the GI tract is incomplete, with only 75% to 80% of a dose entering the blood. Food lowers absorption and may prevent effective concentrations from reaching the blood. *Peak* serum concentrations are reached in 2 to 4 hours in fasting adults. Excretion of tetracycline involves both renal and hepatic mechanisms. The elimination *half-life* in healthy adults is 6 to 12 hours but is extended in renal failure up to 120 hours.

## ☙ NURSING CONSIDERATIONS

### Side effects, toxicities, and associated nursing actions
- See entry for drug class (p. 316).

### Nursing interventions related to drug administration
- See entry for drug class (p. 317).
- Read labels carefully. Preparations with procaine hydrochloride are for IM use only.
- For IV use, dilute as directed on vial to make a solution of 50 mg/ml. Further dilute this solution with 100 to 1000 ml of compatible IV solution. Administer IV solution over 8 to 12 hours. Avoid giving IV solutions IM or subcutaneously. Infuse slowly and avoid extravasation.
- Panmycin brand capsules contain FD & C coloring #5 (tartrazine), which may cause an allergic response in some individuals. Although rare, this response is seen more often in persons with aspirin hypersensitivity.

### Patient and family education
- See entry for drug class (p. 318).
- Tetracycline should be taken 1 hour before or 2 hours after meals or after consuming milk products.
- Review with diabetics the possibility that taking this drug may interfere with accurate results of urine glucose determinations (see Diagnostic Test Interference). Instruct patients to monitor blood glucose levels.

---

## chloramphenicol    (klor-am-FEN-i-kol)    antibiotic

- chloramphenicol palmitate, chloramphenicol sodium succinate, chloramphenicol: Chloromycetin, Mychel

**MECHANISM OF ACTION**    • See entry for drug class (p. 315).

**INDICATIONS**    **Typhoid fever** Acute infections caused by *Salmonella typhi* can be controlled by chloramphenicol. The carrier state is not eliminated by chloramphenicol but is prevented by aminopenicillins such as ampicillin or amoxicillin.    **Infections caused by Hemophilus influenzae** Serious infections, including meningitis, septicemia, septic arthritis, cellulitis, or epiglottitis, may be caused by *H. influenzae*. Chloramphenicol is often used as initial therapy because resistance to chloramphenicol is less common than resistance to ampicillin.    **Infections of the CNS** Chloramphenicol is well distributed to the CNS and is effective for meningitis and cerebral abscesses. Susceptible organisms contributing to these infections include *Hemophilus influenzae, Streptococcus pneumoniae,* or *Neisseria meningitidis*.    **Anaerobic infections** Chloramphenicol is effective against many anaerobic bacteria that contribute to abscesses or to infections of bone, the abdominal cavity, soft tissues, or the mouth.
- For other indications, see entry for drug class (p. 315).

**CONTRAINDICATIONS**    **Prior reaction to chloramphenicol** These patients may be more at risk of serious reactions.    **Neonates** Although neonates may receive chloramphenicol, they cannot tolerate doses adjusted simply by weight of the infant because they excrete the drug much more slowly than adults. If chloramphenicol must be used in this age group, blood concentrations of the drug should be monitored to guide therapy and prevent dangerous or fatal drug accumulation.    **Mild or moderate infections responsive to safer antibiotics** Because chloramphenicol can cause fatal side effects, the drug should be reserved for those infections where safer antibiotics are ineffective. The incidence of fatal complications is estimated as 1 in 30,000 patients.

**DOSAGE**   PO, IV:   **ADULT:** 50 mg/kg daily in equal doses every 6 hours. Doses up to 100 mg/kg may be used if concentrations in the blood are monitored to prevent dangerous accumulation.   **CHILDREN:** Children over 1 month of age may usually receive adult doses. In neonates or other children with immature renal and hepatic excretion mechanisms, 25 mg/kg daily in four equal doses. Between 2 and 4 weeks of age, doses may be 25 mg/kg every 12 hours. Drug concentrations should be monitored to prevent dangerous or fatal accumulation.   **Topical:**   **ADULTS OR CHILDREN:** Apply to affected area three or four times daily.   **Eye:**   **ADULTS OR CHILDREN:** Apply ointment as a 1 cm strip every 3 hours or less; apply solutions 1 drop every 1 to 4 hours.   **Ear:**   **ADULTS OR CHILDREN:** Two or 3 drops in the ear canal every 6 to 8 hours.   *Special patient populations:*   **PREGNANCY:** Safe use in pregnancy and lactation has not been established. Chloramphenicol crosses the placenta and enters milk. **HEPATIC OR RENAL IMPAIRMENT:** Doses may need to be reduced and serum concentrations monitored to prevent dangerous accumulation of the drug.

**PREPARATIONS**   **Chloramphenicol** *Capsules:* 250 mg; *cream, topical:* 1% cream (Chloromycetin); *ointment, ophthalmic:* 1% (Chloromycetin, Chloroptic, Fenicol, Pentamycetin); *solution, ophthalmic:* 0.5% (Chloroptic, Isopto Fenicol, Ophthochlor, Pentamycetin) or 25 mg with 15 ml sterile water for reconstitution (Chloromycetin); *solution, otic:* 0.5%.   **Chloramphenicol palmitate** *Suspension, oral:* 150 mg in 5 ml.   **Chloramphenicol sodium succinate** *Powder to prepare solution for injection:* 1 g. To prepare a 10% (100 mg/ml) solution, add 10 ml sterile water or 5% dextrose solution.

**DRUG INTERACTIONS**   **Phenobarbital** induces liver microsomal enzymes that contribute to metabolism of chloramphenicol. As a result, chloramphenicol is eliminated faster than normally and lower blood concentrations are achieved with standard doses.   **Chlorpropamide, dicumarol, phenytoin, and tolbutamide** are metabolized by liver enzymes that are inhibited by chloramphenicol. As a result, the concentrations of these four drugs may increase, and their effects may be prolonged.   **Folic acid, vitamin B$_{12}$, or iron preparations** may have delayed actions in the presence of chloramphenicol. **Myelosuppressive agents** may have dangerous additive myelosuppressive effects with those of chloramphenicol.

**FATE**   Chloramphenicol is rapidly and completely absorbed from the GI tract, producing *peak* serum concentrations within 1 to 3 hours. Chloramphenicol palmitate must be hydrolyzed to release free chloramphenicol for absorption. Chloramphenicol sodium succinate, which is administered parenterally, must also be hydrolyzed to release the active free chloramphenicol. The rate of hydrolysis varies greatly from patient to patient, causing considerable differences in blood levels achieved with standard doses. Chloramphenicol preparations should not be administered IM because absorption is much worse than for oral or IV doses. Chloramphenicol is well distributed to most body sites, including into the CNS. The drug is chemically combined (conjugated) in the liver with glucuronic acid to form the more water-soluble chloramphenicol glucuronide, which is then excreted by the kidneys. The elimination *half-life* is 1.5 to 4.1 hours if hepatic and renal function are normal. The *half-life* in neonates is 24 hours or longer, because hepatic and renal mechanisms for elimination are immature.

## ❦ NURSING CONSIDERATIONS

### Side effects, toxicities, and associated nursing actions

**CNS** Chloramphenicol is neurotoxic, occasionally causing peripheral neuritis or optic neuritis. Optic neuritis may cause loss of visual acuity in both eyes, central scotomas or, rarely, blindness. These effects usually follow long-term use of high doses. Other effects occasionally reported include headache, confusion, depression, and delirium.
- Ideally, an assessment of visual acuity would be done before therapy. Question patients about subjective changes in vision during drug therapy.
- Be alert to changes in mood or affect. Monitor level of consciousness.

**CV** Cardiovascular collapse is the usual cause of death from gray syndrome. This condition is usually seen in neonates or immature infants who accumulate toxic concentrations of the drug because they lack the capacity to eliminate chloramphenicol as quickly as adults. Symptoms of gray syndrome include failure of the infant to feed, abdominal distention, progressive pallid cyanosis, and irregular respiration.

- Note that gray syndrome can occur in the neonates of a mother who received chloramphenicol during labor or the last few days of pregnancy.
- Assess newborns at risk for gray syndrome every 2 to 4 hours for signs of this syndrome. Monitor the respiratory rate.

**Blood** Chloramphenicol depresses bone marrow function in two ways. The first is a dose-dependent process and is to be expected in any patient receiving more than 4 g daily or whose plasma concentration exceeds 25 μg/ml. Signs include anemia, vacuolation of erythroid cells, reticulocytopenia, leukopenia, thrombocytopenia, and increased serum iron and iron-binding capacity. This form of bone marrow depression is usually reversible. The second form of bone marrow depression is very rare (estimated at 1 in 30,000 patients) but is irreversible. This reaction is not related to dose and progresses to fatal aplastic anemia. Unlike the dose-dependent process, this anemia does not necessarily appear during therapy but may become evident weeks or months after administration of the drug.

- Monitor serum drug levels. Monitor hematocrit and hemoglobin, reticulocyte count, white blood cell differential, platelet count, and serum iron and iron-binding capacity.
- Monitor for signs of aplastic anemia: fever, sore throat, fatigue, bruising, symptoms of a cold or symptoms of urinary tract infection. Teach the patient to report these symptoms should they develop even after discontinuing the medication.

**GI** Nausea, vomiting, diarrhea, irritations of the GI tract, and unpleasant taste are uncommon side effects of chloramphenicol.

- Assess the patient for GI symptoms. If symptoms are persistent or severe, notify the physician.
- A bitter taste that accompanies IV injection usually only lasts 2 to 3 minutes.

**Allergic** Urticaria, rashes, fever, angioedema, hemorrhages in skin and on mucosal surfaces, or anaphylaxis have been reported.

- Before administering any antibacterial agent, assess the patient for a history of allergy to any drug.
- Have drugs, equipment, and personnel readily available to treat acute allergic responses in any setting where antibacterial agents are administered.
- Note clearly and prominently any drug allergy on patient's chart, Kardex, or other records.
- Visually inspect the patient regularly for rashes or skin changes. Assess for other signs or symptoms (see preceding) that may indicate an allergic response.
- Monitor vital signs.

### Nursing interventions related to drug administration
- See entry for drug class (p. 317).
- Systemic effects and toxicities can occur with topical or ophthalmic preparations. Assess patients carefully.
- For IV administration, dilute each gram with 10 ml of sterile water for injection or 5% dextrose injection to make a 10% solution. Administer ordered dose direct IV push over at least 1 minute. The dose may be further diluted in 50 to 100 ml of 5% dextrose in water and administered over 30 to 40 minutes.
- Patients should be switched to oral doses as soon as possible.

### Patient and family education
- See entry for drug class (p. 318).

# Chapter Eighteen
# Macrolides

erythromycin  
erythromycin estolate  
erythromycin ethylsuccinate  
erythromycin gluceptate  

erythromycin lactobionate  
erythromycin stearate  
troleandomycin  

**OVERVIEW OF THE DRUG CLASS**  Erythromycins and other macrolides are used in much the same way as the narrow-spectrum penicillins. Erythromycins are often called penicillin substitutes for this reason. Macrolides are especially effective against atypical pneumonias such as those caused by *Mycoplasma* and *Legionnella* (Legionnaire's disease).

**MECHANISM OF ACTION**  Erythromycins and other macrolides are usually bacteriostatic. These drugs inhibit bacterial protein synthesis by binding to bacterial ribosomes. Macrolides bind to the same general site as other classes of drugs, such as chloramphenicol, clindamycin, or lincomycin. Therefore, when bacteria become resistant to any of these drugs, resistance is often gained toward all. Resistance usually involves altered ribosomes, which prevent the drugs from binding.

**INDICATIONS**  **Preventing infections caused by Streptococcus** To prevent infection in patients who have had rheumatic fever or in patients with artificial heart valves, erythromycins may substitute for penicillins. This substitution is appropriate if the patient is allergic to penicillins.  **Syphilis, gonorrhea, chlamydial infections of the genitourinary tract** Erythromycins may substitute for tetracyclines or penicillins in treating these diseases. This substitution is appropriate if patients are allergic to penicillins, cannot tolerate tetracyclines, or if the organisms are resistant to these drugs.  **Legionnaire's disease** Erythromycins may be used alone or in combination with rifampin.  **Atypical pneumonia** Erythromycins may be effective against *Mycoplasma pneumoniae,* an organism responsible for certain atypical pneumonias.  **Diphtheria** In treating acute cases, erythromycins are as effective as penicillins and are more effective than penicillins in eradicating the carrier state.  **Acne** Erythromycins may be used topically.  **Presurgical prophylaxis** Erythromycins may be part of a regimen to lower intestinal bacterial counts before abdominal surgery.

**CONTRAINDICATIONS**  **Allergy to any erythromycin-type drug** Allergy to any erythromycin preparation is reason to withhold all forms of the drug. • For specific contraindications, see individual agents.

**DRUG INTERACTIONS**  **Carbamazepine** serum concentrations may increase because erythromycin blocks hepatic destruction of carbamazepine. Accumulation of carbamazepine causes ataxia, drowsiness, dizziness, and vomiting.  **Warfarin** anticoagulant may be potentiated, which may lead to bleeding. Erythromycin may block the hepatic metabolism of warfarin, causing accumulation of the anticoagulant and development of symptoms.  **Theophylline** metabolism by the liver may be blocked by erythromycin. Because the safety margin with theophylline is so narrow, blood levels of the drug may need to be monitored when erythromycin and theophylline are given concurrently.

## ❦ NURSING CONSIDERATIONS

### Side effects, toxicities, and associated nursing actions

**GI** Intestinal and stomach cramping are common because erythromycin stimulates smooth muscle of the intestinal tract. Nausea, vomiting, and diarrhea also occur. These reactions are dose-related and are the most common of those experienced with erythromycins.

- If GI symptoms are severe or persistent, notify the physician. Monitor intake, output, and weight.
- Erythromycins should usually be taken on an empty stomach, 1 hour before or 2 hours after eating will a full glass (8 ounces) of water. Exceptions include certain enteric-coated erythromycin preparations, as well as the estolate and ethylsuccinate forms, which may be taken without regard to meals. If GI symptoms are severe, a switch to a different form that could be taken with meals may help; consult the physician.

**Liver** Because erythromycins are metabolized in the liver, the accumulation of the drug may produce some hepatic dysfunction. In some patients jaundice accompanies other signs of impaired hepatic function.

- Instruct patients to report the development of jaundice, malaise, fever, right upper quadrant abdominal pain, or change in the color or consistency of stools.
- Monitor liver function tests.

**Ototoxicity** Very large doses of erythromycins may produce tinnitus, vertigo, or hearing loss. These signs may be reversible when the drug is discontinued.

- Monitor the patient for signs of ototoxicity.
- Instruct patients to report the development of these symptoms.

**Local effects** IV preparations of erythromycins may cause irritation, pain, and phlebitis. For this reason, they are given by slow infusion rather than by IV push.

- Ascertain that the IV line is patent before administering IV doses. Instruct the patient to report the development of pain or irritation in the vein. If discomfort occurs, inspect the vein for signs of phlebitis and slow the infusion. If phlebitis is present, discontinue the infusion and restart in another site.

**Allergy** Urticaria, rashes and, rarely, anaphylaxis have occurred.

- Obtain a history of allergic responses to erythromycins before administering doses.
- Have drugs, equipment, and personnel available to treat acute allergic responses in settings where any erythromycins are administered.
- Note clearly and prominently any drug allergy on the patient's chart, Kardex, or other records.
- Inspect the patient for development of skin changes.

### Nursing interventions related to drug administration

- Review with patients information about taking the prescribed drug with meals if desired (see GI side effects).
- Teach patients that enteric-coated tablets or capsules containing enteric-coated pellets must be swallowed whole, not crushed or chewed.
- Remind patients that chewable tablets must be crushed or chewed for several minutes before swallowing.
- Remind patients to shake suspension forms vigorously before pouring the dose to ensure correct dose.

### Patient and family education

- Review with patients the anticipated benefits and possible side effects of drug therapy.
- Review with patients the need to take the medication as ordered for the specified period of time (usually 7 to 10 days), even if symptoms disappear. Unused medications should be discarded. Tell patients not to share medications with others.
- Teach patients to check expiration dates on medications and not to use them if the expiration date has passed, as the drug may not work as well as desired.
- Instruct patients to read medication labels carefully. Store liquid forms in the refrigerator, but avoid freezing them.
- Encourage patients with a history of allergic response to a drug wear a medication identification tag or bracelet noting their allergy.

**Table 18-1.**

### Clinical summary of macrolides

| Antibacterial agent | Oral | IV | Topical |
|---|---|---|---|
| Erythromycin | + | | + |
| Erythromycin estolate | + | | |
| Erythromycin ethylsuccinate | + | | |
| Erythromycin gluceptate | | + | |
| Erythromycin lactobionate | | + | |
| Erythromycin stearate | + | | |
| Troleandomycin | + | | |

- Caution patients to keep these and all medications out of the reach of children.
- Many antibacterials are excreted through breast milk. Instruct lactating women to check with their physicians before breast-feeding while taking antibacterials.

## erythromycin  (eh-ree-thro-MY-sin)                    macrolide antibiotic

- erythromycin: E-Mycin, ERYC, Ery-Tab, Ilotycin, PCE, Robimycin, RP-mycin

**MECHANISM OF ACTION**   See entry for drug class (p. 327).

**INDICATIONS**   **Intestinal amebiasis** Erythromycin can be useful in controlling amebic infections restricted to the intestinal tract.   **Pertussis** Erythromycin is a drug of choice for this infection. • For other indications, see entry for drug class (p. 327).

**CONTRAINDICATIONS**   • See entry for drug class (p. 327).

**DOSAGE**   PO:   ADULT: 250 to 500 mg every 6 hours or 333 to 666 mg every 8 hours; daily doses should not exceed 4 g.   **CHILDREN:** 30 to 50 mg/kg divided into four equal doses daily; daily doses should not exceed 100 mg/kg. Doses of 0.9 to 3 mg/M$^2$ may also be used in children.   **Topical:**   ADULTS AND CHILDREN: For acne, apply twice daily to affected skin.   *Special patient populations:*   PREGNANCY: Safe use in pregnancy and lactation is not established, although the drug has been used to treat venereal disease in pregnant women without apparent harm.

**PREPARATIONS**   *Tablets, film-coated:* 250 or 500 mg; *tablets, enteric-coated:* 250, 333, or 500 mg; *capsules:* 125 or 250 mg; *ointment, topical:* 2%; *pledgets, topical:* 2% solution saturating pledgets (swabs); *solution, topical:* 1.5% and 2%.

**DRUG INTERACTIONS**   • See entry for drug class (p. 327).

**DIAGNOSTIC TEST INTERFERENCES**   **Catecholamine** assays in urine may be falsely elevated.   **17-hydroxycorticosteroid and 17-ketosteroid** assays in urine may be falsely elevated.   **AST (SGOT) and ALT (SGPT)** colorimetric assays are falsely increased.   **Folate** assays on serum may be falsely lowered by interference with the microbiologic assay. Assays based on chromatographic procedures (Landon) are unaffected.   **Diagnostic procedures for Mycoplasma pneumoniae** may be falsely negative if the serum contains erythromycin.

**FATE**   Erythromycin is absorbed from the GI tract, but *bioavailability* is low unless the drug is protected from the acid in the stomach. Commercially available preparations are therefore enteric-coated to prevent dissolution until the drug enters the duodenum, where it may readily be absorbed. *Peak* serum concentrations are achieved within 1 to 4 hours of oral doses. Distribution to tissues is high with erythromycin; tissue levels often exceed serum levels. Exceptions to this rule include the CNS, where levels are much below serum concentrations; fluids such as breast milk and exudates from the middle ear attain about 50% of the serum concentration. The primary route of elimination of erythromycin is in the bile as active drug. In addition, some of the drug is metabolized by the liver. Very little drug is eliminated by the kidneys. The serum *half-life* of erythromycin is 0.8 to 3 hours and is marginally affected by renal failure. Hepatic failure may modify and prolong the elimination of erythromycin.

## 🕏 NURSING CONSIDERATIONS

### Side effects, toxicities, and associated nursing actions
- See entry for drug class (p. 327).

### Nursing interventions related to drug administration
- See entry for drug class (p. 328).

### Patient and family education
- See entry for drug class (p. 328).

## erythromycin estolate    (eh-ree-thro-MY-sin ESS-toh-late)    macrolide antibiotic

● erythromycin estolate: Ilosone

**MECHANISM OF ACTION**    • See entry for drug class (p. 327).

**INDICATIONS    Intestinal amebiasis** Erythromycin estolate can be useful in controlling amebic infections restricted to the intestinal tract. • For other indications, see entry for drug class (p. 327).

**CONTRAINDICATIONS**    • See entry for drug class (p. 327).

**DOSAGE    PO:    ADULT:** 250 mg erythromycin equivalent every 6 hours; daily doses should not exceed 4 g. **CHILDREN:** 30 to 50 mg/kg divided into four equal doses daily; daily doses should not exceed 100 mg/kg. Doses of 0.9 to 3 mg/M$^2$ may also be used in children.    *Special patient populations:* **PREGNANCY:** Erythromycin estolate should not be used in pregnancy.

**PREPARATIONS**    *Tablets:* 500 mg equivalent of erythromycin; *tablets, chewable:* 125 or 250 mg equivalent of erythromycin; *capsules:* 125 or 250 mg equivalent of erythromycin; *suspension, oral:* 125 or 250 mg in each 5 ml or 100 mg in each milliliter.

**DRUG INTERACTIONS**    • See entry for drug class (p. 327).

**DIAGNOSTIC TEST INTERFERENCE**    • See Erythromycin (p. 329).

**FATE**    Erythromycin estolate is more acid-stable than erythromycin and survives passage through the stomach. Erythromycin estolate is absorbed in the upper intestine and hydrolyzed in the blood to release the free, fully active erythromycin. Hydrolysis rates may vary among patients. The free erythromycin released by hydrolysis is distributed and eliminated in the same way as erythromycin administered as the free base (see Erythromycin, p. 329).

🐾 **NURSING CONSIDERATIONS**

**Side effects, toxicities, and associated nursing actions**
• See entry for drug class (p. 327).

**Nursing interventions related to drug administration**
• See entry for drug class (p. 328).

**Patient and family education**
• See entry for drug class (p. 328).

## erythromycin ethylsuccinate
(eh-ree-thro-MY-sin eth-ill-SUK-sin-ate)    macrolide antibiotic

● erythromycin ethylsuccinate: E.E.S., E-Mycin E, Pediamycin, Wyamycin

**MECHANISM OF ACTION**    • See entry for drug class (p. 327).

**INDICATIONS    Intestinal amebiasis** Erythromycin can be useful in controlling amebic infections restricted to the intestinal tract.    **Pertussis** Erythromycin is a drug of choice for this infection. • For additional indications, see entry for drug class (p. 327).

**CONTRAINDICATIONS**    • See entry for drug class (p. 327).

**DOSAGE    PO:    ADULT:** 400 mg equivalent of erythromycin every 6 hours; rarely, maximum doses may exceed 4 g daily.    **CHILDREN:** 30 to 50 mg/kg divided into four equal doses daily; daily doses should not exceed 100 mg/kg. Doses of 0.9 to 3 mg/M$^2$ may also be used in children.    *Special patient populations:*    **PREGNANCY:** Safe use in pregnancy and lactation is not established, although the drug has been used to treat venereal disease in pregnant women without apparent harm.

**PREPARATIONS**    *Tablets, film-coated:* 400 mg equivalent of erythromycin; *Tablets, chewable:* 200 mg equivalent of erythromycin; *Suspension, oral:* 100 mg equivalent of erythromycin in each 2.5 ml; 200 or 400 mg equivalent of erythromycin in each 5 ml, as powder to be suspended or as preformed suspension.

**DRUG INTERACTIONS**    • See entry for drug class (p. 327).

**DIAGNOSTIC TEST INTERFERENCE**    • See Erythromycin (p. 329).

**FATE**    • See Erythromycin (p. 329).

❦ **NURSING CONSIDERATIONS**
### Side effects, toxicities, and associated nursing actions
   - See entry for drug class (p. 327).
### Nursing interventions related to drug administration
   - See entry for drug class (p. 328).
### Patient and family education
   - See entry for drug class (p. 328).

## erythromycin gluceptate   (eh-ree-thro-MY-sin gloo-SEP-tate)   macrolide antibiotic

   - erythromycin gluceptate: Ilotycin Gluceptate

**MECHANISM OF ACTION**   See entry for drug class (p. 327).
**INDICATIONS**   • See entry for drug class (p. 327).
**CONTRAINDICATIONS**   • See entry for drug class (p. 327).
**DOSAGE**   IV:   ADULTS AND CHILDREN: 15 to 20 mg/kg daily by continuous or intermittent infusion. Daily doses should not exceed 4 g. Pediatric doses may also be calculated by surface area, 300 to 600 mg/M$^2$. *Special patient populations:*   PREGNANCY: Safe use in pregnancy and lactation is not established, although the drug has been used to treat venereal disease in pregnant women without apparent harm.
**PREPARATIONS**   *Solution, injection:* 250 mg, 500 mg, or 1 g to dissolve for infusion.
**DRUG INTERACTIONS**   • See entry for drug class (p. 327).
**DIAGNOSTIC TEST INTERFERENCE**   • See Erythromycin (p. 329).
   **FATE**   Erythromycin gluceptate is hydrolyzed to release active erythromycin, which is then distributed and eliminated from the body just as the free base would be (see Erythromycin, p. 329).

❦ **NURSING CONSIDERATIONS**
### Side effects, toxicities, and associated nursing actions
   - See entry for drug class (p. 327).
### Nursing interventions related to drug administration
   - Reconstitute with sterile water for injection without preservatives, then dilute further with solutions of appropriate pH and compatibility (see manufacturer's literature) to a concentration of 1 g in at least 100 ml.
   - Administer at the rate of 1 g over 20 to 60 minutes. The rate should be slow enough to prevent pain in the vein.
   - See entry for drug class (p. 328).
### Patient and family education
   - See entry for drug class (p. 328).

## erythromycin lactobionate
### (eh-ree-thro-MY-sin lak-toh-BYE-oh-nate)                                                   macrolide antibiotic

   - erythromycin lactobionate: Erythrocin

**MECHANISM OF ACTION**   • See entry for drug class (p. 327).
**INDICATIONS**   • See entry for drug class (p. 327).
**CONTRAINDICATIONS**   • See entry for drug class (p. 327).
**DOSAGE**   IV:   ADULTS AND CHILDREN: 15 to 20 mg/kg daily by continuous or intermittent infusion. Daily doses should not exceed 4 g. Pediatric doses may also be calculated by surface area, 300 to 600 mg/M$^2$. *Special patient populations:*   PREGNANCY: Safe use in pregnancy and lactation is not established, although the drug has been used to treat venereal disease in pregnant women without apparent harm.

**PREPARATIONS** *Tablets, film-coated:* 250 or 500 mg equivalent or erythromycin.
**DRUG INTERACTIONS** • See entry for drug class (p. 327).
**DIAGNOSTIC TEST INTERFERENCE** • See Erythromycin (p. 329).
**FATE** Erythromycin lactobionate is hydrolyzed to release active erythromycin, which is then distributed and eliminated from the body just as the free base would be (see Erythromycin, p. 329).

**❦ NURSING CONSIDERATIONS**

**Side effects, toxicities, and associated nursing actions**
- See entry for drug class (p. 327).

**Nursing interventions related to drug administration**
- Reconstitute with sterile water for injection without preservatives, then dilute further with solutions of appropriate pH and compatibility (see manufacturer's literature) to a concentration of 1 g in at least 100 ml.
- Administer at a rate of 1 g over 20 to 60 minutes. The rate should be slow enough to prevent pain in the vein.
- See entry for drug class (p. 328).

**Patient and family education**
- See entry for drug class (p. 328).

---

## erythromycin stearate   (eh-ree-thro-MY-sin stee-AIR-ate)     macrolide antibiotic

- erythromycin stearate: Eramycin, Erypar, Erythrocin stearate, Ethril, Pfizer-E, SK-erythromycin, Wintrocin, Wyamycin S

**MECHANISM OF ACTION** • See entry for drug class (p. 327).
**INDICATIONS** **Intestinal amebiasis** Erythromycin can be useful in controlling amebic infections restricted to the intestinal tract. **Pertussis** Erythromycin is a drug of choice for this infection. • For additional indications, see entry for drug class (p. 327).
**CONTRAINDICATIONS** • See entry for drug class (p. 327).
**DOSAGE** **PO:** **ADULT:** 250 to 500 mg every 6 hours; daily doses should not exceed 4 g. **CHILDREN:** 30 to 50 mg/kg divided into four equal doses daily; daily doses should not exceed 100 mg/kg. Doses of 0.9 to 3 mg/M$^2$ may also be used in children. *Special patient populations:* **PREGNANCY:** Safe use in pregnancy and lactation is not established, although the drug has been used to treat venereal disease in pregnant women without apparent harm.
**PREPARATIONS** *Tablets, film-coated:* 250 or 500 mg equivalent of erythromycin.
**DRUG INTERACTIONS** • See entry for drug class (p. 327).
**DIAGNOSTIC TEST INTERFERENCE** • See Erythromycin (p. 329).
**FATE** Erythromycin stearate, like erythromycin, may be inactivated by stomach acid. After hydrolysis, free erythromycin is released. See Erythromycin (p. 329).

**❦ NURSING CONSIDERATIONS**

**Side effects, toxicities, and associated nursing actions**
- See entry for drug class (p. 327).

**Nursing interventions related to drug administration**
- See entry for drug class (p. 328).

**Patient and family education**
- See entry for drug class (p. 328).

---

## troleandomycin   (troh-lee-an-doh-MY-sin)     macrolide antibiotic

- troleandomycin: TAO

**MECHANISM OF ACTION** • See entry for drug class (p. 327).

**INDICATIONS**   **Infections caused by gram-positive organisms** Troleandomycin is often effective against staphylococci and certain streptococci, but other less toxic drugs are the drugs of choice and troleandomycin is rarely used.

**CONTRAINDICATIONS**   **Infections caused by organisms susceptible to penicillins or erythromycins** Troleandomycin should not be substituted for effective, less toxic agents.   **Hepatic damage** Troleandomycin is metabolized by the liver and may accumulate if liver function is impaired.

**DOSAGE**   **PO:**   **ADULT:** 250 to 500 mg every 6 hours.   **CHILDREN:** 125 to 250 mg every 6 hours; doses may also be calculated by weight, 6.6 to 11 mg/kg four times daily.   *Special patient populations:* **PREGNANCY:** Safe use in pregnancy has not been established.

**PREPARATIONS**   *Capsules:* 250 mg.

**DRUG INTERACTIONS**   Few interactions are reported because troleandomycin is rarely used. As a macrolide, the drug might be expected to cause the same types of interactions as other macrolides (see Erythromycin, p. 329).

**DIAGNOSTIC TEST INTERFERENCE**   • May be similar to other macrolides (see Erythromycin, p. 329).

**FATE**   Troleandomycin is incompletely absorbed from the GI tract but *peak* serum concentrations are achieved by 2 hours. Troleandomycin is metabolized to release the active compound, oleandomycin, Distribution and elimination are similar to erythromycin (p. 329).

## 🐝 NURSING CONSIDERATIONS

### Side effects, toxicities, and associated nursing actions

**GI** The most common reactions are abdominal cramping and pain. Nausea, vomiting, and diarrhea are also reported.

• If GI symptoms are severe or persistent, notify the physician. Monitor intake, output, and weight.

• See entry for drug class (p. 327).

**Liver** Like erythromycin estolate, troleandomycin can cause cholestatic hepatitis.

• See entry for drug class (p. 327).

**Allergy** Urticaria, rashes, and anaphylaxis are possible.

• Obtain history of allergic response to erythromycins before administering doses.

• See entry for drug class (p. 327).

### Patient and family education

• Review with patients the anticipated benefits and possible side effects of drug therapy.

• See entry for drug class (p. 328).

# Chapter Nineteen

# Miscellaneous antibacterial agents

bacitracin
bacitracin zinc
ciprofloxacin
clindamycin hydrochloride
clindamycin palmitate hydrochloride
clindamycin phosphate
colistimethate sodium
colistin sulfate
lincomycin
methenamine

methenamine hippurate
methenamine mandelate
nalidixic acid
nitrofurantoin
nitrofurantoin sodium
norfloxacin
phenazopyridine hydrochloride
polymyxin B sulfate
trimethoprim
vancomycin

**OVERVIEW OF THE DRUG CLASS**  The drugs covered in this section come from a variety of chemical families and have varied clinical uses (Table 19-1). Because some of these agents accumulate to effective concentrations only in the urinary tract, their clinical application is limited to treatment of urinary tract infections. Examples include nitrofurantoin and nalidixic acid. Other agents are too toxic for routine use systemically and serve as reserve drugs or topical agents. Polymyxin B sulfate and bacitracin are examples of this type of agent. A few drugs in this section are widely used systemically in treating specific infections, such as clindamycin for anaerobic infections.

**MECHANISM OF ACTION**  • See individual drug monographs.

**INDICATIONS**  • See Table 19-1 and the individual drug monographs.

**CONTRAINDICATIONS**  • See individual drug monographs.

**DRUG INTERACTIONS**  • See individual drug monographs.

**❧ NURSING CONSIDERATIONS**

• See individual drug monographs.

| Table 19-1. | Summary of uses of miscellaneous antibacterial agents | | |
|---|---|---|---|
| | **Primary clinical use of antibacterial agent** | | |
| **Antibacterial agent** | **Systemic infections** | **Urinary tract infections** | **Topical** |
| Bacitracin | | | + |
| Ciprofloxacin | + | + | |
| Clindamycin HCl | + | | + |
| Colistimethate sodium | + | | |
| Colistin sulfate | + | | |
| Lincomycin | + | | |
| Methenamine | | + | |
| Nalidixic acid | | + | |
| Nitrofurantoin | | + | |
| Norfloxacin | | + | |
| Phenazopyridine HCl | | + | |
| Polymyxin B sulfate | | | + |
| Trimethoprim | | + | |
| Vancomycin | + | | |

# bacitracin    (baa-see-TRAY-sin)                          polypeptide antibiotic

- bacitracin: Baciguent, ✸Bactin
- bacitracin zinc

**MECHANISM OF ACTION**    Bacitracin alters the bacterial cell membrane and prevents normal transport across the membrane of precursors of the bacterial cell wall. At low concentrations the action of the drug may only inhibit bacterial growth, but at higher concentrations the damaged cell wall may cause the death of the bacteria.

**INDICATIONS**    **Pneumonia and empyema in infants** This parenteral use of bacitracin is indicated only when the staphylococci causing the infection are known to be susceptible to bacitracin and resistant to safer alternate drugs such as penicillins or cephalosporins.    **Infections of the conjunctiva or cornea** Short-term use is common, but concrete proof of effectiveness is lacking.    **Superficial infections of the skin** Topical use is common, but concrete proof of effectiveness is lacking.

**CONTRAINDICATIONS**    **Renal disease** Parenteral bacitracin may damage the kidneys, leading to further drug accumulation and renal damage. Renal excretion is the primary route of elimination for bacitracin.

**DOSAGE**    **IM:**    **ADULT:** 10,000 to 25,000 units every 6 hours, not to exceed 100,000 units daily.    **INFANTS:** Below 2.5 kg, 900 units/kg daily, divided into two or three doses. Infants weighing more than 2.5 kg receive 1000 units/kg daily divided into two or three doses. Doses should not exceed those listed and should not be given longer than 12 days.    **OPHTHALMIC:** Ophthalmic ointments containing 500 units of bacitracin per gram may be applied to the eye one or more times daily. For ophthalmic use, bacitracin may be combined with other agents (see Preparations).    **TOPICAL:** Ointment (500 units/g) or solutions (250 to 100 units/ml) may be applied directly to cleansed superficial wounds. For topical use, bacitracin is often combined with other agents (see Preparations).    *Special patient populations:* **ELDERLY:** Bacitracin is not recommended for systemic use in this age group.    **PREGNANCY:** Bacitracin should be avoided during pregnancy.

**PREPARATIONS**    **Bacitracin** • *Powder for parenteral use:* 10,000 or 50,000 units. The drug should be dissolved in 0.9% sodium chloride containing 2% procaine hydrochloride; 2 ml to 10,000 units or 9.8 ml to 50,000 units produces solutions of 5000 units/ml. • *Ophthalmic ointment:* 500 units/g with chlorobutanol 0.65%. • *Topical ointment:* 500 units/g.    **Combination products containing bacitracin or bacitracin zinc:    OPHTHALMIC OINTMENT:** • Bacitracin 500 units/g with neomycin sulfate 0.5% and polymyxin B sulfate 10,000 units/g (Mycitracin R). • Bacitracin zinc 400 units/g with neomycin sulfate 0.5% and polymyxin B sulfate 10,000 units/g (Ak-Spore, Biotic-O, Neosporin, Neotal, Ocu-Spor-B, Ocusporin, Ocu-Tracin). • Bacitracin zinc 500 units/g with polymyxin B sulfate 10,000 units/g (Ak-Poly-Bac, Polysporin).    **TOPICAL OINTMENTS:** • Bacitracin 400 units/g with neomycin sulfate 0.5% and polymyxin B sulfate 5000 units/g (Clinicydin, N.B.P.). • Bacitracin 500 units/g with neomycin sulfate 0.5% and polymyxin B sulfate 5000 units/g (Mycitracin Triple Antibiotic). • Bacitracin zinc 400 units/g with neomycin sulfate 0.5% and polymyxin B sulfate 5000 units/g (Neomixin, Neosporin). • Bacitracin zinc 500 units/g with polymyxin B sulfate 10,000 units/g (Polysporin).    **TOPICAL AEROSOL:** • Bacitracin zinc 10,000 units/90 g with polymyxin B sulfate 200,000 units/90 g (Polysporin aerosol).

**DRUG INTERACTIONS**    **Nephrotoxic drugs** such as aminoglycoside or polymyxin antibiotics should not be combined with bacitracin because bacitracin is itself nephrotoxic. This interaction is of concern only when the drugs are administered or absorbed systemically and is not ordinarily a danger when polymyxin and bacitracin are combined for topical use.    **Neuromuscular blocking agents** for surgery may produce unexpectedly severe or prolonged paralysis in patients who also receive parenteral bacitracin.

**FATE**    Bacitracin is not absorbed orally. If administered parenterally, the drug is eliminated by glomerular filtration in the kidneys, but substantial amounts of drug are apparently metabolized or destroyed in the body by unknown mechanisms. Absorption from topical sites is not normally observed.

## ❦ NURSING CONSIDERATIONS
### Side effects, toxicities, and associated nursing actions
**Blood** Bone marrow toxicity and blood dyscrasias have occurred following IM injection.

- Visually inspect the patient for bruising, bleeding, or petechiae, when the drug is used parenterally.
- Instruct the patient to report the development of unexplained bruising or bleeding, sore throat, fever, or malaise.
- Monitor complete blood count, white blood cell differential, and platelet count in patients receiving the parenteral form.

**GI** Anorexia, diarrhea, nausea, rectal irritation, and vomiting may follow IM injection.
- Monitor weight. If vomiting or diarrhea appear, monitor intake and output. If GI symptoms are severe or persistent, notify the physician.

**Renal** Renal tubular and glomerular necrosis is the primary limitation to IM use of bacitracin. Early signs include albuminuria, cylindruria, and hematuria. Late signs include azotemia, oliguria, and renal failure. These toxic effects are related to the age of the patient and the dose received. Infants are less sensitive to these effects of bacitracin than are adults.
- Force fluids during parenteral therapy, up to 2500 ml/day. Keeping urinary pH above 6 may lessen renal irritation; sodium bicarbonate or other alkalinizing agent may be prescribed concurrently.
- Inspect color of urine; test for blood if indicated.
- Monitor intake and output.
- Monitor serum creatinine, BUN, and urinalysis.

**Allergic** Urticaria, itching, fever, eosinophilia, and anaphylaxis have occurred.
- Question the patient about previous allergic reactions to antibacterial agents before administering the drug.
- Assess for development of allergic symptoms. Have drugs, equipment, and personnel available for resuscitation in settings where antibacterials are administered.

**Other** Neuromuscular blockade is a special risk for patients receiving other neuromuscular blocking agents for surgery. Patients with myasthenia gravis are also at increased risk because they have less than normal numbers of receptors at the neuromuscular junction.
- Caution patients to keep all health care providers informed of all medications being taken.
- Assess carefully postoperative patients, patients with myasthenia gravis, or other patients who have received neuromuscular blockade agents who have received parenteral bacitracin.

### Nursing interventions related to drug administration
- For IM administration, large muscle masses should be used, such as the dorsogluteal site or rectus femoris muscle in adults or the vastus lateralis in infants and small children. Use anatomic landmarks to choose sites. Aspirate before injecting drug to avoid inadvertent IV administration. Record sites and rotate sites. IM injection is painful.
- For IM use, dilute as directed in manufacturer's literature. For example, dissolve powder in 0.9% sodium chloride injection containing 2% procaine hydrochloride (must be prescribed; consult the physician). Add 9.8 ml of diluent to a vial containing 50,000 units to provide a concentration of 5000 units of bacitracin per milliliter. For additional information, consult a pharmacist.

### Patient and family education
- Review with patients the anticipated benefits and possible side effects of drug therapy.
- Topical administration of bacitracin is rarely associated with side effects, but caution patients to report any unexpected sign or symptom.
- Remind patients to use antibacterial preparations only as directed.

---

## cinoxacin    (sin-OX-uh-sin)                                            antibiotic*

- cinoxacin: Cinobac

**MECHANISM OF ACTION**    Cinoxacin and other quinolone antibiotics (Table 19-2) inhibit the enzyme called DNA gyrase, thereby interfering with reproduction of bacteria. At concentrations achieved in urine, the drug is bactericidal.

**INDICATIONS**    **Urinary tract infections** Initial or recurrent infections caused by susceptible strains of *Escherichia coli, Enterobacter, Klebsiella,* and *Proteus* may be treated.

**CONTRAINDICATIONS**   **Renal disease** Cinoxacin is normally eliminated in urine and may accumulate when renal function fails.   **Prepubertal children** Cinoxacin may damage cartilage in weight-bearing joints in immature patients.

**DOSAGE**   **PO:**   **ADULTS:** 250 mg every 6 hours or 500 mg twice daily for 7 to 14 days for uncomplicated urinary tract infections.   *Special patient populations:*   **CHILDREN:** Cinoxacin should not be used in prepubertal children.   **RENAL IMPAIRMENT:** Patients with creatinine clearance rates between 20 and 80 ml/min/1.73M$^2$ should receive reduced doses (250 mg every 8 to 24 hours).   **PREGNANCY:** FDA pregnancy category B.

**PREPARATIONS**   *Capsules:* 250 and 500 mg.

**DRUG INTERACTIONS**   Not fully established.

**FATE**   Cinoxacin is very well absorbed following oral administration. The drug is eliminated almost exclusively by the kidneys, where concentrations are high. Serum concentrations are relatively low.

## ❦ NURSING CONSIDERATIONS

### Side effects, toxicities, and associated nursing actions

**CNS** Headache, dizziness, insomnia, depression, and visual disturbances occur in less than 1% of patients.
- Teach patients to avoid driving or operating hazardous equipment if dizziness or visual disturbances occur; notify physician.
- Assess for signs of depression: insomnia, withdrawal, lack of interest in personal appearance, and anorexia; notify physician.

**GI** Nausea is the most common side effect (less than 3%), with fewer patients reporting vomiting, anorexia, abdominal cramps, and diarrhea.
- Suggest that patients take ordered doses with meals or snack to lessen gastric side effects.
- If GI side effects are severe, monitor intake and output and weight; notify physician.

**Allergic** Rash and erythema are reported by less than 3% of treated patients.
- Question patients about a history of allergy before administering drug.
- Assess for rash and signs of allergic response.

**Liver** AST and ALT may be elevated.
- Monitor liver function tests.
- Instruct patient to notify physician if jaundice, right upper quadrant abdominal pain, malaise, fever, or change in color or consistency of stools develops.

### Patient and family education
- Review the anticipated benefits and possible side effects of drug therapy with patient and family.
- Remind patients to take antibiotics only as directed. Erratic use of this drug will lessen its effectiveness.
- Encourage patients with urinary tract infections to push fluids to 2500 to 3000 ml per day.
- Remind patients to keep these and all medications out of the reach of children. Point out to parents that this drug should not be used in prepubertal children. Remind parents to avoid sharing with children any medications not specifically prescribed for children.
- Review measures with female patients that may prevent future urinary tract infections, including wiping from front to back after voiding, urinating immediately after sexual intercourse, washing the urethral area with water only, and avoiding bubble baths.

---

## ciprofloxacin   (sip-roh-FLOX-uh-sin)   antibiotic*

- ciprofloxacin: Cipro

**MECHANISM OF ACTION**   Ciprofloxacin is a quinolone antibiotic. Like other members of this class (Table 19-2), ciprofloxacin inhibits the enzyme called DNA gyrase, thereby interfering with reproduction of bacteria. At concentrations achieved in urine, the drug is bactericidal.

**INDICATIONS**   **Infections of the bones and joints, lower respiratory tract, skin and skin structures, and urinary tract** Initial or recurrent infections caused by susceptible strains of *Escherichia coli, Enterobacter,*

*DNA gyrase inhibitor.

Klebsiella, Pseudomonas, Staphylococcus aureus, and *Proteus* may be treated. • Methicillin-resistant *S. aureus* may be susceptible.

**CONTRAINDICATIONS** **Allergy to other quinolones** Patients allergic to norfloxacin, cinoxacin, nalidixic acid, or oxolinic acid may also react to ciprofloxacin. **Prepubertal children** Norfloxacin may damage cartilage in weight-bearing joints in immature patients.

**DOSAGE** **PO:** **ADULTS:** 250 mg twice daily for 7 to 10 days for uncomplicated urinary tract infections. More severe infections require 500 or 750 mg twice daily. *Special patient populations* **CHILDREN:** Ciprofloxacin should not be used in prepubertal children. **RENAL IMPAIRMENT:** Ciprofloxacin may accumulate in patients with impaired renal function. Doses must be reduced accordingly. **PREGNANCY:** FDA pregnancy category C.

**PREPARATIONS** *Tablets:* 250, 500, and 750 mg.

**DRUG INTERACTIONS** **Antacids** may lower absorption of ciprofloxacin and should be avoided while the patient is taking the antibiotic. **Theophylline** may accumulate because ciprofloxacin slows the elimination of theophylline, increasing risk of toxicity. Theophylline levels may need to be monitored. **Probenecid** may cause accumulation of ciprofloxacin by slowing renal excretion of the antibiotic.

**FATE** Ciprofloxacin is very well absorbed following oral administration. The drug is eliminated almost exclusively by the kidneys.

## ❦ NURSING CONSIDERATIONS

### Side effects, toxicities, and associated nursing actions

**CNS** Headache and restlessness, observed in 1.1% to 1.2% of patients, are the most common CNS side effects. Less common signs include anorexia, ataxia, blurred vision, convulsive seizures, depression, diplopia, dizziness, drowsiness, hallucinations, insomnia, irritability, lethargy, lightheadedness, malaise, paresthesia, tinnitus, tremors, and weakness.

- Teach patients to avoid driving or operating hazardous equipment if dizziness, blurred vision, diplopia, lightheadedness, or visual disturbances occur; notify physician.
- Assess for signs of depression: insomnia, withdrawal, lack of interest in personal appearance, and anorexia; notify physician.
- Assess for history of seizures before administering.

**GI** Nausea is the most common side effect (5.2%), followed by diarrhea (2.3%), vomiting (2.0%), and abdominal pain (1.7%).

- Suggest that patients take ordered doses with meals or snack to lessen gastric side effects.
- If GI side effects are severe, monitor intake and output and weight; notify physician.

**Allergic** Rash and erythema are reported by 1.1% of treated patients. Less common reactions include angioedema, edema of face and hands, fever, flushing, photosensitivity, and pruritus.

- Question patients about a history of allergy before administering drug.
- Assess for rash and signs of allergic response.
- If photosensitivity develops, instruct patients to avoid prolonged exposure to the sun, to wear a wide-brimmed hat, to keep extremities covered, and to use a maximum-strength sunscreen on exposed skin surfaces.

**Musculoskeletal** Achiness, back pain, joint pain, and joint stiffness may occur.

- Warn patients about these side effects. If pain and stiffness are severe, notify physician.

**Blood** Eosinophilia (0.6%) and lowered WBC (0.4%) may occur.

- Monitor complete blood cell count and WBC differential.

**Renal** Crystalluria, cylindruria, and hematuria have been reported. Nephritis and renal failure have also occurred.

- Encourage patient to push fluids to 2500 to 3000 ml per day.
- Monitor urinalysis and, for hospitalized patients, intake and output.
- Instruct patients to report any changes in the appearance of urine, or amount of urine output.

**Liver** ALT and AST are elevated in 1.8% of patients; alkaline phosphatase rises in 0.8%.

- Monitor liver function tests.
- Instruct patient to notify physician if jaundice, right upper quadrant abdominal pain, malaise, fever, or change in color or consistency of stools develops.

### Nursing interventions related to drug administration
- Note drug interactions: antacids should be administered 1 hour before or 2 hours after doses of ciprofloxacin.

### Patient and family education
- Review the anticipated benefits and possible side effects of drug therapy with patient and family.
- Remind patients to take antibiotics only as directed. Erratic use of this drug will lessen its effectiveness.
- Encourage patients with urinary tract infections to push fluids to 2500 to 3000 ml per day.
- Remind patients to keep these and all medications out of the reach of children. Point out to parents that this drug should not be used in prepubertal children. Remind parents to avoid sharing with children any medications not specifically prescribed for children.
- Review measures with female patients that may prevent future urinary tract infections, including wiping from front to back after voiding, urinating immediately after sexual intercourse, washing the urethral area with water only, and avoiding bubble baths.

## clindamycin hydrochloride (klin-dah-MY-sin) antibiotic*

- clindamycin: Cleocin, ♣Dalacin C
- clindamycin palmitate hydrochloride
- clindamycin phosphate

**Table 19-2.**

### Quinolone and related antibacterial agents

| Generic name | Trade name | Comments |
| --- | --- | --- |
| Cinoxacin | Cinobac | An older quinolone less potent than newer agents |
| Ciprofloxacin | Cipro | A potent new fluorinated quinolone with the potential for broad clinical use (Table 19-1) |
| Enoxacin | * | A potent drug closely related to nalidixic acid, but with high bioavailability and good serum levels |
| Nalidixic acid | NegGram | An older drug producing low serum levels |
| Norfloxacin | Noroxin | A potent new fluorinated quinolone currently indicated for urinary tract infections |
| Ofloxacin | * | A potent new fluorinated quinolone with a high bioavailability, producing higher serum levels than most other quinolones |
| Pefloxacin | * | A potent new fluorinated quinolone with a high bioavailability, producing higher serum levels than most other quinolones |

*Not available in the United States as of April, 1988.

*Bacterial protein synthesis inhibitor.

**MECHANISM OF ACTION**   Clindamycin inhibits bacterial protein synthesis by actions on the 50S ribosomal subunit. The mechanism of action is similar to that of erythromycin, although the drugs are not chemically related.

**INDICATIONS**   **Infections caused by anaerobic bacteria** Clindamycin is a primary choice against *Bacteroides fragilis* and other anaerobic bacteria that may cause a variety of serious infections.   **Acute pelvic inflammatory disease (PID)** Clindamycin may be combined with gentamicin for this conditon.   **Acute hematogenous osteomyelitis** Staphylococci that cause this infection are usually susceptible to clindamycin, and the drug penetrates well to this site.   **Serious infections caused by staphylcocci or streptococci** Clindamycin is an alternate drug that is especially useful in patients allergic to penicillins or cephalosporins, which would be the first choices for therapy.   **Acne** Clindamycin may be used topically.

**CONTRAINDICATIONS**   **Allergy to lincomycin or clindamycin** Because lincomycin and clindamycin are chemically related, patients allergic to one drug will be likely to react to the other drug as well.

**DOSAGE**   **PO:**   **ADULT:** 150 to 450 mg every 6 hours.   **CHILDREN:** 8 to 25 mg/kg daily in three or four divided doses.   **IM, IV:**   **ADULT:** 600 mg to 2.7 g daily in two to four equally divided doses not to exceed 600 mg in one IM injection or not to exceed 1.2 g IV in 1 hour.   **CHILDREN OLDER THAN 1 MONTH OF AGE:** 15 to 40 mg/kg or 350 to 450 mg/M$^2$ daily in three or four equal doses.   **Topical: ADULTS AND CHILDREN:** Apply to affected areas twice daily to control acne.   *Special patient populations:*   **INFANTS YOUNGER THAN 1 MONTH:** Clindmamycin is usually avoided. If necessary, 15 to 20 mg/kg in three or four equal doses may be given cautiously.   **PREGNANCY:** FDA pregnancy category B.

**PREPARATIONS**   **Clindamycin hydrochloride** *Capsules:* 75 or 150 mg.   **Clindamycin palmitate hydrochloride** *Oral solution:* 75 mg/5 ml.   **Clindamycin phosphate** *Solution for injection:* 150 mg/ml, with 9.45 mg/ml benzyl alcohol and 0.5 mg/ml disodium edetate; *solution, topical:* 1%.

**DRUG INTERACTIONS**   **Neuromuscular blocking agents** such as tubocurarine and pancuronium may be potentiated by the weak neuromuscular blocking activity of clindamycin.

**FATE**   Clindamycin hydrochloride is well absorbed following oral administration, producing peak serum concentrations within 1 hour. Clindamycin palmitate hydrochloride must be hydrolyzed in the intestine to release clindamycin, which is then freely absorbed. Food has little effect on absorption. Clindamycin distributes well into bone and most fluids and tissues, with the exception of the CNS, where clindamycin levels are quite low. Clindamycin is eliminated primarily by metabolism of the drug in the liver. Metabolites and small amounts of active drug are excreted in bile, feces, and urine. The elimination half-life of clindamycin is 2 to 3 hours in healthy adults and only slightly increased in patients with renal or hepatic impairment.

### ❦ NURSING CONSIDERATIONS

#### Side effects, toxicities, and associated nursing actions

**CV** Cardiac arrest can occur if clindamycin is administered too rapidly intravenously.
- Do not administer this drug undiluted, direct IV push.
- Dilute each 300 mg or less with at least 50 ml of diluent, such as 5% dextrose in water, normal saline for injection, or other compatible solution. Administer the diluted dose over 10 to 60 minutes. The rate should not exceed 300 mg/10 min, or 1200 mg/60 min.

**Blood** Agranulocytosis, eosinophilia, neutropenia, thrombocytopenia, and transient leukopenia are reported rarely.
- Inspect patients for development of brusing or petechiae.
- Instruct the patient to report the development of unexplained bruising or bleeding from any site, sore throat, fever, malaise.
- Monitor complete blood count, white blood cell differential, and patelet count.

**GI** GI effects are often severe enough to require stopping clindamycin therapy. Abdominal pain, anorexia, bloating, diarrhea, esophagitis, flatulence, tenesmus, vomiting, and weight loss have been reported. Nonspecific colitis or the potentially fatal pseudomembranous colitis are associated with abdominal cramping and severe diarrhea with blood and mucus in the stool. This reaction is caused by toxins produced by *Clostridium dificile* in the bowel. Successful control requires discontinuing clindamycin and treatment with vancomycin to eliminate the *Clostridium* or with cholestyramine to bind the toxins. Antidiarrheal medications such as opiates or diphenoxylate worsen the condition and should be avoided.

- Caution patients to report the development of any unexpected sign or symptom, but emphasize the need to report immediately the development of diarrhea or the appearance of blood or mucus in the stool. Instruct patients to avoid self-medicating in treating diarrhea and to seek medical assistance.
- If GI symptoms appear, monitor intake, output, weight, and assess skin turgor. Monitor electrolytes.

**Renal** Rarely, azotemia, oliguria, and/or proteinuria have been reported.
- Monitor intake and output.
- Monitor serum creatinine and BUN. Monitor urinalysis.

**Allergic** Generalized morbilliform rash is commonly observed. Less common are maculopapular rash, urticara, pruritis, fever, hypotension, and polyarthritis. Anaphylaxis and erythema multiforme are rare but have been observed.
- Question patients about history of allergic response to clindamycin or lincomycin before administering the first dose.
- Visually inspect patients for allergic manifestations.
- Monitor blood pressure, especially when administering parenteral doses.
- Administer antibacterials only in settings where drugs, equipment, and personnel for resuscitation are available.

**Other** Benzyl alcohol contained in parenteral solutions of clindamycin may cause toxicity in neonates, especially if large doses are used.
- Monitor neonates carefully. Assess vital signs, blood pressure, level of consciousness at regular intervals.

### Nursing interventions related to drug administration
- Instruct patients to take oral doses with meals or a snack to lessen gastric irritation; food will not affect absorption. All oral doses should be taken with a full glass (8 ounces) of water to prevent esophagitis.
- Parenteral doses may cause hypotension. Instruct patient to remain recumbent for 30 minutes following drug administration. Monitor blood pressure and supervise ambulation.
- For IV administration, see CV effects. The use of microdrip tubing and/or an infusion control device may lessen the possibility of a too rapid infusion.
- For IM injection, use anatomic landmarks to choose injection sites. Use large muscle masses such as the dorsogluteal site or the rectus femoris muscle in adults or the vastus lateralis in infants and small children. Aspirate carefully before injecting the dose to avoid inadvertent IV administration. Record sites and rotate sites. Pain at the injection site is common.
- Cleocin HCl brand capsules in 75 mg and 150 mg dosages contain FD & C yellow dye #5 (tartrazine), which may cause an allergic reaction in susceptible individuals. Although rare, this side effect is seen more commonly in persons with aspirin hypersensitivity.

### Patient and family education
- Review with patients the anticipated benefits and possible side effects associated with therapy. Instruct patients to report the development of any unexpected sign or symptom.
- Caution patients to take antibacterials only as ordered and for as long as ordered.

## colistimethate sodium  (ko-liss-tee-METH-ate; ko-LISS-tin)  polymyxin antibiotic

- colistimethate sodium: Coly-Mycin
- colistin sulfate

**MECHANISM OF ACTION**  Colistin is the active form of the drug. Colistin binds to bacterial cell membranes, disrupting membrane function by a detergentlike action that kills the cells.

**INDICATIONS**   **Infections caused by gram-negative bacteria** Infections caused by susceptible strains of *Enterobacter aerogenes, E. coli, K. pneumoniae,* and *P. aeruginosa* may be successfully treated, but other safer drugs of equal efficacy are usually preferred.

**CONTRAINDICATIONS**   **Renal impairment** Drug concentrations must be monitored to allow adjustment of dosage and prevent acute, dangerous accumulation of toxic concentrations of the drug.

**DOSAGE**   **PO:**   **ADULTS AND CHILDREN:** 5 to 15 mg/kg daily in three equal doses.   **IM, IV:**   **ADULTS AND CHILDREN:** 2.5 to 5 mg/kg daily in two to four divided doses.   *Special patient populations:*   **ELDERLY:** Colistin should be avoided if possible in geriatric patients.   **RENAL IMPAIRMENT:** Doses must be reduced in renal impairment.   **PREGNANCY:** Safe use in pregnancy and lactation is not established.

**PREPARATIONS**   **Colistimethate sodium** *Powder, for parenteral use:* 150 mg, to be reconstituted with 2 ml of sterile water for injection to produce a solution of 75 mg/ml.   **Colistin sulfate** *Oral suspension:* 25 mg/5 ml.   **Combination products**   **OTIC SUSPENSION:** 0.3% colistin (as sulfate) with 0.5% neomycin sulfate, 1% hydrocortisone acetate, and 0.05% thonzonium bromide.   **OTIC SUSPENSION:** 0.3% colistin (as sulfate) with 0.5% neomycin sulfate and 0.05% thonzonium bromide.

**DRUG INTERACTIONS**   **Nephrotoxic and neurotoxic agents** such as aminoglycosides, polymyxin B sulfate, capreomycin, amphotericin B, and vancomycin may cause additive toxic effects with colistimethate sodium.   **Neuromuscular blocking agents** such as tubocurarine, succinylcholine, gallamine, and decamethonium may be potentiated by the weak neuromuscular blocking activity of colistimethate sodium.

**FATE**   Colistin sulfate and colistimethate sodium are not absorbed significantly following oral administration. Oral use of the agents is limited to treatment of intestinal infections. Both drugs are highly bound to many tissues in the body and persist in muscle and organs after the drug is discontinued. Colistimethate sodium is hydrolyzed in the body to colistin. Elimination is mainly renal, with an elimination *half-life* of 1.5 to 8 hours.

### ☙ NURSING CONSIDERATIONS

#### Side effects, toxicities, and associated nursing actions

**CNS** Transient effects that usually appear in the first four days of therapy include paresthesia, numbness, tingling, formication of the extremities or tongue, dizziness, vertigo, giddiness, ataxia, blurred vision, and slurred speech. More severe reactions include mental confusion, coma, psychosis, and seizures.

• Instruct patients to avoid driving or operating hazardous equipment if side effects affecting balance or vision occur (such as vertigo, blurred vision, ataxia), and to notify the physician.

• Obtain a baseline assessment before initiating drug therapy. Assess for development of CNS symptoms. If CNS side effects are severe or persistent, notify the physician.

**Peripheral nervous system** Blockade of the neuromuscular junction is possible. Patients especially at risk include those receiving neuromuscular blocking agents for surgery and patients with myasthenia gravis, who lack adequate receptors at the neuromuscular junction.

• Assess carefully postoperative patients or patients with myasthenia gravis who have also been receiving colistin or colistimethate.

• Monitor respirations, auscultate breath sounds, assess for dyspnea, restlessness, and ability to handle secretions. Have a suction machine at the bedside.

• Have oxygen, equipment, and personnel available to provide ventilatory support if apnea occurs.

**Blood** Granulocytopenia and leukopenia are rare.

• Monitor for fever, malaise, and signs of infection.

• Monitor complete blood cell count and white blood cell differential.

**GI** GI effects can occur but are not common or severe.

• Instruct patients to report the development of any gastrointestinal symptoms.

**Renal** Proteinuria, hematuria, and casts in the urine as well as increased serum concentrations of BUN and creatinine may signal renal toxicity. Acute renal tubular necrosis has occurred.

• Monitor intake and output, and weight.

• Monitor serum creatinine and BUN. Monitor urinalysis.

#### Nursing interventions related to drug administration

• Monitor serum drug levels if available.

- Question the patient about a history of allergic response to colistin, colistimethate, or polymyxin B before administering the ordered dose.
- For IM administration, reconstitute with sterile water for injection as directed on the vial. After adding diluent, rotate the vial gently to avoid frothiness. Use anatomic landmarks to choose injection sites. Aspriate before injecting dose to avoid inadvertent IV administration. Rotate sites and record sites. IM injection may be painful.
- For IV administration, the drug may be administered as diluted for IM administration over a 3 to 5 minute period. It may also be further diluted in 20 ml of sterile water for injection and administered at a rate of 75 mg/min. It may also be further diluted in 50 ml of compatible IV solution (see manufacturer's literature) and administered over 1 to 2 hours.
- Use solutions prepared for infusion within 24 hours.

### Patient and family education
- Review with patients the anticipated benefits and possible side effects associated with therapy.
- Remind patients to use medications only as ordered for as long as ordered.

---

## lincomycin hydrochloride    (link-oh-MY-sin)    antibiotic*

- lincomycin hydrochloride: Lincocin

**MECHANISM OF ACTION**    Lincomycin is a close chemical relative of clindamycin and has the same mechanism of action, inhibiting bacterial protein synthesis by actions on the 50S ribosomal subunit.

**INDICATIONS**    **Serious infections caused by gram-positive bacteria** Lincomycin may be effective against staphylococci or streptococci but in general is less effective than clindamycin or the preferred drugs such as penicillins or cephalosporins.

**CONTRAINDICATIONS**    **Allergy to lincomycin or clindamycin** Because lincomycin and clindamycin are chemically related, patients allergic to one drug will be likely to react to the other drug as well.

**DOSAGE**    PO:    ADULT: 500 mg or more every 6 to 8 hours.    CHILDREN OVER 1 MONTH OF AGE: 30 to 60 mg/kg daily in three or four equal doses.    IV:    ADULT: 600 mg every 12 to 24 hours.    CHILDREN OVER 1 MONTH OF AGE: 10 mg/kg every 12 to 24 hours.    IM:    ADULT: 600 mg to 1 g every 8 to 12 hours up to a maximum of 8 g daily.    CHILDREN OVER 1 MONTH OF AGE: 10 to 20 mg/kg daily divided into two or three equal doses. *Special patient populations:* PREGNANCY: Safe use in pregnant or lactating women not established.

**PREPARATIONS**    *Capsules:* 250 or 500 mg; *solution for injection:* 300 mg/ml with benzyl alcohol 9.45 mg/ml.

**DRUG INTERACTIONS**    **Kaolin** prevents adequate absorption of oral doses of lincomycin.    **Neuromuscular blocking agents** such as tubocurarine and pancuronium may be potentiated by the weak neuromuscular blocking activity of lincomycin.    **Cyclamates** used as sweeteners in foods or beverages should not be given with lincomycin.

**FATE**    Lincomycin is absorbed from the GI tract, but absorption is poor and is impaired by food. Absorption from IM sites is adequate. Lincomycin distributes well through most body fluids and tissues but does not enter the CNS well. Lincomycin is metabolized by the liver, and both active drug and metabolites appear in urine. The elimination *half-life* of lincomycin is 4 to 6 hours in healthy adults but increases greatly with renal impairment.

### ☙ NURSING CONSIDERATIONS
#### Side effects, toxicities, and associated nursing actions
CNS Headache, tinnitus, or vertigo occur rarely.
- If vertigo develops, caution patients to avoid driving or operating hazardous equipment until vertigo disappears.
- If vertigo or tinnitus occurs, notify the physician.
CV Cardiac arrest can occur if lincomycin is administered too rapidly intravenously.
- Do not administer this drug undiluted by direct IV push.

*Bacterial protein synthesis inhibitor.

- Dilute each 1 g or less with at least 100 ml of diluent such as 5% dextrose in water, normal saline for injection, or other compatible solution. Administer diluted dose as an infusion. The rate should not exceed 100 ml/h (1 g/hr).

**Blood** Agranulocytosis, eosinophilia, neutropenia, thrombocytopenia, and transient leukopenia are reported rarely.

- Visually inspect patients for development of bruising or petechiae.
- Instruct the patient to report the development of unexplained bruising or bleeding from any site, sore throat, fever, malaise.
- Monitor complete blood count, white blood cell differential, and platelet count.

**GI** GI effects are often severe enough to require stopping lincomycin therapy. Abdominal pain, anorexia, bloating, diarrhea, esophagitis, flatulence, tenesmus, vomiting, and weight loss have been reported. Nonspecific colitis or the potentially fatal pseudomembranous colitis are associated with abdominal cramping and severe diarrhea with blood and mucus in the stool. This reaction is caused by toxins produced by *Clostridium dificile* in the bowel. Successful control requires discontinuing lincomycin and treatment with vancomycin to eliminate the *Clostridium* or with cholestyramine to bind the toxins. Antidiarrheal medications such as opiates or diphenoxylate worsen the condition and should be avoided.

- Caution patients to report the development of any unexpected sign or symptom, but emphasize the need to report immediately the development of diarrhea or the appearance of blood or mucus in the stool. Instruct patients to avoid self-medicating in treating diarrhea but to seek medical assistance.
- If GI symptoms appear, monitor intake, output, weight, and assess skin turgor. Monitor electrolytes.

**Renal** Rarely, azotemia, oliguria, and/or proteinuria have been reported.

- Monitor intake and output.
- Monitor serum creatinine and BUN. Monitor urinalysis.

**Allergic** Rash, urticaria, pruritis, myalgia, tinnitus, exfoliative and vesiculobullous dermatitis have been reported. Anaphylaxis and erythema multiforme are rare but have been observed.

- Question patients about a history of allergic response to clindamycin or lincomycin before administering the first dose.
- Visually inspect patients for allergic manifestations.
- Monitor blood pressure, especially when administering parenteral doses.
- Administer antibacterials only in settings where drugs, equipment, and personnel for resuscitation are available.

**Other** Benzyl alcohol contained in parenteral solutions of lincomycin may cause toxicity in neonates, especially if large doses are used.

- Monitor neonates carefully. Assess vital signs, blood pressure, and level of consciousness at regular intervals.

### Nursing interventions related to drug administration

- Instruct patients to take oral doses 1 hour before or 2 hours after meals. All oral doses should be taken with a full glass (8 ounces) of water to help prevent esophagitis.
- Parenteral doses may cause hypotension. Instruct the patient to remain recumbent for 30 minutes following drug administration. Monitor blood pressure and supervise ambulation.
- For IV administration, see CV effects. The use of microdrip tubing and/or an infusion control device may lessen the possibility of a too rapid infusion.
- For IM injection, use anatomic landmarks to choose injection sites. Use large muscle masses such as the dorsogluteal site or the rectus femoris muscle in adults or the vastus lateralis in infants and small children. Aspirate carefully before injecting the dose to avoid inadvertent IV administration. Record sites and rotate sites. Pain at the injection site is common.

### Patient and family education

- Review with patients the anticipated benefits and possible side effects associated with therapy. Instruct patients to report the development of any unexpected sign or symptom.
- Caution patients to take antibacterials only as ordered and for as long as ordered.

## methenamine    (me-THEEN-uh-meen)                                    urinary antiseptic

- methenamine (methenamine hippurate, methenamine mandelate): Hexamine (see Preparations)

**MECHANISM OF ACTION**    Methenamine breaks down in acidic media to release formaldehyde. Formaldehyde released in the urine by this mechanism may be bactericidal.

**INDICATIONS**    **Prophylaxis or suppression of recurrent urinary tract infections** The nonspecific antibacterial effect of formaldehyde suppresses gram-positive and gram-negative organisms so long as the urinary pH remains sufficiently acidic.

**CONTRAINDICATIONS**    **Renal insufficiency** Patients must produce sufficient urine to eliminate methenamine and its products. **Hepatic impairment** Methenamine hippurate is contraindicated in these patients.

**DOSAGE**    **PO:**    **ADULTS OR CHILDREN OVER 12 YEARS:** 1 g of methenamine or methenamine mandelate four times daily administered after meals and at bedtime. Methenamine hippurate, 1 g twice daily. **CHILDREN:** Ages 6 to 12 receive 500 mg methenamine or methenamine mandelate four times daily or 50 mg/kg daily in three equal doses. Children younger than 6 years receive 18.4 mg/kg four times daily. For methenamine hippurate, children ages 6 to 12 receive 500 mg to 1 g twice daily. Doses are not established for younger children. *Special patient populations:* **ELDERLY:** Special geriatric doses have not been established, but care should be taken when administering methenamine mandelate oral suspension to debilitated, elderly patients. **PREGNANCY:** FDA pregnancy category C.

**PREPARATIONS**    **Methenamine** *Tablets:* 500 mg (Hexamine).    **Methenamine hippurate** *Tablets:* 1 g (Hiprex [with tartrazine] or Urex)    **Methenamine mandelate** *Tablets:* 500 mg or 1 g; *tablets, enteric coated:* 250 or 500 mg (Mandameth, Mandelets); *tablets, film-coated:* 500 mg or 1 g (Mandelamine); *granules for suspension:* 500 mg or 1 g (Mandelamine); *oral suspension:* 250 or 500 mg in 5 ml (Mandelamine).

**DRUG INTERACTIONS**    **Sulfamethizole** will form an insoluble precipitate with formaldehyde in the acidic pH of urine. To avoid damage to the kidney, these two drugs should never be combined.

**DIAGNOSTIC TEST INTERFERENCE**    **Tests for urinary catecholamines and vanillylmandelic acid (VMA)** using fluorometric procedures are falsely increased by formaldehyde. **Tests for urinary estriol** are falsely elevated when nonenzymatic methods are used. **Tests for 17-hydroxycorticosteroids** are falsely elevated when the Porter-Silber test is used. **Tests for 5-hydroxyindoleacetic acid (5HIAA)** are falsely lowered when nitrosonaphthol procedures are used.

**FATE**    Methenamine and its salts are well absorbed from the GI tract, although a significant proportion of an oral dose can be hydrolyzed to formaldehyde and ammonia in the acidic environment of the stomach unless an enteric-coated product is used. Methenamine crosses the placenta and enters milk. The drug and its salts are concentrated in the urine where hydrolysis to formaldehyde takes place. Hydrolysis is promoted when urinary pH is below 5.5. Peak urinary concentrations of formaldehyde are attained within 2 hours following an oral dose; enteric-coated products delay the peak to 3 to 8 hours.

## ☙ NURSING CONSIDERATIONS

### Side effects, toxicities, and associated nursing actions

**GI** Abdominal cramps, anorexia, diarrhea, nausea, and vomiting are the most common side effects.
- Instruct patients to take oral doses with a snack, meal, or large volume (240 ml) of fluid to lessen gastric irritation.
- If GI symptoms are severe or persistent, notify the physician.
- Changing the patient from suspension or tablets to enteric-coated or film-coated tablets may decrease gastric irritation; consult the physician.

**Renal** Albuminuria, bladder irritation, hematuria, and painful or frequent micturition may occur.
- Monitor intake, output, and urinalysis.
- Having patients increase their intake of oral fluids will lessen bladder irritation but will dilute the drug, which acts by concentrating formaldehyde in the bladder. Some physicians prefer that patients limit fluid intake while taking this drug.

- This drug works best when urinary pH is below 5.5. Instruct patients how to monitor urine pH if appropriate; consult the physician.
- If bladder irritation is persistent or severe, notify the physician.

**Allergic** Rash pruritis, stomatitis, and urticaria may develop.

- Visually inspect the patient for allergic manifestations.
- Instruct patients to report the development of any unexpected sign or symptom.

**Other** Dyspnea, edema, headache, muscle cramps, and tinnitus have been reported.

- Instruct patients to report the development of any unexpected sign or symptom.

### Nursing interventions related to drug administration

- Administer methenamine mandelate suspension cautiously in elderly or immobilized patients. This drug form is oil based and may contribute to the development of lipid pneumonia in these two populations.
- Hiprex brand tablets contain FD & C yellow dye #5 (tartrazine), which may cause an allergic reaction in susceptible individuals. Although rare, this side effect is seen more commonly in persons with aspirin hypersensitivity.

### Patient and family education

- Review with patients the anticipated benefits and possible side effects of therapy.
- Review with patients the need to take antibacterials on a consistent basis; erratic use of this drug will reduce its effectiveness.
- Instruct patients about dietary changes that may affect urine pH. Meat, fish, fowl, shellfish, eggs, cheese, peanut butter, corn, lentils, cranberries, plums, prunes, the juices of these fruits, breads, and pasta may increase the acidity (lower the pH) of the urine. Increased intake of these acid-ash foods may increase the effectiveness of methenamine. Intake of alkaline-ash foods such as milk, cream, buttermilk, vegetables except corn and lentils, and fruit, except the three previously listed, may increase the alkalinity (increase the pH) of the urine and decrease the effectiveness of methenamine.
- Review with female patients measures that prevent future urinary tract infections, including wiping from front to back after voiding, urinating immediately after sexual intercourse, washing the urethral area with water only, and avoiding bubble baths.

---

## nalidixic acid   (nal-i-DIX-ic)                                                    antibiotic*

- nalidixic acid: NegGram, ♣Nogram

**MECHANISM OF ACTION**   Nalidixic acid inhibits DNA gyrase, an enzyme required for replication of bacteria. The mechanism of action is similar to the related drug, cinoxacin.

**INDICATIONS**   **Urinary tract infections caused by gram-negative bacteria** Not all gram-negative bacteria respond, and resistance arises readily during therapy.

**CONTRAINDICATIONS**   **Convulsive disorders** Because nalidixic acid may cause seizures, the drug should not be given to patients with a history of convulsive disorders.

**DOSAGE**   PO:   ADULT: 1 g four times daily for 1 to 2 weeks.   CHILDREN 3 MONTHS TO 12 YEARS: 55 mg/kg or 2.25 g/M$^2$ daily administered in four equal doses. *Special patient populations:*   PREGNANCY: Nalidixic acid has been used in the last two trimesters without obvious harm, but safe use in the first trimester is not established.   INFANTS YOUNGER THAN 3 MONTHS: Avoid nalidixic acid.

**PREPARATIONS**   *Tablets:* 250 mg, 500 mg, or 1 g; *oral suspension:* 250 mg/5 ml.

**DRUG INTERACTIONS**   **Coumarin anticoagulants** may have enhanced anticoagulant effects with nalidixic acid. Because the antibacterial agent displaces coumarins from serum proteins, the free and active coumarin concentration is increased.

**DIAGNOSTIC TEST INTERFERENCE**   **Urinary glucose determinations** using cupric sulfate produce false-positives in the presence of nalidixic acid.   **Tests for urinary 17-ketosteroids and 17-ketogenic steroids** are falsely elevated when the method using m-dinitrobenzene is employed but not when the

Porter-Silber test is used.    **Tests for vanillylmandelic acid (VMA)** may be falsely elevated by nalidixic acid.

**FATE**    Nalidixic acid is completely absorbed from the GI tract following oral administration. The drug does not accumulate in tissues, although it may appear in milk and may cross the placenta. Nalidixic acid is partially metabolized in the liver, but virtually all of the drug and metabolites are excreted by the kidneys. The elimination *half-life* in healthy adults is 1.12 to 2.5 hours.

## ☙ NURSING CONSIDERATIONS

### Side effects, toxicities, and associated nursing actions

**CNS** A variety of neurologic reactions have been reported, including confusion, depression, dizziness, drowsiness, excitement, hallucinations, headache, insomnia, malaise, myalgia, peripheral neuritis, sensory abnormalities, syncope, and vertigo. Visual abnormalities have been reported, including changes in color perception, blurred vision, decreased visual acuity, and nystagmus. Increased intracranial pressure with bulging anterior fontanelles, papilledema, and headache may occur. Brief convulsions, sixth cranial nerve palsy, and acute toxic psychoses have also been reported.

- Obtain a careful baseline assessment before initiating drug therapy. Obtain a careful history of previous or existing medical problems, such as epilepsy, parkinsonism, or cerebrovascular disease, which may predispose the patient to toxicity (see Contraindications).
- Inform patients that a variety of side effects have been reported but are usually associated with overdose or are seen more often in infants or the elderly. Caution patients to report the development of any unexpected sign or symptom.
- Caution patients to avoid driving or operating hazardous equipment if dizziness, syncope, drowsiness, or visual disturbances occur.

**Blood** Leukopenia and thrombocytopenia may occur. Hemolytic anemia can occur, especially in patients with glucose-6-phosphate dehydrogenase deficiency.

- Monitor complete blood count, white blood cell differential, and platelet count.
- Caution the patient to avoid exposure to individuals with known infections, colds, bronchitis, and so on.
- Instruct patients to report the development of any new fever, sore throat, malaise, or cough.
- Caution patients to report any sign of bleeding such as bleeding gums, nosebleeds, change of color of the urine that might indicate kidney or bladder bleeding, rectal bleeding, unexplained bruising.

**GI** Nausea and vomiting can occur; less frequent reactions include diarrhea and abdominal pain.

- Blood concentrations of nalidixic acid are higher if the drug is taken on an empty stomach 1 hour before meals. However, if GI symptoms are a problem, instruct patients to take the drug with meals or a snack.
- If GI symptoms are severe or persistent, notify the physician.
- If vomiting or diarrhea occur, monitor intake and output.

**Metabolic** Metabolic acidosis occurs especially in premature infants. Nonketotic hyperglycemia and dyspnea can occur.

- Obtain a careful baseline assessment before starting therapy and at regular intervals throughout therapy. Monitor the respiratory rate and level of consciousness.
- Monitor blood glucose and arterial blood gases.

**Allergic** Rash, urticaria, eosinophilia, pruritis, and photosensitivity reactions occur. Arthritis, arthralgia, and anaphylaxis are rare.

- If photosensitivity occurs, caution patients to avoid exposure to direct sunlight or other sources of ultraviolet light. Caution patients to wear long-sleeved clothing and a hat, to keep legs covered, and to use a maximum-protection sunscreen on exposed skin surfaces. Photosensitivity may persist for several months following discontinuation of therapy.
- Visually inspect the patient for signs of skin manifestations.
- Have drugs, equipment, and personnel available for resuscitation in settings where antibacterials are administered.

### Nursing interventions related to drug administration

- Remain with the patient for several minutes following administration of the first several doses to monitor for the development of allergic or CNS effects. Check on the patient again within 30 minutes of dose.

### Patient and family education

- Review with patients anticipated benefits and possible effects of therapy. Caution patients to report the development of any unexpected sign or symptom.
- Caution patients to take this drug as ordered. Erratic use of nalidixic acid may predispose to the development of bacterial resistance.
- Instruct patients with urinary tract infections to increase fluid intake to 2500 to 3000 ml/day.
- Remind patients to keep these and all medications out of the reach of children. Remind patients not to share drugs with children; this drug should not be used in prepubertal children unless specifically prescribed.
- Review with female patients measures that may prevent future urinary tract infections, including wiping from front to back after voiding, urinating immediately after sexual intercourse, washing the urethral area with water only, and avoiding bubble baths.

## nitrofurantoin　(nitro-fyoor-AN-toyn)　　　urinary antiseptic

- nitrofurantoin (nitrofurantoin sodium): Furadantin, Furalan, Macrodantin, ✿Nephronex, ✿Novofuran

**MECHANISM OF ACTION**　Nitrofurantoin has multiple inhibitory actions against bacterial enzymes. The drug is often bactericidal at acidic pH.

**INDICATIONS**　**Urinary tract infections** Nitrofurantoin is effective against a wide array of gram-positive and gram-negative bacteria but only if the infection is limited to the urinary tract. Soft tissue infections, including abscesses of the kidney, are not responsive.

**CONTRAINDICATIONS**　**Renal impairment** Patients with anuria, oliguria, or significant renal impairment cannot excrete the drug to achieve adequate concentrations in urine and therefore should not receive nitrofurantoin.　**Glucose-6-phosphate dehydrogenase deficiency** These patients may be at increased risk of hemolytic anemia.　**Peripheral neuritis** These patients may be more at risk from dangerous　　　　　　　　　　　　　　　　　　　　　　　　　　　　　　　　　　　　　or permanent nerve impairment.

**DOSAGE**　**PO:**　**ADULT:** 50 to 100 mg four times daily 1 week or more for therapy; 50 to 100 mg once in the evening for suppression of chronic infections.　**CHILDREN OVER 1 MONTH OF AGE:** 5 to 7 mg/kg daily in four equal doses 1 week or more for therapy; 1 mg/kg once or twice daily for suppression of infections.　*Special patient populations:* **PREGNANCY:** Nitrofurantoin should be avoided in women near term to avoid the possibility of hemolytic anemia in the neonate.

**PREPARATIONS**　*Tablets:* 50 and 100 mg, microcrystalline form; *oral suspension:* 25 mg/5 ml, microcrystals; *capsules:* 50 or 100 mg, microcrystals (Furadantin); *capsules:* 25, 50, or 100 mg, macrocrystals (Macrodantin).

**DRUG INTERACTIONS**　**Probenecid** blocks urinary excretion of nitrofurantoin, which lowers the effective concentrations of antibacterial drug in the urine and increases the concentration of nitrofurantoin in the plasma, increasing the potential for side effects.　**Antacids containing magnesium trisilicate** lower oral absorption of nitrofurantoin.　**Nalidixic acid** is less effective in the presence of nitrofurantoin; the combination is considered antagonistic and is avoided.

**DIAGNOSTIC TEST INTERFERENCE**　Tests for glucose using cupric sulfate are falsely positive in the presence of nitrofurantoin.

**FATE**　Nitrofurantoin is readily absorbed following oral administration. The macrocrystals are more slowly absorbed than the microcrystalline forms of the drug. Distribution is limited, although some drug is found in milk and bile. Renal excretion of nitrofurantoin is extremely rapid; the drug has a *half-life* in plasma of only 20 minutes. *Peak* concentrations of drug in the urine are achieved within 30 minutes with microcrystalline preparations. Patients with significant renal impairment cannot concentrate nitrofurantoin in the urine and cannot therefore receive therapeutic benefit from the drug.

## ❧ NURSING CONSIDERATIONS
### Side effects, toxicities, and associated nursing actions

**CNS** Rare effects include cerebellar dysfunction, dizziness, drowsiness, headache, intracranial hypertension, nystagmus, retrobulbar neuritis, and trigeminal neuralgia.
- Obtain careful baseline assessment before starting drug therapy.
- Caution the patient to avoid driving or operating hazardous equipment if dizziness or drowsiness occur; notify the physician.

**Peripheral nervous system** Peripheral polyneuropathy is a serious side effect of nitrofurantoin. Early signs include paresthesia and dysesthesia, usually starting in the legs. Muscle weakness and wasting may follow. Ultimately peripheral nerve fibers may be demyelinated; spinal cord and striated muscles may be affected. This side effect is not dose related. A deficiency of B vitamins increases the likelihood of suffering this reaction.
- Question the patient carefully and regularly about the development of tingling, weakness, dysesthesia, or any unusual sensations of arms or legs.
- Instruct patients to report immediately the development of any unusual sensations in the extremities.

**Blood** Hemolytic anemia is possible, especially in neonates or in persons deficient in glucose-6-phosphate dehydrogenase. Granulocytopenia, leukopenia, and megaloblastic anemia occur rarely.
- Monitor complete blood count and white blood cell differential.
- Caution the patient to avoid exposure to crowds or individuals with known colds, fevers, or infections.
- Instruct the patient to report the development of a new fever, sore throat, or cough.

**GI** Anorexia, nausea, and vomiting are the most common side effects with nitrofurantoin. These effects are related to the dose received and the form; macrocrystals are tolerated better by some patients than are the microcrystalline forms (see Preparations).
- Instruct the patient to take the dose with meals, snack, or milk.
- If vomiting is severe or persistent, notify the physician.

**Renal** The urine is discolored by nitrofurantoin. The dark yellow or brown discoloration is harmless. Crystalluria is rare.
- Instruct the patient about the anticipated change in urine color.
- This drug is contraindicated in persons with renal failure. Monitor serum creatinine and BUN.

**Allergic** Anaphylaxis or asthmatic attacks have been reported rarely.
- Obtain a history of previous allergic response or asthma before administering the first dose.
- Drugs, equipment, and personnel for resuscitation should be readily available in settings where antibacterials are administered.

**Lung** Pulmonary function may be permanently impaired by nitrofurantoin. Acute reactions occur within a few hours of the start of therapy and may be allergic in origin. Signs include chest pain, chills, cough, eosinophilia, fever, myalgia, pruritis, skin rashes, and urticaria. Subacute reactions occur usually within a month of the start of therapy. Signs include cough, dyspnea, fever, interstitial penumonitis, and/or fibrosis and dyspnea. Chronic reactions occurring after prolonged therapy include nonproductive cough, dyspnea on exertion, malaise, and interstitial pneumonitis and/or fibrosis. Recovery from these reactions is favored if nitrofurantoin is discontinued at the first signs of pulmonary toxicity.
- Obtain a thorough pulmonary assessment before starting drug therapy, and monitor at regular intervals.
- Monitor respiratory rate, breath sounds, temperature, and white blood cell differential.
- Instruct the patient to report the development of fever, cough, shortness of breath, difficulty breathing, chest pain, rashes, or any unexpected sign or symptom.

**Liver** Rare hepatotoxicity may be fatal. Acute hepatitis or cholestasis may be self-limiting, but chronic active hepatitis or hepatic necrosis may occur, especially with long-term use of nitrofurantoin.
- Instruct patients to report the development of jaundice, right upper quadrant abdominal pain, change in the color or consistency of stools, malaise, or fever. Monitor liver function tests if available.

**Other** Photosensitization and transient hair loss (alopecia) have occurred.

- If photosensitivity occurs, instruct the patient to avoid exposure to the sun or other sources of ultraviolet light, to keep extremities covered and wear a hat, and to use maximum-protection sunscreen on exposed skin surfaces.
- Instruct the patient to notify the physician if alopecia or photosensitivity occur.

### Patient and family education

- Review with patients the anticipated benefits and possible side effects associated with drug therapy.
- Instruct patients to report the development of any unexpected sign or symptom.
- Remind patients to return for follow-up visits with the health care provider; this is especially important with drugs that have long-term side effects.
- The oral suspension may be mixed with milk, formula, fruit juice, or water. The suspension may discolor teeth if in direct, undiluted contact with the teeth. When the suspension is used, it should be diluted or the patient should carefully rinse the mouth following the dose of medication. The discoloration is not permanent.
- Remind patients using the suspension form to shake the drug vigorously before pouring the ordered dose in order to resuspend the drug.
- Patients with urinary tract infections should be instructed to increase fluid intake to 2500 to 3000 ml/day.
- Remind patients to use antibacterials only as directed.
- Remind patients to keep these and all medications out of the reach of children.
- Review with female patients measures that may prevent future urinary tract infections, including wiping from front to back after voiding, urinating immediately after sexual intercourse, washing the urethral area with water only, and avoiding bubble baths.
- To avoid vitamin B deficiency, encourage patients to maintain a regular intake of meat, legumes, milk and milk products, and whole grains.

---

## norfloxacin   (nor-FLOX-uh-sin)                                  antibiotic*

- norfloxacin: Noroxin

**MECHANISM OF ACTION**   Norfloxacin and related drugs such as nalidixic acid inhibit the enzyme called DNA gyrase, thereby interfering with reproduction of bacteria. At concentrations achieved in urine, the drug is bactericidal.

**INDICATIONS**   Urinary tract infections Initial or recurrent infections caused by susceptible strains of *E. coli, Enterobacter, Klebsiella, Pseudomonas,* and *Proteus* may be treated.

**CONTRAINDICATIONS**   Renal disease Norfloxacin is normally eliminated in urine and may accumulate when renl function fails.   Prepubertal children Norfloxacin may damage cartilage in weight-bearing joints in immature patients.

**DOSAGE**   **PO:**   **ADULT:** 400 mg twice daily for 7 to 10 days for uncomplicated urinary tract infections or up to 21 days for complicated infections. *Special patient populations:*   **CHILDREN:** Norfloxacin should not be used in prepubertal children.   **RENAL IMPAIRMENT:** Patients with creatinine clearance rates less than 30 ml/min/1.73M$^2$ should receive one 400 mg tablet daily.   **PREGNANCY:** FDA pregnancy category C.

**PREPARATIONS**   *Tablets:* 400 mg.

**DRUG INTERACTIONS**   Nitrofurantoin antagonizes the antibacterial action of norfloxacin.   **Antacids** should be avoided while taking norfloxacin.

**FATE**   Norfloxacin is very well absorbed following oral administration. The drug is eliminated almost exclusively by the kidneys.

### ❦ NURSING CONSIDERATIONS

#### Side effects, toxicities, and associated nursing actions

**CNS** Headache (2.7%) and dizziness (1.8%) are among the most common side effects. Fewer report insomnia, depression, and visual disturbances.

*DNA gyrase inhibitor.

- Caution patients to avoid driving or operating hazardous equipment if dizziness occurs.
- Taking the last dose of the day before 7 pm may lessen insomnia.
- Assess for signs of depression: change in affect, lack of interest in personal appearance, loss of appetite.

**GI** Nausea is the most common side effect (2.8%), with fewer patients reporting vomiting, anorexia, abdominal cramps, and diarrhea.

- If GI symptoms appear, monitor intake, output, and weight.
- If GI symptoms are severe or persistent, notify the physician.
- Instruct the patient to take ordered doses 1 hour before or 2 hours after meals, with a full glass (8 ounces) of water.

**Allergic** Rash and erythema were reported by fewer than 1% of treated patients.

- Assess patients for development of allergic reactions.

**Blood** Eosinophilia (1.8%) and lowered WBC (1.2%) may occur.

- Assess for signs of infection: fever and malaise.
- Monitor white blood cell differential.

**Liver** ALT and AST are elevated in 1.8% of patients; alkaline phosphatase rises in 1.4%.

- Monitor liver function tests.
- Instruct the patient to report signs of possible liver dysfunction: jaundice, fever, malaise, right upper quadrant abdominal pain, change in color or consistency of stools.

### Patient and family education

- Review with patients the anticipated benefits and possible side effects associated with therapy. Caution patients to report the development of any unexpected sign or symptom.
- Remind patients to take antibacterials only as directed. Erractic use of this drug will lessen its effectiveness.
- Encourage patients with urinary tract infections to push fluids to 2500 to 3000 ml/day.
- Remind patients to keep these and all medications out of the reach of children. Caution parents that this drug should not be used in prepubertal children. Caution parents to avoid sharing with children any medications not specifically prescribed for children.
- Review with female patients measures that may prevent future urinary tract infections, including wiping from front to back after voiding, urinating immediately after sexual intercourse, washing the urethral area with water only, and avoiding bubble baths.

---

## phenazopyridine hydrochloride (fen-azo-PEER-i-deen)   urinary analgesic

- phenazopyridine hydrochloride: Azo-standard, Baridium, Di-Azo, ✿Phenazo, Phenazodine, Pyridiate, Pyridium, Pyronium

**MECHANISM OF ACTION**   Although phenazopyridine hydrochloride has a weak antibacterial action in vitro, the only documented action in treated patients is an analgesic or anesthetic action the urinary tract. This action minimizes the symptoms associated with urinary tract infections.

**INDICATIONS**   **Urinary tract infections** Phenazopyridine must be combined with an effective antibacterial agent. Phenazopyridine should be used only for the first 2 days of therapy to reduce the symptoms associated with the infection.   **Symptomatic relief of pain following urinary tract procedures** Catheterization, surgery, endoscopy, or other medical procedures may irritate the mucosa of the lower urinary tract.

**CONTRAINDICATIONS**   **Renal impairment** Patients with glomerulonephritis, pyelonephritis, uremia, or significant renal impairment or disease should not receive phenazopyridine.   **Hepatitis** Patients with severe hepatitis should not receive phenazopyridine.

**DOSAGE**   **PO:**   ADULT: 200 mg three times daily after meals.   CHILDREN: 12 mg/kg daily in three equal doses.   *Special patient populations:*   PREGNANCY: Phenazopyridine hydrochloride is possibly carcinogenic and should be avoided if possible in pregnancy. Nevertheless, for short-term use, the drug is listed as FDA pregnancy category B.

**PREPARATIONS** *Tablets:* 100 or 200 mg. **Combination products** • *Capsules:* 50 mg with 250 mg oxytetracycline hydrochloride and 250 mg sulfamethizole (Urobiotic-250). • *Tablets:* 50 mg with 250 mg sulfamethizole (Thiosulfil-A, Uremide). • *Tablets, film-coated:* 50 mg with sulfisoxazole (Azo Gantrisin, Azo-Sulfisocon, Suldiazo); 50 mg with 100 mg sulfamethoxazole (Azo Gantanol).

**DRUG INTERACTIONS** None reported.

**FATE** The pharmacokinetics of phenazopyridine are not well studied, but the drug is believed to cross the placenta. Some drug is probably metabolized in the liver, but most of a dose is excreted by the kidneys. *Peak* excretion occurs within 5 to 6 hours of a dose.

## ❦ NURSING CONSIDERATIONS

### Side effects, toxicities, and associated nursing actions

**CNS** Headache and vertigo are rare.
• Caution the patient to avoid driving or operating hazardous equipment if vertigo develops and to notify the physician.

**Blood** Hemolytic anemia and methemoglobulinemia are possible, especially with overdoses of the drug.
• Monitor complete blood count and white blood cell differential.
• Assess for jaundice, fever, fatigue, and abdominal pain.

**GI** Mild GI effects may occur.
• Instruct patients to take ordered doses after meals.
• If GI symptoms are severe or persistent, notify the physician.

**Renal** Acute renal failure may occur with high doses or with normal doses in patients with pre-existing renal impairment. Phenazopyridine can precipitate in urine to form stones when concentrations are high. Because phenazopyridine is an azo dye, it will appear in urine as an orange or red discoloration. The drug or urine containing the drug will stain fabrics. Stains may be removed by soaking fabric in a 0.25% solution of sodium dithionate or sodium hydrosulfite.
• Assess BUN and serum creatinine before starting drug therapy.
• Encourage patients to increase fluid intake to 2500 to 3000 ml/day.
• Instruct the patient to notify the physician if urinary output diminishes or weight gain or edema occur.
• Review with patients the anticipated change in color of urine and possible staining of fabric.

**Allergic** Jaundice and hepatitis arising from allergic reactions have rarely occurred.
• Instruct patients to report the development of jaundice, malaise, fever, or upper quadrant abdominal pain.

### Patient and family education

• Review with patients the anticipated benefits and possible side effects of drug therapy. Caution patients to report the development of any unexpected sign or symptom.
• Review with female patients measures that may prevent future urinary tract infections, including wiping from front to back after voiding, urinating immediately after sexual intercourse, washing the urethral area with water only, and avoiding bubble baths.

---

## polymyxin B sulfate   (polly-MIX-in)                    polypeptide antibiotic

• polymyxin B sulfate: Aerosporin

**MECHANISM OF ACTION** Polymyxin binds to phospholipids in bacterial cell membranes and disrupts membrane function by a detergentlike action. This mechanism is similar to that of colistin (p. 341).

**INDICATIONS** **Serious systemic infections caused by organisms resistant to safer drugs** Polymyxin B is seldom indicated for systemic use but can be used in the rare instance when infections caused by *P. aeruginosa, H. influenzae, E. coli, E. aerogenes,* or *K. pneumoniae* cannot be treated with safer agents.   **Bacteremia and bacteriuria with indwelling catheters** Polymyxin B can be used with neosporin as an irrigant in the bladder to prevent bacteremia or bacteriuria when an indwelling catheter must remain in place.   **Superficial infections of the skin** Polymyxin B alone or in combination with other agents can be used topically to prevent or treat superficial infections, although clear evidence of effectiveness is lacking.

**CONTRAINDICATIONS**   **Allergy to polymyxin antibiotics** Polymyxin B is chemically related to colistin and colistimethate sodium. Patients allergic to any of these drugs will be likely to react to all.

**DOSAGE**   IM:   **ADULTS AND CHILDREN OVER 2 YEARS:** 25,000 to 30,000 units/kg daily in four to six equal doses.   **INFANTS:** 40,000 units/kg daily in divided doses.   IV:   **ADULTS AND CHILDREN OVER 2 YEARS:** 15,000 to 25,000 units/kg daily in two doses.   **INFANTS:** 40,000 units/kg daily in divided doses.   *Special patient populations:*   **RENAL IMPAIRMENT:** Doses must be reduced if renal function is impaired.   **PREGNANCY:** Polymyxin B should be avoided if possible in pregnancy.

**PREPARATIONS**   *Powder for parenteral use:* 500,000 units, to be reconstituted in 5% dextrose, sterile water, 0.9% sodium chloride, or 1% procaine hydrochloride to the concentration required. **Combination products** *Irrigating solution:* 200,000 units/ml of polymyxin B with 57 mg/ml neomycin sulfate. *Ophthalmic ointments:* 10,000 units/g of polymyxin B with 500 units/g bacitracin and 0.5% neomycin sulfate (Mycitracin); • 10,000 units/g of polymyxin B with 400 units/g bacitracin zinc and 0.5% neomycin sulfate (Ak-spore, Biotic-O, Neosporin); • 10,000 units/g of polymyxin B with 500 units/g bacitracin zinc (Ak-Poly-Bac, Ocumycin, Polysporin); • 10,000 units/g of polymyxin B with chloramphenicol 1% (Chloromyxin); • 10,000 units/g of polymyxin B with neomycin sulfate 0.5% (Statrol); • 10,000 units/g of polymyxin B with oxytetracycline hydrochloride 5 mg/g (Terramycin Ophthalmic ointment. • *Topical ointments (OTC);* • 5000 units/g of polymyxin B with 400 units/g bacitracin and 5 mg/g neomycin sulfate (Triple Antibiotic Ointment; Clinicydin; Lanabiotic; Mycitracin); • 10,000 units/g of polymyxin B with bacitracin zinc 500 units/g (Double Antibiotic Ointment; Polysporin); • 5000 units/g of polymyxin B with 400 units/g bacitracin zinc and 5 mg/g neomycin sulfate.

**DRUG INTERACTIONS**   **Neuromuscular blocking agents** used in conjunction with surgery may be potentiated by the weak neuromuscular blocking activity of polymyxin B. The combinations should be avoided when possible or, if used together, the patients should be closely watched for excessive blockade resulting in respiratory paralysis.   **Aminoglycoside antibiotics, sodium citrate, quinine, or quinidine** should be avoided because the renal and/or neurotoxicity of these agents may be additive with same reactions caused by polymyxin B.

**FATE**   Polymxin B is not significantly absorbed from the GI tract or from skin or mucous membranes. IM administration of polymyxin B produces *peak* serum concentrations within 2 hours. The drug does not appear in significant concentrations in the CNS, aqueous humor, synovial fluid, or amnionic fluid. Polymyxin B is excreted primarily by the kidneys, with an elimination *half-life* of 4 to 6 hours in patients with normal renal function.

## 🐝 NURSING CONSIDERATIONS

### Side effects, toxicities, and associated nursing actions

**CNS** Ataxia, blurred vision, circumoral and peripheral paresthesia or numbness, coma, confusion, dizziness, drowsiness, flushing of the face, giddiness, irritability, muscle weakness, nystagmus, seizures, or slurred speech have all been reported with parenteral polymyxin B.
• Obtain careful baseline assessment before administering the drug.
• Caution the patient to avoid driving or operating hazardous equipment until the effects of the medication can be evaluated.
• Caution the patient to report the development of any unusual sign or symptom.
**Blood** Thrombophlebitis may occur with IV administration.
• Dilute as directed before administering (see Nursing Interventions).
• Check for patency of IV line before administering.
**Renal** Albuminuria, azotemia, cylindruria, electrolyte loss, hematuria, leukocyturia, and increased urinary concentration of the drug have all been reported with parenteral polymyxin B.
• Monitor intake, output, and weight.

- Monitor serum creatinine, BUN, and urinalysis.

**Allergic** Polymyxin B itself is not a strong sensitizing agent, but some OTC ointments contain other chemicals that can lead to contact dermatitis.

- Instruct patients to report the development of any unexpected sign or symptom.

### Nursing interventions related to drug administration
- Before administering the first dose, ask the patient about a history of allergic response to polymyxin B, colistin, or colistimethate.
- Respiratory arrest has been reported with parenteral therapy. Monitor respiratory rate. Assess for dyspnea, restlessness, or inability to handle secretions. Auscultate breath sounds. Have oxygen, a suction machine, and drugs, equipment, and personnel available to provide ventilatory support.
- For IM administration, dilute as directed on vial with 2 ml of diluent. Use anatomic landmarks to choose injection sites. Aspirate before injecting dose to prevent inadvertent IV administration. Record sites and rotate sites. IM administration is especially painful; 1% procaine hydrochloride may be used as a diluent; consult the physician.
- For IV administration, dilute the reconstituted dose in 300 to 500 ml of 5% dextrose in water and administer over 60 to 90 minutes. Do *not* use procaine hydrochloride as a diluent.
- For intrathecal administration, dissolve 500,000 units in 10 ml sodium chloride injection to produce a concentration of 50,000 units per milliliter. Do *not* use procaine hydrochloride as a diluent.

### Patient and family education
- Review with patients the anticipated benefits and possible side effects of therapy. Instruct patients to report the development of any unexpected sign or symptom.
- Review with patients the importance of using this medication only as ordered for as long as ordered.

## trimethoprim   (tri-METH-oh-prim)                                    antibiotic*

- trimethroprim: Proloprim, Trimpex

**MECHANISM OF ACTION**   Trimethoprim is an inhibitor of the enzyme dihydrofolate reductase. This enzyme converts one form of folate to the biologically active form required to make thymidine. Without thymidine, bacterial cells cannot make DNA and they slowly die. Trimethoprim is not as potent an inhibitor of the enzyme in mammalian cells and therefore does not significantly affect folate metabolism in humans.

**INDICATIONS**   **Urinary tract infections** Initial, acute infections caused by susceptible strains of *E. coli, Proteus, Klebsiella, Enterobacter,* and *Staphylococcus* may be successfully treated with trimethoprim. • See co-trimoxazole for other indications (p. 367).

**CONTRAINDICATIONS**   **Folate deficiency** The antifolate action of trimethoprim is normally insignificant but may become a problem for patients with pre-existing folate deficiency.   **Megaloblastic anemia** Megaloblastic anemia arising from folate deficiency may be worsened by the antifolate action of trimethoprim.

**DOSAGE**   **PO:**   **ADULT:** 100 mg every 12 hours or 200 mg daily. Doses must be reduced if renal function is impaired.   *Special patient populations:*   **PREGNANCY:** Trimethoprim is teratogenic and can interfere with folate metabolism in pregnant women and their fetuses (FDA pregnancy category C).

**PREPARATIONS**   *Tablets:* 100 0r 200 mg.

**DRUG INTERACTIONS**   **Phenytoin** may have some antifolate activity that, when added to the effects of trimethoprim, can cause folate deficiency.

**FATE**   Trimethoprim is readily absorbed from the intestinal tract. *Peak* serum concentrations occur within 1 to 4 hours of an oral dose. Trimethoprim is distributed well to most tissues in the body, entering milk and crossing the placenta. Elimination from the body is almost entirely by renal excretion, but metab-

*Dihydrofolate reductase inhibitor.

olism does occur in the liver. The serum *half-life* for the drug is 8 to 11 hours in patients with normal renal function.

### ❦ NURSING CONSIDERATIONS

#### Side effects, toxicities, and associated nursing actions

**Blood** Megaloblastic anemia, neutropenia, and thrombocytopenia can arise from the antifolate effects of trimethoprim. The risk of these effects is increased in patients with pre-existing folate depletion, e.g., geriatric, malnourished, alcoholic, pregnant, or debilitated patients.

- Monitor complete blood count, white blood cell differential, and platelet count.
- Assess for weakness, pallor, dyspnea, jaundice (signs of possible megaloblastic anemia). Caution patients to report the development of fever, pallor, or sore throat.
- Caution patients to report the development of unexplained bruising, bleeding from gums, nosebleeds, change in the color or urine that might suggest bleeding from bladder or kidneys, or blood in stools.

**GI** About 6% of treated patients report epigastric discomfort, glossitis, nausea, vomiting, or abnormal tastes.

- If GI symptoms are severe or persistent, notify the physician.
- Instruct patients to take oral doses with meals or snacks to lessen gastric irritation.

**Other** Skin rashes are common dose-dependent reactions to trimethoprim. Up to 7% of patients receiving doses of 200 mg or less suffer rashes appearing 7 to 14 days after beginning therapy. The incidence climbs to 24% when doses are increased to 400 mg.

- Inspect the patient for the development of rashes.
- Instruct patients to report the appearance of any skin changes.

#### Patient and family education

- Review with patients the anticipated benefits and possible side effects of drug therapy.
- Instruct patients to report the development of any unexpected sign or symptom.
- Encourage patients with urinary tract infections to increase fluid intake to 2500 to 3000 ml/day.
- Remind patients to take medications as ordered; erratic use of antibacterial agents will lessen their effectiveness.
- Remind patients who may also have vitamins or folate preparations prescribed of the importance of taking all prescribed medications.
- Caution patients to keep these and all medications out of the reach of children.
- Review with female patients measures that may prevent future urinary tract infections, including wiping from front to back after voiding, urinating immediately after sexual intercourse, washing the urethral area with water only, and avoiding bubble baths.

---

## vancomycin hydrochloride (van-co-MY-sin) antibiotic*

- vancomycin hydrochloride: Vancocin

**MECHANISM OF ACTION** vancomycin inhibits one step in bacterial cell wall biosynthesis. The site of action is different from penicillins, cephalosporins, bacitracin, or other antibiotics that also inhibit cell wall biosynthesis. The action of vancomycin is usually rapidly bactericidal.

**INDICATIONS** **Severe infections caused by gram-positive bacteria** Infections caused by bacterial strains resistant to penicillins, cephalosporins, or other antibiotics may be successfully treated with vancomycin. Because the mechanism of action of vancomycin is different from that of other clinically used antibiotics, cross-resistance is not a problem. **Suprainfections caused by C. dificile** Overgrowth of *C. dificile* and other clostridia can cause a syndrome called antibiotic-induced colitis, in which toxins produced by the *Clostridium* damage the intestinal lining. This condition can progress to pseudomembranous colitis, which can be fatal. Treatment includes discontinuing the original antibiotic and starting therapy with vancomycin, which eliminates the *Clostridium*.

*Cell wall inhibitor.

**CONTRAINDICATIONS**    **Hearing loss** Vancomycin can cause hearing loss and should be avoided if possible in patients with pre-existing impairment.    **Renal impairment** Vancomycin can be nephrotoxic and should be avoided in patients with pre-existing impairment or in neonates whose renal function is undeveloped.

**DOSAGE**    **PO:**    **ADULT:** 500 mg every 6 hours or 1 g every 12 hours for the control of intestinal suprainfections with *Clostridium dificile*.    **CHILDREN:** 44 mg/kg daily in divided doses for the control of intestinal suprainfections with *C. dificile*.    **IV:**    **ADULT:** 500 mg every 6 hours or 1 g every 12 hours. **CHILDREN:** 10 mg/kg daily for neonates in divided doses. Older infants and children may receive 44 mg/kg daily in divided doses.    *Special patient populations:*    **ELDERLY:** Although special geriatric doses have not been established, geriatric patients may be more at risk of ototoxicity because of previous hearing loss.    **RENAL IMPAIRMENT:** Doses must be reduced if renal function is impaired. **PREGNANCY:** Safe use of vancomycin during pregnancy has not been established.

**PREPARATIONS**    *Powder for oral solution:* 1 or 10 g, to be dissolved in distilled or deionized water. *Powder for parenteral use:* 500 mg, to be reconstituted in sterile water and further diluted as necesssary in 5% dextrose or 0.9% sodium chloride.

**DRUG INTERACTIONS**    **Gentamicin, kanamycin, neomycin, netilmicin, streptomycin, tobramycin, and paromycin (aminoglycosides), as well as polymyxin B and colistin** all have ototoxic and nephrotoxic actions that can be additive with those same effects by vancomycin. The combinations should be avoided.

**FATE**    Vancomycin is not significantly absorbed following oral administration. When administered by that route, the intent is to treat infections within the intestinal lumen. Following IV administration, vancomycin distributes well through most tissues and fluids but is present in low concentrations in bile and CSF. The drug does cross the placenta. Elimination from the body is almost exclusively by renal excretion. The elimination *half-life* is about 6 hours but is elevated when renal function is impaired.

## ☙ NURSING CONSIDERATIONS

### Side effects, toxicities, and associated nursing actions

**Ototoxicity** Vancomycin can damage the auditory branch of the eighth cranial nerve, causing permanent deafness. Early signs of toxicity include tinnitus. If tinnitus develops, the drug should be discontinued.
- Obtain a careful baseline assessment of hearing before starting drug therapy.
- Instruct the patient to report the development of tinnitus or changes in hearing.

**CV** Rapid IV administration of vancomycin can cause acute hypotension, accompanied by maculopapular or erythematous rash of the face, head, chest, and arms. This syndrome is referred to as the "red man's syndrome" or the "red-neck syndrome." The reaction is more common when infusions are given too rapidly. The symptoms usually resolve, but cardiac arrest has occurred.
- Dilute 500 mg or dry powder with 10 ml sterile water for injection. Further dilute this solution with sodium chloride solution of 5% dextrose in water to make a final dilution of 500 mg in 100 to 200 ml. Administer at a rate of 500 mg over 30 minutes. The use of an infusion control device or volume control device and microdrip tubing may lessen the chance of a too rapid infusion.
- Monitor the vital signs. Have personnel, drugs, and equipment available in settings where vancomycin is administered intravenously.

**Blood** Transient leukopenia and neutropenia have been reported.
- Monitor the complete blood count and white blood cell differential.
- Instruct the patient to report the development of fever, malaise, sore throat, cough, or infection.

**GI** Nausea can occur.
- Instruct patients to take the dose with meals or a snack if nausea occurs. If nausea is persistent or severe, notify the physician.

**Renal** Albuminuria, elevations in BUN concentration, and hyaline or granular casts in the urine have been observed. Fatal uremia can occur.
- Monitor urinalysis, serum creatinine, and BUN.

- Monitor intake, output, and weight.
- Monitor serum drug levels if available.

**Allergic** Chills, fever, urticaria, macular rashes, eosinophilia, and anaphylaxis have occurred. Some allergic reaction is reported in up to 10% of patients.

- Have personnel, drugs, and equipment available for resuscitation in settings where antibacterials are administered.
- Remain with the patient for several minutes after administering doses, and check the patient again after 30 minutes.

**Other** Vancomycin is a highly irritating chemical that can cause local necrosis if allowed to seep into tissues surrounding the IV infusion site. Thrombophlebitis and pain can result even from properly administered IV injections.

- Inspect the IV insertion site carefully during drug administration.
- Instruct the patient to report the development of pain, burning, and redness around the IV insertion site.
- Ascertain that the IV is patent before infusing the drug.

## Nursing interventions related to drug administration

- See CV side effects.

## Patient and family education

- Review with patients the anticipated benefits and possible side effects of drug therapy.
- Instruct patients to report the development of any unexpected sign or symptom.
- Instruct patients with urinary tract infections to increase fluid intake to 2500 to 3000 ml/day. Caution patients to notify the physician if urinary output decreases, edema, or swelling develops or weight increases.
- Remind patients to take medications as ordered. Erratic use of antibacterials will lessen their effectiveness.
- Remind patients to keep these and all medications out of the reach of children.

# Chapter Twenty
# Sulfonamides

mafenide acetate
silver sulfadiazine
sulfacetamide
sulfabenzamide
sulfacytine
sulfadiazine
sulfamerazine
sulfamethazine
sulfamethizole
sulfamethoxazole
sulfapyridine
sulfasalazine
sulfathiazole
sulfasoxazole

**Fixed combinations for systemic use**
co-trimazine
co-trimoxazole
sulfadiazine and trimethoprim (see co-trimazine)
sulfadiazine, sulfamerazine, and sulfamethazine
sulfamethizole and phenazopyridine
sulfamethizole, oxytetracycline, and phenazopyridine
sulfamethoxazole and phenazopyridine
sulfamethoxazole and trimethoprim (see co-trimoxazole)
sulfisoxazole and erythromycin succinate

**OVERVIEW OF THE DRUG CLASS** Sulfonamides are broad-spectrum antimicrobial agents that have been in use for over 50 years. Early representatives of this class were not very potent and were rather insoluble, which led to renal side effects as the drugs actually crystallized in urine. Newer sulfonamides are more soluble and avoid many of the complications of the earlier agents (see Table 20-3). Introduction of much more potent antibiotics such as penicillins and cephalosporins has diminished the usefulness of sulfonamides, although they may be indicated for specific diseases. The most common current use is in treating urinary tract infections. For this indication, sulfonamides are inexpensive and effective therapy for many patients. Sulfonamides are also used as topical antibacterial agents (Table 20-1) and are common antibacterials in fixed combination products (Table 20-2).

**MECHANISM OF ACTION** Sulfonamides block the formation of dihydrofolate in susceptible bacteria. This metabolic blockade deprives the bacteria of folate products required for biosynthesis of thymidine and certain amino acids. Thymidine is required for synthesis of DNA, and amino acids are required for production of proteins. By depriving bacteria of these required metabolites, sulfonamides inhibit growth and reproduction of the microorganism. Human cells do not synthesize dihydrofolate but absorb it from external sources. Therefore human cells are not affected by sulfonamides in the same way as are bacteria.

**INDICATIONS** **Urinary tract infections** Sulfonamides may be effective against infections caused by *Escherichia, Klebsiella, Enterobacter, Proteus,* and *Staphylococcus.* • The newer, highly water-soluble sulfonamides are preferred for this indication (Table 20-3). **Nocardiosis** Sulfonamides are drugs of choice for this uncommon infection. **Toxoplasmosis** Sulfadiazine or sulfamethoxazole is often combined with pyrimethamine for treating this unusual infection. **Malaria** Sulfadoxine or sulfadiazine with pyrimethamine and quinine is used for uncomplicated malaria caused by chloroquine-resistant strains of *Plasmodium.* **To eliminate the meningococcal carrier state** *Neisseria meningitidis* can be spread by healthy individuals who carry the organism in the nasopharynx. • Sulfonamides eradicate the organism and prevent the spread of meningitis within populations at high risk. • Resistant strains exist, and alternative drugs may be required. • For specific indications, see individual agents.

**CONTRAINDICATIONS** **Allergy to sulfonamides or related drugs** Previous allergic reactions to any sulfonamide or the chemically related sulfonylureas (Chapter 34) or thiazide diuretics (Chapter 9) are an absolute contraindication to the use of a sulfonamide. **Deficiency of glucose-6-phosphate dehydrogenase** Sulfonamides and other drugs can cause acute hemolytic anemia in patients lacking normal concentrations of the enzyme G-6-PD in their red blood cells. • People of African or Mediterranean ancestry are more likely to have this genetically determined trait. • Newborn infants are developmentally deficient in G-6-PD during the first few days of life. **Newborn state** Neonates lack adequate mechanisms for eliminating a variety of compounds. • Sulfonamides may complicate this problem by displacing bilirubin from protein binding sites. • The accumulated bilirubin may produce serious

Table
20-1.

## Sulfonamides used as topical agents*

| Generic names of components | Trade name | Application form | Clinical use | Comments |
|---|---|---|---|---|
| Mafenide acetate | Sulfamylon | Cream: 85 mg mafenide acetate in each gram | For second- and third-degree burns | Broad spectrum includes *Pseudomonas aeruginosa* |
| Silver sulfadiazine | Flamezine, Silvadene | Cream: 10 mg/g | For second- and third-degree burns | Broad spectrum includes *Pseudomonas aeruginosa* |
| Sulfabenzamide, sulfacetamide, sulfathiazole, urea | Femguard, Sulfa-gyn, Sultrin, Triple sulfa, Trysul | Cream: 3.7% sulfabenzamide, 2.86% sulfacetamide, 3.42% sulfathiazole, 0.64% urea | Vaginal use only | Substantial evidence of effectiveness at this site is lacking |
| Sulfacetamide | Bleph liquifilm, Sulamyd, Sulf-10 | Solution: 10%, 15%, or 30%; ointment: 10% | Ophthalmic only: for conjunctivitis, corneal ulcer, trachoma | Drug allergy may develop in sensitive patients |
| Sulfisoxazole | Cantri, Vagilia | Cream: 10%; suppositories: 600 or 700 mg | Vaginal use only | Substantial evidence of effectiveness at this site is lacking |
| Sulfisoxazole diolamine | Gantrisin ophthalmic | Solution: 4%; ointment: 4% | Ophthalmic only: for conjunctivitis, corneal ulcer, trachoma | Drug allergy may develop in sensitive patients |

*Note that some drug may be absorbed through topical application, resulting in allergic reactions or occasionally other side effects.

toxicity or kernicterus.    **Impaired renal function** Sulfonamides may accumulate to dangerous concentrations in patients lacking adequate renal function. • These drugs may also directly damage the kidneys.    **Impaired hepatic function** Sulfonamides may accumulate to dangerous concentrations in patients lacking adequate hepatic function. • These drugs may also worsen existing hepatic disease. • For specific contraindications, see individual agents.

**DRUG INTERACTIONS**    **Trimethoprim** Sulfonamides interfere with the incorporation of PABA into dihydrofolate, and trimethoprim interferes with the conversion of dihydrofolate into the active form, tetrahydrofolate. By combining trimethoprim with a sulfonamide, a synergistic antibacterial action is achieved. This mechanism is the basis for the fixed combination product co-trimoxazole (Table 20-2). **Coumarin anticoagulants** Sulfonamides potentiate the anticoagulant activity of the coumarins. Coumarins, which are normally almost completely bound to plasma proteins, may be displaced so that more free, active coumarin is available. Sulfonamides may also interfere with normal metabolism of the coumarins, which may further intensify the anticoagulant effect.    **Sulfonylurea hypoglycemic agents** Sulfonamides may potentiate the hypoglycemic action of the sulfonylureas by displacing these

**Table 20-2.**

## Clinical summary of sulfonamides: fixed combinations for oral use

| Components of combination | Drug form | Trade name | Dosage | Clinical use |
|---|---|---|---|---|
| Sulfadiazine 410 mg, trimethoprim 90 mg | Tablet | ♣Coptin | Adults: 1 tablet every 12 hrs; Children 5 to 12 yr: 1/2 to 1 tablet every 12 hr | Urinary tract infections only |
| Sulfadiazine 167 mg, sulfamerazine 167 mg, sulfamethazine 167 mg | Tablet or per 5 ml of suspension | Neotrizine, Terfonyl, Triple Sulfa suspension | Adults: 2 to 4 g initially, then 2 to 4 g daily in 3 to 6 equal doses | Urinary tract infections only |
| Sulfamethizole 250 or 500 mg, Phenazopyridine 100 mg | Tablet | Azo-Gamazole, Azo-Gantanol | Adults: 2 to 4 tablets 2 or 3 times daily; Children: 30 to 45 mg of sulfamethizole per kg daily in 4 doses | Urinary tract infections only, for the first 2 days of therapy |
| Sulfamethizole 250 mg, phenazopyridine 50 mg, oxytetracycline 250 mg | Capsules | Urobiotic 250 | Adults: 0.5 to 1 g, 3 or 4 times daily; Children: 30 to 45 mg of sulfamethizole per kg daily in 4 equal doses | Urinary tract infections, for first 2 days of therapy |
| Sulfamethoxazole 500 mg, phenazopyridine 100 mg | Tablet | Azo-Gamazole, Azo-Gantanol | Adults only: 4 tablets to load, then 2 tablets every 12 hr for 2 days | Urinary tract infections only, for first 2 days of therapy |
| Sulfamethoxazole 400 mg, trimethoprim 80 mg | Tablet | Bactrim, Septra | See co-trimoxazole | |
| Sulfisoxazole 600 mg, erythromycin 200 mg (ethyl succinate) | In each 5 ml of suspension | Pediazole | Children: 12.5 mg/kg erythromycin 4 times daily or 37.5 mg/kg sulfisoxazole every 6 hr | Otitis media caused by susceptible strains of *influenzae* |
| Sulfisoxazole 500 mg, phenazopyridine 50 mg | Tablet | Azo-Gantrisin, Suldiazo | Adults: 4 to 6 tablets every 12 hr for 2 days; Children: doses as for sulfisoxazole alone | Urinary tract infections only, for the first 2 days of therapy |

compounds from protein binding sites and by blocking their normal metabolism by the liver. **Methotrexate** Sulfonamides may increase the toxicity of the anticancer agent methotrexate. **PABA** PABA can block the action of sulfonamides and should not be used when sulfonamides are being taken. **Local anesthetics** Chloroprocaine, piperocaine, procaine, propoxycaine, and tetracaine are derivatives of PABA and have the potential to interfere with sulfonamide action. For specific interactions, see individual agents.

**Table 20-3.**

### Relative solubilities of selected sulfonamides

| | Solubility (mg/dl) | | | |
|---|---|---|---|---|
| | pH 5* | pH 6 | pH 7 | pH 8 |
| Sulfacytine | 109 | 130 | 230 | — |
| Sulfadiazine | 13 | 18 | 68 | 570 |
| Sulfamethizole | 154 | 724 | 8250 | 63500 |
| Sulfamethoxazole | 60 | 100 | 500 | 5000 |
| Sulfapyridine | 79 | 79 | 83 | 116 |
| Sulfisoxazole | 43 | 196 | 1700 | 17000 |

*The pH of normal urine is about 5.5 but may vary considerably.

## 🐾 NURSING CONSIDERATIONS

### Side effects, toxicities, and associated nursing actions

**CNS** Ataxia, acute psychosis, confusion, depression, drowsiness, headache, insomnia, and restlessness are uncommon but may occur.
- Instruct patient to avoid driving or operating hazardous equipment if drowsiness or ataxia occurs; notify the physician.
- Instruct patient to take last dose before 7 PM if insomnia develops.
- Instruct patient and family to notify physician if any change in mood or affect occurs.

**GI** Nausea and vomiting are common reactions. Abdominal pain, anorexia, pharyngitis, glossitis, gastroenteritis, diarrhea, and pancreatitis are possible but uncommon.
- Instruct patients to take oral preparations with meals or snacks to lessen gastric irritation.
- Monitor weight. If GI symptoms are prominent, monitor intake and output.
- If vomiting or diarrhea is severe or persistent, notify physician.

**Renal** Anuria, oliguria, hematuria, proteinuria, renal colic, and urolithiasis may occur if the sulfonamide crystallizes in the urine. Increasing urinary output and alkalinizing the urine are mechanisms that reduce renal side effects (Table 20-3).
- Monitor urinalysis, serum creatinine, and BUN. Monitor urine pH daily.
- Instruct patients to increase fluid intake to 2500 to 3000 ml per day.
- To alkalinize the urine, the physician may prescribe sodium bicarbonate. Emphasize to the patient the need to take both drugs as ordered for best effect.
- It is difficult to achieve urinary alkalinization through dietary means alone. Instruct patients to avoid excessive amounts of vitamin C, which may acidify urine.

**Liver** Signs of liver damage, including jaundice and histologic changes, may occur 3 to 5 days after therapy is started.
- Instruct patients to report the development of jaundice, malaise, fever, right upper quadrant abdominal pain, or change in the color or consistency of stools.
- Monitor liver function tests if available.

**Blood** Acute hemolytic anemia may be triggered by sulfonamides, especially in those patients lacking adequate G-6-PD. Agranulocytosis, aplastic anemia, eosinophilia, hypoprothrombinemia, leukopenia, and methemoglobinemia may also occur. Blood counts are required in patients receiving these drugs for longer than 2 weeks.
- Question patients about history of G-6-PD deficiency before administering first dose. Question mothers who may be breastfeeding if this deficiency has been diagnosed in their infants. Breastfeeding mothers should not take sulfonamides and continue breastfeeding if the infant has G-6-PD deficiency.
- Emphasize to patients the importance of returning for regular follow-up care.
- Monitor the complete blood count, white blood cell differential, and prothrombin time or coagula-

tion factors.
- Instruct patient to report the development of fever, sore throat, malaise, jaundice, fatigue, infection, unexplained bruising, bleeding from gums, nosebleeds, and blood in urine or stool.
- Monitor serum drug levels if available.

**Allergy** Allergic symptoms include rash, pruritis, fever, headache, joint pain, Stevens-Johnson syndrome, Lyell's syndrome, and Behcet's syndrome. High fever, headache, stomatitis, conjunctivitis, rhinitis, urethritis, and balantitis (inflammation of the glans penis) may signal the beginning of Stevens-Johnson syndrome.
- Question patients about known drug allergies to other sulfonamides, sulfonylureas, thiazide diuretics, and acetazolamide before administering first dose.
- Assess patient systematically and frequently for the development of unexpected signs or symptoms. Instruct patients to report the development of symptoms of Stevens-Johnson syndrome listed above.

**Other** Rare side effects include hypothyroidism, goiter production, hypoglycemia, periorbital edema, and infection of the sclera and conjunctiva.
- Instruct patients to report the development of any unexpected sign or symptom.

### Nursing interventions related to drug administration
- Tablets may be crushed before administration. Film-coated tablets must not be crushed or chewed but must be swallowed whole. Tablets should be taken with a full glass (8 oz) of fluid.

### Patient and family education
- Review with patients the anticipated benefits and possible side effects of therapy. Instruct patients to report the development of any unexpected sign or symptom.
- Remind patients to take antibacterials as directed for best effect.
- Remind patients to keep all health care providers informed of all medications being taken.
- Instruct patients who are also taking sulfonylureas that hypoglycemia may be potentiated. Patients taking both drugs may need to monitor blood glucose levels carefully and increase caloric intake while taking both drugs.
- Review with female patients measures that may prevent future urinary tract infections: wiping from front to back after voiding, urinating immediately after sexual intercourse, washing the urethral area with water only, and avoiding bubble baths.
- Remind patients to keep these and all medications out of the reach of children.

---

## sulfacytine   (sul-fa-SYE-teen)                                    sulfonamide

- sulfacytine: Renoquid

**MECHANISM OF ACTION**   See entry for drug class (p. 358)

**INDICATIONS**   **Acute, nonobstructive urinary tract infections** Like other sulfonamides, sulfacytine may be effective against infections caused by *E. coli, Klebsiella, Enterobacter, Proteus,* and *S. aureus.*

**CONTRAINDICATIONS**   See entry for drug class (p. 358)

**DOSAGE**   PO:   ADULT: 500 mg initial dose, followed by 250 mg four times daily for 10 days.   *Special patient populations:*   PREGNANCY: Safe use during pregnancy and lactation has not been established. Use in the mother immediately before delivery may cause kernicterus in the newborn. CHILDREN: Children under 14 years of age should not receive sulfacytine.   RENAL IMPAIRMENT: Doses may need to be reduced.

**PREPARATIONS**   *Tablets:* 250 mg.

**DRUG INTERACTIONS**   See entry for drug class (p. 359).

**FATE**   Sulfacytine is rapidly and almost completely absorbed following oral dosage, producing *peak* levels within 2 to 3 hours. Sulfacytine is extensively metabolized by the liver; unchanged drug and its derivatives are rapidly eliminated by the kidneys. The elimination *half-life* for sulfacytine is 4 to 4.5 hours. Concentrations of the drug in the blood are too low for successful therapy of systemic infections, but the more than twentyfold higher concentrations found in urine are adequate for antibacterial action.

## ☙ NURSING CONSIDERATIONS
### Side effects, toxicities, and associated nursing actions
- See entry for drug class (p. 361).
### Nursing interventions related to drug administration
- See entry for drug class (p. 362).
### Patient and family education
- See entry for drug class (p. 362).

---

## sulfadiazine (sul-fa-DYE-uh-zeen) sulfonamide

- sulfadiazine: Microsulfon

**MECHANISM OF ACTION** See entry for drug class (p. 358).

**INDICATIONS** **Urinary tract infections** Sulfadiazine may be effective against infections caused by *Escherichia*, *Klebsiella*, *Enterobacter*, *Proteus*, and *Staphylococcus*, but sulfadiazine is one of the least soluble sulfonamides currently in use (Table 20-3). **Nocardiosis** Sulfonamides are drugs of choice for this uncommon infection. **Toxoplasmosis** Sulfadiazine is often combined with pyrimethamine for treating this unusual infection. **Malaria** Sulfadiazine with pyrimethamine and quinine is used for uncomplicated malaria caused by chloroquine-resistant strains of *Plasmodium*. **To eliminate the meningococcal carrier state** *Meningitidis* can be spread by healthy individuals who carry the organism in the nasopharynx. • Sulfadiazine may eradicate the organism and prevent the spread of meningitis within populations at high risk. • Resistant strains exist, and alternative drugs may be required.

**CONTRAINDICATIONS** See entry for drug class (p. 358).

**DOSAGE** **PO:** **ADULTS:** 2 to 4 g initially, followed by a daily dose of 2 to 4 g given as 3 to 6 equal doses. For nocardiosis or toxoplasmosis, doses may be as high as 8 g daily and may continue for weeks or months, based on the immune status of the patient. For malaria, doses are 500 mg four times daily for 5 days. For asymptomatic meningococcal carriers, 1 g twice daily for 2 days is sufficient. **CHILDREN OVER 2 MONTHS OF AGE:** 75 mg/kg or 2 g/M$^2$ as an initial dose, followed by a daily dose of 150 mg/kg or 4 g/M$^2$ given as 4 to 6 equal doses up to a daily maximum of 6 g. For toxoplasmosis, the pediatric dose is 100 to 200 mg/kg daily for weeks or months, based on the immune status of the patient. For malaria, doses are 25 to 50 mg/kg four times daily (not to exceed 2 g daily) for 5 days. For asymptomatic meningococcal carriers, 500 mg once daily for 2 days in children from 2 to 12 months; 500 mg twice daily for 2 days in children from 1 to 12 years. *Special patient populations:* **RENAL IMPAIRMENT:** Doses may need to be reduced. **PREGNANCY:** Safe use during pregnancy and lactation has not been established. Use in the mother immediately before delivery may cause kernicterus in the newborn.

**PREPARATIONS** *Tablets:* 500 mg. Combination products include trisulfapyrimidines (see Table 20-2). *Suspension:* sulfadiazine (167 mg/5 ml) with sulfamerazine (167 mg/5 ml) and sulfamethazine (167 mg/5 ml). *Tablets:* sulfadiazine 167 mg with sulfamerazine 167 mg and sulfamethazine 167 mg.

**DRUG INTERACTIONS** See entry for drug class (p. 359).

**FATE** Sulfadiazine is absorbed from the GI tract, producing *peak* serum concentrations within 6 hours. The drug is well distributed to most tissues but is present in relatively low concentrations in the normal CNS. Sulfadiazine is metabolized by the liver, and both the metabolites and unchanged drug are eliminated by the kidneys. The solubility of sulfadiazine is poor at the acidic pH of normal urine, but the major metabolite of sulfadiazine is somewhat more soluble than the parent compound.

## ☙ NURSING CONSIDERATIONS
### Side effects, toxicities, and associated nursing actions
- See entry for drug class (p. 361).
### Nursing interventions related to drug administration
- See entry for drug class (p. 362).
### Patient and family education
- See entry for drug class (p. 362).

## sulfamethizole (sul-fa-METH-i-zole) sulfonamide

- sulfamethizole: Proklar, Thiosulfil, Urobiotic

**MECHANISM OF ACTION** See entry for drug class (p. 358).

**INDICATIONS** **Urinary tract infections** Sulfamethizole may be effective against infections caused by *Escherichia, Klebsiella, Enterobacter, Proteus,* and *Staphylococcus.*

**CONTRAINDICATIONS** See entry for drug class (p. 358).

**DOSAGE** **PO:** **ADULTS:** 0.5 to 1 g given three or four times daily (total daily dose 1.5 to 4 g). **CHILDREN OVER 2 MONTHS OF AGE:** 30 to 45 mg/kg daily, administered in 4 equal doses. *Special patient populations:* **RENAL IMPAIRMENT:** Doses may need to be reduced. **PREGNANCY:** Safe use during pregnancy and lactation has not been established. Use in the mother immediately before delivery may cause kernicterus in the newborn.

**PREPARATIONS** *Tablets:* 500 mg. Combination products (Table 20-2) include *tablets:* sulfamethizole (250 mg) with oxytetracycline hydrochloride (250 mg) and phenazopyridine hydrochloride (50 mg). *Tablets:* sulfamethizole (250 mg) with phenazopyridine hydrochloride (50 mg).

**DRUG INTERACTIONS** See entry for drug class (p. 359).

**FATE** Sulfamethizole is easily absorbed following oral administration and produces *peak* serum concentrations within 2 hours. About 10% of a dose of sulfamethizole is metabolized by the liver, with both the metabolites and the unchanged drug being eliminated rapidly by the kidneys. Concentrations of sulfamethizole in the blood are too low to be useful in systemic infections, but the concentrations in urine are adequate for antibacterial effect. Sulfamethizole is more soluble in urine than any other sulfonamide currently available (Table 20-3).

### ❦ NURSING CONSIDERATIONS

#### Side effects, toxicities, and associated nursing actions
- See entry for drug class (p. 361).

#### Nursing interventions related to drug administration
- See entry for drug class (p. 362).

#### Patient and family education
- See entry for drug class (p. 362).

## sulfamethoxazole (sul-fa-meth-OX-uh-zole) sulfonamide

- sulfamethoxazole: Apo-Sulfamethoxazole, Gamazole, Gantanol, Methoxanol

**MECHANISM OF ACTION** See entry for drug class (p. 358).

**INDICATIONS** **Urinary tract infections** Sulfamethoxazole may be effective against infections caused by *Escherichia, Klebsiella, Enterobacter, Proteus,* and *Staphylococcus.* **Nocardiosis** Sulfonamides are drugs of choice for this uncommon infection. **Toxoplasmosis** Sulfamethoxazole is often combined with pyrimethamine for treating this unusual infection. **To eliminate the meningococcal carrier state** *N. meningitidis* can be spread by healthy individuals who carry the organism in the nasopharynx. • Sulfamethoxazole may eradicate the organism and prevent the spread of meningitis within populations at high risk. • Resistant strains exist, and alternative drugs may be required.

**CONTRAINDICATIONS** See entry for drug class (p. 358).

**DOSAGE** **PO:** **ADULTS:** 2 g initially, followed by 1 g twice or three times daily. **CHILDREN OVER 1 MONTH OF AGE:** 50 to 60 mg/kg (maximum 2 g) initially, followed by 25 to 30 mg/kg twice daily, not to exceed 75 mg/kg daily for maintenance. Alternative dosage is 1.2 mg/$M^2$ initially, followed by 0.6 mg/$M^2$ twice daily. *Special patient populations:* **RENAL IMPAIRMENT:** Doses may need to be reduced. **PREGNANCY:** Safe use during pregnancy and lactation has not been established. Use in the mother immediately before delivery may cause kernicterus in the newborn.

**PREPARATIONS**    *Tablets:* 500 mg and 1 g. *Suspension:* 500 mg/5 ml. Combination products (Table 20-2) include *tablets, film-coated:* sulfamethoxazole 500 mg with phenazopyridine hydrochloride 100 mg. Sulfamethoxazole with trimethoprim, see listing for co-trimoxazole.

**DRUG INTERACTIONS**    See entry for drug class (p. 359).

**FATE**    Sulfamethoxazole is absorbed following oral administration and produces *peak* serum concentrations within 3 to 4 hours. Sulfamethoxazole crosses the placenta and is distributed to most body tissues. About 80% of a dose of sulfamethoxazole is metabolized by the liver, with both the metabolites and the unchanged drug being eliminated rapidly by the kidneys. The elimination *half-life* of the drug is 7 to 12 hours. The acetylated derivative of sulfamethoxazole, which is the major metabolite, is not an active antibacterial substance but does contribute to nephrotoxicity.

## ☙ NURSING CONSIDERATIONS

### Side effects, toxicities, and associated nursing actions
- See entry for drug class (p. 361).

### Nursing interventions related to drug administration
- See entry for drug class (p. 362).
- Read orders and labels carefully; Gantanol DS brand is twice the dose of Gantanol.
- Remind patients to shake suspensions well before preparing dose.

### Patient and family education
- See entry for drug class (p. 362).

---

## sulfapyridine    (sul-fa-PEER-i-deen)    sulfonamide

- sulfapyridine: Sold under generic name in U.S.; ✿Dagenan

**MECHANISM OF ACTION**    See entry for drug class (p. 358).

**INDICATIONS**    Dermatitis herpetiformis Sulfapyridine may be substituted for sulfones when these safer drugs are contraindicated. • Sulfapyridine is too toxic for routine use as an antibacterial agent.

**CONTRAINDICATIONS**    See entry for drug class (p. 358).

**DOSAGE**    PO:    ADULTS: 500 mg four times daily. For long-term maintenance, dosage may be reduced to 500 mg daily at 3-day intervals.    *Special patient populations:*    RENAL IMPAIRMENT: Doses may need to be reduced.    PREGNANCY: Safe use during pregnancy and lactation has not been established. Use in the mother immediately before delivery may cause kernicterus in the newborn.

**PREPARATIONS**    *Tablets:* 500 mg.

**DRUG INTERACTIONS**    See entry for drug class (p. 359).

**FATE**    Sulfapyridine is incompletely absorbed following oral administration, producing *peak* levels at 5 to 7 hours. Sulfapyridine is metabolized by the liver, with both the metabolites and unchanged drug being eliminated by the kidneys. Sulfapyridine has low solubility in urine, and, unlike other sulfonamides, alkalinizing the urine does not greatly improve solubility (Table 20-3).

## ☙ NURSING CONSIDERATIONS

### Side effects, toxicities, and associated nursing actions
- See entry for drug class (p. 361).

### Nursing interventions related to drug administration
- See entry for drug class (p. 362).

### Patient and family education
- See entry for drug class (p. 362).

---

## sulfasalazine    (sul-fa-SAL-uh-zeen)    sulfonamide

- sulfasalazine: Azaline, Azulfidine, ✿Salazopyrin, SAS-500

**MECHANISM OF ACTION**  See entry for drug class (p. 358).

**INDICATIONS**  **Ulcerative colitis** Steroids or surgery may be required, but sulfasalazine is possibly effective as adjunct therapy for acute attacks and for the prevention of relapses. • Although less well-documented, sulfasalazine is also used occasionally for Crohn's disease.

**CONTRAINDICATIONS**  See entry for drug class (p. 358).

**DOSAGE**  **PO:**  **ADULTS:** 3 to 4 g daily for initial therapy, followed by 2 g daily in 4 equal doses for maintenance. Maintenance doses may be continued for months or years.  **CHILDREN OVER 2 YEARS OF AGE:** 40 to 60 mg/kg daily in 3 to 6 equal doses for initial therapy, followed by 30 mg/kg daily in 4 equal doses for maintenance. *Special patient populations:*  **ELDERLY AND RENAL IMPAIRMENT:** Doses may need to be reduced.  **PREGNANCY:** Safe use during pregnancy and lactation has not been established. Use in the mother immediately before delivery may cause kernicterus in the newborn.

**PREPARATIONS**  *Tablets:* 500 mg. *Tablets, enteric-coated:* 500 mg. *Suspension:* 250 mg/5ml.

**DRUG INTERACTIONS**  See entry for drug class (p. 359).

**FATE**  Sulfasalazine is slowly absorbed from the GI tract, producing *peak* serum levels within 6 to 12 hours, depending on the dosage form. Sulfasalazine is converted to sulfapyridine by the action of bacteria in the gut, accounting for a large percentage of the total dose of sulfasalazine. Peak levels of sulfapyridine absorbed from the gut occur within 6 to 24 hours of an oral dose of sulfasalazine. Sulfapyridine is metabolized by the liver. Sulfasalazine, sulfapyridine, and metabolites are eliminated by the kidneys.

### ☙ NURSING CONSIDERATIONS

#### Side effects, toxicities, and associated nursing actions
- See entry for drug class (p. 361).

#### Nursing interventions related to drug administration
- See entry for drug class (p. 362).
- When possible, this drug should be administered after meals or with food.
- Remind patients to shake suspensions well before preparing dose.

#### Patient and family education
- See entry for drug class (p. 362).
- Sulfasalazine may impart an orange-yellow color to the urine. Reassure patients that this discoloration is harmless.

---

## sulfisoxazole  (sul-fe-SOX-uh-zole)  sulfonamide

- sulfisoxazole, sulfisoxazole acetyl, sulfisoxazole diolamine: Gantrisin, Gulfasin, ✿Novosoxazole, SK-Soxazole, Sulfasox

**MECHANISM OF ACTION**  See entry for drug class (p. 358).

**INDICATIONS**  **Urinary tract infections** Sulfisoxazole may be effective against infections caused by *Escherichia, Klebsiella, Enterobacter, Proteus,* and *Staphylococcus.*  **Nocardiosis** Sulfonamides are drugs of choice for this uncommon infection.  **Acute pelvic inflammatory disease** Sulfisoxazole along with a third-generation cephalosporin may be indicated for prepubertal children.  **Lymphogranuloma venereum or chancroid** Therapy may be prolonged.

**CONTRAINDICATIONS**  **Dehydration** Adequate fluid intake must be maintained to prevent crystallization of drug in urine. • For other contraindications, see entry for drug class (p. 358).

**DOSAGE**  **PO:**  **ADULTS:** 2 to 4 g daily for initial therapy, followed by 4 to 8 g daily in 4 to 6 equal doses for maintenance.  **CHILDREN OVER 2 MONTHS OF AGE:** 60 to 75 mg/kg every 12 hours, not to exceed 6 g daily.  **IM, IV:**  **ADULTS OR CHILDREN OVER 2 MONTHS OF AGE:** 50 mg/kg or 1.125 mg/M$^2$ initially, followed by 100 mg/kg or 2.25 mg/M$^2$ daily for maintenance. *Special patient populations:*  **PREGNANCY:** Safe use during pregnancy and lactation has not been established. Use in the mother immediately before delivery may cause kernicterus in the newborn.  **RENAL FAILURE:** Doses must be adjusted in cases of renal failure.

**PREPARATIONS:**  Sulfisoxazole, *tablets:* 500 mg. Sulfisoxazole acetyl, *oral solution:* 500 mg/ml; *oral suspension:* 500 mg/ml; *oral suspension, extended-release:* 1 g/ml (Lipo-Gantrisin). Sulfisoxazole diolamine, *solution for injection:* 400 mg/ml. Combination products include *tablets, film-coated:* sulfisoxazole 500 mg with phenazopyridine hydrochloride 50 mg (Table 20-2). *Cream:* sulfisoxazole 10% with allantoin 2% and aminacrine hydrochloride 0.2% (Table 20-1). *Suppositories:* sulfisoxazole 600 mg with allantoin 120 mg and aminacrine hydrochloride 12 mg; sulfisoxazole 700 mg with allantoin 140 mg and aminacrine hydrochloride 14 mg (Table 20-1). *Oral suspension:* sulfisoxazole acetyl 600 mg/5ml with erythromycin ethylsuccinate 200 mg/5 ml (Table 20-2).

**DRUG INTERACTIONS**  See entry for drug class (p. 359).

**FATE**  Sulfisoxazole is easily absorbed following oral administration and produces *peak* serum concentrations within 2 hours. Sulfisoxazole acetyl is deacetylated to form free sulfisoxazole, delaying absorption of the drug. Sulfisoxazole is less well distributed to tissues than are other sulfonamides. Sulfisoxazole is metabolized in the liver, and the metabolites along with unchanged drug are eliminated by the kidneys. The *half-life* of the drug is 5 to 8 hours. Solubility of sulfisoxazole in urine is high, especially at pH 7 to 8 (slightly alkaline).

## ❦ NURSING CONSIDERATIONS

### Side effects, toxicities, and associated nursing actions
- See entry for drug class (p. 361).

### Nursing interventions related to drug administration
- See entry for drug class (p. 362).
- For IM use, dissolve with sterile water for injection, as directed on the ampule, and administer. There may be pain at the injection site.
- For IV use, further dilute the dissolved drug to a 5% solution (e.g., combine a 5 ml ampule with 35 ml sterile water for injection; only this diluent should be used). Administer slowly, about 1 ml per minute, or through slow infusion.
- Remind patients to shake suspension well before preparing dose.

### Patient and family education
- See entry for drug class (p. 362).

---

## co-trimoxazole  (co-tri-MOX-uh-zole)  fixed combination*

- co-trimoxazole: Apo-sulfatrim, Bactrim, Bethaprim, Comoxol, Cotrim, ✿Novotrimel, ✿Protrin, ✿Roubac, Septra, SMZ-TMP, Sulfamethoprim

**MECHANISM OF ACTION:**  Sulfamethoxazole inhibits incorporation of PABA into dihydrofolate; trimethoprim inhibits conversion of dihydrofolate into tetrahydrofolate, the active form of folic acid. The combined action of these two agents is synergistic, and the bacteria depleted of tetrahydrofolate cannot grow or reproduce. Human cells lack the target of sulfonamide action and resist the action of trimethoprim, thereby remaining relatively unharmed while bacterial growth is inhibited.

**INDICATIONS**  **Urinary tract infections** Co-trimoxazole may be effective against infections caused by *Escherichia, Klebsiella, Enterobacter,* and *Proteus.*  **Nocardiosis** Co-trimoxazole is an effective choice for this uncommon infection.  **Otitis media** Co-trimoxazole is an effective choice, especially when ampicillin-resistant strains of *H. influenzae* are common.  **Pneumocystis carinii pneumonia** Co-trimoxazole and pentamidine are currently drugs of choice for this opportunistic infection most often found in immune suppressed patients.  **Enteritis caused by Shigella** Co-trimoxazole and ampicillin are drugs of choice.

**CONTRAINDICATIONS**  **Allergy to sulfonamides or related drugs** Previous allergic reactions to trimethoprim or any sulfonamide or the chemically related sulfonylureas (Chapter 34) or thiazide diuretics (Chapter 9) are a contraindication to the use of co-trimoxazole.  **Deficiency of G-6-PD** Sulfamethoxazole and other drugs can cause acute hemolytic anemia in patients lacking normal concentrations of the enzyme glucose-6-phosphate dehydrogenase in the red blood cells. • People of African or Mediterranean ancestry are more likely to have this genetically determined trait. • Newborn infants are developmen-

*Sulfamethoxazole and trimethoprim.

tally deficient in G-6-PD during the first few days of life.   **Newborn state** Neonates lack adequate mechanisms for eliminating a variety of compounds. • Sulfamethoxazole may complicate this problem by displacing bilirubin from protein binding sites. • The accumulated bilirubin may produce serious toxicity or kernicterus.   **Impaired renal function** Sulfamethoxazole and trimethoprim may accumulate to dangerous concentrations in patients lacking adequate renal function. • These drugs may also directly damage the kidneys.   **Impaired hepatic function** Sulfamethoxazole may accumulate to dangerous concentrations in patients lacking adequate hepatic function.   **Megaloblastic anemia or folate deficiency** Co-trimoxazole may induce mild folate deficiency, which could harm patients with a preexisting depletion of folate.

**DOSAGE**   **PO:**   **ADULTS:** 160 mg of trimethoprim (with 800 mg sulfamethoxazole) every 12 hours. For treatment of *Pneumocystis carinii* pneumonia, 20 mg/kg daily in 4 equal doses.   **CHILDREN OVER 2 MONTHS OF AGE:** 7.5 to 8 mg/kg of trimethoprim (with 37.5 to 40 mg/kg sulfamethoxazole) daily, divided into 2 equal doses.   **IV:**   **ADULTS OR CHILDREN OVER 2 MONTHS OF AGE:** 8 to 10 mg/kg trimethoprim (with 40 to 50 mg/kg sulfamethoxazole) daily, divided into 2 to 4 equal doses. For treatment of *P. carinii* pneumonia, 15 to 20 mg/kg daily, divided into 3 or 4 equal doses.   *Special patient populations:*   **PREGNANCY:** Safe use during pregnancy and lactation has not been established. Use in the mother immediately before delivery may cause kernicterus in the newborn.   **RENAL FAILURE:** Doses must be adjusted in cases of renal failure.

**PREPARATIONS:**   *Tablets:* 80 mg trimethoprim with 400 mg sulfamethoxazole or 160 mg trimethoprim with 800 mg sulfamethoxazole. *Oral suspension:* 40 mg/5 ml of trimethoprim with 200 mg/5 ml of sulfamethoxazole. *Solution for preparation of infusions:* 16 mg/ml trimethoprim with 80 mg/ml sulfamethoxazole.

**DRUG INTERACTIONS**   See entry for drug class (p. 359).

**FATE**   Both components of co-trimoxazole are well absorbed following oral administration. *Peak* concentrations of both trimethoprim and sulfamethoxazole are achieved within 1 to 4 hours of an oral dose. Co-trimoxazole should not be administered intramuscularly. Trimethoprim is well-distributed to most tissues; sulfamethoxazole enters tissues less readily. The drugs are both metabolized in the liver and eliminated by the kidney. The *half-life* for trimethoprim is 8 to 11 hours and for sulfamethoxazole is 10 to 13 hours.

## ☙ NURSING CONSIDERATIONS

### Side effects, toxicities, and associated nursing actions

**CNS** Apathy, ataxia, fatigue, hallucinations, headache, insomnia, mental depression, muscle weakness, peripheral neuritis, tinnitus, and vertigo are rare adverse reactions.
• See entry for drug class (p. 361).
• Instruct patient and family to notify physician if any change in mood, affect, hearing, or activity level occurs.

**Renal** Anuria or oliguria with toxic nephrosis and diuresis are rare side effects.
• Monitor serum creatinine and BUN.
• Monitor intake and output and weight.
• Instruct the patient to increase fluid intake to 2500 to 3000 ml per day.

**Liver** Hepatitis is rare but possible.
• See entry for drug class (p. 361).

**Blood** These serious side effects occur in about 0.5% of patients. Reactions include agranulocytosis, aplastic anemia, hemolytic anemia, hypoprothrombinemia, megaloblastic anemia, methemoglobinemia, or neutropenia.
• See entry for drug class (p. 361).

**GI** Nausea, vomiting, and other GI effects are among the most common reactions to co-trimoxazole, occurring in 3.5% of treated patients.
• Instruct patients to take oral preparations with meals or snacks to lessen gastric irritation.
• If vomiting or diarrhea is severe or persistent, notify the physician.

**Allergy** Rashes are common side effects. More serious allergic reactions include the potentially fatal Stevens-Johnson syndrome and erythema multiforme.
• See entry for drug class (p. 362).

## Nursing interventions related to drug administration

- Tablets may be crushed before administration. Tablets should be taken with a full glass of fluid.
- Read orders carefully; most brands are available in a lower dose and a double-strength dose.
- For IV administration, dilute each 5 ml ampule in 125 ml of 5% dextrose in water and use within 6 hours. If fluid restriction is required, the amount of diluent per ampule may be reduced to 75 ml; use within 2 hours. Administer a single dose over 60 to 90 minutes.
- Do not mix IV preparations with other drugs or solutions.
- Remind patients to shake suspensions well before administering dose.

## Patient and family education

- Review with patients the anticipated benefits and possible side effects of therapy. Caution patients to report the development of any unexpected sign or symptom.
- See entry for drug class (p. 362).

# Chapter Twenty-one

# Drugs to treat tuberculosis and leprosy

| | |
|---|---|
| aminosalicylic acid | ethionamide |
| aminsalicylate sodium | isoniazid |
| capreomycin sulfate | kanamycin sulfate |
| clofazimine (investigational) | pyrazinamide |
| cycloserine | rifampin |
| dapsone | streptomycin sulfate |
| ethambutol hydrochloride | sulfoxone sodium |

**OVERVIEW OF THE DRUG CLASS**    The drugs covered in this section share only one feature—the ability to effectively control infections caused by mycobacteria. Four species of mycobacteria cause tuberculosis, which is easily spread by patients with the active pulmonary form of the disease. Once known as the white plague, tuberculosis is now curable with proper drug therapy. Prophylactic drug treatment can also prevent active disease in exposed persons.

Infection with *Mycobacterium leprae* causes leprosy, also known as Hansen's disease. This disease was once thought to be highly contagious but is not now considered to be easily spread. If untreated, infection causes a slowly progressive disease in which disfigurement may accompany the long approach to death. Leprosy is now controlled with drug therapy. Sulfones have proven to be most effective, although other agents are also employed successfully today.

**MECHANISM OF ACTION**    The drugs listed above have varied mechanisms by which they inhibit or kill mycobacteria. Resistance can easily develop against many of these drugs. For successful chemotherapy of tuberculosis, combinations of drugs are often required. Combining drugs with different mechanisms of action lowers the likelihood that the mycobacteria will mutate simultaneously to resistance against both drugs. The most common combinations include isoniazid with rifampin. When resistance to one of these agents is suspected, ethambutol is often added to the regimen. See individual agents for details of the mechanisms.

**INDICATIONS**    All of the drugs listed above are used to treat infections caused by mycobacteria. Specific indications are summarized in Table 21-1.

**CONTRAINDICATIONS**    See individual agents.

**Table 21-1.**

| Summary of clinical uses of agents effective against mycobacteria | | | |
|---|---|---|---|
| **Drug** | **Treatment of leprosy** | **Treatment of tuberculosis** | **Prophylaxis of tuberculosis** |
| Aminosalicylic acid | | 2 | |
| Capreomycin sulfate | | 2 | |
| Clofazimine | 2* | | |
| Cycloserine | | 2 | |
| Dapsone | 1† | | |
| Ethambutol HCl | | 1 | |
| Ethionamide | 2 | 2 | |
| Isoniazid | | 1 | 1 |
| Kanamycin sulfate | | 2 | |
| Pyrazinamide | | 2 | |
| Rifampin | 2 | 1 | |
| Streptomycin sulfate | | 2 | |
| Sulfoxone sodium | 2 | | |

*2 Designates second-line or reserve drugs.
†1 Designates drugs of choice or first-line drugs.

**DRUG INTERACTIONS**    See individual agents.

---

### 🐞 NURSING CONSIDERATIONS
#### Patient and family education
- Review with patients and families the anticipated benefits and possible side effects of drug therapy.
- Reinforce the importance of continuing prescribed drugs on a long-term basis, as directed by the physician.
- Encourage patients to return as directed for follow-up visits with the physician, both to monitor drug effectiveness and to monitor for drug side effects.
- Refer patients as needed to the local visiting nurse association, local health department, American Lung Association for tuberculosis, and the Centers for Disease Control in Atlanta, Georgia.
- Remind patients to keep all health care providers informed of chronic diagnoses, as well as current medications being used.
- Remind patients to keep these and all medications out of the reach of children.

---

## aminosalicylic acid    (uh-meen-oh-SAL-i-sill-ik)    antituberculosis agent

- aminosalicylic acid, aminosalicylic acid sodium: ✦Nemasol, P.A.S. sodium, Teebacin

**MECHANISM OF ACTION**    As an analog of para-aminobenzoic acid (PABA), aminosalicylic acid is thought to inhibit bacterial synthesis of dihydrofolate. This mechanism is similar to that of sulfonamides. This inhibition, which ultimately prevents the synthesis of adequate amounts of thymidine and DNA, is usually bacteriostatic in its effect on mycobacteria.

**INDICATIONS**    **Combination chemotherapy of active tuberculosis** Aminosalicylic acid is only indicated when a more effective drug such as ethambutol cannot be used in a combination regimen for active tuberculosis. The most common case in which the drug is currently used is in children under 2 years of age who cannot be tested for ocular side effects caused by ethambutol. For children of this age, aminosalicylic acid may be a safer alternative.

**CONTRAINDICATIONS**    **Gastric ulcer** The irritating effects of aminosalicylic acid can contribute to ulcer formation and worsen existing gastric ulcers.    **Congestive heart failure or hypertension** Patients with these conditions often cannot tolerate the high sodium content of aminosalicylate sodium.    **Renal impairment** Aminosalicylic acid accumulates in patients with inadequate renal function.    **Hepatic impairment** The drug is metabolized in the liver.

**DOSAGE**    **PO:** **ADULTS:** This drug should not be used alone in the treatment of tuberculosis. For aminosalicylic acid, 10 to 12 g daily in 2 or 3 equal doses. For aminosalicylate sodium, 12 to 15 g daily in 2 to 4 equal doses.    **CHILDREN:** This drug should not be used alone in the treatment of tuberculosis. For aminosalicylic acid, 200 to 300 mg/kg daily in 3 or 4 equal doses. For aminosalicylate sodium, 240 to 360 mg/kg daily in 3 or 4 equal doses.    *Special patient populations:*    **ELDERLY:** Special geriatric doses have not been established. Toxic reactions are more likely to occur in geriatric patients. **PREGNANCY:** Safe use has not been established.

**PREPARATIONS**    Aminosalicylic acid, *powder:* for preparation of oral solutions. Aminosalicylate sodium, *tablets:* 500 mg; *powder:* for preparation of oral solutions. These preparations are not chemically stable. Deteriorated drug will show brown or purple discoloration. Discolored powder or tablets should be discarded. Solutions should not be stored longer than 24 hours and should be discarded if they darken at all.

**DRUG INTERACTIONS**    **Probenecid** blocks the renal excretion of aminosalicylic acid or the sodium salt. The increased serum concentrations may cause toxicity.    **Ammonium chloride** may cause crystal formation in the urine when given with aminosalicylic acid.    **Diphenhydramine** interferes with absorption of aminosalicylic acid from the GI tract.    **Oral anticoagulants** may be potentiated by the hypoprothrombinemic effect of aminosalicylic acid.    **Rifampin** absorption from the GI tract can be impaired by bentonite, an excipient (vehicle) used in certain preparations of aminosalicylic acid available abroad but not in the United States.

**DIAGNOSTIC TEST INTERFERENCE**   **Tests for urinary glucose** using cupric sulfate may be falsely positive in the presence of aminosalicylic acid.   **Tests for urobilinogen** using Erhlich's reagent may be falsely elevated by aminosalicylic acid.

**FATE**   Aminosalicylic acid and the sodium salt are both absorbed readily from the GI tract, but absorption of the sodium salt is faster and more complete. *Peak* plasma concentrations of aminosalicylic acid are achieved in 3 to 4 hours, but *peaks* following administration of aminosalicylate sodium occur within about an hour. The drug is metabolized both in the liver and in intestinal mucosa. The capacity for metabolism is sufficient to alter about half of the drug normally administered. Both metabolites and unaltered drug are excreted by the kidneys.

## ❧ NURSING CONSIDERATIONS

### Side effects, toxicities, and associated nursing actions

**CNS** Encephalopathy and psychotic symptoms have been reported rarely.

- Review with patients and families these unusual symptoms. Instruct families to bring to the emergency care setting any patient receiving this drug who exhibits unusual changes in affect.

**Blood** Hemolytic anemia and hematuria are possible in patients with deficiency of G-6-PD.

- Question patients about this deficiency before instituting drug therapy.
- Monitor hematocrit and hemoglobin. Inspect urine for evidence of hematuria and test for the presence of blood if indicated.
- Instruct patients to report any change (dark or reddish) in the color of urine.

**GI** up to 15% of patients suffer severe gastrointestinal side effects that require cessation of therapy. Abdominal pain, anorexia, diarrhea, gastric hemorrhage, nausea, peptic ulcer, and vomiting are all possible reactions. Some of these effects may be minimized by taking the drug with meals or with aluminum hydroxide gel. These reactions are so common among adult patients that any patients reporting no problems with the drug should be carefully watched for evidence of noncompliance (not taking prescribed doses of the medication).

- Support patients who find this drug difficult to take: a 12 g dose requires taking 24 tablets.
- Encourage patients to take each dose with a full glass (240 ml) of fluid; taking doses with milk or meals may lessen gastric irritation.
- Instruct patients to report any worsening of the usual GI symptoms.
- Instruct patients to inspect stools for signs of bleeding: dark, tarry stools. Test stools for occult blood if indicated.
- Teach patients to avoid taking aspirin or other drugs that may also cause gastric irritation while they are taking aminosalicylic acid.

**Renal** Albuminuria and crystalluria occur occasionally.

- Monitor urinalysis.
- Encourage patients to maintain a good urinary output by maintaining an intake of 2500 to 3000 ml per day.

**Metabolic** Hypokalemia and acidosis can occur.

- Monitor serum electrolytes and blood gases if appropriate.
- Instruct the patient to report the development of signs of hypokalemia: abnormal fatigue, lethargy, vertigo, hypotension, nausea, vomiting, muscle weakness, and leg cramps.
- Instruct patients to report signs of metabolic acidosis: headache and metal dullness, and disorientation.

**Allergic** Agranulocytosis, eosinophilia, fever, hepatitis, jaundice, joint pain, leukopenia, pruritis, skin eruptions, thrombocytopenia, and vasculitis have all been reported. These reactions require cessation of therapy in about 4 % of patients, and deaths have occurred.

- Inspect patient for signs of allergic response.
- Instruct patients to report signs of agranulocytosis (fever, sore throat, fatigue, pallor), hepatitis (jaundice, right upper quadrant abdominal pain, anorexia, malaise, change in the color or consistency of stools), thrombocytopenia (unexplained bleeding or bruising, nosebleed, bleeding gums), or any other unexpected sign or symptom.
- Monitor complete blood cell count, white blood cell differential, and platelet count.

### Patient and family education
- Review with patients and families the anticipated benefits and possible side effects of drug therapy.
- Instruct patients to discard discolored powder or tablets; this drug deteriorates rapidly. Teach patients to store medications in a dry, cool place, but not in the bathroom, as the heat and moisture may cause drugs to break down more rapidly.
- Teach patients that this drug may cause urine to turn red when the urine comes in contact with chlorine bleaches (such as might be used to clean a toilet bowl). See side effects above: the drug may also cause blood to appear in the urine. Tell the patient to contact the physician if there are questions about discoloration of urine.
- Tell patients using the powder forms of the drug to dissolve the prescribed dose in water just before taking. The patient should drink all of the fluid to ensure that the whole dose has been taken.

## capreomycin sulfate    (cap-ree-oh-MY-sin)    antituberculosis agent

- capreomycin sulfate: Capastat

**MECHANISM OF ACTION**    Although capreomycin is bacteriostatic, the precise action on mycobacteria is unknown.

**INDICATIONS**    **Combination chemotherapy of active tuberculosis** Capreomycin sulfate is only indicated when parenteral therapy is necessary, as in retreatment regimens.

**CONTRAINDICATIONS**    **Hearing impairment** Because capreomycin causes toxicity to the eighth cranial nerve, the risk of total hearing loss is great in patients taking this drug.    **Renal impairment** Because capreomycin causes nephrotoxicity, the risk of severe renal damage is increased in patients with preexisting renal damage or disease.

**DOSAGE**    IM:    **ADULTS:** This drug should not be used alone to treat tuberculosis. Dosage is 15 mg/kg or 1 g daily for 60 to 120 days, followed by 1 g 2 or 3 times weekly. Daily doses should not exceed 20 mg/kg. *Special patient populations:*    **ELDERLY:** Special geriatric doses have not been established. Side effects are more likely in geriatric patients.    **RENAL IMPAIRMENT:** Doses may need to be reduced.    **CHILDREN:** Safe use in children has not been established.    **PREGNANCY:** Safe use has not been established. Animal tests show evidence of fetal abnormality when high doses are used.

**PREPARATIONS**    *Powder:* 1 g for preparations of solution for deep IM injection. The drug is reconstituted in 0.9% sterile saline solution to produce the desired concentration of drug. Two or three minutes may be required to allow complete dissolution of the drug.

**DRUG INTERACTIONS**    **Ototoxic and nephrotoxic drugs** such as aminoglycoside antibiotics, polymyxin B, colistin, or vancomycin may have additive effects with capreomycin sulfate. The result can be severe hearing loss or dangerous renal damage.    **Neuromuscular blocking agents** may be potentiated by high doses of capreomycin, resulting in temporary partial or complete paralysis.

**FATE**    Capreomycin is not absorbed from the GI tract but is absorbed after injection deep into large muscle masses, producing *peak* plasma concentrations within 1 to 2 hours. The plasma *half-life* of the drug is 4 to 6 hours. Most of the drug is excreted by the kidneys.

## ❦ NURSING CONSIDERATIONS
### Side effects, toxicities, and associated nursing actions
**Ototoxicity** Capreomycin may damage both auditory and vestibular functions of the eighth cranial nerve. Headache, vertigo, and tinnitus, as well as hearing loss, can occur.
- Assess eighth cranial nerve function before the start of therapy and at regular intervals. Refer selected patients for periodic audiometric testing.
- Instruct patients to report the development of hearing loss, headache, tinnitus, and vertigo.
- Instruct patients to avoid driving or operating hazardous equipment if vertigo develops.

**Blood** Eosinophilia is common. Leukocytosis and leukopenia have also occured.
- Monitor white blood cell differential.

**Renal** Renal tubular function may be altered, causing a variety of electrolyte disturbances, decreased creatinine clearance, and increased BUN. Urine may contain casts, erythrocytes, and leukocytes. Rare fatal reactions have occurred.

- Monitor urinalysis, serum BUN, creatinine, and electrolytes.
- Instruct patients to report symptoms of hypokalemia: muscle weakness, apathy, abdominal distention, anorexia, and vomiting.

**Allergic** Eosinophilia is common. Skin rashes of various types arise, with or without fever. Rare fatal reactions have occurred.

- Inspect patients at regular intervals. Instruct patients to report the development of any skin changes.
- Monitor white blood cell differential.

**Other** Excessive bleeding at the injection site and pain, induration, and sterile abscesses have occurred.

- Use anatomic landmarks to choose injection sites. Use large muscle masses, such as the dorsogluteal site or rectus femoris in adults and vastus lateralis in children. Avoid the deltoid muscle, as induration or abscesses there may be cosmetically unattractive.
- Aspirate before injecting medication to prevent inadvertent IV injection. Record and rotate sites.
- Avoid administering a volume larger than 5 ml in any injection site in an adult, and less in a child. Apply firm pressure to the injection site after withdrawing the needle.

**Nursing interventions related to drug administration**
- Reconstitute as directed on the vial. Use careful administration technique as described above (see other side effects above).

**Patient and family education**
- Review with patients and families the anticipated benefits and possible side effects of drug therapy.
- See entry for drug class (p. 371).

---

## clofazimine* (klo-FAZ-i-meen) antileprosy agent

- clofazimine: Lamprene

**MECHANISM OF ACTION**    Clofazimine has a bactericidal effect against *Mycobacterium leprae,* but the exact mechanism of action is unknown. In addition to this bactericidal action, clofazimine possesses antiinflammatory properties that are beneficial in treating reactions such as erythema nodosum leprosum in patients with leprosy.

**INDICATIONS    Leprosy caused by dapsone-resistant mycobacteria** Clofazimine is as effective as the first-line drug for leprosy, dapsone. • When mycobacteria are resistant to dapsone, clofazimine may be substituted.    **Erythema nodosum leprosum** This reaction arising in leprosy patients may respond to the antiinflammatory action of clofazimine.

**CONTRAINDICATIONS**    None have been established.

**DOSAGE    PO:    ADULTS:** 100 mg daily to treat leprosy or 100 mg three times daily for erythema nodosum leprosum.    *Special patient populations:*    **CHILDREN:** Safe use has not been established.    **PREGNANCY:** Safe use has not been established.

**PREPARATIONS**    *Tablets:* 100 mg.

**DRUG INTERACTIONS**    None yet reported.

**FATE**    Clofazimine is a lipid-soluble red dye that may be administered in capsules as a microsuspension in an oil-detergent base. Oral absorption is incomplete, with only about half of the administered drug being absorbed. Clofazimine distributes to tissues, especially fatty tissues, and remains for very long periods. The elimination *half-life* in patients is about 70 days.

**☙ NURSING CONSIDERATIONS**

**Side effects, toxicities, and associated nursing actions**

**GI** Nausea, vomiting, and diarrhea may occur but are not common unless doses in excess of 100 mg daily are used.

- Warn patients about possible GI side effects. If these side effects are severe or persistent, notify physician.

*Investigational.

• If vomiting and diarrhea occur, monitor intake and output and weight.

**Renal** Clofazimine discolors the urine. The red color should not be confused with hematuria.

• Warn patients about this discoloration of the urine. If there is doubt about the source of discoloration, test the urine for the presence of blood.

**Other** The most striking reaction to clofazimine is the red to brown pigmentation imparted to the skin and eyes of all patients receiving the drug. The degree of pigmentation varies from patient to patient. The lesions produced by leprosy are also darkened, becoming mauve, slate-gray, or black. This pigmentation disappears after the drug is discontinued.

• Forewarn patients about this unusual reaction. Provide emotional support to those patients who find this change in pigmentation to be troublesome.

### Patient and family education

• Review with patients and families the anticipated benefits and possible side effects of drug therapy.
• See entry for drug class (p. 371).

---

## cycloserine  (sye-klo-SEER-een)    antituberculosis agent

• cycloserine: Seromycin

**MECHANISM OF ACTION**  Cycloserine inhibits an early step in formation of precursors for cell wall synthesis in bacteria. The action may be either bacteriostatic or bactericidal.

**INDICATIONS**  **Combination chemotherapy of active tuberculosis** Cycloserine may be especially useful in tuberculosis affecting the urinary tract or in retreatment protocols.

**CONTRAINDICATIONS**  **Epilepsy** Cycloserine should not be used in epileptics because the drug can induce seizures.  **Anxiety, depression, or psychosis** Cycloserine should not be used in patients with a history of severe mental illness because the drug can induce or worsen these conditions.  **Renal impairment** Severe renal impairment may cause the drug to accumulate to toxic concentrations.  **Alcohol abuse** Alcohol increases the risk of seizures with cycloserine. • The two drugs should not be combined. • Cycloserine should not be given to patients unable to avoid alcohol use.

**DOSAGE**  **PO:**  **ADULTS:** This drug should not be used alone to treat tuberculosis. Dosage is 250 mg every 12 hours for the first 2 weeks, after which the dosage is adjusted to produce serum concentrations below 30 μg/ml. Daily doses should not exceed 1 g.  *Special patient populations:*  **CHILDREN:** Safe use has not been established.  **PREGNANCY:** Safe use has not been established.  **RENAL IMPAIRMENT:** Doses may need to be reduced.

**PREPARATIONS**  *Capsules:* 250 mg.

**DRUG INTERACTIONS**  **Isoniazid and ethionamide** produce some CNS toxicity that may be additive with the CNS side effects caused by cycloserine.  **Phenytoin** metabolism is inhibited by cycloserine. The result may be accumulation of phenytoin to toxic concentrations.

**FATE**  Cycloserine is well absorbed following oral administration, producing *peak* serum concentrations within 3 to 4 hours. Cycloserine is readily distributed to most tissues and the CNS. The primary route of elimination is excretion by the kidneys. The elimination *half-life* is about 10 hours.

### ❦ NURSING CONSIDERATIONS

#### Side effects, toxicities, and associated nursing actions

**CNS** CNS reactions are the most common side effects of cycloserine. Signs include anxiety, confusion, clonic seizures, convulsions, coma, depression, disorientation, dizziness, drowsiness, dysarthria, headache, hyperreflexia, lethargy, loss of memory, nervousness, paresthesia, paresis, tremor, and vertigo. CNS effects are dose dependent and occur in up to 30% of patients who receive more than 500 mg daily.

• Obtain a complete baseline assessment, including mental status examination, before the start of therapy.
• Review with patients and families the kinds of signs and symptoms that may indicate CNS side effects. Instruct patients and families to notify the physician of any unusual sign or symptom.

- Instruct patients to avoid driving or operating hazardous equipment if dizziness, vertigo, drowsiness, or other serious CNS effects occur.

**CV** Rapidly developing congestive heart failure and cardiac dysrhythmias are reported rarely.

- Monitor daily weight, blood pressure, and pulse; auscultate lung sounds; inspect patient for jugular vein distention and edema of dependent areas.
- Instruct patient to report the development of edema, fluid retention, and shortness of breath.

**Allergic** Rash and photosensitivity are possible.

- Inspect patients for skin changes at regular intervals.
- If photosensitivity occurs, instruct patients to avoid exposure to the sun and other sources of ultraviolet light, to wear a hat and long-sleeve clothing, and to use maximum-protection sunscreens on exposed skin surfaces.
- Instruct patients to report skin changes to the physician.

**Patient and family education**

- Review with patients and families the anticipated benefits and possible side effects of drug therapy.
- Instruct patients to avoid the use of alcohol.
- See entry for drug class (p. 371).

---

## dapsone   (DAP-sone)                                          sulfone*

- dapsone: Avlosulfon

**MECHANISM OF ACTION**   Dapsone seems to inhibit dihydrofolate synthesis in much the same way as sulfonamides. Dapsone is usually bacteriostatic against mycobacteria.

**INDICATIONS**   **Leprosy** All forms of leprosy are effectively controlled by dapsone, either alone or in combination with other agents.   **Dermatitis herpetiformis** Dapsone is the drug of choice to suppress symptoms of this condition.

**CONTRAINDICATIONS**   **Severe anemia** Dapsone may cause dangerous blood dyscrasias, especially in patients with prior abnormalities.   **Allergy to sulfoxone** Dapsone is formed by breakdown of sulfoxone in the body; patients allergic to sulfoxone are likely also to react to dapsone.

**DOSAGE**   **PO:**   **ADULTS:** For leprosy, 50 to 100 mg daily. Patients often receive rifampin or clofazimine with dapsone for the first 3 to 5 years of treatment and receive dapsone alone thereafter for life. For dermatitis herpetiformis, 50 mg daily for initial therapy with doses adjusted as necessary for control. Daily doses may range up to 400 mg.   **CHILDREN:** For leprosy, 1 to 1.5 mg/kg daily for therapy. For prophylaxis in contacts of patients with leprosy, children age 6 to 12 years receive 25 mg daily; ages 2 through 5 years, 25 mg three times weekly; ages 6 to 24 months, 12 mg three times weekly; younger than 6 months, 6 mg three times weekly.   *Special patient populations:*   **PREGNANCY:** FDA pregnancy category A. Women have been treated for leprosy throughout their pregnancy without obvious harm to mother or infant.

**PREPARATIONS**   *Tablets:* 25 or 100 mg.

**DRUG INTERACTIONS**   **Aniline, naphthalene, niridazole, nitrite, nitrofurantoin, phenylhydrazine, and primaquine** are all agents known to cause hemolysis in persons with G-6-PD deficiency. Risk of hemolysis may be increased with dapsone.

**FATE**   Dapsone is completely absorbed following oral administration, producing *peak* serum concentrations within 2 to 8 hours. The drug is widely distributed in body fluids and tissues; it is retained in tissues for up to 3 weeks after therapy stops. The eye seems an exception, for dapsone does not adequately control lesions in ocular tissue, and concentrations of drug are low in the eye. Dapsone is eliminated in bile and undergoes enterohepatic circulation. The drug is also metabolized extensively in the liver. ranges from 10 to 50 hours in normal adults.

*Antileprosy agent.

## ✿ NURSING CONSIDERATIONS

### Side effects, toxicities, and associated nursing actions

**CNS** Blurred vision, headache, insomnia, nervousness, psychosis, tinnitus, and vertigo can occur.
- Instruct patients about possible CNS side effects.
- Instruct patients to avoid driving or operating hazardous equipment if blurred vision or vertigo occurs.
- If insomnia occurs, instruct patient to take the last dose of the day several hours before bedtime. If the patient is receiving once-a-day therapy, ascertain that the patient is taking the dose in the morning (assuming the patient sleeps at night).

**Peripheral nervous system** At high doses, peripheral neuropathy leading to muscle weakness and muscle loss can occur. If signs appear, the drug should be discontinued. This side effect is rare with doses used to treat leprosy.
- Monitor muscle strength at regular intervals.
- Instruct patients to report the development of muscle weakness or tingling of the extremeties.

**CV** Tachycardia can occur with very high, toxic doses.
- Monitor the pulse.

**Blood** Hemolytic anemia and methemoglobinemia are common side effects of dapsone and may be seen when sulfoxone is used; these reactions are more common and severe at higher doses. Patients with deficiency of G-6-PD suffer more severe reactions.
- Question patients about G-6-PD deficiency before administering first doses.
- Monitor complete blood cell count.
- Instruct patients to report the development of fatigue, weakness, pallor, and jaundice.

**GI** Abdominal pain, anorexia, nausea, and vomiting can occur.
- Warn patient about these GI side effects. If side effects are severe or persistent, notify physician.
- If vomiting occurs, monitor intake and output.
- Monitor weight.
- Suggest that the patient take ordered doses with meals or a snack to lessen gastric irritation.

**Renal** Albuminuria, nephrotic syndrome, and renal papillary necrosis are rare.
- Monitor weight and blood pressure.
- Monitor urinalysis, serum BUN, and creatinine.

**Other** Effective treatment of leprosy often precipitates reactions that may include sensitization of the lesions, skin reactions, fever, or more severe signs. Patients may require hospitalization and support with steroids or other drugs, but sulfoxone should be continued.
- Instruct the patient to report any skin changes, fever, or any unexpected sign or symptom.

### Patient and family education

- Review with patients and families the anticipated benefits and possible side effects of drug therapy.
- See entry for drug class (p. 371).
- Patients with dermatitis herpetiformis may also be placed on a gluten-free diet. Emphasize to the patients the need to follow this regimen. Foods to avoid on a gluten-free diet are cereal grains including wheat, barley, oats, rye, bran, graham, millet, wheat germ, bulgar and malt; and foods that contain these grains, such as root beer, pastas, and macaroni products. Instruct patients to read labels carefully. Corn and rice products are permitted on this diet.

---

## ethambutol   (eh-THAM-byoo-tol)                              antituberculosis agent

- ethambutol hydrochloride: ✦Etibi, Myambutol

**MECHANISM OF ACTION**   Ethambutol hydrochloride is bacteriostatic, probably because the drug inhibits synthesis of mycolic acids, which are essential metabolites in mycobacteria.

**INDICATIONS**    **Combination chemotherapy of active tuberculosis** Ethambutol is combined with isoniazid and rifampin in patients with a high likelihood of harboring drug-resistant mycobacteria. • Ethambutol may be combined with other drugs in retreatment programs.

**CONTRAINDICATIONS**    **Optic neuritis** Ocular damage is an expected side effect with ethambutol. • Patients with preexisting damage risk unacceptable visual impairment.    **Cataracts, diabetic retinopathy, or chronic inflammatory disease of the eye** These conditions may impede detection of progressive ocular damage caused by ethambutol.

**DOSAGE**    **PO:**    **ADULTS:** This drug should not be used alone in the treatment of tuberculosis. For standard combinations, 15 mg/kg daily in a single dose. Higher doses may be required in retreatment schedules.    *Special patient populations:*    **CHILDREN:** Safe use has not been established.    **PREGNANCY:** Safe use has not been established.    **RENAL IMPAIRMENT:** Doses must be reduced.

**PREPARATIONS**    *Tablets*: 100 mg. *Tablets, film-coated*: 400 mg.

**DRUG INTERACTIONS**    None have been reported.

**FATE**    Ethambutol is rapidly absorbed following oral administration, producing *peak* plasma concentrations within 2 to 4 hours. The drug penetrates many tissues and fluids but is concentrated in red blood cells. Some metabolism of ethambutol occurs in the liver, but the bulk of a dose is eliminated by the kidneys. The plasma *half-life* of the drug is about 3.3 hours but may be greatly increased in renal failure.

## 🐦 NURSING CONSIDERATIONS

### Side effects, toxicities, and associated nursing actions

**CNS** Confusion, disorientation, dizziness, fever, hallucinations, headache, and malaise are uncommon.
- Instruct patients about these side effects. Instruct patients to avoid driving or operating hazardous equipment if disorientation, dizziness, or hallucinations occur; notify physician.

**GI** Abdominal pain, anorexia, nausea, and vomiting are possible.
- If GI symptoms are severe or persistent, notify physician.
- Suggest that patients take doses with meals or snacks to lessen gastric irritation.
- Monitor weight.

**Renal** Uric acid clearance by the kidney may be blocked, occasionally causing acute gout.
- Monitor serum uric acid levels.
- Be especially alert to gout in persons with preexisting renal disease.

**Allergic** Anaphylaxis is rare. Dermatitis can also occur.
- Have drugs, equipment, and personnel available to treat acute allergic reactions in settings where ethambutol is administered.
- Instruct patients to report the development of skin changes.

**Eye** Ethambutol causes optic neuritis. The degree of damage is greater with higher doses and longer treatment. Any changes in vision or visual acuity should be reported and may necessitate halting therapy.
- Obtain complete ophthalmic examination before the start of therapy and monitor visual acuity at regular intervals. Instruct patients to report the development of any changes in vision.

**Other** Peripheral neuritis can occur, usually marked by numbness and tingling of the extremities.
- Instruct patients to report the development of unusual sensations, numbness, and tingling of the extremities.

### Nursing interventions related to drug administration
- Serum drug levels are best achieved when the drug is taken as a single dose each day; instruct patients about the importance of taking the ordered dose once daily rather than in divided doses. Encourage the patient to try to take the medication at the same time each day for best effect.

### Patient and family education
- Review with patients and families the anticipated benefits and possible side effects of drug therapy.
- See entry for drug class (p. 371).

## ethionamide  (eh-thee-ON-uh-mide)

- ethionamide: Trecator

**MECHANISM OF ACTION**   Ethionamide can inhibit protein synthesis in susceptible mycobacteria. This action may be the basis of the bacteriostatic or bactericidal effect of ethionamide.

**INDICATIONS**   **Combination chemotherapy of active tuberculosis** Ethionamide is combined with one or more other antituberculosis drugs. Ethionamide is not usually considered a first-line drug.   **Leprosy resistant to dapsone** Ethionamide may be combined with clofazimine or rifampin.

**CONTRAINDICATIONS**   **Hepatic impairment** Ethionamide is metabolized by the liver, primarily to inactive metabolites.

**DOSAGE**   **PO:**   **ADULTS:** This drug should not be used alone in the treatment of tuberculosis. Dosage is 500 mg to 1 g daily in 1 to 3 equal doses.   *Special patient populations:*   **CHILDREN:** Safe use has not been established.   **PREGNANCY:** Safe use has not been established.

**PREPARATIONS**   *Tablets:* 250 mg.

**DRUG INTERACTIONS**   **Cycloserine, isoniazid, and ethionamide** all have CNS effects that may be additive when the drugs are combined.

**FATE**   Ethionamide is well absorbed from the GI tract following oral administration, producing *peak* serum concentrations within 3 hours. The drug is well distributed to most tissues and fluids of the body, including the CSF. Ethionamide is extensively metabolized by the liver, with only 1% to 5% of a dose appearing in urine as active drug. The plasma *half-life* of ethionamide is approximately 3 hours.

## 🐾 NURSING CONSIDERATIONS

### Side effects, toxicities, and associated nursing actions

**CNS** Asthenia, depression, dizziness, drowsiness, headache, postural hypotension, and restlessness occur occasionally. Less common effects include blurred vision, diplopia, hallucinations, olfactory disturbances, optic neuritis, pellagra-like syndrome, peripheral neuritis, paresthesia, seizures, and tremors. Pyridoxine hydrochloride may be administered to prevent or treat the neurotoxic side effects of ethionamide.

- Review these side effects with patients and families. Instruct patients to report the development of any unusual sign or symptom.
- Obtain thorough ophthalmic assessment before the start of therapy and monitor vision and eye changes at regular intervals.
- Instruct patients to report the development of tingling, numbness, or unusual sensations of fingers and toes, which may signal a need for pyridoxine.
- Instruct patients to report signs of pellagra: fatigue, anorexia, muscle weakness, headache, indigestion, milky skin eruptions, weight loss, and back pain.
- If postural hypotension occurs, instruct patients to move slowly from lying to sitting or standing. Supervise ambulation. Keep siderails up.

**Blood** Thrombocytopenia can occur.

- Monitor complete blood cell count and platelet count.
- Instruct patients to report the development of bruising, bleeding, petechiae, nosebleeds, and bleeding gums.

**GI** GI problems are the most common side effects with ethionamide. Effects include abdominal pain, anorexia, diarrhea, excessive salivation, metallic taste, nausea, and weight loss. These effects are more common at higher doses. Patients may be able to tolerate lower doses of the drug. The dose may be administered at different times of day to find the treatment schedule best tolerated by an individual patient.

- If GI side effects are severe or persistent, notify physician. Try dividing doses and administering at different times during the day or with meals or snacks to lessen gastric irritation.
- Monitor weight.

**Allergic** Rare reactions include photosensitivity, purpura, rash, stomatitis, and thrombocytopenia.

- If photosensitivity occurs, instruct patients to avoid exposure to the sun or other sources of ultraviolet light, to wear a hat and long-sleeve clothing, and to use maximum-protection sunscreens on exposed skin surfaces.

- Instruct patients to report the development of any skin changes to the physician.

**Liver** Signs of liver dysfunction (increased serum bilirubin, AST, and ALT), jaundice, and hepatitis may occur rarely.

- Instruct patients to report the development of jaundice, right upper quadrant abdominal pain, malaise, fever, and change in the color or consistency of stools.
- Monitor liver function tests.

**Other** Rare reactions include goiter, hypothyroidism, hypoglycemia, gynecomastia, impotence, and menorrhagia. Acne, joint pain, and acute rheumatic symptoms have also occurred.

- Visually inspect patients for signs such as gynecomastia and acne. Obtain careful history of problems the patient may fail to volunteer: impotence, menorrhagia, and joint pain.
- Instruct diabetic patients to monitor blood glucose levels carefully when starting therapy with ethionamide or during periods of dosage adjustment; a change in insulin dosage or diet may be necessary.

### Patient and family education

- Review with patients and families the anticipated benefits and possible side effects of drug therapy.
- If other drugs are prescribed concomitantly, such as pyridoxine, emphasize the importance of taking both drugs for best effect and reduced side effects.
- See entry for drug class (p. 371).

## isoniazid (INH)  (eye-so-NYE-uh-zid)  antituberculosis agent

- isoniazid (INH): ✦Isotamine, Izonid, Laniazid, Nydrazid, Panazid, ✦Rimifon, Teebaconin

**MECHANISM OF ACTION**  Isoniazid has many effects on bacterial metabolism, including inhibition of mycolic acid synthesis, essential metabolites for mycobacteria. The action of the drug may be bacteriostatic or bactericidal.

**INDICATIONS**  **Prophylaxis of tuberculosis** Persons exposed to active cases of tuberculosis or persons converting from negative to positive on the standard Mantoux tuberculin skin test may receive isoniazid for several months to a year.  **Combination chemotherapy of active tuberculosis** Isoniazid is one of the most effective antituberculosis agents available. • The drug should be used with at least one other agent such as rifampin or ethambutol to treat active cases. • When resistance to one of the standard drugs is likely, three or more drugs may be employed.

**CONTRAINDICATIONS**  **Acute liver disease** Isoniazid should not be used in patients with significant liver disease because of the danger of acute liver failure with isoniazid.

**DOSAGE**  **PO:**  **ADULT:** This drug should not be used alone to treat tuberculosis but may be used alone for prophylaxis. For treatment, 5 to 10 mg/kg once daily, not to exceed 300 mg daily. For prophylaxis, 300 mg once daily for 6 months to a year.  **CHILDREN:** This drug should not be used alone to treat tuberculosis but may be used alone for prophylaxis. For treatment, 10 to 20 mg/kg daily, not to exceed 500 mg daily. For prophylaxis, 10 to 15 mg/kg daily, not to exceed 300 mg daily.  **IM:**  **ADULTS AND CHILDREN:** The IM route is only used when oral doses cannot be given. IM doses are the same as oral. *Special patient populations:*  **ELDERLY:** Special geriatric doses have not been established. Nevertheless, older individuals have a greater risk of the hepatotoxicity caused by isoniazid. **PREGNANCY:** Safe use has not been established. In spite of some evidence that isoniazid is carcinogenic and embryocidal in animals, the drug has been used in combination with ethambutol to control tuberculosis in pregnant women.

**PREPARATIONS**  *Tablets*: 50, 100, and 300 mg. *Oral solution*: 50 mg/ml, syrup in 70% sorbitol. *Parenteral solution*: 100 mg/ml. Combination products include *tablets*: isoniazid 100 mg with 5 mg pyridoxine hydrochloride (P-I-N Forte); isoniazid 100 mg with 10 mg pyridoxine hydrochloride or 300 mg isoniazid with 30 mg pyridoxine hydrochloride (Teebaconin and vitamin B 6 [contains tartrazine]). *Solution*: 50 mg/5 ml isoniazid with 2.5 mg/5 ml pyridoxine hydrochloride. *Capsules*: 150 mg isoniazid with 300 mg rifampin (Rifamate).

**DRUG INTERACTIONS**    **Cycloserine, isoniazid, and ethionamide** all have CNS effects that may be additive when the drugs are combined.   **Phenytoin** metabolism in the liver is inhibited by isoniazid. As a result, phenytoin may accumulate to toxic concentrations. This reaction is most common in slow acetylators of isoniazid. Patients receiving both isoniazid and aminosalicylic acid are also at higher risk.   **Aluminum hydroxide gel** lowers absorption of isoniazid unless the antacid is administered at least 1 hour after the isoniazid.   **Disulfiram** may increase the risk of CNS effects of isoniazid. Psychotic reactions and coordination difficulties have been observed.   **BCG vaccine** may be ineffective when given to patients receiving isoniazid because isoniazid blocks multiplication of BCG.

**DIAGNOSTIC TEST INTERFERENCE**    **Tests for urinary glucose** using cupric sulfate may yield false-positive results when patients are receiving isoniazid.

**FATE**    Isoniazid is well absorbed from IM sites and from the GI tract. *Peak* serum concentrations are usually achieved within an hour of oral administration. Distribution of the drug is excellent through all body tissues and fluids and the CNS. Isoniazid appears in the milk of nursing mothers and crosses the placenta easily. Hepatic metabolism is the primary route of elimination of isoniazid. The major metabolite is an acetylated form of isoniazid. The rate of drug acetylation differs markedly among populations, and two genetically determined subtypes are usually identified. The so-called rapid acetylators inactivate isoniazide two to three times as rapidly as the slow acetylators. As expected, the rapid acetylators have lower blood concentrations of drug following standard oral doses. The significance of these differences for response to therapy or development of toxic reactions is unclear.

## ❦ NURSING CONSIDERATIONS

### Side effects, toxicities, and associated nursing actions

**CNS** Ataxia, euphoria, dizziness, encephalopathy, muscle twitching, stupor, tinnitus, memory impairment, optic neuritis, loss of self-control, and toxic psychosis have occurred. Persons especially at risk include malnourished or diabetic patients. Neurotoxic effects can be reduced by administration of pyridoxine hydrochloride.

* Obtain careful mental status examination before the start of therapy and repeat at regular intervals.
* Instruct patients to avoid driving or operating hazardous equipment if ataxia, dizziness, or visual problems occur.

**Peripheral nervous system** The most common side effect of isoniazid is peripheral neuritis. Early signs are paresthesia of the feet and hands. Persons especially at risk include malnourished or diabetic patients. Neurotoxic effects can be reduced by administration of pyridoxine hydrochloride.

* Assess patients regularly for development of numbness, tingling, or unusual sensations of fingers or toes, as these symptoms may signal a need for pyridoxine therapy.

**Blood** Agranulocytosis, aplastic anemia, eosinophilia, hemolytic anemia, methemoglobinemia, sideroblastic anemia, and thrombocytopenia have occurred.

* Instruct patients to report the development of fever, sore throat, malaise, fatigue, pallor, petechiae, unexplained bruising or bleeding, nosebleed, and bleeding gums.
* Monitor complete blood cell count, white blood cell differential, and platelet count.

**GI** Epigastric distress, dry mouth, nausea, and vomiting can occur.

* If GI symptoms are severe or persistent, notify the physician.
* Instruct the patient to take ordered doses with meals or snacks to lessen gastric irritation. The drug should not be taken within 1 hour of the taking of an antacid containing aluminum hydroxide gel (see drug interactions).
* If dry mouth occurs, suggest that the patient rinse the mouth frequently with water, suck on sugarless hard candy or chew sugarless gum, and perform regular oral hygiene but avoid drying mouthwashes. Some patients may wish to try commercially available saliva substitutes.

**Renal** Urinary retention has been reported.

* Monitor intake and output in elderly or immobilized patients.

- Suggest that patients void before taking each dose.
- Instruct patients to report the sensation of incomplete bladder emptying.

**Metabolic** Metabolic acidosis and hyperglycemia are possible.

- Instruct diabetic patients to monitor blood glucose carefully when beginning therapy with isoniazid or during periods of dosage adjustment.

**Allergic** Fever, skin eruptions of various kinds, lymphadenopathy, and vasculitis have all occurred. These are delayed reactions, appearing 3 to 7 weeks after therapy is started.

- Instruct patients to report the development of any skin changes or fever.
- Emphasize the importance of returning to the physician for follow-up visits.

**Liver** Up to 20% of treated patients show mild signs of hepatic stress (increased serum bilirubin, AST, ALT). Rarely patients develop progressive liver disease with jaundice and hepatitis, which is occasionally fatal. The risk of serious hepatic toxicity is increased over age 35 years and is low in patients younger than 20. Daily users of alcohol have increased risk, regardless of age.

- Instruct patients to report the development of fever, malaise, jaundice, right upper quadrant abdominal pain, and change in the color or consistency of stools.
- Monitor liver function tests.
- Instruct patients to avoid the use of alcohol while taking isoniazid.

**Other** Gynecomastia in males, a syndrome resembling lupus erythematosus, and a rheumatic syndrome have occurred rarely.

- Inspect male patients regularly for development of gynecomastia. Question patients about the development of any unexpected sign or symptom.

### Nursing interventions related to drug administration

- Teebaconin and vitamin B6 combination tablets containing isoniazid 100 mg with pyridoxine 10 mg and isoniazid 300 mg with pyridoxine 30 mg contain FD & C yellow dye #5 (tartrazine), which may cause an allergic reaction in susceptible individuals. Although rare, this reaction is seen more commonly in persons with aspirin hypersensitivity.
- For IM use, reconstitute as directed on the vial. If the solution crystallizes, warm to room temperature by running the vial under warm water. Administer into a large muscle mass, such as the dorsogluteal site or rectus femoris muscle in adults or the vastus lateralis in children. Aspirate before injecting the drug to avoid inadvertent IV administration. Record and rotate injection sites.

### Patient and family education

- Review with patients and families the anticipated benefits and possible side effects of drug therapy.
- See entry for drug class (p. 371).
- If pyridoxine is ordered concomitantly, emphasize the importance of taking both drugs as ordered.
- Instruct patients to avoid the use of alcohol.
- Instruct patients to avoid ingestion of fish or cheese while taking isoniazid, as hypertension, headache, palpitations, skin flushing, nausea, vomiting, and pruritis have been reported when these food items are taken concurrently with isoniazid.

## kanamycin   (kan-uh-MY-sin)                                           aminoglycoside*

- kanamycin sulfate: ✿Anamid, Kantrex, Klebcil

**MECHANISM OF ACTION**   Kanamycin inhibits bacterial protein synthesis. Also see listing for kanamycin under aminoglycosides (p. 309).

**INDICATIONS**   **Combination chemotherapy of active tuberculosis** Kanamycin can be used for short-term therapy for strains of mycobacteria shown to be susceptible. • For other indications, see p. 309.

*Antibiotic.

**CONTRAINDICATIONS**  **Renal impairment** Because kanamycin can cause renal tubular necrosis, the drug should be avoided if possible in patients with renal impairment. • If kanamycin must be used, doses should be reduced and the patient monitored for accumulation of drug.  **Hearing loss** Because kanamycin can cause hearing loss, it should be avoided if possible in patients with preexisting hearing problems.

**DOSAGE**  **IM, IV:**  ADULTS, CHILDREN, AND INFANTS: This drug should not be used alone to treat tuberculosis. Dosage is 15 mg/kg daily, in equally divided doses every 8 to 12 hours. Daily dosage must not exceed 1.5 g.  *Special patient populations:*  ELDERLY: Special geriatric doses have not been established, but doses are adjusted for the degree of renal impairment that accompanies aging. RENAL IMPAIRMENT: Doses must be reduced according to the degree of renal failure.  PREGNANCY: FDA pregnancy category D.

**PREPARATIONS**  *Solution, injection:* 36.5, 250, or 333 mg/ml.

**DRUG INTERACTIONS**  **Nephrotoxic drugs** such as amphotericin B, capreomycin, cephalosporins, colistin, cisplatin, methoxyflurane, polymyxin B, or vancomycin may increase the risk of renal damage from kanamycin.  **Ethacrynic acid or furosemide** may increase the risk of hearing loss with kanamycin. **Succinylcholine, tubocurarine** and other neuromuscular blocking agents may have additive effects with kanamycin, causing unexpectedly profound or prolonged paralysis.

**FATE**  Kanamycin is not absorbed orally. *Peak* serum concentrations are achieved within 1 hour following IM administration. Elimination is almost exclusively by glomerular filtration in the kidney. The elimination *half-life* is normally 2 to 4 hours but may be as high as 27 to 80 hours in patients with severe renal impairment.

## ❦ NURSING CONSIDERATIONS

### Side effects, toxicities, and associated nursing actions

**Peripheral nervous system** Neuromuscular blockade is possible with kanamycin, especially when the neuromuscular junction is already depressed by neuromuscular blocking agents, general anesthetics, or diseases such as myasthenia gravis. Rarely patients suffer respiratory paralysis.

• Monitor respiratory rate of patients at risk; do not leave patients who have received neuromuscular blocking agents unattended.

• Have neostigmine and calcium available in settings where kanamycin is used with high-risk patients, such as in the operating room, recovery room, and intensive care units.

**Ototoxicity** Hearing loss is a dose-related side effect of kanamycin.

• Be alert to diminished hearing in patients. Be especially alert in elderly patients and patients with preexisting tinnitus, vertigo, hearing loss, or those who have previously received ototoxic drugs. Question patients about perceived hearing loss.

• Obtain audiologic examination before the start of therapy. If hearing loss is suspected, repeat audiologic examination should be performed.

• Be alert to loss of balance in ambulatory patients. Question patients about dizziness.

**Renal** Nephrotoxicity is a dose-related side effect of kanamycin. Signs of renal damage include proteinuria, cells or casts in urine, decreased urine specific gravity, decreased creatinine clearance, increased serum creatinine, and increased BUN.

• Monitor urinalysis, serum creatinine and creatinine clearance, and BUN.

• Monitor intake and output, daily weight, and blood pressure. If urinary output begins to fall or weight increases by more than 2 lb/day, notify physician.

• Keep patients adequately hydrated. Analyze daily intake and output to determine if patient is adequately hydrated for age and size. Assess skin turgor and mucous membranes for signs of dehydration.

• Inspect urine on a regular basis to note possible development of proteinuria, cells, or casts in urine.

**Blood** Anemia, granulocytopenia, leukopenia, thrombocytopenia, or changes in reticulocyte count may rarely be seen.

• Monitor complete blood cell count, white blood cell differential, platelet count, and reticulocyte count.

- Instruct patient to report the development of fever, sore throat, unexplained bruising or bleeding, petechiae, bleeding gums, and nosebleeds.

**Allergic** A few patients suffer rash, urticaria, pruritis, fever, and eosinophilia. Less common is transient agranulocytosis and anaphylaxis.
- Have available drugs, equipment, and personnel to treat an acute allergic response in settings where this drug is administered.
- Instruct patients to report the development of any skin changes.

### Nursing interventions related to drug administration
- Administer IM doses in a large muscle mass such as the dorsogluteal site or rectus femoris muscle in adults or the vastus lateralis muscle in infants and small children. Aspirate carefully before injecting medication to avoid inadvertent IV injection. Record and rotate injection sites.
- For IV administration, dilute each 500 mg of drug in 100 to 200 ml of usual IV fluid. Infuse dose over 30 to 60 minutes.
- For infants and small children, total volume for IV dose will be reduced, but dose should be infused over 30 to 60 minutes.

### Patient and family education
- Review with patients and families the anticipated benefits and possible side effects of drug therapy.
- Teach patients to weigh themselves daily and record weights. Instruct patients to notify physician if weight increases by more than 2 lb/day or 5 lb/week.

---

## pyrizinamide (peer-i-ZIN-u-mide) antituberculosis agent

- pyrizinamide: Sold under generic name

**MECHANISM OF ACTION** Pyrizinamide may be either bacteriostatic or bactericidal. The mechanism by which these effects are produced is unknown.

**INDICATIONS** **Combination chemotherapy of active tuberculosis** Pyrizinamide may be combined with other agents in some treatment regimens.

**CONTRAINDICATIONS** **Severe hepatic damage** Pyrizinamide is metabolized by the liver and causes hepatotoxicity. • Patients with severely compromised liver function cannot tolerate pyrizinamide.

**DOSAGE** **PO:** **ADULTS:** This drug should not be used alone to treat tuberculosis. Dosage is 20 to 35 mg/kg daily in 3 or 4 equal doses, not to exceed 3 g daily. *Special patient populations:* **CHILDREN:** Safe use has not been established. **PREGNANCY:** Safe use has not been established.

**PREPARATIONS** *Tablets*: 500 mg.

**DRUG INTERACTIONS** None reported to date.

**FATE** Pyrizinamide is well absorbed following oral administration, producing *peak* serum concentrations within 2 hours. The drug distributes well to most body tissues and fluids, and the CNS. Pyrizinamide is hydrolyzed in the liver, as well as in other tissues, to an active metabolite. Metabolites appear in the urine, but little unchanged drug is excreted by the kidneys. The elimination *half-life* is 9 to 10 hours in normal patients but may increase if renal or hepatic function is impaired.

### ❧ NURSING CONSIDERATIONS

#### Side effects, toxicities, and associated nursing actions
**Blood** Thrombocytopenia and sideroblastic anemia are rare effects.
- Instruct patients to report signs of thrombocytopenia: unexplained bleeding or bruising, appearance of petechiae, nosebleeds, and bleeding gums.

- Instruct patients to report signs of possible sideroblastic anemia: anemia, fatigue, dizziness, and pallor.
- Monitor platelet count and complete blood cell count.

**GI** Anorexia, nausea, and vomiting are possible.
- If GI symptoms are severe or persistent, notify physician.
- Suggest that patients take ordered doses with meals or a snack to lessen gastric irritation.

**Renal** Renal excretion of uric acid is inhibited by pyrizinamide, which occasionally causes gout. Porphyria and dysuria occur rarely.
- Encourage patients to maintain a daily intake of 2500 to 3000 ml.
- Instruct patients to report urinary problems.

**Liver** At maximum doses, up to 15% of patients show signs of hepatotoxicity. Signs include anorexia, fever, malaise, liver tenderness, hepatomegaly, and splenomegaly. Jaundice occurs in 2% to 3% of patients. Rarely patients suffer fatal liver damage. Damage is generally worse with larger doses.
- Instruct patients to report the signs and symptoms listed.
- Monitor liver function tests.

**Metabolic** Diabetic control is difficult to maintain when pyrizinamide is given.
- Instruct diabetic patients to monitor blood glucose carefully when initiating drug therapy with pyrizinamide or during periods of dosage adjustment.

**Allergic** Acne, arthralgia, fever, photosensitivity, and maculopapular rash may occur.
- Inspect patients for skin changes. Instruct patients to report the development of skin changes.
- If photosensitivity occurs, instruct patients to avoid exposure to the sun or other sources of ultraviolet light, to wear a hat and long-sleeve clothing, and to use maximum-protection sunscreen on exposed skin surfaces. Instruct patients to report this side effect, as it may be a symptom of porphyria.

### Patient and family education
- Review with patients and families the anticipated benefits and possible side effects of drug therapy.
- See entry for drug class (p. 371).

## rifampin  (reh-FAM-pin)                                           antibiotic*

- rifampin: Rifadin, Rimactane

**MECHANISM OF ACTION**  Rifampin inhibits DNA-dependent RNA polymerase in susceptible bacteria. This enzyme forms RNA, which is the intermediate in producing proteins from the genes carried in DNA. Rifampin may be either bactericidal or bacteriostatic.

**INDICATIONS**  **Combination chemotherapy of active tuberculosis** Rifampin is usually combined with isoniazid. • Other drugs may be added or substituted in the regimen as needed.  **Leprosy** Rifampin is combined with dapsone for certain types of leprosy. • For dapsone-resistant leprosy, rifampin is combined with clofazimine and ethionamide.  **Meningococcus carrier state** Persons who carry *Neisseria meningitidis* in the nasopharynx but show no symptoms of disease may be treated to eliminate this carrier state when the risk of meningitis is high.  **Prophylaxis of Haemophilus influenzae type B infection** Contacts of patients with *H. influenzae* type B infections who are themselves in contact with children under the age of 4 years may be treated with rifampin to eliminate the carrier state and prevent spread of the infection.

**CONTRAINDICATIONS**  **Allergy to rifampin** Patients who have experienced allergic reactions to rifampin should not receive the drug again.

*Broad spectrum.

**DOSAGE**    **PO:**    **ADULTS:** For tuberculosis, 600 mg once daily for months or years. This drug should not be used alone to treat tuberculosis. For prophylaxis of *N. meningitidis* or *H. influenzae* type B, 20 mg/kg up to 600 mg daily for 4 days. For leprosy, 600 mg once monthly with 100 mg dapsone daily for 6 months or longer.    **CHILDREN OVER 5 YEARS:** For tuberculosis, 10 to 20 mg/kg daily, not to exceed 600 mg daily. This drug should not be used alone to treat tuberculosis. For prophylaxis of *N. meningitidis* or *H. influenzae* type B, 10 to 20 mg/kg for 4 days.    *Special patient populations:* **PREGNANCY:** Safe use has not been established.

**PREPARATIONS:**    *Capsules*: 150 or 300 mg. Combination products include *capsules*: 300 mg rifampin with 150 mg isoniazid (Rifamate).

**DRUG INTERACTIONS**    **Aminosalicylic acid** preparations containig bentonite as excipient (vehicle) may interfere with the absorption of rifampin. These preparations are not available in the United States. **Anticoagulants** such as the orally administered coumadins are metabolized by hepatic enzymes induced by rifampin. As a result, the coumadins may be metabolized too rapidly. Doses should be checked and adjusted as necessary.    **Estrogens** are metabolized by hepatic enzymes induced by rifampin. Oral contraceptives containing estrogens may not be effective when rifampin is also given because the increased rate of metabolism may destroy the estrogen before it has time to produce the desired effect.    **Chloramphenicol, cyclosporine, corticosteroids, digitalis, and related drugs, methadone, quinidine, and sulfonylureas** are all metabolized by hepatic enzymes induced by rifampin. The result may be to reduce the effectiveness of these agents.

**DIAGNOSTIC TEST INTERFERENCE**    **Microbiologic assays for serum folate and vitamin B 12** are inhibited by rifampin.    **Sulfobromophthalein tests** are falsely positive unless the test is completed before the daily dose of rifampin    **Total serum bilirubin tests** using the modified Malloy method (with diazotized sulfanilic acid) may be falsely elevated by rifampin.

**FATE**    Rifampin is well absorbed following oral administration, producing *peak* serum concentrations within 2 to 4 hours. Peak serum concentrations are slightly lowered by taking the drug with food. Rifampin is widely distributed in the body, but concentrations in the CNS are lower than in plasma. The drug enters milk and crosses the placenta. Rifampin is metabolized in the liver to an active metabolite. Both the drug and the metabolite are excreted in bile. Minor amounts of the drug appear in urine. The elimination *half-life* for rifampin ranges from 1.7 to 3 hours, decreasing as the metabolizing enzymes are induced.

## ☙ NURSING CONSIDERATIONS

### Side effects, toxicities, and associated nursing actions

**CNS** Ataxia, dizziness, drowsiness, confusion, fatigue, headache, inability to concentrate, fever, muscular weakness, numbness, and visual disturbances have occurred, especially in the early stages of therapy.
- Review with patients these side effects, and caution patients to report their development.
- Caution patients to avoid driving or operating hazardous equipment if ataxia, dizziness, drowsiness, confusion, or visual disturbances occur.
- Reassure patients that side effects may diminish with continued use of the medication.

**Blood** Acute hemolytic anemia has occurred with intermittent therapy only. Hematuria, hemoglobinuria, purpura, thrombocytopenia, and other blood dyscrasias are possible.
- Monitor the complete blood cell count, white blood cell differential, platelet count, and urinalysis.
- Instruct patients to report the development of petechiae, unexplained bruising or bleeding, nosebleeds, bleeding gums, and blood-tinged or orangish urine.
- Instruct patients to report the development of fatigue, pallor, and malaise.

**GI** GI disturbances are the most frequently observed reactions. Signs include anorexia, abdominal cramps, diarrhea, epigastric distress, heartburn, nausea, and vomiting.
- If GI symptoms are severe or persistent, notify physician.
- For best effect, doses should be taken 1 hour before or 2 hours after meals or snack. For ease in

taking, the capsule may be opened and the contents mixed with a small amount of food such as applesauce. A suspension can also be made; consult the pharmacist.
- If GI symptoms produce anorexia, vomiting, or diarrhea, monitor intake and output and weight.

**Liver** Transient liver impairment may occur. Signs include increases in serum concentrations of bilirubin, alkaline phosphatase, AST, and ALT. More serious reactions including jaundice are less common, but fatal reactions have occurred.
- Instruct patients to report the development of right upper quadrant abdominal pain, jaundice, fever, malaise, and change in the color or consistency of stools.
- Monitor liver function tests.

**Allergic** A flulike syndrome is the most common allergic reaction, occurring in about 1% of patients who receive intermittent therapy. The incidence is less with continuous therapy. Other allergic reactions sometimes observed include dyspnea, wheezing, pruritis, urticaria, rash, eosinophilia, sore mouth, pemphigoid reactions, and exudative conjunctivitis.
- Instruct patients to report the development of any unexplained signs or symptoms.

**Other** Rifampin and its metabolites are red-orange in color and discolor urine, feces, sputum, sweat, and tears. Soft contact lenses will be permanently discolored.
- Warn patients about this unusual side effect before initiating drug therapy.

### Patient and family education
- Review with patients and families the anticipated benefits and possible side effects of drug therapy.
- See entry for drug class (p. 371).

---

## streptomycin   (strep-toh-MY-sin)                                         aminoglycoside*

- streptomycin: Sold under generic name

**MECHANISM OF ACTION**   Streptomycin inhibits bacterial protein synthesis and may be bactericidal, especially against extracellular organisms.

**INDICATIONS**   **Combination chemotherapy of active tuberculosis** Streptomycin is used with one or more other drugs for initial therapy of serious cases of active tuberculosis. • For other indications, see listing under aminoglycosides (p. 312).

**CONTRAINDICATIONS**   **Renal impairment** Because streptomycin can cause renal tubular necrosis, doses should be reduced and the patient monitored for accumulation of drug.   **Hearing loss** Because streptomycin can cause hearing loss and vestibular damage, it should be avoided if possible in patients with preexisting hearing problems.

**DOSAGE**   **IM:**   **ADULTS:** 20 mg/kg daily in a single dose for up to 3 weeks. Doses may then be reduced to 1 g two or three times a week. This drug should not be used alone to treat tuberculosis.   **CHILDREN:** 20 mg/kg daily, with adjustment as necessary to prevent drug accumulation.   *Special patient populations*   **ELDERLY:** Doses must be reduced in elderly patients to prevent drug accumulation.   **RENAL IMPAIRMENT:** Doses must be reduced according to degree of renal impairment.   **PREGNANCY:** FDA pregnancy category D.

**PREPARATIONS**   *Solution, injection*: 400 or 500 mg/ml, with sodium bisulfite, sodium citrate, and phenol; 1 or 5 g powder to dissolve for injection.

**DRUG INTERACTIONS**   **Nephrotoxic drugs** such as amphotericin B, capreomycin, cephalosporins, colistin, cisplatin, methoxyflurane, polymyxin B, or vancomycin may increase the risk of renal damage from streptomycin.   **Ethacrynic acid or furosemide** may increase the risk of hearing loss with streptomycin.   **Succinylcholine, tubocurarine,** and other neuromuscular blocking agents may have additive effects with streptomycin, causing unexpectedly profound or prolonged paralysis.

*Antibiotic.

**DIAGNOSTIC TEST INTERFERENCE**   **Glucose** assays using cupric sulfate may yield false-positive results in the presence of streptomycin.

**FATE**   Streptomycin is not absorbed orally. *Peak* serum concentrations are achieved within 1 to 2 hours following IM administration. Distribution is generally good, but the drug does not readily enter the CNS. Elimination is almost exclusively by glomerular filtration in the kidney. The elimination *half-life* is normally 2 to 3 hours but may be as high as 110 hours in patients with severe renal impairment.

## ❦ NURSING CONSIDERATIONS

### Side effects, toxicities, and associated nursing actions

**Peripheral nervous system** Neuromuscular blockade is possible with streptomycin, especially when the neuromuscular junction is already depressed by neuromuscular blocking agents, general anesthetics, or diseases such as myasthenia gravis. Rarely patients suffer respiratory paralysis.

- Monitor respiratory rate of patients at risk; do not leave unattended patients who have received neuromuscular blocking agents.
- Have neostigmine and calcium available in settings where streptomycin is used with high-risk patients, such as in the operating room, recovery room, and intensive care units.

**Ototoxicity** Vestibular damage is a dose-related side effect of streptomycin. Hearing loss is also possible.

- Be alert to diminished hearing in patients. Be especially alert in elderly patients and patients with preexisting tinnitus, vertigo, hearing loss, or patients who have previously received ototoxic drugs. Question patients about perceived hearing loss.
- Obtain audiologic examination before the start of therapy. If hearing loss is suspected, repeat audiologic examination should be performed.
- Be alert to loss of balance in ambulatory patients. Question patients about dizziness.

**Renal** Nephrotoxicity is a dose-related side effect of streptomycin, although other aminoglycosides are more nephrotoxic. Signs of renal damage include proteinuria, cells or casts in urine, decreased urine specific gravity, decreased creatinine clearance, increased serum creatinine, and increased BUN.

- Monitor urinalysis, serum creatinine and creatinine clearance, and BUN.
- Monitor intake and output, daily weight, and blood pressure. If urinary output begins to fall or weight increases by more than 2 lb/day or 5 lb/week, notify physician.
- Keep patients adequately hydrated. Analyze daily intake and output to determine if patient is adequately hydrated for age and size. Assess skin turgor and mucous membranes for signs of dehydration.
- Inspect urine on a regular basis to note possible development of proteinuria, cells, or casts in urine.

**Blood** Anemia, granulocytopenia, leukopenia, thrombocytopenia, or changes in reticulocyte count may rarely be seen.

- Monitor complete blood cell count, white blood cell differential, platelet count, and reticulocyte count.
- Instruct patient to report the development of fever, sore throat, unexplained bruising or bleeding, petechiae, bleeding gums, and nosebleeds.

**Allergic** A few patients suffer rash, urticaria, pruritis, fever, and eosinophilia. Less common is transient agranulocytosis and anaphylaxis.

- Have drugs, equipment, and personnel available to treat an acute allergic response in settings where this drug is administered.
- Instruct patients to report the development of any skin changes.

### Nursing interventions related to drug administration

- Administer IM doses in a large muscle mass such as the dorsogluteal site or rectus femoris muscle in adults or the vastus lateralis muscle in infants and small children. Aspirate carefully before injecting medication to avoid inadvertent IV injection. Record and rotate injection sites.

### Patient and family education

- Review with patients and families the anticipated benefits and possible side effects of drug therapy.
- See entry for drug class (p. 371).

# sulfoxone    (sul-FOX-one)    sulfone*

- sulfoxone sodium: Diasone sodium

**MECHANISM OF ACTION**    Because sulfoxone is hydrolyzed to release dapsone in the body, sulfoxone is presumed to have the same mechanism of action. Sulfones inhibit synthesis of dihydrofolate in susceptible bacteria, an action similar to that of sulfonamides.

**INDICATIONS**    **Leprosy** Sulfoxone sodium may be substituted for dapsone, although dapsone is usually preferred because it is less expensive and more reliably absorbed.

**CONTRAINDICATIONS**    As for dapsone (p.376).

**DOSAGE**    PO:    **ADULTS:** 330 mg daily.    *Special patient populations:*    **CHILDREN:** Safe use has not been established.    **PREGNANCY:** Safe use has not been established.

**PREPARATIONS**    *Tablets, enteric-coated:* 165 mg, equivalent to 25 mg dapsone on average.

**DRUG INTERACTIONS**    As for dapsone.

**FATE**    Sulfoxone sodium is hydrolyzed in the gut to release dapsone. Absorption of sulfoxone sodium is less reliable than for dapsone, but once it is absorbed the pharmacokinetics are similar (see dapsone , p. 376).

## ☙ NURSING CONSIDERATIONS

### Side effects, toxicities, and associated nursing actions

**CNS** Blurred vision, headache, insomnia, nervousness, psychosis, tinnitus, and vertigo can occur.
- Instruct patients about possible CNS side effects.
- Instruct patients to avoid driving or operating hazardous equipment if blurred vision or vertigo occurs.
- If insomnia occurs, instruct patient to take the last dose of the day several hours before bedtime. If the patient is receiving once-a-day therapy, ascertain that the patient is taking the dose in the morning (assuming the patient sleeps at night).

**Peripheral nervous system** At high doses, peripheral neuropathy leading to muscle weakness and muscle loss can occur. If signs appear, the drug should be discontinued. This side effect is rare with doses used to treat leprosy.
- Monitor muscle strength at regular intervals.
- Instruct patients to report the development of muscle weakness or tingling of the extremeties.

**CV** Tachycardia can occur with very high, toxic doses.
- Monitor the pulse.

**Blood** Hemolytic anemia and methemoglobinemia are common side effects of dapsone and so may be seen when sulfoxone is used; these reactions are more common and severe at higher doses. Patients with deficiency of G-6-PD suffer more severe reactions.
- Question patients about G-6-PD deficiency before administering first doses.
- Monitor complete blood cell count.
- Instruct patients to report the development of fatigue, weakness, pallor, and jaundice.

**GI** Abdominal pain, anorexia, nausea, and vomiting can occur.
- Warn patient about these GI side effects. If side effects are severe or persistent, notify physician.
- If vomiting occurs, monitor intake and output.
- Monitor weight.
- Suggest that the patient take ordered doses with meals or a snack to lessen gastric irritation.

**Renal** Albuminuria, nephrotic syndrome, and renal papillary necrosis are rare.
- Monitor weight and blood pressure.
- Monitor urinalysis, serum BUN, and creatinine.

**Other** Effective treatment of leprosy often precipitates reactions that may include sensitization of the lesions, skin reactions, fever, or more severe signs. Patients may require hospitalization and support with steroids or other drugs, but sulfoxone should be continued.
- Instruct the patient to report any skin changes, fever, or any unexpected sign or symptom.

*Antileprosy agent.

### Patient and family education
- Review with patients and families the anticipated benefits and possible side effects of drug therapy.
- See entry for drug class (p. 371).

# ANTIFUNGAL, ANTIVIRAL, AND ANTIPARASITIC AGENTS

**INTRODUCTION**    Agents used to treat infections caused by fungi, viruses, or parasites are selective poisons designed to eliminate the pathogen from the body. Unfortunately, selectivity of action has been more difficult to achieve against these organisms than against bacteria. The best systemic antifungal agents take advantage of differences in sterol composition between human and fungal cells. Amphotericin B damages membranes containing the fungal sterol ergosterol; ketoconazole and related drugs block synthesis of ergosterol. Antiviral agents interfere with viral replication within human cells. These drugs therefore resemble in mechanism the antiproliferative drugs used in cancer chemotherapy. Acyclovir adds some specificity by being readily activated by an enzyme found only in virus-infected cells. Antiparasitic agents are frequently effective because they are specific to the body compartment hosting the parasite. For example, antimalarial compounds such as chloroquine are concentrated within the red blood cell where one form of the malaria parasite is produced. Another example of drug localization is the use of nonabsorbed drugs such as pyrantel pamoate, which is intended to remain in the GI tract and combat intestinal infestations.

VI

# Chapter Twenty-two

# Antifungal agents

amphotericin B
benzoic and salicylic acids
butoconazole
calcium undecylenate
carbol-fuchsin
ciclopirox
clioquinol
clotrimazole
econazole nitrate
flucytosine
gentian violet

griseofulvin
haloprogin
ketoconazole
miconazole
miconazole nitrate
nystatin
sodium thiosulfate
tolnaftate
triacetin
undecylenic acid

**OVERVIEW OF THE DRUG CLASS**  Infections caused by fungi take several forms. In many cases the conditions are superficial dermatophytic infections involving only the skin or mucous membranes. More serious illness may follow pulmonary infection; systemic infections may be life-threatening, with fungi in the bloodstream and invading various tissues. Antifungal agents ideally attack the invading pathogens without directly harming human tissues. Just as with antibacterial drugs, the success of this strategy depends upon the existence of biochemical differences between the pathogen and the human host. A few classes of effective antifungal agents have been developed, but therapy of serious systemic fungal infections is still inadequate (Table 22-1). Agents that are too toxic for internal use may still be used effectively as topical agents to control superficial fungal infections (Table 22-2).

**Table 22-1.**

### Summary of clinical use of antifungal agents

| | Systemic mycoses* | Dermato-phytoses† | Vaginal candidiasis | Other candidiasis‡ |
|---|---|---|---|---|
| Amphotericin B | + | | | + |
| Butoconazole | | | + | |
| Calcium undecylenate | | + | | |
| Carbol-fuchsin | | | | |
| Ciclopirox olamine | | + | | |
| Clioquinol | | + | | |
| Clotrimazole | | + | + | + |
| Econazole nitrate | | + | | + |
| Flucytosine | + | | | |
| Gentian violet | | | + | + |
| Griseofulvin | | + | | |
| Haloprogin | | + | | |
| Ketoconazole | + | + | | |
| Miconazole | | + | + | + |
| Nystatin | | | + | + |
| Sodium thiosulfate | | + | | |
| Tolnaftate | | + | | |
| Triacetin | | + | | |
| Undecylenic acid | | + | | |
| Zinc undecylenate | | + | | |

*Systemic mycoses treated by these drugs include those caused by *Aspergillus, Blastomyces, Coccidioides, Cryptococcus, Histoplasma, Mucor, Paracoccidioides,* and *Rhizopus.*
†Dermatophytoses include the following conditions: tinea corporis (ringworm of the body), tinea cruris (jock itch), tinea pedis (athlete's foot), tinea unguium (onychomycosis), and tinea versicolor.
‡Other forms of candidiasis include cutaneous, mucocutaneous, oral, or intestinal disease.

Table
22-2.

## Summary of drugs used to treat topical fungal infections

| Generic name | Trade name | Administration/dosage | Clinical use | Principal side effects | Comments |
|---|---|---|---|---|---|
| Amphotericin B | Fungizone | TOPICAL: *Adults and children*—3% cream, lotion, or ointment applied two to four times daily | Rx—*Candida* infections of skin or mucous membranes | Local tissue irritation | Allergic reactions may rarely occur |
| Benzoic and salicylic acids | Whitfield's ointment | TOPICAL: *Adults and children*—6% benzoic and 3% salicylic acids, or double strength, applied two or three times daily | OTC—Ringworm | Local tissue irritation | Ointment is also keratolytic |
| Butoconazole | Femstat | INTRAVAGINAL: *Adults*—2% cream applied once daily for 3 days | Rx—Vaginal infections caused by *Candida* | Vaginal burning is possible | Can be used by pregnant women |
| Calcium undecylenate | Caldesene Cruex | TOPICAL: *Adults and children*—10% powder applied as needed | OTC—Tinea cruris (jock itch); also used for diaper rash or other skin irritations of groin area | Powder should not be inhaled or allowed to contact eyes or mucous membranes | Diabetics and others with impaired circulation should use only with physician's advice |
| Carbol-fuchsin | Castellani paint | TOPICAL: *Adults and children*—Solution swabbed over affected area one or two times daily | Rx—Tinea pedis (athlete's foot) and ringworm | Contact sensitivity may cause reactions | Carbol-fuchsin is poisonous if ingested |
| Ciclopirox olamine | Loprox | TOPICAL: *Adults*—1% cream applied twice daily | Rx—Tinea infections including tinea versicolor | Redness, itching, burning, and stinging of skin | Avoid contact with eyes; do not use occlusive dressing |
| Clioquinol (iodochlorhydroxyquin) | Vioform | TOPICAL: *Adults and children*—3% cream, ointment or powder applied several times daily | OTC—Localized dermatophytoses | Irritation of skin usually mild, but eyes must be avoided | Can cause a false-positive result in the ferric chloride test for phenylketonuria (PKU) |

*Continued.*

**Table 22-2.**

## Summary of drugs used to treat topical fungal infections—cont'd

| Generic name | Trade name | Administration/dosage | Clinical use | Principal side effects | Comments |
|---|---|---|---|---|---|
| Clotrimazole | Gyne-Lotrimin Lotrimin Mycelex Myclo♣ | TOPICAL: *Adults and children*—1% cream, lotion, or solution applied twice daily INTRAVAGINAL: *Adults*—tablets or creams containing 100 mg inserted once daily ORAL: *Adults and children over 3*—10 mg lozenge dissolved in mouth five times daily | Rx—Broad spectrum of antifungal activity, including *Candida* | Skin irritation, pruritus, urticaria; general irritation may be severe enough to cause drug to be discontinued | Do not use around eyes |
| Gentian violet | — | TOPICAL: *Adults and children*—1% or 2% solution two or three times daily for 3 days INTRAVAGINAL: *Adults*—One tampon (Genapax) inserted once or twice daily for 12 days | Rx—*Candida* infections of skin or vagina | Irritation of vagina can be damaging | This dye will stain skin and clothing |
| Haloprogin | Halotex | TOPICAL: *Adults and children*—1% cream or solution applied twice daily | Rx—Tinea and other superficial fungal infections | Local tissue irritation or maceration | Do not use around eyes |
| Ketoconazole | Nizoral | TOPICAL: *Adults and children*—2% cream applied once daily | Rx—Tinea and other superficial fungal infections | Irritation is rare | See drug listing (p. xxx) |
| Miconazole nitrate | Micatin Monistat-Derm | TOPICAL: *Adults and children*—2% cream, lotion, or aerosol applied twice daily INTRAVAGINAL: *Adults*—2% cream or suppositories once daily | Rx—Dermatophytoses or *Candida* infections | Local tissue irritation or maceration | Do not use around eyes |

Table 22-2.

## Summary of drugs used to treat topical fungal infections—cont'd

| | | | | | |
|---|---|---|---|---|---|
| Nystatin | Candex<br>Mycostatin<br>Nilstat<br>O-V Statin | ORAL: *Adults and children*—0.5 to 1 million units three times daily. *Infants*—0.1 to 0.2 million units four times daily | Rx—*Candida* infections of intestinal tract | Nausea, vomiting, or diarrhea | Drug is not absorbed from intestinal tract |
| | | TOPICAL: *Adults and children*—ointments, creams, lotions (0.1 million units/g) applied twice daily | Rx—*Candida* infections of skin | Irritation of skin | — |
| | | INTRAVAGINAL: *Adults*—tablets, 0.1 to 0.2 million units daily | Rx—*Candida* infections of vagina | Irritation is rare | Relief of symptoms is rapid, but dosage should be continued for 2 weeks or longer if necessary |
| Sodium thiosulfate | — | TOPICAL: *Adults and children*—25% lotion or solution applied twice daily for weeks | OTC—Tinea versicolor | Irritation is possible | Avoid the eyes |
| Tolnaftate | Aftate<br>Tinactin | TOPICAL: *Adults and children*—1% cream, gel, solution, powder, or aerosol applied twice daily | OTC—Tinea infections only; not effective against *Candida* | Rarely causes irritation or sensitization | Avoid eyes; 2 to 3 weeks of therapy is usually sufficient |
| Triacetin | Enzactin<br>Fungacetin | TOPICAL: *Adults and children*—25% cream or ointment applied twice daily | OTC—Tinea pedis and other dermatophytoses | Not irritating to skin but may harm eyes | Destroys rayon fabric |
| Undecylenic acid | Desenex<br>Ting<br>Undecylenic compound<br>Unde-Jen | TOPICAL: *Adults and children*—ointment (5%, with 20% zinc undecylenate), powder (2%, with 20% zinc undecylenate), 10% solution, 2% soap applied twice daily | OTC—Tinea pedis and ringworm in areas other than around nails or hairy areas | Should not be allowed to contact eyes or mucous membranes | Diabetics and others with impaired circulation should use only with physician's advice |

**MECHANISM OF ACTION**    Many antifungal agents take advantage of the presence of ergosterol in fungal membranes. Cholesterol rather than ergosterol is found in mammalian membranes. The polyene antifungal agents, such as nystatin and amphotericin B, bind to ergosterol and disrupt fungal membrane function. The imidazole antifungal agents, such as ketoconazole, miconazole, clotrimazole, econazole, and butoconazole, interfere with the synthesis of ergosterol. See individual drug listings for specific mechanisms.

**INDICATIONS**    • See Table 22-1 and the listings for individual drugs.

**CONTRAINDICATIONS**    • See listings for individual drugs.

**DRUG INTERACTIONS**    • See listings for individual drugs.

## amphotericin B    (am-foh-TAIR-i-sin)    polyene antifungal

● amphotericin B: Fungizone

**MECHANISM OF ACTION**    Amphotericin B and other polyene compounds bind to ergosterol, the primary sterol found in fungal membranes. In this way amphotericin B disrupts membrane function, allowing potassium and other cell constituents to be lost. The action is usually fungistatic. Mammalian cells are less sensitive to amphotericin B than are fungal cells because mammalian cells contain cholesterol rather than ergosterol.

**INDICATIONS**    **Life-threatening infections caused by fungi**  Amphotericin B is considered the drug of choice for serious systemic infections or meningitis caused by a variety of fungi, e. g., *Aspergillus, Blastomyces, Candida, Coccidioides, Cryptococcus, Histoplasma, Mucor, Rhizopus,* and others.    **Candida infections of skin or mucous membranes**  Amphotericin B may be used topically for these conditions (Table 22-2).

**CONTRAINDICATIONS**    **Allergy to amphotericin B**  For most drugs, allergic responses would contraindicate the use of the drug, but because amphotericin B is used for potentially life-threatening infections, serious side effects may be tolerated. Even serious allergic reactions may have to be accepted as the price of therapy unless an alternate agent can be found.

**DOSAGE**    IV:    ADULT: Doses are adjusted according to severity of the infection and the tolerance of the patient. Initial therapy is usually 0.25 mg/kg over a 2 to 6 hour period. Daily doses should never exceed 1.5 mg/kg. Treatment may continue for months, with the total IV dosage over that period ranging from 2 to 4 g.    *Special patient populations:*    CHILDREN: Safe use is not established. PREGNANCY: Safe use is not established.

**PREPARATIONS**    *Powder to prepare parenteral solutions:* 50 mg. Reconstitute with 10 ml of sterile water without bacteriostatic agent. For IV infusion, add 500 ml of 5% dextrose solution that has been adjusted to a pH above 4.2. The powder should be stored between 2° and 8° C and protected from light or moisture. Solutions should be protected from light and used within 24 hours.    **Combination products** *Capsules:* 50 mg amphotericin B with 250 mg tetracycline hydrochloride or 25 mg amphotericin B with 125 mg tetracycline hydrochloride (Mysteclin-F). *Suspension:* 25 mg/5 ml with 125 mg tetracycline hydrochloride (Mysteclin syrup). • See Table 22-2 for topical preparations.

**DRUG INTERACTIONS**    **Corticosteroids** may worsen potassium depletion caused by amphotericin B.    **Digitalis** toxicity may be worsened because the potassium depletion caused by amphotericin B sensitizes cells to digitalis and increases toxic reactions.    **Nephrotoxic drugs** such as aminoglycoside antibiotics, capreomycin, colistin, cisplatin, methoxyflurane, polymyxin B, or vancomycin may worsen the renal damage caused by amphotericin B.    **Potassium-wasting drugs** such as thiazides, thiazidelike diuretics, and loop diuretics may seriously worsen the potassium depletion caused by amphotericin B. **Skeletal muscle relaxants** are more effective during potassium depletion. Their action may therefore be synergistic with amphotericin B.

**FATE**    Amphotericin B is not absorbed from the GI tract. Because the drug has such low solubility in water, very dilute preparations are administered by slow IV infusion. Distribution is poor into many body compartments, including the CNS, however, the drug crosses the placenta. The metabolism and fate of amphotericin B in the body are not understood. Some drug appears in urine, but elimination is very slow.

### ❦ NURSING CONSIDERATIONS

#### Side effects, toxicities, and associated nursing actions

**CNS** CNS effects are most common with intrathecal administration of the drug. Signs include headache, pain along lumbar nerves, paresthesias, vision changes, and arachnoiditis.

- Perform neurologic assessment at regular intervals. If CNS effects are severe, work with the physician to provide appropriate symptomatic treatment.
- If vision changes occur, caution the patient to avoid driving or operating hazardous equipment.

**CV** Hypotension, ventricular fibrillation, and cardiac arrest can occur if the drug is administered too rapidly.

- Monitor blood pressure and pulse during drug administration.
- Administer daily dose over at least 6 hours.
- Use an infusion control device to help monitor the rate of flow.

**Blood** Anemia (normocytic, normochromic) occurs in most patients receiving amphotericin B but is reversible. Rarely, agranulocytosis, coagulation defects, eosinophilia, leukocytosis, leukopenia, or thrombocytopenia may develop.

- Monitor complete blood cell count, white blood cell differential, and platelet count.
- Inspect the patient for the development of petechiae or bruises. Instruct patients to report the development of sore throat, malaise, bleeding gums, nosebleeds, and unexplained bruising.
- Avoid IM injections in patients with thrombocytopenia.

**GI** Nausea and vomiting may occur.

- Monitor weight. If vomiting is severe, monitor intake and output; notify the physician.

**Renal** About 80% of the patients receiving amphotericin B show signs of renal toxicity, including azotemia, hypokalemia, elevated BUN, lowered creatinine clearance. Urine concentrations of uric acid, potassium, and protein increase.

- Monitor BUN and serum creatinine, serum electrolytes, and urinalysis. Monitor urinary uric acid and urinary electrolytes if available.
- Monitor fluid intake and output, weight, and blood pressure.

**Metabolic** Hypokalemia occurs in most patients receiving the drug.

- Monitor serum potassium level.
- Assess the patient for signs of hypokalemia: dizziness, hypotension, arrhythmias, nausea, vomiting, diarrhea, abdominal distention, decreased bowel sounds, muscle weakness, and leg cramps.

**Allergic** Anaphylactoid reactions are rare.

- Have drugs, equipment, and personnel available to treat acute allergic reactions in settings where amphotericin B is administered.
- Remain with patients for several minutes after beginning daily infusion of the drug; monitor vital signs every 2 hours.

**Other** Most patients experience anorexia, chills, cramping, dyspepsia, epigastric pain, malaise, muscle and joint pain, and weight loss.

- Assess patients for these side effects and any others that develop. If side effects are severe or persistent, work with the physician to develop treatment plans to improve patient comfort.

#### Nursing interventions related to drug administration

- Review the manufacturer's instructions. Reconstitute the drug by adding 10 ml of sterile water for injection without bacteriostatic agent to a vial containing 50 mg of drug. For IV administration, further dilute to a concentration of 0.1 mg/ml by adding the 50 mg/10 ml dilution to 500 ml of 5% dextrose injection, which must have a pH greater than 4.2.
- Inspect for discoloration or particulate matter; if either is present, discard the solution and prepare a fresh solution.
- Do not use an inline filter unless filter is 1 μg or larger. Reconstituted solutions may be stored in the refrigerator for up to 1 week. Use solutions further diluted for IV administration immediately after preparing.
- Monitor vital signs and temperature during infusion.
- Protect infusion from light. Covering the bag or bottle is usually sufficient; it is not necessary to cover the tubing, but follow institutional policy.

- The diluted infusion is a suspension. Gently agitate the IV bag or bottle at regular intervals to promote uniform suspension of the drug.
- Avoid mixing drugs or IV fluid with infusing amphotericin B. A small amount of heparin may be added to the infusion to lessen the possibility of thrombophlebitis; consult the physician and pharmacist.

**Patient and family education**

- Review with patients the anticipated benefits and possible side effects of drug therapy.
- Provide support to patients and families. A course of therapy may require weeks to months of hospitalization.

---

## flucytosine   (floo-SYE-toh-seen)                                     antifungal agent

- flucytosine: Ancobon, ✦ Ancotil

**MECHANISM OF ACTION**   Flucytosine is converted to fluorouracil by the enzyme cytidine deaminase in fungal cells. Fluorouracil is a potent antimetabolite that may interfere with protein, RNA, and DNA synthesis. Mammalian cells are relatively insensitive to flucytosine because they lack sufficient cytidine deaminase activity to form the cytotoxic metabolite fluorouracil.

**INDICATIONS**   Infections caused by Candida or Cryptococcus Strains should be tested for susceptibility before therapy begins. Some physicians combine flucytosine with amphotericin B for certain serious infections such as cryptococcal meningitis.

**CONTRAINDICATIONS**   Bone marrow suppression Flucytosine causes bone marrow depression, which may become profound in patients with compromised bone marrow.   Renal impairment Flucytosine may cause renal toxicity, which can be profound in patients with pre-existing renal impairment.

**DOSAGE**   PO:   ADULTS AND CHILDREN: 50 to 150 mg/kg daily in divided equal doses every 6 hours. CHILDREN BELOW 50 KG: 1.5 to 4.5 g/$M^2$ daily in divided doses.   *Special patient populations:* RENAL IMPAIRMENT: Doses must be reduced according to degree of impairment.   PREGNANCY: Safe use is not established. The drug is teratogenic in animals.

**PREPARATIONS**   *Capsules:* 250 or 500 mg.

**DRUG INTERACTIONS**   Amphotericin B may be synergistic with flucytosine against certain fungi. The membrane effects of amphotericin B are thought to increase the uptake of flucytosine into fungal cells.

**DIAGNOSTIC TEST INTERFERENCE**   Serum creatinine values determined with the Ektachem analyzer are falsely elevated. The Jaffe and alkaline picrate methods are not affected.

**FATE**   Flucytosine is well absorbed orally, with up to 90% of the dose appearing in the bloodstream. Peak concentrations in serum occur from 2 to 6 hours after dosage. The drug is well distributed throughout the body, including the CNS, where concentrations approach or equal serum concentrations. Flucytosine is eliminated by the kidneys and concentrated in urine as the unchanged drug. The elimination *half-life* is 2.5 to 6 hours in healthy patients but increases greatly when renal function is impaired.

❧ **NURSING CONSIDERATIONS**

**Side effects, toxicities, and associated nursing actions**

CNS Confusion, hallucinations, headache, sedation, and vertigo have been reported infrequently.

- Assess patients for these side effects.
- Caution patients to avoid driving or operating hazardous equipment if sedation or vertigo develop; notify the physician.

Blood Bone marrow function is suppressed by flucytosine, resulting in anemia, leukopenia, pancytopenia, or thrombocytopenia. Aplastic anemia has resulted in death in rare cases.

- Monitor complete blood cell count, white blood cell differential, and platelet count.
- Visually inspect the patient for pallor, bruising, and petechiae.
- Instruct the patient to report the development of fever, malaise, sore throat, unexplained bruising, nosebleeds, bleeding gums, and hematuria.
- Avoid IM injections in patients with thrombocytopenia.

**GI** Abdominal bloating, anorexia, diarrhea, nausea, perforation of the bowel, and vomiting occur because flucytosine or its metabolites damage the epithelial cells lining the GI tract.
- Assess for GI complaints. Monitor weight, auscultate bowel sounds, and check stool for occult blood. If GI symptoms are severe or persistent, monitor intake and output.
- Instruct the patient to report the development of changes in bowel habits, the development of severe abdominal pain, or the appearance of blood in the stools.
- Encourage patients to take doses with meals or a snack and to take the dose over 15 to 20 minute period to lessen gastric irritation and nausea.

**Renal** BUN and serum creatinine may be elevated.
- Monitor BUN and serum creatinine.
- Monitor weight and blood pressure.

**Liver** AST, ALT, and alkaline phosphatase are elevated in a dose-dependent manner. Liver enlargement is rare.
- Monitor liver function tests.
- Instruct patients to report the development of fever, malaise, jaundice, right upper quadrant abdominal pain, and change in the color or consistency of stools.
- Monitor serum drug levels if available.

**Nursing interventions related to drug administration**
- Suggest that patients take doses over a 15 to 20 minute period to lessen gastric irritation (see GI).

**Patient and family education**
- Review with patients the anticipated benefits and possible side effects of drug therapy.
- Provide support to patients and families; weeks to months of therapy may be required for treatment of the patient's problem.

---

## griseofulvin   (griz-ee-oh-FULL-vin)                                              antifungal agent

- griseofulvin: Fulvicin, Grisactin,♣ Grisovin

**MECHANISM OF ACTION**   Griseofulvin is thought to disrupt the mitotic spindle in fungal cells, preventing completion of mitosis. Griseofulvin is unusual because it is administered systemically for treatment of superficial fungal infections. The drug concentrates in the keratin precursor cells, thereby preventing these deeper skin layers from being infected. As these cells mature and move toward the surface, they displace infected cells. Eventually the fungal infection is eliminated as the infected cells slough off in the natural renewal process of the skin.

**INDICATIONS**   **Dermatophytoses** Griseofulvin should not be substituted for topical antifungals for minor infections but should be reserved for more resistant infections of the skin, nails, and scalp. • Conditions that respond include tinea corporis, tinea pedis, tinea cruris, tinea barber, tinea capitis, and tinea unguium. • These conditions are known by several common names, including ringworm, athlete's foot, and jock itch. • Griseofulvin is not effective against tinea versicolor.

**CONTRAINDICATIONS**   **Hepatocellular failure** Griseofulvin is normally metabolized in the liver and may dangerously accumulate in patients unable to carry out these reactions.   **Porphyria** Griseofulvin blocks metabolism of porphyrins and may precipitate an acute attack of porphyria, with accumulation of porphyrins in erythrocytes, urine, and feces.

**DOSAGE**   **PO:**   **ADULT:** Dosage varies according to the formulation used. For ultramicrosize preparations, doses range from 330 to 375 mg daily for tinea corporis, tinea cruris, or tinea capitis and up to 660 to 750 mg daily for tinea pedis or tinea unguium. For microsize griseofulvin preparations, doses range from 500 mg daily for tinea corporis, tinea cruris, or tinea capitis and up to 1 g daily for tinea pedis or tinea unguium. Duration of therapy is for weeks or months, depending on the site and severity of infection.   **CHILDREN OVER 2 YEARS:** For ultramicrosize preparations, 7.3 mg/kg daily. For microsize griseofulvin, 10 to 11 mg/kg daily or 300 mg/$M^2$ daily.   *Special patient populations:* **PREGNANCY:** Safe use is not established. Griseofulvin is embryotoxic in rats.

**PREPARATIONS:**    *Tablets:* 250 or 500 mg microsize; *tablets:*125, 165, 250, or 330 mg ultramicrosize; *capsules:* 125 or 250 mg; *suspension:* 125 mg/5 ml.

**DRUG INTERACTIONS**    **Alcohol** may cause tachycardia and flushing when used with griseofulvin. The effects of alcohol may be potentiated.    **Coumarin anticoagulants** may be metabolized more rapidly in the presence of griseofulvin because griseofulvin may induce enzymes in the liver that destroy the coumarins. The result can be loss of adequate anticoagulation effect.    **Oral contraceptives** may be less effective when given with griseofulvin because griseofulvin may induce enzymes in the liver that destroy the steroid hormones.    **Phenobarbital** lowers the amount of active griseofulvin in the blood by inducing enzymes in the liver that destroy griseofulvin and possibly by impairing absorption of griseofulvin.

**FATE**    The absorption of griseofulvin depends on the formulation administered. Ultramicrosize preparations are completely absorbed in the duodenum, but only 30% to 70% of a microsize preparation will be absorbed. A 500 mg dose of microsize griseofulvin is usually considered equivalent to a 250 mg dose of an ultramicrosize preparation. The distribution of griseofulvin accounts for much of the effectiveness of the drug. Griseofulvin accumulates in keratin precursor cells, binding tightly to new keratin. High concentrations may be found in skin, hair, and nails as well as in liver, fat, and muscle. Griseofulvin is metabolized in the liver to form an inactive demethylated product and a glucuronide, both of which are eliminated in urine. The elimination *half-life* is 9 to 24 hours.

## 🦋 NURSING CONSIDERATIONS

### Side effects, toxicities, and associated nursing actions

**CNS** Headache is a common early symptom, often disappearing as therapy continues. Extended therapy rarely causes paresthesias. Large doses can cause confusion, impaired performance or judgement, or symptoms of psychosis.
- Review these side effects with patients and families.
- Caution patients to avoid driving or operating hazardous equipment if confusion develops.
- Instruct the patient to report the development of CNS side effects.

**Blood** Leukopenia (reversible) is rare.
- Monitor white blood cell differential.

**GI** Diarrhea, epigastric distress, flatulence, nausea, and vomiting have been reported.
- Review GI side effects with the patient. Instruct the patient to notify the physician if symptoms are severe or persistent.
- Monitor weight.
- Suggest that patients take oral doses with meals or a high-fat snack to lessen gastric irritation and improve absorption.
- The drug may alter taste sensation; question the patient about changes in food intake.

**Renal** Proteinuria is rare.
- Monitor urinalysis.

**Allergic** Rashes or urticaria may occur. Angioedema or serum sickness is more rare.
- Instruct patients to report the development of rashes or urticaria.
- Have drugs, equipment, and personnel available to treat acute allergic reactions in settings where antifungal agents are administered.
- Review with patients the signs and symptoms of serum sickness: arthralgia, skin eruptions, lymphadenopathy, and pruritis. Abdominal pain, fever, headache, and malaise occur in more serious cases. Instruct the patient to report the development of these or unexpected signs or symptoms.

**Other** Photosensitivity may occur.
- If photosensitivity occurs, instruct patients to avoid exposure to the sun or other sources of ultraviolet light. Caution patients to wear a hat and long-sleeved clothing and to use a maximum-protection sunscreen on exposed skin surfaces.

### Patient and family education
- Review with the patient the anticipated benefits and possible side effects of drug therapy. Provide emotional support to patients and families, as weeks to months of therapy with this drug may be required.
- Caution patients to avoid the use of alcohol while taking griseofulvin (see Drug Interactions).

## ketoconazole (kee-toh-KON-uh-zole)

- ketoconazole: Nizoral

**MECHANISM OF ACTION**  Ketoconazole, like other imidazole derivatives, inhibits the synthesis of ergosterol in fungal cell membranes. Purine transport and other membrane functions are impaired. Ketoconazole also prevents yeast cells from developing hyphae and converting to mycelia. Because yeast cells are more easily phagocytized than are mycelia, this action also contributes to clearing of fungal infections.

**INDICATIONS**  **Systemic and subcutaneous mycoses** Chronic mucocutaneous candidiasis, pulmonary or disseminated histoplasmosis, and paracoccidioidomycosis usually respond to ketoconazole. • The drug may also be used in blastomycosis, chromomycosis, and pulmonary or disseminated coccidioidomycosis. • Treatment of many other types of fungal infections has been attempted with uncertain results. **Dermatophytoses** Tinea corporis, tinea cruris, and tinea versicolor may be treated with topical ketoconazole (Table 22-2).

**CONTRAINDICATIONS**  **Significant liver disease** Patients with diminished liver function may be at great risk from ketoconazole-induced hepatotoxicity.

**DOSAGE**  PO:  ADULT: 200 to 400 mg daily in a single dose.  CHILDREN OVER 2 YEARS: 3.3 to 6.6 mg/kg daily in a single dose.  *Special patient populations:*  PREGNANCY: Safe use is not established.

**PREPARATIONS**  *Tablets:* 200 mg, scored.

**DRUG INTERACTIONS**  **Antacids, antimuscarinic agents, and H-2 receptor blockers (cimetidine and ranitidine)** diminish acid secretion in the stomach. This action diminishes the dissolution and absorption of ketoconazole.  **Coumarin anticoagulants** have enhanced activity in the presence of ketoconazole. Dosage adjustment may be required.  **Cyclosporine** concentrations in plasma increase when ketoconazole is also given. Dosage of cyclosporine may require adjustment.  **Isoniazid** may decrease serum concentrations of ketoconazole. In addition, isoniazid is potentially hepatotoxic, as is ketoconazole. This increased risk of liver damage may preclude use of the drug concomitantly.  **Phenytoin** interferes with the metabolism of ketoconazole, and vice versa. Serum concentrations must be monitored for both drugs to assure adequate therapy.  **Rifampin** may decrease serum concentrations of ketoconazole. A dosage adjustment may be required.

**FATE**  Ketoconazole is well absorbed orally unless gastric pH is increased. In healthy fasting adults, *peak* serum concentrations are achieved within 1 to 4 hours of an oral dose. Absorption tends to vary among individuals. Distribution in the body is generally good, but entry to the CNS is variable. Elimination of ketoconazole from the body is complex. Several metabolites are formed in the liver and excreted in bile, along with unchanged drug. A lesser proportion of drug is eliminated by the kidneys.

### ☙ NURSING CONSIDERATIONS

#### Side effects, toxicities, and associated nursing actions

**CNS** Asthenia, abnormal dreams, dizziness, headaches, insomnia, lethargy, nervousness, paresthesia, and somnolence are reported by less than 1% of patients.

- Review these side effects with patients. Instruct patients to report the development of CNS side effects.
- Caution patients to avoid driving or operating hazardous equipment if dizziness, lethargy, or somnolence occur.

**GI** Nausea and/or vomiting may occur in 3% to 10% of patients. Abdominal pain, constipation, diarrhea, flatulence, and GI bleeding are less common.

- Monitor weight.
- Review GI symptoms with patients. Instruct patients to report persistent or severe side effects.
- Caution the patient to avoid the use of antacids or H-2 receptor blockers for gastric irritation (see Drug Interactions) and to keep all health care providers informed of all medications.

**Allergic** Fever, chills, or anaphylactic reactions are rare.

- Have drugs, equipment, and personnel available to treat acute allergic reactions in settings where antifungal agents are administered.
- Instruct patients to report the development of fever or chills.

**Liver** Serum AST, ALT, and alkaline phosphatase may increase. Less common are more serious signs of hepatotoxicity: dark urine, fatigue, pale feces, and jaundice.
- Monitor liver function tests.
- Instruct patients to report the development of jaundice, fatigue, fever, right upper quadrant abdominal pain, and change in the color or consistency of stools.

**Other** Bilateral breast tenderness and gynecomastia have occurred in males because ketoconazole influences steroid metabolism in several tissues.
- Caution male patients about these side effects, and instruct patients to notify the physician if they occur.

### Nursing interventions related to drug administration
- Absorption of this drug requires an acid pH in the stomach. For patients with achlorhydria, dissolve each 200 mg of ketoconazole in 4 ml of 0.2N HC1 solution. Administer the resulting solution through a straw to avoid contact with the teeth. Follow the dose with a full glass of water.

### Patient and family education
- Review with patients anticipated benefits and possible side effects of drug therapy.
- Review with patients the list of drug interactions. Remind patients to keep all health care providers informed of all medications being used.
- Provide support to patients and families, as weeks to months of drug therapy may be required.

---

## miconazole   (my-KON-uh-zole)                                    imidazole antifungal

- miconazole: Monistat

**MECHANISM OF ACTION**   Miconazole, like other imidazole derivatives, inhibits the synthesis of ergosterol in fungal cell membranes. Purine transport and other membrane functions are impaired. Miconazole also inhibits peroxisomal enzymes, causing accumulation of peroxide within the fungal cell, which can contribute to cell death.

**INDICATIONS**   **Severe mycoses** Miconazole can be effective in disseminated candidiasis, chronic mucocutaneous candidiasis, coccidioidomycosis, pulmonary or disseminated cryptococcosis, pulmonary or disseminated paracoccidioidomycosis, or petriellidiosis.   **Dermatophytoses and superficial mycoses** Miconazole nitrate may be used topically for these conditions (Table 22-2).   **Vaginal candidiasis** miconazole nitrate may be used intravaginally for this condition (Table 22-2).

**CONTRAINDICATIONS**   **Liver disease** Miconazole may accumulate in patients unable to normally metabolize the drug.

**DOSAGE**   **IV:**   **ADULT:** Doses are highly variable, depending on the organism causing the infection. Initial therapy is usually with 200 mg. Dosages range from 200 mg to 3.6 g daily, usually given in three infusions.   **CHILDREN OVER 1 YEAR:** 20 to 40 mg/kg daily in divided doses not to exceed 15 mg/kg.   **Intrathecal** 20 mg may be given at various intervals in conjunction with IV dosage for fungal meningitis.   *Special patient populations:*   **PREGNANCY:** Safe use is not established.

**PREPARATIONS**   *Parenteral solution:* 10 mg/ml. *Topical preparations:* See Table 22-2.

**DRUG INTERACTIONS**   **Coumarin anticoagulants** are more effective when miconazole is given, perhaps because miconazole interferes with the hepatic metabolism of the coumarins.

**DIAGNOSTIC TEST INTERFERENCE**   **Lipoprotein and immunoelectrophoretic patterns** are altered by the carrier used in miconazole preparations.

**FATE**   Oral absorption of miconazole is poor, and the drug is administered IV for treatment of systemic mycoses. Miconazole distributes well throughout the body, except for certain body fluids. Distribution to the CNS is variable. Elimination of the drug is complex and primarily through liver metabolism and biliary excretion of metabolites and unchanged drug. Urinary excretion is minimal.

### ☙ NURSING CONSIDERATIONS
#### Side effects, toxicities, and associated nursing actions
**CNS** Anxiety, increased libido, dizziness, and blurred vision may occur. With intrathecal administration the drug may cause arachnoiditis, transient saddle numbness, twelfth cranial nerve palsy, and

mild ventricular hemorrhage.
* Monitor neurologic assessment.

**CV** Transient tachycardia and cardiac arrhythmias may occur, especially if the undiluted drug is administered.
* Monitor pulse.
* Dilute IV doses as directed and administer slowly.

**Blood** Anemia and a decrease in hematocrit may occur. Hyponatremia and hyperlipidemia are also occasionally observed.
* Monitor complete blood cell count and serum electrolytes.
* Inspect for pallor. Instruct the patient to report the development of fatigue.

**GI** Anorexia, bitter taste, diarrhea, nausea, and vomiting occur.
* Monitor weight. If GI symptoms are severe or persistent, monitor intake and output.

**Allergic** Phlebitis and pruritis at the injection site are the most common reaction to miconazole. Rashes may also be present. An antihistamine such as diphenhydramine may be used to control pruritis.
* Assess for allergic responses. If responses are severe or persistent, consult the physician for symptomatic treatment.

### Nursing interventions related to drug administration
* For IV use, dilute the ordered dose in at least 200 ml of fluid, preferably 0.9% sodium chloride, although 5% dextrose may be used if necessary. Infuse the dose over 30 to 60 minutes.
* It has been suggested that a physician be present for first IV dose in the event the patient develops a hypersensitivity reaction.

### Patient and family education
* Review with patients the anticipated benefits and possible side effects of drug therapy.
* Provide support to patients and families, as weeks to months of hospitalization may be required for the full course of therapy.

# Chapter Twenty-three

# Antiviral agents

acyclovir
acyclovir sodium
amantadine hydrochloride
idoxuridine

ribavirin
trifluridine
vidarabine
zidovudine

**OVERVIEW OF THE DRUG CLASS**    Viral infections are common, usually causing minor symptoms we describe as a "cold" or the "flu." Many of the childhood diseases such as measles, mumps, and chickenpox are also caused by viruses. Herpesviruses can cause minor infections such as cold sores but also cause genital lesions that can infect infants in the birth canal. A virus has also been identified as the agent causing acquired immune deficiency syndrome (AIDS). This virus, known as HTLV-III or HIV (human immunodeficiency virus), is transmitted through contact with blood or semen of infected persons. The virus can be transmitted by anal intercourse between homosexual males or by heterosexual vaginal intercourse. Drug therapy for AIDs is in the early stages of development.

Viral diseases are often more difficult to treat than illnesses caused by bacteria. Symptoms of viral diseases frequently appear late in the course of the illness, which means that the infection progresses without clinical signs during the early phases when therapy might be most appropriate and productive. Although a few effective therapeutic agents have been developed to treat established viral disease (Table 23-1), the most effective control has been from prophylaxis with vaccines (Chapter 25) or drugs. Vaccines have greatly reduced childhood viral diseases and have eliminated smallpox.

**MECHANISM OF ACTION**    Viruses reproduce within mammalian cells, making use of many of the enzymes normally present in dividing cells. The most effective and specific antiviral agent, acyclovir, is specifically activated by a viral enzyme in an infected human cell. Other antiviral drugs are more generally cytotoxic, affecting many normal rapidly growing cells.

**INDICATIONS**    • See Table 23-1 and the listings for individual drugs.

**CONTRAINDICATIONS**    • See listings for individual drugs.

| Table 23-1. | Summary of clinical use of antiviral agents | | |
|---|---|---|---|
| **Drug** | **Viral disease** | | **Route of administration** |
| Acyclovir | Herpes simplex (HSV) type 1 | | PO, topical, IV |
| | Herpes simplex (HSV) type 2 | | PO, topical, IV |
| | Varicella zoster | | PO, IV |
| Amantadine HCl | Influenza Type A | | PO |
| Azidothymidine | Human immunodeficiency virus (HIV) | | PO |
| Idoxuridine | Herpes simplex keratitis | | Ophthalmic |
| Ribavirin | Human syncytial virus | | Inhalation |
| Trifluridine | Herpes simplex keratitis | | Ophthalmic |
| Vidarabine | Herpes simplex keratitis | | Ophthalmic |
| | Herpes simplex encephalitis | | IV |
| | Herpes zoster | | IV |

# acyclovir (a-SYE-klo-veer)

- acyclovir: (acyclovir sodium) Zovirax

**MECHANISM OF ACTION**  Acyclovir is a guanine derivative that must be phosphorylated before it is active. Cells infected with herpesvirus or varicella-zoster virus produce an enzyme called thymidine kinase from viral genes. This enzyme efficiently converts acyclovir from its inactive to its active form, which inhibits viral DNA production and prevents formation of viable virus. Uninfected cells lack an efficient mechanism to activate acyclovir. In this way the drug is directed to be specifically cytoxic toward virus-infected cells.

**INDICATIONS**  **Mucosal and cutaneous herpes simplex** Herpes virus type I (HSV-1) may cause lesions of mouth, esophagus, nose, lips, or face. • Acyclovir reduces symptoms, lessens viral shedding from the lesions, and promotes healing. • Acyclovir does not eradicate the infection, nor does it lessen the number of subsequent recurrent lesions.  **Genital herpesvirus** Herpes virus type II (HSV-2) causes ulcerative or vesicular lesions of the genitalia. • Acyclovir reduces symptoms, lessens viral shedding from the lesions, and promotes healing. • Acyclovir does not eradicate the infection, nor does use of the drug to treat active infections lessen the number of subsequent recurrent lesions.  **Recurrent genital HSV-2** Acyclovir may be used continuously as a prophylactic agent to lessen the frequency and duration of recurrent infections. • Long-term toxicity may limit this use.  **Varicella zoster infections** Acyclovir has been used in limited numbers of patients to control extensive disease caused by varicella zoster (chickenpox) virus.

**CONTRAINDICATIONS**  **Significant renal disease** Acyclovir can be nephrotoxic and should be avoided if possible by patients with pre-existing renal impairment.  **Dehydration** Dehydration increases the risk of nephrotoxicity with acyclovir. • The patient should be well hydrated during the 2 hours following IV infusion.  **Neurological disorders** Acyclovir can cause encephalopathy and should be avoided if possible in patients with neurologic disease or damage caused by drug therapy.

**DOSAGE**  PO:  **ADULT:** For initial genital herpes infections, 200 mg every 4 hours for five doses daily. Treatment should start promptly when lesions appear and continue for 10 days. For prophylaxis of recurrent episodes, 200 mg doses three times daily for up to 6 months have been tested.  **IV: ADULTS AND CHILDREN OVER 12:** 5 mg/kg every 8 hours for 5 to 7 days. Doses must be adjusted, based on renal function.  **CHILDREN:** 250 mg/$M^2$ every 8 hours has been suggested, but data are limited.  **Topical:**  **ADULTS:** Apply 0.5 inch (1.2 cm) ribbon of 5% ointment per 4 inch$^2$ (25 cm$^2$) of skin surface. Use gloves or a finger cot.  *Special patient populations:*  **ELDERLY:** Special geriatric doses have not been established, but doses must be adjusted for renal function, which may be decreased in the elderly.  **RENAL IMPAIRMENT:** Doses must be adjusted, based on renal function. **PREGNANCY:** Safe use is not established. In animals, acyclovir increases fetal resorption in females and diminishes sperm count in males.

**PREPARATIONS**  Acyclovir *Capsules:* 200 mg; *ointment:* 5% ointment for topical use.  **Acyclovir sodium** *Powder for IV solution:* 500 mg (acyclovir). The powder for IV infusion is reconstituted with sterile water for injection or bacteriostatic water to produce a clear, colorless solution. If reconstituted with concentrated dextrose solutions, a harmless yellow discoloration may result. Refrigeration causes a harmless precipitate to form, which may be redissolved by warming to room temperature. Solutions containing parabens are not compatible with acyclovir and cause precipitation of drug.

**DRUG INTERACTIONS**  **Probenecid** slows the renal elimination of acyclovir, increasing the elimination half-life of the antiviral agent.  **Methotrexate** administered intrathecally causes signs of neurologic damage that may mask the signs of damage caused by acyclovir or may worsen the reaction to acyclovir.

**FATE**  Acyclovir is poorly absorbed following oral doses, with only 15% to 30% of the drug entering the blood, producing *peak* plasma concentrations within 1.5 to 2.5 hours. Infusion of acyclovir sodium IV produces predictable peak plasma concentrations. Acyclovir distributes well throughout the body, including the CNS. The drug is excreted by tubular secretion and glomerular filtration in the kidneys, mostly as unchanged drug. The elimination *half-life* ranges from 2.1 to 3.5 hours in patients with normal renal function but is greatly increased in patients with impaired renal function.

## ❦ NURSING CONSIDERATIONS

### Side effects, toxicities, and associated nursing actions

**CNS** Oral acyclovir commonly causes headache (13% of patients) when used longer than 10 days. Therapy of acute disease may cause depression, dizziness, fatigue, headache, insomnia, irritability, and vertigo. About 1% of patients may experience more serious side effects indicating encephalopathy: agitation, coma, confusion, convulsions, hallucinations, lethargy, obtundation, and tremors.

• Review with patients these CNS effects; caution patients to report their appearance.
• Instruct patients to avoid driving or operating hazardous equipment if dizziness, fatigue, vertigo, or confusion develop.

**Blood** Parenteral acyclovir may irritate the vein and surrounding tissues, producing phlebitis, erythema, and pain. Bone marrow hypoplasia, hematopoiesis, leukopenia, lymphopenia, thrombocytopenia, and thrombocytosis are rare and usually reversible.

• Ascertain that the IV line is patent before administering the dose. Use microdrip tubing and an infusion monitoring device to regulate the rate of infusion.
• Inspect the IV insertion site and extremity for signs of irritation, and ask the patient to report irritation or pain.
• Monitor complete blood cell count, white blood cell differential, and platelet count.
• Visually inspect the patient for bruising and petechiae. Instruct the patient to report the development of unexplained bruising or bleeding: nosebleeds, bleeding gums, and hematuria.
• Avoid IM injections in patients with thrombocytopenia.

**GI** Nausea and vomiting occur in about 8% of patients receiving oral acyclovir; diarrhea occurs in about 9%. These reactions are less common with short-term use of acyclovir.

• Assess for the development of GI symptoms. If they are severe or persistent, notify the physician.
• Monitor weight.
• Teach patients to take oral doses with meals or snacks to lessen gastric irritation.

**Renal** Acyclovir can precipitate in the collecting ducts of the kidney, impairing renal function. Because this is a concentration-dependent event, any intervention that decreases the concentration of drug at that site will lessen this complication. Increasing hydration will improve drug solubility. Administering the drug by slow rather than rapid IV infusion also lowers the concentration of the drug in the collecting duct. Renal impairment can be observed in about 10% of patients who receive a parenteral infusion rapidly, but 5% are affected if the infusion is slowed to an hour or longer.

• Encourage a daily fluid intake of 2500 to 3000 ml.
• Use microdrip tubing for IV infusions and an infusion control device.

**Allergic** Rash or urticaria is an occasional complication.

• Instruct patients to report the development of skin rashes.

**Other** Edema, leg cramps, muscle pain, arthralgia, and palpitation have been reported rarely.

• Instruct patients to report the development of any new sign or symptom.

### Nursing interventions related to drug administration

• For IV use, dilute sterile powder per manufacturer's instructions. Further dilute to a concentration of approximately 7 mg/ml or lower; more concentrated solutions are more likely to cause venous irritation and phlebitis. Administer the diluted dose over at least 1 hour.
• For topical use, apply sufficient ointment to cover the lesions at the ordered frequency. For best results, instruct the patient to avoid omitting applications or stopping therapy before the prescribed course has been completed. A finger cot or rubber glove should be worn on the hand of the individual applying the ointment to reduce the possibility of spreading the infection.

### Patient and family education

• Review with patients the anticipated benefits and possible side effects of drug therapy.
• Refer patients with recurrent genital herpes to local support groups if appropriate.
• Review with patients the general measures needed to decrease the spread of the disease. It is possible to transmit herpes even if no visible lesions are present, but it is more likely to be spread if lesions are present. Instruct patients to avoid sexual activity if either partner has any lesions or scabs present. Use of a condom can probably help prevent the spread, although use of a diaphragm and/or sper-

micidal jelly does not limit the spread of genital herpes. Point out that acyclovir does not limit the spread of genital herpes.

- Keep areas of infection clean and dry, and wear loose-fitting garments. Use acyclovir as ordered. Do not use other creams or ointments unless prescribed by the physician.
- Teach female patients that women with genital herpes may be more likely to get cancer of the cervix. Encourage women to get an annual Pap smear to check for this cancer.
- Acyclovir works best when treatment is begun as soon as possible after the symptoms of herpes appear. Instruct patients to keep an adequate supply on hand or to contact the physician as soon as symptoms appear in order to obtain more medication.

## amantadine hydrochloride    (uh-MAN-ta-deen)    antiviral

- amantadine hydrochloride: Symmetrel

**MECHANISM OF ACTION**    Amantadine is primarily a prophylactic agent because the drug must be present to prevent infection of mammalian cells; it does not act on cells that are already actively infected. Amantadine may interfere with penetration of viruses into cells or may prevent uncoating of the virus within the cell. Either of these actions could block clinically significant infection.

**INDICATIONS**    **Prophylaxis of influenza type A infections** The prevention rate is reported to be 50% to 70%.
- Prophylactic use of amantadine may also lessen the severity of illness in those patients who do develop disease.    **Therapy of influenze type A infections** If administered within 24 hours of the onset of disease, amantadine may lessen the severity of illness for some patients.

**CONTRAINDICATIONS**    **CNS disease** Epilepsy, seizures, or uncontrolled psychoses may mask signs of amantadine CNS toxicity.

**DOSAGE**    **PO:**    **CHILDREN OVER 10 AND ADULTS TO AGE 64:** 200 mg daily in two divided doses. Doses must be reduced to 100 mg daily in two divided doses in patients with a history of seizure disorders or with renal impairment.    **CHILDREN 1 TO 9:** 4.4 to 8.8 mg/kg daily in two doses, not to exceed 150 mg total daily. Doses must be reduced in renal failure or in patients with a history of seizure disorders. *Special patient populations:*    **ELDERLY:** Doses should not exceed 100 mg daily in two divided doses; adjustment based on renal function may be necessary.    **RENAL IMPAIRMENT:** Doses must be adjusted, based on renal function.    **PREGNANCY:** Safe use is not established. Amantadine is embryotoxic and teratogenic in rats at high doses. Amantadine is found in breast milk.

**PREPARATIONS**    *Capsules:* 100 mg; *solution:* 50 mg/5 ml syrup.

**DRUG INTERACTIONS**    **CNS stimulants** may increase the CNS side effects of amantadine. Patients may find it difficult to concentrate or to perform hazardous activities such as driving a car.    **Anticholinergic agents** (e.g., atropine) may be potentiated by the anticholinergic effects of amantadine. One sign may be nocturnal confusion and hallucinations.

**FATE**    Amantadine hydrochloride is well absorbed following oral administration, producing *peak* plasma concentrations within 1 to 4 hours. Amantadine distribution in humans is not thoroughly known, but in animals the drug distributes to the CNS (50% plasma concentrations) and lungs, where concentrations exceed plasma concentrations. Amantadine is excreted unchanged in urine, with a *half-life* in young adults of about 24 hours. The half-life is prolonged in older, healthy adults and in any age patient with significant renal impairment.

### ☙ NURSING CONSIDERATIONS
#### Side effects, toxicities, and associated nursing actions
**CNS** Amantadine causes amphetaminelike stimulation of the CNS, which may increase the risk of seizures and worsen psychotic disorders. In addition the drug may cause ataxia, anxiety, confusion, dizziness, depression, forgetfulness, inability to concentrate, insomnia, irritability, lethargy, slurred speech, and weakness.
- Review CNS side effects with patients and families. Instruct patients to notify the physician if these symptoms develop.

- Caution patients to avoid driving or operating hazardous equipment if ataxia, dizziness, or confusion develop.
- If insomnia occurs, suggest that the patient take the last dose of the day several hours before retiring.
- Instruct the patient to try taking the prescribed amount in two or more divided doses daily to lessen side effects.

**CV** Congestive heart failure, edema, and orthostatic hypotension have been reported.

- Monitor blood pressure, pulse, and weight. Auscultate breath sounds. Monitor dependent areas for development of edema.
- If orthostatic hypotension develops, instruct patients to move slowly from lying to sitting or standing. Supervise ambulation, especially of elderly patients, when drug therapy is first begun. Keep side rails up at night.

**GI** Abdominal discomfort, anorexia, constipation, nausea, and vomiting have been reported.

- Assess patients for development of GI side effects. If side effects are persistent or severe, notify the physician.
- Monitor weight.

**Renal** Urinary retention or increased frequency of urination have both been reported.

- Be alert to urinary retention, especially in the elderly or the immobilized. Instruct the patient to report sensation of inadequate bladder emptying or difficulty voiding. Suggest the patient void before taking a dose of amantadine.
- If urinary frequency develops, assist the patient to rule out other causes; notify the physician.

**Skin** Livedo reticularis may occur when amantadine is given for prolonged periods. This condition is characterized by a reddish blue network mottling of the skin, usually on the legs. The cause of livedo reticularis is related to the passive congestion of the superficial capillaries of the skin; the severity is relieved by elevating the legs.

- Review this side effects with patients.

**Other** Visual disturbances have rarely been reported.

- Instruct the patient to report visual disturbances to the physician. Caution patients to avoid driving or operating hazardous equipment if visual disturbances develop.

### Patient and family education
- Review with patients the anticipated benefits and possible side effects of therapy.

---

## idoxuridine  (eye-dox-YOO-reh-deen)                                                    antiviral

- idoxuridine: Herplex, Stoxil

**MECHANISM OF ACTION**  Idoxuridine is incorporated in viral DNA, making the DNA more prone to UV damage and strand breakage. The result may be death or inhibition of the virus. Idoxuridine can be incorporated into certain rapidly growing human cells, damaging bone marrow and GI epithelium. These actions prevent the systemic use of the drug.

**INDICATIONS**  Herpes simplex keratitis Initial epithelial infections respond better to topical idoxuridine than deeper infections or recurrent infections. • Corneal scarring is not reversed by idoxuridine.

**CONTRAINDICATIONS**  Deep corneal ulceration Idoxuridine may delay healing and cause corneal perforation.

**DOSAGE**  Ophthalmic Apply the ointment to the conjuntival sac every 4 hours for five doses, with the last dose at bedtime. Instill one drop of the solution every hour during waking periods and every 2 hours during sleep periods. Therapy should continue for about 21 days.  *Special patient populations:*  CHILDREN: Doses are not established.  PREGNANCY: Safe use is not established.

**PREPARATIONS**  *Ointment:* 0.5% (petrolatum base); *solution:* 0.1% (Herplex Liquifilm: with 1.4% polyvinyl alcohol, benzalkonium chloride, and EDTA, or Stoxil, with 1:50,000 thimerosal).

**DRUG INTERACTIONS**  Corticosteroids may accelerate the spread of infections in the eye and should not be used for superficial keratitis. Rarely, corticosteroids and idoxuridine are combined for treating more serious keratic lesions.  Boric acid is excessively irritating when used with idoxuridine.

**FATE**  Some uptake of drug into the blood occurs in animals receiving ophthalmic preparations.

## ☙ NURSING CONSIDERATIONS
### Side effects, toxicities, and associated nursing actions
**Allergic** Allergic reactions are rare.

**Eye** Irritation, inflammation, pain, and pruritis are possible reactions. Mild edema of the eyelids and cornea may occur. Photophobia is rare. Corneal stippling, corneal clouding, or the formation of small punctate defects in the corneal epithelium can be caused by the drug.
- Review these possible side effects with patients. Instruct patients to report the development of any new sign or symptom. If side effects in the eye are severe or persistent, notify the physician.
- Reinforce to patients the need to use the drug only as ordered and to return as directed for follow-up visits.

### Nursing interventions related to drug administration
- Ascertain that the patient can correctly administer dose into lower conjunctival sac.
- Avoid having the applicator touch any part of the eye itself. Each patient should have a separate applicator.

### Patient and family education
- Review with patients the anticipated benefits and possible side effects of therapy.
- Reinforce to patients that the best effect of this drug will be achieved by using it as directed and not omitting any doses.

---

## ribavirin  (rye-ba-VYE-rin)                                               antiviral

- ribavirin: Virazole

**MECHANISM OF ACTION**  Ribavirin is enzymatically converted to an activated metabolite that inhibits formation of guanine monophosphate. As a result, viral RNA synthesis is inhibited. Ribavirin has a very broad spectrum of antiviral activity, including human respiratory syncytial virus (RSV), influenza types A and B, and herpes.

**INDICATIONS**  **Respiratory syncytial virus (RSV) infections** RSV infections, causing bronchiolitis and pneumonia, are especially dangerous for infants and other youngsters with additional cardiopulmonary disorders.

**CONTRAINDICATIONS**  None yet established.

**DOSAGE**  **Inhalation:**  **INFANTS AND CHILDREN ONLY:** 20 mg/ml delivered as an aerosol by Viratex Small Particle Aerosol Generator (SPAG). Administration is for 12 to 18 hours daily for 3 to 7 days, starting within 3 days of the onset of symptoms. *Special patient populations:*  **ELDERLY:** Not yet indicated for this age group.  **PREGNANCY:** Not yet indicated for this age group.

**PREPARATIONS**  *Powder for preparation of sterile solution:* 6 g, to be reconstituted with 300 ml of sterile water.

**DRUG INTERACTIONS**  None yet established.

**FATE**  Although ribavirin may be effective against some infections when administered orally, the only current indication for the agent is for pulmonary infections. Inhalation of aerosolized drug achieves better drug delivery to the site of infection with lower incidence of side effects.

## ☙ NURSING CONSIDERATIONS
### Side effects, toxicities, and associated nursing actions
**CNS** Mild frontal headaches have been noted in adults taking oral doses.
- Assess patients for development of headache; if they are severe or persistent, notify the physician.

**Other** Little toxicity is noted with administration by inhalation to infants.
- Monitor patients for side effects or any unexpected sign or symptom.

### Nursing interventions related to drug administration
- Review manufacturer's instructions for correct use of inhalation delivery device.

### Patient and family education
- Review with parents the anticipated benefits and possible side effects of drug therapy.

## trifluridine    (try-FLOO-reh-deen)    antiviral

- trifluridine: Viroptic

**MECHANISM OF ACTION**    Trifluridine is incorporated into defective DNA and may inhibit viral DNA synthesis. The drug is effective against herpes virus types 1 and 2, as well as vaccinia.

**INDICATIONS**    **Herpes simplex keratitis and keratoconjunctivitis** Trifluridine is applied topically to treat infections caused by herpesvirus type 1 or 2. • Trifluridine may also be successfully used in infections resistant to vidarabine or idoxuridine.

**CONTRAINDICATIONS**    **Allergy to trifluridine** Sensitivity to trifluridine or components of the formulation may preclude use.

**DOSAGE**    **Ophthalmic** One drop of 1% solution is applied every 2 hours, up to nine drops daily. Healing should start by 7 days and be apparent by 14 days. Avoid use for longer than 21 days.    *Special patient populations:*    **CHILDREN:** Doses are not established.    **PREGNANCY:** Safe use is not established.

**PREPARATIONS**    *Solution:* 1% with 0.001% thimerosal.

**DRUG INTERACTIONS**    None established.

**FATE**    Little trifluridine is absorbed systemically from ocular administration.

### 🐦 NURSING CONSIDERATIONS

#### Side effects, toxicities, and associated nursing actions

**Allergic** Sensitization is rare.

**Eye** Mild burning or stinging can occur on instillation into the eye. Palpebral edema may also occur. Superficial punctate keratopathy, stromal edema, and increased intraocular pressure are less common.

- Review these possible side effects with patients. Instruct patients to report the development of any new sign or symptom. If side effects in the eye are severe or persistent, notify the physician.
- Reinforce to patients the need to use the drug only as ordered and to return as directed for follow-up visits.

#### Nursing interventions related to drug administration

- Ascertain that the patient can correctly administer the dose into the lower conjunctival sac.
- Avoid having the applicator touch any part of the eye itself. Each patient should have a separate applicator.

#### Patient and family education

- Review with patients the anticipated benefits and possible side effects of therapy.
- Reinforce to patients that the best effect of this drug will be achieved by using it as directed and not omitting any doses.

## vidarabine    (vi-DARE-uh-been)    antiviral

- vidarabine (adenine arabinoside): Vira-A

**MECHANISM OF ACTION**    Vidarabine may inhibit DNA polymerase, blocking replication of viruses. Vidarabine is effective against herpes virus types 1 and 2, varicella zoster, cytomegalovirus, vaccinia, and hepatitis B.

**INDICATIONS**    **Herpes simplex keratitis and keratoconjunctivitis** Topical vidarabine is often effective in treating this infection, even in patients whose condition has failed to respond to idoxuridine.    **Herpes simplex encephalitis** Patients may respond if treated very early in the course of the disease.    **Herpes zoster (shingles)** When used in immunocompromised patients, symptoms are diminished and the disease course is shortened.

**CONTRAINDICATIONS**    **Water retention** Patients prone to fluid overload because of renal impairment or patients with cerebral edema may not be able to tolerate the large volumes of fluid required to dissolve vidarabine.

**DOSAGE**    IV:    ADULTS AND CHILDREN: For herpetic encephalitis, 15 mg/kg daily for 10 days. For varicella zoster, 10 mg/kg for 5 days. Doses must be adjusted for renal status.    **Ophthalmic** Apply 7 cm of 3% ointment every 3 hours for five doses daily, up to 21 days. *Special patient populations:* PREGNANCY: Safe use is not established.

**PREPARATIONS**    *Solution:* 200 mg/ml concentrate to dilute for IV infusion; *ophthalmic ointment:* 3%.

**DRUG INTERACTIONS**    Allopurinol may interfere with the metabolism of vidarabine. When given together, anemia, nausea, pain, pruritus, and tremors have occurred in a few patients.

**FATE**    Vidarabine is inadequately absorbed with oral or IM administration. When administered IV, the drug is rapidly but incompletely converted to a less potent derivative. Vidarabine and its major metabolite are well distributed to body tissues and fluids, with adequate penetration of the CNS. Excretion is mainly by the kidneys, but little unchanged vidarabine is eliminated.

## ☙ NURSING CONSIDERATIONS

### Side effects, toxicities, and associated nursing actions

**CNS** Ataxia, confusion, dizziness, hallucinations, malaise, psychosis, tremors, and weakness have been reported with parenteral use of vidarabine.

- Obtain a careful baseline neurologic examination, and monitor closely.
- Review with patients and families the possible CNS side effects. Instruct patients to report the development of these side effects.
- Caution patients to avoid driving or operating hazardous equipment if confusion or dizziness occur.

**Blood** Lowered leukocyte, platelet, and reticulocyte counts may occur, along with lowered hemoglobin and hematocrit. Pain and thrombophlebitis at the infusion site can also occur.

- Monitor complete blood cell count, white blood cell differential, and platelet count.
- Assess patients for pallor, fatigue, bruising, and petechiae.
- Instruct patients to report unexplained bruising or bleeding, bleeding gums, nosebleeds, hematuria, sore throat, fever, or malaise.
- Inspect the infusion site frequently for signs of thrombophlebitis. Instruct patients to report irritation or pain at the infusion site. Ascertain that the IV line is patent before administering IV doses.

**GI** Anorexia, diarrhea, nausea, vomiting, and weight loss are among the most common symptoms of parenteral vidarabine.

- Monitor weight.
- If GI symptoms are severe or persistent, notify the physician.

**Eye** Burning, itching, and transient irritation are common with ophthalmic administration. Lacrimation, conjunctival injection, superficial punctate keratitis, and stromal edema may occur.

- Review these possible side effects with the patient. Instruct patients to report the development of any new sign or symptom. If side effects in the eye are severe or persistent, notify the physician.
- Reinforce to patients the need to use the drug only as ordered and to return as directed for follow-up visits.

### Nursing interventions related to drug administration

- For IV use, shake the drug carefully to promote uniform suspension before preparing an IV dose. Dilute each 1 mg of drug with 2.22 ml of infusion solution (1 l of infusion solution will dilute 450 mg of vidarabine.) Any IV solution can be used except blood, blood products, or protein solutions. Thoroughly agitate the diluted solution to promote uniform suspension. Infuse the total dose over 12 to 24 hours. Use an inline filter of 45 μm or smaller. Use an infusion controlling device to help ensure an even infusion rate.
- For ophthalmic use, ascertain that the patient can correctly administer the dose into the lower conjunctival sac.
- Avoid having the applicator of ophthalmic doses touch any part of the eye itself. Each patient should have a separate applicator.

### Patient and family education

- Review with patients the anticipated benefits and possible side effects of drug therapy.

## zidovudine   (zee-doh-VUE-deen)   antiviral

- zidovudine: Retrovir; also known as azidothymidine, or AZT

**MECHANISM OF ACTION**   Zidovudine may be effective against retroviruses such as HIV (human immunodeficiency virus) because reverse transcriptase uses zidovudine instead of normal thymidine to form defective DNA. Without active DNA, the rest of the life cycle of the retrovirus cannot proceed.

**INDICATIONS**   **AIDS and AIDS-related complex (ARC)** Zidovudine was initially tested in AIDS patients with pneumonia caused by *Pneumocystis carinii;* it has subsequently been shown to prolong the lives of AIDS patients and patients with ARC as well. • As of 1988, this drug is the only agent available for AIDS therapy, but a number of other drugs are under development. • Consult the current literature for information about this rapidly changing field.

**CONTRAINDICATIONS**   Although significant toxicity results from the use of zidovudine, no contraindications are cited because of the invariable fatal outcome of HIV infections.

**DOSAGE**   **PO:**   **ADULT:** 200 mg every 4 hours around the clock. Doses may be reduced if bone marrow is depressed. Therapy is continued for life. *Special patient populations:* **CHILDREN:** Pediatric doses are not completely established.   **PREGNANCY:** Safe use not established.

**PREPARATIONS**   *Capsules:* 100 mg.

**DRUG INTERACTIONS**   **Cytotoxic agents** such as those used in cancer chemotherapy may severely depress bone marrow, adding to the suppression produced by zidovudine.

**FATE**   Azidothymidine is well absorbed orally and distributes well to most tissues, including the CNS. The oral bioavailability is 60% to 70% because the first pass through the liver results in significant metabolism to inactive products. The drug has a *half-life* in plasma of only 1 hour, requiring that doses be given frequently (every 4 hours) in order to maintain effective drug concentrations in the body.

### ❦ NURSING CONSIDERATIONS

#### Side effects, toxicities, and associated nursing actions

**CNS** Headaches have been reported in roughly 30% of patients. Anxiety and confusion may also occur.

- Review these side effects with patients; if symptoms are severe or persistent, notify the physician.

**Blood** Bone marrow suppression is the dose-limiting toxicity for azidothymidine. Doses may be lowered based on the amount of suppression produced by standard doses of the drug. Blood transfusions may be required in up to 25% of patients.

- Monitor complete blood cell count, white blood cell differential, and platelet count.
- Monitor temperature, and pulse.
- Assess patients for pallor and fatigue. Instruct patients to report the development of fever, malaise, or sore throat.

**Allergic** A few patients have reported rashes.

- Instruct patients to report the development of rashes.

#### Patient and family education

- Review with patients the anticipated benefits and possible side effects of drug therapy.
- Instruct patients to report the development of any unexpected sign or symptom. As more information becomes available on this drug, it should be possible to provide patients with more information about possible side effects.

# Chapter Twenty-four

# Drugs used to treat diseases caused by protozoans and helminths

carbarsone
chloroquine hydrochloride
chloroquine phosphate
clotrimazole
co-trimoxazole (see Chapter Twenty, p. 332)
emetine hydrochloride
furazolidone
hydroxychloroquine sulfate
iodoquinol
mebendazole
metronidazole
metronidazole hydrochloride
niclosamide
oxamniquine

paromomycin sulfate (see Chapter Sixteen, p. 283)
pentamidine isethionate
piperazine citrate
praziquantel
primaquine phosphate
pyrantel pamoate
pyrimethamine
quinacrine hydrochloride
quinine sulfate
sulfadiazine (see Chapter Twenty, p. 328)
sulfadoxine with pyrimethamine
tetracycline (See Chapter Seventeen, p. 293)
thiabendazole

**OVERVIEW OF THE DRUG CLASS**   Diseases caused by protozoans and helminths may often be prevented by proper sanitation because many of the parasites are passed from host to host in fecally contaminated food or water. Examples of diseases transmitted in this way include amebiasis, ascariasis, cestodiasis, giardiasis, enterobiasis, and toxoplasmosis (Table 24-1). Some parasitic infestations are passed from person to person through other hosts. For example, malaria is transmitted by the bite of the infected mosquito, and schistosomiasis is passed to humans by snails. Although many of the diseases discussed in this chapter are relatively rare in North America, they cause suffering and death in untold millions of people worldwide.

**MECHANISM OF ACTION**   Treatment of these varied diseases depends on the site of infestation and the life cycle of the parasite. Parasites that are restricted to the intestinal lumen are often easily treated by drugs that are not absorbed systemically (e.g., iodoquinol or mebendazole). Parasites that invade the bloodstream or tissues require specific systemic agents.

**INDICATIONS**   Treatment of the diseases listed in Table 24-1 A few drugs are effective against several pathogenic parasites, but many are quite specific and are employed for only one disease. • See individual drug listings.

**CONTRAINDICATIONS**   • See individual drug listings.

## ☙ NURSING CONSIDERATIONS
### Patient and family education
- Remind patients to keep these and all medications out of the reach of children. Many of the medications in this class are available in pleasant-tasting syrups or chewable tablets, which may tempt young children.
- Remind patients to keep all health care providers informed of all drugs being used or that have been used in the preceding 6 months.
- Most of these drugs are not recommended for use in pregnancy unless absolutely necessary and should not be used during lactation. Question female patients about possible pregnancy before administering.
- Reinforce to patients the need to continue the course of medication for as long as prescribed and to avoid discontinuing medication without notifying the physician. Remind patients to consult the physician about signs, symptoms, or concerns that develop.
- Remind the patient to use medications only as directed.
- Review with patients and families appropriate ways to treat or prevent the disease being treated. Review as appropriate such activities as handwashing, sanitation, and care of infected bedding or clothing. Information about diseases caused by protozoa and helminths may be obtained from

**Table 24-1.  Drugs used to treat diseases caused by protozoans or helminths**

| Diseases | Symptoms | Causative organism | Transmission | Therapy |
| --- | --- | --- | --- | --- |
| Amebiasis | Diarrhea, dysentery, organ abscesses | Amebae (*Entamoeba histolytica*) | Ingestion of fecally contaminated food or water containing cyst forms of amebae | Carbarsone, chloroquine, emetine, iodoquinol, metronidazole, paromomycin |
| Ascariasis | Colicky intestinal pains, organ damage | Roundworms (*Ascaris lumbricoides*) | Ingestion of fecally contaminated food or water containing eggs of *Ascaris* | Mebendazole, piperazine, pyrantel pamoate, thiabendazole |
| Cestodiasis | Often without symptoms, except when larvae of *T. solium* invade tissues and damage organs | Tapeworms (*Taenia saginata, T. solium, Hymenolepis nana. Diphyllobothrium latum*) | Ingestion of fecally contaminated food or water containing eggs of cestode | Niclosamide, paromomycin, praziquantel, quinacrine |
| Cutaneous larva migrans | Skin inflammation often called creeping eruption | Dog or cat hookworm (*Ancylostoma braziliense*) | Exposure to soil containing cat or dog feces produced by infected animals | Thiabendazole |
| Enterobiasis | Anal or perianal itching; pruritus ani or pruritus vulvae | Pinworms (*Enterobius vermicularis*) | Ingestion of eggs that adhere to bedding, towels and clothing of infected persons | Mebendazole, piperazine, pyrantel pamoate |
| Giardiasis | Intestinal distress, diarrhea, or malabsorption | Protozoan (*Giardia lamblia*) | Ingestion of fecally contaminated soil or water containing cysts of *Giardia* | Furazolidone, metronidazole, quinacrine |
| Malaria | Fever, chills, malaise | Protozoan (*Plasmodium falciparum, P. ovale, P. vivax, P. malariae*) | Bite of infected mosquito of the genus *Anopheles* | Chloroquine, hydroxychloroquine, primaquine, pyrimethamine, quinacrine, quinine sulfadoxine with pyrimethamine (Fansidar) |
| Necatoriasis | Skin eruptions, abdominal pain, colic, diarrhea, or anemia | Hookworms (*Necator americanus, Ancylostoma duodenale*) | Contact with fecally contaminated soil containing larvae that can burrow through the skin to begin the life cycle | Mebendazole, thiabendazole |

| Disease | Symptoms | Organism | Transmission | Drugs |
|---|---|---|---|---|
| Pneumocystosis | Interstitial pneumonia | *Pneumocystis carinii* | Ubiquitous organism usually produces disease only in immune-compromised patients | Co-trimoxazole, pentamidine |
| Schistosomiasis | Destruction of tissues, fibrosis, congestion in veins, bladder or intestinal damage | Flukes (*Schistosoma mansoni, S. japonicum, S. haematobium*) | Contact with water containing larval forms that penetrate the skin and migrate to various body sites; the intermediate hosts are fresh-water snails | Oxamniquine, praziquantel |
| Strongyloidiasis | Diarrhea, hemorrhage in the lung, and intestinal perforation | Threadworm (*Strongyloides stercoralis*) | Contact with fecally contaminated soil containing larva of the threadworm, which may penetrate through exposed skin | Thiabendazole |
| Toxoplasmosis | Mild mononucleosislike symptoms in adults; fetal infections lead to severe CNS damage | Protozoan (*Toxoplasma gondii*) | Contact with soil containing oocysts passed by infected cats. | Pyrimethamine |
| Trichinosis | Diarrhea, colic, fever, nausea, muscle pain or stiffness, blood dyscrasias, and insomnia | Pork worm or nematode (*Trichinella spiralis*) | Eating pig or bear meat cooked insufficiently to kill encysted organisms. | Mebendazole |
| Trichomoniasis | Intractable vaginal discharge, irritation of bladder, urethra, or vagina | Protozoan (*Trichomonas vaginalis*) | Sexual contact with an infected person | Clotrimazole, metronidazole |
| Trichuriasis | Diarrhea, vomiting, or rectal prolapse; may also be asymptomatic | Whipworm (*Trichuris trichiura*) | Ingestion of fecally contaminated food or water | Thiabendazole |

the local health department or the Centers for Disease Control in Atlanta.
- Individuals contemplating international travel may wish to contact the Centers for Disease Control about health hazards in countries they will be visiting.
- Refer patients and families as needed to the local public health department.

## carbarsone (KAR-bar-zone) amebicide

- carbarsone: Carbarsone

**MECHANISM OF ACTION** Carbarsone is a rarely used organic arsenical that selectively inhibits sulfhydryl enzymes in parasitic ameba. The drug is a contact amebicide with little effect outside the lumen of the intestine.

**INDICATIONS** **Amebiasis** Carbarsone is used only in intestinal amebiasis, usually with other drug theray.

**CONTRAINDICATIONS** **Liver or renal disease** Patients with pre-existing damage to these organs may not be able to tolerate this toxic drug. **Visual field changes** Carbarsone may damage the retina. **Sensitivity to arsenicals** Carbarsone is an arsenical and may precipitate severe reactions in allergic patients.

**DOSAGE** **PO:** **ADULTS:** 250 mg two or three times daily for 10 days. Retreatment should begin no sooner than 10 days after the end of a course of therapy. **CHILDREN:** The total dosage is 75 mg/kg; this dosage is divided into three daily doses over 10 days. *Special patient populations:* **PREGNANCY:** Safe use in pregnancy and lactation is not established.

**PREPARATIONS** *Capsules:* 250 mg.

**DRUG INTERACTIONS** None have been established.

**FATE** Carbarsone is absorbed from the intestinal tract following oral administration. The drug may be metabolized and slowly excreted by the kidneys. Accumulation of the drug occurs.

### NURSING CONSIDERATIONS

#### Side effects, toxicities, and associated nursing actions

**CNS** Hemorrhagic encephalitis may occur as evidence of arsenic toxicity, as may the signs listed below.
- Obtain a baseline neurologic examination, and repeat as needed.
- Instruct patients and families to report the development of any new sign or symptom.

**Blood** Agranulocytosis and aplastic anemia can occur.
- Monitor the complete blood cell count and white blood cell differential.
- Instruct patients to report the development of fever, malaise, or sore throat.

**GI** Anorexia, constipation, cramps, diarrhea, epigastric pain, gastritis, nausea, vomiting, and weight loss may occur.
- Instruct patients to report GI symptoms if severe or persistent.
- If GI symptoms are prominent, monitor weight, intake and output, and serum electrolytes.

**Renal** Polyuria and albuminuria may occur.
- Monitor urinalysis.
- Instruct patients to report excessive urination.

**Liver** Hepatitis, jaundice, and liver necrosis can occur.
- Assess the patient for jaundice, malaise, fever, right upper quadrant abdominal pain, or change in the color or consistency of stools.
- Monitor liver function tests.

**Other** Edema, splenomegaly, dermatoses, neuritis, fever, and the signs listed previously may all be manifestations of arsenic toxicity.
- Instruct patients to report fever that persists longer than 24 hours.
- Instruct patients to report the development of tight rings, shoes, or clothing. Inspect for development of edema.
- Arsenic toxicity may be treated with dimercaprol (BAL).

#### Nursing interventions related to drug administration
- The capsule may be opened, if necessary, and the contents mixed with a small amount of milk,

orange juice, 1% sodium bicarbonate solution, jelly, or other food for ease in administration.
- The drug has also been administered rectally as a retention enema; consult the manufacturer's literature.

**Patient and family education**
- Review with patients the anticipated benefits and possible side effects of drug therapy.
- See Dosage. Reinforce to patients that at least 10 days should elapse before retreatment; caution patients to keep health care providers informed of drugs that have been taken.
- See entry for drug class (p. 413).

---

## chloroquine hydrochloride
## chloroquine phosphate    (KLOR-oh-kwin)    antimalarial

- chloroquine: Aralen

**MECHANISM OF ACTION**  Chloroquine may interfere with the ability of plasmodia to digest hemoglobin; the drug also binds to DNA of the parasite and may prevent nucleic acid synthesis. Chloroquine is a 4-amino-quinoline and, like other related drugs, possesses a variety of antiinflammatory actions. For this reason, the drug has occasionally been tried in rheumatoid arthritis and lupus erythematosus.

**INDICATIONS**  **Malaria, suppression, or chemoprophylaxis of disease caused by Plasmodium malariae, P. ovale, P. vivax, or susceptible strains of** *P. falciparum* The addition of other drugs (pyrimethamine and sulfadoxine) may be required when exposure is prolonged or when risk of chloroquine-resistant *P. falciparum* is great.  **Malaria, treatment of mild or moderate disease caused by** *Plasmodium malariae, P. ovale, P. vivax,* or susceptible strains of *P. falciparum* Chloroquine is effective only against the asexual erythrocytic forms of plasmodia.  **Amebiasis** Chloroquine can be effective against amebic disease that has spread beyond the intestine but is not useful for disease limited to the intestinal lumen or wall.

**CONTRAINDICATIONS**  **Glucose-6-phosphate-dehydrogenase deficiency (G-6PDH)** Patients with this genetic condition may be more prone to hematologic toxicity, including hemolysis.  **Porphyria** Chloroquine may exacerbate this condition.  **Psoriasis** Chloroquine may worsen this chronic skin condition.  **Visual field or retinal changes** Chloroquine and related drugs may directly damage vision and should be avoided when possible in patients with pre-existing damage.

**DOSAGE**  **PO:**  **ADULTS:** For chemoprophylaxis of malaria, 300 mg chloroquine (500 mg chloroquine phosphate) once weekly for 2 weeks preceding and during exposure and for 6 to 8 weeks following exposure. For treatment of malaria, 600 mg chloroquine (1 g chloroquine phosphate) initially, followed by 300 mg chloroquine 6, 24, and 48 hours later. For treatment of amebiasis, 600 mg chloroquine (1 g chloroquine phosphate) is administered once daily for 2 days, followed by 300 mg chloroquine once daily for 1 to 2 weeks.  **CHILDREN:** For chemoprophylaxis of malaria, 5 mg/kg chloroquine once weekly on the same schedule as for adults. For treatment of malaria, 10 mg/kg chloroquine (16.7 mg/kg chloroquine phosphate) initially, followed by 5 mg/kg chloroquine 6, 24, and 48 hours later. For treatment of amebiasis, 10 mg/kg chloroquine (16.7 mg/kg chloroquine phosphate) once daily for 2 to 3 weeks.  **IM:**  **ADULTS:** For treatment of malaria, 200 mg chloroquine (250 mg chloroquine hydrochloride) every 6 hours. Oral doses should be substituted as soon as possible.  **CHILDREN:** Chloroquine should not be administered parenterally to this age group. *Special patient populations:*  **CHILDREN:** Chloroquine and the other 4-aminoquinolines are especially toxic to children. The drugs should be avoided unless the benefits clearly outweigh the risks.  **PREGNANCY:** Safe use in pregnancy and lactation has not been established. Chloroquine may cause CNS toxicity and may accumulate in fetal eyes.

**PREPARATIONS**  Chloroquine hydrochloride *Solution for injection:* 40 mg of chloroquine per milliliter  Chloroquine phosphate *Tablets:* 150 and 300 mg chloroquine.  **Combination products** *Tablets:* 300 mg chloroquine with 45 mg primaquine as the phosphate.

**DRUG INTERACTIONS**  **Hepatotoxic drugs** may increase liver damage, which is a possible side efect of chloroquine. **Chronic alcohol use** may cause liver damage that can predispose a patient to toxicity from chloroquine.

**FATE** Chloroquine is rapidly and completely absorbed following oral administration, producing *peak* blood concentrations within 1 to 2 hours. Bioavailability is increased by taking the drug with food. The drug is widely distributed and concentrates heavily in tissues such as lung, liver, and spleen, where concentrations are 200 to 700 times those in plasma. The drug also concentrates in brain and eye tissues, as well as in red blood cells. The plasma *half-life* of chloroquine is 72 to 120 hours. Elimination is by metabolism in the liver and slow excretion by the kidneys. Acidification of the urine speeds excretion by the kidneys.

## ❦ NURSING CONSIDERATIONS

### Side effects, toxicities, and associated nursing actions

**Eye** Ocular toxicity is the most common serious reaction to chloroquine. Damage is most severe with long-term administration of large doses. Retinopathy may progress after the drug is discontinued and has resulted in blindness.
• Instruct patients to report any visual changes.
• Encourage patients on long-term therapy to have regular ophthalmic examinations.

**CNS** Aggressiveness, agitation, anxiety, apathy, confusion, depression, fatigue, headache, irritability, nervousness, personality changes, psychotic episodes, seizures, and toxic psychosis may occur. Neuromyopathy may occur, usually with high doses over long periods, and is reversible.
• Obtain a baseline assessment of neurologic function and mental status; repeat at regular intervals.
• Caution the patient to report the development of personality changes or other CNS side effects.
• Assess for signs of depression: withdrawal, lack of interest in personal appearance, insomnia, or anorexia.

**CV** Hypotension and ECG changes may occur, especially with high doses.
• Monitor blood pressure and ECG, especially in patients on long-term therapy.
• Monitor blood pressure before and after parenteral doses.

**Blood** Agranulocytosis, aplastic anemia, neutropenia, and thrombocytopenia may occur. Hemolysis and acute renal failure are more likely in G-6-PD deficiency.
• Question the patient about G-6-PD deficiency before administering the drug. This deficiency is more common in American blacks, Sardinians, and Kurdish Jews.
• Instruct patients to notify the physician if the following signs develop: pallor, malaise, sore throat, fever, unexplained bleeding or bruising, or darkening of the color of urine.
• Monitor complete blood cell count, white blood cell differential, platelet count, serum creatinine, and BUN.

**GI** Abdominal cramps, anorexia, diarrhea, epigastric distress, nausea, and vomiting may occur but are lessened when the drug is given with meals.
• Instruct patients to notify the physician if GI symptoms are severe or persistent.
• Teach the patient to take doses with meals or snack.

**Hearing** Nerve deafness is a rare complication of therapy.
• Monitor hearing acuity.
• Instruct the patient to report any hearing loss.

### Patient and family education
• Review with the patient how to take medication (see Dosage).
• See entry for drug class (p. 413).

---

## clotrimazole  (klo-TRY-ma-zole)                                      antifungal agent

• clotrimazole: Gyne-Lotrimin, Lotrimin, Mycelex, ✤Myclo

**INDICATIONS** **Trichomoniasis** Clotrimazole is an alternative to metronidazole for this condition. • For clinical data and uses of clotrimazole as an antifungal agent, see Chapter 22 (p. 392).

## 🐦 NURSING CONSIDERATIONS

- See Table 22-2.
- See entry for drug class (p. 413).
- Ascertain that patients can apply vaginal creams correctly or insert other vaginal forms correctly, if available.
- Vaginal medication should be used as ordered, even if during menstrual period, for best effect. If applying vaginal medications during menstrual periods, teach the patient that sanitary napkins should be used instead of tampons.

## co-trimoxazole (ko-try-MOX-uh-zole) antibacterial

- co-trimoxazole (sulfamethoxaxole and trimethoprim): Bactrim, Bethaprim, Comoxol, Co-trim, ✤Protrin, ✤Roubac, Septra, SMZ-TMP, Sulfatrim

**INDICATIONS** **Pneumocystis carinii pneumonia** Co-trimoxazole or pentamidine isethionate are listed as drugs of choice in this infection, which is found most commonly in immune-suppressed patients. • For other uses of co-trimoxazole, see Chapter 20 (p. 332).

## 🐦 NURSING CONSIDERATIONS

- See listing in Chapter 20 (p. 332).
- See entry for drug class (p. 413).

## emetine hydrochloride (EM-eh-teen) amebicide

- emetine hydrochloride

**MECHANISM OF ACTION** Emetine directly attacks amebae, destroying their nuclei. Emetine is effective only in those tissues where the drug concentrates, especially liver, and is not effective for disease limited to the intestinal lumen.

**INDICATIONS** **Amebiasis** Severe cases, including those involving liver abscesses, are controlled by emetine, but other drugs must be added to eradicate infection or prevent development of the carrier state.

**CONTRAINDICATIONS** **Heart disease** Additional cardiac toxicity caused by emetine may not be tolerated in these patients. **Kidney disease** Additional renal toxicity caused by emetine may not be tolerated in these patients. **Muscle disease or polyneuropathy** Patients with recent disease may be unable to tolerate additional damage caused by emetine. **Emetine therapy within the preceding 6 to 8 weeks** The toxic effects of emetine are cumulative.

**DOSAGE** **IM:** **ADULTS:** 1 mg/kg daily for 3 to 10 days, not to exceed 65 mg during any one 24 hour period and not to exceed 650 mg for the 10 day period. **Subcutaneous, deep injection:** **CHILDREN:** If all other amebicides are ineffective, emetine can be used with caution in children, 1 mg/kg daily in two divided doses for 4 to 6 days. Maximum daily doses are 10 mg daily for children under 8 years and 20 mg daily for children over 8 years. *Special patient populations:* **ELDERLY:** Geriatric patients generally receive half the normal adult dose. **CHILDREN:** Use is contraindicated in children unless other therapy for serious disease has failed. **PREGNANCY:** Emetine is contraindicated in pregnancy because of direct fetal harm.

**PREPARATIONS** *Solution for injection:* 65 mg/ml.

**DRUG INTERACTIONS** **Drugs toxic to the heart, liver, or kidneys** may not be tolerated by patients receiving emetine because emetine also causes direct toxicity to those tissues.

**FATE** Emetine must be administered parenterally because the drug is irritating to gastric tissue and is erratically absorbed. Emetine concentrates in tissues, especially liver, kidneys, lungs, and spleen. The drug is slowly released from these tissue sites and continues to be excreted in urine up to 60 days after the end of therapy.

## ❦ NURSING CONSIDERATIONS

### Side effects, toxicities, and associated nursing actions

**CNS** Depression, encephalitis, Herxheimerlike reactions, paralysis, paresthesia, and peripheral neuropathy occur, mostly at high doses. Neuromuscular effects are more common and often occur as an early sign of impending serious toxicity. Symptoms include aches, fatigue, listlessness, stiffness, tenderness, and tremors.

- Obtain carefully a baseline assessment of mental status and neurologic function and repeat regularly.
- Assess for signs of depression: withdrawal, change in affect, lack of interest in personal appearance, insomnia, and anorexia.
- Assess for tingling in fingers and toes.

**CV** Up to 54% of patients show signs of cardiac toxicity with emetine, manifested by arrhythmias, precordial pain, hypotension, myocarditis, pericarditis, congestive heart failure, or death.

- Monitor pulse, blood pressure, and weight. Auscultate lung and heart sounds. Assess for development of edema and distended jugular veins. Perform these assessments several times a day.
- Monitor continuous electrocardiogram, if available, or serial ECGs. Changes indicating cardiovascular effects may include inverted T waves, prolonged QT interval, widening of the QRS, prolonged PR interval, premature beats, transient atrial fibrillation, and other changes. ECG changes may not be evident until several days after the first dose is administered.

**GI** Cramps, nausea, vomiting, and diarrhea may occur, often with dizziness or headache.

- If GI symptoms are severe or persistent, monitor weight, intake, and output. Monitor serum electrolytes.

**Renal** Degenerative changes may occur if doses are high or prolonged. Serum potassium levels may also fall in some patients.

- Monitor serum BUN and creatinine and serum electrolytes.
- Assess for signs of hypokalemia: apathy, abdominal distention, paralytic ileus, ECG changes (flattened or inverted T waves, prolonged QT segment, prominent U wave).

**Liver** Degenerative changes may occur if doses are high or prolonged.

- Assess for signs of liver dysfunction: malaise, fever, jaundice, right upper quadrant abdominal pain, change in color or consistency of stools. Monitor liver function tests.

**Other** Local reactions to emetine include urticaria, eczema, or other dermatoses. Pain and tissue necrosis at the injection site may also occur.

- Assess for skin changes.
- As with all injections, record and rotate injection sites.

### Patient and family education

- Review with patients the anticipated benefits and possible side effects of drug therapy.
- Consult with the physician about any limitations of activity for the patient, and review these in detail with the patient and family.
- See entry for drug class (p. 413).

---

## furazolidone   (fyoor-uh-ZOL-i-dohn)                    antiprotozoal agent

- furazolidone: Furoxone

**MECHANISM OF ACTION**   Furazolidone inhibits several microbial enzyme systems.

**INDICATIONS**   **Enteritis caused by Giardia lamblia** Other drugs may be preferred for this condition in ordinary circumstances.

**CONTRAINDICATIONS**   **Glucose-6-phosphate dehydrogenase deficiency** Patients with this genetic condition may suffer hemolysis when given furazolidone, although the condition is usually mild and reversible.

**DOSAGE**   **PO:**   **ADULTS:** 100 mg four times daily for 7 to 10 days.   **CHILDREN:** Above 5 years, 25 to 50 mg four times daily. Ages 1 to 4 years, 17 to 25 mg four times daily. Ages 1 month to 1 year, 8 to 17 mg four times daily. Doses should not exceed 8.8 mg/kg daily.   *Special patient populations:*   **PREG-**

NANCY: Safe use in pregnancy and lactation is not established.

**PREPARATIONS**    *Oral suspension:* 16.7 mg/5 ml; *tablets:* 100 mg.

**DRUG INTERACTIONS**    **Alcohol** use in a patient taking furazolidone may cause a disulfiramlike effect, with flushing, hypotension, and dyspnea.    **MAO inhibitors** may add to the inhibition produced by furazolidone and lead to hypertensive episodes.    **Sympathomimetic compounds** such as amphetamines, cyclopentamine, dopamine, ephedrine, metaraminol, methylphenidate, phenylephrine, pseudoephedrine, or tyramine can lead to hypertensive episodes because furazolidone inhibits MAO, a major enzyme used in inactivating these compounds in the body.

**DIAGNOSTIC TEST INTERFERENCE**    **Urinary glucose tests** using cupric sulfate reagent may yield false-positive reactions because metabolites of furazolidone interfere.

**FATE**    Furazolidone is largely unabsorbed following oral administration. The small amount of absorbed drug may be metabolized and excreted in the urine as metabolites or unchanged drug.

## ☙ NURSING CONSIDERATIONS

### Side effects, toxicities, and associated nursing actions

**CNS** Headache, malaise, partial deafness, and dizziness have been reported.
- Caution patients to avoid driving or operating hazardous equipment if dizziness occurs; notify the physician.
- Assess for hearing loss. Instruct the patient to report the development of hearing loss.

**Blood** Mild hemolysis may occur, especially in persons with genetic G-6-PD deficiency.
- Question the patient about G-6-PD deficiency before administering the first dose.
- Instruct the patient to notify the physician if jaundice or darkening of the color of the urine occurs.
- Monitor complete blood count.

**GI** Abdominal pain, diarrhea, nausea, and vomiting are among the most common side effects of furazolidone. Reducing the dose may lessen the severity of the side effects.
- Instruct the patient to notify the physician if GI symptoms are severe or persistent.

**Allergic** Angioedema, arthralgia, fever, hypotension, and rashes may occur.
- Be alert to these side effects. Instruct patients to report the development of any new sign or symptom.

**Other** Furazolidone may be tumorigenic when administered for long periods. At high doses the drug may inhibit spermatogenesis.

### Patient and family education

- Caution patients to avoid the use of alcohol while taking furazolidone and for several days afterward, as the combination may produce a disulfiramlike reactions, with flushing, hypotension, and dyspnea.
- Counsel patients to avoid foods high in tyramine while taking furazolidone and for several days afterward. Foods to avoid include broad beans, yeast extracts, strong unpasteurized cheeses, beer, wine, pickled herring, chicken livers, and fermented products.
- See Drug Interactions. Caution patients to avoid all medications while taking furazolidone unless the drugs are first approved by the physician.
- See Diagnostic Test Interference. Caution diabetic patients to monitor blood glucose while taking furazolidone.
- See entry for drug class (p. 413).

## hydroxychloroquine sulfate    (hi-drox-ee-KLOR-oh-kwin)    antimalarial agent

- hydroxychloroquine sulfate: Plaquenil

**MECHANISM OF ACTION**    Hydroxychloroquine sulfate is expected to have the same action as chloroquine (p. 417).

**INDICATIONS**    **Malaria** Hydroxychloroquine sulfate is used for suppression, chemoprophylaxis, or treatment of uncomplicated malaria caused by *Plasmodia malariae, P. ovale, P. vivax,* and susceptible strains of

*P. falciparum.* • Hydroxychloroquine sulfate has no advantages over the parent drug, chloroquine. **Rheumatoid arthritis** Hydroxychloroquine sulfate is an alternate to gold compounds or penicillamine in patients requiring medication in addition to nonsteroidal antiinflammatory agents. **Lupus erythematosus** Hydroxychloroquine sulfate can be an adjunct to topical or systemic corticosteroid therapy.

**CONTRAINDICATIONS** **Glucose-6-phosphate-dehydrogenase deficiency (G-6PD)** Patients with this genetic condition may be more prone to hematologic toxicity, including hemolysis. **Porphyria** Hydroxychloroquine sulfate may exacerbate this condition. **Psoriasis** Hydroxychloroquine sulfate may worsen this chronic skin condition. **Visual field or retinal changes** Hydroxychloroquine sulfate may directly damage vision and should be avoided when possible in patients with pre-existing damage. **Hypersensitivity to chloroquine** Because chloroquine and hydroxychloroquine are both 4-aminoquinolines, cross-reactivity is expected.

**DOSAGE** **PO:** **ADULTS:** For suppression or chemoprophylaxis of malaria, 310 mg hydroxychloroquine (400 mg hydroxychloroquine sulfate) weekly, for 1 to 2 weeks before and during exposure and 6 to 8 weeks following exposure. For treatment of uncomplicated malaria, 620 mg initially of hydroxychloroquine (800 mg hydroxychloroquine sulfate), followed by 310 mg at 6, 24, and 48 hours after the first dose. For rheumatoid arthritis, 310 to 465 mg hydroxychloroquine daily (400 to 600 mg hydroxychloroquine sulfate) initially, with dosage gradually increased to achieve optimal effect. After the condition is controlled, the maintenance doses should be reduced to 155 to 310 mg hydroxychloroquine daily. For lupus erythematosus, 310 mg hydroxychloroquine (400 mg hydroxychloroquine sulfate) once or twice daily for weeks or months, as the condition of the patient demands. Maintenance may be achieved with doses of 155 to 310 mg. **CHILDREN:** For suppression or chemoprophylaxis of malaria, 5 mg/kg (6.5 mg/kg hydroxychloroquine sulfate) once weekly as for adults. The total weekly dose should not exceed 310 mg hydroxychloroquine. For treatment of uncomplicated malaria, 10 mg/kg initially of hydroxychloroquine (13 mg/kg hydroxychloroquine sulfate), followed by 5 mg/kg at 6, 24, and 48 hours after the first dose. *Special patient populations:* **CHILDREN:** Children may be especially sensitive to toxicity with 4-aminoquinolines. **PREGNANCY:** Safe use in pregnancy and lactation is not established.

**PREPARATIONS** *Tablets:* 155 mg equivalent of hydroxychloroquine.

**DRUG INTERACTIONS** **Hepatotoxic drugs** may increase the liver damage that may occur with chloroquine. **Chronic alcohol use** may cause liver damage that can predispose a patient to toxicity from chloroquine.

**FATE** The fate of hydroxychloroquine seems to be similar to that of chloroquine. Metabolites are formed that are slowly eliminated from the body by the kidneys. Hydroxychloroquine and its metabolites may accumulate in specific tissues such as in eyes.

### ❦ NURSING CONSIDERATIONS

#### Side effects, toxicities, and associated nursing actions

**Eye** Ocular toxicity is the most common serious reaction to hydroxychloroquine. Damage is most severe with long-term administration of large doses. Retinopathy may progress after the drug is discontinued and has resulted in blindness.
- Instruct patients to report any visual changes.
- Encourage patients on long-term therapy to have regular ophthalmic examinations.

**CNS** Aggressiveness, agitation, anxiety, apathy, confusion, depression, fatigue, headache, irritability, nervousness, personality changes, psychotic episodes, seizures, and toxic psychosis may occur. Neuromyopathy may occur, usually with high doses over long periods, and is reversible.
- Obtain a baseline assessment of neurologic function and mental status; repeat at regular intervals.
- Caution the patient to report the development of personality changes or other CNS side effects.
- Assess for signs of depression: withdrawal, lack of interest in personal appearance, insomnia, or anorexia.

**CV** Hypotension and ECG changes may occur, especially with high doses.
- Monitor blood pressure and ECG, especially in patients on long-term therapy.

**Blood** Agranulocytosis, aplastic anemia, neutropenia, and thrombocytopenia may occur. Hemolysis

and acute renal failure are more likely in G-6-PD deficiency.
- Question the patient about G-6-PD deficiency before administering the drug. This deficiency is more common in American blacks, Sardinians, and Kurdish Jews.
- Instruct patients to notify the physician if the following signs develop: pallor, malaise, sore throat, fever, unexplained bleeding or bruising, darkening of the color of urine.
- Monitor complete blood cell count, white blood cell differential, platelet count, serum creatinine, and BUN.

**GI** Abdominal cramps, anorexia, diarrhea, epigastric distress, nausea, and vomiting may occur but are lessened when the drug is given with meals.
- Instruct patients to notify the physician if GI symptoms are severe or persistent.
- Teach the patient to take doses with meals or snack.

**Hearing** Nerve deafness is a rare complication of therapy.
- Monitor hearing acuity.
- Instruct the patient to report any hearing loss.

**Patient and family education**
- Review with the patient how to take medication (see Dosage).
- See entry for drug class (p. 413).

## iodoquinol  (eye-OH-doh-kwin-ol)                                amebicide

- iodoquinol: Amebaquin, ✿ Diodoquin, Moebiquin, Yodoxin

**MECHANISM OF ACTION**   Iodoquinol is a luminal or contact amebicide that destroys the amebae by an unknown mechanism.

**INDICATIONS**   **Amebiasis** Iodoquinol is useful for treating disease limited to the intestinal tract. • The drug may be effective alone in mild disease or in asymptomatic carriers but is usually combined with other agents when more serious disease is being treated.

**CONTRAINDICATIONS**   **Thyroid disease** Because iodoquinol has a high iodine content, it should be used with caution in patients with thyroid conditions.   **Hepatic or renal disease** Iodoquinol should be avoided in these patients.   **Optic neuropathy** Iodoquinol should be avoided in the presence of this condition.   **Iodoquinol therapy within preceding 3 weeks** Iodoquinol therapy should not be repeated more often than at about 3 week intervals.

**DOSAGE**   **PO:**   **ADULTS:** 630 to 650 mg three times daily for 20 days. Daily doses should not exceed 2 g. **CHILDREN:** 30 to 40 mg/kg daily, administered in two or three doses for 20 days. The total daily dose should not exceed 1.95 g.   *Special patient populations:*   **PREGNANCY:** Safte use in pregnancy and lactation is not established.

**PREPARATIONS**   *Tablets:* 210 or 650 mg; *powder:* for oral use.

**DRUG INTERACTIONS**   None have been documented.

**DIAGNOSTIC TEST INTERFERENCE**   **Protein-bound serum iodine** is increased by iodoquinol. The altered test may persist for up to 6 months following therapy.

**FATE**   Oral absorption is limited, but some iodine from iodoquinol accumulates in the blood. Iodoquinol metabolites appear in low concentrations in tissues and in urine following oral administration.

## ✿ NURSING CONSIDERATIONS
**Side effects, toxicities, and associated nursing actions**

**CNS** Neurotoxicity is the most serious side effect of iodoquinol. Manifestations include agitation, retrograde amnesia, subacute myelo-optic neuropathy (SMON), dysesthesias, and weakness. In children, optic neuritis or atrophy leading to blindness has occurred, especially in malnourished patients.
- Assess and monitor neurologic function.
- Caution patients to avoid driving or operating hazardous equipment until the effects of the medication can be evaluated.
- Instruct patients to report immediately any changes in vision. Observe children closely for changes

in vision; a very young child may not be able to describe changes in vision.

**GI** Abdominal cramps, anorexia, constipation, diarrhea, epigastric distress, gastritis, nausea, and vomiting are common GI effects.

- Monitor weight and keep a record of stools.
- If diarrhea or vomiting is prominent, monitor intake and output and serum electrolytes.
- If constipation occurs, instruct the patient to increase fluid intake to 2500 to 3000 ml/day, increase the intake of fruit, fruit juices, and high-fiber food, and increase daily exercise (if not contraindicated by the general medical condition).
- Instruct patients to notify the physician of persistent or severe GI effects.

**Other** Iodine toxicity may be manifested by a variety of skin reactions, including rashes, eruptions, and discolorations of skin and nails. Enlargement of the thyroid may also occur.

- Assess the patient for skin changes. Instruct patients to report the development of skin changes.
- Monitor thyroid gland size.

### Nursing interventions related to drug administration
- Tablets may be crushed and mixed with applesauce or chocolate syrup.

### Patient and family education
- Review with patients the anticipated benefits and possible side effects of drug therapy.
- Instruct patients to take doses after meals. Review with patients how to crush tablets, if necessary (see preceding section).
- Because iodoquinol can interfere with the protein-bound iodine test, remind the patient to keep all health care providers informed for at least 6 months that this drug has been taken.
- See entry for drug class (p. 413).

---

## mebendazole  (meh-BEN-da-zole)                              antihelminthic agent

- mebendazole: Vermox

**MECHANISM OF ACTION**   Mebendazole inhibits glucose uptake in the intestine of nematodes. Mammalian cells are unaffected.

**INDICATIONS**   **Trichuriasis (whipworm infection)** Mebendazole is the drug of choice, curing 70% of patients and reducing egg formation in over 90% of treated patients.   **Enterobiasis (pinworm infection)** Mebendazole is a drug of choice for this condition, producing cures in over 90% of patients.   **Ascariasis (roundworm infection)** Mebendazole is a drug of choice for this infection, producing cures in over 90% of patients.   **Hookworm infections caused by *Ancylostoma duodenale* or *Necator americanus*** Mebendazole is a drug of choice for this infection, producing cures in over 90% of patients.

**CONTRAINDICATIONS**   **Hypersensitivity to mebendazole** A documented reaction to previously administered mebendazole is the only contraindication to the use of the drug.

**DOSAGE**   PO:   ADULTS AND CHILDREN: 200 mg daily, divided into equal doses in the morning and evening for 3 consecutive days. Treatment may be repeated within 3 to 4 weeks if cure is not achieved. For enterobiasis, a single dose of 100 mg may be repeated routinely after 2 weeks.   *Special patient populations:*   CHILDREN: Children younger than 2 years should not receive the drug until safety for this age group has been established.   PREGNANCY: Safe use in pregnancy and lactation is not established.

**PREPARATIONS**   *Tablets, chewable:* 100 mg.

**DRUG INTERACTIONS**   None have been documented.

**FATE**   Only 2% to 10% of orally administered mebendazole is absorbed. The drug remaining in the intestinal tract is the effective agent. Absorbed drug is metabolized by the liver and excreted by the kidneys.

### ❦ NURSING CONSIDERATIONS
#### Side effects, toxicities, and associated nursing actions
**CNS** Dizziness was reported in a single patient.

- Caution patients to avoid driving or operating hazardous equipment if dizziness occurs; notify the physician.

**GI** Abdominal cramping and transient diarrhea are probably caused by expulsion of massive numbers of helminths.

- Have the patient notify the physician if GI symptoms are severe.

**Patient and family education**

- Inform patients that the tablets may be chewed, swallowed whole, or crushed and mixed with food.
- Review with patients appropriate methods for preventing reinfestation.
- See entry for drug class (p. 413).

---

## metronidazole, metronidazole hydrochloride    (meh-troh-NID-uh-zole)    antiprotozoal agent

- metronidazole, metronidazole hydrochloride: Femazole, Flagyl, Metric, Metronid, Metryl, Protostat, Satric

**MECHANISM OF ACTION**    Metronidazole is metabolized in anaerobic organisms to cytotoxic products that disrupt DNA synthesis. Metronidazole is active systemically, being considered a tissue and a contact amebicide. The drug is also widely active against obligative anaerobic bacteria.

**INDICATIONS**    **Amebiasis** Metronidazole is the drug of choice for acute intestinal amebiasis (in combination with a luminal amebicide) and for amebic liver abscesses caused by *Entamoeba histolytica*.    **Anaerobic bacterial infections** Infections of abdominal or pelvic structures, bones or joints, lower lung, and CNS may be caused by anaerobic bacteria. • Septicemia and endocarditis may also be caused by susceptible anaerobic organisms. • When mixed anaerobic and aerobic infections occur, an antibiotic effective against the aerobic organisms must be added because metronidazole is effective only against anaerobes.    **Giardiasis** Metronidazole is usually considered as an alternative to quinacrine hydrochloride.    **Trichomoniasis** Metronidazole is used in symptomatic or asymptomatic cases and in the sexual contacts of those diagnosed with the disease.

**CONTRAINDICATIONS**    **Edema** Patients predisposed to edema or intolerant of sodium may not be able to tolerate the 28 mEq of sodium in each gram of metronidazole.

**DOSAGE**    **PO:**    **ADULTS:** For amebiasis, 500 to 750 mg three times daily for 5 to 10 days. For anaerobic bacterial infections, 7.5 mg/kg every 6 hours for up to 3 weeks. Therapy should be initiated with IV administration, using oral doses as soon as the condition of the patient allows. For giardiasis, 250 mg three times daily for 5 to 7 days. For trichomoniasis, 2 g as a single dose or 250 mg three times daily for 7 days.    **CHILDREN:** For amebiasis, 35 to 50 mg/kg divided into three equal doses a day for 5 to 10 days. For giardiasis, 15 mg/kg daily in three divided doses for 5 days. For trichomoniasis, 15 mg/kg daily in three divided doses for 7 to 10 days.    **IV:**    **ADULTS:** For anaerobic bacterial infections, 15 mg/kg as a single loading dose, followed by 7.5 mg/kg every 6 hours until the patient is able to tolerate oral dosing.    *Special patient populations:*    **HEPATIC DISEASE:** The dosage may need to be reduced if hepatic disease is severe.    **CHILDREN:** Safe IV use in children not established.    **PREGNANCY:** Safe use in pregnancy and lactation is not established.

**PREPARATIONS**    **Metronidazole** *Tablets:* 250 or 500 mg; *tablets, film-coated:* 250 or 500 mg; *solution for IV infusion:* 5 mg/ml.    **Metronidazole hydrochloride** *Powder:* 500 mg to prepare solution for IV use.

**DRUG INTERACTIONS**    **Alcohol** metabolism may be inhibited by metronidazole, occasionally causing a disulfiramlike reaction.    **Coumarin anticoagulants** are more effective than expected when administered with metronidazole and may cause prolonged prothrombin times or bleeding episodes.    **Disulfiram** may cause acute psychoses or confusion when given with metronidazole.    **Phenobarbital** may increase the metabolism of metronidazole, which shortens the half-life and lowers the plasma concentration of metronidazole.

**FATE** Metronidazole is well absorbed following oral administration, but the rate of absorption is diminished by the presence of food in the stomach. The drug is widely distributed to fluids and tissues, including the CNS, where concentrations range from 43% to 100% of concurrent plasma concentrations. The liver metabolizes 30% to 60% of a dose of metronidazole; metabolites and unchanged drug are excreted primarily in urine but also in feces. The elimination *half-life* of metronidazole is 6 to 8 hours. The half-life is unaltered by renal disease but is increased in hepatic failure.

## ☙ NURSING CONSIDERATIONS

### Side effects, toxicities, and associated nursing actions

**CNS** Ataxia, confusion, dizziness, depression, incoordination, insomnia, irritability, vertigo, and weakness have been reported with oral dosing. IV administration may cause dizziness, headache, and syncope. Peripheral neuropathy may also occur with the drug, causing paresthesia of an extremity or convulsive seizures.

- Caution patients to avoid driving or operating hazardous equipment if dizziness, incoordination, vertigo, or syncope occur.
- Assess for signs of depression: withdrawal, change in affect, insomnia, anorexia, or lack of interest in personal appearance.
- Obtain a baseline neurologic assessment, and repeat at regular intervals.

**CV** Flattening of the T-wave on the ECG is a rare observation.

**Blood** Leukopenia is a rare and usually mild, reversible side effect. Bone marrow aplasia is rare. Thrombophlebitis may occur with IV administration if catheters are allowed to remain in place too long.

- Instruct the patient to report pallor, fatigue, sore throat, fever, or unexplained bleeding, or bruising.
- Inspect the IV insertion site and extremity for signs of thrombophlebitis.

**GI** Nausea is the most common side effect with metronidazole. Anorexia, dry mouth, headache, and a metallic taste in the mouth may also occur. Abdominal distress, constipation, diarrhea, and vomiting are less common. GI effects of metronidazole may occur even after IV administration of the drug.

- Instruct patients to notify the physician if GI side effects are severe or persistent.

**Renal** The urine may be discolored by metabolites of metronidazole, but this condition is harmless. The drug may also cause cystitis, dysuria, dryness of the vagina or vulva, dyspareunia, incontinence, pelvic pressure, polyuria, or urethral burning and discomfort. Libido has been reduced in some patients.

- Warn patients of the reddish brown discoloration of the urine.
- If vaginal dryness is a problem, suggest that women obtain a commercially available lubricant designed for sensitive vaginal mucosa.
- Instruct patients to notify the physician if polyuria, burning on urination, frequency, urgency, bladder-area pain, or fever occur, as these may indicate urinary tract infection.
- Assess tactfully for changes in libido. Provide emotional support as needed. Remind patients to not stop taking medication without notifying the physician. Reinforce to patients the need to take medications as ordered for best effect.

**Allergic** Erythematous rash, fever, flushing, joint pain, nasal congestion, pruritis, and urticaria may occur.

**Other** Superinfections can occur when metronidazole is given. *Candida* overgrowth may cause glossitis, stomatitis, or vaginitis. *Clostridium difficile* overgrowth in the bowel may lead to antibiotic-associated colitis.

- Instruct patients to report the development of any new sign or symptom. Review symptoms of superinfection with patients.

### Nursing interventions related to drug administration

- See the manufacturer's literature for information about reconstitution of IV doses. If prepared for intermittent infusion, the drug must be neutralized first. Do not use syringes with aluminum needles or hubs.
- Administer dose, as prepared and neutralized, over at least 1 hour.
- Ascertain that the IV line is patent before administering the drug.

- Instruct the patient to report the development of redness or pain in the extremity.

**Patient and family education**

- Caution the patient to avoid the use of alcohol while taking this drug, as a disulfiramlike reaction may occur, characterized by vomiting, headache, and flushing.
- Discuss with female patients the need to treat sexual partners for trichomoniasis.
- See entry for drug class (p. 413).

---

## niclosamide   (neh-KLO-suh-mide) antihelminthic agent

- niclosamide: Niclocide ✤

**MECHANISM OF ACTION**   Niclosamide inhibits energy production in tapeworms (cestodes) by its effects on the mitochondria. The drug also alters glucose uptake by tapeworms, further compromising energy production. In the intestinal tract of hosts, the action of the drug is enhanced by the action of digestive enzymes on the damaged worms. Niclosamide does not kill eggs, which may be released when the worms are killed and digested inside the host.

**INDICATIONS**   **Cestodiasis** Infestation caused by *Taenia saginata* (beef tapeworm) and *Diphyllobothrium latum* (fish tapeworm) is eliminated in 80% to 100% of treated patients. • *Hymenolepis nana* (dwarf tapeworm) may also be treated effectively.

**CONTRAINDICATIONS**   **Taenia solium infestations** Infestations caused by *T. solium* (pork tapeworm) are not usually treated with niclosamide because the viable eggs that are released from digested worms of this species can hatch and cause invasive disease.   **Cysticercosis** Helminthic disease caused by larval forms are unresponsive to niclosamide.

**DOSAGE**   **PO:**   **ADULTS:** A single 2 g dose administered after a light meal is sufficient for most infections. For *H. nana* (dwarf tapeworm), administer 2 g as a single daily dose for 7 days, using special hygienic precautions to prevent reinfection.   **CHILDREN:** For children weighing 11 to 34 pounds, 1 g as a single dose; over 34 pounds, 1.5 g as a single dose. For *H. nana* (dwarf tapeworm), children over 34 pounds receive 1.5 g as a single dose on the first day and 1 g as a single daily dose for the next 6 days. Children between 11 and 34 pounds receive 1 g as a single dose on the first day and 500 mg as a single daily dose for the next 6 days.   *Special patient populations:*   **CHILDREN:** Safe use in children under 2 years of age is not established.   **PREGNANCY:** Safe use in pregnancy and lactation is not established.

**PREPARATIONS**   *Tablets, chewable:* 500 mg.

**DRUG INTERACTIONS**   None have been reported.

**FATE**   Niclosamide is not absorbed from the GI tract; it remains in the lumen and exerts its antihelminthic activity there. Some metabolism of the drug may occur in the intestine.

## ❦ NURSING CONSIDERATIONS

### Side effects, toxicities, and associated nursing actions

**GI** Abdominal discomfort, anorexia, diarrhea, dizziness, drowsiness, headache, nausea, and vomiting occur in 1% to 4% of patients receiving niclosamide.

- Caution patients to avoid driving or operating hazardous equipment if dizziness or drowsiness occur.
- Instruct patients to notify the physician if GI symptoms are severe or persistent.

**Other** Rarely, patients report alopecia, backache, constipation, edema of extremities, fever, pruritis ani, oral irritation, rash, rectal bleeding, sweating, or weakness.

- Instruct patients to report the development of any new sign or symptom.

### Patient and family education

- Instruct patients to take the dose after a light meal. Instruct patients to chew tablets thoroughly, then swallow with a sufficient amount of water. For small children, the tablet may be crushed and mixed with enough water to form a paste.

- Instruct patients to take a dose of laxative if they become constipated after the dose of niclosamide.
- See entry for drug class (p. 413).

## oxamniquine   (ox-AM-ni-kwin)                                    antischistosomal agent

- oxamniquine: Vansil

**MECHANISM OF ACTION**   Oxamniquine paralyzes adult forms of schistosomes, causing the worms to be carried by blood flow to the liver, where phagocytes destroy them. Egg production in surviving females is greatly reduced.

**INDICATIONS**   Schistosomiasis (bilharziasis) Infections caused by *Schistosoma mansoni* can be cured in 70% to 100% of patients treated with oxamniquine. • Other species of *Schistosoma* are not affected.

**CONTRAINDICATIONS**   Seizure disorders Patients predisposed to seizures may be more likely to suffer oxamniquine-induced seizures.

**DOSAGE**   PO:   ADULTS: For infections acquired in the western hemisphere, 12 to 15 mg/kg, given as a single dose. For infections acquired in Africa or the Middle East, 15 mg/kg is given twice daily for 1 or 2 days.   CHILDREN: For infections acquired in the western hemisphere, 20 mg/kg total dose, administered in two equal doses 2 to 8 hours apart. For infections acquired in Africa or the Middle East, 15 mg/kg is given twice daily for 1 or 2 days. *Special patient populations:*   PREGNANCY: FDA pregnancy category C.

**PREPARATIONS**   *Capsules:* 250 mg.

**DRUG INTERACTIONS**   Praziquantel may have synergistic antischistosomal activity with oxamniquine.

**DIAGNOSTIC TEST INTERFERENCE**   Urinalysis for various substances using spectrophotometry may be inaccurate because of the orange-red discoloration of the urine caused by oxamniquine.

**FATE**   Oxamniquine is well absorbed following oral administration, producing *peak* serum concentrations within 1 to 3 hours. Food interferes with absorption. The drug is metabolized in the intestine. Unchanged drug and metabolites are excreted mainly by the kidneys. The plasma *half-life* of oxamniquine is 1 to 2.5 hours.

### ☙ NURSING CONSIDERATIONS

#### Side effects, toxicities, and associated nursing actions

**CNS** Dizziness, drowsiness, and headache occur in 30% to 50% of patients. Behavioral changes, excitation, hallucinations, insomnia, malaise, and transient amnesia have occurred less frequently. Generalized seizures are a rare occurrence, being more likely in patients with a predisposition to these disorders.
- Caution patients to avoid driving or operating hazardous equipment if dizziness or drowsiness occur.
- Obtain a health history from the patient. If the patient has a history of seizures, consult with the physician. Instruct the family to be alert for the possibility of seizures.
- Instruct patients and families to notify the physician if other CNS side effects occur.

**Blood** Eosinophilia may result from the disease or possibly from the drug. Oxamniquine may also elevate the erythrocyte sedimentation rate, reticulocyte count, and the leukocyte count.
- Monitor blood work if available.

**Renal** Orange-red discoloration of the urine is a harmless side effect. Reversible proteinuria and hematuria may occur.
- Warn the patient about this side effect. If discoloration is pronounced or persistent, have the patient notify the physician.
- Monitor urinalysis if available.

**Allergic** Joint pain, pruritis, rash, and urticaria have occasionally occurred.
- Instruct patients to report the development of new signs and symptoms.

**Other** Pulmonary condensations have been observed in the radiographs of a few patients.

#### Patient and family education
- Instruct patients to take doses with a meal or snack to lessen gastric irritation.
- See entry for drug class (p. 413).

# paromomycin sulfate aminoglycoside

- paromomycin: Humatin

**INDICATIONS**   **Amebiasis and cestodiasis** • See listing under aminoglycosides (p. 283).

**☙ NURSING CONSIDERATIONS**
- See listing under aminoglycosides (p. 277).
- See entry for drug class (p. 413).

# pentamidine isethionate   (pen-TAM-i-deen eye-seh-THY-oh-nate)   antiprotozoal

- pentamidine isethionate: Pentam

**MECHANISM OF ACTION**   Pentamidine has multiple effects on DNA, RNA, and protein synthesis. The exact mechanism is unknown and may vary for each of the types of organisms against which the drug is used. Pentamidine is directly lethal to several protozoans.

**INDICATIONS**   **Pneumocystis carinii pneumonia** This opportunistic infection occurs in AIDS patients, in patients receiving immunosuppressive drugs for cancer chemotherapy or organ transplantation, and in malnourished low-birth-weight infants. • Pentamidine is an alternative to co-trimoxazole (p. 419), especially in those patients failing therapy with co-trimoxazole.   **Trypanosoma brucei infections** Pentamidine isethionate is an alternative to suramin.   **Leishmaniasis** Pentamidine isethionate is an alternative to stibogluconate sodium.

**CONTRAINDICATIONS**   None noted for treatment of *Pneumocystis carinii* pneumonia because of the high mortality rate associated with this condition.

**DOSAGE**   **IV:**   **ADULTS:** By slow IV infusion (60 minutes or longer) for *P. carinii* pneumonia, 4 mg/kg once daily for 14 days. Longer treatment may be required in AIDS patients.   **CHILDREN:** By slow IV infusion (60 minutes or longer) for *P. carinii* pneumonia, 150 mg/M$^2$ once daily for 5 days followed by 100 mg/M$^2$ for the remainder of the treatment period. Adult doses as previously listed have also been used.   **IM:**   **ADULTS:** By deep injection; doses are as for IV route.   **CHILDREN:** By deep injection; doses are as for IV route.   *Special patient populations:*   **PREGNANCY:** Safe use in pregnancy and lactation is not established.   **RENAL IMPAIRMENT:** Doses may need to be reduced.

**PREPARATIONS**   *Powder to prepare solution for parenteral injection:* 300 mg.

**DRUG INTERACTIONS**   **Nephrotoxic drugs** such as amphotericin B, capreomycin, cisplatin, gentamicin, methoxyflurane, polymyxin B, streptomycin, or vancomycin may increase the renal damage caused by pentamidine isethionate alone.

**FATE**   Pentamidine isethionate is administered only by parenteral routes. The drug appears to bind to tissues but is not thought to penetrate into the CNS. Excretion is by the kidneys, but only a small fraction of the dose appears in urine. The fate of the remainder of the dose is unknown.

**☙ NURSING CONSIDERATIONS**
### Side effects, toxicities, and associated nursing actions
**CV** Sudden hypotensive reactions occasionally leading to death may occur with IM or IV doses, but the risk is increased with rapid IV administration. Arrhythmias, ECG abnormalities, and flushing have also occurred.
- Have patients in a supine position before administering the drug. Monitor blood pressure before administering the drug or beginning infusion. Monitor blood pressure every 5 to 15 minutes until stable.
- Monitor blood pressure and pulse every 4 hours.
- Administer IV doses over at least 1 hour.

**Blood** Phlebitis can occur following IV administration. Leukopenia and thrombocytopenia can occur; anemia is rare.
- Instruct the patient to report redness or pain near the IV insertion site.

- Instruct the patient to report the development of unexplained bleeding or bruising.
- Monitor the complete blood count, white blood cell differential, and platelet count.

**GI** Abdominal discomfort, anorexia, diarrhea, nausea, vomiting, and unpleasant tastes may occur.
- Assess the patient for GI symptoms; if severe or persistent, notify the physician.
- Monitor weight.

**Renal** Renal side effects are those most commonly associated with pentamidine, affecting 25% of patients treated for *P. carinii* pneumonia. Serum creatinine and BUN may gradually increase during therapy, signaling the onset of mild to moderate renal failure. Acute renal failure is rare.
- Monitor intake, output, weight, and blood pressure.
- Monitor serum creatinine and BUN.

**Metabolic** Severe hypoglycemia may occur in up to 10% of patients. This reaction may occur during or after therapy and can be severe enough to cause death. Hypocalcemia and hyperkalemia have also occurred.
- Assess for signs and symptoms of hypoglycemia: pallor, perspiration, tachycardia, palpitations, nervousness, irritibility, weakness, trembling, hunger, headache, blurred vision, diplopia, incoherent speech, emotional changes, and fatigue. If hypoglycemia is suspected, administer carbohydrates, which can be in the form of fruit juice or sweetened soft drinks, sugar, syrup, or hard candy. Review these symptoms with patients, and enlist their aid in identifying possible hypoglycemic episodes.
- Assess for hyperkalemia: nausea, colic, diarrhea, skeletal muscle spasms, or ECG changes.
- Assess for signs of hypocalcemia: numbness and tingling of the nose, ears, fingertips, or toes.
- Monitor serum glucose and electrolyte levels.

**Allergic** Pruritis, rash, and urticaria can occur. Stevens-Johnson syndrome is rare, as is anaphylaxis, but deaths have occurred.
- Visually inspect the patient for skin changes, and instruct patients to report any skin changes.
- Have drugs, equipment, and personnel available to treat acute allergic reactions in settings where pentamidine is administered.

**Other** IM administration is associated with severe local effects in up to 20% of patients. Reactions include erythema, induration, pain, sterile abscess, and tenderness at the site.
- As with all IM injections, use careful technique to prevent contamination, and record and rotate injection sites.
- Inspect injection sites for signs of abscess, and avoid using sites that are suspect.

### Nursing interventions related to drug administration
- Review manufacturer's literature before administring the drug.
- Review Side Effects.

### Patient and family education
- See entry for drug class (p. 413).

---

## piperazine citrate  (PIP-er-uh-zeen)                    antihelminthic agent

- piperazine: Antepar, Vermazine

**MECHANISM OF ACTION**  Piperazine blocks the action of acetylcholine at the neuromuscular junction, causing paralysis of intestinal worms. The worms are eliminated from the body by normal peristalsis.

**INDICATIONS**  **Ascariasis (roundworm infestation)** Cure rates are 80% to 90% with piperazine citrate. **Enterobiasis (pinworm infestation)** Cure rates are 80% to 90%, but piperazine is usually considered an alternative to mebendazole or pyrantel pamoate because multiple doses of piperazine are required for efficacy.

**CONTRAINDICATIONS**  **Renal or hepatic impairment** Piperazine should be avoided if possible in these patients.  **Seizure disorders** Predisposition to these disorders increases the likelihood of suffering CNS toxicity with piperazine.

**DOSAGE**  **PO:**  **ADULTS:** For ascariasis, 3.5 g once daily for 2 days. Severe infestations may require therapy for 4 days. For enterobiasis, 65 mg/kg in a single daily dose, not to exceed 2.5 g, for 7 days. **CHILDREN:** For ascariasis, 2 g/M$^2$ daily for 2 days. For enterobiasis, 1 g/M$^2$ daily for 7 days. *Special patient populations:* **PREGNANCY:** Safe use in pregnancy and lactation is not established.

**PREPARATIONS**    *Solution, oral use:* 500 mg of piperazine hexahydrate/5 ml; *tablets:* 250 or 500 mg piperazine hexahydrate.

**DRUG INTERACTIONS**    **Pyrantel pamoate** antagonizes the action of piperazine.    **Chlorpromazine** effects on the CNS may be altered by piperazine; one patient recently treated with piperazine developed seizures when given chlorpromazine.

**DIAGNOSTIC TEST INTERFERENCE**    **Uric acid** measurements are lowered by piperazine.

**FATE**    Piperazine is absorbed from the intestine. The metabolic fate and rate of elimination seems to vary among individuals. Piperazine is found in the urine of treated patients.

## 🐦 NURSING CONSIDERATIONS

### Side effects, toxicities, and associated nursing actions

**CNS** Ataxia, choreiform movements, EEG abnormalities, hyporeflexia, memory defect, muscular weakness, myoclonus, paresthesia, nystagmus, seizures, and tremors have occurred but are uncommon. **Blood** Hemolytic anemia.
- Instruct patients to report the development of any new sign or symptom.
- Obtain a health history before administering the drug; if the patient has a history of seizures, consult with the physician. Caution families of patients with a history of seizures to be alert for the appearance of seizures.

**GI** Abdominal cramps, diarrhea, nausea, and vomiting may occur.
- Instruct patients to notify the physician if GI symptoms are severe or persistent.

**Allergic** Arthralgia, bronchospasm, cough, erythema multiforme, eczematous skin reactions, photodermatitis, purpura, rhinorrhea, and urticaria can occur.
- Instruct patients to report the development of any new sign or symptom.

### Patient and family education
- Instruct patients to take doses after a meal or snack to lessen gastric irritation.
- See entry for drug class (p. 413).

---

# praziquantel    (pra-zee-KWAN-tell)                                 antihelminthic agent

- praziquantel: Biltricide

**MECHANISM OF ACTION**    Praziquantel paralyzes the musculature of schistosomes, causing them to be dislodged and transported by blood flow to the liver, where they are phagocytized. In addition, praziquantel causes changes in the integument of the worms that ultimately leads to their lysis. Trematodes and cestodes also suffer some of the effects seen in schistosomes.

**INDICATIONS**    **Schistosomiasis (bilharziasis)** Praziquantel is effective against all pathogenic schistosomes.
- Cure rates are 75% to 95%, and egg production may be inhibited as much as 98%. • Oxamniquine is an alternative to praziquantel only for *S. mansoni* infestations.    **Trematodes** Infestations caused by various species of flukes may respond to prazinquantel.    **Cestodiasis** Praziquantel may be effective against adult and larval stages of these organisms.

**CONTRAINDICATIONS**    **Allergy to praziquantel** Allergies are the only direct contraindication to this drug.

**DOSAGE**    **PO:**    **ADULTS AND CHILDREN OVER 4 YEARS:** For schistosomiasis, 60 mg/kg total, given as three equal doses 4 to 6 hours apart. *Special patient populations:* **CHILDREN:** Safe use in children under 4 years is not established.    **PREGNANCY:** FDA pregnancy category B. Breast feeding should be discontinued for 72 hours after administration of praziquantel.

**PREPARATIONS**    *Tablets, film-coated:* 600 mg.

**DRUG INTERACTIONS**    None yet documented.

**FATE**    Praziquantel is well absorbed following oral administration but is extensively degraded by first-pass metabolism in the liver, lowering the amount of active drug available for distribution to other sites.

The drug passes into milk. Praziquantel is eliminated from serum with a *half-life* of 0.8 to 1.5 hours; metabolites persist longer, but it is not known if they possess any antihelmintic activity. About 80% of a dose of praziquantel is eliminated in urine but mostly as metabolites formed by the liver.

## ❦ NURSING CONSIDERATIONS

### Side effects, toxicities, and associated nursing actions

**CNS** Activities demanding mental alertness and motor coordination may be difficult because praziquantel can impair functioning on the day of and the day after therapy. About 90% of treated patients experience dizziness, headache, and malaise. When used for cerebral cysticercosis, intense CNS symptoms, including seizures, may occur as a result of inflammatory reactions to damaged larvae.
- Warn patients about these side effects. Caution patients to avoid driving or operating hazardous equipment until the effects of the medication can be evaluated.

**Blood** Mild eosinophilia may occur, possibly as an immune reaction to parasites damaged by praziquantel.

**Liver** Liver enzymes (AST or ALT) may be mildly elevated in up to 27% of patients, but there is no evidence of serious or permanent liver damage.
- Monitor complete blood count, white blood cell differential, and liver function tests if indicated by patient condition.

**GI** About 90% of treated patients experience abdominal pain or discomfort; a significant proportion also suffer nausea. Anorexia, diarrhea, and vomiting are less common.
- Instruct patients to notify a physician if GI symptoms are severe or persistent.

**Allergic** Urticaria, pruritis, and fever have been reported.
- Instruct patients to report skin changes or fever that persists longer than 24 hours.

### Patient and family education
- Instruct patients to take doses with meals or snacks. Tablets may be cut into halves or quarters but should not be chewed. Whole or part tablets should be immediately swallowed with sufficient water.
- See entry for drug class (p. 413).

---

## primaquine phosphate (PRIM-uh-kwin) antimalarial agent

- Sold under generic name

**MECHANISM OF ACTION** Primaquine has multiple effects that may contribute to its antiplasmodial action. The drug binds to DNA and may interfere with synthesis of nucleic acids. Mitochondria are also damaged, possibly as a result of drug interference with oxidation-reduction reactions used for energy production. Primaquine is schizonticidal and gametocidal, with activity against pre-erythrocytic and exoerythrocytic forms.

**INDICATIONS** **Malaria** Malaria caused by *Plasmodia vivax* or *P. ovale* is characterized by relapses occurring up to 4 years after the initial infection; The relapses are caused by latent organisms in the liver. • Primaquine can produce a radical cure of these types of malaria by eliminating the liver forms of the plasmodia.

**CONTRAINDICATIONS** **Deficiency of glucose-6-phosphate dehydrogenase (G-6-PD) or NADH methemoglobin reductase** Persons deficient in these enzymes are more prone to hematologic reactions to primaquine, including hemolytic anemia. **Acute malaria in patients with rheumatoid arthritis or lupus erythematosus** These patients have a tendency toward granulocytopenia, increasing the risk of hematologic reactions to primaquine.

**DOSAGE** **PO:** **ADULTS:** 15 mg primaquine (26.3 mg of primaquine phosphate) once daily for 14 days. An alternate dosing schedule is 45 mg primaquine (79 mg primaquine phosphate) once a week for 8 weeks. **CHILDREN:** 0.3 mg/kg primaquine (0.5 mg/kg primaquine phosphate) once daily for 14 days. An alternate dosing schedule is 0.9 mg/kg primaquine (1.5 mg/kg primaquine phosphate) once a week for 8 weeks. *Special patient populations:* **PREGNANCY:** Safe use in pregnancy and lactation is not established.

**PREPARATIONS**    *Tablets:* 15 mg.    **Combination products** *Tablets:* 45 mg primaquine with 300 mg of chloroquine as the phosphate.

**DRUG INTERACTIONS**    **Quinacrine** increases the toxicity of antimalarial drugs related to primaquine and probably should not be used in combination with primaquine.

**FATE**    Primaquine is well absorbed following oral administration, producing *peak* serum concentrations within 6 hours. Primaquine is quickly metabolized by the liver, and the metabolites are eliminated by the kidneys. The plasma *half-life* for primaquine is 4 to 10 hours.

### ☙ NURSING CONSIDERATIONS

#### Side effects, toxicities, and associated nursing actions

**CNS** Headache and difficulties with visual accommodation are uncommon reactions.
- Caution patients to avoid driving or operating hazardous equipment if visual difficulties occur.

**CV** Hypertension and cardiac arrhythmias occur rarely.
- Monitor blood pressure and ECG, especially in patients on long-term therapy.

**Blood** Acute hemolytic anemia is a special risk with very high doses or in patients with genetic defects causing deficiencies in G-6-PD. Patients lacking NADH methemoglobin reductase are at special risk of methemoglobinemia. Mild anemia, leukocytosis, leukopenia, or rare agranulocytosis are not associated with any particular genetic pattern.
- Question the patient about G-6-PD deficiency or problems with NADH methemoglobin reductase before administering the first dose.
- Instruct patients to notify the physician if the following signs develop: pallor, malaise, sore throat, fever, unexplained bleeding or bruising, or darkening of the color of the urine.
- Monitor complete blood cell count, white blood cell differential, and platelet count.

**GI** Abdominal cramps, epigastric distress, nausea, and vomiting occur occasionally but may be reduced by taking the drug with meals.
- Instruct patients to notify the physician if GI symptoms are severe or persistent.
- Teach the patient to take doses with meals or snacks.

#### Patient and family education
- Review with the patient how to take the medication (see above).
- See entry for drug class (p. 413).

---

## pyrantel pamoate    (pi-RAN-tell PAM-oh-ate)                    antihelminic agent

- pyrantel pamoate: Antiminth, ♣ Combantrin

**MECHANISM OF ACTION**    Pyrantel pamoate paralyzes helminths by depolarizing blockade of ganglionic nicotinic receptors normally responsive to acetylcholine. Paralyzed worms are not killed but are eliminated from the body by peristalsis.

**INDICATIONS**    **Ascariasis (roundworms)** Pyrantel pamoate cures 85% to 100% of patients.    **Enterobiasis (pinworms)** Pyrantel pamoate cures 90% to 100% of patients.

**CONTRAINDICATIONS**    **Liver dysfunction** Pyrantel pamoate can alter liver function, which may not be well tolerated in patients with pre-existing liver dysfunctions.    **Anemia, dehydration, or malnutrition** These conditions may need to be treated before administering pyrantel pamoate.

**DOSAGE**    **PO:**    **ADULTS AND CHILDREN OVER 2 YEARS OF AGE:** 11 mg/kg, up to a maximal dose of 1 g, as a single dose; the dose is repeated in 2 weeks for enterobiasis. *Special patient populations:* **PREGNANCY:** Safe use in pregnancy and lactation not established.

**PREPARATIONS**    *Suspension for oral use:* 250 mg/5 ml.

**DRUG INTERACTIONS**    **Piperazine** antagonizes the action of pyrantel pamoate.

**FATE**    Pyrantel pamoate is largely unabsorbed from the intestinal tract, with over 50% of a dose appearing unchanged in the feces.

## ❧ NURSING CONSIDERATIONS
### Side effects, toxicities, and associated nursing actions

**CNS** Dizziness, drowsiness, headache, and insomnia are rarely reported.
- Caution patients to avoid driving or operating hazardous equipment if dizziness or drowsiness occur.

**GI** Abdominal cramps, anorexia, diarrhea, gastralgia, tenesmus, and vomiting are among the most common reactions. These side effects are usually mild and disappear after therapy.
- Instruct patients to notify the physician if GI side effects are severe or persistent.

### Patient and family education
- Inform patients that the drug may be mixed with milk or fruit juice if needed for ease of administration. The drug may be taken with meals if desired.
- See entry for drug class (p. 413).

---

## pyrimethamine (pi-reh-METH-uh-meen) antimalarial agent

- pyramethamine: Daraprim

**MECHANISM OF ACTION** Pyrimethamine inhibits dihydrofolate reductase, thereby interfering with folic acid metabolism in much the same way as the antibacterial agent trimethoprim.

**INDICATIONS** **Malaria** Pyrimethamine is used primarily in combination with quinine sulfate and sulfadiazine to treat malaria caused by chloroquine-resistant *P. falciparum*. • Pyrimethamine with sulfadoxine is used for prophylaxis of malaria caused by chloroquine-resistant *P. falciparum*. **Toxoplasmosis** Pyrimethamine with sulfadiazine, sulfamethoxazole, or another sulfonamide is a treatment of choice.

**CONTRAINDICATIONS** **Megaloblastic anemia** Pyrimethamine may worsen the folate deficiency that causes this blood disorder. **A history of seizure disorders** The CNS toxicity of pyrimethamine may induce seizures in these patients.

**DOSAGE** **PO:** **ADULTS:** For malaria, 25 mg once weekly for suppression or prophylaxis, to continue up to 10 weeks following exposure. For therapy of malaria, 25 mg once daily for 2 or 3 days. Chloroquine-resistant *P. falciparum* requires treatment with additional agents. For toxoplasmosis, high doses in combination with a sulfonamide are required. Initial therapy is 50 to 75 mg daily for 1 to 3 weeks, followed by 25 to 37.5 mg daily for the next 4 to 5 weeks. Dosage may be adjusted as required to minimize toxic reactions. **CHILDREN:** For malaria, 0.5 mg/kg once weekly for suppression or prophylaxis. For therapy of malaria, 12.5 mg (10 to 20 kg child) or 6.25 mg (child under 10 kg) daily for 3 days. For toxoplasmosis, high doses in combination with a sulfonamide are required. Initial therapy is 2 mg/kg daily for 3 days, followed by 1 mg/kg daily for 4 weeks. Dosage should not exceed 25 mg daily. *Special patient populations:* **PREGNANCY:** Safe use in pregnancy and lactation is not established.

**PREPARATIONS** *Tablets:* 25 mg. **Combination products** *Tablets:* 25 mg pyrimethamine with 500 mg sulfadoxine (Fansidar).

**DRUG INTERACTIONS** **Sulfonamides** block folic acid metabolism at the enzymatic step immediately preceding the one blocked by pyrimethamine. The result is synergistic action against sensitive organisms.

**FATE** Pyrimethamine is well absorbed following oral administration, producing *peak* serum concentrations within 2 hours. Pyrimethamine is distributed to internal organs with high blood flow but not to the CNS. The drug passes into milk. Pyrimethamine persists in the body and has an average elimination *half-life* of 111 hours. Metabolites and unchanged drug appear in urine.

## ❧ NURSING CONSIDERATIONS
### Side effects, toxicities, and associated nursing actions

**CNS** Ataxia, respiratory failure, seizures, and tremors may be associated with high doses of pyrimethamine, such as those required for toxoplasmosis. Fatigue, irritability, malaise, and photosensitivity are also rarely reported.
- Caution patients to avoid driving or operating hazardous equipment if fatigue is prominent.
- Obtain a baseline neurologic evaluation and repeat at regular intervals.

- If photosensitivity develops, instruct patients to avoid exposure to the sun and other sources of ultraviolet light, to wear a large-brimmed hat, to keep extremities covered with clothing, and to use a maximum-protection sunscreen on exposed skin surfaces.

**Blood** Agranulocytosis, leukopenia, megaloblastic anemia, pancytopenia, and thrombocytopenia are associated with high doses of pyrimethamine, such as those required for toxoplasmosis. These reactions are usually reversible and may arise from folate depletion. Leucovorin administration may supply folate and reverse some of these effects. Hemolysis can occur if pyrimethamine is given to patients with deficiency of G-6-PD.

- Question the patient about G-6-PD deficiency before administering the first dose. This deficiency is more common in American blacks, Sardinians, and Kurdish Jews.
- Instruct the patient to notify the physician if any of the following signs develop: pallor, malaise, sore throat, fever, or unexplained bleeding or bruising.
- Monitor the complete blood cell count, white blood cell differential, and platelet count.

**GI** Abdominal cramps, anorexia, atrophic glossitis, gastritis, and vomiting are possible, especially with higher doses of pyrimethamine.

- Instruct patients to notify the physician if GI symptoms are severe or persistent.

**Allergic** Fatal allergic reactions involving skin and internal organs are rare and usually involve the combination product Fansidar (pp. 414, 439).

- Instruct patients to report immediately the development of skin changes or any new sign or symptom.

### Patient and family education

- Instruct patients that oral doses may be taken with meals. Pyrimethamine tablets may be crushed to prepare a suspension (consult a pharmacist). If the drug is dispensed as a suspension, teach patients to shake the bottle well before pouring the ordered dose.
- See entry for drug class (p. 413).

## quinacrine hydrochloride (KWIN-uh-krin) antiprotozoal agent

- quinacrine hydrochloride: Atabrine

**MECHANISM OF ACTION** Quinacrine has several biochemical actions that may contribute to its activity against cestodes and protozoans. The drug interacts with DNA and may block DNA or RNA synthesis. The action against cestodes may also involve interactions with DNA. The worms are not killed but the scolex is dislodged, allowing it to be eliminated.

**INDICATIONS** **Giardiasis** Quinacrine hydrochloride cures 80% to 95% of patients with intestinal infections caused by *Giardia lamblia*. **Cestodiasis** Although quinacrine hydrochloride can be used for tapeworm infestations, other drugs are more effective and require less patient preparation before treatment. **Malaria** Quinacrine hydrochloride has no advantage over chloroquine, which is the current drug of choice. Quinacrine is usually not effective in chloroquine-resistant malaria caused by *P. falciparum*.

**CONTRAINDICATIONS** **Severe renal or cardiovascular disease** Shock and cardiac arrhythmias have occurred. **Hepatic dysfunction** Quinacrine concentrates in the liver and may contribute to pre-existing damage. **Deficiency of G-6-PD (glucose-6-phosphate dehydrogenase)** Hemolysis may be more likely in these patients. **Psoriasis** Quinacrine may induce severe attacks. **Porphyria** Quinacrine may exacerbate this condition.

**DOSAGE** **PO:** **ADULTS:** For giardiasis, 100 mg three times daily for 5 to 7 days. The dosage should be taken after meals and followed with a full glass of water, tea, or fruit juice. Treatment may be repeated after 2 weeks, if required. For malaria, 200 mg quinacrine hydrochloride with 1 g sodium bicarbonate every 6 hours for five doses, followed by 100 mg quinacrine hydrochloride three times daily for 6 days. For suppression of malaria, 100 mg once daily for 1 to 3 months. **CHILDREN:** For giardiasis, 2 mg/kg three times daily for 5 days, with the daily dose not to exceed 300 mg. For malaria, children 4 to 8 years of age receive 200 mg three times in 1 day, followed by 100 mg twice daily for 6 days. Children 1 to 4 years of age receive 100 mg three times in one day, followed by 100 mg once daily for 6 days.

For suppression of malaria, 50 mg daily for 1 to 3 months. *Special patient populations:* ELDER-LY: Patients older than 60 years should not receive quinacrine hydrochloride. PREGNANCY: Safe use in pregnancy and lactation is not established.

**PREPARATIONS** *Tablets:* 100 mg.

**DRUG INTERACTIONS** **Hepatotoxic drugs** may add to the damaging effects of quinacrine on the liver. **Primaquine** concentrations are increased in patients also receiving quinacrine, because quinacrine displaces primaquine from tissues. The result is increased toxicity from primaquine.

**DIAGNOSTIC TEST INTERFERENCE** **Cortisol** concentrations in urine and plasma are falsely increased by the fluorescence of quinacrine or its metabolites. **Plasma 11-hydroxycorticosteroid** concentrations are falsely elevated when the Mattingly method is used.

**FATE** Quinacrine hydrochloride is well absorbed following oral administration, producing *peak* serum concentrations within 8 hours. The drug is distributed to most body tissues and highly concentrated in liver, where concentrations may be 2000 times those in plasma. Quinacrine also appears in fetal tissues. Because quinacrine is tightly bound to tissues, it persists for long periods after therapy is discontinued. The drug can be detected in urine for as long as 2 months after the last dose.

## ☙ NURSING CONSIDERATIONS

### Side effects, toxicities, and associated nursing actions

**CNS** Dizziness and headache may occur. A few patients have experienced transient toxic psychoses lasting 2 to 4 weeks. With long-term administration of quinacrine, signs of CNS stimulation may occur: aggressive behavior, anxiety, confusion, emotional lability, euphoria, nervousness, nightmares, restlessness, and seizures.
- Obtain a baseline assessment of mental status and repeat at regular intervals.
- Caution patients to avoid driving or operating hazardous equipment if dizziness occurs.

**Blood** Blood dyscrasias, including aplastic anemia, can occur, especially with long-term use.
- Assess for signs of aplastic anemia: pallor of skin and mucous membranes, fatigue, dyspnea on exertion, unexplained bleeding from gums, nose, vagina, and rectum.
- Monitor complete blood cell count.

**GI** Large single doses of quinacrine used to treat cestodiasis cause severe abdominal cramps, nausea, and vomiting; a duodenal tube may reduce GI distress. Doses used in malaria usually cause milder symptoms, including abdominal cramps, anorexia, diarrhea, nausea, and vomiting.
- Instruct the patient to notify the physician if GI symptoms are severe or persistent.
- Monitor weight in persons on long-term therapy.

**Liver** Hepatitis can occur.
- Assess patients for liver dysfunction: jaundice, malaise, fever, right upper quadrant abdominal pain, change in color or consistency of stools.
- Monitor liver function tests in persons on long-term therapy.

**Allergic** Exfoliative dermatitis can occur, as well as contact dermatitis. Other skin reactions such as blue-black pigmentation or lichen planus-like eruptions may occur but are not allergic responses to quinacrine.
- Instruct the patient to notify the physician of any skin changes.

**Eye** Blurred vision, difficulty in focusing, and visual halos may result from reversible corneal edema or corneal deposits. Retinopathy is possible with long-term administration of doses in excess of those used typically in suppressing malaria.
- Caution patients to avoid driving or operating hazardous equipment if changes in vision occur; notify the physician.
- Encourage patients on long-term therapy to have regular ophthalmic examinations.

### Patient and family education
- See Dosage. Tablets may be crushed and mixed with jelly or honey.
- See the manufacturer's literature about preparation of the patient for treatment of cestodiasis (tapeworms). Treatment involves diet restriction and use of cathartics and enemas.
- Reinforce to patients on long-term therapy the need to have regular medical follow-up.
- See entry for drug class (p. 413).

## quinine sulfate    (KWI-nine)                          antimalarial agent

- quinine sulfate: Quin, Quine, Quinamm, Quindan, Quinite, Quiphile

**MECHANISM OF ACTION**    Quinine interferes with function of plasmodial DNA by an unknown mechanism. The drug is considered a blood schizonticidal agent, being active against the asexual erythrocytic forms of plasmodia but not active against sporozoites, pre-erythrocytic forms. Some gametocytes are susceptible to quinine.

**INDICATIONS**    **Malaria** Quinine may be used with tetracycline or with a sulfonamide to treat chloroquine-resistant strains of *Plasmodium falciparum*. • Severe malaria, including cerebral malaria, caused by *P. falciparum* is treated with IV quinine.    **Nocturnal leg cramps** Quinine sulfate has been used effectively in some patients, but controlled studies to establish the safety of such use have not been done.

**CONTRAINDICATIONS**    **Glucose-6-phosphate dehydrogenase (G-6-PD) deficiency** Thrombocytopenic purpura may occur with quinine.    **Tinnitus** Tinnitus is a symptom of cinchonism, the toxic syndrome caused by quinine.    **Optic neuritis** This reaction can also be caused by quinine.    **Atrial fibrillation** Quinine has the same actions on the heart as the related drug quinidine.

**DOSAGE**    **PO:**    **ADULTS:** For treatment of uncomplicated chloroquine-resistant *P. falciparum* malaria, 600 mg quinine sulfate three times daily for 3 days.    **CHILDREN:** For treatment of uncomplicated chloroquine-resistant *P. falciparum* malaria, 25 mg/kg daily given as three equal doses for 3 days.    **IV:** **ADULTS:** For severe malaria, 600 mg quinine dihydrochloride infused over 2 to 4 hours; repeat at 8 hour intervals until oral dosage can be instituted.    **CHILDREN:** For severe malaria, 25 mg/kg quinine dihydrochloride daily; one third of the dose is infused over 2 to 4 hours. Infusions are repeated every 8 hours. Total daily dosage should not exceed 1.8 g.    *Special patient populations:*    **PREGNANCY:** Quinine causes fetal harm and should be avoided in pregnant women. The drug passes into milk and should therefore be avoided by breast-feeding mothers.

**PREPARATIONS**    *Powder:* for oral use; *tablets:* 250 or 325 mg; *capsules:* 130, 200, 300, or 325 mg.

**DRUG INTERACTIONS**    **Digoxin or digitoxin** concentrations in serum may be increased by quinine.    **Pancuronium, succinylcholine, and tubocurarine** may be more effective at neuromuscular blockade when quinine is also given because quinine itself has neuromuscular effects. The result may be respiratory difficulties.    **Warfarin and other oral anticoagulants** may be more effective in the presence of quinine because quinine depresses the synthesis of vitamin K–dependent coagulation factors by the liver. **Acetazolamide, sodium bicarbonate** and other urinary alkalinizing agents may increase plasma concentrations of quinine by slowing renal elimination. Quinine toxicity can result.    **Antacids containing aluminum** (usually as the hydroxide) can interfere with absorption of quinine.

**DIAGNOSTIC TEST INTERFERENCE**    **Urinary catecholamines** determined by the Sobel and Henry modification of the trihydroxyindole method may be falsely increased in the presence of quinine.    **Urinary 17-ketogenic steroids** determined by the Zimmerman method may be falsely increased in the presence of quinine.    **Urinary 17 hydroxycorticosteroids** determined by the Reddy-Jenkins-Thorn method are falsely increased in the presence of quinine. The modified Porter-Silber method is unaffected.

**FATE**    Quinine sulfate is well absorbed following oral administration, producing *peak* serum concentrations within 1 to 3 hours. The drug is metabolized by the liver, and the metabolites are excreted in urine. Excretion is improved in acidic urine. The elimination *half-life* of quinine is 7 to 12 hours. Malaria alters the metabolic fate of quinine, in part because of effects of the disease on liver function.

## ❦ NURSING CONSIDERATIONS
### Side effects, toxicities, and associated nursing actions

**CNS** Headache, tinnitus, and visual disturbances may be early signs of cinchonism, a syndrome arising from direct toxicity from quinine. More advanced signs include confusion, deafness, fever, headache, restlessness, sweating, syncope, and vertigo.

- Caution patients to avoid driving or operating hazardous equipment if vertigo, visual disturbances, or syncope occur.
- Obtain careful neurologic assessment before starting therapy and at regular intervals.

- Review these signs and symptoms with patients and instruct patients to report their development.
**CV** Angina, conduction disturbances, and ventricular tachycardia can occur during long-term therapy. Rapid IV administration of quinine dihydrochloride can cause acute circulatory failure and arrhythmias.
- Monitor pulse and blood pressure. Assess for signs of angina. See Nursing Interventions for discussion of IV administration.
**Blood** Hypoprothrombinemia and thrombocytopenia purpura occur with quinine. Hemolysis is likely when quinine is given to patients with G-6-PD deficiency.
- Instruct patients to report the appearance of unexplained bleeding or bruising or jaundice.
- Question patients about a history of G-6-PD deficiency before administering the first dose.
- Monitor complete blood cell count, platelet count, prothrombin time, and partial thromboplastin time.
**GI** Epigastric pain, nausea, and vomiting may occur. CNS effects of the drug may contribute to the nausea and vomiting.
- Instruct patients to notify the physician if GI symptoms are severe or persistent.
**Metabolic** Hypoglycemia can occur, perhaps as a result of quinine-induced insulin secretion. The condition can be severe and may recur.
- Be alert to symptoms of hypoglycemia: pallor, perspiration, piloerection, tachycardia, palpitation, nervousness, irritability, weakness, trembling, hunger, headache, blurred vision, diplopia, incoherent speech, emotional changes, or fatigue. Review signs and symptoms with the patient, and instruct the patient to eat or drink some sweetened fruit juice if symptoms develop.
- Caution diabetic patients about this side effect. Caution diabetics to monitor blood sugar closely while on quinine; an adjustment in diet or insulin dose may be necessary.
- Monitor blood glucose levels.
**Allergic** Quinine allergies can occur, with typical hypsensitivity reactions.
- Instruct patients to report the development of any new sign or symptom.
**Liver** Granulomatous hepatitis is a rare reaction.
- Instruct patients to report signs of hepatic dysfunction: malaise, fever, jaundice, right upper quadrant abdominal pain, or change in the color or consistency of stools.
- Monitor liver function tests.
**Eye** The retina and optic nerves can be damaged by quinine. Blurred vision, constricted visual fields, diplopia, disturbed color perception, photophobia, and scotomata.
- Assess visual acuity regularly.
- Reinforce to patients on long-term therapy the need for regular ophthalmic examinations.
- Caution patients to avoid driving or operating hazardous equipment if blurred vision, diplopia, or disturbed color perception occurs; notify the physician.

### Nursing interventions related to drug administration
- For IV administration, dilute 600 mg in 300 ml, and infuse over 2 to 4 hours.
- Monitor blood pressure and pulse. Administer IV doses with the patient in the supine position only, and keep the patient recumbent until blood pressure is stable.

### Patient and family education
- Inform patients that doses may be taken with meal or snacks to lessen gastric irritation.
- See entry for drug class (p. 413).

---

## sulfadiazine    sul-fa-DYE-a-zeen                                           sulfonamide

- sulfadiazine: Microsulfon

**MECHANISM OF ACTION**  • See listing in Chapter Twenty, p. 328.
**☙ NURSING CONSIDERATIONS**
- See listing in Chapter 20 (p. 327).
- See entry for drug class (p. 293).

# sulfadoxine with pyrimethamine
(sul-fa-DOX-een; pi-reh-METH-uh-meen)    antimalarial

- sulfadoxine with pyrimethamine: Fansidar

**MECHANISM OF ACTION**    Pyrimethamine inhibits dihydrofolate reductase in a manner similar to that of trimethoprim. Sulfadoxine inhibits an earlier stage of folic acid metabolism, as do other sulfonamides. The combination results in a synergistic blockade of folic acid metabolism in susceptible organisms.

**INDICATIONS**    **Malaria** Suppression or prophylaxis of chloroquine-resistant malaria caused by *Plasmodium falciparum* may be accomplished with the fixed combination of sulfadoxine and pyrimethamine. • Treatment of uncomplicated mild to moderate malaria caused by chloroquine-resistant *P. falciparum* may be accomplished with pyrimethamine and sulfadoxine. • Additional therapy may be required if the infection is severe.

**CONTRAINDICATIONS**    **Megaloblastic anemia** Folate deficiency may be worsened by this fixed drug combination.    **Allergies to pyrimethamine or to sulfonamides** Allergic reactions may be expected if patients have shown hypersensitivity to either component of the fixed combination.

**DOSAGE**    **PO:**    **ADULTS:** For suppression of malaria, 1 tablet (500 mg sulfadoxine and 25 mg pyrimethamine) once weekly during exposure and for 4 to 6 weeks thereafter. For treatment of malaria, 2 or 3 tablets may be taken as a single dose.    **CHILDREN:** For suppression of malaria, children 2 to 11 months of age receive 1/8 tablet weekly; 1 to 3 years, 1/4 tablet weekly; 4 to 8 years, 1/2 tablet weekly; 9 to 14 years, 3/4 tablet weekly. For treatment of malaria, children under 4 years receive 1/2 tablet as a single dose; 4 to 8 years, 1 tablet; 9 to 14 years, 2 tablets.    *Special patient populations:*    **CHILDREN:** Safe use in children under 2 months of age is not established.    **PREGNANCY:** The drugs should be avoided if possible during pregnancy and lactation.

**PREPARATIONS**    *Tablets:* 500 mg sulfadoxine with 25 mg pyrimethamine.

**DRUG INTERACTIONS**    **Sulfonamides or co-trimoxazole** should be avoided when Fansidar is being taken. The sulfonamide component in all these preparations may cause additive toxicity.

**FATE**    Both components of the fixed combination product Fansidar are well absorbed following oral administration. *Peak* concentrations in serum of pyrimethamine are achieved within 1.5 to 8 hours and *peak* concentrations of sulfadoxine are achieved within 2.5 to 6 hours. Sulfadoxine is more widely distributed through the body than is pyrimethamine. Both drugs appear in milk. Both drugs are metabolized to some extent by the liver and are excreted in urine. The elimination *half-life* of pyrimethamine is 111 hours, and the *half-life* of sulfadoxine is 169 hours.

## NURSING CONSIDERATIONS

### Side effects, toxicities, and associated nursing actions

**Blood** Agranulocytosis, aplastic anemia, and other blood dyscrasias can occur. Megaloblastic anemia may be the result of folate deficiency.
- Instruct the patient to notify the physician if any of the following signs develop: pallor, malaise, sore throat, fever, or unexplained bleeding or bruising.
- Monitor the complete blood cell count, white blood cell differential, and platelet count.

**Liver** Hepatocellular necrosis has occurred, which may be fatal.
- Instruct patients to report signs of liver dysfunction: malaise, fever, right upper quadrant abdominal pain, jaundice, or change in the color or consistency of stools.
- Monitor liver function tests.

**Allergic** Hypersensitivity reactions may be fatal, even when the drug combination is used for prophylaxis of malaria.

**Other** Toxic epidermal necrolysis, erythema multiforme, and Stevens-Johnson syndrome are serious and potentially fatal reactions that have occurred.
- Instruct patients to report immediately the development of any skin changes or rashes.
- Remind patients to notify the physician of any new sign or symptom.

### Patient and family education
- Suggest to patients that doses may be taken with meals or a snack.

- Encourage patients to maintain good fluid intake to ensure good fluid output to prevent crystalluria, which may accompany therapy with sufonamides.
- See entry for drug class (p. 413).

## tetracycline  (tet-ra-SYE-kleen)  antibiotic

- sold under generic name

**MECHANISM OF ACTION**  • See listing under Tetracycline, Chapter Seventeen, p. 293.

**NURSING CONSIDERATIONS**
- See listing under Tetracycline (p. 293).
- See entry for drug class (p. 413).

## thiabendazole  (thy-uh-BEN-da-zole)  antihelmintic agent

- thiabendazole: Mintezol

**MECHANISM OF ACTION**  Thiabendazole inhibits the enzyme fumarate reductase, which is important in the metabolism of helminths. Thiabendazole has analgesic, antipyretic, and anti-inflammatory actions in humans.

**INDICATIONS**  **Strongyloidiasis** Thiabendazole is a drug of choice, curing over 90% of treated patients. **Cutaneous larva migrans (creeping eruption) or visceral larva migrans (toxocariasis)** Thiabendazole is a drug of choice, effectively controlling the disease within 2 days in most patients.  **Ascariasis** Thiabendazole is an alternate to the preferred drugs piperazine, pyrantel pamoate, and mebendazole. **Hookworm** Thiabendazole is generally less effective than pyrantel pamoate or mebendazole.  **Trichuriasis (whipworm)** Thiabendazole is less effective than mebendazole.

**CONTRAINDICATIONS**  **Anemia or malnutrition** These conditions should be treated before using thiabendazole if possible.  **Hepatic or renal dysfunction** Thiabendazole should be avoided if possible or used with careful monitoring of organ function.

**DOSAGE**  **PO:**  **ADULTS:** 1.5 g for patient weighing over 70 kg. The maximum daily dose is 3 g. For strongyloidiasis, the dose is repeated on 2 consecutive days. For cutaneous larva migrans, the dose is given twice daily for 2 consecutive days. For toxocariasis, the dose is given twice daily for 5 to 7 days. **CHILDREN:** Children receive 22 to 25 mg/kg as a dose. For strongyloidiasis, the dose is repeated on 2 consecutive days. For cutaneous larva migrans, the dose is given twice daily for 2 consecutive days. For toxocariasis, the dose is given twice daily for 5 to 7 days. Children weighing less than 13.6 kg should not receive the drug.  *Special patient populations:* **PREGNANCY:** Safe use in pregnancy and lactation is not established.

**PREPARATIONS**  *Tablets, chewable:* 500 mg; *suspension for oral use:* 500 mg/5 ml.

**DRUG INTERACTIONS**  **Theophylline** concentrations in blood may rise when thiabendazole is also used, resulting in toxicity.

**FATE**  Thiabendazole is well absorbed following oral administration, producing *peak* serum concentrations within 1 to 2 hours. Metabolism is principally in the liver, with metabolites of the drug being excreted in urine. The drug does not persist in the body for prolonged periods.

**NURSING CONSIDERATIONS**
**Side effects, toxicities, and associated nursing actions**
**CNS** Dizziness is the most frequent CNS effect. Drowsiness, giddiness, headache, psychic disturbance, seizures, and weariness also occur. Changes in vision, hyperirritability, numbness, and tinnitus are less common.
- Caution patients to avoid driving or operating hazardous equipment if dizziness, drowsiness, weariness, or changes in vision occur.

- Instruct patients to report the development of any new sign or symptom.

**CV** Hypotension and bradycardia are possible side effects.
- Monitor pulse and blood pressure if the patient is remaining in the health care setting.

**Blood** Transient leukopenia has occurred.

**Renal** Nephrotoxicity can occur.
- Monitor white blood cell differential, serum creatinine, and BUN if indicated by patient's condition.

**GI** Anorexia, nausea, and vomiting are common. Diarrhea and epigastric distress occur less frequently.
- Instruct the patient to notify the physician if GI symptoms are severe or persistent.

**Liver** Cholestasis, jaundice, increased AST in serum, and parenchymal liver damage can occur.
- Instruct the patient to report signs of liver dysfunction: fever, malaise, jaundice, change in color or consistency of stools, or right upper quadrant abdominal pain.
- Monitor liver function tests if indicated by patient condition.

**Metabolic** Hyperglycemia is rare.
- Monitor serum and urine glucose if indicated by patient condition.
- Caution diabetic patients about this side effect. Instruct diabetics to monitor blood glucose levels carefully for several days. A temporary adjustment in diet or insulin may be necessary.

**Allergic** Angioedema, anaphylaxis, chills, erythema multiforme, fever, flushing, lymphadenopathy, pruritis, and rashes can occur and are rarely fatal.
- Have drugs, equipment, and personnel available to treat acute allergic reactions in settings where this drug is administered.
- Caution patients to report the development of any unexpected sign or symptom.

**Other** *Ascaris* may migrate when thiabendazole is used, resulting in live worms appearing in the nose or mouth of the patient.
- Warn patients of this unpleasant possibility.

## Patient and family education

- Instruct patients to take doses after meals and to chew tablets before swallowing them.
- See entry for drug class (p. 413).

# IMMUNE MODULATORS

**INTRODUCTION** Enhancing the function of the immune system has been a powerful weapon in the long struggle to control infectious diseases. Vaccines have been in use for over 200 years, although the scientific basis for the effectiveness of vaccines was not understood until much later. Vaccines promote the same type of antibody production that can be triggered by natural infection. Moreover, the antibody production can be reinstituted rapidly if exposure occurs subsequently. Toxoids also promote this type of active immunity. Immunoglobulins and antivenins give passive immunity and are intended as short-term control for specific exposure.

Suppression of the immune system is often a medical problem. Immune suppression is an undesirable side effect of many drugs, such as glucocorticoids or anticancer agents, and human immunodeficiency virus (HIV) causes an apparently irreversible immune suppression that leads to death. In a few medical situations, however, immune suppression is a desired therapeutic goal. For example, patients with autoimmune diseases, such as rheumatoid arthritis or lupus erythematosus, may be helped by curbing overactive immune processes. Immune suppression is also necessary in patients receiving organ transplants; without these powerful immunosuppressive agents, transplanted organs would be rapidly rejected.

VII

# Chapter Twenty-five

# Enhancing agents: vaccines, toxoids, and sera

antirabies serum
BCG vaccine
cholera vaccine
crotaline antivenin polyvalent
digoxin immune Fab
diphtheria antitoxin
diphtheria toxoid
diphtheria and tetanus toxoids
diphtheria and tetanus toxoids and pertussis
vaccine
Haemophilus B vaccine
hepatitis B immune globulin
hepatitis B vaccine
immune globulin
influenza virus vaccine
measles virus vaccine live
mumps virus vaccine live
pertussis immune globulin

plague vaccine
pneumococcal vaccine (polyvalent)
poliovirus vaccine inactivated
poliovirus vaccine live oral
rabies immune globulin
rabies vaccine
$Rh_o$ (D) immune globulin
rubella virus vaccine live
smallpox vaccine
tetanus antitoxin
tetanus immune globulin
tetanus toxoid
typhoid vaccine
varicella-zoster immune globulin
widow spider species antivenin (*Latrodectus mactans*)
yellow fever vaccine

**OVERVIEW OF THE DRUG CLASS**  Enhancing the action of the immune system has allowed control of many diseases that once caused devastating epidemics. This control has been possible because of the amazing capacity of the immune system to produce specific antibodies toward a very large number of antigens. This specificity in immune responses makes it necessary to develop vaccines against each individual organism causing disease. For example, the vaccine that protects against measles does not protect against mumps. In some cases the specificity is so great that it defeats medical attempts to develop a vaccine. For example, an effective vaccine against the rhinoviruses that cause colds would have to develop immunity toward all 100 or more serotypes of that virus. This task is impractical.

**MECHANISM OF ACTION**  Immunologic agents used to protect patients from disease are of several types. *Toxoids* are modified bacterial toxins, changed to eliminate their toxicity but retain their ability to induce formation of antitoxin by the patient. *Globulins* are protein mixtures that contain antibodies directed toward various organisms. *Antivenins* contain globulins that absorb and neutralize toxic agents, such as the venoms of snakes or spiders. *Vaccines* contain attenuated or killed microorganisms that provoke an antibody response in a patient without causing the active disease. Toxoids and vaccines promote active immunity that may last years, whereas globulins provide passive immunity that lasts only as long as the globulins remain in circulation, which is usually about 3 weeks.

**INDICATIONS**  See listings for individual drugs.

**CONTRAINDICATIONS**  See listings for individual drugs.

**DRUG INTERACTIONS**  **Corticosteroids** may interfere with the generation of active immunity by toxoids or vaccines. **Immunosuppressive agents** used in cancer chemotherapy may interfere with the generation of active immunity by toxoids or vaccines.

## ❧ NURSING CONSIDERATIONS
### Side effects, toxicities, and associated nursing actions

**Allergic**  Any serum product containing proteins such as immunoglobulins can cause an allergic reaction called serum sickness. Symptoms include arthralgia, skin eruptions, lymphadenopathy, and pruritis. Abdominal pain, fever, headache, and malaise occur in more serious cases. Vaccines and toxoids may also cause allergic reactions that are occasionally severe. Anaphylaxis is rare but possible.

• Review with patients the signs and symptoms of serum sickness. Instruct patients to report the development of serum sickness. Note that serum sickness may not develop for up to 6 to 12 days after immunization.

• Have available epinephrine solution 1:1000 in settings where protein-containing products are administered. Have drugs, equipment, and personnel available to treat acute allergic responses.

**Local effects** Injection of serum products, vaccines, or toxoids may cause local tissue irritation with pain, erythema, and urticaria.

- Caution patient to avoid scratching injection site. Brief application of an ice pack may lessen irritation; have patient consult physician about local irritation.

### Nursing interventions related to drug administration

- Question patients about history of allergy before administering. Many of these drugs are contraindicated in persons with a history of allergy to horse serum, egg protein, or other diluents. Report allergy to the physician, as desensitization may be necessary.
- Question female patients about the possibility of pregnancy before administering drug. Several drugs are contraindicated in pregnant women because of potential damage to the fetus, and women should be counseled to avoid pregnancy for several months after receiving other vaccines. See individual monographs.
- For IM administration, use anatomical landmarks to choose injection sites. Use the deltoid muscle for administration of most vaccines and similar medications for older children and adults. Usually, avoid the injection sites in the gluteal area unless large-volume doses must be divided into two or more injections or the patient is receiving two or more drugs that cannot be administered in the same site. Use the vastus lateralis in infants and small children. Aspirate before injecting drug to avoid inadvertent IM administration; if blood is aspirated, withdraw needle, discard syringe and needle, and prepare a fresh dose. Record and rotate injection sites for subsequent doses.
- Review manufacturer's instructions when preparing unfamiliar medications.

### Patient and family eduction

- Review with patients and families the anticipated benefits and possible side effects of drug therapy.
- Instruct patients to maintain current records of vaccines, toxoids, and other medications that modify the immune system.
- When appropriate, review with patients the schedule for additional doses of immune-modifying medications.
- Refer patients to the local health department if appropriate.
- Instruct patients who manifest allergic response to wear a medical identification tag or bracelet listing the allergic response and to be cautious in taking vaccines or other immune modulators without consultation with the physician.

---

## antirabies serum   (an-ti-RAY-bees)                              serumglobulins*

- antirabies serum: Sold under generic name

**MECHANISM OF ACTION**   Antirabies serum contains antibodies to the rabies virus and confers passive immunity by neutralizing the free virus. Rabies immune globulin (p. 460) is usually preferred for this use. The antibodies are probably not effective once the virus has penetrated nerves.

**INDICATIONS**   **Rabies exposure** The antirabies serum can be used to neutralize rabies virus in the wound before the virus penetrates nerves and begins to cause irreversible disease.

**CONTRAINDICATIONS**   **Allergy to equine serum** Because this product is derived from equine serum, allergic reactions are common.

**DOSAGE**   **IM:**   **ADULTS AND CHILDREN:** 40 IU/kg, administered at the same time as the first dose of rabies vaccine. Half of the dose should be infiltrated immediately around the wound.

*Special patient populations:*   **PREGNANCY:** The risk from untreated exposure to rabies is so high that the risk from use of antirabies serum is negligible by comparison.

**PREPARATIONS**   *Solution for injection:* 1000 IU/8 ml.

**DRUG INTERACTIONS**   **Rabies vaccine** may have a reduced effect if higher than standard doses of antirabies serum are used.

**FATE**   Antirabies serum confers short-term protection. Permanent immunity is not conferred.

## ☙ NURSING CONSIDERATIONS

### Side effects, toxicities, and associated nursing actions
- See entry for drug class (p. 444).

### Nursing interventions related to drug administration
- Before administering prescribed dose, perform sensitivity test on patient (consult physician). Inject intradermally 0.1 ml of a 1:100 dilution of antirabies serum in 0.9% sodium chloride solution. For individuals with a history of allergic response, use only 0.05 ml. Inject a control test of 0.1 ml of 0.9% sodium chloride solution in another site. The skin test is interpreted in 10 to 30 minutes. A positive reaction consists of an urticarial wheal of 10 mm or more, surrounded by an erythematous flare 20 by 20 mm. If the skin test is positive, a course of desensitization injections should be administered.
- For IM injection in adults, the buttocks should be avoided unless large volumes of the drug necessitate multiple injections; the deltoid muscle may be used.

### Patient and family education
- See entry for drug class (p. 445).

---

## BCG vaccine*  (bee-cee-GEE)                                                    vaccine

- BCG vaccine: Sold under generic name

**MECHANISM OF ACTION**   BCG vaccine is prepared from live, attenuated *Mycobacterium bovis*. Vaccination induces development of active immunity against mycobacteria, including strains causing tuberculosis.

**INDICATIONS**   **Repeated exposure to active tuberculosis** Prophylaxis with isoniazid is preferred in the United States for patients with a single exposure; however, active immunity may be preferable when exposure is chronic.

**CONTRAINDICATIONS**   **Positive Mantoux skin test for tuberculosis** The vaccine should not be given to anyone with a positive skin test.   **Recent smallpox immunization** The vaccine should not be given to anyone immunized against smallpox within the past 3 weeks.

**DOSAGE**   **SC:**   ADULTS AND CHILDREN OVER 1 MONTH: Percutaneous, 0.2 to 0.3 ml.   NEONATES: 0.2 to 0.3 ml of a 50% dilution of the adult strength.   **Intradermal:**   ADULTS AND CHILDREN OVER 1 MONTH: 0.1 ml.   NEONATES: 0.05 ml.   *Special patient populations:*   PREGNANCY: Safe use in pregnancy and lactation has not been established.

**PREPARATIONS**   Solution: for injection by percutaneous multiple-puncture only (Antigen Supply House) or for intradermal use only (Glaxo).

**DRUG INTERACTIONS**   **Isoniazid** may diminish the response to BCG vaccine. For other interactions, see entry for drug class (p. 444).

**FATE**   BCG vaccine confers active immunity, but the effect is variable and is not permanent.

## ☙ NURSING CONSIDERATIONS

### Side effects, toxicities, and associated nursing actions
**Skin** Up to 10% of patients may suffer ulceration at the site of injection.
- Inform patients about this side effect. Remind patients not to scratch injection site.

**Allergic** Anaphylactic shock in neonates has occurred rarely.
- Monitor vital signs; do not leave infant unattended for 30 minutes following injection.
- For other side effects, see entry for drug class (p. 444).

### Nursing interventions related to drug administration
- Read labels carefully for information about reconstitution.
- Avoid shaking after reconstituting. Administer immediately following reconstitution.
- Administer dose only by route specified on label.
- For intradermal injection, administer over the insertion of the deltoid muscle in adults.

*Bacillus Calmette-Guerin.

**Patient and family education**
- See entry for drug class (p. 445).
- Instruct patients that lesion will develop over injection site within 7 to 10 days. Area should be completely healed within 3 to 6 months.

---

## cholera vaccine   (KOL-er-ah)       vaccine

- cholera vaccine: Sold under generic name

**MECHANISM OF ACTION**   Cholera vaccine prepared from inactivated *Vibrio cholerae* develops active immunity by causing the development of vibriocidal antibodies.

**INDICATIONS**   **To prevent cholera** Cholera vaccine is used to protect persons who will be exposed to cholera by traveling in areas where the disease is endemic (India, Africa, Far East, Middle East) or persons who have close contact with patients suffering from cholera.

**CONTRAINDICATIONS**   **Previous allergic reactions to cholera vaccine** These patients may be at risk of serious or fatal allergic reactions.

**DOSAGE**   **IM or SC:**  **ADULTS:** 0.5 ml as a single dose.  **CHILDREN:** Ages 6 months to 4 years receive 0.2 ml. Ages 5 to 10 years receive 0.3 ml. Children over 10 years receive adult doses.  **Intradermal: ADULTS AND CHILDREN OVER 2 YEARS:** 0.2 ml.  *Special patient populations:*  **PREGNANCY:** Safe use in pregnancy and lactation has not been established, but the vaccine has been used in pregnant women without apparent harm.

**PREPARATIONS**   *Suspension:* sterile, for injection.

**DRUG INTERACTIONS**   **Yellow fever vaccine** should not be administered within 3 weeks of cholera vaccine. Responses to both vaccines are diminished if given together. For other interactions, see entry for drug class (p. 444).

**FATE**   Only 25% to 50% of vaccinated individuals develop active immunity to cholera. Those persons who do develop active immunity are not permanently protected. Boosters may be required after 6 months to restimulate the waning immunity.

### ❦ NURSING CONSIDERATIONS

**Side effects, toxicities, and associated nursing actions**
- See entry for drug class (p. 444).

**Nursing interventions related to drug administration**
- See entry for drug class (p. 445).

**Patient and family education**
- See entry for drug class (p. 445).

---

## crotaline antivenin, polyvalent   (KRO-ta-lin)       serumglobulins*

- crotaline antivenin: Antivenin (crotalidae) polyvalent, Snakebite (pit vipers) antivenin

**MECHANISM OF ACTION**   Crotaline antivenin contains globulins capable of neutralizing the venoms of the pit vipers native to the Americas. Snakes included are rattlesnakes, copperheads, cotton mouth moccasins, fer-de-lance, and bushmasters. This antivenin does not protect against the bite of the coral snake.

**INDICATIONS**   **Bites of pit vipers** The crotaline antivenin should be administered as soon as possible after the snakebite (see above).

**CONTRAINDICATIONS**   **Allergy to equine serum** If it is necessary to administer the antivenin to patients with allergies, desensitization may be performed.

**DOSAGE**   **IV:**  **ADULTS AND CHILDREN:** Dosage is based on the estimated amount of venom injected. For best results, the first dose should be administered within 4 hours of the bite.  **IM:**  **ADULTS AND CHILDREN:** IV dosage is preferred, but if necessary the antivenin may be injected into a large muscle mass.  *Special patient populations:*  **PREGNANCY:** Safe use in pregnancy and lactation has not been established, but the high risk of untreated snake bite may outweigh the potential risk from the antivenin.

**PREPARATIONS**   *Serum for injection:* antivenin with 0.25% phenol and 0.005% thimerosal. Bacteriostatic water for injection (10 ml) and a separate vial of equine serum (1 ml) are supplied. The antivenin is diluted with water. Before the dose is administered, the patient should be tested for sensitivity to equine serum and desensitization performed if necessary.

**DRUG INTERACTIONS**   See entry for drug class (p. 444).

**FATE**   The antivenin is short-term therapy and does not confer long-term protection.

## ❧ NURSING CONSIDERATIONS

### Side effects, toxicities, and associated nursing actions
- See entry for drug class (p. 444).

### Nursing interventions related to drug administration
- Before administering prescribed dose, perform sensitivity test on patient (consult physician). Inject intradermally 0.02 to 0.03 ml of a 1:10 dilution of normal equine serum or antivenin in 0.9% sodium chloride solution. For individuals with a history of allergic response, use a dilution of 1:100. Inject a control test of 0.9% sodium chloride solution in the other extremity. The skin test is interpreted in 5 to 30 minutes. A positive reaction consists of a urticarial wheal of 10 mm or more, surrounded by an erythematous flare 20 by 20 mm. If the skin test is positive, a course of desensitization injections should be administered.
- For IV administration, a 1:1 to 1:10 dilution of reconstituted antivenin in 0.9% sodium chloride or 5% dextrose solution is prepared; avoid shaking the bottle. Administer 5 to 10 ml over 3 to 5 minutes. Observe patients carefully and monitor vital signs. If no serious problems occur, administer remaining portion of dose.

### Patient and family education
- See entry for drug class (p. 445).

---

## digoxin immune Fab   (di-JOX-in)                    antibody fragments

- digoxin immune Fab: Digibind

**MECHANISM OF ACTION**   Digoxin immune Fab is a preparation containing fragments of antibodies generated in sheep toward digoxin bound to human albumin. When injected into patients overdosed with digoxin, these fragments are able to bind digoxin and remove it from circulation.

**INDICATIONS**   **Acute toxicity from digoxin or digitoxin** Life-threatening overdoses may be treated, but less serious overdoses should be treated with standard medical support.

**CONTRAINDICATIONS**   **Allergy to sheep products or serum products** Although most patients do not require sensitivity testing before use of digoxin immune Fab, certain patients with an increased likelihood to react should be tested before the product is administered.

**DOSAGE**   **IV:**   **ADULTS:** Dosage is adjusted according to the amount of digoxin or digitoxin to be adsorbed. Each mole of digoxin immune Fab adsorbs one mole of digoxin or digitoxin; converted to a weight basis, this relationship predicts that 60 mg of immune Fab will bind 1 mg of digoxin or digitoxin. Rapid treatment for life-threatening toxic reactions in which the total digoxin dose is unknown may be undertaken with 800 mg of immune Fab (twenty 40 mg vials). Refer to manufacturer's literature for charts indicating estimation of dose of immune Fab from patient's body weight and serum concentration of digoxin.   **CHILDREN:** Dosage is carefully calculated to adsorb the amount of digoxin or digitoxin estimated to be present in the whole body as for adults.   **Intradermal:**   **ADULTS AND CHILDREN:** For sensitivity testing, 0.1 ml of a 1:100 dilution of immune Fab in 0.9% sodium chloride solution may be injected. The appearance of a urticarial wheal and surrounding edema constitutes a positive test.   *Special patient populations:*   **PREGNANCY:** Safe use has not been established.

**PREPARATIONS**   *Powder* for reconstitution: 40 mg vial. Add 4 ml sterile water to the 40 mg vial. Gently agitate to dissolve. The resulting 10 mg/ml solution may be used directly but is often diluted further in 0.9%

sodium chloride solution for administration by IV infusion. An in-line 0.22 μm filter removes the small amount of protein aggregates that often remains after reconstitution.

**DRUG INTERACTIONS**    **Cardiac glycosides** are ineffective for as long as the immune Fab remains in the body. Several days are required to clear the immune Fab in normal patients. The process may take over a week in patients with renal impairment.

**FATE**    Binding of digoxin or digitoxin to immune Fab is rapid, and reversal of toxicity may begin within minutes of IV infusion. Digoxin immune Fab with attached digoxin or digitoxin is cleared from the body by glomerular filtration. Clearance requires several days when renal function is normal.

## 🐝 NURSING CONSIDERATIONS

### Side effects, toxicities, and associated nursing actions

**CV** Worsening of heart failure and reduction of cardiac output are probable results of binding cardiac glycosides and prevent the actions of these drugs on the diseased heart.
- Monitor vital signs and blood pressure. Perform continuous ECG monitoring while this drug is being used.
- Monitor weight and intake and output. Auscultate breath sounds. Assess for signs of dependent edema and jugular venous distention.

**Metabolic** Hypokalemia may result as cardiac glycosides are bound and $Na^+$, $K^+$–ATPase inhibition is released, resulting in movement of potassium into cells.
- Assess for signs of hypokalemia: muscle weakness, apathy, abdominal distention, and paralytic ileus. ECG changes include inverted T waves, prolonged QT segments, and prominent U waves.
- Monitor serum electrolytes.

**Allergic** Fever or other reactions are theoretically possible but have not yet been documented. The Fab fragment should be less immunogenic than the entire immunoglobulin molecule.
- Monitor temperature.

### Nursing interventions related to drug administration
- Consult manufacturer's literature for guidelines about dilution, rate of administration, and skin testing.
- Monitor vital signs and ECG tracing. Have drugs, equipment, and personnel available to treat cardiac arrest.

### Patient and family education
- Review with patients and families the anticipated benefits and possible side effects of drug therapy. Provide emotional support to families as needed. Keep patients and families informed of changes in the patient's condition.

---

## diphtheria antitoxin    (dif-THEE-ree-uh)                                          globulins

- diphtheria antitoxin: Sold under generic name

**MECHANISM OF ACTION**    Diphtheria antitoxin is a purified and concentrated form of immunoglobulins prepared from equine serum. The antitoxin neutralizes the tissue-damaging toxin released by *Corynebacterium diphtheriae* during acute diphtheria.

**INDICATIONS**    **Acute diphtheria** Antitoxin should be given as soon as possible after diphtheria is diagnosed.

**CONTRAINDICATIONS**    **Allergy to equine serum** Use should be avoided unless a desensitization test is performed.

**DOSAGE**    **IV:** **ADULTS AND CHILDREN:** 20,000 to 120,000 units by slow infusion, with dosage determined by severity of the disease.    **IM:** **ADULTS AND CHILDREN:** 20,000 to 120,000 units, with dosage determined by severity of the disease. *Special patient populations:* **PREGNANCY:** Safe use in pregnancy and lactation has not been established.

**PREPARATIONS**    *Solution for injection:* 10,000 or 20,000 units, with 0.3% m-cresol.

**DRUG INTERACTIONS**    None established.

**FATE**    Diphtheria antitoxin is for short-term therapy of diphtheria and does not confer long-term protection.

❦ **NURSING CONSIDERATIONS**

**Side effects, toxicities, and associated nursing actions**
- See entry for drug class (p. 444).

**Nursing interventions related to drug administration**
- Before administering prescribed dose, perform sensitivity test on patient (consult physician). Inject intradermally 0.1 ml of a 1:100 dilution of diphtheria antitoxin in 0.9% sodium chloride solution. For individuals with a history of allergic response, a dilution of 1:1000 should be used. Inject a control test of 0.1 ml of 0.9% sodium chloride sodium in the opposite extremity. The skin test is interpreted in 20 minutes. A positive reaction consists of a urticarial wheal of 10 mm or more, surrounded by an erythematous flare 20 by 20 mm. If the skin test is positive, a course of desensitization injections should be administered. A scratch test may be substituted for the intradermal test.
- In addition to the intradermal or scratch test, a conjunctival test should also be performed. Place one drop of a 1:10 dilution of diphterhia antitoxin in the lower conjunctival sac of one eye; administer a control test of 0.9% sodium chloride solution in the other eye. The test is interpreted in 15 minutes. A positive test reaction consists of itching, burning, redness, and lacrimation. When sensitivity tests are positive, a course of desensitization injections should be administered if possible.

**Patient and family education**
- See entry for drug class (p. 445).

---

## diphtheria toxoid adsorbed    (dif-THEE-ree-uh)                                    toxoid

- diphtheria toxoid adsorbed: Sold under generic name

**MECHANISM OF ACTION**    Diphtheria toxoid induces production of specific antitoxins toward the toxin produced by *Corynebacterium diphtheriae*. Immunity to diphtheria may be conferred.

**INDICATIONS**    **Immunization of children 6 weeks to 6 years of age** Three doses several months apart confers immunity to most patients, but the combined product DTP (diphtheria and tetanus toxoids with pertussis vaccine adsorbed; see p. 451) is preferred for most patients.

**CONTRAINDICATIONS**    **CNS disease** Children under 2 years with signs of CNS damage or disease should not receive diphtheria toxoid because of the potential CNS effects of the preparation.

**DOSAGE**    IM:    **CHILDREN 6 WEEKS TO 6 YEARS:** By deep IM injection only, 0.5 ml (15 Lf units). Immunization is with three doses; the second should follow the first by 6 to 8 weeks, and the third dose should come a year after the second dose. *Special patient populations:*    **ELDERLY:** This preparation should not be used in adults because risk of serious side effects is increased.    **PREGNANCY:** This preparation should not be used in adults because risk of serious side effects is increased.

**PREPARATIONS**    Solution for injections: 15 Lf units/0.5 ml. In Canada, diphtheria toxoid is available for SC administration, 50 Lf units/ml. Doses are 0.5 or 1.0 ml for 3 doses at intervals of 3 or 4 weeks.

**DRUG INTERACTIONS**    See entry for drug class (p. 444).

**FATE**    When administered properly in 3 doses as described above, immunity lasting up to 10 years is produced in most patients.

❦ **NURSING CONSIDERATIONS**

**Side effects, toxicities, and associated nursing actions**
- See entry for drug class (p. 444).

**Nursing interventions related to drug administration**
- Read orders and labels carefully; this product is not for use in adults.

**Patient and family education**
- See entry for drug class (p. 445).

## diphtheria and tetanus toxoids (dif-THEE-ree-uh) toxoid

- diphtheria and tetanus toxoids: Diphtheria and tetanus toxoids adsorbed (DT), Tetanus and diphtheria toxoids adsorbed (Td) for adult use

**MECHANISM OF ACTION** This mixture of adsorbed toxoids promotes production of active antitoxins and confers active immunity to diphtheria or tetanus when administered in appropriately spaced doses.

**INDICATION** **Immunization against diphtheria and tetanus** For children, the combined preparation DTP (diphtheria and tetanus toxoids with pertussis vaccine adsorbed) is preferred (p. 451). **Booster for immunization against diphtheria and tetanus** To increase or maintain immunity after age 7 years.

**CONTRAINDICATIONS** **History of neurologic reaction to diphtheria or tetanus toxoid** Risk of subsequent neurologic damage is greater in these patients.

**DOSAGE** **IM:** **ADULTS:** By deep muscle injection only. Adults should receive the tetanus and diphtheria toxoids adsorbed (Td) for adults; 0.5 ml containing 1.4 to 2 Lf units of diphtheria toxoid and 5 to 10 Lf units of tetanus toxoid. Three doses are administered for primary immunization; the second is 4 to 8 weeks after the first, and the third is 6 to 12 months after the second dose. Boosters should be administered every 10 years. **CHILDREN:** By deep muscle injection only. Children should receive the diphtheria and tetanus toxoids adsorbed (DT) for pediatric use; 0.5 ml containing 6.6 to 15 Lf units of diphtheria toxoid and 5 to 10 Lf units of tetanus toxoid. The primary immunization schedule is as described for adults. *Special patient populations:* **PREGNANCY:** Safe use in pregnancy and lactation has not been established, although the preparation has been administered to pregnant women with no apparent harm.

**PREPARATIONS** Diphtheria and tetanus toxoids adsorbed (for pediatric use), *solution for injection:* 6.6, 10, or 12.5 Lf units of diphtheria toxoid with 5 Lf units of tetanus toxoid/.5 ml; 15 Lf units of diphtheria toxoid with 10 Lf units of tetanus toxoid/.5 ml. Tetanus and diphtheria toxoids adsorbed for adult use, *solution for injection:* 5 Lf units of tetanus toxoid with 1.4 or 2 Lf units of diphtheria toxoid/.5 ml; 10 Lf units of tetanus toxoid with 2 units of diphtheria toxoid/.5 ml.

**DRUG INTERACTIONS** See entry for drug class (p. 444).

**FATE** When diphtheria and tetanus toxoids, adsorbed, are administered as primary immunization, most patients are protected for 10 years.

### ☙ NURSING CONSIDERATIONS

#### Side effects, toxicities, and associated nursing actions
- The risk of side effects is increased if adults receive the more concentrated preparation intended for pediatric use.
- Read orders and labels carefully.

#### Nursing interventions related to drug administration
- See entry for drug class (p. 445).

#### Patient and family education
- See entry for drug class (p. 445).

## diphtheria and tetanus toxoids and pertussis vaccine adsorbed (dif-THEE-ree-uh) toxoid/vaccine

- diphtheria and tetanus toxoids and pertussis vaccine adsorbed: Sold under generic name

**MECHANISM OF ACTION** Diphtheria and tetanus toxoids and pertussis vaccine adsorbed (DTP) is a combination product designed to confer active immunity against diphtheria, tetanus, and whooping cough at the same time. The toxoids induce production of specific antitoxins, and the vaccine induces antibodies against *Bordetella pertussis*.

**INDICATIONS** **Immunization against diphtheria, tetanus, and whooping cough** All children are recommended to receive this immunization before the age of 7 years.

**CONTRAINDICATIONS**   **Encephalopathy, seizures, or other signs of CNS damage** Children with these conditions may be at increased risk of neurologic side effects from one or more components of DTP.

**DOSAGE**   IM:   **CHILDREN 6 WEEKS TO 6 YEARS:** By deep muscle injection only. A dose of 0.5 ml contains 6.7 or 12.5 Lf units of diphtheria toxoid, 5 Lf units of tetanus toxoid, and 4 protective units of pertussis vaccine. A total of 4 doses are given for primary immunization. The most common schedule is at 2, 4, 6, and 18 months. Children may receive a booster at age 4 to 6 years. After 7 years of age, DTP should not be used; boosters should be with Td (p. 451). *Special patient populations:* **ELDERLY:** This preparation is not indicated for adults.   **PREGNANCY:** This preparation is not indicated for adults.

**PREPARATIONS**   Solution for injection: each 0.5 ml contains 4 protective units of pertussis vaccine, 5 Lf units of tetanus toxoid, and 6.7 or 12.5 Lf units of diphtheria toxoid.

**DRUG INTERACTIONS**   See entry for drug class (p. 444).

**FATE**   When administered for primary immunization as indicated above, protection lasts up to 10 years, after which boosters may be required.

### ☙ NURSING CONSIDERATIONS

#### Side effects, toxicities, and associated nursing actions

**Fever** Seven percent of inoculated patients develop fever within 24 hours.

- Caution parents about this anticipated side effect. Physician may recommend use of an antipyretic agent; consult physician.

**Encephalopathy** The risk is low in infants up to 12 months of age; incidence is estimated at 1 in 150,000.

- Instruct parents to report the development of any unusual sign or symptom that appears during the first week following injection. Caution parents to be alert to changes in mood, unuusal crying, excessive sleepiness, or any other changes.
- Reinforce to parents the need to remain in contact with the health care team for ongoing immunizations.

#### Nursing interventions related to drug administration

- See entry for drug class (p. 445).

#### Patient and family education

- See entry for drug class (p. 445).

---

## H. influenzae type B vaccine     vaccine

- H. influenzae type B vaccine: b-Capsa I

**MECHANISM OF ACTION**   This vaccine consists of a polysaccharide derived from *H. influenzae*. The preparation induces active immunity against *H. influenzae*, which is a leading cause of childhood meningitis and other serious infections.

**INDICATIONS**   **Immunization against H. influenzae type B** Children under the age of 5 who are in nursery or day-care centers are especially at risk of infection.

**CONTRAINDICATIONS**   **Age** Children younger than 18 months or older than 5 years should not receive the vaccine.

**DOSAGE**   SC:   **CHILDREN 18 MONTHS TO 4 YEARS:** A single 0.5 ml dose confers immunity. Booster schedules have not been established. *Special patient populations:* **ELDERLY:** This preparation is not indicated for adults.   **PREGNANCY:** This preparation is not indicated for adults.

**PREPARATIONS**   *Powder for solution:* 6.5 ml of diluent is supplied for each 10-dose vial of powder.

**DRUG INTERACTIONS**   See entry for drug class (p. 444).

**FATE**   The length of protection conferred by this vaccine has not yet been clearly determined.

### ☙ NURSING CONSIDERATIONS

#### Side effects, toxicities, and associated nursing actions

- See entry for drug class (p. 445).

#### Nursing interventions related to drug administration

- See entry for drug class (p. 445).

**Patient and family education**
- See entry for drug class (p. 445).

---

## hepatitis B immune globulin  (hep-uh-TI-tis)                                globulin

- hepatitis B immune globulin: H-BIG, Hep-B-Gammagee, HyperHep

**MECHANISM OF ACTION**    Hepatitis B immune globulin confers passive immunity. The globulin inactivates the hepatitis virus and prevents or ameliorates infection.

**INDICATIONS**    **Prophylaxis for hepatitis B exposure** Persons who are exposed to patients with hepatitis or who are exposed to blood or blood products contaminated with the hepatitis virus may receive hepatitis B immune globulin to reduce risk of serious infection. • Exposed patients are also treated with hepatitis vaccine (p. 453).

**CONTRAINDICATIONS**    None established.

**DOSAGE**    IM:    ADULTS AND CHILDREN: 0.06 ml/kg. Adult doses may range up to 5 ml. Doses should be administered as soon as possible after exposure.    *Special patient populations:*    PREGNANCY: Safe use in pregnancy and lactation has not been established, but the preparation has been used in pregnant women without apparent harm.

**PREPARATION**    *Solution for injection:* this protein solution also contains 0.3 M glycine and 100 µg/ml thimerosal.

**DRUG INTERACTIONS**    See entry for drug class (p. 444).

**FATE**    Hepatitis B immune globulin confers only transient passive immunity. To be effective, it must be administered within 7 days of exposure.

### ❧ NURSING CONSIDERATIONS

**Side effects, toxicities, and associated nursing actions**
- See entry for drug class (p. 444).

**Nursing interventions related to drug administration**
- In adults, administer IM doses in the deltoid muscle or use sites in the thigh. If the deltoid muscle is used, volumes larger than 3 ml in 1 dose should not be administered; administer divided doses.

**Patient and family education**
- See entry for drug class (p. 445).

---

## hepatitis B virus vaccine inactivated  (hep-uh-TI-tis)                          vaccine

- hepatitis B virus vaccine inactivated: Hepavax-B, Recombivax-HB

**MECHANISM OF ACTION**    Hepatitis B virus vaccine inactivated promotes active immunity by causing production of antibodies directed toward the hepatitis B virus. The preparation called Hepavax-B contains surface antigens of the virus purified from serum of patients who are chronic carriers of the virus. Recombivax-HB is made from surface antigens produced in yeast by recombinant DNA techniques.

**INDICATIONS**    **Immunization of persons at high risk of exposure** Health care personnel or others likely to encounter patients with hepatitis or who are likely to handle blood or blood products contaminated with hepatitis B virus are often routinely immunized.    **Persons exposed to hepatitis B virus** Patients actually exposed to hepatitis may receive the vaccine and hepatitis B immune globulin (p. 453).

**CONTRAINDICATIONS**    **Severe cardiovascular disease with pulmonary dysfunction** These patients may be at high risk from the fever that often develops following injection.

**DOSAGE**    IM, SC:    ADULTS: 20 µg/dose. The second dose follows the first by 1 month; the third dose is 6 months after the first dose. The SC route is used only in patients with bleeding disorders.

**NEONATES AND CHILDREN UP TO 10 YEARS:** 10 µg/dose for 3 doses as described above. The SC route is used only in patients with bleeding disorders. *Special patient populations:* **PREGNANCY:** Safe use in pregnancy and lactation has not been established.

**PREPARATIONS**  *Solution for injection:* 20 µg/ml.

**DRUG INTERACTIONS**  See entry for drug class (p. 444).

**FATE**  The duration of active immunity conferred by this vaccine is unknown but is thought to be at least 5 years.

### ❦ NURSING CONSIDERATIONS

#### Side effects, toxicities, and associated nursing actions
• See entry for drug class (p. 444).

#### Nursing interventions related to drug administration
• Hepatitis B vaccine should be administered into the deltoid muscle of adults and children over the age of 10 years and into the vastus lateralis site in infants and small children.
• Agitate vial well to promote uniform suspension.
• Do not administer hepatitis B vaccine in the same injection site as hepatitis B immune globulin if both are being prescribed for the same patient.

#### Patient and family education
• See entry for drug class (p. 445).
• Reinforce to patients the need to return for the second and third injections in the series.

---

## immune globulin  (im-MUNE GLOB-yoo-lin)  globulins

• immune globulin: Gamastan, Gammar, Immuglobin (immune globulin IM), Gamimune N, Sandoglobulin (immune globulin IV)

**MECHANISM OF ACTION**  Immune globulin is a mixture of antibodies that may be helpful in establishing passive immunity toward a number of infectious diseases.

**INDICATIONS**  **Exposure to hepatitis** Immune globulins may be effective against hepatitis A, hepatitis B, and other nonspecific forms of hepatitis. • Hepatitis B immune globulin may be preferred if the exposure is to hepatitis B (p. 453). **Measles (rubeola)** If the measles virus vaccine live is contraindicated, immune globulin may be substituted for temporary protection (3 to 4 weeks). **Immunodeficiency disease** Patients lacking adequate IgG may be given passive immunity to some acute infectious diseases with immune globulin. **Idiopathic thrombocytopenic purpura** Immune globulin may aid in increasing platelet counts in these patients.

**CONTRAINDICATIONS**  **Selective IgA deficiency** These patients may have an anaphylactic reaction to the IgA in immune globulin. **Thrombocytopenia** Severe bleeding at the infection site may occur in these patients.

**DOSAGE**  **IV:** **ADULTS AND CHILDREN:** For immunodeficiency disease, 100 mg/kg or 2 ml/kg infused at an initial rate of 0.01 to 0.02 ml/kg/min; if no reactions occur the rate can be increased to 0.02 to 0.04 ml/kg/min. Doses are repeated monthly, or more often if necessary. For thrombocytopenic purpura, 400 mg/kg daily for 5 consecutive days. **IM:** **ADULTS AND CHILDREN:** For immunodeficiency disease, 1.2 ml/kg initially, followed by 0.6 ml/kg once every 2 weeks, not to exceed 50 ml as a single dose in adults or 30 ml as a single dose in infants and children. For prophylaxis of infectious disease, doses range from 0.02 ml/kg for hepatitis A exposure to 0.25 ml/kg for measles exposure. *Special patient populations:* **PREGNANCY:** Safe use in pregnancy and lactation has not been established.

**PREPARATIONS**  Immune globulin IM, *solution for IM injection:* serum also contains 0.3 M glycine and 100 µg/ml thimerosal. Immune globulin IV, *solution for IV injection:* 50 mg protein/ml, with 10% maltose. *Powder for reconstitution:* 1, 3, or 6 g protein with sucrose and 0.9% saline for reconstitution (IV use only).

**DRUG INTERACTIONS**  See entry for drug class (p. 444).

**FATE**  Immune globulins confer only short-term passive immunity.

## 🐝 NURSING CONSIDERATIONS

### Side effects, toxicities, and associated nursing actions
- See entry for drug class (p. 444).

### Nursing interventions related to drug administration
- Obtain history of allergic reactions before administering. Immune globulin should not be administered to individuals with a history of allergic response to immune globulin.
- Read orders and labels carefully; IM preparations should not be administered IV, and IV preparations should not be administered IM.
- Monitor vital signs during IV administration.
- Divide large-volume doses into two or more smaller volumes. In the adult, a single injection should not exceed 5 ml, except when the deltoid muscle is used, when volume should not exceed 3 ml. In infants and small children, single-dose volume should not exceed 1 to 3 ml, depending on the size of the child and muscle.

### Patient and family education
- See entry for drug class (p. 445).

---

## influenza virus vaccine (in-floo-EN-zah) vaccine

- influenza virus vaccine: Fluogen, Fluzone

**MECHANISM OF ACTION** Influenza virus vaccine is prepared from inactivated viruses (whole virion) or from inactivated virus particles (subvirion). The vaccine is reformulated each year to cover the specific influenza viruses currently prevalent in North America.

**INDICATIONS** **Immunization against influenza strains** Immunity is conferred only against those strains used in formulating the vaccine. • The vaccine is indicated only for those patients at high risk from influenza (the elderly, children with cardiopulmonary disease) or for health care personnel with frequent exposure.

**CONTRAINDICATIONS** **Allergy to eggs or chickens** Eggs are used as growth media for the viruses used in preparing the vaccine. **A history of Guillain-Barré Syndrome** This type of reversible paralysis is rarely caused by influenza vaccines.

**DOSAGE** **IM:** **ADULTS AND CHILDREN OVER 12 YEARS:** A single dose of 0.5 ml of the whole virion preparation is used. Because this product changes each year, information on the current dosage schedule should be consulted. **CHILDREN:** Ages 3 to 12 years receive 0.5 ml of the subvirion preparation twice, in doses 4 or more weeks apart. Ages 3 weeks to 3 years receive 0.25 ml of the subvirion preparation twice, in doses 4 or more weeks apart. Because this product changes each year, information on the current dosage schedule should be consulted. *Special patient populations:* **PREGNANCY:** Safe use in pregnancy and lactation has not been established.

**PREPARATIONS** Influenza virus vaccine (subvirion), *sterile suspension for injection:* also contains thimerosal 100 µg/ml. Influenza virus vaccine (whole virion), *sterile suspension for injection:* also contains thimerosal 100 µg/ml.

**DRUG INTERACTIONS** **Phenytoin** concentrations are slightly lowered, and seizure control is lost in a few patients who have been previously stabilized on a dosage of phenytoin and receive the influenza vaccine. **Theophylline** concentrations may rise when the influenza vaccine is given. Patients should be watched for signs of theophylline toxicity. **Warfarin** action may be potentiated by vaccination with influenza vaccine. Patients should be observed for signs of bleeding. For other interactions, see entry for drug class (p. 444).

**FATE** Immunity is developed in 70% to 80% of patients receiving the injection. Immunity generally lasts about 1 year.

## 🐝 NURSING CONSIDERATIONS

### Side effects, toxicities, and associated nursing actions
**Fever** Fever may develop in a small percentage of patients.
- Caution patients about this side effect. Instruct patients to notify physician if fever is extremely high

or persistent. Have parents of small children confirm with physician acceptable treatments of fever before leaving treatment site.

**Paralysis** A type of reversible paralysis called Guillain-Barŕe syndrome can rarely be caused by influenza vaccines. The syndrome is occasionally fatal. About 500 cases of Guillain-Barŕe syndrome developed following use of the swine flu vaccine in 1976, but the incidence before and after that time has been much lower.

- Inform patients about this unusual side effect. Review with patients the usual signs and symptoms of the syndrome: muscle weakness, especially of the lower extremeties, and paresthesias (tingling) of the extremities. Instruct patients to report the development of any unexpected sign or symptom.

### Nursing interventions related to drug administration
- Obtain history of allergy before administration. Perform scratch test before administering vaccine to patients with a history of allergy to egg protein (consult physician).
- Administer IM doses into deltoid muscle of adults and children over 10 years. Administer IM doses in vastus lateralis site in infants and small children.

### Patient and family education
- See entry for drug class (p. 445).

---

## measles virus vaccine live (MEE-zuls) vaccine

- measles virus vaccine live: Attenuvax

**MECHANISM OF ACTION** Measles virus vaccine live is prepared from living viruses that have been rendered less pathogenic (attenuated) by multiple passages through cultures of chick embryo cells. The viruses stimulate active immunity.

**INDICATIONS** **Prophylaxis against measles** Immunization is recommended for all individuals unless specific medical conditions prevent it.

**CONTRAINDICATIONS** **Immune deficiencies** Patients with decreased immune function caused by disease or by immunosuppressive drugs should not receive the vaccine. • Replication of the virus may be uncontrolled in these individuals. **Febrile seizures or cerebral trauma** The fever caused by the vaccine may provoke seizure activity in these patients.

**DOSAGE** **SC:** **ADULTS AND CHILDREN:** 1000 $TCID_{50}$ (tissue culture infective dose 50%) units as a single dose. *Special patient populations:* **PREGNANCY:** Pregnant women should not receive the vaccine nor should women become pregnant within 3 months of being vaccinated.

**PREPARATIONS** *Solution for injection:* 1000 $TCID_{50}$, with neomycin sulfate. *Combination products* available include measles and rubella virus vaccine live (M-R-VAX II), *solution for injection:* measles virus vaccine live 1000 $TCID_{50}$ and rubella virus vaccine live 1000 $TCID_{50}$ (with neomycin sulfate). Measles, mumps, and rubella virus vaccine live (M-M-R II), *solution for injection:* 1000 $TCID_{50}$ each of measles virus vaccine live, rubella virus vaccine live with 5000 $TCID_{50}$ of mumps virus vaccine live (with neomycin sulfate).

**DRUG INTERACTIONS** See entry for drug class (p. 444).

**FATE** The active immunity induced by the measles virus vaccine live is developed within 2 to 3 weeks and persists for up to 8 years or longer. The revaccination schedule has not been determined.

### ❦ NURSING CONSIDERATIONS
#### Side effects, toxicities, and associated nursing actions
**Fever** 5% to 15% of infants develop fever within a week of inoculation.
- Review with parents the possibility of this side effect. Provide parents with guidelines about treatment of fever in infants before the parents leave the treatment center.

**Encephalitis** This complication is exceedingly rare, estimated at 1 in 1 million.
- Inform parents about this side effect. Instruct parents to report any unexpected sign or symptom, especially changes in behavior of the infant.

#### Nursing interventions related to drug administration
- Question women about the possibility of pregnancy before administering vaccine (see dosage above).

- Administer this vaccine as SC injection in the upper outer aspect of the arm.
- Read orders and labels carefully. There are available vaccines for measles alone or in combination with mumps and/or rubella.

**Patient and family education**
- See entry for drug class (p. 445).

## mumps virus vaccine live

vaccine

- mumps virus vaccine live: Mumpsvax

**MECHANISM OF ACTION**    Mumps virus vaccine live is prepared from living viruses that have been rendered less pathogenic (attenuated) by multiple passages through cultures of chick embryo cells. The viruses stimulate active immunity.

**INDICATIONS**    **Prophylaxis of mumps** Immunization is recommended for all individuals unless specific medical conditions prevent it.

**CONTRAINDICATIONS**    **Immune deficiencies** Patients with decreased immune function caused by disease or by immunosuppressive drugs should not receive the vaccine. • Replication of the virus may be uncontrolled in these individuals.

**DOSAGE**    **SC:    ADULTS AND CHILDREN:** 5000 $TCID_{50}$ as a single dose.    *Special patient populations:* **PREGNANCY:** Pregnant women should not receive the vaccine nor should women become pregnant within 3 months of being vaccinated.

**PREPARATIONS**    *Solution for injection:* 5000 $TCID_{50}$. *Combination products* include the following. Rubella and mumps virus vaccine live (Biavax II), *solution for injection:* 1000 $TCID_{50}$ rubella virus vaccine live and 5000 $TCID_{50}$ mumps virus vaccine live (with neomycin sulfate). Measles, mumps, and rubella virus vaccine live (M-M-R II), *solution for injection:* 1000 $TCID_{50}$ each of measles virus vaccine live, rubella virus vaccine live with 5000 $TCID_{50}$ of mumps virus vaccine live (with neomycin sulfate).

**DRUG INTERACTIONS**    See entry for drug class (p. 444).

**FATE**    Immunity to mumps is produced in 75% to 90% of patients vaccinated, and the immunity is considered permanent. Protection develops within 2 to 3 weeks of inoculation.

## ❦ NURSING CONSIDERATIONS

**Side effects, toxicities, and associated nursing actions**
- See entry for drug class (p. 444).

**Nursing interventions related to drug administration**
- Question women about the possibility of pregnancy before administering vaccine (see dosage above).
- Administer this vaccine as SC injection in the upper outer aspect of the arm.
- Read orders and labels carefully. There are available vaccines for mumps alone, or in combination with measles and/or rubella.

**Patient and family education**
- See entry for drug class (p. 445).

## pertussis immune globulin    (per-TUSS-iss)

globulin

- pertussis immune globulin: Hypertussis

**MECHANISM OF ACTION**    Pertussis immune globulin is a concentrated preparation of immunoglobulin (IgG) derived from healthy adults. The preparation confers passive immunity for whooping cough.

**INDICATIONS**    **Prophylaxis of pertussis (whooping cough)** This preparation is of no value once infection has occurred.

**CONTRAINDICATIONS**  **Hypersensitivity to IgG** This rarely limits use of the preparation.

**DOSAGE**  IM:  **CHILDREN:** 1.25 ml in infants and 2.5 ml in older children. Special patient populations: **ELDERLY:** This preparation is not indicated for elderly patients.  **PREGNANCY:** This preparation is not indicated for adults.

**PREPARATIONS**  Solution for injection: also contains glycine 0.3 M and thimerosal 100 µg/ml.

**DRUG INTERACTIONS**  See entry for drug class (p. 444).

**FATE**  This preparation offers short-term protection only and may need to be repeated once 1 to 2 weeks after the first dose.

## NURSING CONSIDERATIONS

### Side effects, toxicities, and associated nursing actions
- See entry for drug class (p. 444).

### Nursing interventions related to drug administration
- In adults and children over 3 years, administer into the deltoid muscle. In infants and children under the age of 3, administer into the vastus lateralis muscle.

### Patient and family education
- See entry for drug class (p. 445).

---

# plague vaccine                                                                    vaccine

- plague vaccine: Sold under generic name

**MECHANISM OF ACTION**  Plague vaccine is made from cultures of *Yersinia pestis* (the plague bacillus) inactivated with formaldehyde. This preparation promotes the development of active immunity.

**INDICATIONS**  **Prophylaxis in patients at high risk of plague** Patients at high risk are those exposed to wild rodents or other wild animals likely to carry ectoparasites such as fleas that can transmit the disease to humans.

**CONTRAINDICATIONS**  **Thrombocytopenia** Patients with bleeding disorders may suffer excessive bleeding at the injection site.

**DOSAGE**  IM:  **ADULTS AND CHILDREN OVER 10 YEARS:** The initial dose of 1 ml is followed 4 weeks later by 0.2 ml; the third dose, given 6 months after the first, is also 0.2 ml. Booster doses may be required at 1- to 2-year intervals.  **CHILDREN:** Dosing intervals are as for adults, but doses are reduced according to age: children up to 1 year, doses of 0.2, 0.04, and 0.04 ml with boosters of 0.02 to 0.04 ml; children 1 to 4 years, doses of 0.4, 0.08, and 0.08 ml with boosters of 0.04 to 0.08 ml; children 5 to 10 years, doses of 0.6, 0.12, and 0.12 ml with booters at 0.06 to 0.12 ml.  *Special patient populations:*  **PREGNANCY:** Safe use in pregnancy and lactation has not been established.

**PREPARATIONS**  *Sterile suspension:* suspension for injection is in 0.9% sodium chloride solution with traces of formaldehyde, phenol, beef heart extract, yeast extract, agar, and peptides of soybean and casein.

**DRUG INTERACTIONS**  See entry for drug class (p. 444).

**FATE**  This preparation induces active immunity in 90% of vaccinated individuals but may not prevent infection. Infections that do develop are less severe. Protection only lasts 6 to 12 months, and boosters are required if exposure continues.

## NURSING CONSIDERATIONS

### Side effects, toxicities, and associated nursing actions
- See entry for drug class (p. 444).

### Nursing interventions related to drug administration
- Agitate vial vigorously to promote uniform suspension.

### Patient and family education
- Reinforce the need to return for later injections in the series. • See entry for drug class (p. 445).

## pneumococcal vaccine, polyvalent   (nyoo-moh-KOCK-kul)   vaccine

- pneumococcal vaccine, polyvalent: Pneumovax 23, Pnu-Imune

**MECHANISM OF ACTION**   Pneumococcal vaccine, polyvalent, contains a mixture of the antigenic polysaccharides from *Streptococcus pneumoniae*. Administration of these polysaccharides stimulates active immunity to 23 types of *S. pneumoniae* that may cause pneumonia and other diseases.

**INDICATIONS**   **High risk of morbidity from pneumococcal pneumonia** Patients with chronic diseases that increase the risk of morbidity from pneumococcal pneumonia or bacteremia (splenic dysfunction, Hodgkin's disease, renal failure, multiple myeloma, or cirrhosis) may be protected with the vaccine.

**CONTRAINDICATIONS**   **Recent pneumococcal pneumonia** These patients may have increased local reactions because they already have some antibodies to the pneumococci.

**DOSAGE**   IM or SC:   ADULTS AND CHILDREN OVER 2 YEARS: 0.5 ml as a single injection.   *Special patient populations:*   PREGNANCY: Safe use in pregnancy and lactation has not been established.

**PREPARATIONS**   *Solution for injection:* also contains 0.25% phenol (Pneumovax) or 0.01% thimerosal (Pnu-Imune).

**DRUG INTERACTIONS**   See entry for drug class (p. 444).

**FATE**   The active immunity conferred by this vaccine develops within 2 to 3 weeks and persists for months or years, but the exact duration of protection has not yet been established.

### ❦ NURSING CONSIDERATIONS

#### Side effects, toxicities, and associated nursing actions
- See entry for drug class (p. 444).

#### Nursing interventions related to drug administration
- Administer pneumococcal vaccine into the deltoid muscle of adults and children over the age of 2 years.

#### Patient and family education
- See entry for drug class (p. 445).

## poliovirus vaccine inactivated (IPV)   (POH-lee-oh)   vaccine

- poliovirus vaccine inactivated: Sold under generic name

**MECHANISM OF ACTION**   Poliovirus vaccine inactivated is made from a mixture of types 1, 2, and 3 poliovirus. Active immunity is stimulated.

**INDICATIONS**   **Prevention of poliomyelitis** Poliovirus vaccine inactivated is indicated for persons 18 years or older who are receiving their first immunization against polio. • In children, the oral polio vaccine is preferred (p. 460).

**CONTRAINDICATIONS**   **Acute febrile illnesses** These patients should be allowed to recover before the vaccine is administered. • Minor illnesses are not reason to withhold the vaccine.

**DOSAGE**   SC:   ADULTS: Four 1 ml doses are required for complete immunization. The first 2 doses (1 ml each) are administered at least 4 weeks apart. The remaining doses are administered at intervals of a few months.   CHILDREN: Four 1 ml doses are required for complete immunization. The first 3 doses (1 ml each) are given at 4- to 8-week intervals; the last comes 6 to 12 months after the third dose. *Special patient populations:*   PREGNANCY: Children exposed to an earlier form of poliovirus vaccine inactivated have a higher risk of cancer than normal. The safety of the currently available vaccine has not been established.

**PREPARATIONS**   *Solution for injection:* also contains neomycin, streptomycin, and 2-phenoxyethanol.

**DRUG INTERACTIONS**   See entry for drug class (p. 444).

**FATE**   The active immunity conferred by this vaccine lasts for years, but the exact duration in unknown.

### ☙ NURSING CONSIDERATIONS

**Side effects, toxicities, and associated nursing actions**

- See entry for drug class (p. 444).

**Nursing interventions related to drug administration**

- Administer doses subcutaneously in the upper outer arm near the insertion of the deltoid muscle.

**Patient and family education**

- Reinforce to parents or patients the need to return for subsequent doses in the series.
- See entry for drug class (p. 445).

---

## poliovirus vaccine live oral*    (POH-lee-oh)                    vaccine

- poliovirus vaccine live oral: Orimune Trivalent

**MECHANISM OF ACTION**    Poliovirus vaccine live oral is prepared from cultures of types 1, 2, and 3 polio-viruses. The living viruses have been rendered less pathogenic (attenuated) by multiple passages through cultures of monkey kidney cells. The viruses stimulate active immunity, including intestinal immunity that may lower the incidence of virus carriers and prevent spread of the infection.

**INDICATIONS**    **Prevention of poliomyelitis** This vaccine is preferred over the poliovirus vaccine inactivated (p. 459) for all persons under age 18 years.

**CONTRAINDICATIONS**    **Immune deficiencies** Patients with decreased immune function caused by disease or by immunosuppressive drugs should not receive the vaccine. • Replication of the virus may be uncontrolled in these individuals.

**DOSAGE**    **PO:**    **ADULTS:** A single 0.5 ml dose may be given when rapid immunization is required, but for complete protection adults should receive the poliovirus vaccine inactivated (p. 459).    **CHILDREN:** 0.5 ml given three times. Two currently recommended schedules are 6 to 12 weeks, 8 weeks later, and 8 to 12 months after the second dose; or at 2, 4, and 18 months of age.    *Special patient populations:* **ELDERLY:** All adults are at increased risk of paralytic polio with the oral vaccine.    **PREGNANCY:** Safe use in pregnancy and lactation has not been established, but single doses may be given when rapid immunization is required.

**PREPARATIONS**    *Suspension for oral use:* 0.5 ml in single dose disposable pipette.

**DRUG INTERACTIONS**    See entry for drug class (p. 444).

**FATE**    Poliovirus vaccine live oral confers active humoral and intestinal immunity to the three most common types of poliovirus. Immunity persists for years, but the exact length of protection is unknown.

### ☙ NURSING CONSIDERATIONS

**Side effects, toxicities, and associated nursing actions**

- See entry for drug class (p. 444).

**Nursing interventions related to drug administration**

- This vaccine is administered orally only. Thaw frozen solutions before administering. May be administered via single-dose pipette, mixed with distilled or chlorine-free water, syrup NF, or milk, or may be administered adsorbed on bread, cake, or cube sugar.

**Patient and family education**

- Reinforce to parents or patients the need to return for subsequent doses in the series.
- See entry for drug class (p. 445).

---

## rabies immune globulin    (RAY-bees)                              globulin

- rabies immune globulin: Hyperab, Imogam Rabies

**MECHANISM OF ACTION**    Rabies immune globulin is derived from human serum. This purified preparation contains antibodies to the rabies virus and confers passive immunity by neutralizing the free virus. The antibodies are probably not effective once the virus has penetrated nerves.

*Sabin vaccine.

**INDICATIONS**   Rabies exposure The antirabies serum can be used to neutralize rabies virus in the wound before the virus penetrates nerves and begins to cause irreversible disease.

**CONTRAINDICATIONS**   Thrombocytopenia Patients with bleeding disorders may suffer excessive bleeding at the injection site.

**DOSAGE**   IM:   ADULTS AND CHILDREN: 20 IU/kg. Half the dose may be infiltrated into tissue surrounding the wound. Patients should also receive rabies vaccine (p. 461).   *Special patient populations:* PREGNANCY: Safe use in pregnancy and lactation has not been established, but the preparation has been used without apparent harm.

**PREPARATIONS**   *Solution for injection:* 150 IU/ml (with 0.3 M glycine and 100 µg/ml thimerosal).

**DRUG INTERACTIONS**   See entry for drug class (p. 444).

**FATE**   Rabies immune globulin confers short-term protection. Long-term immunity is not produced.

### ☙ NURSING CONSIDERATIONS

#### Side effects, toxicities, and associated nursing actions
- See entry for drug class (p. 444).

#### Nursing interventions related to drug administration
- Administer doses to adults and older children in the deltoid muscle or rectus femoris site. Administer IM doses to infants and small children into the vastus lateralis site.
- Avoid administering rabies immune globulin and rabies vaccine in the same syringe. Administer these two drugs at different injection sites to avoid having one drug neutralize the other.

#### Patient and family education
- See entry for drug class (p. 445).

---

# rabies vaccine (HDCV)   (RAY-bees)                                    vaccine

- rabies vaccine (HDCV): Imovax

**MECHANISM OF ACTION**   Rabies vaccine is prepared from viruses grown on human diploid cell cultures. The whole viruses are inactivated. This preparation confers active immunity by inducing the formation of immunoglobulins directed toward rabies virus.

**INDICATIONS**   Exposure to rabies virus The bite of an infected animal or exposure of broken skin to saliva of an infected animal carries a high risk of rabies 30 days to 1 year later. • Use of an immunoglobulin (p. 460) is recommended at the same time as the initial dose of the vaccine.   Preexposure prophylaxis Persons at high risk of exposure to the virus may receive vaccine.

**CONTRAINDICATIONS**   None exist because rabies infection is almost invariably fatal. • The vaccine should not be withheld when documented exposure exists.

**DOSAGE**   IM:   ADULTS AND CHILDREN: For preexposure prophylaxis, 1 ml administered on day 1, day 7, and day 28. Boosters may be required every 2 years. For rabies exposure, 1 ml is administered as soon as possible after the exposure (along with rabies immune globulin, p. ●●). Subsequent 1 ml doses are given 3, 7, 14, and 28 days after the first dose.   *Special patient populations:* PREGNANCY: Because of the high mortality of rabies infections, pregnant women who are exposed should receive the vaccine.

**PREPARATIONS**   *Solution for injection:* 2.5 IU, with human albumin, neomycin sulfate, phenolsulfonphthalein, and propiolactone.

**DRUG INTERACTIONS**   See entry for drug class (p. 444).

**FATE**   Rabies vaccine confers active immunity to a high percentage of treated patients. The immunity lasts for years, but boosters may be required in certain circumstances.

### ☙ NURSING CONSIDERATIONS

#### Side effects, toxicities, and associated nursing actions
- See entry for drug class (p. 444).

#### Nursing interventions related to drug administration
- Administer doses to adults and older children in the deltoid muscle or rectus femoris site. Administer IM doses to infants and small children into the vastus lateralis site.

- Avoid administering rabies immune globulin and rabies vaccine in the same syringe. Administer these two drugs at different injection sites to avoid having one drug neutralize the other.
- Consult local public health officials for questions regarding incidence of rabid animals and for other guidelines regarding use of this vaccine.

### Patient and family education
- See entry for drug class (p. 445).

---

# Rh$_o$ (D) immune globulin                                                globulin

- Rh$_o$ immune globulin: Gamulin, HypRho-D, MICRhoGAM, Mini-Gamulin, RhoGam

**MECHANISM OF ACTION**   Rh$_o$ (D) immune globulin is a concentrated form of immunoglobulins directed toward the red blood cell antigen Rh$_o$ (D). Patients lacking the RH$_o$ (D) antigen may mount an immune response if exposed to red blood cells bearing this antigen. This mechanism accounts for hemolytic disease in babies positive for Rh$_o$ (D) antigen born to mothers who lack the antigen. By suppressing this immune reaction in the mother, the attack on the red blood cells of the baby is prevented.

**INDICATIONS**   **Delivery of a Rh$_o$ (D) positive fetus to an Rh$_o$ (D) negative mother** Therapy with Rh$_o$ (D) immune globulin prevents development of active immunity that would threaten future pregnancies. **Transfusion accident** Therapy with Rh$_o$ (D) prevents development of active immunity when a patient negative for Rh$_o$ (D) accidentally receives blood or blood products from Rh$_o$ (D) positive persons.

**CONTRAINDICATIONS**   **Rh$_o$ (D) positive blood type** Patients testing positive for the Rh$_o$ (D) should not receive the Rh$_o$ (D) immune globulin.

**DOSAGE**   **IM:**   **ADULTS:** For obstetric use, one vial is administered within 72 hours of delivery. For use in transfusion accidents, the dose is calculated based on the volume of blood erroneously administered. Each vial of Rh$_o$ (D) immune globulin is sufficient to counteract 15 ml of packed red blood cells. *Special patient populations:*   **ELDERLY:** The preparation is not intended for use in this age group. **PREGNANCY:** Safe use in pregnancy and lactation has not been established, although the preparation has been used without apparent harm.

**PREPARATIONS**   *Solution for injection:* microdose or standard dose preparations.

**DRUG INTERACTIONS**   See entry for drug class (p. 444).

**FATE**   The effects of this preparation are short-lived. Treatment must be repeated after subsequent pregnancies.

### ☙ NURSING CONSIDERATIONS
#### Side effects, toxicities, and associated nursing actions
- See entry for drug class (p. 444).

#### Nursing interventions related to drug administration
- For obstetric use, note that drug is administered to the mother, not the infant.
- Administer IM doses into the deltoid muscle.

#### Patient and family education
- See entry for drug class (p. 445).

---

# rubella virus vaccine live   (roo-BELL-uh)                              vaccine

- rubella virus, vaccine live: Meruvax II

**MECHANISM OF ACTION**   Rubella virus vaccine live is prepared from viruses that have been rendered less pathogenic (attenuated) by multiple passages through cultures of human diploid cells. The viruses stimulate active immunity.

**INDICATIONS**   **Prophylaxis of rubella** Immunization is recommended for all individuals unless specific medical conditions prevent it.

**CONTRAINDICATIONS**   **Immune deficiencies** Patients with decreased immune function caused by disease or by immunosuppressive drugs should not receive the vaccine. • Replication of the virus may be uncontrolled in these individuals.   **Recent treatment with blood products or immune globulins** Patients who have received products containing immune globulins within 3 months should not receive rubella virus vaccine live because development of antibodies may be suppressed.

**DOSAGE**   **SC:**   ADULTS AND CHILDREN: 0.5 ml, equivalent to 1000 TCID$_{50}$ units, is administered as a single dose. *Special patient populations:*   PREGNANCY: Pregnant women should not receive the vaccine nor should women become pregnant within 3 months of being vaccinated.

**PREPARATIONS**   *Solution for injection:* 1000 TCID$_{50}$, with neomycin sulfate. *Combination products* include the following. Measles and rubella virus vaccine live (M-R-VAX II), *solution for injection:* measles virus vaccine live 1000 TCID$_{50}$ and rubella virus vaccine live 1000 TCID$_{50}$ (with neomycin sulfate). Rubella and mumps virus vaccine live (Biavax II), *solution for injection:* 1000 TCID$_{50}$ rubella virus vaccine live and 5000 TCID$_{50}$ mumps virus vaccine live (with neomycin sulfate). Measles, mumps, and rubella virus vaccine live (M-M-R II), *solution for injection:* 1000 TCID$_{50}$ each of measles virus vaccine live, rubella virus vaccine live with 5000 TCID$_{50}$ of mumps virus vaccine live (with neomycin sulfate).

**DRUG INTERACTIONS**   See entry for drug class (p. 444).

**FATE**   Rubella virus vaccine live confers active immunity that develops within 2 to 6 weeks and persists for years. Boosters are not recommended, although the exact duration of protection is unknown.

## NURSING CONSIDERATIONS

**Side effects, toxicities, and associated nursing actions**
- See entry for drug class (p. 444).

**Nursing interventions related to drug administration**
- Question women about the possibility of pregnancy before administering vaccine (see dosage above).
- Administer this vaccine as an SC injection in the upper outer aspect of the arm.
- Read orders and labels carefully. There are available vaccines for rubella alone, or in combination with mumps and/or measles.

**Patient and family education**
- See entry for drug class (p. 445).

# smallpox vaccine   (SMALL-pox)                                         vaccine

- smallpox vaccine: Dryvax

**MECHANISM OF ACTION**   Smallpox vaccine is prepared from live vaccinia virus. Because this virus resembles variola, the virus that causes smallpox, inoculation confers active immunity against smallpox.

**INDICATIONS**   **Persons exposed to smallpox virus** Smallpox is no longer considered a threat because vaccination and treatment programs have eradicated the disease worldwide.

**CONTRAINDICATIONS**   **Viral diseases other than smallpox** Smallpox vaccine should not be used for herpes, warts, or any other viral disease except for verified exposure to smallpox virus.

**DOSAGE**   **Intradermal:**   ADULTS AND CHILDREN: One drop of vaccine is applied to the skin, and pressure punctures are made, according to the manufacturer's directions. *Special patient populations:* PREGNANCY: Smallpox vaccine is strictly contraindicated because the live vaccinia virus may infect the fetus and kill it in utero.

**PREPARATIONS**   *Lyophilized powder:* to be reconstituted with diluent supplied by manufacturer.

**DRUG INTERACTIONS**   See entry for drug class (p. 444).

**FATE**   Smallpox vaccine offers nearly complete protection against smallpox for 1 to 3 years after immunization. Significant protection probably persists for up to 20 years.

## 🐾 NURSING CONSIDERATIONS
### Side effects, toxicities, and associated nursing actions
- See entry for drug class (p. 444).
### Nursing interventions related to drug administration
- Read manufacturer's directions carefully for reconstitution information.
- Cleanse intradermal injection site, preferably over the deltoid region of the upper arm, with soap and water and let dry. Use special needle supplied by manufacturer, and puncture skin as directed on manufacturer's instructions.
- Inspect site 6 to 8 days after administration. A successful primary immunization should usually produce a vesicle within 3 to 5 days. This will become pustular and reach maximum size in 9 days and then form a scab and heal, leaving a small scar. If no vesicle appears, immunization is probably inadequate, and the procedure should be repeated with another lot of vaccine (consult physician).
- Instruct patient to keep the site dry for at least 2 hours and to avoid direct sunlight exposure to site for several days.
- Caution patient to avoid scratching site. Have patient try to avoid covering site, although a small nonocclusive dressing may be applied when the lesion is pustular.
### Patient and family education
- See entry for drug class (p. 445).

---

## tetanus antitoxin   (TE-ta-nus)                                globulins

- tetanus antitoxin: Sold under generic name

**MECHANISM OF ACTION**   Tetanus antitoxin is a preparation of immunoglobulins from equine serum. The antibodies against tetanus that are present in this preparation confer passive immunity to tetanus.

**INDICATIONS**   **Prophylaxis against tetanus after exposure** Tetanus antitoxin can be used after exposure to tetanus via a contaminated wound. • Tetanus immune globulin (p. 465) gives longer lasting protection, has fewer side effects, and should be used if available.

**CONTRAINDICATIONS**   **Allergic reactions to equine serum** Because tetanus antitoxin contains proteins from equine serum, allergic reactions are possible. • Desensitization may be necessary.

**DOSAGE**   **IM or SC:**   **ADULTS AND CHILDREN:** 3000 to 5000 units. Children weighing less than 30 kg receive 1500 units.   *Special patient populations:*   **PREGNANCY:** Safe use in pregnancy and lactation has not been established.

**PREPARATIONS**   *Solution for injection:* 1500 or 20,000 units (with m-cresol).

**DRUG INTERACTIONS**   See entry for drug class (p. 444).

**FATE**   Tetanus antitoxin offers only short-term passive immunity against tetanus. Long-term protection requires administration of tetanus toxoid (p. 465).

## 🐾 NURSING CONSIDERATIONS
### Side effects, toxicities, and associated nursing actions
- See entry for drug class (p. 444).
### Nursing interventions related to drug administration
- Before administering prescribed dose, perform sensitivity test on patient (consult physician). Inject intradermally 0.1 ml of a 1:100 dilution of tetanus antitoxin in 0.9% sodium chloride solution. Inject a control test of 0.1 ml of 0.9% sodium chloride solution in another site. The skin test is interpreted in 10 to 30 minutes. A positive reaction consists of a urticarial wheal of 10 mm or more, surrounded by an erythematous flare 20 by 20 mm. If the skin test is positive, a course of desensitization injections should be administered. A conjunctival test may be performed instead of a skin test if desired.
- Do not administer tetanus antitoxin and tetanus toxoid in the same syringe or in the same injection site, to avoid neutralization of one drug by the other.
### Patient and family education
- See entry for drug class (p. 445).

## tetanus immune globulin   (TE-ta-nus)                                                        globulin

- tetanus immune globulin: Homo-Tet, Hyper-Tet

**MECHANISM OF ACTION**   Tetanus immune globulin is derived from human serum and contains antibodies directed against the toxin formed by *Clostridium tetani*. By neutralizing the toxin, tetanus immune globulin offers some passive immunity to the effect of tetanus.

**INDICATIONS**   **Prophylaxis against tetanus after exposure** Tetanus immune globulin may be used to offer temporary passive immunity to tetanus. • Patients are often also immunized with tetanus toxoid (p. 465) to establish longer-term active immunity.   **Treatment of tetanus** Tetanus immune globulin may be part of the intense therapy required when tetanus has developed. • Patients may also receive antibiotics, sedatives, and muscle relaxants.

**CONTRAINDICATIONS**   **Allergic reaction to immune globulins** Patients may require close attention because anaphylaxis can develop.

**DOSAGE**   **IM:   ADULTS AND CHILDREN OVER 3 YEARS:** For postexposure prophylaxis, 250 units as a single injection. Severly contaminated wounds may require 500 units. For treatment of tetanus, 3000 to 6000 units.   *Special patient populations:*   **PREGNANCY:** Safe use in pregnancy and lactation has not been established.

**PREPARATIONS**   *Solutions for injection:* 250 units, with glycine 0.3 M and thimerosal 100 μg/ml.

**DRUG INTERACTIONS**   See entry for drug class (p. 444).

**FATE**   Tetanus immune globulin confers passive resistance to tetanus. Protection lasts up to 32 days.

### ❦ NURSING CONSIDERATIONS

#### Side effects, toxicities and associated nursing actions
- See entry for drug class (p. 444).

#### Nursing interventions related to drug administration
- Administer IM doses into the deltoid muscle of adults or children over 3 years. Administer doses to infants and small children into the vastus lateralis site
- Do not administer tetanus immune globulin, tetanus antitoxin, or tetanus toxoid in the same injection site.

#### Patient and family education
- See entry for drug class (p. 445).

## tetanus toxoid (adsorbed)   (TE-ta-nus)                                                        toxoid

- tetanus toxoid (adsorbed): Sold under generic name

**MECHANISM OF ACTION**   Tetanus toxoid contains inactivated products of *Clostridium tetani*. Inoculation with this material induces the production of antibodies and confers active immunity.

**INDICATIONS**   **Prophylaxis of tetanus** All children normally are immunized against tetanus in combination with other vaccines (e.g., see diphtheria and tetanus toxoids and pertussis vaccine, p. 451). • Tetanus toxoid or tetanus toxoid adsorbed should be used only when combination products are contraindicated.

**CONTRAINDICATIONS**   **Prior reactions to preparations containing tetanus toxoid** Patients who have had neurologic or other reactions to any preparations containing tetanus toxoid should not receive tetanus toxoid. • Tetanus immune globulins (p. 465) may be given for short-term passive immunity in these patients.

**DOSAGE**   **IM:   ADULTS AND CHILDREN 6 WEEKS OR OLDER:** Tetanus toxoid, 0.5 ml containing 4 or 5 Lf units. Four doses are required, the first 3 spaced 3 to 8 weeks apart and the fourth 6 months to a year later. Tetanus toxoid adsorbed, 0.5 ml containing 5 to 10 units. Three doses are required, the second 4 to 8 weeks after the first; the last follows the second dose by 6 months or a year.   **SC:   ADULTS AND CHILDREN 6 WEEKS OR OLDER:** Tetanus toxoid only, in doses as for IM route. Tetanus toxoid adsorbed should not be given SC.   *Special patient populations:*   PREGNANCY: Safe use in pregnancy and lactation has not been established.

**PREPARATIONS**   Tetanus toxoid, *solution for injection:* 4 or 5 Lf units/.5 ml. Solution also contains 100 μg/ml thimerosal. Tetanus toxoid adsorbed, *solution for injection:* 5 or 10 Lf units/.5 ml. Solution also contains thimerosal 100 μg/ml and aluminum phosphate, aluminum phosphate sulfate, or aluminum hydroxide.

**DRUG INTERACTIONS**   See entry for drug class (p. 444).

**FATE**   Tetanus toxoid and tetanus toxoid adsorbed both confer active immunity to more than 90% of those inoculated. Protection lasts for at least 10 years. Boosters may be required at 10-year intervals.

### ❧ NURSING CONSIDERATIONS

#### Side effects, toxicities, and associated nursing actions

- See entry for drug class (p. 444).

#### Nursing interventions related to drug administration

- Read orders and labels carefully; both tetanus toxoid and tetanus toxoid adsorbed may be administered IM, but tetanus toxoid only may be administered SC.
- Administer IM doses into the deltoid muscle or sites of the anterior thigh (use vastus lateralis site for infants and small children).
- Record and rotate injection sites through the course of injections.

#### Patient and family education

- Reinforce to patients the need to return for subsequent doses of the series.
- See entry for drug class (p. 445).

---

## typhoid vaccine   (TYE-foid)       vaccine

- typhoid vaccine: Sold under generic name

**MECHANISM OF ACTION**   Typhoid vaccine is prepared from killed *Salmonella typhi*. This preparation stimulates production of antibodies toward the organism and therefore confers active immunity against typhoid.

**INDICATIONS**   **Prophylaxis of typhoid** Persons entering an area where typhoid is endemic and sanitation is poor may be protected with the vaccine. • Household contacts of a typhoid carrier may also receive the vaccine.

**CONTRAINDICATIONS**   **Severe febrile illness** Immunization should be postponed.

**DOSAGE**   **SC or intradermal:**   ADULTS AND CHILDREN OVER 10 YEARS: 0.5 ml; dosage is repeated 4 weeks later. Boosters may be administered after 3 years, 0.5 ml SC or 0.1 ml intradermally.   CHILDREN UNDER 10 YEARS: 0.25 ml; dosage is repeated 4 weeks later. Boosters may be administered after 3 years, 0.25 ml SC or 0.1 ml intradermally.   *Special patient populations:*   PREGNANCY: Safe use in pregnancy and lactation has not been established.

**PREPARATIONS**   *Solution for injection:* also contains phenol.

**DRUG INTERACTIONS**   See entry for drug class (p. 444).

**FATE**   When 2 doses are used for primary immunization, 70% to 90% of the persons vaccinated develop active immunity against typhoid. Immunity only lasts about 3 years, after which boosters are required to maintain protection.

### ❧ NURSING CONSIDERATIONS

#### Side effects, toxicities, and associated nursing actions

- See entry for drug class (p. 444).

#### Nursing interventions related to drug administration

- Shake vial thoroughly before preparing dose.
- Administer SC doses to adults and large children in the deltoid area. Administer SC doses to infants and small children in the anterior thigh.
- Administer intradermal injections into the inner aspect of the forearm.

#### Patient and family education

- Reinforce to patients the need to return for subsequent doses in the series.
- See entry for drug class (p. 445).

## varicella-zoster immune globulin   (ver-uh-SEL-uh)   globulins

- varicella-zoster immune globulin: Sold under generic name

**MECHANISM OF ACTION**   Varicella-zoster immune globulin is prepared from the sera of healthy adults with high levels of immunity to varicella (chickenpox). This preparation confers passive immunity toward chickenpox. The same virus is also responsible for the adult disease known as shingles (sometimes also called herpes zoster). It is not known if the varicella-zoster immune globulin protects from shingles.

**INDICATIONS**   **Exposure to varicella zoster in immunocompromised patients** Although chickenpox is a mild disease in normal children, the disease has a greatly increased mortality in immunocompromised patients.   **Neonates at risk** Only those babies born to mothers who develop chickenpox within 5 days before or 2 days after delivery should receive varicella-zoster globulin.

**CONTRAINDICATIONS**   **Allergy to immunoglobulins** Severe reactions may occur.

**DOSAGE**   **IM:**   **ADULTS AND CHILDREN:** Doses are estimated at 125 units/10 kg, up to a maximum dose of 625 units. Adults may require higher doses, depending on degree of exposure and level of immune deficiency.   *Special patient populations:*   **PREGNANCY:** Safe use in pregnancy and lactation has not been established.

**PREPARATIONS**   *Solution for injection:* 125 units per vial (2.5 ml). Preparation also contains 0.3 M glycine and thimerosal 100 µg/ml.

**DRUG INTERACTIONS**   See entry for drug class (p. 444).

**FATE**   Varicella-zoster immune globulin confers passive immunity that persists only 3 to 4 weeks. Infection may still occur, but the severity is often reduced by varicella-zoster immune globulin.

### 🐝 NURSING CONSIDERATIONS
#### Side effects, toxicities, and associated nursing actions
- See entry for drug class (p. 444).

#### Nursing interventions related to drug administration
- Administer IM doses to adults and large children in the deltoid muscle. Administer IM doses to infants and small children in the vastus lateralis site.

#### Patient and family education
- See entry for drug class (p. 445).

---

## widow spider species antivenin   globulins

- widow spider species antivenin: Antivenin (*Latrodectus mactans*)

**MECHANISM OF ACTION**   Widow spider species antivenin is prepared from equine sera and contains specific venom-neutralizing globulins; therefore this preparation can control symptoms of the bite of black widow spiders.

**INDICATIONS**   **Black widow spider bites** Widow spider species antivenin can be helpful in controlling some of the symptoms caused by the venom of the black widow spider and related spiders. • The antivenin must be administered very soon after the bite for maximum effect.

**CONTRAINDICATIONS**   **Allergic reactions to the antivenin** Patients should be tested for allergic reactions before a full dose is given. • If the patient is allergic, treatment should be withheld if possible. • Desensitization should be attempted only if the consequences of the bite are likely to prove fatal.

**DOSAGE**   **IV:**   **ADULTS AND CHILDREN:** Slow IV infusion, 2.5 ml (the contents of one vial), diluted into 10 to 50 ml of 0.9% sodium chloride injection. A second dose is rarely required.   **IM:**   **ADULTS AND CHILDREN:** 2.5 ml (the contents of one vial).   *Special patient populations:*   **PREGNANCY:** Safe use in pregnancy and lactation has not been established.

**PREPARATIONS**   *Solution:* 6000 antivenin units, to be diluted with 2.5 ml sterile water. A vial of equine serum is included for sensitivity testing.

**DRUG INTERACTIONS**   See entry for drug class (p. 444).

   **FATE**   Widow spider species antivenin prevents or lessens the acute symptoms of the spider venom. The effects are short-term. The antivenin does not offer long-term protection.

## ❦ NURSING CONSIDERATIONS
### Side effects, toxicities, and associated nursing actions
   • See entry for drug class (p. 444).

### Nursing interventions related to drug administration
   • Sensitivity testing must be done before administering antivenin; consult physician.
   • Administer IV doses, after dilution, over a 15-minute period.
   • Administer IM injection in muscles of the thigh so that a tourniquet can be applied above the injection site if systemic effects occur. Monitor vital signs.

### Patient and family education
   • See entry for drug class (p. 445).

---

## yellow fever vaccine                                                                         vaccine

   • yellow fever vaccine: YF-Vax

**MECHANISM OF ACTION**   Yellow fever vaccine is prepared from living viruses cultured in chick embryos. This preparation of attenuated virus promotes active immunity against yellow fever.

**INDICATIONS   Prevention of yellow fever** Yellow fever vaccine protects persons who expect to be exposed to the virus by travel through areas where the disease is endemic.

**CONTRAINDICATIONS   Allergy to eggs or chickens** Eggs are used as growth media for the viruses used in preparing the vaccine.   **Immune deficiencies** Patients with decreased immune function caused by disease or by immunosuppressive drugs should not receive the vaccine. • Replication of the virus may be uncontrolled in these individuals.

**DOSAGE   SC:   ADULTS AND CHILDREN:** 0.5 ml as a single dose. Boosters are required at 10-year intervals. *Special patient populations:*   **PREGNANCY:** Safe use in pregnancy and lactation has not been established.

**PREPARATIONS**   *Lyophilized powder:* the powder is reconstituted with 0.9% sodium chloride solution before use.

**DRUG INTERACTIONS**   See entry for drug class (p. 444).

   **FATE**   Following inoculation with yellow fever vaccine, immunity to the disease develops within 7 to 10 days. Significant protection persists for up to 10 years.

## ❦ NURSING CONSIDERATIONS
### Side effects, toxicities, and associated nursing actions
   • See entry for drug class (p. 444).

### Nursing interventions related to drug administration
   • Obtain history of allergy to egg protein before administering this vaccine. If history of allergy to egg is present, an intradermal skin test should be performed before administering dose; consult physician.
   • Administer SC doses to adults and children over 3 years into the deltoid region. Administer SC doses to children under 3 years in the anterolateral thigh.
   • Read manufacturer's instructions for reconstitution and preparation.

### Patient and family education
   • See entry for drug class (p. 445).

# Chapter Twenty-six

# Immune suppressants

| | |
|---|---|
| antilymphocyte globulin | cyclosporine |
| antithymocyte globulin | mercaptopurine (See Chapter Twenty-seven, p. 478) |
| azathioprine | |
| azathioprine sodium | methotrexate (See Chapter Twenty-seven, p. 479) |
| cyclophosphamide (See Chapter Twenty-seven, p. 458) | muromonab-CD3 |

**OVERVIEW OF THE DRUG CLASS**  Suppressing immune responses is necessary in organ transplantation and may be useful in treating certain autoimmune conditions. Many types of drugs have been tested in these situations, including corticosteroids (Chapter Thirty-one) and some antineoplastic drugs (Chapter Twenty-seven). Drugs such as cyclosporine A and muromonab-CD3 are much more specific and powerful than the corticosteroids but the corticosteroids are still useful in certain situations.

**MECHANISM OF ACTION**  The action sought with these agents is inhibition of cell-mediated immune reactions. These reactions are primarily responsible for organ transplant rejection.

**INDICATIONS**  **Organ transplant surgery** These agents are necessary to prevent rejection of the transplanted organ.  **Autoimmune diseases** These agents are becoming more accepted for control of conditions involving autoimmune mechanisms. Azathioprine has been used for rheumatoid arthritis and is being tested in other connective tissue diseases.

**CONTRAINDICATIONS**  **Allergy** Specific allergy to one of these drugs may necessitate using a different drug.

**DRUG INTERACTIONS**  See listing for individual agents.

## ☙ NURSING CONSIDERATIONS

### Side effects, toxicities, and associated nursing actions

**Infections** Infections may increase while patients are receiving immune suppressants. Unusual infections that are difficult to treat are a constant threat to patient survival.

- Inform patients about this side effect. Instruct patients to report to the physician any sign of infection: fever, sore throat, increased malaise, urinary frequency or dysuria, coughing or chest congestion, or skin infections.
- Remind patients to avoid contact with persons with known infections or communicable diseases. This may also require avoiding activities involving large crowds of people.
- Review careful handwashing techniques with patients and families.
- In the hospital setting, it may be appropriate to place patients on immune suppressants in protective isolation. Do not assign caregivers known to have colds or other infections. Reinforce to staff the importance of washing hands before providing direct care to patient. Work with the hospital infection control nurse to develop procedures to limit patient exposure to pathologic organisms.

**Carcinogenesis** Immune suppressants may lessen natural defenses against viral-induced lymphomas. Other types of cancer may also be induced.

- Work with other members of the health care team to ensure that patients are fully informed about advantages and disadvantages of drug therapy, and provide support to patients while decisions about care are being made.

### Patient and family education

- Review anticipated benefits and possible side effects of drug therapy with patients.
- See Drug Interactions for specific drugs. Patients should avoid immunizations with live virus vaccines while receiving immunosuppressant therapy. Warn patients about this hazard.
- These drugs may pose a threat to an unborn fetus. Counsel about birth control as needed. Warn patients to notify the physician immediately if pregnancy is suspected.
- Reinforce to patients the need to remain in close contact with the physician and to report the development of new signs or symptoms.

# antithymocyte globulin
(an-ti-THY-moh-site GLOB-yoo-lin)                                   immunosuppressant antibody

- antithymocyte globuline (equine): Atgam

**MECHANISM OF ACTION**    Antithymocyte globulin is prepared by immunizing horses with human thymus lymphocytes. When injected into humans, the IgG purified from the serum of these horses binds to T-lymphocytes. Because T-lymphocytes are involved in cell-mediated responses such as rejection reactions, antithymocyte globulin may limit such reactions.

**INDICATIONS**    **Renal allotransplantation** Antithymocyte globulin may be used along with other therapy to treat or to prevent rejection reactions.

**CONTRAINDICATIONS**    **Previous allergy to equine materials or serum products** Patients may be cautiously skin-tested if a question arises.

**DOSAGE**    IV:    ADULTS: 10 to 30 mg/kg daily for 14 days, then on alternate days for another 14 days (seven additional doses).    CHILDREN: 5 to 25 mg/kg daily for 14 days, then on alternate days for another 14 days (seven additional doses). Experience with children is limited.    **Intradermal:** ADULTS AND CHILDREN: 0.1 ml of a freshly prepared 1:1000 dilution in 0.9% sodium chloride is injected. A wheal with localized erythema or edema observed within 1 hour is considered a positive test and may preclude safe administration of the drug.    *Special patient populations:*    PREGNANCY: Safe use is not established.

**PREPARATIONS**    *Concentrate for injection*: 50 mg equine IgG/ml.

**DRUG INTERACTIONS**    **Immunosuppressant drugs** may be more effective when given with antithymocyte globulin. Although this interaction is desirable in controlling graft rejections, the additional impairment of host defense mechanisms may increase the risk of infection and blood dyscrasias.    **Live virus vaccines** may cause serious or even fatal disease in immunosuppressed patients.

**FATE**    Equine IgG has a *half-life* of about 6 days in the body. This globulin is presumed to pass the placenta and enter fetuses, as do other immunoglobulins.

## ☙ NURSING CONSIDERATIONS

### Side effects, toxicities, and associated nursing actions

**CNS** Headache, weakness, paresthesia, or seizures are uncommon.

- Discuss these side effects with patients. Instruct patients to notify the physician if any CNS side effects develop.

**CV** Hypotension, hypertension, tachycardia, edema, pulmonary edema, and chest pain have occurred.

- Monitor blood pressure and pulse. Auscultate breath sounds.
- Assess for jugular venous distention.
- Obtain weight before starting therapy and monitor daily. Report to the physician any weight gain in excess of 2 pounds in 1 day or 5 pounds in a week.

**Blood** Leukopenia and/or thrombocytopenia occur in up to 20% of renal transplant patients.

- Assess patients for fever, malaise, or unexplained bleeding or bruising.
- Monitor complete blood cell count and white blood cell differential and platelet count.

**GI** Diarrhea, nausea, vomiting, stomatitis, abdominal distention, hiccups, or epigastric pain have occurred.

- Monitor intake, output, and weight. Monitor serum electrolytes.
- Assess for GI side effects.

**Metabolic** Hyperglycemia is possible.

- Monitor blood glucose levels.
- Instruct diabetic patients to monitor blood glucose levels while on therapy with this drug, as a change in diet or dose of hypoglycemic agent may be necessary.

**Allergic** Fever is the most common reaction, occurring in 33% or more of patients receiving the drug. Chills occur in 14% or more. Serum sickness or anaphylaxis is more rare in renal transplant patients, but the incidence of serum sickness may be higher in certain other classes of patients. Local reactions such as wheal or flare or rash occur in up to 15% of patients.

- Inspect patients for skin changes, and instruct patients to report the development of skin changes.
- Monitor temperature.

- Have drugs, equipment, and personnel available to treat acute allergic attacks in settings where this drug is administered.
- Assess for signs of serum sickness: arthralgia, skin eruptions, lymphadenopathy, and pruritis. Abdominal pain, fever, headache, and malaise occur in more serious cases. Instruct patients to report the development of these signs and symptoms. Point out to patients that serum sickness may not develop for 10 to 14 days following drug therapy.

**Other** Thrombophlebitis is common. Fistulas or shunts may clot in 2% to 5% of patients.

- Assess the IV line for patency before administering IV doses. Instruct the patient to report pain or redness at the IV site.
- Assess fistulas or shunts per agency procedure (through palpation or auscultation) at least every 2 hours while the patient is receiving this drug. If the patient knows to assess clots or fistulas, engage the patient in watching for clotting also.

### Nursing interventions related to drug administration

- Consult the manufacturer's literature for current information regarding dilution and the rate of IV administration.

### Patient and family education

- See entry for drug class (p. 469).

---

## anti-human lymphocyte globulin                  immunosuppressant antibody

- anti-human lymphocyte globulin: Pressimmune

**MECHANISM OF ACTION**    This purified preparation containing IgG and IgT suppresses the activity of human lymphocytes. This action reduces the likelihood of rejection reactions of transplanted organs.

**INDICATIONS**    **Organ transplantation** In renal and other organ transplantation procedures, anti-human lymphocyte globulin may be used along with other immunosuppressant agents to prevent or control rejection reactions.

**CONTRAINDICATIONS**    **Known allergy to equine materials or serum products** Skin testing may be required to assess the likelihood of allergic reactions.

**DOSAGE**    **IM, IV:**  **ADULTS:** Prior to transplantation, 20 to 30 mg/kg by slow infusion, in conjunction with prednisone (two 100 mg doses). After transplantation, 20 to 30 mg/kg for the first 3 days, 10 mg/kg daily for the next 4 weeks, 10 mg/kg every other day for the fifth and sixth weeks, the 10 mg/kg every third day during followup. Other immunosuppressants are also required.  **SC:**  **ADULTS:** 0.1 ml of 1:10 dilution is injected. A wheal developing within 15 minutes constitutes a positive reaction. *Special patient populations:* **PREGNANCY:** Safe use is not established.  **CHILDREN:** Special doses are not established.

**PREPARATIONS**    *Ampule*: 500 mg in 10 ml (50 mg/ml).

**DRUG INTERACTIONS**    **Immunosuppressant drugs** may be more effective when given with anti-human lymphocyte globulin. Although this interaction is desirable in controlling graft rejection, the additional impairment of host defense mechanisms may increase the risk of infection and blood dyscrasias. **Live virus vaccines** may cause serious or even fatal disease in immunosuppressed patients.

**FATE**    Equine IgG has a *half-life* of about 6 days in the body. This globulin is presumed to pass the placenta and enter fetuses, as do other immunoglobulins.

### ☙ NURSING CONSIDERATIONS

#### Side effects, toxicities, and associated nursing actions

**Blood** Lymphocytopenia is a desired effect of the drug, but thrombocytopenia and leukopenia may complicate use of the agent.

- Monitor white blood cell differential and platelet count.
- Assess the patient for fever, malaise, or signs of infection.
- Assess for signs of thrombocytopenia: petechiae or unexplained bleeding or bruising.

**Allergic** Fever is common and expected during the early phase of therapy. Anaphylaxis, serum sickness, urticaria, and pruritis are less common.

- Inspect patients for skin changes, and instruct patients to report the development of skin changes.
- Monitor temperature.
- Have drugs, equipment, and personnel available to treat acute allergic attacks in settings where this drug is administered.
- Assess for signs of serum sickness: arthralgia, skin eruptions, lymphadenopathy, and pruritis. Abdominal pain, fever, headache, and malaise occur in more serious cases. Instruct patients to report the development of these signs and symptoms. Point out to patients that serum sickness may not develop for 10 to 14 days following drug therapy.

### Nursing interventions related to drug administration
- Consult the manufacturer's literature for current information about dilution and rate of administration.

### Patient and family education
- See entry for drug class (p. 469).

---

# azathioprine sodium    (aza-THY-oh-prin)                                    immune suppressant

- azathioprine: Imuran

**MECHANISM OF ACTION**    Azathioprine inhibits cell-mediated immunity and may affect humoral immunity to some extent. Azathioprine is converted in vivo to mercaptopurine (p. 478), an inhibitor of purine synthesis that is also capable of suppressing immune responses.

**INDICATIONS**    **Renal allotransplantation** Azathioprine is used with other drugs to prevent rejection of the transplanted organ.    **Rheumatoid arthritis** Azathioprine should be used only when other therapy has failed.

**CONTRAINDICATIONS**    **Renal impairment** Azathioprine and mercaptopurine may accumulate in patients before renal function is established.

**DOSAGE**    **PO:**    **ADULTS AND CHILDREN:** For renal allotransplantation, 3 to 5 mg/kg daily at the time of transplantation, followed by 1 to 3 mg/kg thereafter for maintenance. For rheumatoid arthritis, 1 mg/kg with 0.5 mg/kg increases after 6 to 8 weeks. After 12 weeks, the response should be evaluated. **IV:**    **ADULTS AND CHILDREN:** For renal allotransplantation, 3 to 5 mg/kg following surgery until the patient is able to tolerate oral doses.    *Special patient populations:*    **PREGNANCY:** Safe use in pregnancy and lactation is not established. The drug is mutagenic and has been linked to fetal abnormalities.

**PREPARATIONS**    **Azathioprine** *Tablets:* 50 mg.    **Azathioprine sodium** *Powder:* 100 mg to be reconstituted for parenteral injection.

**DRUG INTERACTIONS**    **Allopurinol** interferes with the metabolism of azathioprine, causing the drug to accumulate and increasing the risk of bone marrow suppression.    **Immunosuppressants** may aid in controlling rejection reactions but will contribute to side effects, including loss of defense mechanisms against infections.    **Live virus vaccines** may pose a special danger to immunosuppressed patients. Generalized, life-threatening disease may develop.

**FATE**    Azathioprine is easily absorbed following oral administration. The drug distributes rapidly through tissues and is actively metabolized. The metabolites of azathioprine, including the cytotoxic compound mercaptopurine, are excreted by the kidneys.

### ❦ NURSING CONSIDERATIONS
#### Side effects, toxicities, and associated nursing actions
**Blood** Bone marrow suppression is the most common toxic effect of azathioprine, limiting use of the drug. Signs include leukopenia, macrocytic anemia, pancytopenia, and thrombocytopenia. In late stages, patients may hemorrhage.
- Monitor complete blood cell count, white blood cell differential, and platelet count.
- Visually inspect patients for petechiae or bruising. Instruct patients to report the development of unexplained bleeding: bruising, bleeding gums, nosebleeds, or hematuria.
- Avoid IM injections in persons with thrombocytopenia.

- Instruct patients to report the development of any sign of infection: fever, malaise, and sore throat.
- See entry for drug class (page 469).

**GI** Anorexia, diarrhea, nausea, and vomiting occur, especially with large doses. A few patients suffer ulceration of the mouth and esophagus or steatorrhea.

- Monitor weight. If diarrhea or vomiting are severe or persistent, monitor intake and output, and notify the physician.
- Instruct patients to report the development of oral ulceration or pain on eating or swallowing. Instruct patients to report changes in color or consistency of stools.
- Instruct patients to take doses after meals and to try dividing the daily dose in order to take the drug in smaller amounts more frequently; consult the physician.

**Liver** Toxic hepatitis with biliary stasis may cause jaundice in renal transplant patients. The lower doses used for rheumatoid arthritis cause liver toxicity in less than 1% of patients.

- Caution patients to report the development of jaundice, malaise, fever, right upper quadrant abdominal pain, or change in the color or consistency of stools.
- Monitor liver function tests.

**Allergy** Rashes, fever, and serum sickness may occur.

- Instruct patients to report the development of any rashes or skin changes.
- Review with patients the symptoms of serum sickness: arthralgia, skin eruptions, lymphadenopathy, and pruritis. Abdominal pain, fever, headache, and malaise occur in more serious cases. Instruct patients to report the development of these symptoms.

**Other** Rare side effects include alopecia, arthralgia, retinopathy, pulmonary edema, and Raynaud's disease.

- Review these side effects with patients. Instruct patients to report the development of any new signs or symptoms.
- Reinforce to patients the need to return for scheduled follow-up visits to the physician.

### Nursing interventions related to drug administration
- Administer oral doses after meals to lessen gastric irritation.
- For IV administration, reconstitute the drug as directed on the vial. A solution of 10 mg/ml may be given by direct IV injection or further diluted in 0.9% sodium chloride or 5% dextrose. Administer the ordered dose over 30 to 60 minutes.
- Use diluted IV doses within 24 hours.

### Patient and family education
- Review with patients the anticipated benefits and possible side effects of drug therapy.
- See entry for drug class (p. 469).
- Reassure patients taking this drug for rheumatoid arthritis that several weeks or months of therapy may be necessary before improvement is seen.

## cyclophosphamide    (sye-klo-FOSS-fah-mide)    immune suppressant*

- cyclophosphamide: Cytoxan, Neosar, ✿Procytox

**INDICATIONS    Bone marrow transplant** Cyclophosphamide is a potent immunosuppressant that may be used to control rejection of transplants. • For full information on cyclophosphamide, see listing under Cytotoxic Agents (Chapter Twenty-seven, p. 458).

## cyclosporine    (sye-klo-SPOR-in)    immune suppressant

- cyclosporine: Sandimmune

*Antineoplastic.

**MECHANISM OF ACTION**   Cyclosporine inhibits cell-mediated immune reactions, such as those involved in transplant rejection. The drug seems specifically to inhibit T-lymphocytes, especially those called T-helper cells. Unlike other immunosuppressive agents, cyclosporine is not a myelosuppressant, so bone marrow function is retained and blood counts are not significantly altered in most patients.

**INDICATIONS**   **Allotransplantation** Cyclosporine protects transplanted organs from rejection by the host. Used alone, cyclosporine results in 71% to 91% survival of transplanted kidneys at 1 year; cyclosporine with prednisone used in liver transplantation results in a patient survival rate at 1 year of 60% to 80%. Cyclosporine with low doses of corticosteroids used in heart transplantation results in a patient survival rate at 2 years of 77%, as reported in one small study.

**CONTRAINDICATIONS**   **Allergy** Cyclosporine may cause allergic reactions in some patients.

**DOSAGE**   PO:   **ADULTS AND CHILDREN:** 15 mg/kg as a single dose daily, with the first dose preceding the transplantation surgery by 4 to 12 hours. After 1 to 2 weeks, dosage is tapered 5% weekly to a maintenance dosage of 5 to 10 mg/kg. Dosage may be adjusted as necessary based on renal function and plasma concentrations of cyclosporine.   IV:   **ADULTS AND CHILDREN:** 5 to 6 mg/kg as a single dose by infusion. The dose may be repeated daily until the patient can be switched to oral dosage.   *Special patient populations:*   **PREGNANCY:** Safe use in pregnancy and lactation is not established. Cyclosporine is toxic to fetuses in animals.

**PREPARATIONS**   *Solution for oral use:* 100 mg/ml (with 12.5% alcohol, olive oil, and peglicol 5 oleate). *Solution for injection:* 50 mg/ml (with 32.9% alcohol and polyoxyl 35 castor oil, 650 mg/ml).

**DRUG INTERACTIONS**   **Aminoglycoside antibiotics** (e.g., gentamicin; p. 280) are nephrotoxic and should be avoided if possible because the combined nephrotoxicity of cyclosporine and the aminoglycosides could dangerously damage renal function.   **Amphotericin B** is nephrotoxic and also tends to elevate cyclosporine concentrations. Both of these actions tend to increase the risk of serious renal damage. **Corticosteroids** may increase serum concentrations of cyclosporine by blocking normal hepatic metabolism of cyclosporine. This action may increase the risk of renal toxicity from cyclosporine. **Immunosuppressive agents** when used with cyclosporine may result in profound suppression of cell-mediated immunity. The use of multiple agents is associated with increased risk of developing lymphomas.   **Ketoconazole** may increase serum concentrations of cyclosporine by blocking normal hepatic metabolism of cyclosporine. This action may increase the risk of renal toxicity from cyclosporine.   **Live-virus vaccines** may pose a special danger to immunosuppressed patients. Generalized, life-threatening disease may develop.

**FATE**   Oral absorption of cyclosporine is variable, and the bioavailability is only about 30%. *Peak* plasma concentrations of the drug are produced about 3.5 hours after an oral dose. Cyclosporine is relatively lipid soluble and distributes to most tissues and fluids, including fetal tissue and breast milk. The primary route of elimination for cyclosporine is the liver, where the drug is extensively metabolized. A first-pass effect is observed with oral doses of cyclosporine. The elimination *half-life* of cyclosporine is about 19 to 27 hours, with most of the products of metabolism being eliminated in bile. Very little drug appears in urine.

## 🦫 NURSING CONSIDERATIONS

### Side effects, toxicities, and associated nursing actions

**CNS** Up to one half of treated patients may develop tremor. Confusion, flushing, headaches, hyperesthesia, paresthesia, and seizures have also occurred. Psychiatric disorders are rare.

• Review these side effects with patients and instruct patients to report their development.
• Caution patients to avoid driving or operating hazardous equipment if confusion develops.

**CV** Hypertension occurs in up to one half of treated patients. Some may require antihypertensive medication.

• Monitor blood pressure and pulse. If appropriate, teach the patient or other family members to monitor and record blood pressure at home.

**Blood** Blood dyscrasias are rare with cyclosporine, but anemia, leukopenia, and thrombocytopenia have occurred.

• Monitor complete blood cell count, white blood cell differential, and platelet count.
• Instruct patients to report the development of malaise, fatigue, unexplained bleeding or bruising: bleeding gums, nosebleeds, or hematuria.

- Avoid IM injections in persons with thrombocytopenia.

**GI** Anorexia, diarrhea, nausea, and vomiting are common. More serious reactions such as GI bleeding are rare.

- Monitor weight. If diarrhea or vomiting are severe or persistent, notify the physician, and monitor intake and output.

**Skin** Hirsutism occurs in 21% to 45% of patients. Acne may also arise during therapy.

- Warn patients about these side effects. Inspect patients for the development of skin changes. Refer patients to a dermatologist if appropriate.

**Liver** Hepatotoxicity occurs in up to 7% of treated patients during early therapy. Damage appears to be reversed when doses are lowered.

- Instruct the patient to report the development of jaundice, right upper quadrant abdominal pain, fever, malaise, or change in the color or consistency of stools.

**Kidney** Nephrotoxicity is the dose-limiting effect of cyclosporine. Up to 38% of treated patients suffer elevations in BUN and serum creatinine. This reaction is dose dependent.

- Monitor intake, output, and weight.
- Monitor BUN and serum creatinine.

**Cancer** Cyclosporine may induce lymphomas, especially when used with other immunosuppressant drugs.

- Work with other members of the health care team to ensure that patients are fully informed about advantages and disadvantages of drug therapy, and provide support to patients while decisions about care are being made.

**Infections** Because cyclosporine suppresses the immune system, natural defenses against bacterial, viral, fungal, and other types of infections are lowered. Patients receiving cyclosporine suffer increased risk of infection from all causes. See entry for drug class (p. 469).

**Other** Gingival hyperplasia occurs in up to 30% of treated patients.

- Visually inspect teeth and gums at regular intervals.
- Reinforce to patients the importance of regular oral hygiene: brushing, flossing, and regular dental follow-up.
- Refer the patient to a dentist if appropriate.

### Nursing interventions related to drug administration

- Review the manufacturer's instructions. Measure oral doses carefully with the pipette provided, and pour the oral dose into a glass container. Dilute the oral dose with a small amount of milk, chocolate milk, or orange juice, which are at room temperature. Stir the dilution well and administer immediately. Pour a little more of the diluent (e.g., orange juice) into the glass medication cup to rinse the cup, and have the patient drink this also.
- For IV administration, dilute each milliliter of concentrate in 20 to 100 ml if 0.9% sodium chloride or 5% dextrose injection just before administering. Inspect the diluted drug for discoloration or particulate matter, and discard if either is present. Infuse the prescribed dose over 2 to 6 hours. Monitor vital signs. Have drugs, equipment, and personnel available to treat an acute allergic reaction.

### Patient and family education

- Review with patients the anticipated benefits and possible side effects of drug therapy.
- See entry for drug class (p. 469).

---

## mercaptopurine   (mer-kap-toh-PUR-een)   immune suppressant*

- mercaptopurine: Purinethol

**INDICATIONS  Immune suppressant** Mercaptopurine has been used to suppress homograft rejection and to control certain autoimmune diseases, but such use is now rare. • For full information on see listing under Cytotoxic Agents (Chapter Twenty-seven, p. 478).

*Antineoplastic.

## methotrexate   (meth-oh-TREX-ate)                    immune suppressant*

- methotrexate: Folex, Mexate

**INDICATIONS**   **Autoimmune diseases** Conditions such as rheumatoid arthritis may respond to the immune suppressant action of methotrexate. • For full information on methotrexate, see listing under Cytotoxic Agents (Chapter Twenty-seven, p. 479).

## muromonab-CD3   (myoo-roh-MOH-nab)              immunosuppressant antibody

- muromonab-CD3: Orthoclone OKT3

**MECHANISM OF ACTION**   Muromonab is a monoclonal antibody specifically directed against the CD3 molecule linked to an antigen receptor on human T-lymphocytes. This purified IgG molecule is more specific than antibodies prepared by immunization to whole lymphocytes.

**INDICATIONS**   **Acute rejection reactions in renal transplant patients** Muromonab may reverse the rejection reaction without suppressing the entire immune system.

**CONTRAINDICATIONS**   **Recent exposure to chickenpox or herpes zoster** Immune suppression may cause severe generalized disease.   **Fluid overload or pulmonary edema** Risk of life-threatening pulmonary edema is increased.   **Fever above 37.8° C** Must be reduced before giving muromonab.

**DOSAGE**   IV:   ADULTS: 5 mg daily for 10 to 14 days by rapid injection.   *Special patient populations:* PREGNANCY: Safe use is not established.   CHILDREN: Doses are not established.

**PREPARATIONS**   *Solution:* 1 mg/ml.

**DRUG INTERACTIONS**   **Immunosuppressant drugs** may be more effective when given with muromonab. Although this interaction is desirable in controlling graft rejection, the additional impairment of host defense mechanisms may increase risk of infection and blood dyscrasias.   **Live virus vaccines** may cause serious or even fatal disease in immunosuppressed patients. Oral polio vaccine should also be avoided in family members or others in close physical contact with the patient.

**FATE**   Muromonab-CD3 binds T-lymphocytes immediately on administration. The effect persists for about 1 week after discontinuing muromonad-CD3.

## ❧ NURSING CONSIDERATIONS
### Side effects, toxicities, and associated nursing actions
**CNS** Trembling and shaking of hands following the first dose is common but seldom recurs with subsequent doses.
- Forewarn patients about this side effect. Tell patients to notify the physician if it continues after the first dose.

**CV** Chest pain may follow the first dose but is rare thereafter.
- Monitor pulse and blood pressure. Remain with the patient for 15 to 30 minutes after the first dose. If pain is severe or persists, notify the physician.

**GI** Diarrhea, nausea, and vomiting may occur after the first dose but are rare thereafter.
- Monitor intake, output, and weight.

**Allergic** Fever, chills, wheezing, and shortness of breath are not uncommon following the first dose. If these reactions persist, the underlying cause should be sought (e.g., infection, severe pulmonary edema, fluid overload.).
- Monitor temperature and auscultate breath sounds. Assess for jugular venous distention, edema, or weight gain if symptoms persist.

### Nursing interventions related to drug administration
- Review current manufacturer's literature for information about dilution and rate of administration.

### Patient and family education
- See entry for drug class (p. 469).

*Antineoplastic.

# ANTINEOPLASTIC AGENTS

**INTRODUCTION**   Neoplastic diseases arise from many causes, and their development may be promoted in several ways. Risk of some forms of cancer is increased by smoking tobacco and by excessive use of alcoholic beverages. Exposure to certain chemicals also increases risk of specific cancers. The diseases called cancer in fact range from easily treated mild conditions to rapidly progressive fatal diseases. Chemotherapy is successful in a portion of these conditions, either alone or in combination with surgery, radiation, or both (Table 27-2, p. 480). Some selectivity of action toward cancer cells is evident with chemotherapeutic agents, but the degree of selectivity is less than optimal. The toxicity of most anticancer drugs limits their use; most cannot be used at doses required to kill all the cancer cells.

Because toxicity limits the dose of many anticancer drugs and because cure of cancer requires killing all of the cancerous cells in the body, chemotherapeutic regimens often involve combinations of drugs (Table 27-1, p. 479). The combinations are designed to maximize the anticancer activity and minimize toxicity. Research with a group of drugs called radioprotectors may one day allow pretreatment of patients with agents that protect healthy cells from the lethal effects of radiation and chemotherapy, while allowing cancerous tissues to be destroyed.

VIII

# Chapter Twenty-seven
# Cytotoxic agents

asparaginase
bleomycin sulfate
busulfan
carmustine
chlorambucil
cisplatin
cyclophosphamide
cytarabine
dacarbazine
dactinomycin
daunorubicin hydrochloride
doxorubicin hydrochloride
etoposide
floxuridine
fluorouracil
hydroxyurea
lomustine

mechlorethamine hydrochloride
melphalan
mercaptopurine
methotrexate
methotrexate sodium
mitomycin
mitoxantrone hydrochloride (investigational U.S.)
pipobroman
plicamycin
procarbazine hydrochloride
thioguanine
triethylenethiophosphoramide
uracil mustard
vinblastine sulfate
vincristine sulfate
vindesine sulfate (Investigational U.S.)

**MECHANISM OF ACTION** Most drugs used for the chemotherapy of cancer attack proliferating cells, both normal and cancerous, and are therefore called cytotoxic agents. The drugs inhibit proliferation by several mechanisms. One group of drugs directly attacks DNA. By damaging DNA, the drugs prevent successful reading of cellular genes; those cells that cannot rapidly repair the DNA will die. Drugs that act by this mechanism are chemically highly reactive compounds. Alkylating agents directly attack the chemical structure of DNA. Other agents cross-link DNA or cause breaks in the strands. These agents are usually highly mutagenic and may in fact cause cancer as a delayed side effect.

A second class of drugs inhibits DNA synthesis. This group includes agents that are chemically similar to natural purines or pyrimidines. Folate antagonists may also inhibit DNA synthesis. As a group, these agents are often referred to as antimetabolites.

A third class of drugs blocks RNA or protein synthesis. One of these drugs (asparaginase) starves the cancer cell of required amino acids. The other drugs block RNA synthesis from DNA by binding tightly between the strands of double-stranded DNA. Drugs of this second type are called intercalating agents.

A fourth group of drugs blocks mitosis, thereby preventing replication of cancer cells. Drugs of this type include the vinca alkaloids (vincristine, vinblastine, and vindesine).

Drugs from these four categories are often combined with each other and with radiation and/or surgery for optimal therapeutic effect (Table 27-1). The goal of therapy differs, depending on the type of cancer present and the age or condition of the patient. Cure is possible in many situations, and aggressive therapy is aimed at destroying all cancer cells in the body. In some cases, cure is not likely, but appropriate therapy may induce remissions and prolong life. In later stages of many neoplastic diseases the aim of therapy is palliation, or relief of suffering, and not cure or prolongation of life.

**INDICATIONS** • See Table 27-2. **Cure of neoplastic disease** • See specific agents. **Induction of remissions and prolongation of life** • See specific agents. **Palliation of neoplastic disease** • See specific agents.

**CONTRAINDICATIONS** **Chickenpox or herpes zoster infections** Because many anticancer drugs suppress the immune system, active infections of many types may be worsened; among the most dangerous are those caused by herpes zoster (chickenpox, shingles) because this virus can cause generalized systemic infections in immune-suppressed patients.

**DRUG INTERACTIONS** **Myelosuppressive agents** previously administered will influence the tolerance of a patient to the myelosuppressive effects of a specific anticancer drug. A previous history of radiation therapy will also influence tolerance. Doses are often based on the degree of immune suppression produced. **Vaccines containing live viruses** should never be administered to patients with impaired

**Table 27-1.**

| Selected drug combinations used in cancer chemotherapy | | |
| --- | --- | --- |
| **Combination** | **Disease** | **Result of therapy** |
| ABVD (Adriamycin [doxorubicin], bleomycin, vinblastine, dacarbazine) | Hodgkin's disease | Long-term remissions or cures |
| BACOP (bleomycin, Adriamycin [doxorubicin], cyclophosphamide, Oncovin [vincristine], prednisone) | Non-Hodgkin's lymphoma | Long-term remissions |
| CMFVP (cyclophosphamide, methotrexate, fluorouracil, prednisone, vincristine) | Advanced breast carcinoma | Palliation |
| Cytarabine, daunorubicin | Acute myelogenous leukemia | Remissions |
| CYVADIC (cyclophosphamide, vincristine, Adriamycin [doxorubicin], dacarbazine) | Soft tissue sarcoma | Remissions |
| FAM (fluorouracil, Adriamycin [doxorubicin], mitomycin) | Gastric carcinoma | Palliation |
| MAC (methotrexate, Actinomycin-D [dactinomycin], chlorambucil) | Choriocarcinoma | Long-term remissions or cures |
| MOPP (mechlorethamine, Oncovin [vincristine], procarbazine, prednisone) | Hodgkin's disease | Long-term remissions or cures |
| Prednisone, vincristine, and asparaginase for induction; methotrexate, mercaptopurine for maintenance | Acute lymphocytic leukemia | Long-term remissions |
| PVB (Platinol [cisplatin], vinblastine, bleomycin) | Testicular carcinoma | Long-term remissions or cures |
| VA (vincristine, Actinomycin-D [dactinomycin]) | Embryonal rhabdomyosarcoma | Remissions |

immune systems because these patients are at risk of generalized, potentially fatal, disease. Patients on chemotherapy for cancer are almost always immune suppressed to some degree and therefore at risk.

## ❦ NURSING CONSIDERATIONS
### Side effects, toxicities, and associated nursing actions

**Blood** Many of the drugs used to treat cancer suppress those elements of bone marrow that form blood cells. As a result, severe blood dyscrasias are a common side effect with these drugs. Immune suppression may also be severe and can lower the ability of patients to withstand ordinary infections. Specific problems include the following conditions.

ANEMIA: Anemia may be caused by several factors, including anorexia, poor nutrition, and bone marrow depression. These problems can be caused by drug therapy or by the cancer itself.
• Assess for malaise, easy fatigability, pale skin color. Monitor hematocrit and hemoglobin, and monitor stools for occult blood.

| Table 27-2. | Summary of major indications for antineoplastic agents | |
| --- | --- | --- |
| **Disease** | **Drugs** | |
| Carcinoma of breast | Cyclophosphamide, diethylstilbestrol, doxorubicin, fluorouracil, megestrol, methotrexate, prednisone, tamoxifen, testolactone | |
| Carcinoma of colon | Fluorouracil, mitomycin | |
| Carcinoma of lung (small cell) | Cyclophosphamide, doxorubicin, etoposide, lomustine, methotrexate, vincristine | |
| Carcinoma of testes | Bleomycin, cisplatin, cyclophosphamide, dactinomycin, etoposide, vinblastine | |
| Gliomas | Carmustine, lomustine, procarbazine | |
| Leukemia, acute lymphocytic | Asparaginase, daunorubicin, mercaptopurine, methotrexate, prednisone, vincristine | |
| Leukemia, acute myelogenous | Cytarabine, daunorubicin, doxorubicin, thioguanine, vincristine | |
| Leukemia, chronic lymphocyt-ic | Chlorambucil, cyclophosphamide, prednisone, vincristine | |
| Leukemia, chronic myeloge-nous | Busulfan, hydroxyurea | |
| Lymphomas, Hodgkin's dis-ease | Bleomycin, carmustine, cyclophosphamide, dacarbazine, doxorubicin, mechloretham-ine, prednisone, procarbazine, vincristine | |
| Lymphomas, non-Hodgkin's | Bleomycin, chlorambucil, cyclophosphamide, doxorubicin, prednisone, vincristine | |
| Sarcomas | Cyclophosphamide, dacarbazine, doxorubicin, methotrexate, vincristine | |

- Obtain a dietary history. Do dietary teaching and counseling as appropriate, although iron-rich foods may be unappealing if anorexia or nausea is present.
- Encourage frequent, small feedings. See interventions under Anorexia.
- Encourage the use of iron preparations, if prescribed, although they may have limited value until chemotherapy is finished. Fluoxymesterone (Halotestin), an androgen, may also be prescribed to reverse anemia.

**LEUKOPENIA (GRANULOCYTOPENIA):** Reduced white blood cell counts occur 1 to 3 weeks following chemotherapy. Patients are most susceptible to infection during this period.

- Assess for signs of infection: fever (greater than 100° F or 38.3° C), malaise, altered level of consciousness, or the development of new signs or symptoms: cough, sore throat, dyspnea, urinary frequency, or dysuria. Review these signs and symptoms with patients and families, and instruct them to notify the physician if they occur.
- Monitor the white blood cell count and differential.
- Review with patients and families the anticipated nadir for each drug being used with the patient. The *nadir* is the point of greatest bone marrow suppression, or stated differently, point of lowest blood count following administration of each drug.
- Caution patients to avoid contact with anyone with an infection, cold, bronchitis, herpes simplex or zoster, chicken pox, measles, or other infectious disease during the period 1 to 3 weeks following chemotherapy. It may be necessary for patients to limit contact with young children or grandchildren if the youngsters are having frequent colds.
- Assess carefully patients who are receiving steroids, as the usual signs of infection may be masked.

- Be alert to preventing infection in hospitalized patients. Wash hands carefully before providing care and instruct patients to use careful personal hygiene. Assign patients to rooms where the other occupants do not have infections; use private rooms if appropriate. For cases of severe leukopenia, protective isolation may be appropriate; consult with the physician. Protective isolation may contribute to social isolation, which may be emotionally undesirable for the patient.
- Avoid the use of rectal thermometers, which may contribute to development of perirectal abscesses.

**THROMBOCYTOPENIA:** The platelet count may fall as the cells that form platelets are destroyed by chemotherapy. Spontaneous bleeding may be severe and even life-threatening.

- Instruct patients to report the development of signs or symptoms that may signal thrombocytopenia: bleeding gums, nosebleeds, change in the color of urine that might indicate kidney or bladder bleeding, rectal bleeding, change of color of stools, excessive bruising, or the development of petechiae (minute hemorrhagic spots, pinpoint to pinhead size, seen on the skin).
- Monitor stools for occult blood. This is only necessary beginning 3 to 5 days before the nadir of bone marrow suppression.
- Instruct patients to avoid the use of a razor with a blade; have them use an electric razor.
- Monitor the platelet count. Avoid IM or subcutaneous injections if the platelet count is below 60,000.
- Avoid the use of dental floss if gums are bleeding or if the platelet count is below 10,000 to 15,000. Use a water-spraying oral care device only on the low setting. Brush the teeth with a soft-bristle brush until the platelet count drops to 5000 to 10,000, then stop brushing. If teeth are not being brushed, clean the mouth with a swab or 4 by 4 gauze pad wrapped around a tongue blade, using a mouthwash or other solution; a rinse of hydrogen peroxide and water may be used. Avoid the use of lemon-glycerin combinations, as they are drying and may irritate oral mucosa. See nursing actions under Stomatitis (p. 482).
- Instruct patients to limit strenuous activities, based on the platelet count. Consult the physician for personal preference. One regimen from the American Cancer Society is listed below: for platelet counts of 100,000 to 250,000, the patient may engage in tennis, jogging, basketball, and so on, but contact sports should be avoided; for platelet counts of 50,000 to 100,000, the patient may continue with moderate activity, including walking, swimming, and usual activities of daily living; when the platelet count falls below 50,000, the patient should engage in only mild activities such as walking, light housework, or yard work. Clarify with each patient the specific activities that the person engages in, since a general term such as ''light yard work'' may be interpreted differently by each individual.
- Instruct families to notify the physician immediately if symptoms of intracranial bleeding develop: headache, stiff neck, decreasing level of consciousness, pupillary inequality, and increasing blood pressure.
- Have only experienced professionals perform venipunctures on patients with thrombocytopenia. Observe venipuncture sites for hematoma formation. Apply firm pressure for at least 10 minutes to reduce hematoma formation at venipuncture sites.
- Avoid the use of restraints. If restraints must be used, apply loosely and pad well. Inspect the skin under restraints every 2 hours.
- Instruct patients to avoid the use of aspirin or aspirin-containing products. Remind patients to discuss all medications being used with all health care providers.
- Avoid constipation (see below). Avoid enemas.

**GI** Many of the anticancer drugs are cytotoxic toward the rapidly growing normal cells of the GI mucosa. When these cells are damaged by chemotherapy, a variety of symptoms can arise.

**ANOREXIA:** Anorexia may arise from drug therapy or may be caused by the underlying disease.

- Assess dietary intake; monitor weight.
- Avoid foods with a strong odor. Cool or cold foods may be more appealing than foods served hot.
- Encourage small, frequent feedings. Instruct caregivers to fix small portions in an attractive manner to encourage eating.
- If the patient develops a craving for a specific food item, it is usually permissible for the patient to have the item; the alternative may be no intake at all.

- If food preparation is tiring to the patient, suggest that the patient prepare and freeze small portions of food on days the patient feels better, so that when the patient is not feeling well, it is only necessary to thaw and eat the food servings. Encourage interested friends and family members to prepare individual servings for the patient also. Encourage snacking and nibbling during the day. Encourage the patient to keep available in the refrigerator high-protein beverages or snacks that may be appealing; examples include milk shakes, frozen yogurt, and ice cream. Have family members obtain recipes for high-protein snacks from dietitians, the American Cancer Society, and some oncologists' offices. Other patients may wish to purchase commercially prepared high-protein supplements that can be consumed as a drink or frozen and eaten as ice cream.

**CONSTIPATION:** When food intake decreases, some patients develop constipation. This condition may need special attention in patients with other side effects of chemotherapy, such as thrombocytopenia.

- Anticipate that constipation may develop in patients who are less active than usual, who have anorexia, decreased dietary intake, oral or anal stomatitis, or who are receiving narcotic analgesics. Encourage a high fluid intake (2500 ml/day). Encourage intake of fruits, fruit juices, and fiber.
- Monitor weight. Keep a record of bowel movements. Auscultate bowel sounds. Consult with the physician about the use of a stool softener.
- Caution the patient to avoid the use of over-the-counter cathartics or enemas without first consulting with the physician.

**DIARRHEA:** Certain drugs used for chemotherapy of cancer will cause diarrhea. This symptom may appear within 24 to 48 hours of receiving the drug or may be delayed for 5 to 10 days.

- If diarrhea occurs, instruct patients to switch to a clear liquid diet or a low-residue diet high in protein and calories and to maintain an intake of at least 2500 ml/day. Caution the patient to avoid foods known to be irritating to the GI tract, such as fruit, fruit juices, spicy foods, raw vegetables, corn, and coffee.
- Instruct patients to notify the physician if diarrhea persists longer than 2 days.
- Teach the patient that diarrhea can lead to electrolyte imbalance. When possible, monitor serum electrolyte levels. Instruct the patient to consider using a commerically prepared electrolyte replacement solution (e.g., Gatorade) if the diarrhea persists, if the patient can afford the product, and if the physician approves. Rarely, in severe or protracted cases of diarrhea, the patient may need to be admitted to the hospital for intravenous replacement of fluids and electrolytes.
- Instruct the patient to avoid the use of enemas, rectal suppositories, and rectal thermometers.
- If anal irritation occurs, encourage the patient to shower or sit in a warm tub of water two or three times per day. Instruct the patient to wash the anal area with mild soap and water and to dry the area carefully after each loose bowel movement. Some patients may find it easier or more comfortable to wash the area with a prepackaged towelette, such as those used to clean infants during diaper changes, or with preparations such as Tucks.

**STOMATITIS:** Mucosal cells lining the GI tract are sensitive to the cytotoxic drugs used for chemotherapy. As these mucosal cells are destroyed, severe irritation or pain may be experienced all along the GI tract from the mouth to the anus.

- Assess mouth before starting chemotherapy and at regular intervals during chemotherapy. Establish an oral care regimen, including regular brushing and flossing, unless thrombocytopenia is present, and regular rinsing with a solution of baking soda and water; baking soda, salt, and water; or hydrogen peroxide and water. If possible, and if the patient can afford it, dental caries and other oral problems should be treated before starting chemotherapy.
- If oral discomfort is present, suggest that the patient switch to a liquid diet, including such foods as milkshakes and ice cream. During periods of severe stomatitis, patients may stop eating; encourage a fluid intake of at least 2500 ml/day. Encourage intake of high-protein, high-calorie supplements, which can be purchased or made at home (see interventions for anorexia). Chilled food or fluids may decrease discomfort.
- Instruct patients to brush their teeth gently with a soft-bristle brush. If irritation is severe, instruct the patient to forego brushing, using swabs instead to clean the mouth until healing has begun. Avoid flossing when stomatitis is severe. Use water-spraying oral care devices on low setting only.

- Assess the mouth for oral fungal infections (thrush). To avoid fungal infections, instruct patients to rinse their mouths (or brush their teeth) each time they eat. Instruct patients to report to the physician the appearance of white patchy spots in the mouth.
- Caution patients to avoid spicy foods such as pizza or foods that may cause local irritation, such as hard bread crusts.
- Suggest that patients apply petrolatum jelly (Vaseline) or a lip balm as needed to the lips to decrease irritation.
- Instruct patients to wear dentures or bridgework only when eating and to remove them at other times to decrease oral irritation.
- Suggest that patients use a humidifier at the bedside to keep the air less dry, especially if the patient is mouth breathing during sleep.
- Suggest that patients use a local anesthetic gargle or mouthwash 10 minutes before eating to reduce oral irritation. Note that the use of an anesthetic agent may decrease the gag reflex and contribute to aspiration. In addition, too-frequent application of some anesthetic agents to denuded mucosa may contribute to greater systemic absorption and reaction to the drug. A physician's order may be needed for these preparations.
- Suggest that patients paint their oral cavities with substrate of milk of magnesia up to four times per day to prevent or treat stomatitis. Obtain the substrate by allowing the milk of magnesia to settle out of solution. Discard the liquid portion at the top of the dose or bottle, and paint the mouth with the white, pasty portion remaining.
- Encourage the use, if prescribed, of special mouthwashes for treatment of stomatitis. There are many "recipes" available; example ingredients include peroxide, nystatin, tetracycline or other antibiotics, flavoring, and sterile water. Consult the physician, hospital pharmacist, regional medical center, or the American Cancer Society for additional formulas. Use these preparations on a regular basis, not a "prn" or as needed basis, for best results. Avoid the use of lemon-glycerin preparations or mouthwashes containing alcohol, as they may be drying and irritating.
- Be alert to stomatitis in children, in whom it often appears earlier, 2 to 3 days after chemotherapy.
- For anal irritation, instruct the patient to avoid the use of rectal thermometers, suppositories, or enemas. Suggest that soaking in a tub of warm water several times daily may reduce irritation. Recommend that patients clean the anal area well after each bowel movement. Some patients may find the use of a commercially packaged towelette to clean the anal area after defecation to be helpful.
- For vaginal care, instruct female patients to wipe from front to back after voiding or bowel movement. The vaginal-anal area should be kept clean; remind patients to rinse soap off well and gently pat dry. Instruct patients to report to the physician the development of vaginal discharge or change in the color, consistency, odor, or amount of vaginal discharge. Instruct the patient to avoid douching or using tampons unless approved by the physician.
- To decrease irritation during intercourse, suggest that women use one of the commercially available lubricants designed for this purpose. Caution patients to avoid using hand lotion or other substances not designed for sensitive vaginal mucosa.
- If dry mouth or thick saliva is a problem, suggest that patients use a commercially available saliva substitute such as Xero-Lube.

**NAUSEA AND VOMITING:** This side effect of chemotherapy may occur within hours of receiving the dose or may be delayed for 5 to 10 days.
- Monitor carefully each patient's response to chemotherapy. Keep as part of the care plan actions that seem to contribute to or lessen the incidence of nausea and vomiting.
- Administer antiemetics, sedatives, and other drugs to decrease nausea on the schedule ordered.
- Consider the following interventions, which may help individual patients: reschedule chemotherapy time in relation to meal times, either closer to or further away from usual mealtimes. Limit oral intake to clear liquids on the day of or evening before chemotherapy. Keep the environment odor free. Have the patient avoid spicy, fatty, or greasy foods the day of or day before chemotherapy.

- Instruct patients and families in relaxation techniques, hypnotism guided imagery, or distraction techniques if the family is interested.
- Instruct patients to report severe or persistent nausea and vomiting that occur when the patient is home. Excessive vomiting may require intravenous fluid and electrolyte replacement.

**Metabolic** Rapid cancer cell destruction can release large quantities of purines, which are metabolized to uric acid. Accumulation of uric acid may lead to renal damage or gout.

- Instruct patients to force fluids to 3000 ml/day to ensure adequate urinary output.
- Antigout medications and/or drugs to alkalinize the urine may be prescribed; encourage patients to use them as ordered.
- Monitor serum uric acid and weight.
- Encourage patients to increase dietary intake of milk, vegetables, and fruits, except cranberries, prunes, and plums, to promote urinary alkalinzation.

**Reproductive** A wide range of effects on the reproductive system has been produced by cytotoxic drugs, including amenorrhea, ovarian failure, impaired spermatogenesis, azoospermia, and testicular atrophy (see individual drugs).

- Review side effects on the reproductive system with the patient, and provide support as needed.
- Instruct female patients to keep a record of menstrual periods. Advise patients to inform the physician immediately if pregnancy is suspected.
- Counsel male and female patients to use birth control measures during therapy with these drugs and for several months after therapy with cytotoxic agents ends.
- Discuss with male patients the possibility of storing sperm in a sperm bank before starting drug therapy for possible later use. Although this may be expensive, and not always effective, it is an option a male patient may wish to consider.

**Other** Cytotoxic agents may damage many types of normal cells and may be directly irritating to tissues.

**ALOPECIA:** Hair loss occurs when sensitive cells in the hair follicle are damaged by chemotherapy or radiation.

- Before starting chemotherapy, inform patients about the possibility of hair loss. Some patients may wish to invest in a wig resembling their own hair color and style before hair loss begins.
- Point out to patients that hair loss may involve eyebrows, eyelashes, nasal hair, and pubic hair.
- When appropriate, use a head tourniquet or ice cap to reduce alopecia. Both are used during the intravenous infusion of a drug and for 15 to 30 minutes after the infusion. The ice cap is applied 15 minutes before the infusion. These devices should be avoided in patients with leukemia or lymphoma or any cancer that may migrate to or be found in the scalp; check with the physician when in doubt. Inform patients that some hair loss will probably occur, even with the use of the ice cap or tourniquet. These devices are only effective with intravenous drugs.
- Reassure patients that in most cases hair will grow back after chemotherapy is finished, but patients on monthly or 6 week cycles of chemotherapy will often continue to have little hair until the entire course of chemotherapy is completed. For some patients, hair return may begin during chemotherapy. Reassure patients that the resumption of hair growth does not mean the chemotherapy is no longer effective.
- Reassure patients that new hair growth will usually be the same color and texture as hair that was lost. Note that some patients have hair of different color or texture when hair growth returns.
- During hair loss, instruct patients to wash hair as little as possible and to brush and comb it gently. If all hair is gone, suggest that the patient apply a thin layer of baby oil to prevent dryness.
- Instruct patients with hair loss to avoid direct exposure to the sun, either by wearing a hat or using a maximum-protection sunscreen when outside. During cold weather, instruct patients to wear a hat when outside.

**EXTRAVASATION:** Many cytotoxic agents are highly irritating to normal tissues. When these drugs are administered IV, great care must be taken to prevent them from escaping into tissues surrounding the injection site. Pain, tissue damage, and necrosis can result.

- Assess for signs of extravasation when administering intravenous chemotherapy: redness or swelling

at the insertion site, decreased infusion rate, inability to get a blood return, pain, or resistance during the injection of medication.
- Avoid extravasation of any intravenous medication, but be especially alert when the following drugs are administered because of tissue necrosis and sloughing that may occur: dactinomycin, mitomycin, carmustine, cisplatin, dacarbazine, daunorubicin, plicamycin, streptozocin, vincristine, and vinblastine.
- In the ideal situation, perform a fresh venipuncture for administering chemotherapy. In the absence of the ideal situation, ascertain that the infusion line to be used is patent prior to administering chemotherapy.
- Use a forearm infusion site rather than the dorsum of the hand for infusions of drugs that may cause necrosis and sloughing if extravasation occurs. Extravasation in the forearm may be less severe than extravasation in the area of the dorsum of the hand, where muscles and tendons for hand control may be affected. Remain with the patient during the infusion.
- If extravasation occurs, discontinue the infusion. Follow agency procedures for handling the extravasation. A typical procedure would be to administer a corticosteriod subcutaneously or intravenously, cover the area with a topical steroid, then cover with an occlusive dressing. Finally, apply ice compresses for 15 minutes four times a day, and keep the extremity elevated for 48 hours. Notify the physician. Use a fresh venipuncture site for infusion of any remaining chemotherapy drug.
- Medical orders for treatment of extravasation should be written at the time the chemotherapy drugs are ordered. Standing orders should be readily available to all persons who administer chemotherapy. Keep drugs ordered for extravasation readily available.

### Nursing interventions related to drug administration
- Because of the mutagenic and carcinogenic potential of many of the cytotoxic drugs, take special care during the handling and preparation of these drugs. In many agencies, the administration of intravenous cytotoxic drugs is restricted to a few specially trained personnel.
- Prepare intravenous medications using a laminar airflow hood. Wash hands before and after handling the medications.
- Wear disposable gloves and a long-sleeved gown during drug preparation. Wear gloves during drug administration.
- Use good technique to avoid skin contact with prepared dosages. Use Luer-lock fittings whenever possible to avoid inadvertent separation of syringe and needle. Establish and abide by procedures for disposal of drug containers, as well as contaminated gloves, syringes, and tubing.
- After drawing up dosages into the syringe, discard the needle and attach a new sterile needle to avoid skin contact with any traces of medication that might be on the outside of the first needle.

### Patient and family education
- Review with patients and families the anticipated benefits and possible side effects of drug therapy. Provide support to these patients, who may be facing a difficult diagnosis, as well as anticipating alopecia, nausea, stomatitis, or other side effects.
- Encourage patients to return for follow-up visits as directed and to consult the nurse or physician about any unusual sign, symptom, or concern. Point out to patients that many side effects may not become evident for 2 to 3 weeks following the last dose of therapy.
- Remind patients to keep all health care providers informed of all medications being taken. This is especially important because bone marrow suppression, stomatitis, and other side effects may not even appear until days to weeks after the drug has been administered.
- Review with patients appropriate actions for missed doses (consult with the physician). Typical instructions: A missed dose remembered within a few hours of the ordered dose time may be taken; missed doses remembered within 12 hours of the next scheduled dose should be omitted; patients should never double up with cytotoxic drug dosages.
- Review with patients actions to be taken if the patient vomits shortly after taking a dose of medication (consult with the physician). Typical instructions: if particles of the dose are clearly visible in the emesis, the dose may be repeated. If the particles of the dose are not discernible, or an hour or more has passed since the dose was swallowed, no more drug should be taken until the next scheduled dose. When in doubt, the patient should feel free to call the physician for clarification.

**Table 27-3.**

## Summary of side effects of antineoplastic drugs

| Side effect | Drugs most likely to cause side effect |
|---|---|
| Alopecia | Dactinomycin, daunorubicin |
| Cardiotoxicity | Daunorubicin, doxorubicin |
| Nervous system toxicity | Asparaginase, fluorouracil, methotrexate (intrathecal), mitotane, plicamycin, procarbazine, vincristine |
| Emesis | Cisplatin, carmustine, dacarbazine, mechlorethamine, procarbazine, streptozocin |
| Hematologic | Busulfan, carmustine, cisplatin, cyclophosphamide, cytarabine, dacarbazine, dactinomycin, daunorubicin, doxorubicin, etoposide, fluorouracil, hydroxy-urea, mercaptopurine, methotrexate, mitomycin, plicamycin, procarbazine, thioguanine, thiotepa, vinblastine |
| Hepatic | Carmustine, cytarabine, floxuridine, mercaptopurine, methotrexate, plicamycin, thioguanine |
| Immunosuppression | Chlorambucil, cisplatin, cyclophosphamide, cytarabine, dactinomycin, dauno-mycin, doxorubicin, mercaptopurine, methotrexate |
| Mucocutaneous toxicity | Bleomycin, cytarabine, dactinomycin, daunorubicin, doxorubicin, fluorouracil, procarbazine, methotrexate, mitomycin |
| Renal | Carmustine, cisplatin, cyclophosphamide, methotrexate, mitomycin, plicamycin, streptozocin |
| Local tissue necrosis | Dacarbazine, dactinomycin, daunorubicin, doxorubicin, vinblastine |
| Pulmonary toxicity | Bleomycin, carmustine, methotrexate, mitomycin |

Caution patients to avoid the use of over-the-counter preparations without prior clearance of the physician.

- Emphasize to patients the importance of keeping these and all medications out of the reach of children.
- Caution patients to avoid receiving any immunizations while taking cytotoxic drugs, without first consulting the physician. Before starting chemotherapy, some physicians recommend that patients receive flu shots and/or update immunizations; consult the physician.
- Inform patients that ridges in the fingernails may occur during chemotherapy; these reflect the effect of the drugs on the dividing cells of the nails.
- For information about the drugs, drug protocols, protocols to treat extravasation, oral gargles, mouthwashes, dietary supplements, snack recipes, patient teaching aids, and other information for patients, families, and health care providers, contact the chemotherapy department of local medical centers, the American Cancer Society, the Office of Cancer Communications at the National Cancer Institute, Bethesda, MD 20892, the Department of Health and Human Services, or local oncologists' offices. Refer patients as appropriate to the local visiting nurse agencies or hospice.

## asparaginase (uh-SPARE-uh-jin-ase)    antineoplastic*

- asparaginase: Elspar, ♣Kidrolase

**MECHANISM OF ACTION**    Asparaginase is an enzyme that destroys the amino acid asparagine. Whereas normal cells synthesize sufficient asparagine, leukemic cells may require externally supplied asparagine. When asparaginase is present, the external supply of asparagine is destroyed, resulting in starvation of the leukemic cells.

**INDICATIONS**    **Acute lymphocytic leukemia** Asparaginase is used to induce remissions. • The drug should not be used alone and is usually combined with prednisone or with prednisone and vincristine.

Protein synthesis inhibitor.

**CONTRAINDICATIONS** **Previous anaphylatic reaction to asparaginase** The drug should not be used when previous exposure caused severe reactions. **Pancreatitis** Asparaginase impairs pancreatic function, which may be dangerous in patients with pre-existing impairment. **Herpes zoster (chickenpox, shingles) infection or exposure** The risk of severe generalized disease is increased by the immunosuppressive action of asparaginase.

**DOSAGE** **IV:** **CHILDREN:** Asparaginase usually follows prednisone and vincristine, beginning on day 22 of the treatment schedule, 1000 IU/kg daily for 10 successive days. **IM:** **ADULTS OR CHILDREN:** In combination with vincristine and prednisone, 6000 IU/$M^2$ on days 4, 7, 10, 13, 16, 19, 22, 25, and 28. *Special patient populations:* **PREGNANCY:** FDA pregnancy category C. **DIABETES MELLITUS:** Blood glucose concentrations may be increased by asparaginase, requiring adjustment of insulin or oral hypoglycemic dosage. **HEPATIC DYSFUNCTION:** Risk of hepatotoxicity may be increased.

**PREPARATIONS** *Powder for reconstitution:* 10,000 IU with 80 mg mannitol. The powder is reconstituted by adding 5 ml of sterile water or 0.9% sodium chloride injection to the vial containing 10,000 IU. For IV infusion the drug may be further diluted in 0.9% sodium chloride or 5% dextrose.

**DRUG INTERACTIONS** **Methotrexate** anticancer activity may be diminished by concomitant administration of asparaginase. **Vincristine** neuropathy and blood toxicity may be increased when asparaginase is given before or with vincristine. **Vaccines containing live virus** should be avoided because the risk of severe generalized disease is increased.

**DIAGNOSTIC TEST INTERFERENCE** **Total serum thyroxine** concentrations may be decreased because asparaginase inhibits hepatic synthesis of thyroxine-binding globulin. **Uric acid** in blood and urine may increase.

**FATE** Because asparaginase is a protein, it is not adequately absorbed from the GI tract. The large molecular weight of the protein prevents it from diffusing freely from the vascular system. Little drug appears outside blood vessels. The drug is probably destroyed by proteases in the blood. Little active drug appears in urine.

## ☙ NURSING CONSIDERATIONS

### Side effects, toxicities, and associated nursing actions

**CNS** Neurotoxicity is especially prevalent in adults, where 25% may exhibit decreased consciousness. CNS signs may include agitation, coma, confusion, convulsions, depression, dizziness, EEG changes, fatigue, hallucinations, headache, lethargy, and somnolence. Syndromes similar to parkinsonism and delirium tremens have also been reported.

- Review these signs and symptoms with patients and families. Instruct families to notify the physician if CNS side effects appear.
- Caution patients to avoid driving or operating hazardous equipment if fatigue, lethargy, somnolence, or other CNS effects occur.

**Blood** Lowered fibrinogen concentrations commonly prolong thrombin, prothrombin, and partial prothrombin times. Leukopenia may occur early in therapy.

- Monitor prothrombin time and partial prothrombin time and white blood cell count and differential.
- Instruct patients to report the development of signs or symptoms that may signal bleeding: bleeding gums, nosebleeds, change in the color of urine that might indicate kidney or bladder bleeding, rectal bleeding, change of color of stools, excessive bruising, or the development of petechiae.
- Monitor stools for occult blood.
- For nursing interventions related to a low white blood cell count, see entry for drug class (p. 480).

**GI** Abdominal cramps, anorexia, and weight loss may occur, but almost all patients experience nausea and vomiting. Antiemetics may be helpful.

- Monitor the patient's weight.
- Include the patient in the ongoing development of the care plan to treat nausea; the patient may be able to suggest ways to lessen the nausea and vomiting.
- For other nursing interventions related to anorexia, nausea, and vomiting, see entry for drug class (p. 481).

**Renal** Azotemia is common. Acute renal failure can occur.

- Monitor the patient's weight and BUN. If renal involvement is suspected, monitor intake and output.

**Metabolic** Hyperglycemia may signal pancreatic damage. Damage may be mild or severe and has occasionally resulted in death by acute hemorrhagic pancreatitis.

• Monitor blood glucose levels and serum amylase.

• Assess the patient for epigastric or left upper quadrant abdominal pain, fever, nausea and vomiting, tachycardia, and hypotension.

**Allergic** Allergic reactions are common and include anaphylaxis, arthralgia, edema, hypotension, rashes, respiratory distress, and urticaria. Skin tests are not reliable indicators of allergy.

• Be alert to allergic reactions with each course of therapy. Consult the manufacturer's directions for preparing skin test and desensitization injections. A skin test is required before the first dose. Allergic reactions are more common when the interval between doses is longer than 7 days. Previous desensitization does not rule out later allergic reactions.

• Have drugs (epinephrine, steroids), equipment, and personnel readily available to treat acute allergic reactions in settings where asparaginase is administered.

• Monitor blood pressure and pulse. Assess for difficulty breathing, cyanosis, and complaints of tightness in throat or chest. Do not leave the patient unattended during drug administration or for up to 1 hour afterward.

**Liver** Fatty liver changes have occurred. Ammonia, AST, ALT, and bilirubin may increase, whereas cholesterol, albumin, fibrinogen, albumin, and calcium may decrease.

• Assess the patient for signs of liver involvement: right upper quadrant abdominal pain, jaundice, or change in the color or consistency of stools.

• Monitor serum ammonia, AST, ALT, and bilirubin.

### Nursing interventions related to drug administration

• Prepare as directed in the manufacturer's literature or in Preparations. Refrigerate before and after dilution. Use within 8 hours. Do not use cloudy solutions. Do not use a filter smaller than 5.0 μm.

• Administer direct IV over at least 30 minutes.

• For other nursing interventions, see entry for drug class (p. 485).

### Patient and family education

• Review with patients the anticipated benefits and possible side effects of drug therapy.

• See entry for drug class (p. 485).

---

## bleomycin sulfate    (blee-oh-MY-sin)                                antineoplastic*

• bleomycin sulfate: Blenoxane

**MECHANISM OF ACTION**    Bleomycin may interfere with DNA synthesis as well as cause breaks in the strands of DNA. Damaged DNA is unable to serve as a template for RNA synthesis, which leads to death of the cell.

**INDICATIONS**    **Lymphomas** Hodgkin's disease, reticulum cell sarcoma, lymphosarcoma, and other lymphomas may respond to bleomycin. About one fourth of patients with Hodgkin's disease experience more than a 50% reduction in tumor mass; improvements may persist up to 2 years. Better control of Hodgkin's disease is achieved with combination chemotherapy, including doxorubicin, dacarbazine, vinblastine, and bleomycin (Table 27-1).    **Squamous cell carcinomas** Some reduction of tumor mass can be achieved with certain carcinomas, but individual types of carcinomas differ widely in response rates.    **Sarcomas** Responses to bleomycin are generally small and of short duration.    **Choriocarcinoma** This postgestational tumor responds well to chemotherapy and cures are commonly achieved using combinations of drugs, including bleomycin.

**CONTRAINDICATIONS**    **Allergic reactions to bleomycin** Patients with documented prior reactions to bleomycin may not be able to tolerate retreatment with the drug.

**DOSAGE**    **IV, IM, SC** 0.25 to 0.5 units/kg (10 to 20 units/$M^2$) once or twice weekly. Doses may be reduced to 1 unit daily or 5 units once weekly after improvement is noted. A cumulative dose of 400 units of bleomycin is the maximum. High cumulative doses result in excessive toxicity. *Special patient populations:*    **ELDERLY:** Special geriatric doses have not been established, but elderly patients are

---

*Breaks DNA strands.

more susceptible to the pulmonary toxicity associated with bleomycin.  **CHILDREN:** This drug should be avoided if other drugs may be substituted.  **PREGNANCY:** Use of this drug in pregnancy carries substantial risk to the fetus.  **RENAL DISEASE:** Risk of toxicity is increased when renal function is severely compromised.  **SMOKERS OR PATIENTS WITH PULMONARY DISEASE:** Risk of pulmonary toxicity is greatly increased in these patients.

**PREPARATIONS**  *Powder for reconstitution:* 15 units of bleomycin. For reconstitution, use 1 to 5 ml sterile water, 0.9% sodium chloride injection, 5% dextrose injection or bacteriostatic water.

**DRUG INTERACTIONS**  **General anesthetics** may cause rapid pulmonary deterioration in patients who received bleomycin.

**FATE**  Bleomycin is not absorbed from the GI tract and must be given parenterally. Distribution is mainly to skin, lungs, kidneys, peritoneum, and lymphatics. Up to 70% of a dose of bleomycin is excreted in urine; the plasma *half-life* is about 2 hours.

## ☙ NURSING CONSIDERATIONS

### Side effects, toxicities, and associated nursing actions

**CNS** Aggressive behavior and disorientation are rare side effects.
- Review these side effects with the patient and family. Instruct the family to notify the physician if changes in behavior occur.

**CV** Hypotension may occur.
- Monitor blood pressure and pulse. Caution patients to move slowly from sitting to standing positions.

**Blood** Bleomycin is not considered toxic to bone marrow, but occasionally mild thrombocytopenia, leukopenia, and depression of hemoglobin levels occurs. Phlebitis may occur.
- Review nursing interventions for granulocytopenia and thrombocytopenia in entry for drug class (p. 480).
- Monitor hematocrit, hemoglobin, white blood cell count and differential, and platelet count.
- Inspect the infusion site frequently during IV drug administration. If the patient complains of burning, slow the infusion rate. Assess for redness, swelling, and complaints of pain or discomfort.

**GI** Nausea and vomiting may occur. Anorexia and weight loss are common but may be at least partly related to the disease itself.
- See entry for drug class (p. 481).

**Lung** Interstitial pneumonitis, which occurs in 10% of patients, is the most serious reaction to bleomycin. About 1% of patients treated with bleomycin die of this reaction. Patients older than 70 years and those receiving total doses of over 400 units are most at risk.
- Monitor patients for this side effect. Auscultate lung sounds for rales, rhonchi, or pleural friction rubs. Assess the patient for dyspnea or cough. Monitor serial chest x-rays. Monitor serial pulmonary function studies, although these may not be predictive of pneumonitis.

**Renal** Hematuria and cystitis may rarely occur.
- Monitor urinalysis. Instruct the patient to report any change in color of urine.
- Assess the patient for symptoms of cystitis: urinary frequency, burning, or urgency.

**Allergic** Fever and chills may persist 4 to 12 hours. Anaphylactic reactions have occurred, most commonly after the first or second dose. Death is possible.
- Instruct the patient to monitor temperature every 4 hours if fever develops, to maintain adequate fluid intake (2500 ml/day), and to take antipyretics as ordered. Instruct the patient to notify the physician if fever persists longer than 48 hours.
- Have drugs, equipment, and personnel available to treat acute allergic reactions in settings where bleomycin is administered. Assess patient for difficulty breathing and tightness in throat or chest. Monitor blood pressure.
- Premedicate patients with aspirin and diphenhydramine if ordered.
- Anaphylactic reactions are more common in patients with lymphoma; a test dose of drug may be administered 24 hours prior to the therapeutic dose, and the patient's response should be monitored. Consult with the physician, and consult the manufacturer's literature.

**Skin** Alopecia, bleeding, hypoesthesia, hyperesthesia, hyperpigmentation, hyperkeratosis, icthyosis, peeling, rash, stomatitis, striae, swelling, ulcerations of tongue and lips, urticaria, and vesiculation may occur.

**Other** Mucocutaneous toxicity occurs in at least 50% of patients. The effects are usually delayed, appearing 1 to 3 weeks after start of therapy or after a total of 150 to 200 units of drug have been administered.

- Caution the patient about these side effects. See entry for drug class (p. 484) for additional interventions for alopecia and stomatitis.
- Visually inspect the patient before therapy and at regular intervals for skin changes. If skin changes are severe or persistent, a change in drug or dosage may be necessary; consult the physician.

### Nursing interventions related to drug administration

- For IV administration, after initial reconstitution (see Preparations), further dilute with 50 to 100 ml of the same diluent. Administer at a rate of 15 units or less over 10 minutes.
- See entry for drug class (p. 485).

### Patient and family education

- See entry for drug class (p. 485).

---

## busulfan   (byoo-SUL-fan)                                    antineoplastic*

- busulfan: Myleran

**MECHANISM OF ACTION**   Busulfan alters the properties of DNA by chemically changing (alkylating) its structure. Without fully functional DNA, cells eventually die. Rapidly growing cells are most susceptible.

**INDICATIONS**   **Chronic myelogenous leukemia** Remissions are produced in 80% to 90% of treated patients, but cures should not be expected. • Remissions take about 2 months to induce and generally last 9 to 12 months.

**CONTRAINDICATIONS**   **Prior unsuccessful therapy with busulfan** If chronic myelogenous leukemia has failed to respond to prior therapy with busulfan, other drugs should be substituted.   **Herpes zoster (chickenpox, shingles) infection or exposure** The risk of severe generalized disease is increased by the immunosuppressive action of busulfan.

**DOSAGE**   **PO:**   **ADULTS:** Daily doses of 0.065 to 0.1 mg/kg (usual doses 4 to 8 mg) are administered until the leukocyte count falls below a predetermined value (10,000 to 25,000/mm$^3$). Intermittent therapy may be necessary to maintain remissions in some patients.   **CHILDREN:** Daily doses of 0.06 to 0.12 mg/kg (1.8 to 4.6 mg/M$^2$) are selected to maintain a leukocyte count of about 20,000/mm$^3$.   *Special patient populations:*   **CHILDREN:** This carcinogenic drug should be avoided if other drugs may be substituted.   **PREGNANCY:** FDA pregnancy category D.

**PREPARATIONS**   *Tablets:* 2 mg.

**DRUG INTERACTIONS**   **Myelosuppressive drugs or radiation** may not be tolerated because of the potent myelosuppressive action of busulfan.   **Vaccines containing live virus** should be avoided because the risk of severe generalized disease is increased.

**FATE**   Busulfan is rapidly absorbed following oral administration, producing *peak* concentrations in blood within 0.5 to 2 hours. The drug is extensively metabolized.

### ❦ NURSING CONSIDERATIONS

#### Side effects, toxicities, and associated nursing actions

**Blood** Anemia, leukopenia, and thrombocytopenia may be severe. These common reactions are related to dose of the drug and are usually but not always reversible. Agranulocytosis is rare and may progress to fatal pancytopenia.
- See entry for drug class (p. 479) for a discussion of anemia, leukopenia, and thrombocytopenia.

**GI** Anorexia, diarrhea, glossitis, nausea, vomiting, and weight loss are uncommon.
- See entry for drug class (p. 481).

**Renal** Destruction of cancer cells by busulfan increases purine catabolism, releasing large amounts of uric acid. Acute renal failure, renal stones, and uric acid nephropathy may occur.
- See entry for drug class (p. 487).

**Liver** Hepatic dysfunction and jaundice may occur.
- Assess the patient for right upper quadrant abdominal pain, malaise, change in the color or consistency of stools, and jaundice.
- Monitor liver function tests.

*DNA alkylator.

**Lung** Diffuse interstitial pulmonary fibrosis is a rare side effect arising after prolonged therapy with busulfan.
- Monitor patients for this side effect. Auscultate lung sounds for rales, rhonchi, or pleural friction rubs. Assess the patient for dyspnea or cough. Monitor serial chest x-rays. Monitor serial pulmonary function studies, although these may not be predictive.

**Metabolic** A wasting syndrome resembling Addison's disease may occur after prolonged therapy.
- Monitor weight, blood pressure, and mood. Assess the patient for fatigue, anorexia, apathy, and confusion.

**Skin** Alopecia, cheilosis, dry skin, melanoderma, rashes, and urticaria may occur.
- Visually inspect the patient before starting therapy and at regular intervals for skin changes. If changes are severe, it may be necessary to adjust dosage; notify the physician.
- See entry for drug class (p. 484) for a discussion of alopecia.

**Reproductive** Amenorrhea, ovarian suppression, menopausal symptoms, ovarian fibrosis, and atrophy may occur in females; males may suffer azoospermia, impotence, sterility, and testicular atrophy.
- See entry for drug class (p. 484).

**Other** Anhidrosis and gynecomastia may occur.
- Inspect the patient regularly for development of gynecomastia.
- Caution patients to avoid activities in which they would become overheated and to allow for frequent periods of cooling off when engaging in activities that would normally cause them to perspire.

### Nursing interventions related to drug administration
- See entry for drug class (p. 485).

### Patient and family education
- See entry for drug class (p. 485).

---

## carmustine   (kar-MUS-teen)                                          antineoplastic*

- carmustine: BiCNU

**MECHANISM OF ACTION**   Carmustine causes chemical changes in nucleic acids that may lead to inhibition of DNA and RNA synthesis. In addition the drug may alter cellular proteins. The mechanism is the same as the related drug lomustine (p. 512) and cross-resistance occurs.

**INDICATIONS**   **Brain tumors** Carmustine crosses the blood-brain barrier and may therefore be effective in controlling brain tumors. • About 50% of treated patients respond when carmustine is used alone; cures should not be expected. • Carmustine combined with radiation therapy prolongs life in patients with malignant gliomas.   **Multiple myeloma** Carmustine is an alternate to melphalan. • When combined with prednisone (p. 547, 623), carmustine produces objective responses in 39% of patients. **Hodgkin's disease and malignant lymphomas** Carmustine causes objective responses in about 50% of patients with advanced Hodgkin's disease who have failed standard therapy. • Carmustine may also be substituted for mechlorethamine in the MOPP regimen (p. 479). • Response rates are lower for non-Hodgkin's lymphomas.

**CONTRAINDICATIONS**   **Myelosuppression** Patients with low platelet, leukocyte, or erythrocyte counts may be unable to tolerate the additional depression caused by carmustine.   **Herpes zoster (chickenpox, shingles) infection or exposure** The risk of severe generalized disease is increased by the immunosuppressive action of carmustine.

**DOSAGE**   **IV:**   **ADULTS:** Initial therapy, 200 mg/M$^2$ as a single dose or divided into two doses given on successive days. Retreatment must be delayed at least 6 weeks or longer to allow production of leukocytes and platelets to recover. *Special patient populations:*   **CHILDREN:** This drug is carcinogenic and should be avoided if other drugs may be substituted.   **PREGNANCY:** Use of this drug in pregnancy carries substantial risk to the fetus.   **SMOKERS OR PATIENTS WITH PULMONARY DISEASE:** Risk of pulmonary toxicity is greatly increased.   **RENAL OR HEPATIC IMPAIRMENT:** Risk of organ damage may be increased.

*DNA alkylator.

**PREPARATIONS**    *Powder for reconstitution:* 100 mg. Each vial of drug is accompanied by a vial containing 3 ml of sterile absolute alcohol, which is to be added to the powder for reconstitution. An additional 27 ml of sterile water for injection must be added. The final solution is 3.3 mg/ml carmustine and 10% alcohol. Additional dilution may be in 0.9% sodium chloride or 5% dextrose.

**DRUG INTERACTIONS**    **Cimetidine** may cause additive bone marrow suppression when given with carmustine. The combination should be avoided if possible.

**FATE**    Carmustine must be administered parenterally. The drug rapidly crosses the blood-brain barrier, achieving substantial levels in the CNS and other tissues or fluids, including milk. Carmustine is metabolized and eliminated by renal and other routes.

## ❦ NURSING CONSIDERATIONS

### Side effects, toxicities, and associated nursing actions

**CNS** Ataxia, dizziness, and loss of equilibrium are rare.

* Caution the patient to avoid driving or operating hazardous equipment if CNS effects occur.

**Blood** Hematologic toxicity is the dose-limiting side effect of carmustine. Effectively treated patients should be expected to show changes in blood composition. Thrombocytopenia is the most severe change, with lowest platelet counts appearing 4 to 5 weeks after therapy. Leukocyte counts are lowest 5 to 6 weeks after therapy. Anemia may also occur.

* See entry for drug class (p. 480) for a discussion of granulocytopenia, thrombocytopenia, and anemia.

**GI** Nausea and vomiting should be expected with IV carmustine, sometimes occurring during the infusion and persisting for up to 6 hours. Anorexia, diarrhea, dysphagia, and esophagitis are less common.

* See entry for drug class (p. 481) for a discussion of nausea and vomiting, anorexia, diarrhea, and stomatitis.

**Hepatic** High doses of carmustine cause reversible hepatotoxicity in up to 26% of patients. Serum transaminase, alkaline phosphatase, and bilirubin concentrations may be increased; jaundice is less common.

* Assess the patient for right upper quadrant abdominal pain, malaise, fever, change in the color or consistency of stools, and jaundice.
* Monitor liver function tests and serum bilirubin.

**Renal** Large cumulative doses may cause progressive azotemia, decreased kidney size, and even renal failure.

* Monitor weight. Monitor serum BUN and creatinine. If renal involvement is suspected, monitor intake and output. Visually inspect the patient for evidence of edema.

**Lung** Prolonged therapy may cause pulmonary infiltrates and fibrosis.

* Monitor patients for this side effect. Auscultate lung sounds for rales, rhonchi, and pleural friction rubs. Assess the patient for dyspnea and cough. Monitor serial chest x-rays. Monitor serial pulmonary function studies, although these may not be predictive.

**Allergic** Flushing of the skin and suffusion of the conjunctiva may occur with rapid IV administration of carmustine.

* Reduce the rate of infusion if these side effects occur; see Nursing interventions, below.

**Skin** Hyperpigmentation may occur when the drug accidentally contacts skin.

* Wear gloves when preparing or administering carmustine. If contact with the skin occurs, rinse the skin surface immediately with copious amounts of water.

### Nursing interventions related to drug administration

* Burning pain and venospasm at the site of IV administration are common; thrombosis and thrombophlebitis are rare. See Preparations for information about reconstitution. After reconstitution, further dilute in 100 to 500 ml of diluent and administer as an infusion. Administer the ordered dose over at least 1 hour. Slow the rate of infusion for pain, vasospasm, flushing of the skin, or suffusion of the conjunctiva.
* See entry for drug class (p. 485).

### Patient and family education

* See entry for drug class (p. 485).

## chlorambucil   (klor-AM-byoo-sil)                antineoplastic*

- chlorambucil: Leukeran

**MECHANISM OF ACTION**   Chlorambucil changes the properties of DNA by chemically changing (alkylating) its structure. Without fully functional DNA, cells eventually die. Rapidly growing cells are most susceptible. Chlorambucil is also an immunosuppressant, most effective against lymphocytes.

**INDICATIONS**   **Chronic lymphocytic leukemia** Remissions occur in 10% of patients receiving chlorambucil alone; 60% to 70% show objective improvement. • Combining prednisone with chlorambucil leads to a higher percentage of remissions and responses.   **Hodgkin's disease and malignant lymphomas** Chlorambucil alone may produce remissions in 10% to 15% of patients with non-Hodgkin's lymphomas; 40% to 70% may show objective improvement. • A higher percentage of remissions and responses occurs when chlorambucil is combined with other drugs. • Hodgkin's disease is usually treated with the MOPP regimen (p. 479), but chlorambucil is occasionally used in patients intolerant of established therapy.   **Trophoblastic neoplasms** Choriocarcinoma and related conditions may respond well to chemotherapy. • Advanced cases may be treated with chlorambucil, dactinomycin (p. 502), and methotrexate (p. 517); up to 80% will be cured.   **Macroglobulinemia** Chlorambucil with prednisone improves the condition of about 75% of treated patients.

**CONTRAINDICATIONS**   **Non-life-threatening conditions** Chlorambucil can induce acute leukemias. • The drug should be avoided whenever possible in younger patients and in any condition that is not itself life-threatening.   **Myelosuppression** Patients with leukopenia or thrombocytopenia may be unable to tolerate the myelosuppressive action of chlorambucil.   **Herpes zoster (chickenpox, shingles) infection or exposure** The risk of severe generalized disease is increased by the immunosuppressive action of chlorambucil.

**DOSAGE**   **PO:**   **ADULTS:** Usual doses are 0.1 to 0.2 mg/kg (3 to 6 mg/M$^2$) daily as a single dose for 3 to 6 weeks. Daily doses are usually 4 to 10 mg. Doses may be varied for maintenance therapy and reduced when other drugs are also used.   **CHILDREN:** Usual doses are 0.1 to 0.2 mg/kg or 4.5 mg/M$^2$ as a single daily dose for 3 to 6 weeks. Doses may be varied for maintenance therapy and reduced when other drugs are also used.   *Special patient populations:*   **CHILDREN:** This drug is carcinogenic and should be avoided if other drugs may be substituted.   **PREGNANCY:** FDA pregnancy category D.

**PREPARATIONS**   *Tablets:* 2 mg.

**DRUG INTERACTIONS**   **Immunosuppressants** such as azathioprine, corticotropin, cyclophosphamide, cyclosporine, glucocorticoids, mercaptopurine, or muromonab-CD3 may increase the risk of severe infection or later risk of development of cancer.   **Vaccines containing live virus** should be avoided because the risk of severe generalized disease is increased.

**FATE**   Chlorambucil is rapidly absorbed; oral doses produce *peak* plasma concentrations within 1 hour. Active metabolites are formed rapidly and persist longer than chlorambucil; both are excreted primarily by the kidneys with elimination *half-lives* of 1.5 to 2.5 hours. Chlorambucil crosses the placenta.

### ❧ NURSING CONSIDERATIONS

#### Side effects, toxicities, and associated nursing actions

**CNS** Overdosage may produce seizures that usually resolve spontaneously without sequelae.
- Calculate the dosage carefully. Reinforce to patients the importance of taking the drug only in the dose ordered.
- Remind patients to keep all drugs out of the reach of children.
- Caution the family to notify the physician immediately of any seizurelike behavior.

**Blood** Myelosuppression is the most common, dose-limiting side effect of chlorambucil. Leukopenia and thrombocytopenia occur but are usually slowly reversible after therapy ends.
- See entry for drug class (p. 480).

**GI** High doses (more than 20 mg) may cause abdominal pain, anorexia, diarrhea, gastric discomfort, nausea, and vomiting. Ordinary doses are usually well tolerated.
- See entry for drug class (p. 481).

*DNA alkylator.

- Encourage patients to notify the health care provider if side effects occur. Because treatment continues for 3 to 6 weeks, problems that did not occur initially may eventually develop.
- If GI symptoms develop, discuss with the patient and physician the possibility of taking the dose once a day, taking the dose on an empty stomach, and/or taking the dose at bedtime, all of which may lessen GI side effects.

**Liver** Elevated serum alkaline phosphatase and AST may occur; jaundice is rare.

- Assess the patient for development of fever, malaise, right upper quadrant abdominal pain, change in color or consistency of stools, and jaundice.
- Monitor liver function tests.

**Metabolic** Hyperuricemia may occur when large numbers of destroyed cancer cells release purines for catabolism.

- See entry for drug class (p. 484).

**Lung** Bronchopulmonary dysplasia and interstitial pneumonitis or pulmonary fibrosis may occur in rare patients.

- Monitor pulmonary function: auscultate lung sounds for rales, rhonchi, and pleural friction rubs. Assess the patient for dyspnea and cough. Monitor serial chest x-rays, if available. Monitor serial pulmonary function studies, although these may not be predictive.

**Skin** Rashes, pruritis, urticaria, or erythema may occur. Alopecia is rare.

- Visually inspect the patient's skin before starting therapy and at regular intervals.
- Instruct patients to notify the physician about concerns related to skin changes or rashes.
- See entry for drug class (p. 484) for a discussion of alopecia.

**Allergic** Drug fever is rare.

- If fever persists longer than 24 hours or is unresponsive to antipyretics, notify the physician, as it will be necessary to determine the cause of fever.

**Reproductive** Chlorambucil causes infertility in a high percentage of prepubertal or pubertal males receiving the drug. Adult males may also suffer azoospermia, but function occasionally returns. Amenorrhea has occurred in pubertal and adult females.

- See entry for drug class (p. 484).

### Nursing interventions related to drug administration

- See entry for drug class (p. 485).

### Patient and family education

- See entry for drug class (p. 485).

---

## cisplatin (sis-PLA-tin) antineoplastic*

- cisplatin: Platinol

**MECHANISM OF ACTION** Cisplatin changes the properties of DNA by chemically changing (cross-linking) its structure. Without fully functional DNA, cells eventually die. Rapidly growing cells are most susceptible. Cisplatin is also an immunosuppressant.

**INDICATIONS** **Testicular cancers** Testicular carcinomas and related cancers respond well to cisplatin, either alone or in combinations. • Cisplatin with bleomycin (p. 488) and vinblastine sulfate (p. 529) produces complete remissions in 60% to 70% of patients with disseminated nonseminomatous carcinoma or extragonadal germ cell tumors. • Many of these patients are cured. **Ovarian tumors** Cisplatin is combined with other drugs to treat metastatic ovarian tumors that have already been treated by surgery and/or radiation. • Combinations with doxorubicin and cyclophosphamide are effective for palliation, but cures are not ordinarily produced. **Bladder cancer** Cisplatin may arrest the disease or improve the patient's condition in about 67% of the cases; cures should not be expected. **Cervical carcinoma** Cisplatin alone provides objective improvement for about 50% of patients with recurrent or advanced squamous cell carcinoma. **Head and neck cancer** Cisplatin alone may provide palliation of recurrent or metastatic squamous cell carcinomas of the head and neck; objective improvement occurs

*DNA cross-linker.

in about 30% of patients.    **Lung cancer** Non-small cell carcinoma may respond to cisplatin. • Objective improvement is seen in about half the patients receiving combinations of cisplatin with doxorubicin and cyclophosphamide or with cisplatin, etoposide, and vindesine or vinblastine.

**CONTRAINDICATIONS**    **Myelosuppression** Patients with leukopenia or thrombocytopenia may be unable to tolerate the myelosuppressive action of cisplatin.    **Hearing impairment** Patients with pre-existing hearing impairment may suffer hearing loss with cisplatin. • If possible, other agents may be selected. **Herpes zoster (chickenpox, shingles) infection or exposure** The risk of severe generalized disease is increased by the immunosuppressive action of cisplatin.

**DOSAGE**    IV:    **ADULTS:** For testicular cancers, 20 mg/M$^2$ daily for 5 consecutive days every 3 weeks for three or four courses of therapy in combination with other agents; or 120 mg/M$^2$ once every 3 or 4 weeks for three courses of therapy in combination with other agents. For other conditions, doses of 30 to 120 mg/M$^2$ may be used in various combinations. Doses are individualized based on the type and severity of disease and the condition of the patient.    *Special patient populations:*    **ELDERLY:** Special geriatric doses have not been established. The elderly may be more susceptible than younger adults to ototoxicity with cisplatin.    **CHILDREN:** This drug is carcinogenic and should be avoided if other drugs may be substituted. Pediatric doses are not established.    **PREGNANCY:** Use of this drug carries substantial risk to the fetus.    **RENAL IMPAIRMENT:** Doses may need to be reduced. Toxicity and accumulation are possible.

**PREPARATIONS**    *Powder for reconstitution:* 10 mg or 50 mg. For reconstitution, add 10 ml of sterile water to the 10 mg vial or 50 ml of sterile water to the 50 mg vial. The result is a 1 mg/ml solution. Do not refrigerate; the drug precipitates in the cold. Avoid use of aluminum-containing materials such as syringes or needles. Prevent the drug from contacting the skin.

**DRUG INTERACTIONS**    **Aminoglycoside antibiotics** may cause additive renal toxicity and ototoxicity with cisplatin.    **Etoposide** activity against cancers may be potentiated by cisplatin.

**FATE**    Cisplatin is administered parenterally and rapidly distributes to tissues. Highest concentrations are in liver, kidneys, and prostate. The plasma elimination *half-life* of cisplatin is 20 to 30 minutes. Excretion is by the kidneys.

## ✾ NURSING CONSIDERATIONS

### Side effects, toxicities, and associated nursing actions

**CNS** Loss of taste, memory loss, intention tremor, slurred speech, and seizures (focal and grand mal) have been reported.
- Perform a thorough baseline assessment before starting therapy and at regular intervals during the course of therapy. Notify the physician of apparent CNS side effects.
- Since loss of taste may affect nutritional intake, monitor weight.

**CV** Bradycardia, left bundle branch block, and ST-T wave changes with congestive heart failure are rare. Hypertension or hypotension may also occur.
- Monitor blood pressure, pulse, and weight. Auscultate lung sounds. Monitor the electrocardiogram. Visually inspect the patient for development of jugular venous distention and edema, especially in dependent areas.

**Blood** Myelosuppression (leukopenia, thrombocytopenia, and anemia) is cumulative and occurs in about 30% of patients. Thrombocytopenia and leukopenia are dose-dependent; these effects are delayed, the most profound effects occurring between 18 and 23 days. Local phlebitis or severe cellulitis may occur at the site of infusion when the drug is allowed to extravasate.
- See entry for drug class (p. 479) for discussion of leukopenia, thrombocytopenia, anemia, and extravasation.

**GI** Nausea and vomiting occur in almost all patients and may be severe enough to warrant discontinuing therapy. Vomiting usually occurs within 6 hours of administration and may persist longer than 24 hours. Treatment with metoclopramide or other antiemetics may be required.
- Because vomiting is so common when this drug is administered, many physicians use established protocols involving metoclopramide, steroids, sedatives, other antiemetics, or other drugs before each course of therapy; administer these drug regimens as ordered for best effect.
- See entry for drug class (p. 481).

**Renal** Renal toxicity may be cumulative and dose-limiting. Serum creatinine, BUN, and serum uric acid may increase, and the glomerular filtration rate decreases.

- To prevent renal toxicity, the drug is often infused with large volumes of IV fluids, such as 250 to 500 ml/hour for 4 hours; mannitol and/or furosemide may also be administered concomitantly. Monitor intake and output hourly for the first 6 to 8 hours, then every 24 hours. Monitor blood pressure and pulse. Auscultate breath sounds.
- Monitor serum creatinine and BUN.
  Electrolyte disturbances may be severe and require appropriate specific management. Hypomagnesemia and hypocalcemia are especially noteworthy, causing cramps, carpopedal spasm, clonus, muscle irritability and/or tetany. Hypomagnesemia has persisted for long periods in some patients. Uric acid concentration in plasma may increase as a result of renal toxicity.
- Monitor serum electrolytes and uric acid.
- Assess for signs of hypocalcemia: numbness and tingling of the nose, ears, fingertips, or toes. Assess for signs of hypomagnesemia: confusion, hallucinations, convulsions, increased reflexes, tremors, muscle spasms, and paresthesias.

**Ototoxicity** Tinnitus with or without hearing loss occurs in 9% of patients. Audiograms are altered in about 24% of patients. Children and the elderly are more susceptible to this side effect. Hearing loss occurs in about 6% of patients. Vestibular damage is possible. Ototoxicity may be cumulative and dose-related.
- If possible, obtain a baseline audiogram before starting drug therapy and at regular intervals during the course of therapy.
- Assess regularly for the development of tinnitus or changes in hearing acuity. Instruct the patient to report the development of any ringing or noises in the ear or any suspected hearing loss.

**Liver** Serum AST and ALT may be transiently increased.
- Assess the patient for development of malaise, fever, right upper quadrant abdominal pain, and change in the color or consistency of stools.
- Monitor liver function studies.

**Eye** Optic neuritis, papilledema, and cerebral blindness are rare side effects that usually resolve when the drug is discontinued.
- Instruct the patient to report any changes in vision.

**Allergic** Anaphylactoid reactions can occur, with facial edema, flushing, hypotension, wheezing, respiratory difficulty, and tachycardia.
- Monitor blood pressure and pulse. Assess for signs of allergic response, as listed previously.
- Have drugs, equipment, and personnel available to treat acute allergic reactions in settings where cisplatin is administered.

**Reproductive** Aspermia may occur but is often reversible.
- See entry for drug class (p. 484).

**Other** Alopecia, gingival platinum line, pyrexia, and myalgia have all been reported occasionally.
- Instruct patients to report the development of any unexpected sign or symptom.

### Nursing interventions related to drug administration
- See entry for drug class (p. 485).
- See Preparations.
- After reconstituting as directed, further dilute the dosage in 2 liters of 5% dextrose in 0.2% or 0.45% saline. Mannitol or furosemide may also be ordered (see Renal). Administer at a rate of 1 liter every 3 to 4 hours.
- Wash the skin immediately with copious amounts of water if drug comes in direct contact with skin.

### Patient and family education
- See entry for drug class (p. 485).

---

# cyclophosphamide  (sye-kloh-FOSS-fa-mide)　　　　　　antineoplastic*

- cyclophosphamide: Cytoxan, Neosar, ✚Procytox

**MECHANISM OF ACTION**　Cyclophosphamide must be activated by the liver to a form that affects DNA by chemically changing (alkylating) its structure. Without fully functional DNA, cells eventually die.

*DNA alkylator.

Rapidly growing cells are most susceptible. In addition to anticancer action, cyclophosphamide is strongly immunosuppressive.

**INDICATIONS**  **Hodgkin's disease and malignant lymphomas** Cyclophosphamide causes objective improvement in 60% to 90% of patients with Hodgkin's disease, lymphocytic lymphoma, histiocytic lymphoma, or Burkitt's lymphoma. • Cures are achieved by combinations of drugs, including those containing cyclophosphamide.  **Multiple myeloma** Cyclophosphamide with prednisone increases the likelihood of survival in many patients.  **Leukemias** Cyclophosphamide is a drug of choice for chronic lymphocytic leukemia and acute lymphoblastic leukemia; complete remissions and presumed cures of acute lymphoblastic leukemia have been obtained with drug combinations including cyclophosphamide (Table 27-2). • Cyclophosphamide is an alternate in combinations used to treat chronic myelocytic leukemia and acute myeloblastic leukemia.  **Neuroblastoma** Combinations including cyclophosphamide produce objective improvement in more than 65% of patients with disseminated neuroblastoma and may improve survival rates.  **Ovarian carcinoma** Cyclophosphamide alone produces objective improvement in more than 60% of patients; Cures should not be expected.  **Retinoblastoma** Cyclophosphamide is a drug of choice.  **Breast carcinoma** Combinations including cyclophosphamide produce objective improvement in 90% of patients.  **Lung carcinomas** Bronchogenic carcinoma, small cell and non-small cell carinomas may respond to combinations containing cyclophosphamide.  **Bone marrow transplant** Cyclophosphamide is a potent immunosuppressant that may be used to control rejection of transplants.

**CONTRAINDICATIONS**  **Bone marrow suppression** Patients with severe leukopenia, thrombocytopenia, or other signs of bone marrow damage may be unable to tolerate the effects of cyclophosphamide. **Herpes zoster (chickenpox, shingles) infection or exposure** The risk of severe generalized disease is increased by the immunosuppressive action of cyclophosphamide.

**DOSAGE**  **PO:**  **ADULTS:** Usual doses are 1 to 5 mg/kg daily for induction of remissions. Maintenance doses are determined by response and tolerance of the patient.  **CHILDREN:** Usual doses for induction of remission are 2 to 8 mg/kg or 60 to 250 mg/$M^2$ daily. Maintenance doses are usually 2 to 5 mg/kg or 50 to 150 mg/$M^2$ given twice weekly.  **IV:**  **ADULTS:** Doses for induction of remission range from 40 to 100 mg/kg in divided doses over 2 to 5 days. Maintenance doses may be 10 to 15 mg/kg (350 to 550 mg/$M^2$) every 7 to 10 days; alternatively, 3 to 5 mg/kg (110 to 185 mg/$M^2$) may be given twice weekly.  **CHILDREN:** Usual doses for induction of remission are 2 to 8 mg/kg or 60 to 250 mg/$M^2$ daily.  *Special patient populations:*  **CHILDREN:** This drug is carcinogenic and should be avoided if other drugs may be substituted.  **PREGNANCY:** FDA pregnancy category C.  **BREAST-FEEDING MOTHERS:** Cyclophosphamide passes into breast milk; breast-feeding should be avoided while taking this drug.  **RENAL IMPAIRMENT:** Lower doses may be required.  **HEPATIC IMPAIRMENT:** Cyclophosphamide may be less effective because the impaired liver may fail to activate the drug.

**PREPARATIONS**  *Tablets:* 25 or 50 mg for oral use, *powder for reconstitution:* 100 mg, 200 mg, 500 mg, 1 g, or 2 g cyclophosphamide anhydrous, with sodium chloride or lyophilized with mannitol. The powder or lyophilized powder may be reconstituted with sterile water for injection or bacteriostatic water for injection to yield solutions of 20 mg/ml: 5 ml to 100 mg vial, 10 ml to 200 mg vial, 25 ml to 500 mg vial, 50 ml to 1 g vial, and 100 ml to 2 g vial.

**DRUG INTERACTIONS**  **Immunosuppressants** such as azathioprine, corticotropin, cyclophosphamide, cyclosporine, glucocorticoids, mercaptopurine, or muromonab-CD3 may produce intolerable immune suppression.  **Allopurinol** may increase bone marrow suppression and toxicity of cyclophosphamide. **Cardiotoxic drugs** such as doxorubicin should be avoided if possible because the cardiotoxicity of cyclophosphamide may be additive. Doxorubicin may also exacerbate cyclophosphamide-induced hemorrhagic cystitis.  **Barbiturates** induce the enzymes in the liver that activate cyclophosphamide. The combination may result in increased toxicity from the active metabolites.  **Succinylcholine** may have prolonged action in patients receiving high doses of cyclophosphamide because cyclophosphamide may reduce serum pseudocholinesterase, the enzyme that normally rapidly degrades succinylcholine and terminates its action.  **Vaccines containing live virus** should be avoided because the risk of severe generalized disease is increased.

**FATE**  Cyclophosphamide is well-absorbed orally, producing *peak* plasma concentrations within 1 hour. Cyclophosphamide is in an inactive form as administered and must be converted by enzymes in the liver to the active cytotoxic form. Excretion of the drug and its metabolites is almost exclusively by the kidneys.

## ❦ NURSING CONSIDERATIONS

### Side effects, toxicities, and associated nursing actions

**CNS** Headache and dizziness have occurred.
* Review these possible side effects with patients.
* Caution patients to avoid driving or operating hazardous equipment if dizziness occurs; notify the physician.

**CV** High doses of cyclophosphamide have caused hemorrhagic myocardial necrosis and acute myopericarditis; deaths have occurred.
* Assess for changes in cardiovascular functioning; assess pulse, blood pressure, and respiratory rate; auscultate breath and heart sounds, and monitor weight.

**Blood** Depression of leukocyte counts is an expected, dose-limiting side effect of cyclophosphamide therapy. The counts are lowest 8 to 15 days after a dose. Thrombocytopenia is not as common but may occur 10 to 15 days after a dose. Anemia is usually associated with long-term therapy or high doses.
* See entry for drug class (p. 479) for a discussion of leukopenia, thrombocytopenia, and anemia.

**GI** Anorexia, nausea, and vomiting are common and related to dose. Diarrhea, hemorrhagic colitis, mucosal irritation, and oral ulceration are less common.
* See entry for drug class (p. 481) for a discussion of GI side effects.

**Liver** Hepatic dysfunction and jaundice are rare.
* Assess the patient for right upper quadrant abdominal pain, fever, malaise, jaundice, and change in color or consistency of stools.
* Monitor liver function tests.

**Renal** Nephrotoxicity with renal hemorrhage and tubular necrosis may occur. Blood in the urine more commonly arises from sterile hemorrhagic cystitis, which occurs in up to 20% of patients. Metabolites of cyclophosphamide concentrate in urine and irritate the lining of the bladder. Deaths have occurred. Fibrosis of the bladder may also occur. Water retention may occur. Inappropriate secretion of antidiuretic hormones is especially noted in patients receiving higher doses.
* Encourage patients to force fluids by drinking up to eight glasses (8 ounce glasses) of water daily, plus a glass before bedtime and a glass during the night if they must get up.
* Instruct the patients to report any discoloration of the urine or any problems with voiding.
* Monitor weight. Instruct the patient to monitor and record weight at home. Have the patient notify the physician if weight begins to increase (more than 2 pounds in 1 day) or if urinary output seems to be diminishing.
* Monitor serum electrolytes.

**Metabolic** Rapid lysis of cancer cells may release large quantities of potassium and purines. Purines are converted to uric acid, which may accumulate and cause goutlike symptoms. If the kidneys are unable to excrete the excess potassium, hyperkalemia may result.
* Encourage fluid intake (see Renal).
* Assess for signs of hyperkalemia: nausea, colic, diarrhea, and skeletal muscle spasms.
* Monitor serum electrolytes.
* See entry for drug class (p. 484).

**Lung** High doses over prolonged periods may cause pulmonary fibrosis, which can be fatal.
* Monitor patients for this side effect. Auscultate lung sounds for rales, rhonchi, and pleural friction rubs. Assess the patient for dyspnea, and cough. Monitor serial chest x-rays. Monitor serial pulmonary function studies, if available, although these many not be predictive.

**Skin** Changes in skin pigmentation and nail forms may occur.
* Warn patient about these possible, but temporary, skin changes.

**Allergic** Diaphoresis, faintness, facial flushing and a feeling of constriction in the throat have occurred.

- Assess the patient for these side effects. Remain with the patient and provide calm reassurance as needed. If the drug is being administered IV, slow the rate of infusion.

**Reproductive** Gonadal suppression occurs, with more severe effects occurring with higher doses and longer therapy. Up to 30% of patients experience azoospermia, oligospermia, or amenorrhea. Sterility appearing after long use may be permanent. Ovarian failure and testicular atrophy also occur.
- See entry for drug class (p. 484).

**Other** Alopecia occurs in about one third of patients, appearing within 3 weeks of starting the drug.
- See entry for drug class (p. 484).

### Nursing interventions related to drug administration

- For IV administration, after reconstituting as directed, dose may be further diluted in up to 250 ml of 5% glucose or normal saline. If given without dilution, administer each 100 mg over at least 1 minute. If further diluted, administer the total volume at an appropriate rate for the patient's age.
- If the patient has difficulty swallowing tablets, an oral liquid form can be prepared by the pharmacist; inform patients of this option.

### Patient and family education

- See entry for drug class (p. 485).
- Instruct patients to take cyclophosphamide on an empty stomach if possible. If stomach upset occurs, however, the drug can be taken with meals.

## cytarabine   (sye-TARE-uh-been)                                   antineoplastic*

- cytarabine: Cytosar-U, (ARA-C)

**MECHANISM OF ACTION**   Cytarabine mimics a natural pyrimidine and is activated to a form that inhibits DNA synthesis and function. In addition to anticancer action, the drug has strong immunosuppressive activity.

**INDICATIONS**   **Leukemias** Acute myelogenous leukemia may be effectively controlled with cytarabine in combination with other drugs; complete remissions occur in 60% to 85% of patients. Cytarabine may also be useful in the blastic phase of chronic myelogenous leukemia, meningeal leukemia, and acute lymphocytic leukemia.   **Lymphomas** Non-Hodgkin's lymphomas may respond to combinations containing cytarabine.

**CONTRAINDICATIONS**   **Hepatic impairment** Hepatic disease may predispose patients to the hepatotoxic effects of cytarabine.   **Herpes zoster (chickenpox, shingles) infection or exposure** The risk of severe generalized disease is increased by the immunosuppressive action of cytarabine.

**DOSAGE**   **IV:**   **ADULTS AND CHILDREN:** Usual doses for induction of remission are 200 mg/M$^2$ daily by continuous infusion for 5 days. Repeat as appropriate at 2 week intervals. Maintenance usually is with 70 to 200 mg/M$^2$ repeated at monthly intervals. High-dose IV therapy, 3 g/M$^2$ infused over 1 hour every 12 hours for 12 doses.   **SC:**   **ADULTS AND CHILDREN:** For maintenance therapy of acute leukemias, 50 mg/m$_2$ weekly.   **Intrathecal:**   **ADULTS AND CHILDREN:** 50 to 100 mg in 10 ml of saline, one to three times weekly.   *Special patient populations:*   **CHILDREN:** This drug is carcinogenic and should be avoided if other drugs may be substituted.   **PREGNANCY:** FDA pregnancy category C.   **RENAL IMPAIRMENT:** Lower doses may be required.

**PREPARATIONS**   *Powder for reconstitution:* 100 to 500 mg. For IV use in standard doses, reconstitute with bacteriostatic water for injection containing 0.945% benzyl alcohol. Add 5 ml diluent to 100 mg vial to produce 20 mg/ml solution or add 10 ml to 500 mg vial to produce 50 mg/ml solution. For intrathecal use or use in neonates, reconstitute in 0.9% sodium chloride preservative-free.

**DRUG INTERACTIONS**   **Methotrexate** may potentiate the anticancer effect of cytarabine.   **Cytotoxic drugs** may damage the bone marrow, requiring that lower doses of cytarabine be used.

*Pyrimidine antimetabolite.

**FATE**   Absorption of cytarabine from subcutaneous sites is low but adequate for maintenance therapy. Oral absorption is too low to be used. Distribution of the drug is widespread in fluids and tissues, including the placenta. Cytarabine is rapidly metabolized in the liver; the plasma *half-life* is about 10 minutes. Nearly all of the drug and metabolites are excreted in urine.

## ☙ NURSING CONSIDERATIONS
### Side effects, toxicities, and associated nursing actions

**CNS** Intrathecal administration commonly causes nausea, vomiting, fever, and transient headaches. Rare side effects include meningism, paraplegia, paresthesia, seizures, and spastic paraparesis. Benzyl alcohol used as a preservative in some diluents has caused other CNS reactions; such diluents should not be used intrathecally. High-dose therapy may cause cerebral and cerebellar dysfunction, with coma, personality changes, or somnolence.
- Review with the patient and family the possible side effects. instruct the family to report the development of any usual sign or symptom.
- Anticipate possible CNS effects. Keep side rails up. Monitor temperature every 4 hours.

**CV** High-dose therapy may cause pericarditis with tamponade, cardiomegaly, or other cardiomyopathy.
- Monitor pulse and blood pressure. Assess for adequate cardiovascular function: monitor weight, visually inspect feet and ankles for signs of edema, and auscultate breath sounds.

**Blood** Anemia, myelosuppression, and thrombocytopenia may be expected in nearly all patients receiving cytarabine. These side effects are dose-limiting in most patients. Thrombophlebitis, pain, and inflammation at the injection site are common.
- See entry for drug class (p. 479) for a discussion of anemia, granulocytopenia, thrombocytopenia, and extravasation.
- Instruct the patient to report pain or discomfort at the infusion site. For pain during infusion, slow infusion rate, and perform fresh venipuncture if indicated.

**GI** Nausea and vomiting are frequent with rapid IV administration but less troublesome with continuous infusion. Anorexia, diarrhea, and oral or anal inflammation with or without ulceration are less common. Abdominal pain, esophagitis, esophageal ulceration, and GI hemorrhage are possible, especially with high doses.
- See entry for drug class (p. 481) for a discussion of GI side effects.

**Renal** Renal dysfunction and urinary retention may occur.
- Monitor serum electrolytes, creatinine, and BUN.
- If renal dysfunction is suspected or likely based on patient history, monitor intake, output, and weight.

**Liver** Jaundice and elevations in serum bilirubin, transaminases, and alkaline phosphatase may occur. High doses may cause liver abscess or other liver damage.
- Assess the patient for signs of liver dysfunction: jaundice, fever, malaise, right upper quadrant abdominal pain, or change in the color or consistency of stools.
- Monitor liver function tests.

**Metabolic** Rapid cancer cell destruction can release large quantities of purines, which are metabolized to uric acid. Accumulation of uric acid may lead to renal damage or gout.
- See entry for drug class (p. 484).

**Allergic** Rash, fever, and anaphylaxis have occurred.
- Have drugs, equipment, and personnel available to treat acute allergic reactions in settings where cytarabine is administered.
- Instruct patients to notify the physician if fever persists longer than 24 hours.

**Eye** Keratitis and hemorrhagic conjunctivitis can occur with high doses.
- Instruct patients to report changes in eyes or vision.

**Lung** High doses may cause pulmonary edema and acute respiratory failure.
- Monitor pulse, blood pressure, and respiratory rate. Monitor weight. Auscultate breath sounds. Assess for dyspnea.

**Skin** Freckling and skin ulceration may occur.

**Other** Alopecia may occur.

- Instruct patients to report the development of skin changes.
- See entry for drug class (p. 484) for a discussion of alopecia.

### Nursing interventions related to drug administration
- For IV administration, dilute as noted under Preparations. May be given by direct IV injection at a rate of 100 mg over 1 to 3 minutes or further diluted in 50 to 100 ml of normal saline or 5% dextrose in water and infused over 1 to 24 hours.
- For intrathecal use or for use in neonates, reconstitute in 0.9% sodium chloride preservative-free.
- Store in the refrigerator until reconstituted, then use within 48 hours.

### Patient and family education
- See entry for drug class (p. 485).

## dacarbazine  (da-KAR-ba-zeen)   antineoplastic*

- dacarbazine (imidazole carboxamide) DTIC-Dome

**MECHANISM OF ACTION**   Dacarbazine changes the properties of DNA by chemically changing (alkylating) its structure. Without fully functional DNA, cells eventually die. Rapidly growing cells are most susceptible.

**INDICATIONS**   **Malignant melanoma** About 20% of patients with metastatic malignant melanoma obtain a 50% reduction of tumor mass.   **Hodgkin's disease** Advanced forms of the disease may be treated with combinations including dacarbazine (p. 479).

**CONTRAINDICATIONS**   **Herpes zoster (chickenpox, shingles) infection or exposure** The risk of severe generalized disease is increased by the immunosuppressive action of dacarbazine.

**DOSAGE**   **IV:**   **ADULTS:** For malignant melanoma, 2 to 4.5 mg/kg daily for 10 days, repeated at 4-week intervals; alternatively, 250 mg/M$^2$ daily for 5 days, repeated at 3 week intervals. For Hodgkin's disease, 150 mg/M$^2$ daily for 5 days in a schedule with other drugs.   *Special patient populations:* **CHILDREN:** This drug is carcinogenic and should be avoided if other drugs may be substituted. **PREGNANCY:** FDA pregnancy category C.   **RENAL IMPAIRMENT:** Lower doses may be required.

**PREPARATIONS**   *Powder for reconstitution:* 100 or 200 mg vials. Reconstitute by adding 9.9 ml sterile water for injection to the 100 mg vial or 19.7 ml to the 200 mg vial. These reconstituted solutions are 10 mg/ml and may be used directly or further diluted with up to 250 ml 5% dextrose or 0.9% sodium chloride injection.

**DRUG INTERACTIONS**   **Myelosuppressive agents** must be used with care in patients also receiving dacarbazine to avoid excessive bone marrow suppression.   **Vaccines containing live virus** should be avoided because the risk of severe generalized disease is increased.

**FATE**   Dacarbazine must be given IV to assure adequate absorption. The drug is metabolized extensively. The drug and its metabolites are excreted by the kidneys. The elimination *half-life* is 5 hours.

## 🐾 NURSING CONSIDERATIONS
### Side effects, toxicities, and associated nursing actions
**CNS** Blurred vision, confusion, headache, lethargy, and seizures may occur
- Review these possible side effects with patients. Instruct patients to avoid driving or operating hazardous equipment if blurred vision, lethargy, or other unusual symptoms occur; notify the physician.

**Blood** Leukopenia and thrombocytopenia appear 2 to 4 weeks after therapy and should be expected to a degree in all patients. Dacarbazine causes extreme pain along the vein in which it is administered. Extravasation can damage tissue and cause pain.
- See entry for drug class (p. 479) for a discussion of leukopenia, thrombocytopenia, and extravasation.

*DNA alkylator.

- If the patient complains of pain during administration, ascertain that extravasation has not occurred; slow the infusion rate.

**GI** Over 90% of patients suffer anorexia, nausea, and vomiting. Symptoms appear within an hour of starting the drug but often lessen over the first few days of therapy.
- See entry for drug class (p. 481).

**Liver** Hepatic vein thrombosis and hepatocellular necrosis are rare but potentially fatal side effects. Rare increases in serum alkaline phosphatase, AST, ALT, and BUN are usually dangerous.
- Assess the patient for right upper quadrant abdominal pain, malaise, fever, change in color or consistency of stools, and jaundice.
- Monitor liver function tests and BUN.

**Skin** Alopecia, rashes, and photosensitivity may occur.
- See entry for drug class (p. 484) for discussion of alopecia.
- If photosensitivity develops, caution patients to avoid exposure to the sun or other sources of ultraviolet light, to wear a large-brimmed hat when outside, to keep extremities covered, and to use a maximum-protectin sunscreen on exposed skin surfaces.

**Allergic** Anaphylaxis is rare.
- Have drugs, equipment, and personnel available to treat acute allergic reactions is settings where dacarbazine is administered.

**Other** A flulike syndrome with fever, myalgia, and malaise occurs infrequently.
- Instruct patients to report the development of any unusual signs or symptoms. Caution patients to report fever that persists longer than 24 hours.

### Nursing interventions related to drug administration
- See Preparations for information on reconstitution. For direct IV administration, administer the dose over at least 1 minute. For dilute solutions up to 250 ml, administer over 30 minutes.

### Patient and family education
- See entry for drug class (p. 485).

---

## dactinomycin    (dak-tin-oh-MY-sin)    antineoplastic*

- dactinomycin (actinomycin-D): Cosmegan

**MECHANISM OF ACTION**    Dactinomycin binds tightly to double-stranded DNA, thereby preventing RNA formation from the natural genetic template. Cells unable to form RNA eventually die. Dactinomycin is also an immune suppressant.

**INDICATIONS**    **Wilms' tumor** Dactinomycin with vincristine and radiation frees 80% to 90% of patients from the disease for at least 2 years.    **Rhabdomyosarcoma** Dactinomycin with cyclophosphamide and vincristine is adjunctive therapy, along with radiation and surgery. • Two-year disease-free remissions are produced in 80% to 90% of patients.    **Ewing's sarcoma** Combinations including dactinomycin provide 5 year relapse-free survival in 75% of patients (p. 479).    **Trophoblastic neoplasms** Dactinomycin alone can cure 90% to 100% of patients with early choriocarcinoma. For advanced disease, dactinomycin is often combined with methotrexate and chlorambucil.    **Testicular carcinoma** Combinations including dactinomycin may be used to induce remissions in this disease.    **Sarcomas** A variety of sarcomas may respond to regional perfusion with dactinomycin; therapy is palliative, not curative.

**CONTRAINDICATIONS**    **Active chickenpox of herpes zoster** Dactinomycin may induce severe generalized disease in these patients, leading to death.

**DOSAGE**    **IV:** **ADULTS:** Usual doses are 500 μg daily for 5 days. Doses must not exceed 600 μg/m$^2$ daily for 5 days. Doses may be repeated at 2 to 4 week intervals.    **CHILDREN:** Usual doses are 15 μg/kg (up to 500 μg daily) for 5 days; alternatively, 2.5 mg/m$^2$ in divided doses over a week. Doses may be repeated at 2 to 4 week intervals. *Special patient populations:* **CHILDREN:** This drug is carcinogenic and should be avoided if other drugs may be substituted. Infants younger than 6 months

*DNA intercalator.

should not receive the drug.  **PREGNANCY:** FDA pregnancy category C.  **HEPATIC IMPAIR-MENT:** Doses may need to be reduced.

**PREPARATIONS**    *Powder for reconstitution:* 500 μg. Reconstitute by adding 1.1 ml of sterile water for injection without preservatives to the 500 μg vial. Wear protective gloves and avoid direct contact with solutions of dactinomycin.

**DRUG INTERACTIONS**    **Myelosuppressive** agents may impair bone marrow function, making patients unable to tolerate the additional myelosuppressive effects of dactinomycin.    **Vaccines containing live virus** should be avoided because the risk of severe generalized disease is increased.

**FATE**    Dactinomycin must be administered IV to minimize damage to tissues caused by direct contact with this highly irritating drug. The drug concentrates in bone marrow and crosses the placenta, but concentrations in the CNS are low. Elimination is primarily renal, with a *half-life* of about 36 hours.

### ☙ NURSING CONSIDERATIONS

#### Side effects, toxicities, and associated nursing actions

**CV** Congestive heart failure induced by doxorubicin may be exacerbated.
* Monitor weight, blood pressure, pulse, intake, and output. Assess for edema, especially in dependent areas. Auscultate lung sounds, and inspect for jugular venous distention.

**Blood** Myelosuppression is expected following dactinomycin therapy and is the dose-limiting side effect in most patients. Platelet counts decline within a week of therapy and are lowest 2 to 3 weeks after the start of therapy. Leukocyte counts are also lowered. Anemia, pancytopenia, reticulopenia, agranulocytopenia, and aplastic anemia are less common.
* See entry for drug class (p. 479) for discussion of granulocytopenia, thrombocytopenia, and anemia.

**GI** Nausea and vomiting are common early side effects. Stomatitis, cheilitis, glossitis, dysphagia, and oral ulceration are common later side effects. Abdominal pain, anorexia, diarrhea, esophagitis, GI ulceration, pharyngitis, and proctitis are less common.
* See entry for drug class (p. 481) for discussion of GI side effects.

**Skin** Acne, folliculitis, and rashes may occur. Alopecia also often occurs but is reversible. When patients have also received radiation, erythema followed by hyperpigmentation and edema may occur at the site. Desquamation, vesiculation, and necrosis occasionally also occur.
* See entry for drug class (p. 484) for discussion of alopecia.
* Visually inspect skin before therapy and at regular intervals; be especially vigilant in assessing areas of previous radiation. Instruct patients to report the development of any skin changes.

**Allergic** Anaphylactoid reactions may occur.
* Have drugs, equipment, and personnel available to treat acute allergic reactions in settings where dactinomycin is administered.

**Other** Pain and erythema at the injection site are common. Extravasation of the drug causes immediate intense pain; extensive tissue destruction may follow. When dactinomycin is used for regional perfusion, soft tissue damage may include phlebitis, edema, cellulitis, and necrosis.
* Ascertain that the IV is patent before administering this drug. Instruct the patient to report any discomfort during infusion. Do not leave the patient unattended.

#### Nursing interventions related to drug administration
* See Preparations for information about reconstitution. For direct IV injection, administer 0.5 mg or less over 1 minute. Reconstituted drug may be further diluted in 50 ml of 5% dextrose in water or normal saline and administered over 10 to 15 minutes.
* See entry for drug class (p. 485).

#### Patient and family education
* See entry for drug class (p. 485).

---

## daunorubicin hydrochloride    (daw-noh-ROO-bi-sin)    antineoplastic*

* daunorubicin hydrochloride: Cerubidine

DNA intercalator.

**MECHANISM OF ACTION**  Daunorubicin binds tightly to double-stranded DNA, thus preventing RNA formation from the natural genetic template. Cells that cannot form RNA eventually die. The mechanism is similar to that of dactinomycin (p. 502). Daunorubicin is also immunosuppressive.

**INDICATIONS**  Leukemias Daunorubicin is used primarily in acute myelogenous leukemia, inducing remissions in up to 85% of patients when used in combinations with other drugs (Table 27-2). • Daunorubicin alone or with other drugs may also induce remissions in acute lymphocytic leukemia.

**CONTRAINDICATIONS**  **Bone marrow suppression** Patients with pre-existing bone marrow suppression may be unable to tolerate the additional suppression caused by daunorubicin.   **Herpes zoster (chickenpox, shingles) infection or exposure** The risk of severe generalized disease is increased by the immunosuppressive action of daunorubicin.   **Heart disease** Patients with pre-exsiting cardiac disease may be unable to tolerate the direct cardiotoxicity of daunorubicin.

**DOSAGE**  IV:  **ADULTS:** Usual doses are 30 to 60 mg/m$^2$ daily for 3 to 5 days. Doses may be repeated every 3 to 4 weeks when bone marrow function allows.   **CHILDREN:** Usual doses are 25 to 45 mg/m$^2$. Children younger than 2 years or having a body surface area smaller than 0.5 m$^2$ should have doses calculated on the basis of body weight.  *Special patient populations:*  **CHILDREN:** This drug is carcinogenic and should be avoided if other drugs may be substituted.  **PREGNANCY:** FDA pregnancy category D.  **RENAL OR HEPATIC IMPAIRMENT:** Doses may need to be reduced.

**PREPARATIONS**  *Powder for reconstitution:* 20 mg. Reconstitute by adding 4 ml of sterile water for injection to the 20 mg vial. Agitate gently to dissolve. This 5 mg/ml solution may be used to prepare further dilutions in 0.9% sodium chloride. The final dilutions should be injected into a freely flowing IV line. Gloves should be worn to avoid contact with the drug.

**DRUG INTERACTONS**  **Myelosuppressive** agents may impair bone marrow function, making patients unable to tolerate the additional myelosuppressive effects of daunorubicin.   **Vaccines containing live virus** should be avoided because the risk of severe generalized disease is increased.

**FATE**  Daunorubicin must be given IV to minimize damage to tissues caused by direct contact with this highly irritating drug. Concentrations in the CNS are low, but daunorubicin crosses the placenta. Elimination is by renal and hepatic mechanisms, with a *half-life* of 18 to 27 hours.

### ❧ NURSING CONSIDERATIONS

#### Side effects, toxicities, and associated nursing actions

**CV** Daunorubicin causes acute cardiotoxicity with ECG changes and arrhythmias, including sinus tachycardia, heart block, and premature ventricular contractions. These effects are usually insignificant. Serious cardiotoxicity can occur, leading to congestive heart failure. This latter reaction is cumulative and dose-dependent. At a total cumulative dosage of 550 mg/m$^2$, 1% to 2% of treated adults develop congestive heart failure. Children may be more susceptible, as are patients who have received radiation to the heart.

• Monitor pulse and blood pressure. Assess for signs of congestive heart failure: weight gain, edema (especially of dependent areas), dyspnea, and jugular venous distention. Auscultate breath sounds and monitor respiratory rate.

• Obtain a baseline electrocardiogram before starting therapy and monitor serial ECGs, echocardiograms, or other indicators of cardiac function.

**Blood** Leukopenia is to be expected in all patients. Thrombocytopenia also occurs; anemia is less common.

• See entry for drug drug class (p. 479) for discussion of leukopenia, thrombocytopenia, and anemia.

**GI** Nausea and vomiting are early side effects. Stomatitis and esophagitis may occur several days after therapy. Abdominal pain and diarrhea are less common.

• See entry for drug class (p. 481) for a discussion of GI side effects.

**Metabolic** Rapid cancer cell destruction can release large quantities of purines, which are metabolized to uric acid. Accumulation of uric acid may lead to renal damage or gout.

• See entry for drug class (p. 484).

**Skin** Reversible alopecia occurs in over 80% of patients, with hair loss all over the body. Unusual pigmentation of the nails may also occur. Rashes, contact dermatitis, and urticaria are rare.

• See entry for drug class (p. 484) for a discussion of alopecia.

• Instruct the patient to report the development of any skin changes.

**Allergic** Transient fever and chills may occur.

- Instruct the patient to report to the physician any fever that persists longer than 24 hours.
**Other** Extravasation causes painful induration and may produce severe local tissue necrosis.
- Ascertain that IV infusion is patent before administering the drug. Instruct the patient to report any discomfort during infusion. Do not leave the patient unattended during infusion.
- See entry for drug class (p. 484) for further discussion of extravasation.

### Nursing interventions related to drug administration
- See Preparations for information about reconstitution. Further dilute in 10 to 15 ml of normal saline; administer the diluted dose over at least 3 to 5 minutes.

### Patient and family education
- See entry for drug class (p. 485).
- Inform patients that urine may be reddish for 1 to 2 days following drug therapy with daunorubicin.

---

## doxorubicin hydrochloride    (dox-oh-ROO-be-sin)    antineoplastic*

- doxorubicin hydrochloride: Adriamycin

**MECHANISM OF ACTION**    Doxorubicin binds tightly to double-stranded DNA, thereby preventing RNA formation from the natural genetic template. Cells unable to form RNA eventually die. The mechanism of action is similar to dactinomycin (p. 502). Doxorubicin is also immunosuppressive.

**INDICATIONS**    **Carcinomas** Doxorubicin causes clinical improvement in significant numbers of patients with carcinomas of breast, ovary, bladder, lung, and stomach. • Tumors in the kidneys, brain, and colon are usually unresponsive.    **Sarcomas** Soft tissue and osteogenic sarcomas may respond.    **Wilms' tumor** Doxorubicin is an alternative to dactinomycin (p. 502).    **Neuroblastoma** Doxorubicin is an alternative to dactinomycin.    **Leukemias** Acute lymphoblastic and acute myeloblastic leukemias may be treated with combinations including doxorubicin.

**CONTRAINDICATIONS**    **Bone marrow suppression** Patients with pre-existing bone marrow suppression may be unable to tolerate the additional suppression caused by doxorubicin.    **Heart disease** Patients with impaired cardiac function may be unable to tolerate the additional impairment caused by doxorubicin. **Previous therapy with daunorubicin** Patients who have received a full course of therapy ($550 \text{ mg/M}^2$) with daunorubicin or doxorubicin should not receive an additional drug.    **Herpes zoster (chickenpox, shingles) infection or exposure** The risk of severe generalized disease is increased by the immunosuppressive action of daunorubicin.

**DOSAGE**    **IV:    ADULTS OR CHILDREN:** Usual doses are 60 to 75 $\text{mg/M}^2$, given as a single dose at 3 week intervals if bone marrow function allows. An alternate schedule is 20 $\text{mg/M}^2$ once weekly.    *Special patient populations:*    **ELDERLY:** Elderly patients may require reduced doses because bone marrow, liver, and renal function may be reduced.    **CHILDREN:** This drug is carcinogenic and should be avoided if other drugs may be substituted.    **PREGNANCY:** Use of this drug in pregnancy carries substantial risk to the fetus.    **HEPATIC IMPAIRMENT:** Doses must be reduced.

**PREPARATIONS**    *Powder for reconstitution:* 10, 20, or 50 mg with lactose. Reconstitute by adding 5 ml of sterile water for injection to the 10 mg vial, 10 ml to the 20 mg vial, or 25 ml to the 50 mg vial. Agitate gently to dissolve. This 2 mg/ml solution should be further diluted in 0.9% sodium chloride. The final dilutions should be injected into a freely flowing IV line. Gloves should be worn to avoid direct contact with the drug.

**DRUG INTERACTIONS**    **Myelosuppressive** agents may impair bone marrow function, making patients unable to tolerate the additional myelosuppressive effects of doxorubicin.    **Fluorouracil** may cause doxorubicin to precipitate from solution.    **Heparin** may cause doxorubicin to precipitate from solution. **Streptozocin** may prolong the half-life of doxorubicin.    **Vaccines containing live virus** should be avoided because the risk of severe generalized disease is increased.

*DNA intercalator.

**FATE** Doxorubicin must be given IV to minimize damage to tissues caused by direct contact with this highly irritating drug. Concentrations in the CNS are low, but doxorubicin crosses the placenta. Elimination is mostly by hepatic mechanisms, with a *half-life* of 17 to 32 hours. Although little drug is excreted renally, the small amount present causes a harmless red discoloration to urine.

## ☙ NURSING CONSIDERATIONS
### Side effects, toxicities, and associated nursing actions

**CV** Doxorubicin causes acute cardiotoxicity with ECG changes and arrhythmias, including sinus tachycardia, heart block, and premature ventricular contractions. These effects are usually insignificant. Serious cardiotoxicity can occur, leading to congestive heart failure. This latter reaction is cumulative and dose-dependent. At a total cumulative dosage of 550 mg/M$^2$, 1% to 2% of treated adults develop congestive heart failure. Children may be more susceptible, as are patients who have received radiation to the heart.
- Monitor pulse and blood pressure. Assess for signs of congestive heart failure: weight gain, edema (especially of dependent areas), dyspnea, and jugular venous distention. Auscultate breath sounds and monitor respiratory rate.
- Obtain a baseline electrocardiogram before starting therapy and monitor serial ECGs, echocardiograms, or other indicators of cardiac function.

**Blood** Leukopenia is to be expected in all patients. Thrombocytopenia also occurs; anemia is less common.
- See entry for drug class (p. 481) for discussion of leukopenia, thrombocytopenia, and anemia.

**GI** Nausea and vomiting are early side effects. Stomatitis and esophagitis may occur several days after therapy. Abdominal pain and diarrhea are less common.
- See entry for drug class (p. 481) for a discussion of GI side effects.

**Metabolic** Rapid cancer cell destruction can release large quantities of purines, which are metabolized to uric acid. Accumulation of uric acid may lead to renal damage or gout.
- See entry for drug class (p. 484).

**Skin** Reversible alopecia occurs in over 80% of patients, with hair loss all over the body. Unusual pigmentation of the nails may also occur. Rashes, contact dermatitis, and urticaria are rare.
- See entry for drug class (p. 484) for a discussion of alopecia.
- Instruct the patient to report the development of any skin changes.

**Allergic** Transient fever and chills may occur.
- Instruct the patient to report to the physician any fever that persists longer than 24 hours.

**Other** Extravasation causes painful induration and may produce severe local tissue necrosis.
- Ascertain that IV infusion is patent before administering the drug. Instruct the patient to report any discomfort during infusion. Do not leave the patient unattended during infusion.
- See entry for drug class (p. 484) for further discussion of extravasation.

### Nursing interventions related to drug administration
- See Preparations for information about reconstitution. Administer the diluted dose over at least 3 to 5 minutes.

### Patient and family education
- See entry for drug class (p. 485).
- Inform patients that urine may be reddish for 1 to 2 days following drug therapy with doxorubicin.

---

## etoposide (eh-TOH-poh-side)
antineoplastic*

- etoposide: VePesid, VP-16

**MECHANISM OF ACTION** Etoposide inhibits enzymes (topoisomerases) that normally remodel double-stranded DNA, resulting in breaks in the DNA strands. As a result, DNA function is lost, and cells eventually die. Rapidly dividing cells are most susceptible.

*Topoisomerase inhibitor.

**INDICATIONS**    Lung carcinoma Combinations including etoposide are useful in treating small cell carcinoma and may benefit some patients with non-small cell carcinoma.    **Testicular neoplasms** Etoposide with cisplatin and other drugs may be useful in patients with disseminated testicular carcinoma or disseminated seminoma testis. • Up to 50% of treated patients may achieve remission of disease.    **Hodgkin's disease and malignant lymphomas** Advanced Hodgkin's disease or advanced non-Hodgkin's lymphomas may respond to combinations including etoposide. • Improvement may occur in up to 40% of patients.    **Leukemias** Acute myelogenous leukemia refractory to standard therapy may respond to etoposide; complete remissions may be achieved in 10% to 15% of patients. Acute lymphocytic leukemia refractory to initial therapy may respond to etoposide alone or with other drugs; therapy is often effective in children but not effective in adults. Chronic myelogenous leukemia may respond.    **Solid tumors** Etoposide is a relatively new agent that is currently being tested for activity against a large number of solid tumors, including trophoblastic tumors, Wilms' tumor, rhabdomyosarcoma, neuroblastoma, Ewing's sarcoma, and tumors of the brain, ovary, and breast.

**CONTRAINDICATIONS**    **Bone marrow suppression** Patients with pre-existing bone marrow suppression may be unable to tolerate the additional suppression caused by etoposide.    **Herpes zoster (chickenpox, shingles) infection or exposure** The risk of severe generalized disease is increased by the immunosuppressive action of etoposide.

**DOSAGE**    IV:    ADULTS AND CHILDREN: Dosages have not been completely established, but most schedules call for 35 to 100 mg/M$^2$ for 3 to 5 days, repeated every 3 or 4 weeks if bone marrow function allows. *Special patient populations:*    ELDERLY: The elderly are especially vulnerable to hypotension during or after infusion of the drug.    CHILDREN: This drug is carcinogenic and should be avoided if other drugs may be substituted.    PREGNANCY: FDA pregnancy category D.    RENAL IMPAIRMENT: Lower doses may be required.

**PREPARATIONS**    *Solution for dilution to prepare IV infusion:* 20 mg/ml. Dilute before use in 0.9% sodium chloride or 5% dextrose injection. The ratio for dilution should be 50 or 100 ml of diluent for each milliliter of concentrated drug solution. The preparer should wear gloves.

**DRUG INTERACTIONS**    **Myelosuppressive** agents may impair bone marrow function, making patients unable to tolerate the additional myelosuppressive effects of doxorubicin.    **Cisplatin** and etoposide may have synergistic anticancer action.    **Vaccines containing live virus** should be avoided because the risk of severe generalized disease is increased.

**FATE**    Absorption of etoposide following oral administration is erratic with present dosage forms. The drug is distributed to many tissues, including the placenta. Etoposide is metabolized, with the drug and its metabolites being excreted primarily by the kidneys. The elimination *half-life* is about 10 hours.

## ❦ NURSING CONSIDERATIONS

### Side effects, toxicities, and associated nursing actions

**CNS** Somnolence and fatigue occur in about 3% of patients. High doses may lead to mental confusion, an effect at least partially caused by the alcohol content of the diluent.

• Instruct patients to avoid driving or operating hazardous equipment if somnolence or fatigue occur.

**CV** Transient hypotension occurs in 1% to 2% of patients. Geriatric patients are more susceptible than younger adults. A few patients have suffered hypertension, myocardial infarction, or congestive heart failure, an effect at least partially caused by prolonged administration of the drug with associated sodium chloride.

• Monitor pulse, blood pressure, and weight. Assess for congestive heart failure: auscultate breath sounds, assess for dyspnea, development of edema in dependent areas, and jugular venous distention.

• Monitor electrocardiograms at regular intervals.

• If hypotension occurs, instruct patients to move slowly from a lying to a sitting or standing position, supervise ambulation, keep side rails up, and keep a light on at night.

**Blood** Leukopenia occurs in up to 91% of patients and may be severe in up to 17%. Thrombocytopenia and anemia are less common; pancytopenia is rare. Retreatment with etoposide or other myelosuppressive agents must not be undertaken until the bone marrow has recovered.

- See entry for drug class (p. 479) for discussion of granulocytopenia, anemia, and thrombocytopenia.

**GI** Nausea and vomiting occur in about 30% of patients. Anorexia and diarrhea occur in up to 13% of patients. Stomatitis is less common (1% occurrence) but may be increased when doses are very high.

- See entry for drug class (p. 481) for discussion of GI side effects.

**Skin** Rash and pruritis are rare. Reversible alopecia may occur in 8% to 20% of patients.

- Instruct patients to report the development of skin changes.
- See entry for drug class (p. 484) for discussion of alopecia.

**Metabolic** Metabolic acidosis following high-dose therapy may result from components in the drug diluent.

- Assess for symptoms of metabolic acidosis: headache, mental dullness, Kussmaul's respirations.
- Monitor serum electrolytes and blood gases.

**Allergic** Anaphylactoid reactions include bronchospasm, chills, dyspnea, fever, hypotension, hypertension, or tachycardia. Abdominal cramps, body pain, flushing, lacrimation, sneezing, and sweating may also occur.

- Monitor blood pressure, pulse, and respiratory rate. Assess for other signs of allergic response.
- Have drugs, equipment, and personnel available to treat acute allergic reactions in settings where etoposide is administered.

### Nursing interventions related to drug administration

- See preparations for dilution. Administer the dilute solution over at least 30 to 60 minutes, depending on volume of dilute drug and age of patient.

### Patient and family education

- See entry for drug class (p. 485).

---

# floxuridine   (flox-YOO-re-deen)                                      antineoplastic*

- floxuridine: FUDR

**MECHANISM OF ACTION**   Floxuridine mimics a natural pyrimidine and is activated to a form that inhibits DNA synthesis and RNA function. Without functional nucleic acids, cells eventually die. Rapidly growing cells are most susceptible.

**INDICATIONS**   **Carcinomas** Certain types of tumors that cannot be cured by surgery or by standard chemotherapy may be treated with regional intra-arterial infusion of floxuridine. • Treatment is palliative, not curative.

**CONTRAINDICATIONS**   **Bone marrow suppression** Patients with pre-existing bone marrow suppression may be unable to tolerate the additional suppression caused by floxuridine.   **High-dose pelvic irradiation** Patients so exposed are at higher risk of toxicity from floxuridine.   **Malnutrition** Patients who are not well nourished may be at higher risk of toxicity.   **Herpes zoster (chickenpox, shingles) infection or exposure** The risk of severe generalized disease is increased by the immunosuppressive action of floxuridine.

**DOSAGE**   **Intra-arterial:**   **ADULTS:** Usual doses are 0.1 to 0.6 mg/kg daily by infusion directly into the artery supplying blood to the tumor. Drug is administered continuously until toxicity intervenes.   *Special patient populations:*   **CHILDREN:** This drug is carcinogenic and should be avoided if other drugs may be substituted.   **PREGNANCY:** Use of this drug in pregnancy carries substantial risk to the fetus. **RENAL OR HEPATIC DYSFUNCTION:** These patients may be unable to eliminate floxuridine normally and may accumulate toxic levels; doses may be lowered.

**PREPARATIONS**   *Powder for reconstitution:* 500 mg. Reconstitute by adding 5 ml of sterile water for injection to the 500 mg vial. This 100 mg/ml solution is further diluted with 5% dextrose or 0.9% sodium chloride to a volume appropriate for infusion.

*Pyrimidine antimetabolite.

**DRUG INTERACTIONS**   **Alkylating agents** such as chlorambucil or cyclophosphamide may predispose a patient to toxicity from floxuridine.   **Vaccines containing live virus** should be avoided because the risk of severe generalized disease is increased.

**FATE**   Slow infusion of floxuridine allows the drug to be metabolized to an active form, which exerts the anticancer effect. The drug is eventually eliminated by hepatic degradation and renal excretion.

## ☙ NURSING CONSIDERATIONS

### Side effects, toxicities, and associated nursing actions

**CNS** Symptoms may include ataxia, blurred vision, hiccups, hemiplegia, lethargy, malaise, mental depression, nystagmus, seizures, vertigo, and weakness.
- Obtain a thorough baseline assessment before starting drug therapy. Assess for changes in mental status and neurologic status.
- Caution patients to avoid driving or operating hazardous equipment until the effects of the medication can be evaluated.

**Blood** Leukopenia and anemia occur commonly; thrombocytopenia is less common.
- See entry for drug class (p. 479) for a discussion of leukopenia, anemia, and thrombocytopenia.

**GI** Nausea, vomiting, diarrhea, stomatitis, and enteritis are common. Anorexia, cramps, duodenal ulcer, duodenitis, gastritis, glossitis, pain, and pharyngitis may also occur.
- Instruct patients to report the development of any new sign or symptom.
- See entry for drug class (p. 481) for a discussion of GI side effects.

**Skin** Localized erythema is a common sign of floxuridine toxicity. Alopecia, dermatitis, edema, excoriation, maceration, pruritis, rash, and ulceration may also occur.
- Visually inspect the patient's skin before starting therapy and at regular intervals during therapy. Instruct patients to report any skin changes.
- See entry for drug class (p. 484) for a discussion of alopecia.

**Other** Specific damage to organs or tissues receiving regional infusion should be expected.

### Nursing interventions related to drug administration
- The catheter for arterial infusion is inserted by the physician. Inspect the insertion site for local changes: redness, swelling, pain, or irritation. Monitor temperature, blood pressure, pulse, intake, and output. Maintain the pump at the ordered infusion rate. Do not disconnect the tubing between pump and patient, as hemorrhage may occur. Instruct the patient to report pain, discomfort, or other signs or symptoms.

### Patient and family education
- See entry for drug class (p. 485).
- If the patient will be using a portable pump and supervising the infusion, review carefully with patient and family the use of the pump.

---

## fluorouracil   (flue-roh-YOO-rah-sil)                                   antineoplastic*

- fluorouracil: Adrucil, ♣ Efudex, 5 Fluorouracil, 5-F4

**MECHANISM OF ACTION**   Fluorouracil mimics a natural pyrimidine and is activated to a form that inhibits synthesis of DNA and RNA and function of RNA. Without functional nucleic acids, cells eventually die. Rapidly growing cells are most susceptible.

**INDICATIONS**   **Carcinomas** Carcinoma of the colon, rectum, stomach, and other portions of the GI tract may respond to fluorouracil, with remissions observed in 10% to 40% of patients. • Metastatic breast cancer may also be treated. • Treatment with fluorouracil is palliative, not curative, and is reserved for cancers that are not amenable to surgery or irradiation.   **Actinic keratosis** Multiple solar keratoses may be treated with topical fluorouracil.

*Pyrimidine antimetabolite.

**CONTRAINDICATIONS**    **Bone marrow suppression** Patients with pre-existing bone marrow suppression may be unable to tolerate the additional suppression caused by fluorouracil.    **High-dose pelvic irradiation** Patients so exposed are at higher risk of toxicity from fluorouracil.    **Malnutrition** Patients who are not well nourished may be at higher risk of toxicity.    **Herpes zoster (chickenpox, shingles) infection or exposure** The risk of severe generalized disease is increased by the immunosuppressive action of fluorouracil.

**DOSAGE**    IV:    ADULTS: Doses are individualized. A common dose is 12 mg/kg once daily for 4 days, followed by 6 mg/kg on day 6, 8, 10, and 12. Toxicity may require discontinuation before the course is completed. Total daily doses must not exceed 800 mg.    *Special patient populations:*    CHILDREN: This drug is carcinogenic and should be avoided if other drugs may be substituted.    PREGNANCY: Use of this drug in pregnancy carries substantial risk to the fetus.    RENAL OR HEPATIC DYSFUNCTION: These patients may be unable to eliminate fluorouracil normally and may accumulate toxic levels. Doses may need to be reduced.

**PREPARATIONS**    *Solution for IV use:* 50 mg/ml; *cream for topical use:* 5; *solution for topical use:* 2% or 5%.

**DRUG INTERACTIONS**    **Alkylating agents** such as chlorambucil or cyclophosphamide may predispose a patient to toxicity from floxuridine.    **Vaccines containing live virus** should be avoided because the risk of severe generalized disease is increased.

**FATE**    Fluorouracil is poorly absorbed orally and must be administered IV. Distribution through the body is rapid, and the drug may concentrate in tumors. A portion of administered drug is activated, but most of the dose is destroyed by the liver. Metabolites and a small amount of active drug are excreted in urine.

## ❧ NURSING CONSIDERATIONS

### Side effects, toxicities, and associated nursing actions

**CNS** Symptoms include ataxia, euphoria, and acute cerebellar syndrome.
• Monitor balance and ambulation, as well as mental status.
**Blood** Leukopenia is to be expected. Thrombocytopenia and anemia also occur commonly.
• See entry for drug class (p. 479) for discussion of leukopenia, thrombocytopenia, and anemia.
**GI** Nausea, vomiting, diarrhea, stomatitis, and enteritis are common. Anorexia, cramps, duodenal ulcer, duodenitis, gastritis, glossitis, pain, and pharyngitis may also occur. Ulceration and perforation of the GI tract are possible if fluorouracil is not discontinued at the first sign of excessive GI toxicity.
• Reinforce to patients the importance of notifying the physician if any GI symptoms develop.
• See entry for drug class (p. 481) for a discussion of GI side effects.
**Skin** A maculopapular rash is a common sign of fluorouracil toxicity. Alopecia, dermatitis, and diffuse erythema may also occur.
• Visually inspect the patient's skin before starting therapy and at regular intervals.
• Instruct patients to report the development of any skin changes.
• Caution the patient to avoid exposure to the sun or other sources of ultraviolet light, as exposure to light may intensify skin reactions.
**Other** Fever and nosebleed may occur.
• Caution patients to report fever that persists longer than 24 hours.
• Review with the patient the treatment of nosebleeds: pinch nares shut; bend head forward while sitting. If nosebleeds are frequent, severe, or persistent, have the patient notify the physician.

### Nursing interventions related to drug administration
• For IV use, the drug may be given undiluted. Administer the dose over 1 to 3 minutes.
• For topical use, apply with a nonmetallic applicator, clean fingertips, or gloved hand. If fingertips are used, hands should be washed thoroughly immediately after application. Occlusive dressings should be avoided as they may intensify skin reactions; a light gauze dressing may be used for cosmetic reasons.

### Patient and family education
• See entry for drug class (p. 485).

# hydroxyurea  (hye-DROX-ee-yoo-ree-ah)

antineoplastic*

- hydroxyurea: Hydrea

**MECHANISM OF ACTION**   Hydroxyurea inhibits a specific enzyme that forms the precursors of DNA. Without these precursors, DNA synthesis halts, and the cell eventually dies. Rapidly growing cells are most susceptible.

**INDICATIONS**   **Malignant melanoma** Favorable responses may occur in 20% of patients, but cures should not be expected.   **Chronic myelocytic leukemia** Hydroxyurea may be used in those cases refractory to busulfan or mercaptopurine.   **Carcinoma** Advanced ovarian carcinoma and primary squamous cell carcinoma of the head and neck may respond.

**CONTRAINDICATIONS**   **Renal dysfunction** Patients with very poor renal function may suffer excessive toxicity with hydroxyurea.   **Herpes zoster (chickenpox, shingles) infection or exposure** The risk of severe generalized disease is increased by the immunosuppressive action of hydroxyurea.   **Bone marrow suppression** Patients with marked depression may be unable to tolerate hydroxyurea.

**DOSAGE**   **PO:**   **ADULTS:** Intermittent therapy for solid tumors, 80 mg/kg once every third day. For leukemia, 20 to 30 mg/kg as a single dose daily.   *Special patient populations:*   **ELDERLY:** Elderly patients require smaller doses because they are often more sensitive to side effects caused by the drug.   **CHILDREN:** This drug is carcinogenic and should be avoided if other drugs may be substituted.   **PREGNANCY:** Use of this drug in pregnancy carries substantial risk to the fetus.

**PREPARATIONS**   *Capsules:* 500 mg.

**DRUG INTERACTIONS**   **Myelosuppressive** agents may impair bone marrow function, making patients unable to tolerate the additional myelosuppressive effects of hydroxyurea.

**FATE**   Hydroxyurea is rapidly absorbed following oral administration, producing *peak* serum concentrations within 2 hours. The drug is distributed widely, including into the CNS. Hydroxyurea is eliminated by hepatic metabolism and renal excretion.

## ☙ NURSING CONSIDERATIONS

### Side effects, toxicities, and associated nursing actions

**CNS** Convulsions, disorientation, dizziness, drowsiness, hallucinations, and headache have been reported, but the mechanism is unclear.
- Caution patients to avoid driving or operating hazardous equipment if drowsiness, dizziness, or hallucinations occur.
- Obtain careful neurologic and mental status assessment before starting therapy and at regular intervals.

**Blood** Leukopenia appears early and is the most common side effect of hydroxyurea. Thrombocytopenia and anemia may also occur. Megaloblastic erythropoiesis may occur but is self-limiting.
- See entry for drug class (p. 479) for discussion of anemia, leukopenia, and thrombocytopenia.

**GI** Anorexia, constipation, diarrhea, nausea, stomatitis, and vomiting may occur at normal doses. Ulceration of the buccal mucosa or GI epithelium may occur, especially at high doses.
- See entry for drug class (p. 481) for discussion of GI side effects.

**Renal** Renal tubular function may be depressed in some patients. BUN and serum creatinine may be elevated.
- Monitor weight and inspect for development of edema. Monitor serum creatinine and BUN.

**Liver** Hepatic enzymes may be elevated.
- Assess patients for right upper quadrant abdominal pain, jaundice, fever, malaise, and change in color or consistency of stools.
- Monitor liver function tests.

**Metabolic** Rapid cancer cell destruction can release large quantities of purines, which are metabolized to uric acid. Accumulation of uric acid may lead to renal damage or gout.
- See entry for drug class (p. 484).

*Antimetabolite.

**Allergic** Fever and chills have occurred.
- Instruct the patient to notify the physician if fever persists longer than 24 hours.

**Skin** Alopecia is rare. Facial erythema, maculopapular rash, and pruritis may also occur.
- See entry for drug class (p. 484) for discussion of alopecia.
- Instruct the patient to report any skin changes to the physician.

### Nursing interventions to drug administration
- If the patient is unable to swallow the capsule, the capsule may be opened and emptied into a glass of water and administered immediately. Some particles may float on top of the water.

### Patient and family education
- See entry for drug class (p. 485).

## lomustine    (loh-MUSS-teen)                                     antineoplastic*

- lomustine: CeeNU

**MECHANISM OF ACTION**    Lomustine causes chemical changes in nucleic acids, which may lead to inhibition of DNA and RNA synthesis. In addition the drug may alter cellular proteins. The mechanism is the same as the related drug carmustine (p. 491) and cross-resistance occurs.

**INDICATIONS**    **Brain tumors** Lomustine crosses the blood-brain barrier and may therefore be effective in controlling brain tumors. • About 40% of treated patients may respond, but cures should not be expected. **Hodgkin's disease and malignant lymphomas** Lomustine-containing combinations may be substituted when standard therapy has failed.

**CONTRAINDICATIONS**    **Myelosuppression** Patients with low platelet, leukocyte, or erythrocyte counts may be unable to tolerate the additional depression caused by lomustine. **Herpes zoster (chickenpox, shingles) infection or exposure** The risk of severe generalized disease is increased by the immunosuppressive action of lomustine.

**DOSAGE**    **PO:**    **ADULTS AND CHILDREN:** Initial therapy, 130 mg/M$^2$ as a single dose. Retreatment must be delayed at least 6 weeks or longer to allow production of leukocytes and platelets to recover. *Special patient populations:*    **CHILDREN:** This drug is carcinogenic and should be avoided if other drugs may be substituted.    **PREGNANCY:** Use of this drug in pregnancy carries substantial risk to the fetus.

**PREPARATIONS**    *Capsules:* 10, 40, and 100 mg.

**DRUG INTERACTIONS**    **Cimetidine** may cause additive bone marrow suppression when given with lomustine. The combination should be avoided if possible.

**FATE**    Lomustine is rapidly absorbed following oral administration. The drug rapidly crosses the blood-brain barrier, achieving substantial concentrations in the CNS and other tissues or fluids, including milk. Lomustine is rapidly converted to active metabolites that may persist for long periods in the body. The drug is eliminated primarily by renal routes.

### 🐝 NURSING CONSIDERATIONS
#### Side effects, toxicities, and associated nursing actions

**CNS** Ataxia, disorientation, dysarthria, and lethargy are rare.
- Assess for CNS side effects. Caution patients to avoid driving or operating hazardous equipment if ataxia or other CNS effects appear.

**Blood** Hematologic toxicity is the dose-limiting side effect of lomustine. Effectively treated patients should be expected to show changes in blood composition. Thrombocytopenia is the most severe change, with lowest platelet counts appearing 4 to 5 weeks after therapy. Leukocyte counts are lowest 5 to 6 weeks after therapy. Anemia may also occur.
- See entry for drug class (p. 479) for discussion of leukopenia, thrombocytopenia, and anemia.

**GI** Nausea and vomiting should be expected in nearly all patients, occurring within 45 minutes and

*DNA alkylator.

persisting for up to 6 hours. Anorexia may persist for 2 or 3 days thereafter.
- See entry for drug class (p. 481)

**Liver** High doses of lomustine cause reversible hepatotoxocity. Serum transaminase, alkaline phosphatase, and bilirubin concentrations may be increased.
- Assess patients for fever, malaise, jaundice, right upper quadrant abdominal pain, and change in color or consistency of stools.
- Monitor liver function tests.

**Renal** Large cumulative doses may cause progressive azotemia, decreased kidney size, and even renal failure.
- Monitor weight and blood pressure. Assess for development of edema. Monitor intake and output if renal involvement is suspected.
- Monitor serum creatinine and BUN.

**Lung** Prolonged therapy may cause pulmonary infiltrates and fibrosis.
- Monitor respiratory rate. Assess for dyspnea and cough. Auscultate breath sounds.

**Skin** Hyperpigmentation may occur when the drug accidentally contacts skin.
- Wear gloves while preparing doses. If drug contacts skin, wash the area immediately with copious amounts of water.

**Other** Alopecia may occur.
- See entry for drug class (p. 484) for discussion of alopecia.

### Nursing interventions related to drug administration
- See entry for drug class (p. 485).

### Patient and family education
- See entry for drug class (p. 485).
- Point out to patients that in order to prepare the correct dose, the pharmacist may supply the patient with several capsules in varying color and doses; all of the capsules should be taken at the same time to achieve the ordered dose.

## mechlorethamine hydrochloride    (meh-klor-ETH-a-meen)    antineoplastic*

- mechlorethamine hydrochloride: Mustargen

**MECHANISM OF ACTION**    Mechlorethamine changes the properties of DNA by chemically changing (alkylating) its structure. Without fully functional DNA, cells eventually die. Rapidly growing cells are most susceptible. Mechlorethamine is weakly immunosuppressive.

**INDICATIONS**    **Hodgkin's disease and malignant lymphomas** Mechlorethamine is extremely effective in treating Hodgkin's disease, with up to 80% of patients with advanced disease achieving remission when treated with combinations including mechlorethamine (MOPP, p. 479). • Cures are frequent. • Lymphosarcoma may be treated with the MOPP regimen, but therapy is only palliative. **Carcinomas** Bronchogenic, ovarian, and breast carcinomas may respond for short periods. **Leukemias** Chronic myelogenous leukemia is rarely treated with combinations including mechlorethamine. **Mycosis fungoides, polycythemia vera** These unusual neoplastic diseases may respond to mechlorethamine, but treatment is usually palliative.

**CONTRAINDICATIONS**    **Active infections** Mechlorethamine may diminish immune function and exacerbate infections. • Patients with foci of acute or chronic suppurative inflammation may develop amyloidosis. • Normally mild herpes zoster infections may blossom to generalized fatal infections. **Chronic lymphocytic leukemia** These patients are extremely sensitive to the bone marrow suppression produced by mechlorethamine.

**DOSAGE**    **IV:**    **ADULTS:** 0.4 mg/kg as a single dose or equally divided over 2 or 4 days. Treatment must not be repeated until bone marrow function recovers, usually at 3 to 6 weeks. In the MOPP regimen, mechlorethamine doses are 6 mg/$M^2$ on days 1 and 8 of the 28 day schedule. *Special patient*

*DNA alkylator.

*populations:* **ELDERLY:** Elderly patients may be more susceptible to neurotoxicity. **CHILDREN:** This drug is carcinogenic and should be avoided if other drugs may be substituted. **PREGNANCY:** Use of this drug in pregnancy carries substantial risk to the fetus.

**PREPARATIONS** *Powder for reconstitution:* 10 mg. Reconstitute immediately before use by adding 10 ml sterile water for injection of 0.9% sodium chloride injection to the 10 mg vial. With the needle still in the rubber stopper, shake to dissolve. The solution is 1 mg/ml. Do not dilute into large volumes for administration, but administer directly into the tubing or sidearm of a freely flowing IV line. Wear gloves and avoid skin contact or inhalation of drug.

**DRUG INTERACTIONS** **Myelosuppressive** agents may impair bone marrow function, making patients unable to tolerate the additional myelosuppressive effects of mechlorethamine. **Procarbazine or cyclophosphamide** may predispose patients to neurotoxicity with mechlorethamine, especially at high doses. **Vaccines containing live virus** should be avoided because the risk of severe generalized disease is increased.

**FATE** Mechlorethamine is highly irritating and cannot be tolerated by any route except IV and occasionally intracavitary. This highly chemically reactive agent disappears from the blood within 1 minute of administration and is destroyed by tissues.

## ❦ NURSING CONSIDERATIONS

### Side effects, toxicities, and associated nursing actions

**CNS** Cerebral degeneration, coma, convulsions, drowsiness, headache, lightheadedness, progressive muscular paralysis, paresthesia, vertigo, and weakness may occur. High doses are responsible for the more serious side effects, which may include death.

- Assess neurologic function thoroughly and periodically.
- Caution patients to avoid driving or operating hazardous equipment if drowsiness, vertigo, weakness, or other CNS side effects occur.
- Calculate drug dosages carefully.

**Blood** Anemia, severe leukopenia, thrombocytopenia, and hemorrhagic diathesis may occur. One or more of these side effects often limits therapy with mechlorethamine. Mechlorethamine is extremely irritating to tissues and may cause pain, inflammation, and sloughing of tissues if allowed to extravasate.

- See entry for drug class (p. 479).
- Ascertain that the IV is patent before administering doses. Instruct the patient to report any pain or irritation. Do not leave the patient unattended during infusion. If extravasation occurs, discontinue the infusion. Aspirate infiltrated drug if possible. Promptly infiltrate the area with sterile isotonic sodium thiosulfate injection (dilute 4 ml of sodium thiosulfate injection [10%] with 6 ml of sterile water for injection), then apply cold compresses for 6 to 12 hours.
- Wear gloves and goggles while preparing the drug. If the drug comes in direct contact with skin, wash immediately with copious amounts of water for 15 minutes, then rinse with a 2% sodium thiosulfate solution. If the drug comes in contact with the eye, irrigate immediately with 0.9% sodium chloride or balanced salt ophthalmic solution, then promptly consult an ophthalmologist.

**GI** Up to 90% of patients experience nausea and severe vomiting. Violent vomiting has caused vascular accidents in some patients. Anorexia and diarrhea may also occur.

- See entry for drug class (p. 481).

**Metabolic** Rapid cancer cell destruction can release large quantities of purines, which are metabolized to uric acid. Accumulation of uric acid may lead to renal damage or gout.

- See entry for drug class (p. 484).

**Allergic** Topical mechlorethamine sensitizes many patients and may cause dermatitis.

- See Nursing Interventions under Blood. Mechlorethamine may be used in topical ointments or solutions. Patients should wear protective gloves when applying topical drug. Have the patient apply the drug to the entire body (or as ordered), but sparingly to the axillary, perineal, inguinal, and inframammary areas.
- Assess skin condition on a regular, systematic basis.
- Have drugs, equipment, and personnel available to treat acute allergic reactions in settings where mechlorethamine is administered.

**Reproductive** Amenorrhea, azoospermia, and total germinal aplasia have occurred.
- See entry for drug class (p. 484).

**Other** Alopecia, tinnitus, hearing loss, and a metallic taste are rare side effects.
- See entry for drug class (p. 484) for a discussion of alopecia.
- Obtain a baseline evaluation of hearing, and assess for tinnitus, strange noises, and hearing loss at regular intervals.

### Nursing interventions related to drug administration
- See entry for drug class (p. 485).
- For IV use, see Blood. See Preparations. Drug must be prepared immediately before use and administered within minutes of preparation. Administer the dose over 3 to 5 minutes.

### Patient and family education
- See entry for drug class (p. 485).

## melphalan   (MEL-fah-lan)                                    antineoplastic*

- melphalan: Alkeran

**MECHANISM OF ACTION**   Melphalan alters the properties of DNA by chemically changing (alkylating) its structure. Without fully functional DNA, cells eventually die. Rapidly growing cells are most susceptible. Melphalan is weakly immunosuppressive.

**INDICATIONS**   **Multiple myeloma** Melphalan alone or in combinations may prolong life in some patients. **Carcinoma** Ovarian carcinoma unsuitable for surgery may respond to melphalan. • Objective improvement may be seen in up to 50% of patients, but cures should not be expected.

**CONTRAINDICATIONS**   **Myelosuppression** Myelosuppression caused by irradiation or chemotherapy may make patients unable to tolerate the additional myelosuppression caused by melphalan. **Herpes zoster (chickenpox, shingles) infection or exposure** The risk of severe generalized disease is increased by the immunosuppressive action of melphalan. **Allergy to chlorambucil or related drugs** Persons who developed rashes following treatment with chlorambucil may not tolerate the chemically related drug, melphalan.

**DOSAGE**   **PO:** **ADULTS:** Usual doses are 6 mg as a single daily dose for 2 to 3 weeks, as allowed by bone marrow function. Maintenance doses may be 2 mg daily. *Special patient populations:* **CHILDREN:** This drug is carcinogenic and should be avoided if other drugs may be substituted. **PREGNANCY:** Use of this drug in pregnancy carries substantial risk to the fetus.

**PREPARATIONS**   *Tablets:* 2 mg.

**DRUG INTERACTIONS**   **Myelosuppressive** agents may impair bone marrow function, making patients unable to tolerate the additional myelosuppressive effects of melphalan. **Vaccines containing live virus** should be avoided because the risk of severe generalized disease is increased.

**FATE**   Oral absorption of melphalan is extremely variable, but *peak* concentrations in plasma are reached within 2 hours. A portion of the dose is metabolized. Melphalan and its metabolites are eliminated primarily by the kidneys, with elimination *half-lives* ranging from 1.5 to 4.5 hours.

### ☙ NURSING CONSIDERATIONS
#### Side effects, toxicities, and associated nursing actions
**Blood** Leukopenia and thrombocytopenia are the major dose-limiting side effects of melphalan. Anemia, pancytopenia, and agranulocytosis may also occur. Hemolytic anemia has been reported.
- See entry for drug class (p. 479) for a discussion of blood-related side effects.

**GI** Nausea and vomiting are uncommon unless large doses are used. Diarrhea, oral ulceration, and stomatitis have been reported.
- See entry for drug class (p. 481).

**Lung** Bronchopulmonary dysplasia and pulmonary interstitial fibrosis may occur with prolonged therapy.

*DNA alkylator.

- Monitor pulmonary function: auscultate lung sounds for rales, rhonchi, and pleural friction rubs. Assess the patient for dyspnea and cough. Monitor serial chest x-rays if available.

**Skin** Dermatitis, pruritis, maculopapular and urticarial rashes may occur. Alopecia is uncommon.

- See entry for drug class (p. 484) for a discussion of alopecia.
- Instruct patients to report the development of any skin changes.

**Allergic** Anaphylaxis has been reported. Parenteral melphalan seems to have been associated with more frequent allergic reactions.

- Have drugs, equipment, and personnel available to treat acute allergic reactions in settings where melphalan is used.

### Nursing interventions related to drug administration

- See entry for drug class (p. 485).

### Patient and family education

- See entry for drug class (p. 485).

---

## mercaptopurine　(mer-kap-toh-PYOO-reen)　antineoplastic*

- mercaptopurine: Purinethol, 6MP

**MECHANISM OF ACTION**　Mercaptopurine mimics a natural purine and is activated to a form that inhibits synthesis of DNA and RNA. Without functional nucleic acids, cells eventually die. Rapidly growing cells are most susceptible. Mercaptopurine is also a powerful imune suppressant, with greatest effect on humoral responses.

**INDICATIONS**　**Leukemias** Mercaptopurine is used in combinations for acute lymphoblastic leukemia; up to 90% of patients achieve complete remissions. • Mercaptopurine is often a component of maintenance regimens. • Mercaptopurine may also be used in chronic myelocytic leukemia, causing temporary remissions in up to 50% of patients.　**Immune suppression** Mercaptopurine has been used to suppress homograph rejection and to control certain autoimmune diseases, but such use is now rare.

**CONTRANDICATIONS**　**Myelosuppression** Myelosuppression caused by irradiation or chemotherapy may make patients unable to tolerate the additional myelosuppression caused by mercaptopurine.　**Herpes zoster (chickenpox, shingles) infection or exposure** The risk of severe generalized disease is increased by the immunosuppressive action of mercaptopurine.

**DOSAGE**　PO:　**ADULTS AND CHILDREN:** Doses are individualized, but usual doses for induction are 2.5 mg/kg daily. • Maintenance dosage is usually 1.5 to 2.5 mg/kg daily.　**CHILDREN:** Doses of 70 mg/$M^2$ daily have been used.　*Special patient populations:*　**CHILDREN:** This drug is carcinogenic and should be avoided if other drugs may be substituted.　**PREGNANCY:** Use of this drug in pregnancy carries substantial risk to the fetus.　**RENAL OR HEPATIC IMPAIRMENT:** Lower doses may be required.

**PREPARATIONS**　*Tablets:* 50 mg.

**DRUG INTERACTIONS**　**Myelosuppressive** agents may impair bone marrow function, making patients unable to tolerate the additional myelosuppressive effects of mercaptopurine.　**Allopurinol** inhibits metabolism of mercaptopurine, requiring that dosage of mercaptopurine be reduced to avoid toxicity. **Doxorubicin** may enhance hepatotoxicity of mercaptopurine.　**Hepatotoxic** agents may potentiate the liver damage caused by mercaptopurine.　**Vaccines containing live virus** should be avoided because the risk of severe generalized disease is increased.　**Warfarin** action may be altered in the presence of mercaptopurine.

**DIAGNOSTIC TEST INTERFERENCE**　**Serum glucose and uric acid** determinations may be falsely elevated when a sequential multiple analyzer (SMA) is used.

**FATE**　Absorption of mercaptopurine following oral administration is quite variable, but bioavailability is less than 50% for most patients. *Peak* concentrations are achieved within 2 hours. Elimination of urine.

*Purine antimetabolite.

### ☙ NURSING CONSIDERATIONS

#### Side effects, toxicities, and associated nursing actions

**CNS** Headaches occasionally occur.
* Instruct patients to notify the physician if headaches are severe or persistent.

**Blood** Leukopenia, anemia, and thrombocytopenia are to be expected and may occasionally become severe. These reactions are usually dose-limiting. Agranulocytosis and pancytopenia are less common.
* See entry for drug class (p. 479) for blood-related side effects.

**GI** Abdominal pain, anorexia, diarrhea, epigastric distress, mucositis, nausea, oral lesions, spruelike symptoms, ulceration of the intestinal epithelium, and vomiting may occur.
* See entry for drug class (p. 481).

**Renal** Flank pain, hematuria, crystalluria, oliguria, and renal insufficiency are uncommon.
* Assess for flank pain and subjective changes in urinary output or color of urine. Monitor weight.
* Monitor urinalysis, serum creatinine, and BUN.

**Metabolic** Rapid cancer cell destruction can release large quantities of purines, which are metabolized to uric acid. Accumulation of uric acid may lead to renal damage or gout.
* See entry for drug class (p. 484).

**Skin** Cutaneous hyperpigmentation, lichenoid papular eruption, and rash are infrequent.
* Instruct patients to report any skin changes.

**Liver** Deaths from hepatic necrosis have occurred. Ascites, cholestasis, hepatic encephalopathy, and jaundice may arise quickly. Jaundice may occur in up to 40% of patients with leukemia who receive mercaptopurine. The incidence is higher as dosage increases.
* Assess patients for right upper quadrant abdominal pain, fever, malaise, change in color or consistency of stools, and jaundice.
* Monitor liver function tests.

**Other** Fever and excessive weakness have been reported.
* Instruct the patient to report any fever that persists longer than 24 hours.

#### Nursing interventions related to drug administration
* See entry for drug class (p. 485).

#### Patient and family education
* See entry for drug class (p. 485).

---

## methotrexate
## methotrexate sodium    (meth-oh-TREX-ate)                    antineoplastic*

* methotrexate: Folex, Mexate, Amethopterin, or generic

**MECHANISM OF ACTION**    Methotrexate blocks the action of a natural folate required for synthesis of precursors of DNA. Without precursors, DNA synthesis fails, and cells eventually die. Rapidly growing cells are most susceptible. Methotrexate is also an immune suppressant.

**INDICATIONS**    **Trophoblastic neoplasms** Choriocarcinoma, chorioadenoma destruens, and hydatidiform mole respond well. • Over 75% of patients achieve complete remissions; most patients are cured.    **Leukemias** Acute lymphocytic leukemia is well controlled with chemotherapy; methotrexate is a valuable component of maintenance regimens. • Intrathecal methotrexate is used to control CNS leukemia. **Carcinomas** Carcinomas of lung, breast, head, or neck may respond to methotrexate alone or in combinations, but treatment is palliative.    **Burkitt's lymphoma** Burkitt's lymphoma and lymphosarcoma may respond to methotrexate.    **Mycosis fungoides** Advanced cases may respond to methotrexate.    **Psoriasis** Only severe, disabling disease resistant to safer forms of therapy should be treated with methotrexate.

*Folate antagonist.

**CONTRAINDICATIONS    Myelosuppression** Myelosuppression caused by irradiation or chemotherapy may make patients unable to tolerate the additional myelosuppression caused by methotrexate.    **Infections** The immune suppression caused by methotrexate may exacerbate infections. • Normally mild herpes zoster infections may produce severe generalized disease that is potentially fatal.    **Hepatic damage** Patients with liver damage or a history of excessive alcohol intake may be more susceptible to the hepatotoxicity caused by methotrexate.

**DOSAGE    PO:    ADULTS:** For trophoblastic neoplasms, 15 to 30 mg daily for 5 days, to be repeated after at least 1 week if the toxicity level permits. For leukemia, 3.3 mg/M$^2$ daily with prednisone for 4 to 6 weeks to achieve remission or 20 to 30 mg/M$^2$ twice weekly to maintain remission. For Burkitt's lymphoma, 10 to 25 mg/M$^2$ daily for 4 to 8 days. For lymphosarcoma, 0.625 to 2.5 mg/kg daily in combinations with other drugs. For mycosis fungoides, 2.5 to 10 mg daily for weeks or months.    **CHILDREN:** For leukemia, 3.3 mg/M$^2$ daily with prednisone for 4 to 6 weeks to achieve remission or 20 to 30 mg/M$^2$ twice weekly to maintain remission.    **IV:    ADULTS AND CHILDREN:** For leukemia, 2.5 mg/kg every 14 days.    **IM:    ADULTS:** For trophoblastic neoplasms, 15 to 30 mg daily for 5 days, to be repeated after at least 1 week if the toxicity level permits. For leukemia, 20 to 30 mg/M$^2$ twice weekly to maintain remission. For mycosis fungoides, 50 mg once weekly or 25 mg twice weekly.    **CHILDREN:** For leukemia, 20 to 30 mg/M$^2$ twice weekly to maintain remission.    **Intrathecal:    ADULTS AND CHILDREN:** For meningeal leukemia, 12 mg/M$^2$ or 15 mg every 2 to 5 days until the clinical response is adequate. Preservative-free preparations should be used by this route.    *Special patient populations:*    **PREGNANCY:** FDA pregnancy category D.    **IMPAIRED RENAL FUNCTION:** Methotrexate may accumulate dangerously in these patients.

**PREPARATIONS    Methotrexate** *Tablets:* 2.5 mg.    **Methotrexate sodium** *Solution for parenteral use:* 2.5 mg/ml or 25 mg/ml, with benzyl alcohol and sodium chloride; *powder for reconstitution:* 20, 25, 50, 100, or 250 mg without preservatives. To reconstitute, add 0.9% sodium chloride or 5% dextrose injection without preservatives.

**DRUG INTERACTIONS    Aspirin, chloramphenicol, phenylbutazone, phenytoin, salicylates, sulfonamides, and sulfonylureas** may displace methotrexate from plasma proteins, resulting in increased toxicity.    **Salicylates and other weak organic acids** may partially block methotrexate excretion, increasing accumulation and toxicity.    **Indomethacin, ketoprofen,** and other nonsteroidal anti-inflammatory agents can cause a fatal reaction involving elevations in methotrexate concentrations in blood.    **Pyrimethamine and other dihydrofolate reductase inhibitors** act by the same mechanism as methotrexate and may combine to cause folate depletion in patients.    **Live virus vaccines** may cause generalized disease in patients receiving methotrexate because of the immunosuppressive activity of methotrexate.    **High doses of folic acid** may antagonize the anticancer action of methotrexate.    **Leucovorin** may be used to rescue normal cells from the lethal effects of high doses of methotrexate. Leucovorin, which supplies folic acid, may be given some time after a large dose of methotrexate. Normal cells are better able to transport folic acid inside the cell and are rescued; the cancer cells exposed to methotrexate fail to acquire sufficient folic acid and die.

**FATE** Methotrexate is well absorbed following oral administration, producing *peak* plasma concentrations within 1 to 4 hours; peaks are achieved within 0.5 to 2 hours with IM doses. The drug is actively transported into many tissues and remains bound in liver and kidneys for weeks or months. The serum *half-life* is 2 to 4 hours, with excretion by the kidneys as unchanged drug.

## 🐝 NURSING CONSIDERATIONS

### Side effects, toxicities, and associated nursing actions

**CNS** Intrathecal administration may be associated with a variety of symptoms, including chemical arachnoiditis (headache, back pain, nuchal rigidity, or fever), paresis, leukoencephalopathy (confusion, irritability, ataxia, dementia, somnolence, seizures), and increases in CSF pressure. Systemic administration occasionally causes blurred vision, dizziness, drowsiness, headaches, and malaise.

• Obtain a thorough mental status and neurologic assessment before therapy and at regular intervals. Monitor temperature.

- Caution patients to avoid driving or operating hazardous equipment if blurred vision, dizziness, drowsiness, somnolence, or ataxia occur; notify the physician.
- Keep side rails up, supervise ambulation, and keep a night light on as needed.
- Instruct patients and families to notify the physician of any unusual sign or symptom.

**Blood** Leukopenia, thrombocytopenia, anemia, and hemorrhage are common and may arise rapidly.
- See entry for drug class (p. 479).

**GI** Damage to GI epithelium is usually one of the earliest signs of toxicity. Symptoms include abdominal distress, anorexia, diarrhea, gingivitis, glossitis, enteritis, hematemesis, nausea, melena, pharyngitis, stomatitis, ulcerations of the mucous membranes lining the GI tract, and vomiting.
- See entry for drug class (p. 481).

**Renal** Azotemia, hematuria, and acute renal failure leading to death have occurred.
- Monitor weight, and inspect for development of edema.
- Monitor urinalysis, serum creatinine, and BUN.
- Assess the patient for subjective changes in urinary output and changes in color of urine.

**Liver** Atrophy, cirrhosis, fatty changes, fibrosis, and necrosis have all occurred. Incidence seems highest with small, frequent doses administered for prolonged periods.
- Assess patients for right upper quadrant abdominal pain, fever, malaise, change in color or consistency of stools, and jaundice.
- Monitor liver function tests.

**Skin** Alopecia, acne, depigmentation, ecchymoses, folliculitis, furunculosis, hyperpigmentation, petechiae, photosensitivity, pruritis, rashes, and telangiectasia occur in a few patients.
- See entry for drug class (p. 484) for discussion of alopecia.
- Instruct patients to report the development of skin changes.
- If photosensitivity develops, caution patients to avoid exposure to the sun or other sources of ultraviolet light, to wear a large-brimmed hat, to keep extremities covered, and to use a maximum-protection sunscreen on exposed skin surfaces.

**Metabolic** Rapid cancer cell destruction can release large quantities of purines, which are metabolized to uric acid. Accumulation of uric acid may lead to renal damage or gout.
- See entry for drug class (p. 484).

**Allergic** Chills and fever may occur.
- Instruct patients to report fever that persists longer than 24 hours.

**Reproductive** Infertility, with defective oogenesis or spermatogenesis, transient oligospermia, and menstrual dysfunction occur.
- See entry for drug class (p. 484).

**Other** Diabetes may be precipitated.
- Monitor serum and urinary glucose levels.
- Instruct diabetic patients to monitor blood glucose levels on a regular basis. Insulin and/or diet prescriptions may need to be adjusted.

## Nursing interventions related to drug administration
- For IV use, see Preparations. Reconstitute powder to a dilution of 2.5 mg/ml. Administer each 10 mg over at least 1 minute.
- Leucovorin rescue may be used with high-dose methotrexate. The patient is kept well hydrated. The urine may be alkalinized to increase the solubility of the methotrexate; usually sodium bicarbonate is used. Monitor intake, output, and renal function tests.

## Patient and family education
- Note Drug Interactions. Caution patients to avoid the use of any medications unless approved by the physician.
- Instruct the patient to clear the use of vitamin supplements with the physician before use. Preparations containing folic acid may alter the patient's response to methotrexate.
- Caution patients to limit alcohol consumption while receiving methotrexate.
- See entry for drug class (p. 485).

## mitomycin    (my-toh-MY-sin)    antineoplastic*

- mitomycin: Mutamycin, Mitomycin-C

**MECHANISM OF ACTION**    Mitomycin alters the properties of DNA by chemically changing (cross-linking) its structure. Without fully functional DNA, cells eventually die. Rapidly growing cells are most susceptible.

**INDICATIONS**    **Adenocarcinoma** Tumors of the stomach and pancreas may respond to multidrug regimens including mitomycin. • Therapy is palliative, not curative. Adenocarcinoma of the breast also occasionally responds.    **Chronic myelocytic leukemia** Treatment may include a variety of drugs.

**CONTRAINDICATIONS**    **Myelosuppression** Myelosuppression caused by irradiation or chemotherapy may make patients unable to tolerate the additional myelosuppression caused by mitomycin.    **Herpes zoster (chickenpox, shingles) infection or exposure** The risk of severe generalized disease is increased by the immunosuppressive action of mitomycin.

**DOSAGE**    IV:    ADULTS: Usual doses are 20 mg/$M^2$ once every 6 to 8 weeks.    *Special patient populations:* CHILDREN: This drug is carcinogenic and should be avoided if other drugs may be substituted. PREGNANCY: Use of this drug in pregnancy carries substantial risk to the fetus.

**PREPARATIONS**    *Powder for reconstitution:* 5 or 20 mg. Reconstitute by adding 10 ml to the 5 mg vial or 40 ml to the 20 mg vial. The resulting solutions are 0.5 mg/ml. Shake or let stand at room temperature to facilitate dissolution.

**DRUG INTERACTIONS**    **Myelosuppressive** agents may impair bone marrow function, making patients unable to tolerate the additional myelosuppressive effects of mitomycin.    **Vaccines containing live virus** should be avoided because the risk of severe generalized disease is increased.

**FATE**    Mitomycin is rapidly taken into tissues following IV administration but is rapidly inactivated at some sites (brain, spleen, and liver). Tumors have varying capacity to degrade mitomycin. Little drug is eliminated in urine.

### 🐦 NURSING CONSIDERATIONS

#### Side effects, toxicities, and associated nursing actions

**Blood** Cumulative myelosuppression is the common limiting side effect of mitomycin therapy. Thrombocytopenia and leukopenia are much more common than anemia. Up to 40% of patients suffer thrombocytopenia, and leukopenia occurs in about 50%. Pain at the injection site, thrombophlebitis, and necrosis with extravasation also occur.
- See entry for drug class (p. 479).
- Ascertain that the IV is patent before administering the dose.
- Instruct the patient to report the development of pain or irritation. Do not leave the patient unattended during drug administration.

**GI** Anorexia, nausea, or vomiting occur within 2 hours of therapy and may persist for 2 to 3 days. Mouth ulcers may occur in 4% of patients.
- See entry for drug class (p. 481).

**Renal** Increased BUN and/or serum creatinine occur in 2% of patients.
- Monitor serum creatinine and BUN.
- Monitor intake, output, and weight if renal involvement is suspected. Inspect for development of edema.

**Lung** Dyspnea, coughing, hemoptysis, and pneumonia may develop. Acute bronchospasm has occurred in a few patients.
- Assess for pulmonary side effects; auscultate lung sounds.

#### Nursing interventions related to drug administration
- See Preparations for reconstitution. Administer dose over 5 to 10 minutes, or further dilute in normal saline or 5% dextrose and administer as an infusion. Adjust the rate of infusion as appropriate to dose and volume of fluid. Diluted doses are stable at room temperature for 3 hours.

#### Patient and family education
- See entry for drug class (p. 485).

*DNA cross-linker.

# mitoxantrone hydrochloride   (my-TOX-an-trone)   antineoplastic*

● mitoxantrone hydrochloride (investigational U.S.): ✿Novantrone

**MECHANISM OF ACTION**   Mitoxantrone interacts with DNA to block nucleic acid synthesis.

**INDICATIONS**   **Carcinoma of the breast** Advanced or metastatic disease may respond.   **Lymphomas or leukemias** Mitoxantrone may be used in adult patients whose disease has relapsed following conventional therapy.   **Hepatoma** Some patients may respond.

**CONTRAINDICATIONS**   **Hypersensitivity to related drugs** Mitoxantrone is chemically related to doxorubicin and daunorubicin and may be cross-allergic with them.

**DOSAGE**   IV:   ADULTS: 14 mg/M$^2$ as a single dose, repeated at 21 day intervals.   *Special patient populations:*   CHILDREN: Pediatric doses are not established.   PREGNANCY: Use of this drug in pregnancy carries substantial risk to the fetus.

**PREPARATIONS**   Solution, for injection: 2 mg/ml. Solutions of this drug should be clear and dark blue. Dilute to at least 50 ml with sodium chloride for injection or dextrose 5%.

**DRUG INTERACTIONS**   **Myelosuppressive agents** may cause intolerable bone marrow suppression in patients who are also receiving mitoxantrone.

**FATE**   Mitoxantrone is rapidly cleared from plasma and distributed to tissues, where it remains bound for prolonged periods. The drug does not enter the CNS.

## ☙ NURSING CONSIDERATIONS

### Side effects, toxicities, and associated nursing actions

**CV** Congestive heart failure developed in 0.9% of treated patients. Acute arrhythmias, ECG changes, and decreased cardiac function may also occur.
● Monitor intake, output, and weight. Auscultate lung sounds. Inspect for jugular venous distention and development of edema, especially in dependent areas. Monitor pulse, blood pressure, and respiratory rate. Monitor serial electrocardiograms.

**Blood** Leukopenia is common, but it is usually mild.
● See entry for drug class (p. 479).

**GI** About 8% of patients suffer moderate nausea and vomiting; 3.5% suffer severe nausea and vomiting. Diarrhea occurs in up to 13% of patients. Moderate to severe mucositis or stomatitis occurs in up to 29% of patients. Anorexia, constipation, and GI bleeding are uncommon.
● See entry for drug class (p. 481).

**Liver** Moderate or severe jaundice or hepatitis is seen in up to 8% of patients.
● Assess patients for right upper quadrant abdominal pain, fever, malaise, jaundice, and change in color or consistency of stools.
● Monitor liver function tests.

**Skin** Alopecia occurs in up to 11% of patients.
● See entry for drug class (p. 484).

**Other** Amenorrhea, dyspnea, fatigue, and weakness have been reported. Tissue necrosis may rarely occur following extravasation.
● Caution female patients to keep a record of menstrual periods. Counsel about the use of birth control as needed. See entry for drug class (p. 484).
● Ascertain that the IV is patent before administering IV doses. Instruct patients to report the development of pain or discomfort during infusion. Do not leave the patient unattended during drug administration.
● Instruct patients to report the development of any unexpected sign or symptom.

### Nursing interventions related to drug administration
● Check the manufacturer's literature for most current information about this drug.
● See entry for drug class (p. 485).

### Patient and family education
● See entry for drug class (p. 485).

*DNA intercalator.

## pipobroman    (pi-poh-BROH-man)                                    antineoplastic*

- pipobroman: Vercyte

**MECHANISM OF ACTION**    Pipobroman alters the properties of DNA by chemically changing (alkylating) its structure. Without fully functional DNA, cells eventually die. Rapidly growing cells are most susceptible.

**INDICATIONS**    **Polycythemia vera** Pipobroman may be effective in patients failing standard therapy.    **Chronic myelocytic leukemia** Pipobroman may be useful in patients whose disease is refractory to standard therapy.

**CONTRAINDICATIONS**    **Myelosuppression** Myelosuppression caused by irradiation or chemotherapy may make patients unable to tolerate the additional myelosuppression caused by pipobroman.

**DOSAGE**    **PO:**    **ADULTS:** For polycythemia vera, 1 mg/kg daily for 30 days or longer, after which the dose may be increased if toxicity allows. For leukemia, 1.5 to 2.5 mg/kg daily until a response is achieved or toxicity intervenes. Maintenance doses are lower. *Special patient populations:* **CHILDREN:** Pipobroman should not be used in patients younger than 15 years.    **PREGNANCY:** Use of this drug in pregnancy carries substantial risk to the fetus.

**PREPARATIONS**    *Tablets:* 25 mg.

**DRUG INTERACTIONS**    **Myelosuppressive** agents may impair bone marrow function, making patients unable to tolerate the additional myelosuppressive effects of pipobroman.

**FATE**    Pipobroman is well absorbed following oral administration, but the fate of the drug in the body is not yet known.

### ☙ NURSING CONSIDERATIONS

#### Side effects, toxicities, and associated nursing actions

**Blood** Bone marrow suppression is the common dose-limiting side effect, causing leukopenia, thrombocytopenia, and anemia. Hemolysis may also occur.
- See entry for drug class (p. 479).

**GI** Abdominal cramping, anorexia, diarrhea, nausea, and vomiting may occur.
- See entry for drug class (p. 481).

**Allergic** Rashes may occur.
- Instruct patients to report the development of any skin changes.

#### Nursing interventions related to drug administration
- See entry for drug class (p. 485).

#### Patient and family education
- See entry for drug class (p. 485).

## plicamycin    (plik-uh-MY-sin)                                    antineoplastic†

- plicamycin: Mithracin

**MECHANISM OF ACTION**    Plicamycin binds tightly to double-stranded DNA, thereby preventing RNA formation from the natural genetic template. Without functional nucleic acids, cells eventually die. Rapidly growing cells are most susceptible. Plicamycin also has a hypocalcemic effect produced by an unknown mechanism.

**INDICATIONS**    **Testicular tumors** Advanced tumors unresponsive to other therapy may respond to plicamycin. **Hypercalciuria and hypercalcemia** Certain advanced neoplasms cause hypercalcemia and hypercalciuria. • Plicamycin may reduce the calcium concentration, even if no anticancer effect is achieved.

**CONTRAINDICATIONS**    **Myelosuppression** Myelosuppression caused by irradiation or chemotherapy may make patients unable to tolerate the additional myelosuppression caused by plicamycin.    **Renal or**

*DNA alkylator.
†DNA intercalator.

**hepatic impairment** These patients may suffer irreversible toxicity from plicamycin. **Herpes zoster (chickenpox, shingles) infection or exposure** The risk of severe generalized disease is increased by the immunosuppressive action of plicamycin.

**DOSAGE** IV: ADULTS: For testicular cancer, 25 to 30 µg/kg once daily for 8 to 10 days unless toxicity intervenes. For hypercalcemia, 25 µg/kg daily for 3 to 4 days. Intermittent doses may also be used. *Special patient populations:* ELDERLY: Because renal function is often reduced in the elderly, these patients may be very sensitive to toxicity associated with plicamycin. CHILDREN: This drug is carcinogenic and should be avoided if other drugs may be substituted. PREGNANCY: Use of this drug in pregnancy carries substantial risk to the fetus.

**PREPARATIONS** *Powder for reconstitution:* 2.5 mg. Reconstitute by adding 4.9 ml of sterile water for injection to the 2.5 mg vial. This solution is 500 µg/ml. The dose may be diluted into 1 liter of 0.9% sodium chloride or 5% dextrose injection.

**DRUG INTERACTIONS** **Myelosuppressive** agents may impair bone marrow function, making patients unable to tolerate the additional myelosuppressive effects of plicamycin. **Vaccines containing live virus** should be avoided because the risk of severe generalized disease is increased. **Valproic acid** may increase risk of hemorrhage with plicamycin.

**FATE** Plicamycin enters the CNS as well as other tissues and is bound in liver, kidney, and bone. Excretion is through the kidneys.

### ❦ NURSING CONSIDERATIONS

#### Side effects, toxicities, and associated nursing actions

**CNS** Depression, drowsiness, dizziness, fatigue, headache, irritability, lethargy, malaise, and nervousness may occur.
- Obtain a thorough baseline assessment of mental status, and repeat at regular intervals.
- Caution patients to avoid driving or operating hazardous equipment if drowsiness, dizziness, fatigue, or lethargy occur; notify the physician.

**Blood** Thrombocytopenia with bleeding episodes may occur in 5.4% of patients; the mortality rate was 1.6%. The incidence increases with higher doses or longer periods of treatment. Hemorrhage, persistent epistaxis, and prolongation of prothrombin time occur. Leukopenia occurs in about 6% of patients.
- See entry for drug class (p. 479).

**GI** Anorexia, diarrhea, nausea, stomatitis, and vomiting occur, increasing in severity when large doses are given rapidly.
- See entry for drug class (p. 481).

**Renal** Increased BUN, serum creatinine, and proteinuria may occur. Electrolyte imbalance is also possible.
- Monitor serum creatinine, BUN, electrolytes, and urinalysis.

**Other** Intense facial flushing occurs.
- Warn patients of this unusual reaction.

#### Nursing interventions related to drug administration
- Dilute as directed in Preparations. Administer the liter of fluid over 4 to 6 hours; too-rapid administration may increase the severity of some side effects.
- Be alert to prevent extravasation; see entry for drug class (p. 485).

#### Patient and family education
- See entry for drug class (p. 485).

---

## procarbazine hydrochloride  (pro-KAR-ba-zeen)                antineoplastic*

- procarbazine hydrochloride: Matulane, ✽Natulan

*DNA inhibitor.

**MECHANISM OF ACTION**   Procarbazine inhibits a variety of processes that form precursors for nucleic acid synthesis. When precursors are unavailable, nucleic acids cannot be formed normally, and the cells eventually die. Rapidly dividing cells are most susceptible.

**INDICATIONS**   **Hodgkin's disease** Procarbazine is a component of the MOPP regimen (p. 479) used to treat Hodgkin's disease. • Even with advanced disease, 70% to 80% of patients will achieve remission; between 60% and 70% of these will remain free of the disease for 10 years or longer. Many are cured.

**CONTRAINDICATIONS**   **Myelosuppression** Myelosuppression caused by irradiation or chemotherapy may make patients unable to tolerate the additional myelosuppression caused by procarbazine.   **Herpes zoster (chickenpox, shingles) infection or exposure** The risk of severe generalized disease is increased by the immunosuppressive action of procarbazine.   **Cadiovascular disease** Low blood pressure caused by procarbazine may exacerbate angina or cerebrovascular disease.

**DOSAGE**   **PO:**   ADULTS: Initially, 2 to 4 mg/kg daily in single or divided doses; after 1 week, doses may be 4 to 6 mg/kg unless toxicity intervenes. Maintenance doses are 1 to 2 mg/kg daily. Dosage in the MOPP regimen is 100 mg/M$^2$ daily on days 1 through 14 of the 28 day schedule.   *Special patient populations:*   CHILDREN: This drug is carcinogenic and should be avoided if other drugs may be substituted.   PREGNANCY: Use of this drug in pregnancy carries substantial risk to the fetus.   RENAL IMPAIRMENT: Drug may accumulate and increase toxicity. Lower doses may be required.   HEPATIC IMPAIRMENT: Risk of additional damage is increased. Coma may be induced in cirrhotic patients. Lower doses may be required.

**PREPARATIONS**   *Capsules:* 50 mg.

**DRUG INTERACTIONS**   **CNS depressants** such as antihistamines, barbiturates, hypotensive agents, opiates, or phenothiazines may produce additive CNS depression with procarbazine. Doses may need to be reduced or the combination avoided.   **Alcohol** consumption may produce a disulfiramlike reaction. **Insulin or oral hypoglycemic agents** may cause excessive hypoglycemia in the presence of procarbazine.   **Sympathomimetics, tricyclic antidepressants, and dietary tyramine** (e.g., bananas, ripe cheese, red wine, yogurt) may have their actions altered or dangerously potentiated because procarbazine inhibits monoamine oxidase. This enzyme normally terminates the action of sympathomimetics and related compounds.   **Vaccines containing live virus** should be avoided because the risk of severe generalized disease is increased.

**FATE**   Procarbazine is well absorbed following oral administration and rapidly distributed to many tissues, including the CNS. The elimination *half-life* is about 1 hour. The primary route of elimination is metabolism in the liver.

## ☙ NURSING CONSIDERATIONS

### Side effects, toxicities, and associated nursing actions

**CNS** CNS reactions are common with procarbazine, especially in children. Symptoms include apprehension, ataxia, coma, confusion, delirium, disorientation, decreased reflexes, depression, dizziness, falling, footdrop, hallucinations, headache, insomnia, manic reactions, nervousness, neuropathies, nightmares, paresthesia, psychosis, tremors, seizures, or unsteadiness. Altered hearing and slurred speech are rare. Paresthesia, neuropathies, or confusion are cause to discontinue the drug.
* Obtain a thorough baseline evaluation of mental status and neurologic function, and repeat at regular intervals.
* Anticipate CNS side effects: keep side rails up, supervise ambulation, and keep a night light on.
* Caution patients to avoid driving or operating hazardous equipment until the effects of the medication can be evaluated.

**CV** Hypotension and fainting may occur.
* Monitor blood pressure and pulse. Instruct patients to move slowly from a lying to a sitting position. Supervise ambulation.

**Blood** Leukopenia and thrombocytopenia are to be expected. Hemolysis, anisocytosis, poikilocytosis, eosinophilia, lymphocytosis, and Heinz-Ehrlich inclusion bodies in erythrocytes may occur.
* See entry for drug class (p. 480).

**GI** Severe nausea and vomiting are common; anorexia, constipation, diarrhea, dryness of the mouth,

dysphagia, and stomatitis may occur. Diarrhea or stomatitis are cause to discontinue the drug.
- Caution patients to report the development of GI side effects to the physician.
- See entry for drug class (p. 481).

**Renal** Genitourinary disorders including infections may arise, partly from drug-induced leukopenia.
- Instruct the patient to notify the physician if fever, dysuria, frequency, or urgency develop or if there is a change in the color or odor of urine.

**Eye** Diplopia, inability to focus, papilledema, nystagmus, photosensitivity, and retinal hemorrhage are uncommon.
- Caution patients to report the development of any eye changes.

**Lung** Edema, effusion, and cough, or other respiratory disorders are common.
- Auscultate lung sounds. Assess for cough and dyspnea. Monitor the respiratory rate.

**Skin** Alopecia, dermatitis, hyperpigmentation, and pruritis amy occur.
- Instruct patients to report the development of skin changes.
- See entry for drug class (p. 484).

**Reproductive** Marked depression of spermatogenesis and atrophy of the testes may occur.
- See entry for drug class (p. 484).

**Other** Herpes may break out. Arthralgia, myalgia, chills, fever, lethargy, sweating, and weakness have also occurred.
- Instruct patients to report fever that persists longer than 24 hours.
- Caution patients to report the development of any new sign or symptom.

### Nursing interventions related to drug administration
- See entry for drug class (p. 485).

### Patient and family education
- Caution patients to avoid the use of alcohol (including wine or beer) while taking this drug and for at least 2 weeks following the last dose of procarbazine, as a disulfiram type of reaction may occur if alcohol is consumed. The symptoms are flushing, headache, nausea, and hypertension.
- Caution patients to avoid foods high in tyramine (cheeses, sour cream, yogurt, pickled herring, chicken liver, canned figs, raisins, bananas, avocados, soy sauce, broad bean pods [fava beans], yeast extracts, or meats prepared with tenderizers).
- Caution patients to limit intake of caffeine-containing foods such as chocolate, coffee, tea, or colas.
- Caution diabetic patients to monitor blood glucose levels carefully; an adjustment in diet or insulin may be necessary while the patient is receiving procarbazine.
- See entry for drug class (p. 485).

## thioguanine   (thy-oh-GWAH-neen)                          antineoplastic*

- generic

**MECHANISM OF ACTION**   Thioguanine mimics a natural purine and is activated to forms that inhibit nucleic acid synthesis and function. Without functional nucleic acids, cells eventually die. Rapidly growing cells are most susceptible. Thioguanine is weakly immunosuppressive.

**INDICATIONS**   **Leukemias** Acute myelogenous leukemia or acute lymphocytic leukemia may respond to combinations including thioguanine.

**CONTRAINDICATIONS**   **Myelosuppression** Myelosuppression caused by irradiation or chemotherapy may make patients unable to tolerate the additional myelosuppression caused by thioguanine.   **Herpes zoster (chickenpox, shingles) infection or exposure** The risk of severe generalized disease is increased by the immunosuppressive action of thioguanine.

**DOSAGE**   **PO:**   **ADULTS AND CHILDREN:** For induction, 2mg/kg as a single dose daily for 4 weeks or 75 to 200 mg/M² daily for 5 to 7 days or daily until remission is achieved. For maintenance, 2 mg/kg daily is

*Purine antimetabolite.

common, but doses may range from 75 to 400 mg/M$^2$.  *Special patient populations:*  **CHILDREN:** This drug is carcinogenic and should be avoided if other drugs may be substituted.  **PREGNANCY:** Use of this drug in pregnancy carries substantial risk to the fetus.

**PREPARATIONS**  *Tablets:* 40 mg.

**DRUG INTERACTIONS**  **Myelosuppressive** agents may impair bone marrow function, making patients unable to tolerate the additional myelosuppressive effects of thioguanine.  **Vaccines containing live virus** should be avoided because the risk of severe generalized disease is increased.

**FATE**  Thioguanine is poorly absorbed following oral administration, with only 30% of a dose entering the bloodstream. The drug concentrates in bone marrow and crosses the placenta. Thioguanine is metabolized in the liver, and the metabolites are excreted in urine. The elimination *half-life* is about 11 hours.

## NURSING CONSIDERATIONS

### Side effects, toxicities, and associated nursing actions

**CNS** An unsteady gait may be observed.
- Assess gait. Caution patients to avoid driving or operating hazardous equipment if an unsteady gait develops.

**Blood** Leukopenia, thrombocytopenia, and anemia all occur. The first sign of myelosuppression is often leukopenia.
- See entry for drug class (p. 479).

**GI** Anorexia, diarrhea, nausea, stomatitis, and vomiting are more likely at high doses.
- See entry for drug class (p. 481).

**Liver** Jaundice or veno-occlusive hepatic disease is uncommon.
- Assess the patient for right upper quadrant abdominal pain, fever, malaise, jaundice, or change in color or consistency of stools.
- Monitor liver function tests.

**Metabolic** Rapid cancer cell destruction can release large quantities of purines, which are metabolized to uric acid.
- See entry for drug class (p. 484).

**Skin** Dermatitis and rash are infrequent.
- Instruct patients to report the development of any skin changes.

### Nursing interventions related to drug administration
- See entry for drug class (p. 485).

### Patient and family education
- See entry for drug class (p. 485).

## triethylenethiophosphoramide
(tri-eth-ill-een-thy-oh-fos-FOR-a-mide)                                        antineoplastic*

- triethylenethiophosphoramide (thiotepa)

**MECHANISM OF ACTION**  Thiotepa changes the properties of DNA by chemically changing (alkylating) its structure. Without fully functional DNA, cells eventually die. Rapidly growing cells are most susceptible. Thiotepa is weakly immunosuppressive.

**INDICATIONS**  **Bladder tumors** Thiotepa is used intravesically for superficial tumors of the bladder, producing remission in up to two thirds of patients.  **Carcinomas** Adenocarcinoma of the breast or ovary may respond, but therapy is palliative.  **Malignant effusions** Pericardial, pleural, or peritoneal effusions caused by metastatic cancers can be controlled by intracavitary injection of thiotepa.

**CONTRAINDICATIONS**  **Myelosuppression** Myelosuppression caused by irradiation or chemotherapy may make patients unable to tolerate the additional myelosuppression caused by thiotepa.  **Herpes zoster (chickenpox, shingles) infection or exposure** The risk of severe generalized disease is increased by the immunosuppressive action of thiotepa.

*DNA alkylator.

**DOSAGE**    **IV:**    **ADULTS:** Usual doses are 0.3 to 0.4 mg/kg once every 1 to 4 weeks; or 0.2 mg/kg (6 mg/M$^2$) daily for 4 or 5 days, repeated every 2 to 4 weeks, as the toxicity level allows.    **Intracavitary:** **ADULTS:** 0.6 to 0.8 mg/kg at intervals of 1 week or more.    **Intravesical:**    **ADULTS:** 30 to 60 mg in 30 to 60 ml of sterile water to be instilled into the bladder by catheter. Repeat once a week for 4 weeks. *Special patient populations:*    **ELDERLY:** Special geriatric doses have not been established.    **CHILDREN:** This drug is carcinogenic and should be avoided if other drugs may be substituted.    **PREGNANCY:** Use of this drug in pregnancy carries substantial risk to the fetus.    **RENAL OR HEPATIC IMPAIRMENT:** Lower doses may be required.

**PREPARATIONS**    *Powder for reconstitution:* 15 mg. Reconstitute by adding 1.5 ml sterile water to the 15 mg vial. Use directly for IV administration or dilute further into sodium chloride, dextrose, or Ringer's solutions for intracavitary or intravesical administration.

**DRUG INTERACTIONS**    **Myelosuppressive** agents may impair bone marrow function, making patients unable to tolerate the additional myelosuppressive effects of thiotepa.    **Vaccines containing live virus** should be avoided because the risk of severe generalized disease is increased.

**FATE**    Thiotepa may be absorbed across the membranes of the bladder if the membranes are inflamed or extensively damaged. Absorbed drug is metabolized and excreted in urine.

**❦ NURSING CONSIDERATIONS**

**Side effects, toxicities, and associated nursing actions**

**CNS** Headache and dizziness are uncommon.
- Caution the patient to avoid driving or operating hazardous equipment if dizziness develops; notify the physician.
- Instruct the patient to notify the physician if headache is severe or persistent.

**Blood** Leukopenia, anemia, thrombocytopenia, and pancytopenia may occur. Fatalities have resulted.
- See entry for drug class (p. 479).

**GI** Anorexia, nausea, stomatitis, ulceration of the intestinal mucosa, and vomiting may occur.
- See entry for drug class (p. 481).

**Allergic** Rarely, hives, rash, pruritis, and tightness of the throat have occurred.
- Instruct the patient to report the development of skin changes.
- Remain with the patient for several minutes after IV administration to evaluate side effects.

**Reproductive** Amenorrhea and impaired spermatogenesis may occur.
- See entry for drug class (p. 484).

**Other** Lower abdominal pain, vesical irritability, hematuria, and hemorrhagic chemical cystitis may arise infrequently with intravesical administration.
- Assess patient for symptoms related to the urinary tract: urgency, frequency, lower abdominal discomfort, or change in color of urine. Instruct patients to report any changes in urine or urinary output.
- Monitor urinalysis.

**Nursing interventions related to drug administration**
- For IV administration, administer 60 mg or less over 1 minute.
- See entry for drug class (p. 485).

**Patient and family education**
- See entry for drug class (p. 485).

---

## uracil mustard    (YOO-ra-sil)                                    antineoplastic*

- generic

**MECHANISM OF ACTION**    Uracil mustard alters the properties of DNA by chemically changing (alkylating) its structure. Without fully functional DNA, cells eventually die. Rapidly growing cells are most susceptible.

*DNA alkylator.

**INDICATIONS** **Leukemias** Chronic lymphocytic leukemia and chronic myelogenous leukemia may respond, but treatment is palliative. **Lymphomas** Lymphomas, including Hodgkin's disease, may respond, but treatment is palliative. **Mycosis fungoides** Treatment is palliative. **Polycythemia vera** Treatment is palliative

**CONTRAINDICATIONS** **Myelosuppression** Myelosuppression caused by irradiation or chemotherapy may make patients unable to tolerate the additional myelosuppression caused by uracil mustard. **Allergy to tartrazine or aspirin** Uracil mustard capsules contain tartrazine. • Susceptible individuals may suffer bronchial asthma or other signs. **Herpes zoster (chickenpox, shingles) infection or exposure** The risk of severe generalized disease is increased by the immunosuppressive action of uracil mustard.

**DOSAGE** **PO:** **ADULTS:** Single doses of 0.15 mg/kg are administered weekly for 4 weeks or until a relapse occurs. **CHILDREN:** Single doses of 0.3 mg/kg are administered weekly for 4 weeks or until a relapse occurs. *Special patient populations:* **CHILDREN:** This drug is carcinogenic and should be avoided if other drugs may be substituted. **PREGNANCY:** Use of this drug in pregnancy carries substantial risk to the fetus.

**PREPARATIONS** *Capsules:* 1 mg.

**DRUG INTERACTIONS** **Myelosuppressive** agents may impair bone marrow function, making patients unable to tolerate the additional myelosuppressive effects of uracil mustard. **Vaccines containing live virus** should be avoided because the risk of severe generalized disease is increased.

**FATE** The fate in human beings is unknown.

## ☙ NURSING CONSIDERATIONS

### Side effects, toxicities, and associated nursing actions

**CNS** Depression, irritability, mental cloudiness, and nervousness have occurred.
• Assess mental status before therapy and at regular intervals.
• Caution the patient and family to report personality changes to the physician.

**Blood** Leukopenia and thrombocytopenia occur frequently at normal therapeutic doses. Damage to the bone marrow is cumulative; at cumulative doses of 1 mg/kg, irreversible damage begins to appear.
• Calculate drug doses carefully.
• See entry for drug class (p. 479).

**GI** Abdominal pain, anorexia, diarrhea, epigastric distress, nausea, ulceration, and vomiting may occur.
• See entry for drug class (p. 481).

**Metabolic** Rapid cancer cell destruction can release large quantities of purines, which are metabolized to uric acid. Accumulation of uric acid may lead to renal damage or gout.
• See entry for drug class (p. 484).

**Liver** Jaundice and glycogen infiltration are rare.
• Assess patients for right upper quadrant abdominal pain, fever, malaise, change in color or consistency of stools, and jaundice.
• Monitor liver function tests.

**Skin** Alopecia, dermatitis, hyperpigmentation, and pruritis may occur.
• Instruct the patient to report skin changes to the physician.
• See entry for drug class (p. 484) for a discussion of alopecia.

**Reproductive** Amenorrhea and impaired spermatogenesis may occur.
• See entry for drug class (p. 484).

### Nursing interventions related to drug administration
• See entry for drug class (p. 485).

### Patient and family education
• See entry for drug class (p. 485).

# vinblastine sulfate    (vin-BLAS-teen)    antineoplastic*

- vinblastine sulfate: Velban, ✤ Velbe

**MECHANISM OF ACTION**    Vinblastine binds to microtubular proteins, preventing formation of the mitotic spindle. Dividing cells are arrested in metaphase. Vinblastine is weakly immunosuppressive.

**INDICATIONS**    **Hodgkin's disease** Vinblastine is one of the most active drugs against Hodgkin's disease, producing positive responses in up to 90% of patients. • Vinblastine is one component of the ABVD (p. 479) regimen used in advanced cases; it is also effective for non-Hodgkin's lymphomas.    **Testicular carcinoma** Advanced nonseminomatous testicular carcinoma is effectively treated with combinations including vinblastine (p. 480).    **Choriocarcinoma** Vinblastine may be used palliatively.    **Carcinoma** Vinblastine may be used palliatively for advanced breast carcinoma that is unresponsive to standard therapy.

**CONTRAINDICATIONS**    **Cachexia** Debilitated patients are more prone to the leukopenic effects of vinblastine.    **Infections** Vinblastine interferes with normal body defense mechanisms and may greatly worsen infections. They should be resolved before therapy with vinblastine. Normally mild herpes zoster infections may become severe generalized infections that are potentially fatal.    **Myelosuppression** Myelosuppression caused by irradiation or chemotherapy may make patients unable to tolerate the additional myelosuppression caused by vinblastine.

**DOSAGE**    IV:    **ADULTS:** Usual doses are 3.7 mg/M$^2$ as a single dose, not to be repeated for at least 1 week. Further doses are adjusted based on the response of the bone marrow.    **CHILDREN:** Usual doses are 2.5 mg/M$^2$ as a single dose, not to be repeated for at least 1 week. Further doses are adjusted based on the response of the bone marrow.    *Special patient populations:*    **ELDERLY:** Elderly patients who are malnourished or suffer from skin ulcers are more prone to the leukopenic effects of vinblastine.    **PREGNANCY:** Use of this drug in pregnancy carries substantial risk to the fetus.

**PREPARATIONS**    *Powder for reconstitution:* 10 mg. Reconstitute by adding 10 ml of 0.9% sodium chloride injection containing phenol and benzyl alcohol as preservative to the 10 mg vial. The resulting 1 mg/ml solution may be used to inject the appropriate dose into a running IV line.

**DRUG INTERACTIONS**    **Bleomycin** with vinblastine used for testicular carcinoma has caused Raynaud's disease in a few persons.    **Myelosuppressive** agents may impair bone marrow function, making patients unable to tolerate the additional myelosuppressive effects of vinblastine.    **Mitomycin** use in the past may predispose a patient to acute bronchospasm when vinblastine is administered.    **Vaccines containing live virus** should be avoided because the risk of severe generalized disease is increased.

**FATE**    Vinblastine is poorly absorbed from the GI tract and highly irritating to tissues. It therefore must be administered IV. The drug distributes well to most tissues but not to the CNS. Vinblastine is metabolized to active and inactive metabolites. Elimination is in urine and bile.

## ☙ NURSING CONSIDERATIONS

### Side effects, toxicities, and associated nursing actions

**CNS** High doses or prolonged use of vinblastine may cause neurologic toxicity, including depression, dizziness, headache, loss of deep tendon reflexes, neuritis, numbness, malaise, pain of face or jaw, paresthesia, peripheral neuropathy, psychoses, vocal cord paralysis, seizures, sinus tachycardia, urinary retention, and weakness.
- Obtain a thorough baseline assessment, including mental status and neurologic function, and repeat at regular intervals.
- Caution patients to avoid driving or operating hazardous equipment until the effects of the medication can be evaluated.
- Monitor pulse and blood pressure. Monitor intake and output.

**Blood** Leukopenia is the most common and the dose-limiting side effect of therapy. Thrombocytopenia also occurs. Vinblastine also causes phlebitis; local tissue necrosis occurs if the drug is allowed to extravasate.
- See entry for drug class (p. 479).

*Mitotic inhibitor.

- Ascertain that the IV is patent before administering the drug. Caution the patient to report the development of pain or discomfort. Do not leave the patient unattended during infusion. If extravasation occurs, discontinue drug administration, and infiltrate the area of extravasation with hyaluronidase. Apply moist heat for several hours.

**GI** Nausea and vomiting are common. Abdominal pain, adynamic ileus, anorexia, bleeding from old peptic ulcers, constipation, diarrhea, epigastric distress, hemorrhagic enteritis, pharyngitis, rectal bleeding, stomatitis, and vesiculation of the mouth are less common.

- See entry for drug class (p. 481).

**Skin** Alopecia, dermatitis, epilation, photoxicity, or vesiculation may occur.

- Instruct patients to report the development of any skin changes.
- For photosensitivity, instruct patients to avoid exposure to the sun or other sources of ultraviolet light, wear a large-brimmed hat when outside, keep extremities covered, and use a maximum-protection sunscreen on exposed skin surfaces.
- See entry for drug class (p. 484) for a discussion of alopecia.

**Other** Fever is uncommon.

- Instruct patients to notify the physician if fever persists longer than 24 hours.

### Nursing interventions related to drug administration

- Reconstitute as noted in Preparations. Administer the dose over at least 1 minute.
- See entry for drug class (p. 485).

### Patient and family education

- See entry for drug class (p. 485).

---

## vincristine sulfate  (vin-KRIS-teen)                                  antineoplastic*

- vincristine sulfate: Oncovin

**MECHANISM OF ACTION**  Vincristine binds to microtubular proteins, preventing formation of the mitotic spindle. Dividing cells are arrested in metaphase. Vincristine is weakly immunosuppressive.

**INDICATIONS**  **Leukemia** Acute lymphocytic and acute myelogenous leukemias respond well to combinations containing vincristine. Vincristine with prednisone is the treatment of choice in inducing remissions in acute lymphocytic leukemia (p. 480).   **Hodgkin's disease** Combinations including vincristine (e.g., MOPP, p. 479) are very effective against Hodgkin's disease, with remissions in up to 80% of patients; 60% to 70% of those patients remain disease-free for 10 years, and many are cured.   **Malignant lymphomas** Combinations including vincristine may be effective.   **Neuroblastoma** Vincristine with cyclophosphamide may produce objective improvement in most patients.   **Rhabdomyosarcoma** Combinations including vincristine may be a useful adjunct to surgery; up to 90% of patients respond. **Wilms' tumor** Combinations including vincristine may be a useful adjunct to surgery and/or irradiation; up to 90% of patients respond.

**CONTRAINDICATIONS**  **Neuromuscular disease** The neurotoxic effects of vincristine may be most profound in these patients.   **Herpes zoster (chickenpox, shingles) infection or exposure** The risk of severe generalized disease is increased by the immunosuppressive action of vincristine.

**DOSAGE**  IV:   **ADULTS:** Usual doses are 1.4 mg/M$^2$, repeated no more often than weekly. Subsequent doses are determined by response and toxicity.   **CHILDREN:** Usual doses are 2 mg/M$^2$, repeated no more often than weekly. Subsequent doses are determined by response and toxicity. *Special patient populations:*   **ELDERLY:** Geriatric patients are more susceptible to the neurotoxic effects of vincristine.   **PREGNANCY:** Use of this drug in pregnancy carries substantial risk to the fetus.

**PREPARATIONS**   Solution for IV use only: 1 mg/ml.

**DRUG INTERACTIONS**  **Asparaginase** may increase the hematologic or neurologic toxicity of vincristine. **Mitomycin** use in the past may predispose a patient to acute bronchospasm when vincristine is administered.   **Vaccines containing live virus** should be avoided because the risk of severe generalized disease is increased.

*Mitotic inhibitor.

**FATE** Vincristine is poorly absorbed from the GI tract and is highly irritating to tissues. It therefore must be administered IV. The drug distributes well to most tissues but not to the CNS. Vincristine is metabolized to active and inactive metabolites. Elimination is in urine and bile. Patients with impaired hepatic function may have diminished capacity to eliminate vincristine.

## ❦ NURSING CONSIDERATIONS

### Side effects, toxicities, and associated nursing actions

**CNS** Nearly every patient suffers a degree of peripheral neuropathy, the earliest sign being depression of the Achilles' reflex. Peripheral paresthesias are also common. High doses or prolonged therapy may produce ataxia, atrophy, cranial nerve palsy, cramps, difficulty in walking, footdrop, slapping gait, and wrist drop. Autonomic or CNS neurotoxicity is less common. Signs, including abdominal cramps, constipation, obstipation, orthostatic hypotension, myoclonic jerks, and urinary difficulties, arise from autonomic toxicity. Altered consciousness, agitation, depression, hallucinations, insomnia, progressive encephalopathy, respiratory difficulties, and seizures are signs of CNS toxicity. Intrathecal injection of vincristine is invariably fatal because of the high incidence of CNS effects.

* Obtain a thorough baseline assessment, including mental status exam and neurologic function, as well as review of systems; repeat on a regular basis.
* Monitor intake, output, blood pressure, pulse, and respiratory rate. Auscultate bowel sounds and lung sounds. Monitor reflexes and gait. Keep a record of bowel movements. The regular use of a stool softener before and during the course of therapy with this drug is often necessary.
* Instruct patients to report the development of any unusual sign or symptom.

**Blood** Hematologic toxicity at normal doses is rare. At higher doses, mild leukopenia, anemia, or thrombocytopenia may occur. Phlebitis may occur. Extravasation causes pain, cellulitis, and necrosis.

* See entry for drug class (p. 479).
* Ascertain that the IV is patent before administering the drug. Caution the patient to report the development of pain or discomfort. Do not leave the patient unattended during infusion. If extravasation occurs, discontinue drug administration, and infiltrate the area of extravasation with hyaluronidase. Apply moist heat for several hours.

**GI** Abdominal distention, diarrhea, nausea, oral ulceration, stomatitis, and vomiting may occur.

* See entry for drug class (p. 481)

**Renal** Rarely, inappropriate antidiuretic hormone secretion causes increased urinary sodium excretion, leading to hyponatremia.

* Monitor intake, output, and weight.
* Monitor serum electrolytes.

**Metabolic** Rapid cancer cell destruction can release large quantities of purines, which are metabolized to uric acid. Accumulation of uric acid may lead to renal damage or gout.

* See entry for drug class (p. 484).

**Skin** Alopecia occurs in 20% to 70% of patients.

* See entry for drug class (p. 484).

### Nursing interventions related to drug administration

* See entry for drug class (p. 485).
* Administer the dose over at least 1 minute.

### Patient and family education

* See entry for drug class (p. 485).

---

## vindesine sulfate  (VIN-de-seen)                                          antineoplastic*

* vindesine sulfate: ✦Eldisine (investigational, U.S.)

**MECHANISM OF ACTION**    Vindesine binds to microtubular proteins, preventing formation of the mitotic spindle. Dividing cells are arrested in metaphase.

*Antimitotic.

**INDICATIONS** **Acute lymphoblastic leukemia** Combinations including vindesine may be effective. **Lymphomas** Both Hodgkin's and non-Hodgkin's lymphomas may respond to combinations including vindesine. **Breast carcinoma** Vindesine may be palliative. **Malignant melanoma** Vindesine may be helpful in controlling this difficult-to-treat tumor. **Lung cancer** Non-small cell cancers may respond.

**CONTRAINDICATIONS** **Myelosuppression** Patients with pre-existing myelosuppression may be unable to tolerate the additional myelosuppression caused by vindesine. **Herpes zoster (chickenpox, shingles) infection or exposure** The risk of severe generalized disease is increased by the immunosuppressive action of vindesine.

**DOSAGE** IV: ADULTS: 3 to 4 mg/M$^2$ by slow push into a running IV line. To be repeated weekly. *Special patient populations:* PREGNANCY: Use of this drug in pregnancy carries substantial risk to the fetus.

**PREPARATIONS** Powder for reconstitution: 5 mg. Reconstitute by adding the 5 ml diluent supplied with the drug.

**DRUG INTERACTIONS** **Mitomycin** use in the past may predispose a patient to acute bronchospasm when vindesine is administered. **Vincristine or vinblastine** should not be used with vindesine because cumulative neurotoxicity results. **Vaccines containing live virus** should be avoided because the risk of severe generalized disease is increased.

**FATE** Vindesine resembles the other vinca alkaloids. The terminal elimination *half-life* is 24 hours.

## 🐦 NURSING CONSIDERATIONS

### Side effects, toxicities, and associated nursing actions

**CNS** Paresthesias, muscle weakness, and loss of deep tendon reflexes occur frequently and may limit therapy. Vindesine is less neurotoxic than vincristine but more so than vinblastine.
- Monitor deep tendon reflexes and gait.
- Instruct patients to report the development of any unexpected sign or symptom.

**Blood** Neutropenia is the most common dose-limiting side effect of vindesine. Phlebitis and local tissue damage can result at the injection site.
- See entry for drug class (p. 479).
- Ascertain that the IV is patent before administering the drug. Caution the patient to report the development of pain or discomfort. Do not leave the patient unattended during infusion. If extravasation occurs, discontinue drug administration. Apply moist heat for several hours. Consult the manufacturer's literature for current information regarding treatment of extravasation.

**GI** Diarrhea, nausea, and vomiting may occur.
- See entry for drug class (p. 481).

**Skin** Alopecia, dermatitis, and stomatitis occur.
- See entry for drug class (p. 484).

### Nursing interventions related to drug administration
- Administer via slow IV push.
- Consult the manufacturer's literature for current information about drug administration.
- See entry for drug class (p. 485).

### Patient and family education
- See entry for drug class (p. 485).

# Chapter Twenty-eight

# Tissue-specific agents and radiochemicals

alpha-interferon
aminoglutethimide (investigational U.S.)
diethylstilbestrol
diethylstilbestrol diphosphate
dromostanolone propionate
estramustine
leuprolide acetate
medroxyprogesterone acetate
megestrol acetate
mitotane

polyestradiol phosphate
prednisone
sodium iodide I 131
sodium phosphate P 32
streptozocin
tamoxifen
testolactone
zoladex (investigational)

**MECHANISM OF ACTION**   Many anticancer drugs are useful because they directly affect specific tissues. Androgens and estrogens often inhibit tumors arising from reproductive tissues. Antiestrogens and progestins also act on tumors of reproductive tissues. Glucocorticoids suppress lymphoid tissues and tumors arising from those tissues. Radioactive iodine is specifically concentrated in thyroid, allowing ionizing radiation to destroy nearby cells. Radioactive phosphorus is less specific, being taken up by any rapidly growing tissues.

## ❦ NURSING CONSIDERATIONS

### Patient and family education

- Review with patients and families the anticipated benefits and possible side effects of drug therapy. Provide support to these patients, who may be facing a difficult diagnosis, as well as anticipating a variety of serious or unpleasant side effects.
- Encourage patients to return for follow-up visits as directed and to consult the nurse or physician about any unusual sign, symptom, or concern.
- Remind patients to keep all health care providers informed of all medications being taken. This is especially important because many side effects may not appear until days or weeks after the drug has been administered or drug therapy started.
- Review with patients appropriate actions for missed doses (consult with the physician). Typical instructions: a missed dose remembered within a few hours of the ordered dose time may be taken; missed doses remembered within 2 to 4 hours of the next scheduled dose should be omitted (this time span varies with the frequency of doses each day). Patients should never double-up with drug doses unless specifically instructed to do so. If more than two doses, or two day's worth of a drug are missed, the patient should notify the physician.
- Caution patients to avoid the use of over-the-counter preparations without prior approval of the physician.
- Emphasize to the patient the importance of keeping these and all medications out of the reach of children.
- See Overview of Drug Class, Cytotoxic Agents (p. 485) for additional information.

## alpha-interferon   (alfa-in-ter-FEAR-on)                    antineoplastic*

- alpha-interferon: Intron A (interferon alfa-2a, recombinant)
  Referon-A (interferon alfa-2B, recombinant)

Immune modulator.

**Table 28-1.**

## Summary of tissue-specific anticancer agents

| Drug | Classification | Affected tumors |
|---|---|---|
| Alpha-interferon | Interferon | Hairy cell leukemia |
| Aminoglutethimide | Steroid synthesis inhibitor | Breast carcinoma |
| Diethylstilbestrol | Estrogen | Breast carcinoma<br>Prostate carcinoma |
| Dromostanolone propionate | Androgen | Breast carcinoma |
| Estramustine | Estrogen/alkylator | Prostate carcinoma |
| Leuprolide acetate | GnRH analog | Breast carcinoma<br>Prostate carcinoma |
| Medroxyprogesterone acetate | Progestin | Endometrial carcinoma<br>Renal carcinoma |
| Megestrol acetate | Progestin | Endometrial carcinoma<br>Breast carcinoma |
| Mitotane | Antiadrenal | Adrenocortical carcinoma |
| Polyestradiol phosphate | Estrogen | Prostate carcinoma |
| Prednisone | Glucocorticoid | Acute lymphocytic leukemia<br>Lymphomas |
| Sodium iodide I 131 | Antithyroid | Thyroid carcinoma |
| Sodium phosphate P 32 | Antiproliferative | Polycythemia vera<br>Chronic myelogenous leukemia |
| Streptozocin | Anti-beta cell | Pancreatic islet cell carcinoma |
| Tamoxifen | Antiestrogen | Breast carcinoma |
| Testolactone | Androgen | Breast carcinoma |
| Zoladex | GnRH analog | Breast carcinoma<br>Prostate carcinoma |

**MECHANISM OF ACTION**    Interferons are antiviral, antiproliferative, and immunosuppressive agents. The antineoplastic effects may be related to any or all of these actions.

**INDICATIONS**    **Hairy cell leukemia** This relatively rare form of leukemia responds well to alpha-interferons but is difficult to treat by other means.    **Investigational indications** Alpha-interferons are being tested against malignant melanoma, multiple myeloma, Kaposi's syndrome in AIDS patients, renal carcinoma and papilloma, chronic myelocytic leukemia, non-Hodgkin's lymphomas, papillomas, and mycosis fungoides.

**CONTRAINDICATIONS**    **Heart disease** Severe heart disease or recent myocardial infarction renders patients more susceptible to cardiotoxicity produced by the drug.    **Pulmonary disease** Pulmonary function may be compromised by fever and chills accompanying the use of interferon.    **Chickenpox or herpes zoster** Persons exposed to the virus or actively suffering infection run the risk of developing severe generalized infection.    **CNS disease** The risk of severe CNS side effects, including seizures, is greater in the patient with pre-existing disease.

**DOSAGE**    **IM or SC:**    **ADULTS:** Interferon alfa-2a for induction, 3 million units daily for 16 to 24 weeks. For maintenance, 3 million units three times a week. Interferon alfa-2b, 2 million units/$M^2$ three times a week.    *Special patient populations:*    **ELDERLY:** Geriatric patients are more likely to suffer cardiotoxicity or neurotoxicity than younger adults.    **CHILDREN:** Pediatric doses have not been established.    **PREGNANCY:** FDA pregnancy category C.

**PREPARATIONS**    **Interferon alfa-2a, recombinant** *Solution:* 3 and 6 million units/ml; *powder for reconstitution:* 18 million units to be reconstituted with 3 ml diluent supplied.    **Interferon alfa-2b, recombi-**

**nant** *Powder for reconstitution:* 3, 5, 10, and 25 million units to be reconstituted with diluent supplied.

**DRUG INTERACTIONS**    **Vaccines based on living viruses** including oral polio vaccines, may cause generalized disease and death in patients also receiving alph-interferon.    **Myelosuppressive agents** may produce intolerable bone marrow suppression in patients also receiving alpha-interferon.

**FATE**    Both forms of alpha-interferon are absorbed well from IM or SC sites. *Peak* concentrations in blood following IM injections are observed by 4 hours for interferon alfa-2a and between 6 to 8 hours for alfa 2-b. Alpha-interferons are completely metabolized, with very little appearing in the urine.

## ✿ NURSING CONSIDERATIONS

### Side effects, toxicities, and associated nursing actions

**CNS** Confusion, difficulty in thinking, depression, insomnia, and nervousness may occur. High doses may cause coma, obtundation, or stupor. Peripheral neuropathies may also occur, with tingling in face, fingers, and toes.

- Perform a thorough baseline assessment of mental status and neurologic functioning before starting therapy and at regular intervals.
- Be alert to signs of depression: insomnia, weight loss, withdrawal, anorexia, lack of interest in personal appearance. Question family members about changes in affect if appropriate.
- Question the patient about tingling in face, fingers, and toes. Caution the patient to avoid driving or operating hazardous equipment until the effects of the medication can be evaluated.

**CV** Irregular heart beat or chest pain may signal cardiotoxicity.

- Monitor pulse and blood pressure. Auscultate heart and lung sounds.
- Investigate chest pain as indicated, including monitoring electrocardiogram and obtaining cardiac enzyme studies.

**Blood** Leukopenia and thrombocytopenia occur frequently but rarely cause symptoms.

- See entry for drug class, Cytotoxic Agents (p. 479).

**GI** Anorexia, weight loss, diarrhea, nausea, or vomiting are common but usually resolve after discontinuing therapy.

- See entry for drug class, Cytotoxic Agents (p. 481).

**Skin** Alopecia may occur.

- See entry for drug class, Cytotoxic Agents (p 484).

**Other** A flulike syndrome with fever and chills is most prominent in the first week of therapy.

- Alert patients to this possible side effect. If fever persists longer than 24 hours, notify the physician.

### Nursing interventions related to drug administration

- Consult the manufacturer's literature for current administration information.

### Patient and family education

- Review with patients and families the anticipated benefits and possible side effects of drug therapy. Instruct patients to report the development of any new signs or symptoms.
- See entry for drug class (p. 533).

---

## aminoglutethimide    (a-meen-oh-gloo-TETH-i-mide)    *antineoplastic

- aminoglutethimide (investigational U.S.): ✿ Cytadren

**MECHANISM OF ACTION**    Aminoglutethimide inhibits two enzymes that are involved in synthesis of steroids, including estrogens. Adrenal production of estrogens is essentially abolished, which aids in control of estrogen-dependent tumors.

**INDICATIONS**    **Estrogen-responsive breast tumors** Up to 50% of treated patients show objective improvement.

**CONTRAINDICATIONS**    **Myelosuppression** Patients with pre-existing bone morrow suppression may be unable to tolerate the additional myelosuppression caused by aminoglutethimide.

**DOSAGE**    **PO:**    **ADULTS:** 250 mg twice daily for 2 weeks, then 250 mg four times daily.    *Special patient populations:*    **CHILDREN:** Pediatric doses have not been established.    **PREGNANCY:** FDA pregnancy category D.

*Steriod inhibitor.

**PREPARATIONS** *Tablets:* 250 mg.

**DRUG INTERACTIONS** **Dexamethasone** metabolism is hastened by aminoglutethimide, reducing the effectiveness of the glucocorticoid.

**FATE** Absorption of aminoglutethimide is adequate following oral administration. The plasma *half-life* is about 7 hours after therapy is well established. The drug is altered by metabolizing enzymes and excreted in urine as unchanged drug and metabolites.

## ❦ NURSING CONSIDERATIONS

### Side effects, toxicities, and associated nursing actions

**CNS** Ataxia occurs in 10% and lethargy in 40% of patients. Acute soporific effects also occur. Tolerance develops over a period of weeks.

- Assess gait and mental status at regular intervals.
- Caution patients to avoid driving or operating hazardous equipment until lethargy and soporific effects wear off. Reassure patients that these side effects will lessen with time.

**CV** Orthostatic hypotension with dizziness and weakness occurs in about 10% of patients. Tachycardia has also occurred.

- Monitor blood pressure and pulse.
- Instruct patients to move slowly from a lying to a sitting or standing position. Instruct patients to "dangle" feet on the floor before standing, when moving from a lying to a standing position. Supervise ambulation. Keep side rails up. Use night lights.

**Blood** Leukopenia, thrombocytopenia, pancytopenia, and agranulocytosis are possible.

- See entry for drug class, Cytotoxic Agents (p. 479).

**GI** Anorexia and nausea are common early effects, resolving later in therapy. • See entry for drug class, Cytotoxic Agents (p. 481).

**Metabolic** Hypothyroidism, goiters, masculinization and hirsutism in females, and precocious sexual development in males may occur.

- Assess patients for changes in sexual characteristics. Provide support as needed; these changes may be especially difficult for women to tolerate. Reinforce the need to continue the medication as ordered. Caution patients not to discontinue medication without notifying the physician.
- Assess for goiter on a regular basis. Monitor thyroid function tests if available. Assess for signs of hypothyroidism: sluggishness, weight gain, sleepiness, intolerance to cold, constipation, dry skin, or changes in hair.

**Liver** AST and ALT may be elevated.

- Assess the patient for manifestations of liver problems: jaundice, malaise, fever, right upper quadrant abdominal pain, and change in color or consistency of stools.
- Monitor liver function tests.

**Other** Fever, myalgia, and pruritis may occur.

- Assess patients for these side effects. Instruct the patient to notify the physician if fever persists longer than 24 hours or is excessively high.

### Nursing interventions related to drug administration

- See the manufacturer's literature for most current information.

### Patient and family education

- Review with patients and families the anticipated benefits and possible side effects of drug therapy. Instruct patients to report the development of any new sign or symptom.
- See entry for drug class (p. 533).

---

# diethylstilbestrol (DES), diethylstilbestrol diphosphate
(dye-eth-ill-stil-BES-trol)       antineoplastic*

- diethylstilbestrol: ✤Honvol, Stilphostrol

*Estrogen.

**MECHANISM OF ACTION**   Certain reproductive tumors such as breast cancer in postmenopausal women and prostatic cancers in men retain hormone receptors that render them sensitive to estrogens, including diethylstilbestrol.

**INDICATIONS**   **Estrogen-responsive breast cancer** Tumors in postmenopausal women may respond.   **Prostatic cancer** These hormone-responsive tumors may regress when treated with estrogens.

**CONTRAINDICATIONS**   **Liver damage** Estrogen toxicity may be greater because metabolism of the steroids is diminished.   **Thrombophlebitis** This condition may increase the risk from DES.

**DOSAGE**   PO:   **ADULTS:** For breast cancer, 5 to 15 mg three times daily. For prostatic cancer, 1 to 3 mg daily. Diethylstilbestrol diphosphate, for prostatic carcinoma 50 to 200 mg three times daily.   **IV: ADULTS:** Diethylstilbestrol diphosphate, 500 mg infused on the first day, 1 g on days 2 through 5. Maintenance may be with 250 to 500 mg once or twice weekly.   *Special patient populations:* **CHILDREN:** This drug has profound effects on endocrine function and development and should be avoided if possible.   **PREGNANCY:** Use of this drug in pregnancy carries substantial risk to the fetus. Up to 90% of females exposed in utero to diethylstilbestrol develop adenosis of the vagina and cervix in later life and many develop clear cell adenocarcinoma. Males exposed in utero may suffer a variety of genital abnormalities in later life.

**PREPARATIONS**   **Diethylstilbestrol** *Tablets:* 1 and 5 mg; *tablets, enteric coated:* 0.1, 1, and 5 mg.   **Diethylstilbestrol diphosphate** *Tablets:* 50 mg; *solution for parenteral injection:* 50 mg/ml.

**DRUG INTERACTIONS**   **Rifampin** may decrease estrogen activity by hastening metabolism of steroids.   **Corticosteroid** effects may be exaggerated in patients with concomitent estrogen therapy because estrogens may slow metabolism of the corticosteroid.   **Oral anticoagulants** may be less effective in patients receiving estrogens because metabolism of the anticoagulants is hastened.

**FATE**   Diethylstilbestrol is well absorbed following oral administration. The drug is metabolized to glucuronide by the liver and excreted in that form by the kidneys.

### 🐾 NURSING CONSIDERATIONS

#### Side effects, toxicities, and associated nursing actions

**CNS** Dizziness, irritability, and changes in libido may occur.
* Caution patients to avoid driving or operating hazardous equipment if dizziness occurs.
* Warn patients about possible irritability.
* Assess tactfully for changes in libido; many patients may be unwilling to discuss this. Provide emotional support as needed. Caution patients to take the drug only as ordered and to not discontinue the medication without notifying the physician.

**CV** Hypertension occurs during therapy and may persist after the drug is discontinued. Edema may occur with high doses.
* Monitor blood pressure and pulse
* Monitor the weight. Assess for edema. Instruct patients to report tight rings, shoes, or clothing. Have the patient monitor and record weight at home. Instruct the patient to report a weight gain greater than 2 pounds per day or 5 pounds per week.

**Blood** Thrombophlebitis or other thromboembolic disorders may occur with prolonged estrogen therapy. The high doses used in cancer chemotherapy also increase the risk.
* Monitor the patient for this side effect and review signs and symptoms with the patient: pain in an extremity and swelling. The affected limb may be cool and pale, with the area of the affected vein red and warm to touch. Instruct the patient to notify the physician if these symptoms occur.
* Encourage regular ambulation.

**GI** Anorexia, abdominal cramps, and nausea are expected with high doses.
* See entry for drug class, Cytotoxic Agents (p. 481).
* Assess for signs of hypercalcemia: anorexia, nausea, vomiting, and constipation. Monitor serum electrolytes.

**Renal** Women may experience urinary incontinence or urinary frequency.
* Warn patients about this possible side effect.
* Instruct patients to notify the physician if urinary frequency is severe, persistent, or is accompanied by fever, pain in the bladder area, change in the color or clarity of urine, or pain in urination.
* Teach patients to perform perineal exercises to strengthen perineal and gluteal muscles. Examples of exercises follow: Have the patient sit on the toilet with knees wide apart, then, while voiding, start

and stop the urinary stream. Have the patient tighten the perineal muscles as if trying not to void; hold for 3 seconds, then relax; repeat several times.

**Reproductive** Females may experience breast tenderness, uterine bleeding, and anogenital pain and pruritis. Males should expect gynecomastia and impotence.

- Assess patients for these problems. Provide emotional support as needed. Caution patients to not discontinue medications without notifying the physician and to take medications as ordered for best results.
- Instruct patients to notify the physician about uterine bleeding. Although bleeding may be a drug side effect, it should be investigated.

### Nursing interventions related to drug administration

For IV use, dilute the daily dose in 100 ml of normal saline or dextrose for infusion. Administer at a rate of 20 drops per minute for 15 minutes while monitoring the patient. Increase the rate of infusion after 15 minutes to complete the infusion in 1 hour.

- Reclining position during IV administration may reduce dizziness.

### Patient and family education

- Review with patients the anticipated benefits and possible side effects of drug therapy.
- Instruct patients to swallow enteric-coated tablets whole, without crushing or chewing.
- See entry for drug class, Cytotoxic Agents (p. 485).
- See entry for drug class, Drugs Acting on the Female Reproductive System (p. 627).

---

## dromostanolone propionate   (droh-moh-STAN-oh-lone)   antineoplastic*

- dromostanolone propionate: Drolban

**MECHANISM OF ACTION**   Certain reproductive tumors such as breast cancer in postmenopausal women retain hormone receptors that render them sensitive to androgens, including dromostanolone propionate.

**INDICATIONS**   **Breast carcinoma** Inoperable or metastatic carcinoma of the breast in postmenopausal women may respond to androgen therapy, but treatment is palliative, not curative.

**CONTRAINDICATIONS**   **Breast carcinoma in males** Androgens are not indicated for this condition in males. **Premenopausal women** Androgens are not indicated in this age group of women.   **Cardiovascular disease** Fluid retention and cardiovascular symptoms may be worsened.   **Prostatic carcinoma** This condition may be worsened by dromostanolone.

**DOSAGE**   **IM:**   **ADULTS:** Give 100 mg by deep injection three times weekly for 8 to 12 weeks or as long as beneficial results are obtained. *Special patient populations:*   **CHILDREN:** This drug has profound effects on endocrine function and development and should be avoided if possible.   **PREGNANCY:** Use of this drug in pregnancy carries substantial risk to the fetus.

**PREPARATIONS**   *Solution for IM injection:* 50 mg/ml.

**DRUG INTERACTIONS**   Dromostanolone may share interactions that occur with other androgens (p. 645), but documentation is lacking.

**FATE**   Dromostanolone is inadequately absorbed following oral administration and must be administered IM.

### ☙ NURSING CONSIDERATIONS

#### Side effects, toxicities, and associated nursing actions

**CNS** Increased libido is less frequent with dromostanolone than with other anabolic androgens. Anxiety, depression, and paresthesias are uncommon.

- Assess tactfully for changes in libido; some patients may be unwilling to discuss this subject. Provide emotional support as needed. Reinforce to patients the need to take medications as ordered and to not discontinue medications without notifying the physician.
- Monitor for signs of depression: withdrawal, insomnia, anorexia, weight loss, or lack of interest in personal appearance.

*Androgen.

- Assess for tingling of fingers and toes.

**CV** Retention of water may occur.

- Monitor pulse, blood pressure, and weight.
- Instruct patients to report increasing tightness of rings, shoes, or clothing.
- Instruct patients to monitor and record weight at home. Instruct patients to report weight gain in excess of 2 pounds per day or 5 pounds per week.

**Blood** Polycythemia may occur. Leukopenia and suppression of clotting factors has also been observed.

- Monitor hematocrit, hemoglobin, white blood cell differential, and clotting factors.
- See entry for drug class, Cytotoxic Agents (p. 479).

**Metabolic** Hypercalcemia may indicate metastases.

- Assess for signs of hypercalcemia: thirst, polyuria, lethargy, anorexia, nausea, vomiting, or constipation. Monitor serum electrolytes.

**Allergic** These reactions are rare.

- Be alert for allergic reactions. Have the patient remain in the health care setting for at least 15 minutes after receiving an IM dose of medication.

**Reproductive** Females may suffer virilization with hirsutism, deepening of the voice, or other signs. These signs are less common with dromostanolone than with other androgens.

- Assess women for these changes. Provide emotional support as needed. Caution patients not to discontinue medication without notifying the physician. Remind patients to take medications as ordered for best effect.

**Other** Urticaria and inflammation at the injection site may occur.

- Anticipate these reactions. If they are severe, notify the physician.
- Assess the injection site for several minutes after administering the injection.

**Patient and family education** • Review with patients the anticipated benefits and possible side effects of drug therapy. • See entry for drug class (p. 533). • See entry for drug class, Drugs Acting on the Male Reproductive System (p. 646).

---

## estramustine   (es-tra-MUS-teen)

antineoplastic*

- estramustine: Emcyt

**MECHANISM OF ACTION**   Estramustine was designed to link an estrogen with an alkylating agent to take advantage of the activity of both types of compounds against certain tumors of the reproductive tract.

**INDICATIONS**   **Prostatic carcinoma** Advanced cases may be treated palliatively with estramustine.

**CONTRAINDICATIONS**   **Hepatic impairment** Liver function can be further altered by extramustine.   **Allergy to estradiol or mechlorethamine** Because these drugs are related to components of estramustine, there may be cross-allergenicity.   **Thrombophlebotic disorders** Patients with active disease or recent myocardial infarction or stroke may be at greater risk of severe side effects.

**DOSAGE**   **PO:**   **ADULTS:** 1 to 10 capsules daily for 30 to 90 days or longer if the disease does not progress. *Special patient populations:*   **CHILDREN:** Pediatric doses have not been established.   **PREGNANCY:** Use of this drug in pregnancy carries substantial risk to the fetus.

**PREPARATIONS**   *Capsules:* 140 mg. Refrigerate capsules and protect from light.

**DRUG INTERACTIONS**   None yet reported.

**FATE**   Estramustine is well absorbed following oral administration. The drug is metabolized by the liver and excreted in bile.

## ☙ NURSING CONSIDERATIONS

### Side effects, toxicities, and associated nursing actions

**CV** Fluid retention is common. Risk of vascular accidents is increased.

---

*Estrogen/alkylator.

- Monitor blood pressure and pulse. Monitor weight. Assess for edema. Instruct patients to report tight rings, shoes, or clothing. Have the patient monitor and record weight at home. Instruct the patient to report a weight gain greater than 2 pounds per day or 5 pounds per week.

**GI** Diarrhea and nausea are minor common side effects.

- See entry for drug class, Cytotoxic Agents (p. 681).

**Metabolic** Hypercalcemia is uncommon but is a dangerous side effect.

- Assess for signs of hypercalcemia: thirst, polyuria, lethargy, anorexia, nausea, vomiting, and constipation. Monitor serum electrolytes.

**Liver** Liver function tests are altered.

- Monitor liver function tests.
- Assess patients for signs of liver dysfunction: malaise, fever, jaundice, right upper quadrant abdominal pain, and change in color or consistency of stools.

**Reproductive** Gynecomastia is common.

- Assess patients for these problems. Provide emotional support as needed. Caution patients to not discontinue medications without notifying the physician and to take medications as ordered for best results.

**Other** Estramustine is expected to be carcinogenic and teratogenic.

- Advice patients about the use of birth control measures, as indicated. Birth control measures should be continued for several months after cessation of drug therapy. If a female patient taking this drug suspects she is pregnant, caution her to notify the physician immediately.

### Nursing interventions related to drug administration

- Note cautions under preparations.
- See the manufacturer's literature for most current information.

### Patient and family education

- Review with patients the anticipated benefits and possible side effects of drug therapy.
- See entry for drug class, Cytotoxic Agents (p. 485).

## leuprolide acetate   (loo-PRO-lide)                                    antineoplastic*

- leuprolide acetate: Lupron

**MECHANISM OF ACTION**   Leuprolide acetate resembles GnRH (gonadotropin-releasing hormone). Long-term administration of leuprolide inhibits gonadotropin secretion and suppresses steroid synthesis in both ovaries and testes.

**INDICATIONS**   **Prostatic carcinoma** Advanced or inoperable disease may respond to leuprolide, but treatment is palliative.   **Breast carcinoma** Advanced cases in premenopausal women may respond.

**CONTRAINDICATIONS**   **Metastatic vertebral lesions or urinary tract obstruction** These patients may not tolerate the initial worsening of symptoms caused by leuprolide.

**DOSAGE**   **SC:**   **ADULTS:** 1 mg daily.   *Special patient populations:*   **CHILDREN:** Pediatric doses have not been established.   **PREGNANCY:** Use of this drug in pregnancy carries substantial risk to the fetus.

**PREPARATIONS**   *Solution:* 5 mg/ml. Refrigerate unopened vials and protect from light.

**DRUG INTERACTIONS**   None established.

**FATE**   Leuprolide acetate is a polypeptide that must be administered parenterally. Bioavailability is high with subcutaneous administration. The elimination *half-life* of the drug administered IV is about 3 hours, but the fate of leuprolide following SC injection is not yet known.

### ☙ NURSING CONSIDERATIONS

#### Side effects, toxicities, and associated nursing actions

**CNS** Up to 3% of patients report headache, dizziness, pain, and paresthesia. Blurred vision, insomnia, irritability, lethargy, memory disorder, and numbness are less common.

*Gonadotropin synthesis blocker.

- Assess for tingling of face, fingers, and toes.
- Caution patients to avoid driving or operating hazardous equipment if dizziness, blurred vision, lethargy, or memory disorder occur.

**CV** Peripheral edema occurs in about 8% of patients. Less than 3% suffer cardiac arrhythmias or myocardial infarction. Embolic disease and congestive heart failure are less common with leuprolide than with alternative therapy for prostatic carcinoma (e.g., DES, p. 536).

- Monitor pulse, blood pressure, and weight. Assess for development of edema. Auscultate lung and breath sounds.
- Instruct the patient to report development of tight rings, shoes, or clothing. Instruct the patient to monitor and record weight at home. Instruct the patient to report weight gain in excess of 2 pounds per day or 5 pounds per week.

**GI** Anorexia, constipation, nausea, and vomiting may occur in up to 2% of patients. Diarrhea, GI bleeding, or altered taste sensations are less frequent.

- See entry for drug class, Cytotoxic Agents (p. 481).

**Blood** Lowered hematocrit and hemoglobin are uncommon.

- Monitor hematocrit and hemoglobin.
- See Anemia, entry for drug class, Cytotoxic Agents (p. 479).

**Renal** Increased BUN, serum creatinine, and polyuria are uncommon, but the initial flare of the disease at start of therapy may cause urinary tract obstruction in patients with advanced prostatic carcinoma.

- Monitor BUN and serum creatinine.
- Monitor intake and output. Instruct patient to report difficulty in voiding.

**Bone** Bone pain may arise initially in 10% of patients with metastatic disease. About 3% experience myalgia.

- Warn patients about these side effects. Instruct patients to notify the physician for severe to moderate pain so that appropriate analgesics can be prescribed.

**Allergic** Facial swelling, fever, rash, and hives occur in less than 3% of patients.

- Have patients remain in the health care setting for at least 15 minutes after administering the dose.
- Have drugs, equipment, and personnel available to treat acute allergic reactions.
- Assess the patient several times in the first 15 minutes after administering the dose.
- Instruct the patient to notify the physician for fever that persists longer than 24 hours.

**Reproductive** Impotence and decreased libido are frequent. Testicular atrophy may occur in up to 3% of patients. Gynecomastia and/or breast tenderness is infrequent.

- Assess patients tactfully for these side effects; some patients are hesitant to discuss sexual matters. Provide emotional support as needed. Remind patients not to discontinue medications without first notifying the physician. Reinforce to patients the importance of taking medications as prescribed for best effect.

**Other** Up to 77% of patients experience hot flashes, ranging from mild flushing to intense sweating.

- Warn patients of this side effect. Provide emotional support as needed.

### Patient and family education
- Review with patients the anticipated benefits and possible side effects of drug therapy. Instruct patients to notify the physician with any concerns or with any new signs or symptoms.
- Teach patients appropriate technique for subcutaneous injection at home. Remind patients to rotate sites. Syringes are provided by the manufacturer. If a syringe cannot be used, instruct the patient to notify the pharmacist. Provide the patient with the patient instruction sheet supplied by the manufacturer.
- See entry for drug class, Cytotoxic Agents (p. 485).

## medroxyprogesterone acetate   (meh-droxy-pro-JES-ter-one)   antineoplastic*

- medroxyprogesterone acetate: Amen, Curretab, Depo-Provera, Provera

*Progestin.

**MECHANISM OF ACTION**　Medroxyprogesterone acetate, like other progestins (p. 633), transforms the endometrium from a proliferative to a secretory phase when estrogens are also present. Slight anabolic and androgenic actions may exist. The exact mechanism of anticancer action is unknown.

**INDICATIONS**　**Secondary amenorrhea** Medroxyprogesterone acetate may restore proper hormone balance and induce menstruation.　**Abnormal uterine bleeding** Medroxyprogesterone acetate may restore the normal cycle of proliferation and secretory activity of the endometrium.　**Endometrial carcinoma** Inoperable, recurrent, or metastatic disease may respond to medroxyprogesterone, but treatment is palliative.　**Renal carcinoma** Inoperable advanced disease may respond to medroxyprogesterone, but treatment is palliative.

**CONTRAINDICATIONS**　**Pregnancy** Progestins may directly affect the fetus.　**Thromboembolic disease** Progestins increase the risk of this side effect.　**Carcinoma of the breast** Progestins may worsen this condition.　**Liver disease** Progestins are metabolized by the liver.

**DOSAGE**　**PO:**　**ADULTS:** For secondary amenorrhea or abnormal uterine bleeding, 5 to 10 mg daily for 5 to 10 days. In some situations estrogens will also have to be administered.　**IM:**　**ADULTS:** For palliative treatment of advanced endometrial or renal carcinoma, 400 to 1000 mg/week initially. Doses may be reduced to as low as 400 mg/month after the drug effect has been established.　*Special patient populations:*　**CHILDREN:** This drug should be avoided.　**PREGNANCY:** Use of this drug in pregnancy carries substantial risk to the fetus.

**PREPARATIONS**　*Tablets:* 2.5, 5, 10 mg; *suspension for IM injection:* 100 or 400 mg/ml.

**DRUG INTERACTIONS**　**Rifampin** may induce the liver enzymes that metabolize progestins, thereby diminishing the effect of the hormone.

**FATE**　Progestins are metabolized to a variety of compounds in the liver and excreted in urine and bile. Medroxyprogesterone acetate persists for long periods in the body.

### 🦌 NURSING CONSIDERATIONS

#### Side effects, toxicities, and associated nursing actions

**CNS** Dizziness, fatigue, headache, hyperpyrexia, insomnia, mood changes, nervousness, and somnolence may occur. Significant depression may require discontinuing therapy.
- Caution patients to avoid driving or operating hazardous equipment if dizziness, fatigue, or other CNS side effects occur.
- Assess for signs of depression: change in affect, withdrawal, insomnia, anorexia, or lack of interest in personal appearance. Question family members about emotional changes in the patient.

**Blood** Thrombophlebitis, pulmonary embolism, and cerebral embolism or thrombosis may be induced by medroxyprogesterone, especially in patients predisposed to these conditions.
- Monitor pulse, blood pressure, and weight.
- Monitor the patient for thrombophlebitis, and review signs and symptoms with the patient: pain in the extremity and swelling. The affected limb may be cool and pale, with the area of the affected vessel red and warm to touch. Instruct the patient to notify the physician if these symptoms occur.
- Encourage regular ambulation.

**GI** Abdominal discomfort and nausea may occur.
- See Overview of Drug Class, Cytotoxic Agents (p. 481).

**Metabolic** Decreased glucose tolerance may occur.
- Monitor urine and blood glucose levels.
- Caution diabetic patients to monitor urine and blood glucose levels carefully. An adjustment in diet or insulin may be necessary.

**Allergic** Anaphylaxis, angioedema, pruritis, rash, and urticaria may occur.
- Have drugs, equipment, and personnel available to treat an acute allergic reaction in settings where this drug is administered.
- Instruct patients to report the development of any skin changes.

**Skin** Acne, alopecia, chloasma, hirsutism, or melasma are uncommon.
- Warn patients about these possible side effects; provide reassurance as needed.
- See entry for drug class, Cytotoxic Agents (p. 484).
- If skin changes are severe, consult the physician about drug or dosage changes.

**Liver** Jaundice is rare.
- Monitor the patient for jaundice. Monitor liver function tests. Assess the patient for other signs of liver dysfunction: fatigue, malaise, fever, right upper quadrant abdominal pain, and change in color or consistency of stools.

**Reproductive** Amenorrhea, breakthrough bleeding, changes in cervical secretions, changes in menstrual flow, breast tenderness, or galactorrhea are common.
- Review these side effects with patients, and instruct them to report their development.

**Eye** Diplopia, proptosis, retinal vascular lesions, or unexplained loss of vision are grounds for discontinuing therapy.
- Instruct patients to notify the physician immediately of any changes in vision.

**Other** Fluid retention or edema may complicate other conditions such as asthma, heart disease, migraine, or renal disorders.
- Obtain a thorough history of other medical problems before starting therapy. Warn patient with conditions aggravated by fluid retention to be careful about monitoring weight and to notify physician about the development of edema.

### Patient and family education
- Review with patients the anticipated benefits and possible side effects of drug therapy.
- See entry for drug class (p. 533).
- See entry for drug class, Drugs Acting on the Female Reproductive System (p. 627).

## megestrol acetate (meh-GES-trol)    antineoplastic*

- megestrol acetate: Megace, Pallace

**MECHANISM OF ACTION** Megestrol acetate, like other progestins (p. 633), transforms the endometrium from proliferative to secretory phases and inhibits the pituitary. The drug has no anabolic, androgenic, or estrogenic activity. The anticancer effect may be related to these actions or to direct antiproliferative effects on cancerous tissue.

**INDICATIONS** **Endometrial or breast carcinoma** Advanced or metastatic disease may be treated palliatively with megestrol acetate; surgery and radiation are often included in the regimen. • About 50% of patients respond.

**CONTRAINDICATIONS** **Pregnancy** Progestins should not be used during the first 4 months of pregnancy. **Thrombombolic disease** Progestins may increase the risk of these complications.

**DOSAGE** **PO:** **ADULTS:** For advanced breast carcinoma, 160 mg daily in four divided doses. For advanced endometrial carcinoma, 40 to 320 mg daily in divided doses. Therapy should continue for 2 months to allow full evaluation of effect. *Special patient populations;* **CHILDREN:** This drug should be avoided. **PREGNANCY:** Use of this drug in pregnancy carries substantial risk to the fetus.

**PREPARATIONS** *Tablets:* 20 or 40 mg.

**DRUG INTERACTIONS** **Rifampin** may induce the liver enzymes that metabolize progestins, thereby diminishing the effect of the hormone.

**FATE** Megestrol acetate is absorbed well following oral administration, producing *peak* plasma concentrations within 3 hours. The drug is extensively metabolized in the liver. The metabolites are excreted slowly.

### ☙ NURSING CONSIDERATIONS
#### Side effects, toxicities, and associated nursing actions
**Blood** Thrombophlebitis may occur.
- Monitor the patient for this side effect and review signs and symptoms with the patient: pain in the extremity and swelling. The affected limb may be cool and pale, with the area of the affected vessel red and warm to touch. Instruct the patient to notify the physician if these symptoms occur.
- Encourage regular ambulation.

*Progestin.

**Other** Alopecia, carpal tunnel syndrome, and a feeling of coldness have been rarely reported.
- Encourage patients to report the development of any unusual sign or symptom.
- See entry for drug class, Cytotoxic Agents (p. 485).

**Patient and family education**
- Review with patients the anticipated benefits and possible side effects of therapy.
- See entry for drug class (p. 485).
- See entry for drug class, Drugs Acting on the Female Reproductive System (p. 627).

---

## mitotane   (MY-toh-tane)                                    antineoplastic*

- mitotane: Lysodren

**MECHANISM OF ACTION**    Mitotane causes specific degeneration of the zona fasciculata and zona reticularis of the adrenal cortex, resulting in loss of synthesis of glucocorticoids. Mineralocorticoid synthesis is not significantly impaired because mitotane does not damage the zona glomerulosa.

**INDICATIONS**    **Adrenocortical carcinoma** About 50% of patients with inoperable disease experience tumor regression; some may attain long-term remission.

**CONTRAINDICATIONS**    **Stress** Patients receiving mitotane are unable to deal with the stress of injury or infection and require glucocorticoid therapy.

**DOSAGE**    **PO:**    **ADULTS:** Initially, 8 to 10 g daily in three or four divided doses. Doses are increased according to need and tolerance of the patient. Doses up to 16 gm daily have been used. Discontinue after 3 months if the patient does not respond.    *Special patient populations:*    **CHILDREN:** Pediatric doses are not established.    **PREGNANCY:** Use of this drug in pregnancy carries substantial risk to the fetus.

**PREPARATIONS**    *Tablets:* 500 mg.

**DRUG INTERACTIONS**    **Coumarin anticoagulants, barbiturates and phenytoin** may be more rapidly metabolized when mitotane is given because mitotane induces liver microsomal enzymes responsible for eliminating these drugs.    **CNS depressants** may have additive depressant action with mitotane.

**DIAGNOSTIC TEST INTERFERENCE**    **Serum protein-bound iodine** may be reduced because mitotane displaces thyroxin from thyroxine-binding globulin.    **Urinary 17-hydroxycorticosteroids** may be decreased.

**FATE**    Mitotane is incompletely absorbed following oral administration, with only about 40% of a dose ultimately entering the blood. Mitotane distributes to all tissues within about 12 hours. Some metabolism occurs in the liver, and excretion is in urine and bile. Elimination from tissues is slow; the elimination *half-life* from the body therefore ranges from 18 to 159 days.

**NURSING CONSIDERATIONS**
### Side effects, toxicities, and associated nursing actions

**CNS** About 40% of patients suffer CNS side effects. The most common reactions are lethargy and somnolence. Confusion, depression, dizziness, fatigue, headache, irritability, tremors, vertigo, and weakness also may occur. Ataxia, encephalopathy, hallucinations, impaired memory, myelopathy, neuropathy, psychosis, and speech difficulty are uncommon. Prolonged high doses may lead to functional impairment and brain damage.
- Caution patients to avoid driving or operating hazardous equipment until the effects of the medication can be evaluated.
- Obtain a thorough baseline assessment of mental status and neurologic function before starting therapy and at regular intervals.
- Assess for signs of depression: anorexia, insomnia, lack of interest in personal appearance, and withdrawal.

**CV** Hypertension or hypotension may occur.
- Monitor blood pressure and pulse.

*Tissue-specific.

**Blood** Leukopenia or thrombocytopenia.
* See entry for drug class, Cytotoxic Agents (p. 479).

**GI** About 80% of patients suffer GI side effects, including anorexia, diarrhea, nausea, and vomiting.
* See entry for drug class, Cytotoxic Agents (p. 481).

**Renal** Albuminuria, hematuria, and hemorrhagic cystitis may occur.
* Monitor urinalysis. Instruct patients to report changes in the color of urine or the appearance of blood in the urine.

**Metabolic** Serum cholesterol may be elevated.
* Monitor serum cholesterol levels.

**Eye** Blurred vision, diplopia, lens opacities, optic neuritis, papilledema, and retinal hemorrhage occur infrequently.
* Instruct patients to report any changes in vision.
* Refer patients for regular ophthalmic examinations.

**Reproductive** Gynecomastia may occur in males.
* Assess patients for the development of this side effect. Provide emotional support as needed. Encourage patients not to discontinue the medication without first notifying the physician. Remind patients to take drugs as prescribed for best effect.

**Skin** About 15% of patients suffer transient maculopapular rash. Alopecia, chloasma, erythema multiforme, facial or periorbital swelling, hyperpigmentation, perinasal scaling, and urticaria are less common.
* Instruct patients to report the development of any skin changes.

**Other** Arthralgia, myalgia, generalized aching, fever, shortness of breath, wheezing, flushing, excessive salivation, and decreased hearing have all occasionally been reported.
* Instruct patients to notify the physician of any new sign or symptom.

### Patient and family education
* Review with patients the anticipated benefits and possible side effects of drug therapy.
* Instruct patients taking mitotane to wear a medical identification tag or bracelet stating their medications. In the event of trauma or other injury, it would be necessary to administer glucocorticoids to the patient who has been receiving mitotane.
* See entry for drug class (p. 485).
* For a general discussion about adrenal steroids, see p. 606.

---

## polyestradiol phosphate   (poly-ess-tra-DYE-ol)   antineoplastic*

* polyestradiol phosphate: Estradurin

**MECHANISM OF ACTION**   Certain reproductive tumors, including prostatic cancers in men, retain hormone receptors that render them sensitive to estrogens such as polyestradiol phosphate.

**INDICATIONS**   **Carcinoma of the prostate** Advanced, inoperable disease may respond to estrogen therapy. Beneficial effects are obtained in about 75% of treated patients.

**CONTRAINDICATIONS**   **Estrogen-dependent neoplasm** Such tumors may progress rapidly when estrogens are given.   **Thromboembolic disease** Patients with pre-existing conditions may be more at risk of severe episodes when estrogens are given.   **Pregnancy** Polyestradiol phosphate should not be used in pregnant women.

**DOSAGE**   **IM:**   **ADULTS:** A single dose of 40 mg every 2 to 4 weeks until relapse occurs. Up to 80 mg may be given. *Special patient populations:*   **CHILDREN:** This drug is not indicated for children.   **PREGNANCY:** Use of this drug in pregnancy carries substantial risk to the fetus.

**PREPARATIONS**   *Powder for reconstitution:* 40 mg with 2 ml diluent. Swirl gently to dissolve; do not shake vigorously.

*Estrogen.

**DRUG INTERACTIONS**   **Rifampin** may decrease estrogen activity by hastening metabolism of steroids.   **Corticosteroid** effects may be exaggerated in patients with concomitent estrogen therapy because estrogens may slow metabolism of the corticosteroid.   **Oral anticoagulants** may be less effective in patients receiving estrogens because metabolism of the anticoagulants is hastened.

**FATE**   Polyestradiol phosphate is a polymeric form of extradiol phosphate. The low solubility of the polymer in water causes it to be absorbed slowly from IM sites, creating a long-acting depot of drug. The drug is slowly dephosphorylated to yield estradiol, the active form of the drug. Estradiol may be metabolized by the liver and excreted in urine and bile.

## ❦ NURSING CONSIDERATIONS

### Side effects, toxicities, and associated nursing actions

**CNS** Dizziness, irritability, and changes in libido may occur.
- Caution patients to avoid driving or operating hazardous equipment if dizziness occurs.
- Warn patients about possible irritability.
- Assess tactfully for changes in libido; many patients may be unwilling to discuss this. Provide emotional support as needed. Caution patients to take the drug only as ordered and to not discontinue the medication without notifying the physician.

**CV** Hypertension occurs during therapy and may persist after the drug is discontinued. Edema may occur with high doses.
- Monitor the blood pressure and pulse.
- Monitor weight. Assess for edema. Instruct patients to report tight rings, shoes, or clothing. Have the patient monitor and record weight at home. Instruct the patient to report a weight gain greater than 2 pounds per day or 5 pounds per week.

**Blood** Thrombophlebitis or other thromboembolic disorders may occur with prolonged estrogen therapy. The high doses used in cancer chemotherapy also increase the risk.
- Monitor the patient for these side effects, and review signs and symptoms with the patient: pain in the extremity and swelling. The affected limb may be cool and pale, with the area of the affected vein red and warm to touch. Instruct the patient to notify the physician if these symptoms occur.
- Encourage regular ambulation.

**GI** Anorexia, abdominal cramps, and nausea are expected with high doses.
- See entry for drug class, Cytotoxic Agents (p. 481).
- Assess for signs of hypercalcemia: anorexia, nausea, vomiting, and constipation. Monitor serum electrolytes.

**Renal** Women may experience urinary incontinence or urinary frequency.
- Warn patients about this possible side effect.
- Instruct patients to notify the physician if urinary frequency is severe, persistent, or is accompanied by fever, pain in the bladder area, change in the color or clarity of urine, or pain on urination.
- Teach patients to perform perineal exercises to strengthen perineal and gluteal muscles. Two examples of exercises follow: Have the patient sit on the toilet with knees wide apart and then, while voiding, start and stop the urinary stream. Have the patient tighten the perineal muscles as if trying not to void; hold for 3 seconds, then relax; repeat several times.

**Reproductive** Women may experience breast tenderness, uterine bleeding, and anogenital pain and pruritis. Men should expect gynecomastia and impotence.
- Assess patients for these problems. Provide emotional support as needed. Caution patients to not discontinue medications without notifying the physician and to take medications as ordered for best results.
- Instruct patients to notify the physician about uterine bleeding. Although bleeding may be a drug side effect, it should be investigated.

### Patient and family education
- Review with patients the anticipated benefits and possible side effects of drug therapy.
- See entry for drug class, Cytotoxic Agents (p. 485).
- See entry for drug class, Drugs Acting on the Female Reproductive System (p. 627).

# prednisone   (PRED-ni-sone)                                    antineoplastic*

- prednisone: Meticorten, Orasone, Prednicen

**MECHANISM OF ACTION**   Prednisone, like other glucocorticoids, is cytotoxic toward lymphoid tissue. This action allows the drug to be used against cancers arising from lymphoid tissue. For other actions of prednisone, see Chapter 31 (p. 623).

**INDICATIONS**   **Acute lymphocytic leukemia** Prednisone is used with vincristine to induce remissions. **Advanced Hodgkin's disease** Prednisone is part of the MOPP regimen (p. 479).   **Non-Hodgkin's lymphomas** Prednisone is part of the CVP, CHOP, and BACOP regimens (p. 479) used in these diseases.

**CONTRAINDICATIONS**   See entry for prednisone in Chapter 31 (p. 623).

**DOSAGE**   **PO:**   **ADULTS AND CHILDREN:** Doses depend on the severity of the disease and range from 10 to 100 mg daily in divided doses.   *Special patient populations:*   **PREGNANCY:** Use of this drug in pregnancy carries substantial risk to the fetus.

**PREPARATIONS**   *Tablets:* 1, 2.5, 5, 10, 20, 25, and 50 mg; *tablets, film-coated:* 5 and 50 mg; *solution, oral:* 5 mg/5 ml with 5% alcohol; *solution concentrate:* 5 mg/ml with 30% alcohol; syrup: 5 mg/5 ml with 5% alcohol.

**DRUG INTERACTIONS**   **Anticholinesterase agents** such as *ambenonium, neostigmine,* or *pyridostigmine* may produce severe weakness in myasthenia gravis patients also receiving prednisone.   **Anticoagulants** used orally may be less effective when given with glucocorticoids.   **Barbiturates, phenytoin, and rifampin** all induce hepatic microsomal enzymes, increasing the rate of metabolism (inactivation) of glucocorticoids.   **Estrogens** may displace glucocorticoids from the transport protein transcortin, thereby increasing the activity of the glucocorticoid.   **Nonsteroidal anti-inflammatory agents** such as *aspirin* and *indomethacin* may increase risk of GI ulceration with prednisone.   **Potassium-depleting drugs (amphotericin B, ethacrynic acid, furosemide, and thiazides)** enhance potassium loss caused by prednisone.   **Toxoids and vaccines** are less effective when patients also are receiving prednisone because the glucocorticoid inhibits the antibody response.

**DIAGNOSTIC TEST INTERFERENCE**   **Nitro blue tetrazolium (NBT) test** for bacterial infections may be falsely negative in the presence of prednisone.

**FATE**   Prednisone is converted by the liver to the active form prednisolone. Further breakdown to inactive metabolites also occurs in the liver, with most of these forms being eliminated in the urine.

## 🐾 NURSING CONSIDERATIONS

### Side effects, toxicities, and associated nursing actions

**CNS** Euphoria is common. Anxiety, depression, emotional instability, mood swings, and psychoses may also occur.
- Obtain a mental status exam before therapy and at regular intervals. If CNS symptoms are severe or troublesome, notify the physician. Mild euphoria in cancer patients may be well tolerated by some patients.
- Assess for signs of depression: withdrawal, insomnia, anorexia, and lack of interest in personal appearance.

**CV** Sodium retention caused by glucocorticoids may lead to hypertension, edema, and heart failure.
- Monitor pulse, blood pressure, and weight. Auscultate heart and lung sounds.
- Instruct the patient to monitor weight and record weight at home.
- Instruct the patient to report the development of tight rings, shoes, or clothing.

**GI** Anorexia, nausea, and vomiting may occur. Glucocorticoids can also increase the risk of GI ulceration.
- See entry for drug class, Cytotoxic agents (p. 481).
- Instruct patients to take glucocorticoids with meals or a snack. Many physicians prescribe antacids or cimetidine concurrently with glucocorticoids.

*Glucocorticoid.

- Instruct patients to report the development of abdominal pain or bleeding in the stool.
- Monitor stools for occult blood.

**Metabolic** Glucocorticoids decrease glucose tolerance and may induce diabetes mellitus. Glucocorticoids also cause potassium loss, leading to a variety of effects including muscle weakness.

- Monitor urine and blood glucose levels. Instruct diabetic patients to monitor blood glucose levels carefully, as an adjustment in diet or insulin dosage may be necessary.
- Assess for signs of hypokalemia: muscle weakness, apathy, abdominal distention, and paralytic ileus. Auscultate bowel sounds.
- Other signs of hypokalemia include electrocardiographic changes: flattened or inverted T waves, prolonged QT segments, and prominent U waves. Monitor serial ECGs. Be alert to hypokalemia when the patient is receiving other drugs that affect or depend on potassium balance: diuretics, cardiac glycosides, and others.

**Skin** Acne, atrophy of the skin, ecchymoses, facial erythema, and fragility of the skin may arise with long-term therapy.

- Caution patients about these changes. Caution patients to avoid bruising and rough contact activities if possible.

**Reproductive** Amenorrhea and reduced sperm count may occur.

- Warn patients about these side effects. Instruct women to keep a record of menstrual periods. Counsel men and women about birth control measures as appropriate. Instruct women to notify the physican immediately if pregnancy is suspected.

**Endocrine** Long-term use at high doses may produce a cushingoid state.

- Warn patients about this side effect. Provide emotional support as needed.

### Patient and family education

- Review with patients the anticipated benefits and possible side effects of drug therapy.
- For a more detailed discussion of glucocorticoids, see entry for drug class, Adrenal Steroids and Related Agents (p. 606).
- See entry for drug class (p. 533)

---

## sodium iodide I 131                                      antineoplastic*

- sodium iodide I 131: Iodotype

**MECHANISM OF ACTION**  Sodium iodide I 131 is a radioactive form of iodine. Like the common isotope of iodine, this radioactive form is concentrated by the thyroid so that high doses of the short-range ionizing beta radiation are delivered to thyroid tissue. This technique allows nonsurgical destruction of hyperactive or cancerous regions within the thyroid.

**INDICATIONS**  **Hyperthyroidism** Destruction of part of the gland may reduce the production of thyroid hormones.  **Thyroid carcinoma** Hyperactive cancerous regions may receive lethal radiation doses.

**CONTRAINDICATIONS**  **Severe thyrotoxic heart disease** Such patients may not survive the temporary initial thyrotoxic reactions that can occur during therapy.  **Lack of specialized facilities** Use of this radioactive drug is restricted to physicians licensed by the Nuclear Regulatory Commission and to facilities prepared to contain and dispose of the drug properly.

**DOSAGE**  **PO:**  **ADULTS:** For Graves' disease, 4 to 10 mCi. For thyroid carcinoma, 30 to 200 mCi, the dose depending on the extent and site of disease. *Special patient populations:*  **CHILDREN:** This drug is sometimes used in very small doses for diagnostic purposes in children.  **PREGNANCY:** Radioactive iodine should be avoided during pregnancy.

**PREPARATIONS**  *Capsules:* 0.8 to 100 mCi; *solution for oral use:* 3.5 to 150 mCi/ml. This radioactive drug should be used with all precautions decreed by the local radiation safety program. All materials actually in contact with oral solutions require special disposal and handling. Body fluids and waste from patients receiving more than 30 mCi may require careful collection and disposal.

*Antithyroid.

**DRUG INTERACTIONS**   **Antithyroid drugs** given concurrently may block uptake of radioactive iodine into thyroid tissue.

**FATE**   The radioactive form of iodine is absorbed and concentrated in thyroid tissue just as normal dietary iodine. The radioactive *half-life* of the compound is 8 days. The biologic *half-life* is 138 days.

## ☙ NURSING CONSIDERATIONS

### Side effects, toxicities, and associated nursing actions

**Blood** Leukopenia and thrombocytopenia are rare.
* See entry for drug class, Cytotoxic Agents (p. 479).

**GI** Nausea, vomiting, and loss of taste are uncommon.
* See entry for drug class, Cytotoxic Agents (p. 481).
* If vomiting occurs within 6 to 8 hours after administration of drug, the vomitus is highly radioactive; dispose of according to agency guidelines.

**Endocrine** Hypothyroidism will occur in 100% of patients effectively treated for thyroid carcinoma. Appropriate replacement therapy must be given.
* Assess for signs of hypothyroidism: sluggishness, weight gain, sleepiness, intolerance to cold, constipation, dry skin, dry, and sparse hair. Monitor thyroid function tests.

**Other** Tenderness or swelling of the neck or salivary glands is uncommon but may signal radiation damage to tissues surrounding the thyroid.
* Assess for these problems. Instruct the patient to report the development of any new sign or symptom.

### Nursing interventions related to drug administration

* If liquid is administered, add water to the container twice and have the patient drink these rinses to ensure that the total dose was taken.
* Consult agency policies and procedures for handling and administering radioactive drugs.
* Patients may have to fast before taking the drug.

### Patient and family education

* Review with patients the anticipated benefits and possible side effects of drug therapy.
* See entry for drug class (p. 485).

---

## sodium phosphate P 32                                                        antineoplastic*

* generic

**MECHANISM OF ACTION**   Sodium phosphate P 32 is a radioactive form of phosphorous that emits beta radiation. Rapidly proliferating tissues such as bone marrow and neoplastic tissues utilize large amounts of phosphate and therefore concentrate this radioactive isotope. The ionizing radiation destroys the proliferating cells.

**INDICATIONS**   **Polycythemia vera** The proliferative phase of this disease can be controlled with sodium phosphate P 32.   **Chronic myelogenous leukemia** The isotope may be used for palliative treatment in the early stages of this disease.

**CONTRAINDICATIONS**   **Mild disease in patients under 40** Sodium phosphate P 32 may induce leukemia in patients with polycythemia vera. Use should be restricted to more serious disease.   **Lack of specialized facilities** Use of this radioactive drug is restricted to physicians licensed by the Nuclear Regulatory Commission and to facilities prepared to contain and dispose of the drug properly.

**DOSAGE**   PO:   **ADULTS:** For polycythemia vera, 6 mCi as a single dose, followed by a second dose within 6 months if needed to complete remission. IV:   **ADULTS:** For polycythemia vera, 2.3 mCi/ml. *Special patient populations:*   **CHILDREN:** Pediatric doses have not been established.   **PREGNANCY:** FDA pregnancy category C.

**PREPARATIONS**   *Solution:* 0.67 mCi/ml in a 10 ml container.

**DRUG INTERACTIONS**   **Myelosuppressive drugs** may have additive effects with sodium phosphate P 32.

*Radioactive.

**FATE** Sodium phosphate P 32 is taken up readily following oral administration. The drug is distributed well through the body and concentrated in those tissues with most rapid turnover rates because those tissues have the highest requirement for phosphate. The radioactivity of sodium phosphate P 32 diappears with a *half-life* of 14.3 days.

## ☙ NURSING CONSIDERATIONS

### Side effects, toxicities, and associated nursing actions

**Blood** High doses may cause anemia, leukopenia, or thrombocytopenia.

- See entry for drug class, Cytotoxic Agents (p. 479).

**Other** Massive exposure could cause mild radiation poisoning, but this is not a risk with the small doses ordinarily used. The ionizing radiation produced by this isotope may induce leukemia in a few patients.

### Nursing interventions related to drug administration

- Consult agency policies and procedures for handling and administering radioactive drugs.

### Patient and family education

- Review with patients the anticipated benefits and possible side effects of drug therapy.
- See entry for drug class (p. 533).

## streptozocin  (strep-toh-ZOH-sin)  antineoplastic*

- streptozocin: Zanosar

**MECHANISM OF ACTION**  Streptozocin is related to nitrosourea alkylating agents, but because the drug has a sugar included in its structure it is concentrated in the islet cells of the pancreas. The islet cells are therefore specifically destroyed.

**INDICATIONS**  **Pancreatic islet cell carcinoma** Up to 60% of patients improve with streptozocin therapy alone or with other anticancer agents such as fluorouracil.

**CONTRAINDICATIONS**  **Renal disease** Streptozocin is a highly nephrotoxic drug that may destroy renal function, especially in patients with impaired kidneys.

**DOSAGE**  IV:  ADULTS: 1 to 1.5 $g/M^2$ weekly or 500 $mg/M^2$ daily for 5 days repeated every 6 weeks.  *Special patient populations:*  CHILDREN: Pediatric doses have not been established.  PREGNANCY: FDA pregnancy category C.

**PREPARATIONS**  *Solution for parenteral injection:* 1 g.

**DRUG INTERACTIONS**  **Myelosuppressive drugs** given with streptozocin may have synergistic hematologic toxicity.  **Phenytoin** may interfere with the action of streptozocin on beta cells of the pancreas, diminishing the anticancer action.  **Nephrotoxic drugs** may dangerously diminish renal function already damaged by streptozocin.

**FATE**  Streptozocin must be administered IV to achieve adequate concentrations in blood and tissues. The drug is rapidly distributed and metabolized to various products, which are excreted primarily in urine.

## ☙ NURSING CONSIDERATIONS

### Side effects, toxicities, and associated nursing actions

**CNS** Confusion, depression, and lethargy have occurred in patients receiving continuous infusion for 5 days.

- Obtain a thorough assessment of mental status before starting therapy and at regular intervals.
- Assess for signs of depression: withdrawal, anorexia, insomnia, change in affect, and lack of interest in personal appearance.

**Blood** Up to 20% of patients may experience mild myelosuppression (anemia, leukopenia, or thrombocytopenia).

- See entry for drug class, Cytotoxic Agents (p. 479).

**GI** Severe nausea and vomiting occur in most treated patients.

*Tissue specific.

- See entry for drug class, Cytotoxic Agents (p. 481).

**Renal** Up to 75% of patients suffer renal toxicity, which is cumulative and may be fatal. Symptoms may include anuria, azotemia, hypophosphatemia, hyperchloremia, proximal renal tubular acidosis, and proteinuria.

- Push fluids to at least 2500 ml/day.
- Monitor urinalysis, serum electrolytes, BUN, and serum creatinine.
- Monitor weight, intake, and output.

**Metabolic** Some patients may suffer glycosuria or changes in glucose tolerance.

- Monitor serum and urine glucose levels. Have diabetic patients monitor glucose levels carefully: an adjustment in diet or insulin dose may be necessary.

**Liver** Hypoalbuminemia and increased serum bilirubin concentration may occur, but severe or fatal hepatotoxicity is rare.

- Monitor serum albumin, bilirubin, and liver function tests.
- Assess for signs of liver dysfunction: jaundice, malaise, fever, right upper quadrant abdominal pain, and change in color or consistency of stools.

**Other** Extravasation causes tissue damage. Too-rapid IV injection causes burning pain.

- See discussion of IV administration, Cytotoxic Agents (p. 484).

### Nursing Interventions related to drug administration

- Procedures for the handling and administering of cytotoxic agents should also be applied to this drug. See entry for drug class, Cytotoxic Agents (p. 485).
- Dilute as directed, each 1 g with 9.5 ml of 0.9% sodium chloride or 5% dextrose for injection. It may be further diluted in 50 to 250 ml of the same fluid. Administer a dose in minimal diluent over 5 to 15 minutes. If drug has been further diluted, or if needed for patient comfort, infusion time may be increased.

### Patient and family education

- Review with patients the anticipated benefits and possible side effects of drug therapy.
- See entry for drug class (p. 533).
- See entry for drug class, Cytotoxic Agents (p. 485).

---

## tamoxifen citrate    (tam-OX-i-fen)                                   antineoplastic*

- tamoxifen citrate: Nolvadex

**MECHANISM OF ACTION**    Tamoxifen citrate binds to estrogen receptors but prevents estrogenic effects.

**INDICATIONS**    **Carcinoma of the breast** Advanced or disseminated tumors in about 60% of treated postmenopausal women may respond to tamoxifen.

**CONTRAINDICATIONS**    **Leukopenia and thrombocytopenia** Patients with pre-existing impairment may be more susceptible to additional damage by tamoxifen.

**DOSAGE**    **PO:** **ADULTS:** 10 or 20 mg morning and evening. *Special patient populations:* **CHILDREN:** This drug is not indicated for use in children. **PREGNANCY:** Use of this drug in pregnancy carries substantial risk to the fetus.

**PREPARATIONS**    *Tablets:* 50 mg.

**DRUG INTERACTIONS**    **Myelosuppressive agents** may produce more severe effects in the presence of tamoxifen.

**FATE**    Tamoxifen is adequately absorbed following oral administration, with *peak* serum concentrations within 7 hours. The drug tends to concentrate in tissues with estrogen receptors, including tumor tissue. The elimination *half-life* is about 7 days, with most of the drug undergoing hepatic metabolism. Metabolites are excreted primarily in feces, with small amounts in urine.

### ☙ NURSING CONSIDERATIONS

#### Side effects, toxicities, and associated nursing actions

**CNS** Confusion, depression, dizziness, headache, lassitude, and lightheadedness have occurred.

*Antiestrogen.

- Caution the patient to avoid driving or operating hazardous equipment if confusion, dizziness, lassitude, or lightheadedness occur.
- Assess for signs of depression: withdrawal, change in affect, lack of interest in personal appearance, insomnia, and anorexia.
- Assess mental status and neurologic function.

**Blood** Mild leukopenia and thrombocytopenia may occur.
- See entry for drug class. Cytotoxic Agents (p. 479).

**GI** Nausea and vomiting are among the more common side effects. Anorexia or distaste for food can occur.

**Endocrine** Hypercalcemia occurs early in therapy of patients with metastases to the bone.
- Assess for signs of hypercalcemia: anorexia, nausea, vomiting, and constipation. Monitor serum electrolytes.
- Push fluids to 3000 ml/day to foster calcium excretion and help prevent constipation.

**Eye:** Corneal opacities, decreased visual acuity and retinopathy have occurred with high doses over long periods.
- Assess visual acuity regularly. Instruct the patient to report any changes in vision.
- Encourage patients to have regular ophthalmic examinations.

**Reproductive** Hot flashes are a common side effect, vaginal discharge, menstrual irregularities, and pruritis vulvae are less common.
- Warn patients about these side effects. Provide support as needed.
- Instruct female patients to keep a record of menstrual periods. Instruct women to notify the physician if vaginal discharge becomes excessive or if significant vaginal bleeding occurs.

**Other** Peripheral edema and leg cramps may occur. Bone pain can occur, as well as temporary increase in tumor size (flare).
- Warn patients about these possible side effects.
- Instruct patients to notify the physician of moderate to severe pain so analgesics can be prescribed if the patient does not already have sufficient analgesics.
- Instruct the patient to report tight rings or shoes. Have the patient monitor and record weight at home. Instruct the patient to report weight gain in excess of 2 pounds per day or 5 pounds per week.

### Patient and family education
- Review with patients the anticipated benefits and possible side effects of drug therapy.
- See entry for drug class (p. 533).

---

## testolactone   (tes-toh-LAK-tone)                                    antineoplastic*

- Testolactone: Teslac

**MECHANISM OF ACTION**   Testolactone acts similarly to androgens but does not produce virilization at ordinary doses. The exact antineoplastic mechanism is unknown.

**INDICATIONS**   **Carcinoma of the breast** Advanced or disseminated tumors in postmenopausal women may respond.

**CONTRAINDICATIONS**   **Carcinoma of the breast in males** These tumors may not be controlled by androgen action.

**DOSAGE**   **PO:**   **ADULTS:** 250 mg four times daily for 3 months or longer.   *Special patient populations:* **CHILDREN:** This drug is not indicated for use in children.   **PREGNANCY:** Use of this drug in pregnancy carries substantial risk to the fetus.

**PREPARATIONS**   *Tablets:* 50 mg.

*Androgen.

**DRUG INTERACTIONS**    Oral anticoagulants may have enhanced action in the presence of testolactone.

**FATE**    Testolactone is well absorbed following oral administration and is metabolized and excreted in urine.

## 🐾 NURSING CONSIDERATIONS

### Side effects, toxicities, and associated nursing actions

**CNS** Paresthesias may occur.
- Assess for tingling of fingers and toes.

**CV** Hypertension and edema have been noted.
- Monitor pulse, blood pressure, and weight.
- Instruct patients to report development of tight rings, shoes, or clothing.
- Instruct patients to monitor and record weight at home. Instruct patients to report weight gain in excess of 2 pounds per day or 5 pounds per week.

**GI** Anorexia, diarrhea, nausea, and vomiting may occur. Glossitis has also been noted.
- See entry for drug class, Cytotoxic Agents (p. 481).
- Assess for signs of hypercalcemia: anorexia, nausea, vomiting, and constipation. Monitor serum electrolytes.

**Other** Alopecia, glossitis, and nail growth disturbance are rare.
- See entry for drug class, Cytotoxic Agents (p. 484).

### Patient and family education
- Review with patients the anticipated benefits and possible side effects of drug therapy.
- See entry for drug class (p. 533).
- See Overview, Drugs Acting on the Male Reproductive System (p. 646).

---

## goserelin    (GOE-se-rel-in)                                    antineoplastic*

- goserelin (investigational): Zoladex

**MECHANISM OF ACTION**    Zoladex is more potent and longer-acting form of gonadotropin-releasing hormone (GnRH).

**INDICATIONS**    **Carcinoma or the breast or prostate** These conditions may regress after an initial flare.

**CONTRAINDICATIONS**    **Conditions worsened by edema** Heart disease or asthma might be worsened by fluid retention caused by zoladex.

**DOSAGE**    **SC:** **ADULTS:** 3.6 mg every 4 weeks. *Special patient populations:* **CHILDREN:** This drug is not indicated for use in children. **PREGNANCY:** Use of this drug in pregnancy carries substantial risk to the fetus.

**PREPARATIONS**    *Syringe:* 3.6 mg zoladex in a polymer to create a depot.

**DRUG INTERACTIONS**    None yet determined.

**FATE**    Zoladex is a polypeptide that cannot be administered orally but is adequately absorbed when administered as a depot SC.

## 🐾 NURSING CONSIDERATIONS

### Side effects, toxicities, and associated nursing actions

**CV** Edema may occur.
- Monitor pulse, blood pressure, and weight.
- Instruct patients to report the development of tight rings, shoes, or clothing. Have patients monitor and record weight at home. Instruct patients to report weight gain in excess of 2 pounds per day or 5 pounds per week.

**Blood** Thrombophlebitis is infrequent.
- Monitor the patient for this side effect, and review signs and symptoms with the patient: pain in an

*GnRH analog.

extremity and swelling. The affected limb may be cool and pale, with the area of the affected vessel red and warm to touch. Instruct the patient to notify the physician if these symptoms occur.
- Encourage regular ambulation.

**GI** Nausea and vomiting are infrequent.
- See entry for drug class, Cytotoxic Agents (p. 481).

**Endocrine** Hot flashes are common. Loss of libido may occur. Gynecomastia is uncommon.
- Warn patients about these side effects, and assess patients for their development. Provide support as needed. Caution patients not to discontinue medication without notifying the physician. Remind patients to take medications as ordered for best effect.

## Nursing interventions related to drug administration
- See the manufacturer's literature for the most current information.

## Patient and family education
- Review with patients the anticipated benefits and possible side effects of drug therapy.
- Encourage patients to return on a regular basis for subsequent injections.
- See entry for drug class, Cytotoxic Agents (p. 485).

# HORMONES AND DRUGS INFLUENCING THE ENDOCRINE SYSTEM

**INTRODUCTION**  The endocrine system integrates the function of organs and tissues throughout the body. Many of the natural hormones can be used for replacement therapy in patients lacking normal endocrine function; examples of this use include insulin therapy in diabetics (Chapter 34) or thyroxine therapy in myxedemics (Chapter 30).

Natural or synthetic hormones may also be used at supranormal doses to achieve some desired pharmacologic effect; an example of this use is adrenocorticosteroid therapy for inflammatory diseases (Chapter 31).

Many hormones or related compounds may also be used diagnostically; for example, pituitary hormones may be administered to test the capacity of target organs to respond (Chapter 29).

In addition to natural and synthetic forms of hormones, the chapters in this unit also include drugs that may influence synthesis, secretion, or action of natural hormones.

**IX**

# Chapter Twenty-nine

# Pituitary hormones and related agents

**Adrenal effectors**
corticoptropin (ACTH)
cosyntropin
metyrapone

**Growth hormones and antagonists**
bromocriptine
somatrem
somatropin

**Gonadotropins**
chorionic gonadotropin
menotropins

**Oxytocics**
dinoprost tromethamine
dinoprostone
ergonovine maleate
methylergonovine maleate
oxytocin

**Thyroid effectors**
thyrotropin

**Vasopressins**
desmopressin
lypressin
vasopressin
vasopressin tannate

**INTRODUCTION**   The pituitary gland secretes many peptide hormones that modulate the function of other tissues in the body (Table 29-1). Two hormones are released from the posterior pituitary (neurohypophysis)—oxytocin and vasopressin. Oxytocin and related compounds specifically stimulate the myometrium. Vasopressin has more widespread actions, causing water retention by the kidney and constriction of peripheral vasculature. In addition, vasopressin is a neurotransmitter in the CNS.

The anterior pituitary (adenohypophysis) secretes several regulatory hormones, including corticotropin, gonadotropins, growth hormone, and thyrotropin. The target of corticotropin is the adrenal gland, which responds by releasing adrenocorticosteroids. Gonadotropins (LH, FSH) modulate maturation of the sex organs and regulate function in mature individuals. Growth hormone stimulates the liver to release somatomedins, which stimulate body growth in a variety of ways. Thyrotropin stimulates release of thyroxin and thyronine from the thyroid gland.

# Adrenal effectors

corticotropin (ACTH)  ~  cosyntropin  ~  metyrapone

**OVERVIEW OF THE DRUG CLASS**   Corticotropin is a peptide hormone synthesized by cells within the anterior pituitary. Synthesis and release is regulated by corticotropin-releasing factor (CRF) from the hypothalamus. Metyrapone is a synthetic compound that blocks the synthesis of cortisol in the adrenal gland. Both these compounds are used diagnostically to evaluate function of the pituitary and adrenal glands.

**MECHANISM OF ACTION**   Corticotropin stimulates the adrenals to release adrenocorticosteroids. Failure of steroid levels to rise in response to corticotropin implies impairment of the adrenal gland. If the adrenal does respond to exogenous corticotropin, yet shows signs of adrenal insufficiency, a metyrapone test may be performed. Metyrapone blocks synthesis of adrenal steroids, thereby activating the feedback loop, which normally increases pituitary release of corticotropin. The excess corticotropin stimulates the adrenal gland to release additional steroids, which appear in the urine as precursors. When pituitary function is impaired, steroid precursors do not increase because the pituitary fails to release corticotropin to stimulate the adrenals.

Corticotropin is most commonly used diagnostically but may occasionally be used for longer periods when the desired effect is actually caused by the adrenal steroids released in response to corticotropin. In most cases, direct administration of adrenal steroids is preferred.

**Table 29-1.**

| Physiologic action of selected adenohypophyseal hormones* | | | | |
|---|---|---|---|---|
| Descriptive name | Other names | Hypothalamic releasing factor | Target tissue | Target tissue response |
| Adrenocorticotropic hormone | ACTH Corticotropin | Corticotropin-releasing factor (CRF) | Adrenal cortex Pigment cells of skin | Increased steroid synthesis Increased pigmentation |
| Follicle-stimulating hormone | FSH | Gonadotropin-releasing hormone (GnRH); FSH-releasing hormone (FRH, FSH-RH) | Ovary Seminiferous tubules | Increased estrogen production Maturation |
| Growth hormone | GH Somatotropin Somatropin STH | Somatotropin or growth hormone–releasing factor (SRF or GRF); somatostatin or somatotropin-release inhibitory factor (SRIF) | Whole body | Increased anabolism, cell size, cell numbers |
| Luteinizing hormone or interstitial cell–stimulating hormone | ICSH LH | Gonadotropin-releasing hormone (GnRH); luteinizing hormone-releasing factor or hormone (LRF, LRH, LHRF, LHRH) | Ovary Leydig cells | Ovulation; formation of corpus luteum Increased androgen synthesis |
| Prolactin | LTH Luteotropic hormone | Prolactin-inhibiting factor (PIF); prolactin-releasing factor (PRF) | Breast | Milk formation |
| Thyroid-stimulating TSH | Thyrotropin TSH | Thyrotropin-releasing hormone or factor (TRH, TRF) | Thyroid gland | Increased $T_3$, $T_4$ synthesis |

*From Clark JB, Queener SF, Karb VB: Pharmacological Basis of Nursing Practice, ed. 2, St. Louis, 1986, The C.V. Mosby Co.

## corticotropin (ACTH), corticotropin zinc hydroxide

(cor-ti-co-TRO-pin)    adrenal stimulator

- corticotropin (ACTH), corticotropin zinc hydroxide: ACTH, Acthar, ✽Duracton

**MECHANISM OF ACTION**    See entry for drug class (p. 556).

**INDICATIONS**    **Diagnosis of adrenal insufficiency** Corticotropin normally stimulates adrenal production of adrenocorticosteroids. • Failure of stimulation implies primary adrenal disease.    **Acute exacerbation of multiple sclerosis or dermatomyositis** Corticotropin stimulates release of androgens from the adrenal cortex, which tends to offset the muscle-wasting effects of corticosteroids.

**CONTRAINDICATIONS**    **Allergy to corticotropin** Because corticotropin is a peptide, it can cause allergic sensitization. • Patients extremely allergic to porcine proteins may be at risk because the product is derived from hogs.    **Hypothyroidism** These patients may suffer an exaggerated response to corticotropin.    **Cirrhosis** These patients may suffer an exaggerated response to corticotropin.    **Seizures** Corticotropin can trigger seizures, especially in predisposed patients.    **Psychosis** The mood-altering effects may be worse in these patients.    **Ulcerative GI disease** Corticotropin may trigger worsening of these conditions.    **Active infections** Viral, fungal, or bacterial diseases may fulminate when immune defenses are lessened by the action of corticotropin.    **Myasthenia gravis** Muscle strength is initially lowered in these patients. • Respiratory support may be required.    **Thromboembolitic disorders**

Corticotropin may increase risk of thrombosis. **Renal insufficiency** Corticotropin tends to cause water retention, potassium loss, and hypokalemic alkalosis, which may be worsened in patients without full renal function. **Scleroderma** This collagen disorder should not be treated with corticotropin. **Congestive heart failure** Patients with congestive heart failure may not be able to tolerate fluid retention caused by corticotropin.

**DOSAGE** IV: ADULTS: 10 to 25 units of corticotropin infused over 8 hours. IM: ADULTS: 40 units of corticotropin repository or corticotropin zinc hydroxide suspension every 12 hours for 1 to 2 days. SC: ADULTS: 40 units of corticotropin repository. *Special patient populations:* CHILDREN: Pediatric doses are not established. PREGNANCY: Safe use in pregnancy has not been established.

**PREPARATIONS** Corticotropin, *powder for reconstitution:* 25 or 40 units, for IV, IM, or SC use. Reconstitute in sterile saline solution to volumes appropriate for 8-hour infusion or for injection. Corticotropin, repository, *solution:* 40 or 80 units/ml. For IM or SC use only. Corticotropin zinc hydroxide, *suspension:* 40 units/ml. For IM use only.

**DRUG INTERACTIONS** **Cortisone, hydrocortisone, or estrogen** may elevate baseline steroid concentrations, complicating interpretation of the corticotropin stimulation test. **Spironolactone** metabolites interfere with the fluorescent assay for cortisol. **Barbiturates, phenytoin, and rifampin** may increase liver metabolism of glucocorticoids, which diminishes the effect of corticotropin. **Salicylates and indomethacin** may increase risk of GI ulceration with corticotropin. **Amphotericin B, thiazide diuretics, ethacrynic acid, and furosemide** may potentiate potassium loss caused by corticotropin.

**DIAGNOSTIC TEST INTERFERENCE** **Cortisol assays** necessary for analysis of the corticotropin stimulation test may be falsely elevated by bilirubin or hemoglobin free in plasma. **Skin test** reactions are diminished by corticotropin. **Tests for urinary estrogens** may be falsely decreased by corticotropin.

**FATE** Corticotropin is a peptide that must be administered parenterally for adequate absorption. Absorption is rapid for corticotropin but takes 8 to 16 hours for corticotropin zinc hydroxide or corticotropin repository. Many tissues clear corticotropin from plasma. The agent may be destroyed by specific or nonspecific proteases.

## ☙ NURSING CONSIDERATIONS

**Side effects, toxicities, and associated nursing actions** Many of the side effects listed below are caused by the glucocorticoids released by the adrenal gland in response to corticotropin.

**CNS** Depression, EEG abnormalities, euphoria, headache, insomnia, psychosis, seizures, or vertigo may arise.
- Assess for signs of depression: anorexia, withdrawal, lack of interest in personal appearance, and insomnia.
- In patients with a history of seizures, pad siderails and have a suction machine available.
- Caution patients to avoid driving or operating hazardous equipment if vertigo is present.
- If CNS symptoms are severe or persistent, notify physician.

**CV** Congestive heart failure can be triggered by edema, potassium loss, hypokalemic alkalosis, and hypertension.
- Assess for signs of congestive heart failure: edema, weight gain, and distended jugular veins. Monitor skin color and breath sounds.
- Assess for signs of hypokalemia: ECG changes, weakness, apathy, abdominal distention, anorexia, vomiting, and paralytic ileus.
- Monitor blood pressure and pulse. Monitor serum electrolytes.

**GI** Abdominal distention, peptic ulcer, ulcerative esophagitis, and pancreatitis may occur.
- Check stools and emesis for occult blood.
- Ask about GI symptoms.
- Assess for pancreatitis: pain, nausea, vomiting, malabsorption, and weight loss.

**Renal** Calcium excretion rises, occasionally causing hypocalcemia. Anuria and renal cortical necrosis are rare.
- Monitor serum electrolytes. If renal involvement is suspected, monitor intake and output.
- Assess for signs of hypocalcemia: numbness and tingling of the nose, toes, fingertips, and ears.

**Eye** Cataracts, exophthalmos, and increased intraocular pressure may lead to glaucoma or blindness.
- Advise patients receiving long-term therapy to obtain regular ophthalmic examinations.
- Assess vision on a regular basis.

**Skin** Acne, atrophy, bruising, ecchymoses, facial erythema, hirsutism, hyperpigmentation, petechiae, and increased sweating can occur.
- Caution patients to avoid activities that would cause bruising or rough skin contact.
- Visually inspect skin on a regular basis. Refer patients as appropriate to a dermatologist. Review aspects of good skin hygiene with patients with acne.
- Caution patients to report the development of unexplained bleeding, bruising, or petechiae.

**Endocrine** Prolonged administration may cause Cushingoid symptoms (hypercorticism), decreased glucose tolerance, and suppressed hypothalamus-pituitary regulation of adrenal function. Menstrual irregularities may also occur.
- Monitor patients for signs of hypercorticism: truncal obesity, "buffalo hump," moon face, muscle wasting, and poor wound healing.
- Monitor blood glucose levels. Instruct diabetic patients to monitor blood and urine glucose levels carefully for several weeks following initiation of drug therapy or dosage adjustments, as a change in diet or insulin may be necessary.
- Instruct women to keep a record of menstrual periods. If excessive bleeding or possible pregnancy develops, instruct women to notify physician.

**Allergic** Allergic reactions, including anaphylaxis, circulatory collapse, fever, nausea, rashes, vomiting, and wheezing, can occur. These are the only serious reactions associated with short-term diagnostic use of corticotropin.
- Have available drugs, equipment, and personnel to treat an acute allergic reaction in any setting where corticotropin is administered.
- Remain with patients for several minutes following administration of dose and check back frequently during the first 30 minutes following the start of therapy.

**Other** IM or SC use may cause induration, pain, or abscesses at the injection site.
- Use usual careful aseptic technique in administering doses.
- Record and rotate injection site.

### Nursing interventions related to drug administration
- Read orders carefully: only one preparation is safe for IV use.
- Consult with physician about giving a skin test before administering first dose.

### Patient and family education
- Review anticipated benefits and possible side effects of drug therapy with patient and family.
- Encourage patients receiving long-term therapy to return as directed for follow-up visits.
- Instruct patients to report the development of any new signs or symptoms.
- Caution patients to avoid the use of other medications unless first approved by the physician.
- Caution patients to keep all health care providers informed of all medications being used.
- Encourage patients receiving long-term therapy to wear a medical identification tag or bracelet.

---

## cosyntropin    (ko-SIN-tro-pin)                                adrenal stimulator

- cosyntropin: Cortrosyn, ✽Synacthen Depot

**MECHANISM OF ACTION**    See entry for drug class (p. 556).

**INDICATIONS**    **Diagnosis of adrenal insufficiency** Cosyntropin normally stimulates adrenal production of adrenocorticosteroids. • Failure of stimulation implies primary adrenal disease.

**CONTRAINDICATIONS**    **Allergy to corticotropin or cosyntropin** Cosyntropin is less likely to cause allergic reactions than corticotropin, but some patients may react.

**DOSAGE**    **IV, IM:**    **ADULTS:** 0.25 mg IM or IV over a 2-minute period. Alternatively, 0.25 mg infused IV over 6 hours (0.04 mg/hr).    **CHILDREN:** Children under 2 have received 0.125 mg IM or IV; neonates may receive 0.015 mg/kg IM.    *Special patient populations:*    **PREGNANCY:** Safe use in pregnancy has not been established.

**PREPARATIONS**    *Powder,* for reconstitution: 0.25 mg. Reconstitute by adding 1 ml of 0.9% sodium chloride injection to the 0.25 mg vial.

**DRUG INTERACTIONS** **Cortisone, hydrocortisone, or estrogen** may elevate baseline steroid concentrations, complicating interpretation of the cosyntropin stimulation test. **Spironolactone** metabolites inferfere with the fluorescent assay for cortisol.

**DIAGNOSTIC TEST INTERFERENCE** **Cortisol assays** necessary for analysis of the cosyntropin stimulation test may be falsely elevated by bilirubin or hemoglobin free in plasma.

**FATE** Cosyntropin is a peptide that must be administered parenterally for adequate absorption. Absorption is rapid from IM sites. Many tissues clear cosyntropin from plasma. The agent may be destroyed by specific or nonspecific proteases.

## ☙ NURSING CONSIDERATIONS

### Side effects, toxicities, and associated nursing actions

**Allergic** Allergic reactions, including anaphylaxis, circulatory collapse, fever, nausea, rashes, vomiting, and wheezing can occur. These are the only serious reactions associated with short-term diagnostic use of cosyntropin.

- Have available drugs, equipment, and personnel to treat an acute allergic reaction in any setting where cosyntropin is administered.
- Remain with patients for several minutes following administration of dose and check back frequently during the first 30 minutes following the start of therapy.

**Other** IM use may cause induration, pain, or abscesses at the injection site.

- Use usual careful aseptic technique in administering doses.
- Record and rotate injection sites.

### Patient and family education

- Review anticipated benefits and possible side effects of drug therapy with patients and family.

---

## metyrapone (me-TYR-uh-pone) adrenal steroid synthesis inhibitor

- metyrapone: Metopirone

**MECHANISM OF ACTION** See entry for drug class (p. 556).

**INDICATIONS** **Diagnosis of hypopituitarism** Metyrapone blocks synthesis of cortisol, thereby increasing CRF and ACTH release. • Under the influence of ACTH, the normal adrenal gland synthesizes increased amounts of cortisol precursors (17-OHCS, 17-KGS). • If the pituitary is impaired, ACTH levels do not rise, and the adrenal is not stimulated. **Differential diagnosis of adrenal hyperplasia and adrenal adenoma** Many, but not all, adrenal adenomas fail to respond to metyrapone, whereas hyperplastic tissues usually respond.

**CONTRAINDICATIONS** **Adrenocortical insufficiency** Acute adrenal insufficiency, which can be fatal, may be triggered by metyrapone.

**DOSAGE** PO: **ADULTS:** 750 mg every 4 hours for 6 doses, with urine collected for the 24 hours following the last dose. Therapy should not be started until baseline 17-OHCS and 17-KGS concentrations have been determined on a 24-hour urine specimen and adrenal insufficiency has been demonstrated. **CHILDREN:** 15 mg/kg on the same schedule as for adults. *Special patient populations:* **PREGNANCY:** Safe use in pregnancy has not been established.

**PREPARATIONS** *Tablets:* 250 mg.

**DRUG INTERACTIONS** **Phenytoin** enhances liver metabolism of metyrapone, preventing adequate inhibition of cortisol synthesis and invalidating any conclusions based on the metyrapone test. Phenytoin must be discontinued at least 2 weeks before a metyrapone test. **Amitriptyline, chlordiazepoxide, chlorpromazine, corticosteroids, estrogens, methysergide, phenobarbital, phenothiazines, and progestins** may lower the effectiveness of metyrapone.

**FATE** Metyrapone is erratically absorbed following oral administration, but inhibition of cortisol synthesis is observed within 4 hours of administration. The plasma *half-life* is 20 to 26 minutes. Metabolism is in both liver and kidneys.

## ❦ NURSING CONSIDERATIONS

### Side effects, toxicities, and associated nursing actions

**CNS** Dizziness, headache, sedation, and vertigo are uncommon.
- Caution patients to avoid driving or operating hazardous equipment if dizziness, sedation, or vertigo develops.

**CV** Blood pressure and heart rate may increase in some patients.
- Monitor blood pressure and pulse.

**GI** Abdominal discomfort and nausea can occur.
- Encourage patients to take doses with milk or food to lessen gastric irritation.

**Allergic** Rashes have been reported.
- Visually inspect patient for rashes.

### Patient and family education
- Review with patients the anticipated benefits and possible side effects associated with this drug.

---

# Growth hormones and antagonists

bromocriptine  ~  somatrem  ~  somatropin

**OVERVIEW OF THE DRUG CLASS**  Growth hormone or somatropin is required for replacement therapy in patients lacking sufficient endogenous hormone to promote full body growth. Because only the human form of the hormone is active in humans, the original product was purified from cadavers. That preparation has recently become suspect because some patients receiving it developed Jakob-Creutz-feldt disease. To replace the natural hormone, products have been developed using either synthetic somatropin or somatropin produced by recombinant DNA techniques.

Overproduction of somatropin occurs in rare circumstances, producing either gigantism or acromegaly. Treatment of these conditions often requires surgery, but bromocriptine may be helpful in antagonizing the effects of excessive somatropin in some patients.

**MECHANISM OF ACTION**  Growth hormone is synthesized by cells within the anterior pituitary, then released into systemic circulation. In response, somatomedins are released by the liver. The end result is an overall increase in many anabolic processes, enabling the body to grow. Bromocriptine inhibits release of prolactin (p. 557) and growth hormone in the anterior pituitary.

**INDICATIONS**  **Hypopituitarism** Growth failure, which is caused by lack of endogenous somatropin, can often be at least partially reversed by treatment with preparations of somatropin.  **Acromegaly** In addition to surgery or radiation, bromocriptine may be useful in antagonizing the action of excess somatropin.

---

## bromocriptine mesylate  (broh-moh-KRIP-teen)  somatropin suppressant

- bromocriptine mesylate: Parlodel

**MECHANISM OF ACTION**  See entry for drug class (p. 561).

**INDICATIONS**  **Acromegaly** Bromocriptine inhibits release of somatropin, which may aid in controlling acromegaly • Surgery or radiation is the preferred definitive therapy. • For other uses of bromocriptine, see Chapter 43.

**CONTRAINDICATIONS**  **Hepatic impairment** Metabolism of bromocriptine may be diminished, leading to higher drug concentrations.  **Psychiatric disease** Bromocriptine may exacerbate such conditions.

**DOSAGE**  **PO:**  ADULTS: For acromegaly, initially, 1.25 to 2.5 mg once daily with milk or with meals. Doses are increased at 2- or 3-day intervals to an effective maintenance dosage. Maintenance doses normally range from 15 to 30 mg daily in divided doses but may go as high as 100 mg. *Special patient populations:* CHILDREN: Pediatric doses for patients younger than 15 years are not established. PREGNANCY: Safe use has not been established. Bromocriptine inhibits lactation (Chapter 32).

**PREPARATIONS**  *Tablets:* 2.5 mg. *Capsules:* 5 mg.

**DRUG INTERACTIONS**   **Antihypertensive medications** may have additive hypotensive effects with bromo-criptine. Doses of antihypertensives may require reduction.

**FATE**   Bromocriptine bioavailability is low because only about 28% of an oral dose of the drug is absorbed, and most of the absorbed drug is destroyed on first pass through the liver. With proper doses, inhibition of somatropin release can be detected within 2 hours, but full clinical effect is not observed until 4 to 8 weeks of continuous therapy has been completed. Almost all elimination of bromocriptine is by hepatic metabolism.

## ☙ NURSING CONSIDERATIONS

### Side effects, toxicities, and associated nursing actions

**CNS** Confusion, depression, drowsiness, hallucinations, or uncontrolled body movements may occur, especially at high doses. Seizures are possible.

- Assess for signs of depression: lack of interest in personal appearance, withdrawal, anorexia, and insomnia.
- Monitor mental status.
- In patients with a history of seizures, pad siderails and have a suction machine available.
- **GI** Constipation, loss of appetite, nausea, stomach pain, tarry stools, and vomiting are possible. Up to 60% of patients may report one or more of these symptoms.
- Instruct patients to notify physician if GI symptoms are severe or persistent.
- Monitor stools and emesis for occult blood.
- If GI symptoms are prominent, monitor intake and output.
- If constipation occurs, instruct patients to increase fluid intake to 2500 to 3000 ml/day; to increase dietary intake of fruits, fruit juices, and roughage; and to increase daily exercise.
- Instruct patients to take doses with meals or snacks to reduce gastric irritation.

**Other** Dry mouth, nocturnal leg cramps, stuffy nose, and Raynaud's phenomenon (tingling in fingers and toes when cold) may occur in up to 60% of patients.

- If dry mouth occurs, instruct patients to suck on ice chips or sugarless hard candy or to chew sugarless gum. Some patients may wish to try a commercially available saliva substitute.
- Warn patients to notify physician if any new sign or symptom develops.

### Patient and family education

- Review the anticipated benefits and possible side effects of drug therapy with patients and family.
- Encourage patients to take drugs as ordered; full effects of this drug may not be seen for 4 to 8 weeks.
- Encourage patients to return for follow-up as directed.
- Remind patients to keep these and all medications out of the reach of children.

---

## somatrem   (SOH-muh-trem)   human growth hormone*

- somatrem: Protropin

**MECHANISM OF ACTION**   See entry for drug class (p. 561).

**INDICATIONS**   **Pituitary dwarfism** Growth failure caused by deficiency of somatropin can often be partially reversed by treatment with a form of human growth hormone.

**CONTRAINDICATIONS**   **Intracranial malignancy** Patients treated for such conditions within the previous year should not receive somatrem.   **Diabetes mellitus** Somatrem is diabetogenic and may precipitate or worsen diabetes mellitus.   **Hypothyroidism** Unless treated, hypothyroidism interferes with response to somatrem.

**DOSAGE**   **IM, SC:   CHILDREN:** Initially, 0.05 to 0.1 IU/kg on alternate days or three times weekly. Doses should be spaced at least 48 hours apart. Therapy is continued until adult height is reached or until the epiphyses close.   *Special patient populations:* Patients above the age of 14 to 16 years should not receive somatrem.

**PREPARATIONS**   *Powder,* for reconstitution: 5 mg (10 IU) per vial. Reconstitute by adding 10 ml of bacte-

*\*Synthetic.*

riostatic water for injection (with benzyl alcohol). Swirl but do not shake to dissolve. The resulting clear solution is 1 IU/ml. Use within 7 days.

**DRUG INTERACTIONS** **Adrenocorticoids or corticotropin** may inhibit the growth response to somatrem. Avoid concurrent use if possible. **Anabolic steroids, androgens, estrogens, or thyroid hormones** may hasten closure of epiphyses, thereby limiting the response to somatropin.

**FATE** Somatrem is a polypeptide and therefore would be destroyed if administered orally. The *half-life* of the drug is 20 to 30 minutes, with almost all of the drug being destroyed by the liver. The effects of the dose are prolonged beyond the time somatrem can be detected in the bloodstream.

### ❦ NURSING CONSIDERATIONS

#### Side effects, toxicities, and associated nursing actions

**Endocrine** Hypothyroidism is rare. Acromegalic signs or gigantism may occur with overdosage or with use in patients not deficient in somatropin.
- Monitor weight and height.
- Encourage patients to return for regular follow-up for best results.

**Allergic** Antibodies form in up to 40% of patients early in therapy, but neutralizing antibodies are found in only about 5% and rarely interfere with therapy.

**Other** Pain and swelling rarely occur at the injection site.
- Use usual careful aseptic technique in adminsitering drug.
- Record and rotate injection sites.

#### Patient and family education
- Review anticipated benefits and possible side effects of drug therapy with patient and family.
- Caution diabetic patients to monitor blood and urine glucose levels carefully, as an adjustment in diet or insulin may be necessary.
- Consult with physician, then teach family to monitor and record patient's weight, height, and other necessary parameters on a weekly basis.
- If patients or patients' families are self-administering this drug, teach injection administration technique and to record and rotate injection sites.

---

## somatropin (soh-muh-TRO-pin) human growth hormone*

- somatropin: Humatrope, Crescormon

**MECHANISM OF ACTION** See entry for drug class (p. 561).

**INDICATIONS** **Pituitary dwarfism** Growth failure caused by deficiency of somatropin can often be partially reversed by treatment with a form of human growth hormone.

**CONTRAINDICATIONS** **Intracranial malignancy** Patients treated for such conditions within the previous year should not receive somatropin. **Diabetes mellitus** Somatropin is diabetogenic and may precipitate or worsen diabetes mellitus. **Hypothyroidism** Unless treated, hypothyroidism interferes with response to somatropin.

**DOSAGE** **IM:** **CHILDREN::** Up to 0.06 mg/kg three times weekly, with at least 48 hours between doses. *Special patient populations:* Use in patients older than 14 to 16 years is not indicated.

**PREPARATIONS** *Powder,* for reconstitution: 5 mg (13 IU) per vial.

**DRUG INTERACTIONS** **Adrenocorticoids or corticotropin** may inhibit the growth response to somatropin. Avoid concurrent use if possible. **Anabolic steroids, androgens, estrogens, or thyroid hormones** may hasten closure of epiphyses, thereby limiting the response to somatropin.

**FATE** Somatropin is a polypeptide and therefore would be destroyed if administered orally. The *half-life* of the drug is 20 to 30 minutes, with almost all of the drug being destroyed by the liver. The effects of the dose are prolonged beyond the time somatropin can be detected in the bloodstream.

*\*Natural form by recombinant technology.*

## ❦ NURSING CONSIDERATIONS

### Side effects, toxicities, and associated nursing actions

**Endocrine** Hypothyroidism is rare. Acromegalic signs or gigantism may occur with overdosage or with use in patients not deficient in somatropin.
- Monitor weight and height.
- Encourage patients to return for regular follow-up for best results.

**Allergic** Antibodies form in up to 40% of patients early in therapy, but neutralizing antibodies are found in only about 5% and rarely interfere with therapy.

**Other** Pain and swelling rarely occur at the injection site.
- Use usual careful aseptic techniques in administering drug.
- Record and rotate injection sites.

### Patient and family education
- Review anticipated benefits and possible side effects of drug therapy with patient and family.
- Caution diabetic patients to monitor blood and urine glucose levels carefully, as an adjustment in diet or insulin may be necessary.
- Consult with physician, then teach patient's family to monitor and record patient's weight, height, and other necessary parameters on a weekly basis.
- If patients or patients' families are self-administering this drug, teach injection administration technique and to record and rotate injection sites.

# Gonadotropins

chorionic gonadotropin  ～  menotropins

**OVERVIEW OF THE DRUG CLASS**    The gonadotropins are proteins purified from urine of postmenopausal women (menotropins) or pregnant women (chorionic gonadotropin).

**MECHANISM OF ACTION**    Three gonatropins function in humans: follicle-stimulating hormone (FSH), luteinizing hormone (LH), and chorionic gonadotropin (CG). FSH promotes development of the ovaries, and LH stimulates development of the corpus luteum in females and stimulates spermatogenesis in males. CG acts the same as LH but has only weak FSH-like activity. Because of these actions, menotropins and CG may overcome certain types of infertility.

## chorionic gonadotropin    (kor-i-ON-ik goh-NAD-oh-tro-pin)         gonadotropin

- chorionic gonadotropin: Antuitrin, ♣ A.P.L., Chorex, Corgonject, Glukor, Profasi HP

**MECHANISM OF ACTION**    See entry for drug class (p. 564).

**INDICATIONS**    **Prepubertal cryptorchidism** CG promotes temporary or permanent testicular descent in boys without anatomical obstruction.    **Hypogonadism** Males failing to develop sexually because of pituitary deficiency may respond to CG.    **Failure of spermatogenesis** CG may be used as part of a two-step treatment, with menotropins as the second stage.    **Anovulation** Anovulation caused by pituitary deficiency may respond to CG, after menotropins pretreatment.    **Infertility caused by corpus luteum failure** CG therapy may replace hormone normally produced by the corpus luteum.

**CONTRAINDICATIONS**    **Precocious puberty** The androgen production induced by CG intensifies preococious puberty in boys.    **Prostate carcinoma** This or other androgen-dependent neoplasms are worsened by the androgens produced in response to CG.

**DOSAGE**    **IM:**    **ADULTS:** For hypogonadism, 500 to 1000 USP units three times weekly for 3 weeks, then twice weekly for an additional 3 weeks; therapy for longer periods is possible. For stimulation of spermatogenesis, 5000 USP units three times weekly until secondary sex characteristics develop and serum testosterone concentrations are normal; when these criteria are met (usually within 4 to 6 months), menotropins are added (75 IU each of FSH and LH activity three times weekly with 2000 USP units of

CG twice weekly). For induction of ovulation and pregnancy, 5000 to 10,000 USP units is given on the last day of menotropin therapy (9 to 12 days, 75 IU each FSH and LH). **CHILDREN:** For prepubertal cryptorchidism, 4000 USP units three times weekly for 3 weeks, or 5000 USP units every other day for 4 doses, or 15 doses of 500 to 1000 USP units given over 6 weeks. *Special patient populations:* **PREGNANCY:** During normal pregnancies the corpus luteum produces CG. The only indication for use during pregnancy is when the corpus luteum has failed, and exogenous sources of CG are required to maintain pregnancy.

**PREPARATIONS** *Powder,* for reconstitution: 2000, 5000, 10,000, or 20,000 USP units. The diluent for reconstitution supplied by the manufacturer contains benzyl alcohol (0.9% to 2%).

**DRUG INTERACTIONS** None documented.

**FATE** CG is a protein and must be administered parenterally to achieve useful concentrations in blood. CG concentrates in ovarian and testicular tissues. CG is slowly eliminated from the body, with less than 20% being excreted in urine.

## 🦋 NURSING CONSIDERATIONS

### Side effects, toxicities, and associated nursing actions

**CNS** Depression, fatigue, headache, irritability, and restlessness may occur but are usually mild.
- Assess for signs of depression: insomnia, anorexia, withdrawal, and lack of interest in personal appearance.
- If CNS side effects are severe or persistent, have patient notify physician.

**Renal** Edema is not uncommon.
- Monitor weight and assess for edema.

**Endocrine** Gynecomastia may occur.
- Assess for gynecomastia; this may be very troubling to young male patients.

**Allergic** Because CG is a protein, some patients may develop allergies.
- Question patients about the development of new signs and symptoms.
- Have available drugs and equipment to treat acute allergic reactions.

**Other** Pain at the injection site may occur.
- Use usual careful aseptic technique.
- Record and rotate injection sites.

### Patient and family education
- Review with patients and the family the anticipated benefits and possible side effects of drug therapy.
- Encourage patients to return for scheduled follow-up visits to monitor drug effectiveness.

---

# menotropins (min-oh-TRO-pins)                                    gonadotropins

- menotropins: Pergonal

**MECHANISM OF ACTION** See entry for drug class (p. 564).

**INDICATIONS** **Anovulation** Menotropins with CG may be used to induce ovulation and allow pregnancy to occur. **Stimulation of spermatogenesis** Males must be pretreated with CG for menotropins to be effective. • Therapy is indicated only for those males lacking adequate pituitary function.

**CONTRAINDICATIONS** **Primary ovarian failure** Such patients do not ovulate in response to menotropins. **Ovarian cysts or enlargement** Menotropins may cause overstimulation and rupture of ovarian cysts, with bleeding into the peritoneum. **Pregnancy** Menotropins are not indicated for use during pregnancy. **Primary testicular failure** These patients do not respond to menotropins.

**DOSAGE** **IM:** **ADULTS:** For stimulation of spermatogenesis, 5000 USP units of CG three times weekly until secondary sex characteristics develop and serum testosterone concentrations are normal. When these criteria are met (usually within 4 to 6 months), menotropins are added (75 IU each of FSH and LH activity three times weekly with 2000 USP units of CG twice weekly). For induction of ovulation and pregnancy, 5000 to 10,000 USP units of CG given on the last day of menotropin therapy (9 to 12 days,

75 IU each FSH and LH). *Special patient populations:* **CHILDREN:** Menotropins are not indicated for use in childhood. **PREGNANCY:** Safe use in pregnancy has not been established.

**PREPARATIONS** *Powder,* for reconstitution: 75 or 150 IU each of FSH and LH activity. Reconstitute in 1 to 2 ml of 0.9% sterile sodium chloride injection and use immediately. Do not store.

**DRUG INTERACTIONS** None documented.

**FATE** Menotropins must be administered parenterally because the proteins are destroyed in the GI tract. Disposition of the drug is unknown, but little appears in urine.

### ❦ NURSING CONSIDERATIONS

#### Side effects, toxicities, and associated nursing actions

**CV** Arterial thromboembolism is rare.
- Monitor peripheral pulses.
- Instruct patient to report the development of pain in an extremity or if the extremity is cool to touch or bluish in color.

**Blood** Erythrocytosis is rare.
- Monitor complete blood count.

**GI** Diarrhea, nausea, and vomiting.
- If GI symptoms are severe, instruct patient to notify physician.
- Monitor intake and output in hospitalized patients.

**Allergic** Fever or other allergic reactions are possible.
- Have available drugs, equipment, and personnel to treat an acute allergic reaction in settings where menotropins are administered.
- Instruct patients to report the development of any unexpected sign or symptom.

**Other** Overstimulation of the ovaries may cause development of cysts, loss of fluid into the peritoneum, or bleeding into the peritoneum. This reaction is more common at higher doses.
- Instruct women to report the development of lower abdominal pain and fever.

#### Patient and family education

- Review anticipated benefits and possible side effects of drug therapy with patient.
- Encourage patient to return for scheduled follow-up visits to monitor drug effectiveness.
- Discuss with patients the possibility of multiple births.

---

# Oxytocics

dinoprost tromethamine ~ dinoprostone ~ ergonovine maleate ~ methylergonovine maleate ~ oxytocin

**OVERVIEW OF THE DRUG CLASS** Three types of drugs are used to stimulate contractions of the myometrium. Dinoprost tromethamine and dinoprostone are prostaglandins. Ergonovine and methylergonovine maleate are ergot alkaloids. Oxytocin is a peptide normally produced by the posterior pituitary.

**MECHANISM OF ACTION** Oxytocic drugs stimulate contractions of myometrium, the smooth muscle of the uterus. Vascular smooth muscle may also be stimulated to contract by dinoprost tromethamine, dinoprostone, ergonovine maleate, and methylergonovine maleate. In contrast, oxytocin causes vasodilation.

**INDICATIONS** **Induction of abortion** Abortions in the second trimester may be induced with dinoprost tromethamine or dinoprostone because the uterus is more sensitive to the prostaglandins than to oxytocin at this stage of pregnancy. **Postpartum hemorrhage** Postpartum hemorrhage caused by uterine involution or atony may be controlled with ergonovine or methylergonovine maleate because these agents induce powerful, sustained contractions of the uterus. **Induction of labor** Patients at or near full term may have labor induced by oxytocin. • None of the other oxytocics are indicated for this purpose.

**CONTRAINDICATIONS** **Conditions that preclude safe vaginal delivery** Patients receiving oxytocic drugs must fulfill adequate medical criteria to avoid damage to the uterus and surrounding structures or to the fetus.

## dinoprost tromethamine   (dye-no-prost tro-METH-uh-meen)   oxytocic

- dinoprost tromethamine: Prostin $F_2$ alpha

**MECHANISM OF ACTION**   See entry for drug class (p. 566).

**INDICATIONS**   See entry for drug class (p. 566).

**CONTRAINDICATIONS**   **Asthma** Contraction of bronchiolar smooth muscle may precipitate attacks.   **Cardiovascular disease** Blood pressure and heart rate may be elevated, which may not be tolerated in patients with preexisting disease.   **Epilepsy** Dinoprost tromethamine may increase risk of seizures.   **Glaucoma** Pressure inside the eye may be elevated.   **Hypertension** These patients may be unable to tolerate further increases in pressure caused by dinoprost tromethamine.

**DOSAGE**   **Intra-amniotic:**   ADULTS: 40 mg slowly by transabdominal intra-amniotic catheter.   *Special patient populations:*   CHILDREN: This drug is not indicated for use in children.   PREGNANCY: If abortion by dinoprost tromethamine fails, it should be completed by another method. Teratogenic effects of the drug and the anoxia produced by its use cause grave fetal damage.

**PREPARATIONS**   *Solution:* 5 mg/ml.

**DRUG INTERACTIONS**   **Oxytocin** administered with dinoprost tromethamine may cause tearing of the cervix or other tissues.

**FATE**   Dinoprost tromethamine slowly diffuses from the uterus. The drug is rapidly metabolized in lung and liver. The Plasma *half-life* is less than 1 minute.

### 🐾 NURSING CONSIDERATIONS

#### Side effects, toxicities, and associated nursing actions

**CNS** Anxiety, diplopia, drowsiness, headache, paresthesia, and seizures may occur.
- Remain with patient during therapy or check patient frequently.
- Keep siderails up. Have a suction machine available.

**CV** Arrhythmias, bradycardia, heart block, hypotension, and hypertension have been reported.
- Monitor blood pressure and pulse. If woman has a history of heart disease, have patient attached to a cardiac monitor during drug use.

**GI** Up to 20% of patients suffer diarrhea, and up to 50% experience nausea and vomiting. Abdominal distress and epigastric pain have also been reported.
- Monitor intake and output.
- Notify physician if GI symptoms are severe.

**Lung** Bronchoconstriction, bronchospasm, dyspnea, hyperventilation, rales, and wheezing occur.
- Monitor respiratory rate and auscultate breath sounds.

**Other** Cervical laceration or uterine rupture is possible.
- Palpate fundus at regular intervals.
- Assess vaginal bleeding. Be alert for excessive bleeding or continued bleeding after fetus has been expelled. Monitor blood pressure and assess for lower abdominal pain.

#### Patient and family education
- Review with patient the anticipated effects and possible side effects of drug therapy.
- Provide emotional support as appropriate. If indicated, refer patient for counseling.

## dinoprostone   (dye-no-PROS-tone)   oxytocic

- dinoprostone: Prostin $E_2$

**MECHANISM OF ACTION**   See entry for drug class (p. 566).

**INDICATIONS**   See entry for drug class (p. 566).

**CONTRAINDICATIONS**   See entry for drug class (p. 566).

**DOSAGE**   **Intravaginal:**   ADULTS: 20 mg every 2 to 3 hours until abortion occurs.   *Special patient populations:*   CHILDREN: This drug is not indicated for use in children.   PREGNANCY: Patients failing to abort with dinoprostone should be aborted by other methods.

**PREPARATIONS**    *Vaginal suppositories:* 20 mg.

**DRUG INTERACTIONS**    Oxytocin administered with dinoprostone may cause tearing of the cervix or other tissues.

**FATE**    Maternal absorption of dinoprostone does occur through the vaginal walls. The drug is rapidly metabolized and destroyed by several organs.

❦ **NURSING CONSIDERATIONS**

### Side effects, toxicities, and associated nursing actions

**CNS** Chills, headache, paresthesia, shivering, tension, and tremor have occurred in up to 10% of patients.
- Remain with patient during therapy, or check patient frequently.
- Keep siderails up. Have a suction machine available.

**CV** Cardiac arrhythmias, hypotension, dizziness, or fainting may occur.
- Monitor blood pressure and pulse. If woman has a history of heart disease, have patient attached to cardiac monitor during drug use.
- Supervise ambulation and keep siderails up.

**GI** Up to 40% of patients suffer diarrhea and up to 60% suffer nausea and vomiting, even when they have been premedicated to lessen these reactions.
- Monitor intake and output.
- Notify physician if GI symptoms are severe.

**Lung** Bronchoconstriction, bronchospasm, coughing, dyspnea, and wheezing may occur.
- Monitor respiratory rate and auscultate breath sounds.

**Other** Cervical tearing or uterine rupture is possible with powerful contractions induced by dinoprostone.
- Palpate fundus at regular intervals.
- Assess vaginal bleeding. Be alert for excessive or continued bleeding after fetus has been expelled. Monitor blood pressure and assess for lower abdominal pain. Fever without endometritis occurs in up to 70% of patients. Vaginal discomfort, vaginitis, and vulvitis may occur.
- Monitor temperature every 4 hours.
- Inspect vagina and vulva at regular intervals, especially if patient complains of discomfort; notify physician if symptoms are severe.
- Allow suppository to warm to room temperature before inserting.

### Patient and family education
- Review with patient the anticipated effects and possible side effects of drug therapy.
- Provide emotional support as appropriate. If indicated, refer patient for counseling.

---

## ergonovine maleate    (er-GON-oh-veen)                                    oxytocic

- ergonovine maleate: Ergotrate maleate

**MECHANISM OF ACTION**    See entry for drug class (p. 566).

**INDICATIONS**    See entry for drug class (p. 566).

**CONTRAINDICATIONS**    See entry for drug class (p. 566).

**DOSAGE**    PO:    **ADULTS:** For postpartum bleeding, 0.2 to 0.4 mg every 6 to 12 hours.    **IV:**    **ADULTS:** For severe uterine bleeding, 0.2 mg administered over a minute or more. No more than 5 doses should be given by this route, and the doses should be 2 to 4 hours apart.    **IM:**    **ADULTS:** For initial therapy of postpartum bleeding, 0.2 mg. Oral dosing should follow.    *Special patient populations:*    **CHILDREN:** This drug is not indicated for use in children.    **PREGNANCY:** Use of this drug during pregnancy carries substantial risk to the fetus.

**PREPARATIONS**    *Tablets:* 0.2 mg. *Solution for injection:* 0.2 mg/ml.

**DRUG INTERACTIONS**    **Propranolol** may block processes that offset some of the vasoconstrictor action of ergonovine. The result can be excessive vasoconstriction.    **Sympathomimetic agents** such as dopamine or methoxamine may have additive vasoconstrictor activity with ergonovine.

**FATE** Ergonovine stimulates uterine contractions within 15 minutes when given orally, within 2 to 5 minutes following IM dosage, or immediately following IV dosage. The effects persist for 45 minutes after IV dosage but up to 3 hours with IM or oral dosage.

## ❦ NURSING CONSIDERATIONS

### Side effects, toxicities, and associated nursing actions

**CNS** Dizziness, headache, and tinnitus have occurred with routine doses. Toxic overdosage causes seizures and loss of consciousness.
- Question patient about the development of these side effects.
- If dizziness occurs, supervise ambulation; keep siderails up.

**CV** Arrhythmias, chest pain, palpitations, and hypertension can occur and are more severe with toxic overdosage.

**Blood** Hypercoagulability occurs with toxic overdosage.
- Monitor blood pressure and pulse.
- Consider continuous cardiac monitoring if patient has a history of heart disease.
- Calculate dosage carefully and administer IV doses at recommended rate.
- Monitor uterus: palpate fundus and assess lochia.

**GI** Nausea and vomiting are common side effects.
- If GI symptoms are severe or persistent, notify physician.

**Lung** Dyspnea.
- Monitor respiratory rate and auscultate breath sounds.
- Remain calm and reassuring with patient.

**Allergic** Allergic reactions may include shock.
- Monitor vital signs.
- Have available drugs, equipment, and personnel to treat acute allergic reactions in settings where this drug is administered.

**Other** Toxic overdosage of ergonovine causes gangrene of the extremities because the drug produces potent and prolonged vasoconstriction, shutting off blood supply.
- As noted, calculate dosage carefully. If overdose is suspected, notify physician immediately.

### Nursing interventions related to drug administration
- Oral or IM administration is preferred to IV.
- Check expiration date before preparing dose.
- For IV use, may administer undiluted. Administer at a rate of 0.2 mg or less over 1 minute.
- Do not confuse this drug with ergotamine.

### Patient and family education
- Review with patient the anticipated benefits and possible side effects of drug therapy.
- Instruct patient to report the development of any new symptoms.

---

## methylergonovine maleate  (meth-ill-er-GON-oh-veen)  oxytocic

- methylergonovine maleate: Methergine

**MECHANISM OF ACTION** See entry for drug class (p. 566).

**INDICATIONS** See entry for drug class (p. 566).

**CONTRAINDICATIONS** See entry for drug class (p. 566).

**DOSAGE** **PO: ADULTS:** For postpartum bleeding, 0.2 to 0.4 mg every 6 to 12 hours. **IV: ADULTS:** For severe uterine bleeding, 0.2 mg administered over a minute or more. No more than 5 doses should be given by this route, and the doses should be 2 to 4 hours apart. **IM: ADULTS:** For initial therapy of postpartum bleeding, 0.2 mg. Oral dosing should follow. *Special patient populations:* **CHILDREN:** This drug is not indicated for use in children. **PREGNANCY:** Use of this drug in pregnancy carries substantial risk to the fetus.

**PREPARATIONS** *Tablets:* 0.2 mg. *Solution for injection:* 0.2 mg/ml.

**DRUG INTERACTIONS**    **Propranolol** may block processes that offset some of the vasoconstrictor action of methylergonovine. The result can be excessive vasoconstriction.    **Sympathomimetic agents** such as dopamine or methoxamine may have additive vasoconstrictor activity with methylergonovine.

**FATE**    Methylergonovine stimulates uterine contractions within 15 minutes when given orally, within 2 to 5 minutes following IM dosage, or immediately following IV dosage. The effects persist for 45 minutes after IV dosage but up to 3 hours with IM or oral dosage.

## ❦ NURSING CONSIDERATIONS

### Side effects, toxicities, and associated nursing actions

**CNS** Dizziness, headache, and tinnitus have occurred with routine doses. Toxic overdosage causes seizures and loss of consciousness.
* Question patient about the development of these side effects.
* If dizziness occurs, supervise ambulation and keep siderails up.

**CV** Arrhythmias, chest pain, palpitations, and hypertension can occur and are more severe with toxic overdosage.

**Blood** Hypercoagulability occurs with toxic overdosage.
* Monitor blood pressure and pulse.
* Consider continuous cardiac monitoring if patient has a history of heart disease.
* Calculate dosage carefully and administer IV doses at recommended rate.
* Monitor uterus: palpate fundus and assess lochia.

**GI** Nausea and vomiting are common side effects.
* If GI symptoms are severe or persistent, notify physician.

**Lung** Dyspnea.
* Monitor respiratory rate and auscultate breath sounds.
* Remain calm and reassuring with patient.

**Allergic** Allergic reactions may include shock.
* Monitor vital signs.
* Have available drugs, equipment, and personnel to treat acute allergic reactions in settings where this drug is administered.

**Other** Toxic overdosage of methylergonovine causes gangrene of the extremities because the drug produces potent and prolonged vasoconstriction, shutting off blood supply.
* As noted, calculate dosage carefully. If overdose is suspected, notify physician immediately.

### Nursing interventions related to drug administration
* Oral or IM administration is preferred to IV.
* Check expiration date before preparing dose.
* For IV use, may administer undiluted. Administer at a rate of 0.2 mg or less over 1 minute.

### Patient and family education
* Review with patient the anticipated benefits and possible side effects of drug therapy.
* Instruct patient to report the development of any new symptoms.

---

## oxytocin    (oxy-TOH-sin)                                        oxytocic

* oxytocin: Pitocin, Syntocinon

**MECHANISM OF ACTION**    See entry for drug class (p. 566).

**INDICATIONS**    See entry for drug class (p. 566).

**CONTRAINDICATIONS**    See entry for drug class (p. 566).

**DOSAGE**    IV:    **ADULTS:** To induce labor, 1 mU/min. To augment labor, 2 to 20 mU/min with gradual increases to the higher dose. To control postpartum bleeding, 10 units delivered at 20 to 40 mU/min.    **Intranasal:**    **ADULTS:** To promote milk ejection, 1 spray or 3 drops of nasal solution into one or both nostrils 2 to 3 minutes before nursing.    *Special patient populations:*    **CHILDREN:** This drug is not indicated for use in children.    **PREGNANCY:** Use of this drug in pregnancy, except for induction of labor in full-term pregnancies, carries substantial risk to the fetus.

**PREPARATIONS**   *Solution for injection:* 10 units/ml. *Nasal solution:* 40 units/ml.

**DRUG INTERACTIONS**   **Sympathomimetic agents** such as dopamine or methoxamine may have additive vaso-constrictor activity with oxytocin.

**FATE**   Because oxytocin is a peptide, it is destroyed in the GI tract. Oxytocin is absorbed from IM sites, but control of the strength and duration of action is difficult. When used IV, the effect is immediate, and the duration is usually less than 1 hour. Intranasal absorption is adequate to stimulate milk ejection within 2 or 3 minutes; the action persists for up to 20 minutes.

## ☙ NURSING CONSIDERATIONS

### Side effects, toxicities, and associated nursing actions

**CNS** Seizures, coma, and death may follow water intoxication if large volumes of oxytocin are administered IV over prolonged periods.
- Monitor level of consciousness.
- Monitor weight and intake and output. Monitor serum electrolytes.

**CV** Overdosage causes hypotension and arrhythmias.
- Monitor blood pressure and pulse.
- Caution patients using nasal spray to use only as directed.

**Blood** Oxytocin may cause thrombocytopenia, afibrinogenemia, and hypoprothrombinemia. The result may be excessive bleeding.
- Instruct patients to report the development of unexplained bleeding or bruising: petechiae, bruises, nosebleeds, bleeding gums, or bleeding into urine.
- Monitor platelet, hematocrit, and hemoglobin counts and prothrombin time.

**GI** Nausea and vomiting may occur.
- If GI symptoms are severe, notify physician.

**Allergic** Allergic reactions may rarely include anaphylaxis.
- Have available drugs, equipment, and personnel to treat acute allergic reactions in settings where this drug is administered.

**Other** Cervical tearing, uterine rupture, and other signs of overstimulation may occur.
- Remain with patient during infusion of this drug.
- Monitor fetal heart tones; notify physician of significant changes in rate or rhythm; follow agency protocol.
- Palpate uterus and monitor uterine contractions.
- Monitor vaginal bleeding. Be alert to excessive bleeding or bright red bleeding.
- Assess vital signs. Be alert to severe lower abdominal pain.

### Nursing interventions related to drug administration
- For IV use, dilute as ordered or according to agency protocol. Use a microdrip infusion set and an infusion monitoring device. Titrate dose according to physician order and patient response. Monitor mother and fetus, as noted above.
- For intranasal use, instruct patient to sit upright to use as nasal spray or to tilt head back to administer nasal drops.

### Patient and family education
- Review anticipated benefits and possible side effects of drug therapy with patient.
- If intranasal spray is used to promote milk ejection, review with mother other actions that may promote milk ejection, such as relaxation, breast massage, keeping well hydrated, and cuddling with infant before trying to nurse.

# Thyroid effectors

thyrotropin

## thyrotropin   (thy-roh-TRO-pin)                                               vasopressin

- thyrotropin: Thytropar

**MECHANISM OF ACTION**    Thyrotropin is a peptide hormone synthesized by cells within the anterior pituitary gland. Synthesis and release is regulated by thyrotropin-releasing factor (TRF) from the hypothalamus. Thyrotropin stimulates the thyroid to release thyroxine and triiodothyronine.

**INDICATIONS**    **Diagnosis of hypothyroidism** Normal thyroid tissue responds to thyrotropin by increasing uptake of iodine and by releasing thyroxine and triiodothyronine. • Administration of thyrotropin can therefore be used to demonstrate ability of the thyroid to respond to appropriate stimulation.

**CONTRAINDICATIONS**    **Cardiac disease** These patients may be unable to tolerate the metabolic stimulation produced in response to thyrotropin.    **Hypopituitarism or untreated Addison's disease** In both conditions, patients may lack sufficient adrenal steroid reserves to be able to tolerate the metabolic stimulation produced in response to thyrotropin.

**DOSAGE**    **IM, SC:**    ADULTS: 10 IU daily for varying periods, depending on the exact diagnosis being sought. *Special patient populations:*    CHILDREN: Pediatric doses have not been established.    PREGNANCY: Safe use in pregnancy has not been established.

**PREPARATIONS**    *Powder,* for reconstitution: 10 IU. Reconstitute by adding 2 ml 0.9% sodium chloride diluent from the manufacturer.

**DRUG INTERACTIONS**    **Sympathomimetics** that increase heart rate may have additive effects with thyrotropin.

**FATE**    Thyrotropin is rapidly cleared from the body, once absorbed from IM or SC sites.

☙ **NURSING CONSIDERATIONS**

**Side effects, toxicities, and associated nursing actions**

**CV** Atrial fibrillation and tachycardia may occur. Overdosage can induce angina pectoris or congestive heart failure.
• Question patient about any history of heart disease before administering.
• Monitor blood pressure and pulse. Instruct patients to report any subjective complaints.
**GI** Nausea and vomiting.
• Instruct patient to notify physician if GI symptoms are severe or persistent.
**Endocrine** Thyroid swelling may occur.
• Assess thyroid gland size before administering thyrotropin, then monitor size on a daily basis.
• Instruct patient to report the development of thyroid discomfort or difficulty in swallowing.
**Allergic** Fever, hypotension, postinjection flare, urticaria, and anaphylactic reactions may occur.
• Monitor temperature, pulse, and blood pressure. Inspect injection sites.
• Have available drugs, equipment, and personnel to treat anaphylactic reactions in settings where this drug is administered.
• If patient is being treated on an outpatient basis, have patient remain in the agency for at least 30 minutes following the injection to assess for the development of serious allergic response.
**Other** Menstrual irregularities.
• Have female patients keep a record of menstrual periods. If pregnancy is suspected, instruct patient to notify physician immediately.

**Patient and family education**
• Review with patients the expected benefits of drug use and possible side effects that may occur.
• Instruct patients to report the development of any new sign or symptom.

---

# Vasopressins

desmopressin ~ lyopressin ~ vasopressin ~ vasopressin tannate

**OVERVIEW OF THE DRUG CLASS**    Vasopressin is a peptide hormone released by the posterior pituitary gland. Synthesis takes place in the hypothalamus within the brain. In its native form, vasopressin is very rapidly destroyed when taken orally or injected. Depot forms such as vasopressin tannate in oil prolong the duration of action by slowing absorption. Desmopressin and lyopressin are synthetic forms of vasopressin, differing from the natural product in ways that create higher potency, longer duration of action, and/or more specificity.

**MECHANISM OF ACTION**    Vasopressin increases permeability of collecting ducts in the kidney to water, resulting in water retention. Vasopressin is also called antidiuretic hormone (ADH) because of this action. Other actions of vasopressin include stimulation of contraction of vascular smooth muscle and neuromodulator activity in the CNS.

**INDICATIONS**   **Diabetes insipidus** Polyuria and polydipsia in this condition are caused by lack of vasopressin.
• Replacement therapy with vasopressin or one of its analogs controls these symptoms. Other drugs useful for this condition are summarized in Table 29-2.

**CONTRAINDICATIONS**   **Water intoxication** Any of the vasopressins may worsen this condition by preventing water excretion.   **Cardiac disease** Vasopressin may increase blood pressure and induce arrhythmias.
• Angina attacks may be induced. • Desmopressin is less likely to lead to difficulties than are the other forms of vasopressin.

---

## desmopressin acetate   (dez-moh-PRESS-sin)

vasopressin

● desmopressin acetate: DDAVP

**MECHANISM OF ACTION**   See entry for drug class (p. 572).

**INDICATIONS**   **Diabetes insipidus** See entry for drug class (p. 573).   **Bleeding in patients with hemophilia A or type I Von Willebrand's disease** Desmopressin can assist in maintaining hemostasis.

**CONTRAINDICATIONS**   **Water intoxication** Any of the vasopressins may worsen this condition by preventing water excretion.   **Cardiac disease** Vasopressins may increase blood pressure and induce arrhythmias.
• Angina attacks may be induced. • Desmporessin is less likely to lead to difficulties than are the other forms of vasopressin.   **Type IIB Von Willebrand's disease** Desmopressin increases the risk of platelet aggregation and thrombocytopenia.

**DOSAGE**   **Intranasal:**   ADULTS: For diabetes insipidus, 10 μg (0.1 ml of 0.01% solution) once in the evening. Doses are increased in 2.5 μg increments until nocturia is controlled. Additional morning doses are added if total urine volume remains above 2 liters. Maintenance doses usually range from 5 to 40 μg daily.   **CHILDREN:** For diabetes insipidus, 5 μg (0.05 ml of a 0.01% solution) once in the evening. Doses are increased in 2.5 μg increments until nocturia is controlled. Additional morning doses of 5 μg are added if needed. Maintenance doses usually range from 5 to 30 μg daily.   **IV, SC:**   ADULTS: For diabetes insipidus, 2 to 4 daily in 2 divided doses. For Von Willebrand's disease, 0.3 μg/kg (or 10 μg/M$^2$) by slow infusion.   **CHILDREN:** For Von Willebrand's disease, 0.3 μg/kg by slow infusion. *Special patient populations:*   CHILDREN: Safe use in children younger than 3 months of age is not established.   PREGNANCY: Safe use in pregnancy has not been established.

**PREPARATIONS**   *Solution for injection:* 4 μg/ml. *Nasal solution:* 100 μg/ml.

**DRUG INTERACTIONS**   **Alcohol, demeclocycline, epinephrine, heparin, and lithium** may decrease the antidiuretic action of desmopressin.   **Clofibrate, chlorpropamide, fludrocortisone, and urea** may potentiate the antidiuretic action of desmopressin.

**FATE**   Desmopressin is not absorbed following oral administration. Intranasal instillation results in absorption of 10% to 20% of the dose, with antidiuretic action resulting within 1 hour. *Peak* effects occur between 1 and 5 hours; antidiuresis persists for up to 20 hours. *Onset* and *duration* are both shorter when the drug is given IV. Desmopressin enters breast milk. The metabolic *fate* of the drug is not fully understood.

## ☙ NURSING CONSIDERATIONS

### Side effects, toxicities, and associated nursing actions

**CNS** Headache is a rare, transient side effect.
• Instruct patient to notify physician if headache is severe or persistent.
**CV** Blood pressure may increase with large doses. Large IV doses may cause flushing, hypotension, and tachycardia.
• With IV administration, monitor pulse and blood pressure.
**GI** Mild abdominal cramps and nausea may occur.
• Instruct patient to notify physician if GI symptoms are severe or persistent.
**Renal** Water intoxication is possible with large parenteral doses.

**Table 29-2.**

## Clinical summary of drugs to treat diabetes insipidus*

| Generic name | Trade name | Drug class | Administration | Properties | Uses | Side effects |
|---|---|---|---|---|---|---|
| Desmopressin acetate | DDAVP | Synthetic derivative of neurohypophyseal hormone | Nasal | Peptide with longer serum half-life than vasopressin; increases renal reabsorption of water | Replacement therapy in diabetes insipidus | Vasoconstriction; smooth muscle contraction |
| Lypressin | Diapid | Synthetic derivative of neurohypophyseal hormone | Nasal | Peptide with short serum half-life; increases real reabsorption of water | Replacement therapy in diabetes insipidus | Vasoconstriction; smooth muscle contraction |
| Vasopressin | Pitressin | Neurohypophyseal hormone | Parenteral | Peptide with short serum half-life; increases renal reabsorption of water | Tests ADH response of kidney; short-term maintenance of unconscious patient | Vasoconstriction; smooth muscle contraction |
| Vasopressin tannate in oil | Pitressin Tannate in oil | Neurohypophyseal hormone | Intramuscular depot | Peptide derivative slowly absorbed; increases renal reabsorption of water | Replacement in diabetes insipidus | Vasoconstriction; smooth muscle contraction |
| Chlorothiazide | Diuril | Thiazide diuretic | Oral | Promotes sodium, chloride excretion | Control of diuresis in diabetes insipidus | Hyponatremia; hypokalemia |
| Chlorpropamide | Diabinese | Sulfonylurea hypoglycemic agent | Oral | Increases release of ADH from posterior pituitary and increases ADH action in kidney | Control of diuresis in diabetes insipidus | Hypoglycemia |
| Clofibrate | Atromid S | Hypolipidemic agent | Oral | Increases release of ADH from posterior pituitary | Control of diuresis in diabetes insipidus | Nausea, weakness, muscle cramps |
| Carbamazepine | Tegretol | Tricyclic antidepressant | Oral | Increases release of ADH from posterior pituitary | Control of diuresis in diabetes insipidus | Dizziness, confusion, drowsiness |

*From Clark JB, Queener SF, Karb VB: Pharmacological Basis of Nursing Practice, ed. 2, St. Louis, 1986, The C.V. Mosby Co.

- Monitor intake and output and weight.
- Monitor serum electrolytes.
- Monitor urine specific gravity.
- Monitor level of consciousness.

**Other** Nasal congestion and rhinitis may occur with intranasal dosing. Erythema, swelling, and burning pain may occur at injection sites.

- Assess degree of nasal irritation, which may lessen with continued use. If nasal irritation is severe, it may interfere with adequate drug absorption; consult physician.
- Assess injection sites. Record and rotate sites. If irritation is severe, patient may require another route of administration; consult physician.

### Nursing interventions related to drug administration

- For IV use, dilute dose in 0.9% sodium chloride diluent before administering. Dilute the doses for a child under 10 kg in 10 ml and the doses for larger children and adults in at least 50 ml. Infuse diluted solution over at least 15 to 30 minutes. Monitor vital signs.
- For intranasal administration, consult literature supplied by the manufacturer for use of the drug administration device.

### Patient and family education

- Review anticipated benefits and possible side effects of drug therapy with patient.
- For patients using intranasal administration, review correct application of dose (see above). Review parameters patient may be instructed to monitor or record at home: frequency of nocturia, urine specific gravity, and intake and output. Instruct patient to notify physician if intranasal route cannot be used, as might occur with sinusitis, bad cold, or nasal surgery.
- If dose is missed, instruct patient to take dose as soon as it is remembered, unless close in time to next dose, in which case patient should omit missed dose completely and resume regular schedule with next dose. Instruct patient not to double up for missed doses. Reinforce to patient to consult physician for questions about doses.
- Suggest that patient wear a medical identification tag or bracelet indicating that desmopressin is being used.
- Remind patients to keep all health care providers informed of all medications being used.
- Caution patients to avoid the use of alcohol unless alcohol use is approved by physician.
- Note Drug interactions. Caution patients to consult with physician before using new medications.

## lypressin    (lye-PRES-sin)                                           vasopressin

- lypressin: Diapid

**MECHANISM OF ACTION**    See entry for drug class (p. 572).
**INDICATIONS**    See entry for drug class (p. 573).
**CONTRAINDICATIONS**    See entry for drug class (p. 573).
**DOSAGE**    Intranasal:    **ADULTS AND CHILDREN:** For diabetes insipidus, one of two sprays in each nostril four times daily. Additional doses may be added if control of polyuria is not adequate.    *Special patient populations:*    **PREGNANCY:** Safe use during pregnancy has not been established.
**PREPARATIONS**    *Nasal solution:* 185 μg/ml.
**DRUG INTERACTIONS**    Not fully documented but expected to be similar to desmopressin (p. 573).
**FATE**    Lypressin is destroyed in the GI tract but may be adequately absorbed following intranasal administration. *Onset* of action is within 2 hours and persists for 3 to 8 hours. Nasal congestion or rhinitis lowers absorption. The plasma *half-life* of lypressin is 15 minutes. Drug is inactivated in liver and kidneys, with the inactive metabolites being excreted in urine.

### ❦ NURSING CONSIDERATIONS

#### Side effects, toxicities, and associated nursing actions

**CNS** Dizziness and headache are mild.

- Caution patients to avoid driving or operating hazardous equipment if dizziness occurs.
- Instruct patient to notify physician if dizziness or headache is severe or persistent.

**CV** Cardiovascular pressor effects are rare and usually mild.

- Monitor blood pressure and pulse.

**GI** Abdominal cramps and increased bowel movements may occur.

- Instruct patient to notify physician if GI symptoms are severe or persistent.

**Allergy** Allergy may develop.

**Other** Nasal irritation, congestion, rhinorrhea, nasal ulceration, and pruritis may occur.

- Assess degree of nasal irritation, which may lessen with continued use. If nasal irritation is severe, it may interfere with adequate drug absorption; consult physician.

### Nursing interventions related to drug administration

- To self-administer, instruct patient to blow nose gently. Then, while sitting upright, patient should spray ordered number of sprays into each nostril. Patient should not lie down while administering dose.
- Keep applicator bottle clean by washing off tip and wiping dry after each use.

### Patient and family education

- Review anticipated benefits and possible side effects of drug therapy with patient.
- Review correct appication of dose (see above). Review parameters patient may be instructed to monitor or record at home: frequency of nocturia, urine specific gravity, and intake and output. Instruct patient to notify physician if intranasal route cannot be used, as might occur with sinusitis, bad cold, or nasal surgery.
- If dose is missed, instruct patient to take dose as soon as it is remembered, unless close in time to next dose, in which case patient should omit missed dose completely and resume regular schedule with next dose. Instruct patient not to double up for missed doses. Reinforce to patient the need to consult physician for questions about doses.
- Suggest that patient wear a medical identification tag or bracelet indicating that lypressin is being used.
- Remind patients to keep all health care providers informed of all medications being used.
- Caution patients to avoid the use of alcohol unless alcohol use is approved by physician.
- Note drug interactions. Caution patients to consult with physician before using new medications.

---

## vasopressin, vasopressin tannate   (VA-soh-pres-sin)                    vasopressin

- vasopressin, vasopressin tennate: Pitressin

**MECHANISM OF ACTION**   See entry for drug class (p. 572).

**INDICATIONS**   **Diabetes insipidus** See entry for drug class (p. 573).   **Abdominal distention** Vasopressin stimulates smooth muscle, thereby increasing peristalsis.   **Abdominal radiographic procedures** By increasing peristalsis, vasopressin will eliminate gas and concentrate the contrast media.

**CONTRAINDICATIONS**   **Water intoxication** See entry for drug class (p. 573).   **Cardiac disease** See entry for drug class (p. 573).   **Chronic nephritis** Patients with nitrogen retention may be intolerant of vasopressin.

**DOSAGE**   **IM:**   **ADULTS:** For diabetes insipidus, 5 to 10 units two to four times daily of vasopressin injection or 1.5 to 5 units once every 2 to 3 days of vasopressin tannate in oil. For radiographic procedures of vasopressin injection, 5 to 15 units 2 hours and 30 minutes before the procedure.   **CHILDREN:** For diabetes insipidus, 2.5 to 10 units two to four times daily of vasopressin injection or 1.25 to 2.5 units once every 2 to 3 days vasopressin tannate in oil.   **SC:**   **ADULTS:** For diabetes insipidus, 5 to 10 units two to four times daily of vasopressin injection. For abdominal distention, 5 units of vasopressin injection every 3 to 4 hours.   **CHILDREN:** For diabetes insipidus, 2.5 to 10 units two to four times daily of vasopressin injection.   *Special patient populations:*   **ELDERLY:** Elderly patients are much more susceptible to the side effects of vasopressin than are younger adults. These patients may need to be monitored very carefully to prevent life-threatening reactions.   **PREGNANCY:** Vasopressin may cause uterine stimulation at high doses or in sensitive persons.

**PREPARATIONS**   Vasopressin, *solution for injection:* 20 units/ml. Vasopressin tannate in oil, *suspension:* 5 units/ml. For IM use only.

**DRUG INTERACTIONS**   **Alcohol, demeclocycline, epinephrine, heparin,** and **lithium** may decrease the antidiuretic action of vasopressin.   **Clofibrate, chlorpropamide, fludrocortisone,** and *urea* may potentiate the antidiuretic action of vasopressin.   **Ganglionic blocking agents** increase sensitivity to the pressor effects of vasopressin.

**FATE**   Vasopressin is destroyed in the GI tract. Absorption from IM sites may be erratic when vasopressin tannate in oil is used. SC absorption is also erratic when the aqueous vasopressin preparation is used. Absorbed vasopressin is quickly destroyed in the liver and kidneys; duration of action therefore depends mostly on speed of absorption. The duration of action of vasopressin tannate in oil is up to 72 hours, whereas the duration of the more rapidly absorbed aqueous solution is from 2 to 8 hours.

## ❦ NURSING CONSIDERATIONS

### Side effects, toxicities, and associated nursing actions

**CNS** Tremor, vertigo, and pounding in the head have occurred.
* Caution patients to avoid driving or operating hazardous equipment if vertigo develops.
* If CNS symptoms are severe or persistent, notify physician.

**CV** Large doses may cause angina, arrhythmias, peripheral vascular collapse, coronary insufficiency, and myocardial infarction.
* Obtain history of cardiac problems before administering first dose.
* Calculate dosages carefully.
* Monitor blood pressure and pulse. Instruct patient to report the development of new symptoms.

**GI** Abdominal cramps, diarrhea, intestinal hyperactivity, nausea, vomiting, and gas may occur.
* Instruct patient to notify physician if GI symptoms are severe or persistent, as they may indicate the need to lower the dosage.
* Monitor intake and output and weight.
* Instruct patient to drink one or two glasses of water when taking a dose of medication to limit side effects.

**Renal** Water intoxication may occur especially with large doses.
* Monitor weight, intake and output, and urine specific gravity.
* Monitor serum electrolytes.
* Monitor level of consciousness.

**Endocrine** Plasma concentrations of cortisol and growth hormone may increase.
* Monitor serum levels of cortisol and growth hormone, if available. Monitor serum and urine glucose levels.

**Allergic** Angioedema, bronchoconstriction, circulatory collapse, dyspnea, fever, rash, and wheezing may occur.
* Monitor respiratory rate and blood pressure and pulse, auscultate breath sounds, and monitor temperature.
* Have available drugs, equipment, and personnel to treat acute allergic reactions in settings where this drug is administered.

**Other** Pallor and uterine contractions may occur.
* Assess whether patient is pregnant before administering dose. Palpate uterus after administering dose, if uterus is palpable.

### Nursing interventions related to drug administration

* Read orders carefully to prepare correct preparation.
* To administer any IM preparation that is suspended in oil (as is vasopressin tannate in oil), do the following. Heat unopened vial in warm water for several minutes to decrease the viscosity of the oil. Vigorously agitate the ampule to resuspend the drug, which is usually an inconspicuous spot on the side of the vial. Resuspension is adequate when no particles of medication remain visible on the sides or bottom of the vial. Draw up correct dose in a syringe fitted with a 19 to 21 gauge, 1½ in needle.

Administer immediately, before oil cools completely. Inject medication with slow, even pressure. Attempts to inject too rapidly may cause needle and syringe to separate, causing spilling of the medication and inaccurate dosage administration. Appropriate injection sites in adults include the buttocks, thigh, or ventrogluteal site. Because the drug leaves palpable lumps at injection sites, avoid the deltoid muscles. Record and rotate injection sites. Oil-based medications should never be given IV.

### Patient and family education

- Review anticipated benefits and possible side effects of drug therapy with patients.
- Teach patient correct administration technique if patient is to self-administer drug at home (see above for administration of IM oil-based preparations).
- If dose is missed, instruct patient to take dose as soon as it is remembered, unless close in time to next dose, in which case patient should omit missed dose completely and resume regular schedule with next dose. Instruct patient not to double up for missed doses. Reinforce to patient the need to consult physician for questions about doses.
- Suggest that patient wear a medical identification tag or bracelet indicating that vasopressin is being used.
- Remind patients to keep all health care providers informed of all medications being used.
- Caution patients to avoid the use of alcohol unless alcohol use is approved by physician.
- Note drug interactions. Caution patients to consult with physician before using new medications.

# Chapter Thirty

# Thyroid hormones and related agents

| | |
|---|---|
| **Thyroid hormones** | **Antithyroid drugs** |
| levothyroxine sodium | methimazole |
| liothyronine sodium | propylthiouracil |
| liotrix | **Regulators of calcium homeostasis** |
| thyroglobulin | calcitonin |
| thyroid | calcifediol |
| | calcitriol |
| | dihydrotachysterol |
| | ergocalciferol |

**INTRODUCTION** The thyroid gland regulates basal metabolic rate. When stimulated by thyrotropin (Chapter 29, p. 571), the thyroid gland releases thyroxine ($T_4$) and liothyronine ($T_3$) into general circulation. These two hormones influence metabolism in many tissues of the body.

Thyroid failure or insufficiency may be treated with replacement of the missing thyroid hormones. Overactivity of thyroid may require surgery or drug therapy. Methimazole and propylthiouracil are available to suppress thyroid function and relieve hyperthyroidism.

Parafollicular cells within the thyroid synthesize and release a protein called calcitonin, which may influence calcium metabolism. Calcium metabolism is also regulated by parathyroid hormone from the parathyroid glands and forms of vitamin D from the liver, skin, and kidneys.

---

## Thyroid hormones

levothyroxine sodium ~ liothyronine sodium ~ liotrix ~ thyroglobulin ~ thyroid

**OVERVIEW OF THE DRUG CLASS** Levothyroxine sodium and liothyronine sodium are synthetic forms of the natural thyroid hormones. Liotrix is a synthetic mixture of thyroid hormones in proportions that mimic naturally released hormones. Thyroglobulin, the storage protein from thyroid, contains both thyroid hormones in releasable forms. The preparation designated *thyroid* is a powder prepared from desiccated, defatted bovine and/or porcine thyroids.

**MECHANISM OF ACTION** The active forms in all thyroid hormone preparations are thyroxine ($T_4$) and/or triiodothyronine ($T_3$). Of the two, $T_3$ is the more active. More $T_4$ is present in the thyroid gland and released into blood, but $T_4$ is converted to $T_3$ in many target tissues. $T_3$ is bound to nuclear receptors in target cells, setting off events that alter protein synthesis and change the metabolic activity of the cell. The overall result of these actions is to increase metabolic rates.

**INDICATIONS** **Hypothroidism** Primary, secondary, or tertiary hypothyroidism may be treated with thyroid hormones. Such use constitutes replacement therapy and must be continued for life. **Nontoxic goiter** Thyroid hormones are used as replacement therapy for this condition. • Suppression of thyrotropin release removes the stimulus for thyroid growth. **Hashimoto's disease** This chronic thyroiditis damages thyroid function; replacement therapy may be required. • Suppression of thyrotropin release removes the stimulus for thyroid growth. **Diagnosis of hyperthyroidism** Mild disease may be detected by response to suppression with thyroid hormones (see Table 30-1, p. 580).

**CONTRAINDICATIONS** **Cardiovascular disease** Cardiac arrhythmias may be precipitated by thyroid hormone therapy. **Adrenal insufficiency** Thyroid hormone therapy may precipitate an acute adrenal crisis due to insufficient corticosteroid production. **Euthyroid obesity** Thyroid hormones should not be used for weight control in obesity unless the patient is hypothyroid. The purpose of therapy in the latter case is to reverse hypothyroidism, not to control weight.

**DRUG INTERACTIONS** **Anticoagulants** used orally may be potentiated by thyroid hormones because the thyroid hormones increase catabolism of vitamin K–dependent clotting factors. **Antidiabetic agents** may need to be given at higher doses because tissue demands increase when the hypothyroid state is corrected by thyroid hormones. **Cholestyramine resin** impairs the absorption of thyroid

**Table 30-1.**

| Common tests used to evaluate thyroid function | | | | |
|---|---|---|---|---|
| **Test** | **Procedure** | **Diagnostic use** | **Normal values** | **Comments** |
| Serum $T_4$ | Total serum $T_4$ is measured by competitive protein binding test or radioimmunnoassay. | To distinguish hyperthyroid or hypothyroid conditions from euthyroid state. | 5 to 12 $\mu$g/100 ml serum | Conditions that elevate thyroid-binding globulin (TBG) levels. (e.g., pregnancy or estrogen administration) also elevate total serum $T_4$ levels.  Lowered TBG levels in cirrhosis or nephrotic syndrome also lower total serum $T_4$ levels in both cases, free hormone levels are usually normal, and patients are functionally euthyroid. |
| Free thyroxine ($FT_4$) | Radioimmunoassay or equilibrium dialysis. | To distinguish hyperthyroid or hypothyroid conditions from euthyroid state. | 1 to 2.5 ng/100 ml (0.001 to 0.0025 $\mu$g/100 ml) | Normal values may vary greatly from laboratory to laboratory. |
| $T_3$ uptake ($T_3U$) or resin $T_3$ uptake ($RT_3U$) | Test measures the degree of saturation of patient's TBG with endogenous thyroid hormones. | To distinguish hyperthyroid or hypothyroid conditions from euthyroid state. | 25% to 45%, or 0.82 to 1.35 when expressed as a ratio of $T_3U$ to normal | Hyperthyroidism elevates the ratio; hypothyroidism lowers the ratio. Levels of TBG and $T_4$ in the patient's blood affect the test more than do $T_3$ values. |
| Serum $T_3$ | *Total* serum $T_3$ is measured by specific radioimmunoassay. | To distinguish hyperthyroid conditions from euthyroid state. | 0.08 to 0.20 $\mu$g/100 ml | Test is not useful for hypothyroidism, since $T_3$ may be relatively more abundant than $T_4$ in hypothyroidism. |
| Serum TSH | Serum TSH is measured by specific radioimmunoassay. | To distinguish hypothyroid conditions from euthyroid state; to distinguish primary from secondary hypothyroidism. | 0.5 to 5 $\mu$U/ml | Hypothyroidism caused by thyroid failure (primary) will show elevated TSH levels; hypothyroidism caused by pituitary failure (secondary) will show little or no TSH. |

| | | | | |
|---|---|---|---|---|
| Thyroid-releasing hormone test (TRH test) | Synthetic TRH (500 μg) is given IV, causing a peak release of TSH 30 min later in patients with normal pituitary glands | To distinguish hypothyroidism caused by pituitary failure from other forms of hypothyroidism. | Peak concentrations of TSH produced in normal patients are 5 to 35 μU/ml serum. | No rise is usually observed in serum TSH in hyperthyroid patients. |
| Thyroid uptake of radioiodine | Radioactivity in the thyroid measured 4, 6, and 24 hr after administration of tracer dose of radioactive iodine. | To distinguish hyperthyroid and hypothyroid conditions from euthyroid state. | Normal glands take up 10% to 35% of tracer dose in 24 hr. | This test may be affected by dietary intake of iodine, by administration of iodine-containing medications, or by use of antithyroid drugs. |
| TSH test | Bovine TSH is given IM, after which serum $T_4$ or radioiodine uptake is measured. | To distinguish primary from secondary hypothyroidism. | A normal thyroid gland responds by increasing iodine uptake and $T_4$ release. | This test is rarely used when TSH levels may be measured. |
| Thyroid suppression tests | $T_3$ (75 μg) is given daily for 7 days. Radioiodine uptake by thyroid gland is measured before and after test. | To distinguish hyperthyroid conditions from euthyroid state. | Uptake is 50% or less of the pretest uptake. | This test may be dangerous for elderly patients, weakened patients, or patients with heart disease. |

hormones from the GI tract.    **Sympathomimetic agents** such as epinephrine may precipitate an attack of coronary insufficiency in patients with coronary artery disease, especially if thyroid hormones are also being given.    **Estrogens** may increase thyroxine-binding globulin, thus decreasing free, active thyroxine in the blood. Doses of thyroid hormones may need to be increased.

## ❦ NURSING CONSIDERATIONS

**Side effects, toxicities, and associated nursing actions**    The side effects listed are essentially the same as for hyperthyroidism and result from overdosage with thyroid hormones.
- Monitor thyroid function tests.

**CNS** Headache, insomnia, nervousness, and tremors may result from overdosage.
- Assess patients for CNS side effects. Obtain a thorough history of other health problems. Keep an ongoing record of patient response to thyroid medications.

**CV** Angina pectoris, arrhythmias, cardiac decompensation, cardiac failure, increased blood pressure, increased pulse pressure, palpitations, and tachycardia can occur. Death may follow.
- Monitor blood pressure and pulse. If pulse is greater than 100 beats/min in an adult, withhold the dose and notify the physician.
- Monitor the ECG, which should be obtained before therapy and at regular intervals.
- Assess for signs of cardiac problems: edema, weight gain, pallor, and fatigue.

**GI** Abdominal cramps, diarrhea, increased appetite, and weight loss may occur.
- Monitor weight. Assess for complaints of GI side effects.

**Other** Intolerance to heat, sweating, fever, and menstrual irregularities may occur.
- Instruct women to keep a record of menstrual periods.
- Question patients about heat intolerance.

**Nursing interventions related to drug administration**
- Instruct patients to take doses in the morning to avoid night-time insomnia.

**Patient and family education**
- Review anticipated benefits and possible side effects of drug therapy with the patient. Since side effects may not develop for 4 to 6 weeks after the start of therapy or an increase in dose, caution patients to notify the physician of any new sign or symptom.
- Encourage patients to return for regular follow-up visits for dosage adjustment and monitoring.
- Instruct diabetic patients to monitor blood and urine glucose carefully for several weeks following the start of therapy or dosage change, as an adjustment in diet or insulin may be necessary.
- Remind patients to keep all health care providers informed of all medications being taken. Remind patients to keep these and all medications out of the reach of children.
- Instruct patients to keep thyroid medications dry and in a light-resistant container.
- Encourage patients to wear a medical identification tag or bracelet stating that thyroid medication is being used.
- Caution patients not to switch brands of medications without consulting the physician or pharmacist.

## levothyroxine sodium    (lee-voh-thy-ROX-in)    thyroid hormone

- levothyroxine soduim: ✿Eltroxin, Levothroid, Synthroid

**MECHANISM OF ACTION**   • See entry for drug class (p. 579).
**INDICATIONS**   • See entry for drug class (p. 579).
**DOSAGE**   **PO:**   **ADULTS:** For hypothyroidism, initial doses are 50 μg as a single daily dose for mild disease or 12.5 to 25 μg as a single daily dose for severe disease. The dose is gradually increased by increments of 25 to 50 μg every 2 to 4 weeks until adequate replacement is achieved. Full replacement doses seldom exceed 200 μg daily. Geriatric patients should receive 12.5 to 50 μg daily initially, increased in small increments at 3 to 8 week intervals.   **CHILDREN:** Congenital hypothyroidism is treated with 25 to 50 μg daily as a single dose in full-term infants. Lower doses are used in premature infants or infants with symptoms of cardiac failure. Infants from 6 to 12 months of age receive 50 to 75 μg daily; 1 to 5 years, 75 to 100 μg daily; 6 to 12 years, 100 to 150 μg daily.   **IV:**   **ADULTS:** For myexedemic

coma, 200 to 500 µg initially; 100 to 300 µg on the second day; 50 to 200 µg on subsequent days until oral dosage can begin. Parenteral replacement dosages are about one half the previously established oral doses. **CHILDREN:** Parenteral replacement dosages are about one-half to three-fourths the previously established oral doses. Use only when oral doses are not tolerated. **IM: ADULTS:** Parenteral replacement dosages are about one-half the previously established oral doses. Use only when oral doses are not tolerated. **CHILDREN:** Parenteral replacement dosage are about one-half to three-fourths the previously established oral doses. Use only when oral doses are not tolerated. *Special patient populations:* **ELDERLY:** Thyroid hormones should be used cautiously in geriatric patients because this group of patients is likely to have a degree of undetected heart disease that can make the thyroid hormones acutely dangerous. **PREGNANCY:** Use of thyroid hormones must continue during pregnancy to maintain the mother. The hormones do not cross the placenta in large amounts.

**PREPARATIONS** *Tablets:* 25, 50, 75, 100, 125, 150, 175, 200 and 300 µg; *powder, for reconstitution:* 200 or 500 µg. To reconstitute, add 0.9% sodium chloride injection to achieve the desired concentration. The vial should be shaken to dissolve the powder. The resulting clear solution should be used immediately, should not be mixed with other IV infusion solutions, and any left-over solution should be discarded.

**DRUG INTERACTIONS** See entry for drug class (p. 579).

**FATE** Levothyroxine sodium is normally administered orally, but only 50% to 80% of an oral dose is absorbed. Different preparations may differ in bioavailability. Levothyroxine is tightly bound to thyroxin-binding globulin. The *onset* of action is between 1 and 3 weeks, and the action persists for 1 to 3 weeks following discontinuance. In contrast the plasma *half-life* is 6 to 7 days. Between 20% and 40% of a dose is eliminated by biliary routes into feces. An additional 35% is converted to triiodothyronine by the liver and kidneys.

## ☙ NURSING CONSIDERATIONS

### Side effects, toxicities, and associated nursing actions
- See entry for drug class (p. 582).

### Nursing interventions related to drug administration
- For IV use, dilute as directed under Preparations. Administer at a rate of 0.1 mg or less over 1 minute.
- Synthroid 100 and 300 mg tablets, contain FD & C yellow dye #5 (tartrazine), which may cause an allergic reaction in susceptible individuals. Although rare, this side effect is seen more commonly in persons with aspirin hypersensitivity.
- See entry for drug class (p. 582).

### Patient and family education
- See entry for drug class (p. 582).

---

## liothyronine sodium    (lye-oh-THY-roh-neen)                    thyroid hormone

- liothyronine sodium: Cytomel

**MECHANISM OF ACTION** • See entry for drug class (p. 579).

**INDICATIONS** • See entry for drug class (p. 579).

**CONTRAINDICATIONS** • See entry for drug class (p. 579).

**DOSAGE** **PO:** **ADULTS:** For mild hypothyroidism, initially 25 µg daily as a single dose; increase in increments of 12.5 to 25 µg daily every 1 to 2 weeks until a response is achieved. Usual replacement doses are 25 to 75 µg daily. • For severe hypothyroidism, initially 5 µg daily as a single dose; increase in increments of 5 to 10 µg daily every 1 to 2 weeks until a response is achieved. Usual replacement doses are 50 to 100 µg. • Geriatric patients receive 5 µg daily as an initial dosage, with 5 µg increments added every 1 to 2 weeks until symptoms are controlled. • For simple nontoxic goiter, initially 5 µg daily as a single dose, increased by 5 to 10 µg daily every 1 to 2 weeks up to a dose of 25 µg. Further increases may be 12.5 to 25 µg daily at 1 to 2 week intervals. The usual maintenance dosage is 75 µg daily. • For the T3 suppression test, 75 to 100 µg daily for 7 days, with a radioactive iodine uptake test performed before and after the test (see Table 30-1, p. 580).   **CHILDREN:** For congenital hypothyroidism, initially 5 µg daily as a single dose; increase by increments of 5 µg every 3 to 4 days until the desired response is achieved.   *Special patient populations:*   **ELDERLY:** Thyroid hormones should be used cautiously in geriatric patients because this group is likely to have a degree of undetected heart disease that can make the thyroid hormones acutely dangerous.   **PREGNANCY:** Use of thyroid hormones must be continued during pregnancy to maintain the mother. The hormones do not cross the placenta in large amounts.

**PREPARATIONS**   *Tablets:* 5, 25, and 50 µg.

**DRUG INTERACTIONS**   • See entry for drug class (p. 579).

**FATE**   Liothyronine sodium is almost completely absorbed following oral administration. The drug is bound to thyroxine-binding globulin but much less extensively than is thyroxine. The *onset* of action is 24 to 72 hours, and the effects persist for 72 hours after discontinuing the drug.

## ☙ NURSING CONSIDERATIONS

### Side effects, toxicities, and associated nursing actions
  • See entry for drug class (p. 582).

### Nursing interventions related to drug administration
  • See entry for drug class (p. 582).

### Patient and family education
  • See entry for drug class (p. 582).

---

## liotrix   (LYE-oh-trix)                                    thyroid hormone

  • liotrix: Euthroid, Thyrolar

**MECHANISM OF ACTION**   • See entry for drug class (p. 579).

**INDICATIONS**   • See entry for drug class (p. 579).

**CONTRAINDICATIONS**   • See entry for drug class (p. 579).

**DOSAGE**   **PO:**   **ADULTS AND CHILDREN:** Usual initial doses are single daily doses of Thyrolar-¼, Thyrolar-½, or Euthroid-½. Dosage is increased at 2 week intervals as needed. Children may need higher maintenance doses, and geriatric patient require smaller doses.   *Special patient populations:* **ELDERLY:** Thyroid hormones should be used cautiously in geriatric patients because this group is likely to have a degree of undetected heart disease that can make the thyroid hormones acutely dangerous.   **PREGNANCY:** Use of thyroid hormones must be continued during pregnancy to maintain the mother. The hormones do not cross the placenta in large amounts.

**PREPARATIONS**   *Tablets:* See Table 30-2.

**DRUG INTERACTIONS**   • See entry for drug class (p. 579).

**FATE**   The active ingredients of liotrix are levothyroxine and liothyronine. These are handled by the body as described for those individual agents (Table 30-3).

## ☙ NURSING CONSIDERATIONS

### Side effects, toxicities, and associated nursing actions
  • See entry for drug class (p. 582).

### Nursing interventions related to drug administration
  • See Table 30-1. Euthroid tablets contain FD & C yellow dye #5 (tartrazine), which may cause an allergic reaction in susceptible individuals. Although rare, this side effect is seen more commonly in persons with aspirin hypersensitivity.
  • See entry for drug class (p. 582).

### Patient and family education
  • See entry for drug class (p. 582).

| Table 30-2. | Preparations of liotrix | | |
|---|---|---|---|
| **Preparation (trade name)** | **Levothyroxine sodium (μg)** | | **Liothyronine sodium (μg)** |
| Thyrolar-¼ | 12.5 | | 3.1 |
| Thyrolar-½ | 25 | | 6.25 |
| Euthroid-½* | 30 | | 7.5 |
| Thyrolar-1 | 50 | | 12.5 |
| Euthroid-1* | 60 | | 15 |
| Thyrolar-2 | 100 | | 25 |
| Euthroid-2* | 120 | | 30 |
| Thyrolar-3 | 150 | | 37.5 |
| Euthroid-3* | 180 | | 45 |

*All preparations designated Euthroid contain tartrazine.

## thyroglobulin  (thy-roh-GLOB-yoo-lin)

thyroid hormone

- thyroglobulin: Proloid

**MECHANISM OF ACTION** • See entry for drug class (p. 579).
**INDICATIONS** • See entry for drug class (p. 579).
**CONTRAINDICATIONS** • See entry for drug class (p. 579).
**DOSAGE** **PO:** **ADULTS:** For mild hypothyroidism, initially 60 mg daily as a single dose; increase monthly in 60 mg daily increments to achieve desired effect. For severe hypothyroidism, initially 15 mg daily for 2 weeks; increase to 30 mg daily for 2 weeks, then increase to 60 mg daily and observe for 1 month. Maintenance doses normally range from 32 to 200 mg daily. **CHILDREN:** As for severe hypothyroidism in adults, but increases in dosage can be made at 2-week intervals until full replacement is achieved. *Special patient populations:* **ELDERLY:** Thyroid hormones should be used cautiously in geriatric patients because this group is likely to have a degree of undetected heart disease that can make thyroid hormones acutely dangerous. **PREGNANCY:** Use of thyroid hormones must be continued during pregnancy to maintain the mother. The hormones do not cross the placenta in large amounts.
**PREPARATIONS** *Tablets:* 32, 65, 100, 130, and 200 mg.
**DRUG INTERACTIONS** • See entry for drug class (p. 579).
**FATE** Thyroglobulin contains both thyroxine and triiodothyronine. The absorption of thyroid hormones contained in thyroglobulin is similar to synthetic levothyroxine and liothyronine (Table 30-2, above).

### ☙ NURSING CONSIDERATIONS
**Side effects, toxicities, and associated nursing actions**
- See entry for drug class (p. 582).

**Nursing interventions related to drug administration**
- See entry for drug class (p. 582).

**Patient and family education**
- See entry for drug class (p. 582).

## thyroid  (THY-roid)

thyroid hormone

- thyroid: S-P-T, Thyrar, Thyro-teric

**MECHANISM OF ACTION** • See entry for drug class (p. 579).

**INDICATIONS** • See entry for drug class (p. 579).

**CONTRAINDICATIONS** • See entry for drug class (p. 579).

**DOSAGE**    PO:    ADULTS: For mild hypothyroidism, initially 60 mg daily as a single dose usually taken before breakfast; increase monthly in 60 mg daily increments to achieve the desired effect. For severe hypothyroidism, initially 15 mg daily for 2 weeks; increase to 30 mg daily for 2 weeks, then increase to 60 mg daily and observe for 1 month. Maintenance doses normally range from 32 to 200 mg daily. CHILDREN: As for severe hypothyroidism in adults, but increases in dosage can be made at 2 week intervals until full replacement is achieved. *Special patient populations:*    ELDERLY: Thyroid hormones should be used cautiously in geriatric patients because this group of patients is likely to have a degree of undetected heart disease that can make the thyroid hormones acutely dangerous.    PREGNANCY: Use of thyroid hormones must be continued during pregnancy to maintain the mother. The hormones do not cross the placenta in large amounts.

**PREPARATIONS**    **Thyroid** *Tablets:* 15, 30, 60, 65, 90, 120, 130, 180, 240, and 300 mg. Tablets sold under the trade name of Thyrar contain beef thyroid; all others may contain pork thyroid. *Tablets, enteric coated:* 30, 60, or 120 mg. *Capsules:* 60, 120, 180, and 300 mg pork thyroid powder suspended in soybean oil.    **Thyroid strong** *Tablets:* 32.5, 65, 130, or 200 mg.

**DRUG INTERACTIONS** • See entry for drug class (p. 579).

**FATE**    Thyroid contains both thyroxine and triiodothyronine. The absorption of thyroid hormones contained in thyroglobulin is similar to synthetic levothyroxine and liothyronine (Table 30-3, below).

❧ **NURSING CONSIDERATIONS**

**Side effects, toxicities, and associated nursing actions**
• See entry for drug class (p. 582).

**Nursing interventions related to drug administration**
• See entry for drug class (p. 582).

**Patient and family education**
• Avoid excessive intake of turnips, cabbage, or related vegetables.
• See entry for drug class (p. 582).

Table
30-3.

| Clinical summary of thyroid hormones | | | |
|---|---|---|---|
| **Drug** | **Routes** | **Duration of action** | **Equivalent dosage** |
| Levothyroxine sodium (T4) | PO (50%-80% absorbed) | 1 to 3 weeks | 100 μg or less |
| Liothyronine sodium (T3) | PO (95% absorbed) | 72 hours | 25 μ |
| Liotrix | | | |
|   Thyrolar | PO | 1 to 3 weeks | 50 μg $T_4$/12.5 μg $T_3$ |
|   Euthroid | PO | 1 to 3 weeks | 60 μg $T_4$/15 μg $T_3$ |
| Thyroglobulin | PO | 1 to 3 weeks | 65 mg |
| Thyroid | PO | 1 to 3 weeks | 60–65 mg |

# Antithyroid drugs

methimazole ~ propylthiouracil

**OVERVIEW OF THE DRUG CLASS**    To form thyroxine and triiodothyronine, the thyroid gland must take in iodine from the blood. Iodine is metabolized within cells of the thyroid, ultimately forming the thyroid hormones, which are then stored in colloid within the gland. When the thyroid is overactive, suppression of synthesis and release of thyroid hormones must be achieved to control the hyperthyroidism. Surgery, radiation, and drug therapy are commonly employed (Table 30-3, p. 586).

**MECHANISM OF ACTION**   Methimazole and propylthiouracil interfere with the oxidative processes that allow iodine to be inserted into thyroid hormones. When synthesis is blocked in this way, active hormone fails to be formed or stored. Hormones previously stored in colloid continue to be released for several weeks, but when these stores are depleted, suppression of synthesis is obvious.

**INDICATIONS**   **Hyperthyroidism** Methimazole and propylthiouracil may be used for 1 to 2 years to control hyperthyroidism; some patients undergo spontaneous remission. • Radiation and surgery may ultimately be required in many patients.   **Thyroidectomy in a hyperthyroid patient** Methimazole and propylthiouracil may be used as a pretreatment to protect a patient from the effects of hyperthyroidism during or immediately after thyroidectomy or irradiation of the thyroid.

**CONTRAINDICATIONS**   **Pregnancy** Methimazole and propylthiouracil cross the placenta and may induce goiter or hypothyroidism in the newborn.   **Blood dyscrasias** Methimazole and propylthiouracil may cause agranulocytosis.

**DRUG INTERACTIONS**   **Drugs causing agranulocytosis** should not be given at the same time patients are receiving methimazole and propylthiouracil because damage to the blood-forming tissues may be additive.

## methimazole (thiamazole)   (meth-IM-uh-zole)                    antithyroid

●  methimazole (thiamazole): Tapazole

**MECHANISM OF ACTION**   • See entry for drug class (p. 587).
**INDICATIONS**   • See entry for drug class (p. 587).
**CONTRAINDICATIONS**   • See entry for drug class (p. 587).
**DOSAGE**   **PO:**   **ADULTS:** Initially, 15 to 60 mg daily divided into three doses. After 2 months, dosage may be carefully reduced to maintain control and minimize side effects. Maintenance dosage usually ranges from 5 to 30 mg daily.   **CHILDREN:** Initially, 0.4 mg/kg daily in three doses. Maintenance doses are usually half the initial dose.   *Special patient populations:*   **ELDERLY:** Patients over the age of 40 years have a substantially greater risk of agranulocytosis.   **PREGNANCY:** Use of this drug in pregnancy carries substantial risk to the fetus.
**PREPARATIONS**   *Tablets:* 5 or 10 mg.
**DRUG INTERACTIONS**   • See entry for drug class (p. 587).
   **FATE**   Methimazole is well absorbed following oral administration and distributes to many tissues. The drug crosses the placenta and freely enters milk. The elimination *half-life* is 5 to 13 hours. Excretion is in urine.

### ❦ NURSING CONSIDERATIONS
   #### Side effects, toxicities, and associated nursing actions
   **CNS** Drowsiness, headache, neuritis, paresthesia, and vertigo have been reported but are rare.
   • Assess patients for tingling of fingers and toes.
   • Caution patients to avoid driving or operating hazardous equipment if vertigo or drowsiness develop.
   **Blood** Agranulocytosis is an uncommon but serious side effect that is more likely to occur with daily doses above 40 mg or in patients older than 40 years.
   • Instruct patients to report the development of fever, chills, sore throat, and unexplained bleeding.
   **GI** Epigastric distress, loss of taste, nausea, and vomiting occur in less than 3% of patients.
   • Monitor weight. If GI symptoms are severe or persistent, notify the physician.
   • Instruct patients to take ordered doses with meals or snacks to lessen gastric irritation.
   **Skin** Abnormal hair loss, pruritis, rash, skin pigmentation, and urticaria occur in less than 3% of patients.
   • Assess hair distribution, and visually inspect patients at regular intervals for changes in hair or skin.
   • Instruct patients to report the development of skin changes.

**Other** Arthralgia, myalgia, sialadenopathy (swelling of a salivary gland), and lymphadenopathy are rare.
- Caution patients to report the development of any new sign or symptom.

### Patient and family education
- Review anticipated benefits and possible side effects of drug therapy with patients. Since side effects may not develop for weeks after the start of therapy or an increase in dose, caution patients to notify the physician of any unexpected sign or symptom.
- Doses should be taken in three evenly spaced doses.
- Encourage patients to return for follow-up visits and take medications as ordered for best effect.
- Remind patients to keep all health care providers informed of all medications being taken.
- Encourage patients to wear a medical identification tag or bracelet.
- Remind patients to keep these and all medications out of the reach of children.

---

## propylthiouracil    (pro-pyl-thy-oh-YOO-rah-sill)                                antithyroid

- propylthiouracil: ✽Propyl-Thyracil

**MECHANISM OF ACTION**  • See entry for drug class (p. 587).
**INDICATIONS**  • See entry for drug class (p. 587).
**CONTRAINDICATIONS**  • See entry for drug class (p. 587).
**DOSAGE**    PO:    ADULTS: Initially, 300 to 450 mg daily divided in three equal doses. After 2 months, the dose may be carefully reduced to maintain control and minimize side effects. Maintenance doses range from 100 to 150 mg daily. Higher initial doses may be required for thyrotoxic crisis.    CHILDREN: Neonates, 5 to 10 mg/kg daily. Children 6 to 10 years, initially 50 to 150 mg daily divided in three equal doses. Children over 10 years, 150 to 300 mg or 150 mg/M$^2$.    *Special patient populations:* Patients over the age of 40 years have a substantially greater risk of agranulocytosis.    PREGNANCY: Use of this drug in pregnancy carries substantial risk to the fetus.
**PREPARATIONS**    *Tablets:* 50 mg.
**DRUG INTERACTIONS**    **Anticoagulant drugs** may be potentiated by propylthiouracil. • For other interactions, see entry for drug class (p. 587).
**FATE**    Propylthiouracil is well absorbed following oral administration. The drug concentrates in thyroid tissue, passes into milk, and crosses the placenta. The drug is rapidly metabolized to forms that are readily excreted in urine.

### ☙ NURSING CONSIDERATIONS
#### Side effects, toxicities, and associated nursing actions
**CNS** Drowsiness, headache, neuritis, paresthesia, and vertigo are rare.
- Assess patients for tingling of fingers and toes.
- Caution patients to avoid driving or operating hazardous equipment if vertigo or drowsiness develop.

**Blood** Agranulocytosis is uncommon but is a serious side effect.
- Instruct patients to report the development of fever, chills, sore throat or unexplained bleeding.

**GI** Epigastric distress, loss of taste, nausea, and vomiting occur in less than 1% of patients.
- Monitor weight. If GI symptoms are severe or persistent, notify the physician.
- Instruct patients to take ordered doses with meals or snacks to lessen gastric irritation.

**Renal** Nephritis is uncommon.
- Monitor weight; question about urinary output.
- Monitor urinalysis for hematuria and proteinuria.
- Assess for fever and rash.

**Liver** Jaundice in uncommon.
- Instruct patients to report the development of jaundice.

**Skin** Abnormal hair loss, lightening of hair color, pruritis, rash, skin pigmentation, and urticaria may occur.

Table
30-3.

## Summary of drugs used to treat hyperthyroidism

| Generic name | Trade name | Administration/dosage | Properties | Comments |
|---|---|---|---|---|
| **THIOAMIDES** | | | | |
| Propylthiouracil (PTU) | | ORAL: Adults—50 to 300 mg daily in 3 doses. Initially 300 to 450 mg daily is given in 3 or 4 doses. Children over 10 yr—half the adult dose. Children 6 to 10 yr—one-quarter the adult dose. | Inhibits thyroid hormone synthesis but not release. | See Drug monograph (p. 588). |
| Methimazole | Tapazole | ORAL: Adults—5 to 20 mg 2 or 3 times daily. Children 6 to 10 yr—0.4 mg/kg body weight daily in 3 or 4 doses. | Inhibits thyroid hormone synthesis but not release. | See Drug monograph (p. 587). |
| **BETA ADRENERGIC BLOCKER** | | | | |
| Propranolol hydrochloride | Inderal | ORAL: Adults—40 to 240 mg daily in divided doses. INTRAVENOUS: Adults—5 mg or less administered at 1 mg/min or more slowly. | Controls symptoms of hyperthyroidism but does not lower $T_3$ and $T_4$ release from the thyroid. | Controls palpitations, tremor, sweating, proximal muscle weakness, and cardiac symptoms of hyperthyroidism by competitively blocking beta adrenergic receptors. Bronchospasm may occur in asthmatic patients; may precipitate frank heart failure in patients with heart function maintained by sympathetic tone. |
| **IODINE** | | | | |
| Potassium or sodium iodide | Strong Iodine Solution Lugol's Solution | ORAL: Adults—0.1 to 0.3 ml 3 times daily INTRAVENOUS: Adults—250 to 500 mg daily for thyrotoxic crisis. | Produces short-term inhibition of thyroid hormone synthesis by direct action on the thyroid. | Used as presurgical medication to reduce the size of the thyroid gland after thioamide therapy. Used with thioamide and propranolol for hyperthyroid crisis. May produce iodism. |
| **RADIOACTIVE IODINE** | | | | |
| $^{131}$I as NaI | | ORAL: Adults—4 to 10 mCi as a single dose for Graves' disease. For thyroid carcinoma, single doses of up to 150 mCi may be used. Smaller doses are used for diagnostic purposes (see Table 30.4). | These radionuclides are concentrated in the thyroid and release radiation, which destroys thyroid tissue. | Used to destroy thyroid tissue without surgery for control of Graves' disease or thyroid carcinoma. Hypothyroidism ultimately develops in most patients. |

- Assess hair distribution, and visually inspect patients at regular intervals for changes in hair or skin.
- Instruct patients to report the development of skin changes.

**Other** Arthralgia, myalgia, sialadenopathy (swelling of a salivary gland), and lymphadenopathy are rare.

- Caution patients to report the development of any new sign or symptom.

### Patient and family education

- Review anticipated benefits and possible side effects of drug therapy with patients. Since side effects may not develop for weeks after the start of therapy or an increase in dose, caution patients to notify the physician of any unexpected sign or symptom.
- Medication should be taken in three evenly spaced doses.
- Encourage patients to return for follow-up visits and take medications as ordered for best effect.
- Remind patients to keep all health care providers informed of all medications being taken.
- Encourage patients to wear a medical identification tag or bracelet.
- Remind patients to keep these and all medications out of the reach of children.

---

# Regulators of calcium homeostasis

calcitonin ~ calcitriol ~ calcifediol ~ dihydrotachysterol ~ ergocalciferol

**OVERVIEW OF THE DRUG CLASS**    The metabolism of calcium is carefully regulated by an integrated system involving several tissues. Calcium intake can be modulated by altering absorption from the intestine. Elimination can be regulated by changing excretion in the kidneys. Finally, bone serves as a massive depot of calcium with deposition in new bone and resorption from remodeled bone.

**MECHANISM OF ACTION**    Parafollicular cells of the thyroid produce the peptide hormone calcitonin. Calcitonin can increase excretion of calcium by the kidneys, decrease absorption of calcium in the intestine, and inhibit resorption in bone. The parathyroid glands produce a peptide hormone with opposite effects; parathyroid hormone blocks excretion of calcium by the kidneys, increases absorption of calcium in the intestine, and diminishes deposition in bone.

The vitamin D derivatives are necessary for adequate absorption of calcium from the intestine, for regulating renal excretion, and for proper deposition in bone. Dietary vitamin D is primarily cholecalciferol or ergocalciferol (p. 596). Cholecalciferol is also formed from 7-dehydrocholesterol in skin exposed to ultraviolet light. Dihydrotachysterol is chemically related and similar in action to ergocalciferol. These forms of vitamin D may be thought of as precursors for the more active forms. Liver forms the 25-hydroxy metabolites such as calcifediol (p. 591). The kidneys form 1,25-dihydroxycholecalciferol (calcitriol, p. 593), which is apparently the most active form of vitamin D.

---

## calcitonin    (kal-see-TOH-nin)               calcium regulator

- calcitonin: Cibacalcin, Calcimar

**MECHANISM OF ACTION**    • See entry for drug class (p. 590).

**INDICATIONS**    **Paget's disease** Patients with bone pain and deformation may respond to chronic therapy with calcitonin; relapse occasionally occurs.    **Hypercalcemia** Calcitonin may be useful along with other agents to rapidly lower serum calcium in emergencies.    **Postmenopausal osteoporosis** Successful therapy also includes vitamin D and adequate calcium intake.

**CONTRAINDICATIONS**    **Allergy** Calcitonin salmon occasionally causes allergic reactions and should not be used in a patient who has experienced such reactions.

**DOSAGE**    **IM or SC:**    **ADULTS:** Initially, 0.5 mg daily of calcitonin human or 100 IU daily of calcitonin salmon. Maintenance therapy may be adequate with 0.25 mg daily or 0.5 mg two or three times weekly of calcitonin human or with 50 IU daily or 50 to 100 IU three times weekly.    *Special patient popula-*

*tions:* **CHILDREN:** Pediatric doses have not been established. **PREGNANCY:** Safe use has not been established.

**PREPARATIONS** **Calcitonin,** human *powder for reconstitution:* 0.5 mg, supplied with diluent. **Calcitonin,** salmon *solution:* 200 IU/mL.

**DRUG INTERACTIONS** None established.

**FATE** Calcitonin is a peptide that is destroyed when taken orally. Absorption is adequate from IM or SC sites. Onset of action is within 15 minutes and persists for up to 24 hours. Clinical responses may take months to become visible, as extensive areas of bone may need to be restored. Calcitonin is rapidly metabolized to inactive metabolites that are excreted in urine.

## 🦉 NURSING CONSIDERATIONS

### Side effects, toxicities, and associated nursing actions

**CNS** Dizziness and headache are rare.
- Caution patients to avoid driving or operating hazardous equipment if dizziness occurs.

**GI** Transient nausea is the most common side effect. Abdominal distress, anorexia, diarrhea, epigastric distress, unusual tastes or vomiting may also occur.
- Monitor weight. If vomiting or diarrhea occur, monitor intake and output.
- If GI symptoms are severe or persistent, notify the physician.

**Renal** Diuresis and urinary frequency may occur.
- Assess the patient for urinary frequency; monitor weight and skin turgor.

**Allergic** Flushing, erythema, rashes, urticaria, and swelling can occur.
- Warn patients about possible skin changes, and instruct them to notify the physician for severe reactions.
- Before administering the first dose of calcitonin salmon, consult the physician about administering a test dose. For the test dose, dilute 10 IU with sufficient 0.9% sodium chloride to make 1 ml. After mixing, discard 0.9 ml. Administer 0.1 ml intracutaneously on the flexor surface of the forearm. Monitor the injection site for at least 15 minutes; anything more than a mild erythema reaction or wheal indicates a positive reaction, and calcitonin salmon should not be administered.
- Have drugs, equipment, and personnel available to treat acute allergic reactions.

**Other** Chills, chest pressure, weakness, nasal congestion, and shortness of breath can occur. Hypercalcemia and tetany are rare.
- Remain with patient for several minutes following injection, and check again several times in the next 30 minutes.
- Monitor vital signs following injection.
- Assess for hypercalcemia: thirst, polyuria, anorexia, nausea, vomiting, and constipation.
- Assess for hypocalcemia: tetany and numbness and tingling of nose, ears, fingertips, and toes. Have calcium gluconate available for treatment of tetany.
- Monitor serum electrolytes.

### Patient and family education

- Review anticipated benefits and possible side effects of drug therapy with patient and family.
- Encourage the patient to return for regular follow-up visits.
- For home administration, patients are usually taught to administer the drug subcutaneously. Teach the patient subcutaneous injection technique; include aseptic technique, accurate dosage preparation, recording of injection sites, and rotation of injection sites.
- Refer the patient for public health nurse follow-up if indicated.
- Suggest to patient that taking ordered doses in the evening may minimize problems with flushing.
- Encourage patients on long-term therapy to wear a medical identification tag or bracelet indicating that calcitonin is being used.
- Dietary counseling may be needed to adjust calcium intake.

---

# calcifediol (kal-sif-ee-DYE-ol)

vitamin D analog

- calcifediol (25-hydroxycholecalciferol): Calderol

**MECHANISM OF ACTION**   See entry for drug class (p. 590).

**INDICATIONS**   **Hypocalcemia in chronic renal failure** Calcifediol may be useful in controlling hypocalcemia in patients whose kidneys do not form adequate amounts of 25-hydroxycholecalciferol. (Although calcifediol can substitute in any condition where ergocalciferol is used, calcifediol is much more expensive and is not usually indicated unless patients are unable to convert ergocalciferol to the more active metabolites.)

**CONTRAINDICATIONS**   **Sarcoidosis** These patients are more sensitive to vitamin D analogs and may develop hypercalcemia.   **Hypoparathyroidism** Patients with this disorder may be more sensitive to vitamin D analogs and may develop hypercalcemia.   **Renal impairment** Damaged kidneys may be unable to maintain calcium concentrations in normal ranges. • Renal stones may also form.   **Heart disease** Changes in calcium concentration in the blood may induce arrhythmias or worsen cardiac failure.

**DOSAGE**   **PO:**   ADULTS: Initially, 300 to 350 μg weekly, dividing the dosage into equal daily doses or alternating days. Dosage adjustments must be based upon blood calcium concentrations. Daily doses for most patients range from 50 to 100 μg.   *Special patient populations:*   CHILDREN: Safe use in children has not been established.   PREGNANCY: Safe use has not been established.

**PREPARATIONS**   *Capsules:* 20 and 50 μg.

**DRUG INTERACTIONS**   **Cardiac glycosides** (Chapter 6) may be more likely to cause arrhythmias in patients also receiving vitamin D analogs.   **Thiazide diuretics** may trigger hypercalcemia in patients also receiving vitamin D analogs.

**FATE**   Calcifediol is well absorbed from the intestine, producing *peak* concentrations of active forms within 4 hours. Calcifediol is hydroxylated by the kidneys to form 1, 25-dihydroxycholecalciferol, which is the most active form of vitamin D. The kidneys may also inactivate various forms of cholecalciferol. Excretion is mostly in bile and feces, with minor amounts in urine. The *half-life* of calcifediol is about 16 days.

## ☙ NURSING CONSIDERATIONS

**Side effects, toxicities, and associated nursing actions**   The following side effects are essentially those of hypercalcemia and are a result of overdosage.
* Monitor serum calcium levels.
* Calculate and prepare dosages carefully.
* Review with patients their procedures for taking this drug.
* Caution patients not to double up for missed doses unless specifically directed to do so by the physician.

**CNS** Ataxia, fatigue, headache, irritability, seizures, somnolence, tinnitus, vertigo, and weakness may occur.
* Caution patients to avoid driving or operating hazardous equipment if ataxia, somnolence, vertigo, or weakness occur.
* Assess for CNS effects. Note that ongoing assessment is important, as some symptoms, such as fatigue, weakness, and irritability, may be difficult to distinguish from those accompanying renal failure or other chronic diseases.

**CV** Hypertension and vascular calcification are uncommon.
* Monitor blood pressure and pulse.

**GI** Abdominal cramps, anorexia, constipation, diarrhea, metallic taste, nausea, and vomiting are early signs of toxicity.
* Assess for GI symptoms. As with CNS symptoms, some GI symptoms, such as anorexia or constipation, may be chronic problems for the patient and thus be overlooked as a side effect indicating hypercalcemia.

**Renal** Hyposthenuria, nephrocalcinosis, nocturia, polydipsia, polyuria, and proteinuria are late signs.
* Monitor urinalysis.
* Assess for nocturia, polydipsia, and polyuria. Monitor intake and output.

**Other** Hypotonia in infants, bone pain, muscle pain, photophobia, or psychosis may occur.
* Assess infants carefully for signs of hypercalcemia.
* Instruct the patient to notify the physician if photophobia or other signs and symptoms occur.

**Patient and family education**
- Review anticipated benefits and possible side effects of drug therapy with patients.
- Encourage patients to notify the physician with any new sign or symptom. Encourage patients to return for regular medical follow-up, as titration of the correct dosage may be difficult.
- Instruct the patient to avoid using any medications not first approved by the physician.
- Patients in renal failure should avoid aluminum-containing antacids while taking this drug; consult with the physician.
- Instruct patients taking this drug to avoid sources of vitamin D, which include fish oils, milk, some butter, margarines, certain cereals, and infant formula products. Skin exposure to sunlight also activates vitamin D in the body.

---

## calcitriol    (kal-see-TREE-ol)    vitamin D analog

- calcitriol (1,25-dihydroxycholecalciferol): Calcijex, Rocaltrol

**MECHANISM OF ACTION**    See entry for drug class (p. 590).

**INDICATIONS**    **Hypocalcemia in chronic renal failure** Calcitriol may be useful in controlling hypocalcemia in patients whose kidneys do not adequately activate vitamin D.    **Familial hypophosphatemia** Calcitriol and phosphate supplements may be used to control this condition.    **Vitamin D–dependent rickets** Patients with this disorder are unable to form the active metabolite of vitamin D (1,25-dihydroxycholecalciferol). They therefore respond well to therapy with calcitriol, which is the active form of the vitamin.    **Hypoparathyroidism and pseudohypoparathyroidism** Vitamin D analogs such as calcitriol can elevate serum calcium concentrations in these patients, who lack parathyroid hormone action.

**CONTRAINDICATIONS**    **Sarcoidosis** These patients are more sensitive to vitamin D analogs and may develop hypercalcemia.    **Hypoparathyroidism** Patients with this disorder may be more sensitive to vitamin D analogs and may develop hypercalcemia.    **Renal impairment** Damaged kidneys may be unable to maintain calcium concentrations in normal ranges. Renal stones may also form.    **Heart disease** Changes in calcium concentration in the blood may induce arrhythmias or worsen cardiac failure.

**DOSAGE**    **PO:**    **ADULTS:** Initially 0.25 µg daily, adjusted as necessary to maintain normal blood calcium concentrations. Maintenance doses often range from 0.5 to 2 µg daily.    **CHILDREN:** For hypoparathyroidism or pseudohypoparathyroidism in children over 1 year of age, 0.25 µg daily. Adjust as necessary to maintain normal blood calcium concentrations. Maintenance doses are normally 0.25 to 0.75 µg daily for children 1 to 5 years.    **IV:**    **ADULTS:** In chronic renal failure, 0.5 µg three times weekly. Adjust as necessary to maintain normal blood calcium concentrations. For most patients doses will be between 0.5 and 3 µg three times weekly.    *Special patient populations:*    **CHILDREN:** Safe use in children with renal failure has not been established.    **PREGNANCY:** Safe use has not been established.

**PREPARATIONS**    *Capsules:* 0.25 and 0.5 µg; *solution for IV use only:* 1 or 2 µg/mL.

**DRUG INTERACTIONS**    **Cardiac glycosides** (Chapter 6) may be more likely to cause arrhythmias in patients also receiving vitamin D analogs.    **Thiazide diuretics** may trigger hypercalcemia in patients also receiving vitamin D analogs.

**FATE**    Calcitriol administered orally causes increased calcium absorption from the intestine within 2 hours and maximal effects by 10 hours. The *duration* is 3 to 5 days, which is shorter than that of ergocalciferol. Calcitriol is inactivated by the kidneys. Excretion is mostly in bile and feces, with minor amounts in urine.

### 🕯 NURSING CONSIDERATIONS

**Side effects, toxicities, and associated nursing actions**    The following side effects are essentially those of hypercalcemia and are a result of overdosage.
- Monitor serum calcium levels.
- Calculate and prepare dosages carefully.
- Review with patients their procedures for taking this drug.

- Caution patients not to double up for missed doses unless specifically directed to do so by the physician.

**CNS** Ataxia, fatigue, headache, irritability, seizures, somnolence, tinnitus, vertigo, and weakness may occur.
- Caution patients to avoid driving or operating hazardous equipment if ataxia, somnolence, vertigo, or weakness occur.
- Assess for CNS effects. Note that ongoing assessment is important, as some symptoms, such as fatigue, weakness, and irritability, may be difficult to distinguish from those accompanying renal failure or other chronic diseases.

**CV** Hypertension and vascular calcification are uncommon.
- Monitor blood pressure and pulse.

**GI** Abdominal cramps, anorexia, constipation, diarrhea, metallic taste, nausea, and vomiting are early signs of toxicity.
- Assess for GI symptoms. As with CNS symptoms, some GI symptoms, such as anorexia or constipation, may be chronic problems for the patient and thus be overlooked as a side effect indicating hypercalcemia.

**Renal** Hyposthenuria, nephrocalcinosis, nocturia, polydipsia, polyuria, and proteinuria are late signs.
- Monitor urinalysis.
- Assess for nocturia, polydipsia, and polyuria. Monitor intake and output.

**Other** Hypotonia in infants, bone pain, muscle pain, photophobia, or psychosis may occur.
- Assess infants carefully for signs of hypercalcemia.
- Instruct the patient to notify the physician if photophobia or other signs and symptoms occur.

### Nursing interventions related to drug administration
- Administer the IV dose over 1 minute.

### Patient and family education
- Review anticipated benefits and possible side effects of drug therapy with patients.
- Encourage patients to notify the physician with any new sign or symptom. Encourage patients to return for regular medical follow-up, as titration of the correct dosage may be difficult.
- Instruct the patient to avoid using any medications not first approved by the physician.
- Patients in renal failure should avoid aluminum-containing antacids while taking this drug; consult with the physician.
- Instruct patients taking this drug to avoid sources of vitamin D, which include fish oils, milk, some butter, margarines, certain cereals, and infant formula products. Skin exposure to sunlight also activates vitamin D in the body.

## dihydrotachysterol　(dye-hye-dro-tak-ISS-ter-ole)　vitamin D analog

- dihydrotachysterol: DHT, Hytakerol

**MECHANISM OF ACTION** • See entry for drug class (p. 590).

**INDICATIONS** **Hypocalcemia in chronic renal failure** Dihydrotachysterol may be useful in controlling hypocalcemia in patients whose kidneys do not adequately activate vitamin D. **Familial hypophosphatemia** Dihydrotachysterol and phosphate supplements may be used to control this condition. **Hypoparathyroidism and pseudohypoparathyroidism** Vitamin D analogs such as dihydrotachysterol can elevate serum calcium concentrations in these patients, who lack parathyroid hormone action. **Osteoporosis** Dihydrotachysterol with calcium and fluoride is being tested in osteoporosis.

**CONTRAINDICATIONS** **Sarcoidosis** These patients are more sensitive to vitamin D analogs and may develop hypercalcemia. **Hypoparathyroidism** Patients with this disorder may be more sensitive to vitamin D analogs and may develop hypercalcemia. **Renal impairment** Damaged kidneys may be unable to maintain calcium concentrations in normal ranges. Renal stones may also form. **Heart disease** Changes in calcium concentration in the blood may induce arrhythmias or worsen cardiac failure.

**DOSAGE**   PO:   **ADULTS:** For hypoparathyroidism or pseudohypoparathyroidism, initially 0.75 to 2.5 mg daily; maintenance doses are usually 0.2 to 1 mg daily. In chronic renal failure, 0.1 to 0.6 mg daily. For familial hypophosphatemia, initially 0.5 to 2 mg daily; maintenance is usually with 0.2 to 1.5 mg daily. For osteoporosis, 0.6 mg daily with calcium and fluoride has been tested.   **CHILDREN:** For hypoparathyroidism or pseudohypoparathyroidism, initially 1 to 5 mg daily for 4 days; maintenance doses are usually 0.5 to 1.5 mg daily. In chronic renal failure, 0.1 to 0.5 mg daily.   *Special patient populations:* **PREGNANCY:** Safe use has not been established.

**PREPARATIONS**   *Capsules:* 0.125 mg; *solution for oral use:* 0.2 mg/5 ml; *solution, concentrate:* 0.2 or 0.25 mg/ml; *tablets:* 0.125, 0.2 or 0.4 mg.

**DRUG INTERACTIONS**   **Cardiac glycosides** may be more likely to cause arrhythmias in patients also receiving vitamin D analogs.

**FATE**   Dihydroxytachysterol is well absorbed following oral administration. This form of vitamin D requires activation by the liver. The *onset* of action is within a few hours of dosing, but maximal effects require several weeks of continuous administration. The *duration* of action is about 2 weeks. Elimination is primarily in bile and feces.

## 🐦 NURSING CONSIDERATIONS

### Side effects, toxicities, and associated nursing actions   The following side effects are essentially those of hypercalcemia and are a result of overdosage.
- Monitor serum calcium levels.
- Calculate and prepare dosages carefully.
- Review with patients their procedures for taking this drug.
- Caution patients not to double up for missed doses unless specifically directed to do so by the physician.

**CNS** Ataxia, fatigue, headache, irritability, seizures, somnolence, tinnitus, vertigo, and weakness may occur.
- Caution patients to avoid driving or operating hazardous equipment if ataxia, somnolence, vertigo, or weakness occur.
- Assess for CNS effects. Note that ongoing assessment is important, as some symptoms, such as fatigue, weakness, and irritability, may be difficult to distinguish from those accompanying renal failure or other chronic diseases.

**CV** Hypertension and vascular calcification are uncommon.
- Monitor blood pressure and pulse.

**GI** Abdominal cramps, anorexia, constipation, diarrhea, metallic taste, nausea, and vomiting are early signs of toxicity.
- Assess for GI symptoms. As with CNS symptoms, some GI symptoms, such as anorexia or constipation, may be chronic problems for the patient and thus be overlooked as a side effect indicating hypercalcemia.

**Renal** Hyposthenuria, nephrocalcinosis, nocturia, polydipsia, polyuria, and proteinuria are late signs.
- Monitor urinalysis.
- Assess for nocturia, polydipsia, and polyuria. Monitor intake and output.

**Other** Hypotonia in infants, bone pain, muscle pain, photophobia, or psychosis may occur.
- Assess infants carefully for signs of hypercalcemia.
- Instruct the patient to notify the physician if photophobia or other signs and symptoms occur.

### Patient and family education
- Review anticipated benefits and possible side effects of drug therapy with patients.
- Encourage patients to notify the physician with any new sign or symptom. Encourage patients to return for regular medical follow-up, as titration of the correct dosage may be difficult.
- Instruct the patient to avoid using any medications not first approved by the physician.
- Patients in renal failure should avoid aluminum-containing antacids while taking this drug; consult with the physician.
- Instruct patients taking this drug to avoid sources of vitamin D, which include fish oils, milk, some butter, margarines, certain cereals, and infant formula products. Skin exposure to sunlight also activates vitamin D in the body.

## ergocalciferol (er-goh-kal-SIF-e-role) vitamin D analog

- ● ergocalciferol: Calciferol, Deltalin, Drisdol

**MECHANISM OF ACTION** • See entry for drug class (p. 590).

**INDICATIONS** **Familial hypophosphatemia** Ergocalciferol and phosphate supplements are used occasionally to control this condition. **Hypoparathyroidism and pseudohypoparathyroidism** Ergocalciferol can elevate serum calcium concentrations in these patients, who lack parathyroid hormone action, but the more active analogs (e.g., calcitriol) are preferred. **Rickets or osteomalacia** Ergocalciferol can reverse this condition, which is caused by vitamin D deficiency or by anticonvulsant therapy. **Vitamin D–dependent rickets** Large doses of ergocalciferol are required because these patients cannot metabolically activate this form of vitamin D. **Hypocalcemia of chronic renal disease** Large doses of ergocalciferol are required because the damaged kidneys of these patients may not be able to metabolically activate sufficient amounts of vitamin D. **Osteoporosis** Ergocalciferol has been tested for this condition. **Dietary supplementation** Normal children and adults require up to 10 μg daily. Pregnant or lactating females require up to 15 μg daily. Ergocalciferol is routinely added to milk in the U.S. to provide adequate supplementation for most persons.

**CONTRAINDICATIONS** **Sarcoidosis** These patients are more sensitive to vitamin D analogs and may develop hypercalcemia. **Hypoparathyroidism** Patients with this disorder may be more sensitive to vitamin D analogs and may develop hypercalcemia. **Renal impairment** Damaged kidneys may be unable to maintain calcium concentrations in normal ranges. Renal stones may also form. **Heart disease** Changes in calcium concentration in the blood may induce arrhythmias or worsen cardiac failure.

**DOSAGE** **PO:** **ADULTS:** For rickets and osteomalacia, 25 to 125 μg daily to correct nutritional deficiencies. Patients with malabsorption require 250 μg to 7.5 mg daily. For vitamin D–dependent rickets or familial hypophosphatemia, 250 μg to 1.5 mg daily. For rickets caused by anticonvulsant therapy, 50 μg to 1.25 mg daily. For hypoparathyroidism and pseudohypoparathyroidism, 625 μg to 5 mg daily. For dietary supplementation, 10 μg daily. **CHILDREN:** For rickets and osteomalacia, 25 to 125 μg daily to correct nutritional deficiencies. For vitamin D–dependent rickets, 75 to 125 μg daily. For familial hypophosphatemia, initially 1 to 2 mg daily with phosphate supplements; increase by 250 to 500 μg increments every 3 to 4 months to control condition. **IM:** **ADULTS:** For severe vitamin D deficiency in malabsorption syndrome, 250 μg daily by deep IM injection. *Special patient populations:* **PREGNANCY:** Safe use has not been established.

**PREPARATIONS** *Capsules:* 0.625 mg (25,000 units) and 1.25 mg (50,000 units); *tablets:* 1.25 mg (50,000 units); *solution for oral use:* 200 μg (8000 units)/ml; *solution for injection:* 12.5 mg (500,000 units)/ml.

**DRUG INTERACTIONS** **Cardiac glycosides** may be more likely to cause arrhythmias in patients also receiving vitamin D analogs. **Thiazide diuretics** may trigger hypercalcemia in patients also receiving vitamin D analogs.

**FATE** Ergocalciferol is well absorbed following oral administration and the hypercalcemic effect is observed within 24 hours. Maximal effects require about 4 weeks of continuous therapy, and the *duration* of action is up to 2 months. Ergocalciferol is converted in the body to active metabolites. Elimination is primarily in bile and feces, with limited amounts in urine.

### ☙ NURSING CONSIDERATIONS

**Side effects, toxicities, and associated nursing actions** The side effects listed below are essentially those of hypercalcemia and are a result of overdosage.
- Monitor serum calcium levels.
- Calculate and prepare dosages carefully.
- Review with patients their procedures for taking this drug.
- Caution patients not to double up for missed doses unless specifically directed to do so by the physician.

**CNS** Ataxia, fatigue, headache, irritability, seizures, somnolence, tinnitus, vertigo, and weakness may occur.

Table
30-5.

## Clinical summary of vitamin D analogs

| Drug | Route | Onset | Hypercalcemic duration* | Effect maximal* |
|------|-------|-------|------------------------|-----------------|
| Calcifediol | PO | 4 hrs | 2 weeks | 8 hr |
| Calcitriol | PO | 2 hrs | 3-5 days | 10 hr |
| Dihydrotachysterol | PO | 10-24 hr | 2 weeks | 2 weeks |
| Ergocalciferol | IM, PO | 10-24 hr | 2 months | 4 weeks |

*With continuous therapy.

- Caution patients to avoid driving or operating hazardous equipment if ataxia, somnolence, vertigo, or weakness occur.
- Assess for CNS effects. Note that ongoing assessment is important, as some symptoms, such as fatigue, weakness, and irritability, may be difficult to distinguish from those accompanying renal failure or other chronic diseases.

**CV** Hypertension and vascular calcification are uncommon.
- Monitor blood pressure and pulse.

**GI** Abdominal cramps, anorexia, constipation, diarrhea, metallic taste, nausea, and vomiting are early signs of toxicity.
- Assess for GI symptoms. As with CNS symptoms, some GI symptoms, such as anorexia or constipation, may be chronic problems for the patient and thus be overlooked as a side effect indicating hypercalcemia.

**Renal** Hyposthenuria, nephrocalcinosis, nocturia, polydipsia, polyuria, and proteinuria are late signs.
- Monitor urinalysis.
- Assess for nocturia, polydipsia, and polyuria. Monitor intake and output.

**Other** Hypotonia in infants, bone pain, muscle pain, photophobia, or psychosis may occur.
- Assess infants carefully for signs of hypercalcemia.
- Instruct the patient to notify the physician if photophobia or other signs and symptoms occur.

### Patient and family education
- Review anticipated benefits and possible side effects of drug therapy with patients.
- Encourage patients to notify the physician of any new sign or symptom. Encourage patients to return for regular medical follow-up, as titration of the correct dosage may be difficult.
- Instruct the patient to avoid using any medications not first approved by the physician.
- Patients in renal failure should avoid aluminum-containing antacids while taking this drug; consult with the physician.
- Refer the patient and family to a dietitian for diet counseling regarding sources of calcium, vitamin D, and phosphorus.

# Chapter Thirty-one
# Adrenal steroids and related agents

| | |
|---|---|
| amcinonide | halcinonide |
| beclomethasone dipropionate | hydrocortisone |
| betamethasone | hydrocortisone acetate |
| betamethasone acetate | hydrocortisone butyrate |
| betamethasone benzoate | hydrocortisone cypionate |
| betamethasone dipropionate | hydrocortisone sodium phosphate |
| betamethasone sodium phosphate | hydrocortisone sodium succinate |
| betamethasone valerate | hydrocortisone valerate |
| clobetasol propionate | medrysone |
| clocortolone pivalate | methylprednisolone |
| cortisone acetate | methylprednisolone acetate |
| desonide | methylprednisolone sodium succinate |
| desoximetasone | paramethasone acetate |
| dexamethasone | prednisolone |
| dexamethasone acetate | prednisolone acetate |
| dexamethasone sodium phosphate | prednisolone sodium phosphate |
| diflorasone diacetate | prednisolone tebutate |
| fludrocortisone | prednisone |
| flunisolide | triamcinolone |
| fluocinolone acetonide | triamcinolone acetonide |
| fluocinonide | triamcinolone diacetate |
| fluorometholone | triamcinolone hexacetonide |
| flurandrenolide | |

**OVERVIEW OF THE DRUG CLASS**    Adrenal steroids are used as replacement therapy for endocrine conditions in which one or more natural hormones are lacking. A more common use of the synthetic forms of adrenal steroids is as anti-inflammatory agents. The various members of this large class of drugs differ in route of administration, onset and duration of action, and potency (Tables 31-1 to 31-3).

**MECHANISM OF ACTION**    Steroid hormones enter target cells, bind to receptors, and ultimately alter transcription of genes for certain proteins. The end result may be profound changes in the function of a variety of cell types. The physiologic effects of the steroids are divided into mineralocorticoid and glucocorticoid activities. Mineralocorticoid effects include sodium and fluid retention with potassium loss. Glucocorticoid activities include increasing protein catabolism, increasing gluconeogenesis, and promoting fat deposition on the body trunk while diminishing peripheral fat stores. Glucocorticoids also have direct anti-inflammatory effects and diminish immune responses.

When used at physiologic doses (doses roughly equivalent to 20 mg hydrocortisone) the primary effects are maintenance of normal function. When used at pharmacologic doses, which may be greatly in excess of physiologic doses, anti-inflammatory actions are often sought, but other actions may lead to side effects of varying severity.

Long-term use of corticosteroids suppresses production of the patient's own adrenal steroids. The degree of suppression is more severe with larger doses and longer therapy. Children also tend to be more susceptible to suppression. Recovery of the hypothalmic-pituitary-adrenal system is not immediate when drug therapy is discontinued. Patients may suffer adrenocortical insufficiency unless the corticosteroids are discontinued gradually to allow the hypothalmic-pituitary-adrenal system to recover. Some physicians prefer to use alternate-day rather than continuous therapy when the corticosteroids are used long term. Alternate-day therapy limits adrenal suppression and makes withdrawal less dangerous.

**INDICATIONS    Adrenocortical insufficiency** A steroid with both glucocorticoid and mineralocorticoid activity is required for effective replacement therapy; hydrocortisone or cortisone is often selected. Fludro-

| Table 31-1. | Summary of adrenal steroids in clinical use | | | |
|---|---|---|---|---|
| | | | Application | |
| **Drug** | | **Systemic** | **topical** | **EENT\*** |
| Amcinonide | | | + | |
| Beclomethasone dipropionate | | + | | + |
| Betamethasone | | + | | |
| Betamethasone acetate | | + | | |
| Betamethasone benzoate | | | + | |
| Betamethasone dipropionate | | | + | |
| Betamethasone sodium phosphate | | + | | |
| Betamethasone valerate | | | + | |
| Clobetasol propionate | | | + | |
| Clocortolone pivalate | | | + | |
| Cortisone acetate | | + | | |
| Desonide | | | + | |
| Desoximetasone | | | + | |
| Dexamethasone | | + | + | |
| Dexamethasone acetate | | + | | |
| Dexamethasone sodium phosphate | | + | | + |
| Diflorasone diacetate | | | + | |
| Fludrocortisone acetate | | + | | |
| Flunisolide | | + | | + |
| Fluocinolone acetonide | | | + | |
| Fluocinonide | | | + | |
| Fluorometholone | | | | + |
| Flurandrenoline | | | + | |
| Halcinonide | | | + | |
| Hydrocortisone | | + | + | + |
| Hydrocortisone acetate | | + | + | + |
| Hydrocortisone butyrate | | | + | |
| Hydrocortisone cypionate | | + | | |
| Hydrocortisone sodium phosphate | | + | | |
| Hydrocortisone sodium succinate | | + | | |
| Hydrocortisone valerate | | | + | |
| Medrysone | | | | + |
| Methylprednisolone | | + | | |
| Methylprednisolone acetate | | + | + | |
| Methylprednisolone sodium succinate | | + | | |
| Paramethasone acetate | | + | | |
| Prednisolone | | + | | |
| Prednisolone acetate | | + | | + |
| Prednisolone sodium phosphate | | + | | |
| Prednisolone tebutate | | + | | |
| Prednisone | | + | | |
| Triamcinolone | | + | | |
| Triamcinolone acetonide | | + | + | |
| Triamcinolone diacetate | | + | | |
| Triamcinolone hexacetonide | | + | | |

\*EENT=eye, ear, nose, and throat.

**Table 31-2.**

## Summary of systemic uses of adrenal steroids

| Corticosteroid | Route | Glucocorticoid activity | | Potency | |
|---|---|---|---|---|---|
| | | Onset | Duration | Gluco-corticoid* | Mineralo-corticoid |
| Betamethasone | PO | 1 hr | 3 days | 20–30 | Very low |
| Betamethasone sodium phosphate | IV, IM | Rapid | Short | | |
| Betamethasone acetate/sodium phosphate | IM, IA, ST | 1–3 hr | 1–2 weeks | | |
| Cortisone acetate | PO | Rapid | 1.5 days | 0.8 | High |
| | IM | Slow | Several days | | |
| Dexamethasone | PO | 1 hr | 3 days | 20–30 | Very low |
| Dexamethasone acetate | IM | <8 hr | 6 days | | |
| Dexamethasone acetate | IA, ST, IL | Slow | 1–3 weeks | | |
| Dexamethasone sodium phosphate | IV, IM | Rapid | Short | | |
| Dexamethasone sodium phosphate | IA, IS, IL, ST | Slow | 3 days–3 weeks | | |
| Dexamethasone tebutate | IA | 12 hr | Variable | | |
| Fludrocortisone acetate | PO | Intermed. | Intermed. | | Very high |
| Hydrocortisone | PO | <1 hr | 1.5 days | 1 | High |
| | IM | <4 hr | Days | | |
| | Rectal | 3–5 days | | | |
| Hydrocortisone acetate | IA, IS, IB, IL, ST | <24 hr | 3 days–4 weeks | | |
| Hydrocortisone acetate | Rectal | 5–7 days | | | |
| Hydrocortisone cypionate | PO | <2hr | | | |
| Hydrocortisone sodium phosphate | IV, IM | Rapid | Short | | |
| Hydrocortisone sodium succinate | IV, IM | Rapid | Variable | | |
| Methylprednisolone | PO | <1 hr | 1.5 days | 5 | Very low |
| Methylprednisolone acetate | IM | 6–48 hr | 1-4 weeks | | |
| Methylprednisolone acetate | IA, IL, ST | Very slow | 1-5 weeks | | |
| Methylprednisolone sodium succinate | IV, IM | Rapid | Int. | | |
| Paramethasone acetate | PO | <1 hr | 2 days | 10 | Very low |
| Prednisolone | PO | <1 hr | 1.5 days | 4 | Moderate |
| Prednisolone acetate | IM | Slow | | | |
| Prednisolone acetate/sodium phosphate | IM, IB, IS | Slow | 3 days–4 weeks | | |
| Prednisolone sodium phosphate | IV, IM | <1 hr | Short | | |
| Prednisolone sodium phosphate | IA, IL, ST | Slow | 3 days–3 weeks | | |
| Prednisolone tebutate | IA, IL, ST | 1–2 days | 1–3 weeks | | |
| Prednisone | PO | <2 hr | 1.5 days | 4 | Moderate |
| Triamcinolone | PO | <2 hr | 2 days | 5 | Very low |
| Triamcinolone acetonide | IM | 1–2 days | 1–6 weeks | | |
| Triamcinolone acetonide | IB, IA, IS IL, ST | Slow | Several weeks | | |
| Triamcinolone diacetate | PO | <2 hr | Intermed. | | |
| Triamcinolone diacetate | IM | Slow | 4 days–4 weeks | | |
| Triamcinolone diacetate | IL | Slow | 1–2 weeks | | |
| Triamcinolone diacetate | IA, IS, ST | slow | 1–8 weeks | | |
| Triamcinolone hexacetonide | IA, IL | Slow | 3–4 weeks | | |

*Relative potencies.

| Table 31-3. | Summary of preparations of corticosteroids for nonsystemic use | | |
|---|---|---|---|
| **Use** | **Preparations** | | **Representative trade names** |
| Antiasthmatic: inhalation aerosols | Beclomethasone dipropionate | | Beclovent, Becotide |
| | Dexamethasone sodium phosphate | | Decadron Respihales |
| | | | AeroBid |
| | Flunisolide | | Azmacort |
| | Triamcinolone acetonide | | |
| Dental: paste, pellets | Betamethasone sodium phosphate | | Betnesol |
| | Hydrocortisone acetate | | Orabase-HCA |
| | Triamcinolone acetonide | | Adcortyl in Orabase |
| | | | Kenalog in Orabase |
| Dermatitis: topical creams, gels, ointments, lotions, or sprays | Amcinonide | | Cyclocort |
| | Betamethasone benzoate | | Benisone, Uticort |
| | Betamethasone dipropionate | | Alphatrex, Diprolene, Diprosone |
| | Betamethasone valerate | | Betatrex, Beta-Val, Valisone |
| | Clobetasol propionate | | Dermovate, Temovate |
| | Clocortolone pivalate | | Cloderm |
| | Desonide | | DesOwen, Tridesilon |
| | Desoximetasone | | Topicort |
| | Dexamethasone | | Aeroseb-Dex, Decadern |
| | Dexamethasone sodium phosphate | | Decadron |
| | Diflorasone diacetate | | Florone, Maxiflor |
| | Flumethasone | | ❋ Locacorten |
| | Fluocinolone acetonide | | Fluonid, Flurosyn, Synalar |
| | Fluocinonide | | Lidex |
| | Flurandrenolide | | Cordran |
| | Halcinonide | | Halog |
| | Hydrocortisone | | CaldeCort, Cortaid, Cort-Dome, Cortizone, DermaCort, Dermolate, Dermtex, Hytone, Penecort, Synacort |
| | Hydrocortisone acetate | | CaldeCort, Cortaid, Cortef, Epifoam, Gynecort, Lanacort |
| | Hydrocortisone butyrate | | Locoid |
| | Hydrocortisone valerate | | Westcort |
| | Methylprednisolone | | Medrol |
| | Triamcinolone acetonide | | Aristocort, Flutex, Kenalog, Triacet |
| Nasal: aerosols, solutions | Beclomethasone | | Beconase, Vancenase |
| | Dexamethasone sodium phosphate | | Decadron Turbinaire |
| | | | Nasalide |
| | Flunisolide | | |
| Ophthalmic-otic: solutions, suspensions, ointments | Betamethasone sodium phosphate | | Betnesol |
| | Dexamethasone | | Maxidex |
| | Dexamethasone sodium phosphate | | Ak-dex, Decadron, Dexair, Maxidex |

*Continued.*

**Table 31-3.** Summary of preparations of corticosteroids for nonsystemic use—cont'd.

| Use | Preparations | Representative trade names |
| --- | --- | --- |
| | Fluorometholone | Fluor-OP, FML Forte, FML-Liquifilm, FML S.O.P. |
| | Hydrocortisone | Cortamed |
| | Medrysone | HMS Liquifilm |
| | Prednisolone acetate | A-tate, Econopred, Ocu-Pred-A, Predair-A Pred Forte |
| | Prednisolone sodium phosphate | Ak-Pred, Inflamase, Metreton, Ocu-Pred, Predair |
| Rectal: ointments, suppositories | Hydrocortisone | Dermolate, Rectocort |
| | Hydrocortisone acetate | Cort-Dome, Corticaine |

cortisone may be added if more mineralocorticoid activity is required. **Adrenogenital syndrome** Cortisone or hydrocortisone may control salt-losing forms of this condition. **Neoplastic diseases** Lymphomas and leukemias arising from lymphoid tissue may respond to systemic steroids such as prednisone or prednisolone when used with cytotoxic agents (p. 479); remission or palliation of symptoms arises in part from the lympholytic action of these corticosteroids. **Dermatologic diseases** Systemic glucocorticoids may be required for acute exacerbations of dermatitis herpetiformis, eczema, erythema multiforme, exfoliative dermatitis, lichen planus, mycosis fungoides, and pemphigus. • Intralesional injections may be effective for alopecia areata, discoid lupus erythematosus, granuloma annulare, keloids, and psoriatic plaques. **Allergic states** Systemic steroids are used to control acute episodes of bronchial asthma that are unresponsive to conventional therapy. • Angioedema and serum sickness may require acute therapy with systemic steroids. • Contact dermatitis usually responds to topical therapy. **Cerebral edema** Systemic corticosteroids may be of benefit in controlling edema associated with brain tumors, neurosurgery, or tuberculous meningitis; glucocorticoids such as betamethasone or dexamethasone, which lack mineralocorticoid activity, are preferred. **Collagen diseases** Systemic corticosteroids may be used for acute exacerbations of lupus erythematosus or occasionally for maintenance. **GI diseases** Acute ulcerative colitis may respond to systemic or local application of corticosteroids. • The steroids are not normally indicated for maintenance therapy because risk of side effects is so large. **Hematologic disorders** Certain conditions such as autoimmune hemolytic anemia or thrombocytopenia may respond to systemic corticosteroids. **Hepatic disease** Systemic corticosteroids may be beneficial for subacute hepatic necrosis, chronic active hepatitis, nonalcoholic cirrhosis in women, and alcoholic cirrhosis with hepatic encephalopathy. • Other forms of liver disease may be worsened by corticosteroids. **Myasthenia gravis** High-dose, alternate-day therapy with systemic corticosteroids may be beneficial in patients failing to respond to anticholinesterases. **Nephrotic syndrome** Nephrotic syndrome caused by primary renal disease or lupus nephritis may respond to high-dose, alternate-day therapy with systemic corticosteroids. • Other forms of nephrotic syndrome are less responsive. **Ophthalmic diseases** Allergic conjunctivitis, allergic corneal marginal ulcers, or other superficial conditions may be treated with steroids applied directly to the eye; chorioretinitis, iritis, iridocyclitis, keratitis, and optic neuritis may also respond. • Diseases of the internal structures of the eye may require systemic therapy. **Organ transplantation** High doses of systemic corticosteroids may be used along with other agents to maintain immunosuppression so that the transplanted organ will not be rejected. **Respiratory diseases** Systemic corticosteroids may aid in controlling symptoms of sarcoidosis, Löffler's syndrome, berylliosis, and fulminating tuberculosis. • Systemic corticosteroids such as betamethasone or dexamethasone administered 48 to 72 hours before birth may prevent respiratory distress syndrome in premature infants. **Rheumatoid diseases** Systemic corticosteroids may be used for acute exacerbations of rheumatic carditis, dermatomyositis, polymyositis, polyarteritis nodosa, relapsing polychondritis, or polymyalgia rheumatica arteritis. • Rheumatoid arthritis involving only a few joints may be treated with injections directly into the affected joint (intrabursal, intrasynovial).

**CONTRAINDICATIONS**    **Bacterial fungal or viral infections** Infections should ordinarily be brought under control before steroid therapy is started. • Infections may be greatly worsened in patients receiving steroids because the drugs are immunosuppressive.    **Cirrhosis** Patients with this disorder may show exaggerated responses to glucocorticoids.    **Congestive heart failure** Patients with this condition may be unable to tolerate fluid retention, which can occur with glucocorticoids.    **Hypertension** Hypertensive patients may be unable to tolerate fluid retention, which can occur with glucocorticoids. **Hypothyroidism** Patients with this disorder may show exaggerated responses to glucocorticoids. **Peptic ulcer** Peptic ulcers may fail to heal or may perforate. The condition can worsen dramatically with few obvious symptoms until hemorrhage occurs.    **Pregnancy** Corticosteroids may cause fetal damage, including cleft palate, hydrocephalus, gastroschisis, spontaneous abortions, and stillbirths. **Psychosis** Corticosteroids may induce psychotic episodes, especially in patients predisposed to these conditions.    **Thromboembolitic disease** Corticosteroids may increase risk of thrombosis, thromboembolism, and thrombophlebitis.    **Ulcerative colitis with impending perforation** Infection or impending perforation may be worsened by corticosteroid treatment.

**DRUG INTERACTIONS**    **Amphotericin B, ethacrynic acid, furosemide, and thiazides** may cause potassium depletion, worsening that side effect of corticosteroids.    **Anticholinesterase drugs** interact with corticosteroids to cause profound muscle weakness in patients with myasthenia gravis. • If corticosteroids must by used in myasthenic patients, the anticholinesterases must be discontinued at least 24 hours before.    **Anticoagulants** used orally may rarely be antagonized by cortisone.    **Barbiturates, phenytoin, and rifampin** induce hepatic enzymes, thereby increasing the metabolism of corticosteroids.    **Cyclosporine** levels in renal transplant patients may be increased by prednisolone.    **Estrogens** may potentiate effects of hydrocortisone or prednisolone.    **Nonsteroidal anti-inflammatory agents** when combined with corticosteroids, may influence the concentrations of both drugs and may increase risk of GI ulceration or hypoprothrombinemia.    **Vaccines and toxoids** are less effective when given with corticosteroids because the steroids suppress the immune system. Live vaccines may be more dangerous because the organisms contained in them may replicate. • Neurologic reactions to some vaccines may be aggravated.

**DIAGNOSTIC TEST INTERFERENCE**    **Skin test reactions** may be suppressed by the immune suppressive actions of corticosteroids.    **Nitroblue tetrazolium test** for bacterial infection may be falsely negative in the present of glucocorticoids.    **Uptake of I 131** may be decreased by corticosteroids.

## 🐾 NURSING CONSIDERATIONS
**Side effects, toxicities, and associated nursing actions** The side effects of long-term glucocorticoid therapy are summarized in Table 31-4 (p. 604).

**CNS** Anxiety, depression, EEG changes, emotional lability, euphoria, headache, increased motor activity, insomnia, ischemic neuropathy, mood swings, restlessness, psychosis, seizures, and vertigo.
- Obtain a baseline assessment of mental status and neurologic function before starting therapy and at regular intervals.
- Caution patients to avoid driving or operating hazardous equipment if vertigo occurs; notify the physician.
- Assess for signs of depression: lack of interest in personal appearance, withdrawal, insomnia, and anorexia.
- Be alert for seizures if patient has a history of seizures; pad side rails, and have a suction machine handy.
- Caution patients and family to report changes in mood or affect.

**CV** Glucocorticoids may cause fluid retention, which in turn leads to edema, potassium loss, hypertension, and hypokalemic alkalosis. Congestive heart failure may develop. Thromboembolitic disease, palpitation, and tachycardia are also possible.

**Table 31-4.**

## Summary of toxic reactions to long-term glucocorticoid therapy with pharmacologic doses

| Toxic reaction | Cause | Comments |
|---|---|---|
| Impaired glucose tolerance and/or hyperglycemia | Gluconeogenic action of glucocorticoids | If diabetes develops, it is usually mild and reversible. |
| Fat deposition on trunk of body increased, as are plasma triglyceride levels | Stimulation of lipid synthesis by glucocorticoids | Changes in lipid metabolism produce classic Cushing-type signs of moon face and truncal obesity. |
| Muscle weakness or muscle wasting | Stimulation of protein breakdown by glucocorticoids | This side effect is more pronounced with fluoride derivatives of glucocorticoids, such as triamcinolone. |
| Peptic ulcer or intestinal perforation | Direct irritation and/or protein-wasting effects of glucocorticoids | It is not entirely clear whether steroids induce these conditions or whether they merely mask the symptoms and allow the condition to progress to a serious stage before diagnosis. |
| Pancreatitis | Not known, but may involve effects on lipid metabolism | Glucocorticoids may mask symptoms of disease in early stages. |
| Growth inhibition | Glucocorticoid inhibition of growth hormone action | Glucocorticoids should be given with caution to children; doses below those producing growth inhibition should be used if possible. |
| Mood changes or psychoses | Not known | All patients receiving glucocorticoids should be observed closely for altered mood or behavior, especially those with a history of this type of disorder. |
| Osteoporosis or bone fractures | Glucocorticoids alter several aspects of calcium metabolism, which increase bone resorption | This side effect is noted especially in patients with arthritis, in postmenopausal women, or persons with low calcium intake. |
| Sodium retention and potassium loss | Mineralocorticoid activity associated with some glucocorticoids | Newer, synthetic glucocorticoids minimize these effects. |
| Increased susceptibility to infection | Glucocorticoid inhibition of immune system | Infections are more difficult to eradicate in these patients, even with good antibiotic therapy. |
| Glaucoma | Glucocorticoids interfere with normal aqueous outflow from eye and elevate intraocular pressure | The risk is especially great in genetically predisposed or diabetic patients. |
| Cataracts | Not known | Topical or systemic therapy has been implicated. |

- Monitor blood pressure, pulse, and weight. Monitor serum electrolytes.
- Assess patients for signs of congestive heart failure: shortness of breath, edema, distended neck veins, and fatigue.
- Assess for signs of hypokalemia: ECG changes, including flattened or inverted T waves and prolonged QT segments; apathy, weakness, abdominal distention, anorexia, vomiting, and paralytic ileus.

**Blood** Thrombocytopenia may occur with prolonged use of high doses.

- Assess for unexplained bleeding, bruising, and petechiae. Note skin changes (see Skin).
- Monitor platelet count.

**GI** Abdominal distention, anorexia, constipation, diarrhea, gastric irritation, nausea, pancreatitis, vomiting, weight gain, or weight loss may occur. Risk of peptic ulcer may be increased by high doses, but the incidence is less than 2% of treated patients.

- Monitor weight. Monitor intake and output if GI symptoms are prominent.
- Check stools and vomitus for occult blood; instruct patients to report a change in the color or consistency of stools or the appearance of ''coffee-ground'' emesis.
- Encourage patients to take doses with meals or snack to reduce gastric irritation. Some physicians prescribe antacids on a regular basis to reduce gastric irritation.
- Caution patients to avoid aspirin and other drugs that may cause GI irritation.
- If constipation occurs, instruct the patient to increase daily fluid intake to 2500 to 3000 ml, to increase dietary intake of fruit, fruit juices, and fiber, and increase daily exercise.

**Skin** Acne, atrophy of skin, bruising, ecchymoses, facial erythema, hirsutism, petechiae, striae, and sweating occur with systemic use of corticosteroids. Injection sites may develop induration, pain, or sterile abscesses. Topical application may cause allergic dermatitis, angioedema, or urticaria.

- Caution patients to avoid activities that cause rough skin contact or bruising if possible.
- Use careful sterile technique with injections. Record and rotate injection sites.
- Avoid contact with topical agents by wearing gloves or using an applicator to apply.
- Instruct patients to report skin changes.
- If acne occurs, review measures for careful skin cleansing. If acne is severe, refer the patient to a dermatologist.

**Eye** Prolonged use may cause posterior subcapsular cataracts, exophthalmos, and increased intraocular pressure. Glaucoma may result. Eye infections may also by promoted.

- Refer patients on long-term therapy to an ophthalmologist for regular eye examinations.

**Musculoskeletal** Corticosteroids enhance protein catabolism, which may result in atrophy of the protein matrix of bone, muscle pain, weakness, muscle wasting, or delayed wound healing. Osteoporosis is promoted, with increases in fractures.

- Be alert in moving patients in bed or assisting out of bed if patients have been on long-term steroids.
- Caution patients about measures to reduce the possibility of falling: use night lights and hand rails.

**Endocrine** Doses above the physiologic range suppress production of corticotropin from the pituitary. As a result, adrenal function falls, and if treatment continues for long periods, the adrenals may atrophy. When patients are taken off long-term therapy, gradual reduction of doses are necessary to allow adrenal function to recover.

Corticosteroids may decrease glucose tolerance, produce hyperglycemia, and aggravate diabetes mellitus.

- Reinforce to patients the need to keep track of the supply of drug on hand in order to avoid running out of medication.
- Caution patients to take the medication every day, as ordered. If patient is ill or unable to take the medication, instruct the patient to notify the physician.
- Remind patients to keep all health care providers informed of all medications being used.
- Monitor urine and blood glucose levels.
- Caution diabetic patients to monitor blood glucose levels frequently while on steroids; a change in insulin or diet may be necessary during a course of glucocorticoid therapy.

**Allergic** Acute reactions are possible but uncommon.
- Have available drugs, equipment, and personnel to treat acute allergic reactions in settings where steroids are administered.

**Reproductive** Amenorrhea or menstrual difficulties may arise following long-term therapy. Sperm motility and numbers may be reduced in men.
- Instruct women to keep a record of menstrual periods. Counsel about birth control methods if appropriate. Caution patients to notify the physician if pregnancy is suspected.
- Inform men about possible effects on sperm.
- Provide emotional support as needed.

**Other** Large doses of corticosteroids increase susceptibility to infection and mask the symptoms of infection.
- Warn patients about this side effect. Instruct patients to notify the physician of fever, cough, malaise, sore throat, and injuries that do not heal.
- Instruct patients to avoid exposure to individuals with active infections, even a common cold.

### Nursing interventions related to drug administration
- Glucocorticoids are administered via many routes of administration: IV, IM, IA (intra-articular), IS (intrasynovial), IL (intralesional), ST (soft tissue injection), topically, intranasally, via oral inhalation, orally, and via the ear or eye. Read orders and labels carefully, as not all forms are safe for all routes of administration.
- Review with the patient the directions supplied by the manufacturer for metered dose devices. Instruct patients to keep mouthpieces clean and dry between use and to wash the mouthpiece at least weekly.
- Caution patients using eye medications to administer the dose into the conjunctival sac, never directly on the eye. Each person should have a personal bottle or tube of eye medication; containers should not be shared.
- For topical administration, wear gloves or apply doses with an applicator. If obvious infection is present, do not apply an occlusive dressing. Assess skin for response to steroids; local irritation may necessitate switching to another drug. Caution the patient to use only as ordered.
- Systemic effects from steroids are less common and less severe when the drug is administered via inhalation, topical, or eye routes but can occur. Assess patients for systemic reactions.
- Caution patients who receive an IA injection to avoid joint overuse if joint pain markedly decreases or disappears.

### Patient and family education
- Review the anticipated benefits and possible side effects of drug therapy with patient and family.
- Explain to patients on long-term therapy the importance of continuing steroids as ordered and not stopping them suddenly.
- Caution patients on long-term therapy to wear a medical identification tag or bracelet.
- Review with patients appropriate modifications in diet, based on drug dose, length of therapy, patient response, and usual dietary patterns. Appropriate recommendations might be decreasing sodium intake, increasing intake of potassium-rich foods, and increasing protein intake. Refer to a dietitian as needed.
- Note Drug Interactions. Remind patients to keep all health care providers informed of all medications being used.
- Remind patients not to share medications with others. Remind patients to keep all medications out of the reach of children.

---

## amcinonide   (am-SIN-oh-nide)                                                          corticosteroid*

- amcinonide: Cyclocort

*Topical.

**MECHANISM OF ACTION**   • See entry for drug class (p. 598).

**INDICATIONS   Inflammatory dermatoses** Topical steroids may relieve inflammatory manifestations of certain dermatoses (see Table 31-2 and entry for drug class, p. 602).

**CONTRAINDICATIONS**   • See entry for drug class (p. 603).

**DOSAGE   Topical:   ADULTS AND CHILDREN:** A thin film of ointment is spread or the cream is rubbed on the affected area two or three times daily. *Special patient populations:*  **PREGNANCY:** Safe use has not been established.

**PREPARATIONS**   *Cream:* 0.1%; *ointment:* 0.1%.

**DRUG INTERACTIONS**   • See entry for drug class (p. 603).

**DIAGNOSTIC TEST INTERFERENCE**   • See entry for drug class (p. 603).

**FATE**   Absorption through skin is minimal unless large areas are treated for prolonged periods or unless the skin is broken. Children may be more likely to suffer adrenal suppression than adults.

### 🐚 NURSING CONSIDERATIONS

**Side effects, toxicities, and associated nursing actions**
• See entry for drug class (p. 603).

**Nursing interventions related to drug administration**
• See entry for drug class (p. 606).

**Patient and family education**
• See entry for drug class (p. 606).

---

## beclomethasone dipropionate
(bek-loh-METH-a-zone dye-PRO-pee-oh-nate)                    corticosteroid

• beclomethasone depropionate: Beclovent, Beconase, Vancenase, Vanceril

**MECHANISM OF ACTION**   • See entry for drug class (p. 598).

**INDICATIONS   Asthma** Oral inhalation therapy may relieve symptoms of bronchial asthma; the effect may take 1 to 4 weeks to develop.   **Rhinitis** Seasonal or perennial rhinitis may be controlled with intranasal beclomethasone dipropionate; this therapy may be effective when conventional therapy with decongestants and antihistamines has failed.   **Nasal polyposis** Nasal application of beclomethasone dipropionate may prevent recurrence of polyps removed surgically.

**CONTRAINDICATIONS**   • See entry for drug class (p. 603).

**DOSAGE   Oral inhalation   ADULTS AND CHILDREN OVER 6 YEARS:** Initially, 84 µg (two sprays with the oral inhaler) three or four times daily. Daily dosage should not exceed 840 µg (20 sprays). Children's doses may be lower than for adults; daily dosage should not exceed 420 µg (10 sprays).   **Nasal inhalation:   ADULTS AND CHILDREN OVER 6 YEARS:** Initially, 42 µg (one spray with the nasal inhaler) in each nostril two to four times daily. Children may receive a maximum of three daily doses. *Special patient populations:*  **CHILDREN:** Not recommended for children under 6 years of age. **PREGNANCY:** Safe use has not been established.

**PREPARATIONS**   *Aerosol for oral use* (Beclovent, Vanceril: 42 µg/metered spray; *aerosol for nasal use* (Beconase, Vancenase): 42 µg metered spray.

**DRUG INTERACTIONS**   • See entry for drug class (p. 603).

**DIAGNOSTIC TEST INTERFERENCE**   • See entry for drug class (p. 603).

**FATE**   Beclomethasone dipropionate may be systemically absorbed when administered by intranasal or oral inhalation, creating the possibility of systemic side effects such as suppression of hypothalamic-pituitary-adrenal function. Only 10% to 25% of orally inhaled doses reach the respiratory tract; the remainder is retained in the mouth or pharynx and swallowed. The swallowed portion is metabolized rapidly by the liver, limiting the possibility of serious systemic effects. *Elimination* is primarily through metabolism.

## 🦶 NURSING CONSIDERATIONS
### Side effects, toxicities, and associated nursing actions

**Nasal** When administered intranasally, beclamethasone dipropionate causes irritation or sneezing attacks in about 10% of patients. Intranasal bleeding may occur in up to 15% of patients but is usually ot severe. Atropic rhinitis is possible with long-term therapy.
* Caution patients to report symptoms that are severe or persistent, as it may necessitate a change in drug.
* Ascertain that the patient is using the drug in the frequency ordered, and not more often than ordered, as side effects may be aggravated.

**Endocrine** Adrenal suppression is less likely with nasal than with oral aerosols.
* Caution patients to use drugs only as ordered for best effect.
* Caution patients not to discontinue medication without discussing with the physician.

**Dysphonia** Voice failure may be persistent and severe in some patients receiving oral inhalation therapy.
* Caution patients to report persistent voice failure.

**Suprainfections** *Candida* infections of the mouth, pharynx, larynx, bronchus, or esophagus are frequently observed in patients receiving oral inhalation therapy. Nasal administration is less likely to cause this side effect.
* Instruct patients to report difficulty or pain in swallowing, oral pain, or development of white patchy areas in mouth.
* Caution patients to wash mouth piece on sprayer after each use, and to keep it dry.
* For other possible reactions to adsorbed drug, see entry for drug class (p. 603).

### Nursing interventions related to drug administration
* See entry for drug class (p. 606).
* Read labels carefully: Some forms are for oral use; others are for Nasal use.

### Patient and family education
* See entry for drug class (p. 606).

---

## betamethasone   (bay-ta-METH-a-zone)                                 corticosteroid

* betamethasone (betamethasone acetate, betamethasone benzoate, betamethasone sodium phosphate, betamethasone valerate): Celestone (See also Preparations.)

**MECHANISM OF ACTION**   See entry for drug class (p. 598).
**INDICATIONS**   The immunosuppressive and anti-inflammatory effects of betamethasone are useful for the following conditions. For a full discussion, see entry for drug class (p. 598). • Allergic states. • Cerebral edema. • Collagen diseases. • Dermatologic diseases. • Hematologic disorders. • Hepatic disease. • Myasthenia gravis. • Nephrotic syndrome. • Organ transplantation. • Respiratory diseases. • Rheumatoid diseases.
**CONTRAINDICATIONS**   • See entry for drug class (p. 603).
**DOSAGE**   PO:   ADULTS: Betamethasone initial doses are commonly between 0.6 and 7.2 mg daily, divided into two to four equal doses.   CHILDREN: Betamethasone doses are 0.0175 to 0.25 mg/kg daily or 0.5 to 7.5 mg/M$^2$ divided into three or four equal doses.   IV:   ADULTS: Betamethasone sodium phosphate doses up to 9 mg daily may be given IV, with the actual dose depending on the condition being treated.   IM:   ADULTS: Betamethasone sodium phosphate alone or in the preparation with betamethasone acetate may be used in doses from 0.5 to 9 mg daily, depending on the condition being treated.   IA, IS, IL, ST:   ADULTS: Betamethasone sodium phosphate with betamethasone acetate is injected in doses ranging from 1.2 mg for intralesional injections to 12 mg for injection into large joints. Intralesional and soft tissue injections may be repeated weekly, but injections into joints are repeated less frequently.   **Topical:**   ADULTS: Apply sparingly in a thin film and rub into the affected area one to four times daily. Preparations of betamethasone dipropionate should not be applied more frequently than twice daily, and occlusive dressings should not be used. Avoid use in children under

12. *Special patient populations:* **PREGNANCY:** Use of this drug in pregnancy carries substantial risk to the fetus.

**PREPARATIONS** **Betamethasone** *Tablets:* 0.6 mg; *solution for oral use:* 0.6 mg/5ml. **Betamethasone benzoate** *Topical cream, ointment, gel, or lotion:* 0.025% (Uticort). **Betamethasone dipropionate** *Aerosol, topical:* 60 μg/3-second spray (Diprosone); *topical cream, ointment, or lotion:* 0.05% (Alphatrex, Diprolene, Diprosone). **Betamethasone sodium phosphate** *Solution for IV, IM, IA, IS, IL, or ST injection:* 3 mg/ml. **Betamethasone sodium phosphate with betamethasone acetate** *Suspension for IM, IA, IS, IL or ST injection:* 3 mg/ml. **Betamethasone valerate** *Topical cream:* 0.01% or 0.1% (Betatrex, Beta-Val, Valisone); *topical ointment or lotion:* 0.1% (Betatrex, Beta-Val, Valisone).

**DRUG INTERACTIONS** • See entry for drug class (p. 603).

**DIAGNOSTIC TEST INTERFERENCE** • See entry for drug class (p. 603).

**FATE** Betamethasone is adequately absorbed following oral administration to allow continuous therapy for chronic conditions by this route. Betamethasone sodium phosphate is a soluble form of the drug that may be used IV for rapid action. Betamethasone sodium phosphate is also absorbed from IM sites; betamethasone acetate is absorbed more slowly from IM sites, prolonging the *duration* of action of the drug. Betamethasone is not highly bound to transcortin, the corticosteroid transport protein, and is therefore more available for distribution to tissues than are natural steroids. Betamethasone is metabolized in liver and eliminated in urine. The drug crosses the placenta and enters milk.

## 🐝 NURSING CONSIDERATIONS

### Side effects, toxicities, and associated nursing actions
• See entry for drug class (p. 603).

### Nursing interventions related to drug administration
• Gargling with warm water after each inhalation removes residual medication and may delay onset of hoarseness or dryness.
• For other nursing interventions, see entry for drug class (p. 606).

### Patient and family education
• See entry for drug class (p. 606).

## clobetasol propionate (klo-BAY-tuh-sol PRO-pee-oh-nate) corticosteroid

• clobetasol propionate: 🍁 Dermovate, Temovate

**MECHANISM OF ACTION** • See entry for drug class (p. 598).

**INDICATIONS** **Inflammatory dermatoses** Topical steroids may relieve inflammatory manifestations of certain dermatoses (see Table 31-2).

**CONTRAINDICATIONS** • See entry for drug class (p. 603).

**DOSAGE** **Topical:** **ADULTS:** Ointments and creams are applied sparingly in thin films and rubbed gently into the affected area morning and evening. Weekly doses should not exceed 50 g of cream or ointment. The drug should not be administered longer than 14 days. *Special patient populations:* **CHILDREN:** Not recommended for children under 12 years. **PREGNANCY:** Clobetasol propionate should be avoided because of risk of teratogenic effects.

**PREPARATIONS** *Cream:* 0.05%; *ointment:* 0.05%.

**DRUG INTERACTIONS** • See entry for drug class (p. 603).

**DIAGNOSTIC TEST INTERFERENCE** • See entry for drug class (p. 603).

**FATE** Absorption through skin is detectable in many patients and is enhanced when large areas are treated for prolonged periods or when the skin is broken. Occlusive dressings should not be applied. Clobetasole propionate is among the most potent corticosteroids available.

## 🐝 NURSING CONSIDERATIONS

### Side effects, toxicities, and associated nursing actions
• See entry for drug class (p. 603).

**Nursing interventions related to drug administration**
- Note Fate; occlusive dressings should not be used.
- See entry for drug class (p. 606).

**Patient and family education**
- See entry for drug class (p. 606).

## clocortolone pivalate   (klo-KOR-toh-lone pye-val-ate)            corticosteroid

- clocortolone pivalate: Cloderm

**MECHANISM OF ACTION**   • See entry for drug class (p. 598).

**INDICATIONS**   **Inflammatory dermatoses** Topical steroids may relieve inflammatory manifestations of certain dermatoses (see Table 31-2).

**CONTRAINDICATIONS**   • See entry for drug class (p. 603).

**DOSAGE**   **Topical:**   ADULTS AND CHILDREN: Apply sparingly in a thin film and rub gently into affected area one to four times daily.   *Special patient populations:*   PREGNANCY: Safe use has not been established.

**PREPARATIONS**   *Cream:* 0.1%.

**DRUG INTERACTIONS**   • See entry for drug class (p. 603).

**DIAGNOSTIC TEST INTERFERENCE**   • See entry for drug class (p. 603).

   **FATE**   Absorption through skin is minimal unless large areas are treated for prolonged periods or unless the skin is broken. Children may be more likely to suffer adrenal suppression than adults.

### ❦ NURSING CONSIDERATIONS

**Side effects, toxicities, and associated nursing actions**
- See entry for drug class (p. 603).

**Nursing interventions related to drug administration**
- See entry for drug class (p. 606).

**Patient and family education**
- See entry for drug class (p. 606).

## cortisone acetate   (KOR-te-zone)            corticosteroid

- cortisone acetate: Cortone acetate

**MECHANISM OF ACTION**   • See entry for drug class (p. 598).

**INDICATIONS**   Cortisone, a natural corticosteroid, possesses both glucocorticoid and mineralocorticoid activity (Table 31-2, p. 600); for this reason cortisone acetate is useful in the following conditions: • Adrenocortical insufficiency • Adrenogenital syndrome. • For full discussion, see entry for drug class (p. 598).

**CONTRAINDICATIONS**   • See entry for drug class (p. 603).

**DOSAGE**   **PO:**   ADULTS: Initially 25 to 300 mg daily, depending on the severity of the condition being treated.   CHILDREN: Initially 0.7 to 10 mg/kg or 20 to 300 mg/M$^2$ daily, divided into four equal doses.   **IM:**   ADULTS: Daily doses of 20 to 300 mg are administered, divided into two equal doses.   CHILDREN: Daily doses of 0.2 to 1.25 mg/kg or 7 to 37.5 mg/M$^2$ are given as single injections or divided into two equal doses.   *Special patient populations:*   PREGNANCY: Use of this drug in pregnancy carries substantial risk to the fetus.

**PREPARATIONS**   *Tablets:* 5, 10, or 25 mg; *suspension for parenteral use:* 25 to 50 mg/ml.

**DRUG INTERACTIONS**   • See entry for drug class (p. 603).

**DIAGNOSTIC TEST INTERFERENCE**   • See entry for drug class (p. 603).

   **FATE**   Cortisone acetate is well absorbed orally and slowly absorbed from IM sites. Like other corticosteroids, cortisone is well distributed to most tissues and crosses the placenta. The drug also appears in milk. *Elimination* is primarily by liver metabolism with excretion in urine.

☙ **NURSING CONSIDERATIONS**
    Side effects, toxicities, and associated nursing actions
        • See entry for drug class (p. 603).
    Nursing interventions related to drug administration
        • See entry for drug class (p. 606).
    Patient and family education
        • See entry for drug class (p. 606).

---

## desonide   (DESS-oh-nide)        corticosteroid

• desonide: DesOwen, Tridesilon

**MECHANISM OF ACTION**  • See entry for drug class (p. 598).
**INDICATIONS**  **Inflammatory dermatoses** Topical steroids may relieve inflammatory manifestations of certain dermatoses (see Table 31-2).
**CONTRAINDICATIONS**  • See entry for drug class (p. 603).
**DOSAGE**  **Topical:**  ADULTS AND CHILDREN: Apply sparingly in thin films and rub gently into affected area two to four times daily.  *Special patient populations:*  PREGNANCY: Safe use has not been established.
**PREPARATIONS**  *Cream:* 0.05%; *ointment:* 0.05%.
**DRUG INTERACTIONS**  • See entry for drug class (p. 603).
**DIAGNOSTIC TEST INTERFERENCE**  • See entry for drug class (p. 603).
**FATE**  Absorption through skin is minimal unless large areas are treated for prolonged periods or unless the skin is broken. Children may be more likely to suffer adrenal suppression than adults.

☙ **NURSING CONSIDERATIONS**
    Side effects, toxicities, and associated nursing actions
        • See entry for drug class (p. 603).
    Nursing interventions related to drug administration
        • See entry for drug class (p. 606).
    Patient and family education
        • See entry for drug class (p. 606).

---

## desoximetasone   (dex-ox-ee-MET-uh-zone)        corticosteroid

• desoximetasone: Topicort

**MECHANISM OF ACTION**  • See entry for drug class (p. 598).
**INDICATIONS**  **Inflammatory dermatoses** Topical steroids may relieve inflammatory manifestations of certain dermatoses (see Table 31-2).
**CONTRAINDICATIONS**  • See entry for drug class (p. 603).
**DOSAGE**  **Topical:**  ADULTS AND CHILDREN: Apply sparingly in thin films and rub gently into affected area twice daily.  *Special patient populations:*  PREGNANCY: Safe use has not been established.
**PREPARATIONS**  *Cream:* 0.05%, 0.25%; *ointment:* 0.25%; *gel:* 0.05%
**DRUG INTERACTIONS**  • See entry for drug class (p. 603).
**DIAGNOSTIC TEST INTERFERENCE**  • See entry for drug class (p. 603).
**FATE**  Absorption through skin is minimal unless large areas are treated for prolonged periods or unless the skin is broken. Children may be more likely to suffer adrenal suppression than adults.

☙ **NURSING CONSIDERATIONS**
    Side effects, toxicities, and associated nursing actions
        • See entry for drug class (p. 603).

**Nursing interventions related to drug administration**
• See entry for drug class (p. 606).
**Patient and family education**
• See entry for drug class (p. 606).

## dexamethasone (dex-uh-METH-uh-zone)

corticosteroid

• dexamethasone (dexamethasone acetate, dexamethasone sodium phosphate): Decadron (also see Preparations)

**MECHANISM OF ACTION** • See entry for drug class (p. 598).

**INDICATIONS** **Diagnosis** The dexamethasone suppression test is useful for diagnosing Cushing's syndrome, adrenal hyperplasia, or adrenal adenoma. Dexamethasone inhibits release of ACTH, which will lower corticosteroid production in normal adrenal glands. **Acute allergic reactions** High initial doses are reduced over 6 days and then discontinued. **Shock** Dexamethasone is effective in addisonian shock (adrenal insufficiency) and may be effective in septic shock. **Other** As a potent glucocorticoid with little mineralocorticoid activity, dexamethasone may also be useful in the following conditions: • Dermatologic diseases. • Asthma • Rheumatoid diseases • Respiratory diseases • Cerebral edema • Ophthalmic diseases. • For a full discussion, see entry for drug class (p. 602).

**CONTRAINDICATIONS** • See entry for drug class (p. 603).

**DOSAGE** **PO:** **ADULTS:** Initially 0.75 to 9 mg daily, divided into two to four equal doses. Actual dose is determined by the severity and responsiveness of the condition being treated. **CHILDREN:** Initially 0.024 to 0.34 mg/kg or 0.66 to 10 mg/M$^2$ daily, divided into four equal doses. Actual dose is determined by the severity and responsiveness of the condition being treated. **IV:** **ADULTS:** Dexamethasone sodium phosphate, 0.5 to 24 mg daily. Actual dose is determined by the severity and responsiveness of the condition being treated. Massive IV doses may be administered for shock (40 mg every 2 to 6 hours as needed). **CHILDREN:** Dexamethasone sodium phosphate, 6 to 40 µg/kg or 0.235 to 1.25 mg/M$^2$. Actual dose is determined by the severity and responsiveness of the condition being treated. **IM:** **ADULTS:** Dexamethasone acetate, 8 to 16 mg, repeated every 1 to 3 weeks as necessary. Dexamethasone sodium phosphate, 0.5 to 24 mg daily. Actual dose is determined by the severity and responsiveness of the condition being treated. **CHILDREN:** Dexamethasone acetate is not indicated for children under 12. Dexamethasone sodium phosphate, 6 to 40 µg/kg or 0.235 to 1.25 mg/M$^2$. Actual dose is determined by the severity and responsiveness of the condition being treated. **IL, IA, ST:** **ADULTS:** Dexamethasone acetate or dexamethasone sodium phosphate, 0.8 to 1.6 mg intralesionally or 4 to 16 mg injected into joints. Dexamethasone sodium phosphate may also be injected intrasynovially. *Special patient populations:* **PREGNANCY:** Use of this drug in pregnancy carries substantial risk to the fetus.

**PREPARATIONS** **Dexamethasone** *Tablets:* 0.25, 0.5, 0.75, 1, 1.5, 2, 4, and 6 mg (Decradron, Dexone, Hexadrol); *elixir:* 0.5 mg/5 ml (Decadron, Hexadrol, Mymethasone); *oral solution:* 0.5 mg/5 m; *oral solution concentrate:* 0.5 mg/0.5 ml; *topical aerosol:* 0.01% or 0.04% (Aeroseb-Dex, Decaspray); *topical gel:* 0.1% (Decaderm); ophthalmic suspension: 0.1% (Maxidex). **Dexamethasone acetate** *Suspension for IM, IA, IL, or ST injection:* 8 or 16 mg/ml (Dalalone, Decadron-L.A., Decaject-L.A., Dexacen L.A., Dexasone L.A., Dexone L.S. Solurex L.S.) **Dexamethasone sodium phosphate** *Aerosol, oral inhaler:* 100 µg per metered spray; *solution for IM or IV use:* 4, 10 or 20 mg/ml (Dalalone, Decadrol, Decadron phosphate, Decaject, Dexacen, Dexasone, Dexone, Hexadrol phosphate, Solurex); *topical cream:* 0.1% (Decadron phosphate); *nasal aerosol:* 100 µg per metered spray; *ophthalmic ointment:* 0.05% (Ak-Dex, Decadron phosphate, Dexair, Maxidex, Ocu-Dex); *ophthalmic solution:* 0.1% (Ak-Dex, Decradron phosphate, Dexair). **Combination products** *Ophthalmic suspension or ointment:* neomycin sulfate, 0.1%, and polymyxin B 10,000 units with 0.1% dexamethasone (Ak-Trol, Dexacidin, Dexasporin, Maxitrol, Ocu-Trol); *Solution for injection:* lidocaine hydrochloride, 10 mg/ml, with 4 mg/ml dexamethasone sodium phosphate. *topical cream:* Neomycin sulfate 0.5% with 0.1% dexamethasone phosphate; *ophthalmic ointment:* neomycin sulfate

0.5% with 0.05% dexamethasone phosphate (NeoDecadron); *ophthalmic solution:* neomycin sulfate 0.5% with 0.1% dexamethasone phosphate (Ak-Neo-Dex, NeoDecadron, Neo Dexair).

**DRUG INTERACTIONS** • See entry for drug class (p. 603).

**DIAGNOSTIC TEST INTERFERENCE** • See entry for drug class (p. 603).

**FATE** Dexamethasone is well absorbed orally. The acetate form is slowly absorbed from IM sites. Dexamethasone sodium phosphate is a soluble form, which may be used IV for rapid action. When administered by oral inhalation for respiratory actions, about half the dose is absorbed systemically because much of the dose remains in the oral cavity and is swallowed. Like other corticosteroids, dexamethasone is well distributed to most tissues and crosses the placenta. The drug also appears in milk. Elimination is primarily by liver metabolism with excretion of metabolites in urine.

## NURSING CONSIDERATIONS

### Side effects, toxicities, and associated nursing actions
- See entry for drug class (p. 603).

### Nursing interventions related to drug administration
- Read orders and labels carefully to get correct form for ordered route of administration.
- May be given undiluted or further diluted in IV glucose or saline. Administer direct IV at a rate of one dose over 1 minute.
- See entry for drug class (p. 606).

### Patient and family education
- See entry for drug class (p. 606).

---

## diflorasone diacetate    (dye-FLOR-a-zone)                     corticosteroid

- diflorasone diacetate: Florone, Maxiflor

**MECHANISM OF ACTION** • See entry for drug class (p. 598).

**INDICATIONS** *Inflammatory dermatoses* Topical steroids may relieve inflammatory manifestations of certain dermatoses (see Table 31-2).

**CONTRAINDICATIONS** • See entry for drug class (p. 603).

**DOSAGE** *Topical:* **ADULTS AND CHILDREN:** Apply sparingly in thin films and rub gently into affected area one to three times daily for the ointment or two to four times daily for the cream. *Special patient populations:* **PREGNANCY:** Safe use has not been established.

**PREPARATIONS** *Cream:* 0.05%; *ointment:* 0.05%.

**DRUG INTERACTIONS** • See entry for drug class (p. 603).

**DIAGNOSTIC TEST INTERFERENCE** • See entry for drug class (p. 603).

**FATE** Absorption through skin is minimal unless large areas are treated for prolonged periods or unless the skin is broken. Children may be more likely to suffer adrenal suppression than adults.

## NURSING CONSIDERATIONS

### Side effects, toxicities, and associated nursing actions
- See entry for drug class (p. 603).

### Nursing interventions related to drug administration
- See entry for drug class (p. 606).

### Patient and family education
- See entry for drug class (p. 606).

---

## fludrocortisone acetate    (floo-dro-KOR-ti-zone)              corticosteroid

- fludrocortisone: Florinef

**MECHANISM OF ACTION** • See entry for drug class (p. 598).

**INDICATIONS** **Adrenocortical insufficiency** When this condition is not adequately controlled by cortisone or hydrocortisone, a more potent mineralocorticoid such as fludrocortisone may be required. **Adreno-genital syndrome** In salt-losing forms of this condition, fludrocortisone may be added to cortisone or hydrocortisone therapy to control sodium loss and hypotension.

**CONTRAINDICATIONS** • See entry for drug class (p. 603).

**DOSAGE** PO: ADULTS AND CHILDREN: 0.05 to 2 mg daily, depending on the response of the patient. *Special patient populations:* PREGNANCY: Use of this drug in pregnancy carries substantial risk to the fetus.

**PREPARATIONS** *Tablets:* 0.1 mg.

**DRUG INTERACTIONS** • See entry for drug class (p. 603).

**DIAGNOSTIC TEST INTERFERENCE** • See entry for drug class (p. 603).

**FATE** Fludrocortisone acetate is well absorbed orally. Like other corticosteroids, fludrocortisone is well distributed to most tissues and crosses the placenta. The drug also appears in milk. Elimination is primarily by liver metabolism with excretion of metabolites in urine.

### ❧ NURSING CONSIDERATIONS

**Side effects, toxicities, and associated nursing actions**
- See entry for drug class (p. 603).

**Nursing interventions related to drug administration**
- See entry for drug class (p. 606).

**Patient and family education**
- See entry for drug class (p. 606).

---

## flunisolide (floo-NIS-oh-lide) corticosteroid

- flunisolide: AeroBid, Nasalide, ✦Rhinalar

**MECHANISM OF ACTION** • See entry for drug class (p. 598).

**INDICATIONS** **Asthma** Oral inhalation therapy may relieve symptoms of bronchial asthma. The effect may take 1 to 4 weeks to develop. **Rhinitis** Seasonal or perennial rhinitis may be controlled with intranasal flunisolide. This therapy may be effective when conventional therapy with decongestants and anti-histamines has failed.

**CONTRAINDICATIONS** • See entry for drug class. (p. 603).

**DOSAGE** Intranasal: ADULTS: Initially 50 µg (two sprays) in each nostril twice daily. Maximum daily dosage should not exceed 200 µg (8 sprays) in each nostril. CHILDREN 6 TO 14 YEARS: Initially 25 µg in each nostril three times daily. Maximum daily dosage should not exceed 100 µg (four sprays) in each nostril. **Oral inhalation:** ADULTS: Initially, 500 µg (two sprays of the oral aerosol inhaler) once in the morning and once in the evening. Total daily doses should not exceed 2000 µg. CHIL-DREN 6 TO 15 YEARS: Initially, 500 µg (two sprays of the oral aerosol inhaler) once in the morning and once in the evening. *Special patient populations:* PREGNANCY: Safe use has not been established.

**PREPARATIONS** *Nasal solution:* 25 µg per metered spray; *oral aerosol:* 250 µg per metered spray.

**DRUG INTERACTIONS** • See entry for drug class (p. 603).

**DIAGNOSTIC TEST INTERFERENCE** • See entry for drug class (p. 603).

**FATE** Flunisolide is systemically absorbed following intranasal administration. Absorbed drug is rapidly metabolized in the liver and widely distributed to most tissues. The elimination *half-life* is about 2 hours. Drug metabolites are excreted in bile and urine.

### ❧ NURSING CONSIDERATIONS

**Side effects, toxicities, and associated nursing actions**
**Nasal** Burning is reported by about 45% of patients using nasal preparations of flunisolide. Sneezing, nasal congestion, bloody secretions, nasal dryness, sore throat, hoarseness, and changes in taste or smell are reported by less than 5% of patients.

- Caution patients to report symptoms that are severe or persistent, they may require a change in drug.
- Ascertain that the patient is using drug in the frequency ordered, and not more often than ordered, because side effects may be aggravated.

**Endocrine** Suppression of the adrenal gland is possible if higher than recommended doses are used.

- Caution patients to use drugs only as ordered for best effect.
- Caution patients not to discontinue medication without discussing with the physician.

**Other** Abdominal bloating, dizziness, headache, nausea, vomiting, and watery eyes have also been reported.

- Caution patients to report the development of any unexpected sign or symptom.
- For other possible reactions to adsorbed drug, see entry for drug class (p. 603).

**Nursing interventions related to drug administration**
- See entry for drug class (p. 606).

**Patient and family education**
- See entry for drug class (p. 606)

## fluocinolone acetonide  (floo-oh-SIN-oh-lone a-SEE-toh-nide)  corticosteroid

- fluocinolone acetonide (fluocinolide): Flurosyn, Lidex, Synalar, Synemol

**MECHANISM OF ACTION** • See entry for drug class (p. 598).
**INDICATIONS** **Inflammatory dermatoses** Topical steroids may relieve inflammatory manifestations of certain dermatoses (see Table 31-2).
**CONTRAINDICATIONS** • See entry for drug class (p. 603).
**DOSAGE** **Topical:** **ADULTS AND CHILDREN:** Apply sparingly in thin films and rub gently into affected area two to four times daily for fluocinolone acetonide preparations and three or four times daily for fluocinonide preparations. *Special patient populations:* **PREGNANCY:** Safe use has not been established.
**PREPARATIONS** **Fluocinonide** *Cream:* 0.05% ointment: 0.05%; *solution:* 0.05%; *gel:* 0.05%. **Fluocinolone acetonide** *Cream:* 0.01%, 0.025%, 0.2%; *ointment:* 0.025%. *solution:* 0.01%. **Combination products** *Cream:* 0.025% fluocinolone acetonide with 0.5% neomycin sulfate.
**DRUG INTERACTIONS** • See entry for drug class (p. 603).
**DIAGNOSTIC TEST INTERFERENCE** • See entry for drug class (p. 603).
**FATE** Absorption through skin is minimal unless large areas are treated for prolonged periods or unless the skin is broken. Children may be more likely to suffer adrenal suppression than adults.

**NURSING CONSIDERATIONS**
**Side effects, toxicities, and associated nursing actions**
- See entry for drug class (p. 603).
**Nursing interventions related to drug administration**
- See entry for drug class (p. 606).
**Patient and family education**
- See entry for drug class (p. 606).

## fluorometholone  (floo-roh-METH-oh-lone)  corticosteroid

- fluorometholone: FML, Fluor-Op

**MECHANISM OF ACTION** • See entry for drug class (p. 598).
**INDICATIONS** **Ophthalmic conditions** Inflammation may be reduced by direct application to the eye.
**CONTRAINDICATIONS** • See entry for drug class (p. 603).

**DOSAGE** Ophthalmic: ADULTS AND CHILDREN OVER 2 YEARS: One to two drops of 0.1% or 0.25% suspension or 1.3 cm of ointment are placed in the conjunctival sac two to four times daily. *Special patient populations:* PREGNANCY: Safe use has not been established.

**PREPARATIONS** *Ophthalmic ointment:* 0.1%; *ophthalmic suspension:* 0.1% or 0.25%.

**DRUG INTERACTIONS** • See entry for drug class (p. 603).

**DIAGNOSTIC TEST INTERFERENCE** • See entry for drug class (p. 603).

**FATE** Insignificant absorption is expected when used as directed.

☙ **NURSING CONSIDERATIONS**

**Side effects, toxicities, and associated nursing actions**
• See entry for drug class (p. 603).

**Nursing interventions to drug administration**
• See entry for drug class (p. 606).

**Patient and family education**
• See entry for drug class (p. 606).

---

## flurandrenolide  (floo-an-DREN-oh-lide)                 corticosteroid

• flurandrenolide: Cordran, ♣Drenison

**MECHANISM OF ACTION** • See entry for drug class (p. 598).

**INDICATIONS** Inflammatory dermatoses Topical steroids may relieve inflammatory manifestations of certain dermatoses (see Table 31-2).

**CONTRAINDICATIONS** • See entry for drug class (p. 603).

**DOSAGE** Topical: ADULTS AND CHILDREN: Apply sparingly in thin films and rub gently into affected area two or three times daily. *Special patient populations:* PREGNANCY: Safe use has not been established.

**PREPARATIONS** *Cream:* 0.025%, 0.05%; *ointment:* 0.025%, 0.05%; *lotion:* 0.05%; *dressing:* 4 µg/cm$^2$ of tape.

**DRUG INTERACTIONS** • See entry for drug class (p. 603).

**DIAGNOSTIC TEST INTERFERENCE** • See entry for drug class (p. 603).

**FATE** Absorption through skin is minimal unless large areas are treated for prolonged periods or unless the skin is broken. Children may be more likely to suffer adrenal suppression than adults.

☙ **NURSING CONSIDERATIONS**

**Side effects, toxicities, and associated nursing actions**
• See entry for drug class (p. 603).

**Nursing interventions related to drug administration**
• Caution patients to avoid excessive exposure to sunlight.
• For other Nursing Interventions, see entry for drug class (p. 606).

**Patient and family education**
• See entry for drug class (p. 606).

---

## halcinonide  (hal-SIN-oh-nide)                 corticosteroid

• halcinonide: Halog

**MECHANISM OF ACTION** • See entry for drug class (p. 598).

**INDICATIONS** Inflammatory dermatoses Topical steroids may relieve inflammatory manifestations of certain dermatoses (see Table 31-2).

**CONTRAINDICATIONS** • See entry for drug class (p. 603).

**DOSAGE** Topical: ADULTS AND CHILDREN: Apply sparingly in thin films and rub gently into affected area two or three times daily.   *Special patient populations:*   PREGNANCY: Safe use has not been established.

**PREPARATIONS**   *Cream:* 0.025%, 0.1%; *ointment:* 0.1% *solution:* 0.1%.

**DRUG INTERACTIONS**   • See entry for drug class (p. 603).

**DIAGNOSTIC TEST INTERFERENCE**   • See entry for drug class (p. 603).

**FATE**   Absorption through skin is minimal unless large areas are treated for prolonged periods or unless the skin is broken. Children may be more likely to suffer adrenal suppression than adults.

## ❦ NURSING CONSIDERATIONS

### Side effects, toxicities, and associated nursing actions
   • See entry for drug class (p. 603).

### Nursing interventions related to drug administration
   • See entry for drug class (p. 606).

### Patient and family education
   • See entry for drug class (p. 606).

---

## hydrocortisone   (hy-dro-KOR-ti-sone)                              corticosteroid

   • hydrocortisone (hydrocortisone acetate, hydrocortisone butyrate, hydrocortisone cypionate, hydrocortisone sodium phosphate, hydrocortisone sodium succinate, hydrocortisone valerate): Cortef (also see Preparations)

**MECHANISM OF ACTION**   • See entry for drug class (p. 598).

**INDICATIONS**   **Adrenocortical insufficiency** Systemic hydrocortisone supplies both glucocorticoid and mineralocorticoid activity.   **Adrenogenital syndrome** Systemic hydrocortisone may control salt-losing forms of this disease.   **Shock** Life-threatening shock may be treated initially with massive IV doses of hydrocortisone sodium succinate.   **Rheumatoid arthritis** Hydrocortisone acetate may be injected into affected joints, but synthetic steroids with less mineralocorticoid activity are preferred.   **Dermatitis** Topical hydrocortisone may be used to control minor irritations.   **Ulcerative colitis or rectal inflammation** Hydrocortisone suppositories or enemas may be used for symptomatic relief.   **Ophthalmic conditions** Hydrocortisone in combination with antiinfectives may be used to control inflammations of the eye.   **Otic inflammations** Hydrocortisone in combinations with antiinfectives may be effective. • For a full discussion, see entry for drug class (p. 602).

**CONTRAINDICATIONS**   • See entry for drug class (p. 603).

**DOSAGE**   PO:   ADULTS: Hydrocortisone or hydrocortisone cypionate, 10 to 320 mg daily divided into three or four doses. Take with meals or with low-salt snack to minimize gastric irritation.   CHILDREN: Hydrocortisone or hydrocortisone cypionate, 0.56 to 8 mg/kg or 16 to 240 mg/M$^2$ daily.   IM,IV: ADULTS: Hydrocortisone sodium phosphate 15 to 240 mg daily as an IV infusion or by injection every 12 hours. Hydrocortisone sodium succinate 100 mg to 8 g daily, given as 100 to 500 mg doses every 20 to 10 hours as needed.   CHILDREN: Hydrocortisone sodium phosphate or hydrocortisone sodium succinate, 0.16 to 1 mg/kg or 6 to 30 mg/M$^2$ IM in one or two injections daily.   IA, IS, IB, IL, ST: ADULTS: Hydrocortisone acetate, 5 to 75 mg, depending upong the site. Injections into joints may be repeated every 1 to 4 weeks.   **Topical:**   ADULTS OR CHILDREN: Apply sparingly in thin film and rub into affected area one to four times daily.   **Rectal:**   ADULTS: 100 mg nightly as a retention enema or 90 mg in aerosol foam once or twice daily or 25 mg suppository two or three times daily. **Ophthalmic:**   ADULTS AND CHILDREN: 1 to 2 drops every 3 or 4 hours or more often if necessary. **Otic:**   ADULTS: 4 or 5 drops three or four times daily.   CHILDREN: 3 drops three or four times daily.   *Special patient populations:*   PREGNANCY: Use of this drug in pregnancy carries substantial risk to the fetus.

**PREPARATIONS**   Combination products are covered in Tables 31-5 and 31-6.   **Hydrocortisone** *Tablets:* 5, 10, 20 mg (Cortef, Hydrocortone). • *Topical aerosol:* 0.5% (Aeroseb HC). • *Topical cream:* 0.25%, 0.5%, 1%, 2.5% (Cort-Dome, Cortifair, Cortizone-5, DermiCort, Dermolate, Hi-Cor, Hydro-Tex, Penecort, Prepcort, Racet SE, Synacort). • *Topical lotion:* 0.25%, 0.5%, 1%, and 2.5% (Cetacort,

Cort-Dome, Dermolate, Hytone, Nutracort). • *Topical ointment:* 0.5%, 1%, or 2.5% (Cortil, Hytone, Penecort). • *Topical powder:* 0.1% (Lexocort). • *Topical solution:* 0.5%, 1% (Cortaid, Dermolate, Penecort, Texacort). • *Rectal cream:* 1% (Proctocort). • *Rectal ointment:* 0.5% (Dermolate Anal-Itch). • *Rectal suspension:* 100 mg/60 ml (Cortenema).   **Hydrocortisone acetate** • *Suspension for parenteral injection:* 25 or 50 mg/ml. • *Topical aerosol:* 0.5% (CaldeCort). • *Topical cream:* 0.5% (CaldeCort, Cortaid, Gynecort, Lanacort, Pharma-Cort, Rhulicort). • *Topical lotion:* 0.5% (Cortaid). • *Topical ointment:* 0.5% or 1% (Cortaid, Cortef). • *Topical paste:* 0.5% (Orabase HCA). • *Rectal aerosol foam suspension:* 10% (Cortiform). • *Rectal suppositories:* 10 or 25 mg (Corticaine, Cort-Dome).   **Hydrocortisone butyrate** • *Topical cream:* 0.1% (Locoid). • *Topical ointment:* 0.1% (Locoid).   **Hydrocortisone cypionate** • *Suspension for oral use:* 10 mg/5 ml.   **Hydrocortisone sodium phosphate** • Solution for IM or IV use: 50 mg/ml.   **Hydrocortisone sodium succinate** • *Solution for IM or IV use:* 100, 250, 500, or 1 g vials (A-hydroCort, Solu-Cortef).   **Hydrocortisone valerate** • *Topical cream:* 0.2% (Westcort). • *Topical ointment:* 0.2% (Westcort).

**DRUG INTERACTIONS** • See entry for drug class (p. 603).

**DIAGNOSTIC TEST INTERFERENCE** • See entry for drug class (p. 603).

**FATE**   Hydrocortisone or hydrocortisone cypionate is adequately absorbed following oral administration. Hydrocortisone sodium phosphate or sodium succinate is used IV or IM for rapid action. Hydrocortisone acetate is slowly absorbed from joints or soft tissue sites, where it is injected for direct anti-inflammatory actions. Hydrocortisone, hydrocortisone acetate, hydrocortisone butyrate, and hydrocortisone valerate are also used topically. Once absorbed, hydrocortisone is transported to many tissues in the body. It is metabolized in the liver, and the inactive metabolites are excreted in urine.

## ❧ NURSING CONSIDERATIONS

### Side effects, toxicities, and associated nursing actions
• See entry for drug class (p. 603).

| Table 31-5. | Summary of topical combination products containing hydrocortisone | | | |
|---|---|---|---|---|
| **Form of hydrocortisone** | **Strength (%)** | **Other ingredients** | | **Trade names** |
| **Topical ointments** | | | | |
| Hydrocortisone | 1 | Neomycin sulfate 0.5% | | Sold as generic |
| Hydrocortisone | 1 | Bacitracin zinc, 400 units/g; neomycin sulfate, 0.5%; and polymyxin B sulfate 5000 units/g | | Cortisporin |
| Hydrocortisone acetate | 0.5, 1, or 2.5 | Neomycin sulfate 0.5% | | Neo-Cortef |
| **Topical creams** | | | | |
| Hydrocortisone | 1 | Urea 10% | | Alphaderm |
| Hydrocortisone acetate | 0.5 | Dibucaine 0.5% | | Corticaine |
| Hydrocortisone acetate | 0.5 | Neomycin sulfate, 0.5%; polymyxin B sulfate, 10,000 units/g | | Cortisporin |
| Hydrocortisone acetate | 1 | Neomycin sulfate 0.5% | | Neo-Cortef |
| Hydrocortisone acetate | 1 | Urea 10% | | Carmol HC |
| **Topical aerosol foam** | | | | |
| Hydrocortisone acetate | 1 | Pramoxine HC1 | | Epifoam |

**Table 31-6.**

## Summary of ophthalmic and otic preparations of hydrocortisone

| Form of hydrocortisone | Strength (%) | Other ingredients | Trade names |
|---|---|---|---|
| **Ophthalmic ointments** | | | |
| Hydrocortisone | 1 | Bacitracin zinc, 400 units/g; neomycin sulfate, 0.5%; and polymyxin B sulfate, 10,000 units/g | Ak-Spore, Cortisporin, Ocu-cort, Ocutricin HC, Triple Antibiotic Hydrocortisone Ophthalmic ointment, Tri-Thalmic HC Ophthalmic Ointment |
| Hydrocortisone acetate | 0.5 | Chloramphenicol, 1%; polymyxin B sulfate, 10,000 units/g | Ophthocort |
| Hydrocortisone acetate | 1 | Bacitracin zinc, 400 units/g; neomycin sulfate, 0.5%; polymyxin B sulfate, 10,000 units/g | Coracin |
| **Ophthalmic suspensions** | | | |
| Hydrocortisone | 1 | Neomycin sulfate, 0.5%; polymyxin B sulfate, 10,000 units/g | Ak-Spore HC, Bacticort Ophthalmic, Cortisporin, Ocutricin |
| Hydrocortisone acetate | 0.5 | Neomycin sulfate, 0.5% | Neo-Cortef |
| Hydrocortisone acetate | 1.5 | Neomycin sulfate, 0.5% | Ak-Neo-Cort |
| Hydrocortisone acetate | 1.5 | Oxytetracycline HCl 0.5% | Terra-Cortril |
| Hydrocortisone acetate | 2.5 | Chloramphenicol 1.25% | Chloromycetin hydrocortisone ophthalmic |
| **Otic solutions** | | | |
| Hydrocortisone | 0.5 | Polymyxin B sulfate, 10,000 units/ml | Otobiotic, Pyocidin-Otic |
| Hydrocortisone | 1 | Acetic acid, 2% | Acetasol HC, VoSol |
| Hydrocortisone | 1 | Acetic acid, 2%; pramoxine HCl, 1% | Otic-HC |
| Hydrocortisone | 1 | Antipyrine, 5%; dibucaine HCl, 0.25%; neomycin sulfate, 0.5%, and polymyxin B sulfate, 2000 units/ml | My-Cort-Otic |
| Hydrocortisone | 1 | Neomycin sulfate, 0.5%; polymyxin B sulfate, 10,000 units/ml | Ak-Spore, Cortisporin, Drotic, Octicair, Ortega Otic M, Oti-Sone, Otocidin, Otocort, Otomycin-HPN, Otoreid-HC |
| **Otic suspensions** | | | |
| Hydrocortisone | 1 | Neomycin sulfate, 0.5%; polymyxin B sulfate, 10,000 units/ml | Ak-Spore HC, Cortisporin, Hydromycin, Octicair, Oti-Sone |
| Hydrocortisone acetate | 1 | Colistin sulfate, 0.3%; neomycin sulfate, 0.5%; thonzonium bromide 0.05% | Coly-Mycin S Otic |

### Nursing interventions related to drug administration
- Read orders and labels carefully to prepare correct drug for ordered route of administration.
- For direct IV administration, administer each 500 mg over at least 1 minute.
- See entry for drug class (p. 606).

### Patient and family education
- See entry for drug class (p. 606).

---

## medrysone   (MED-ree-zone)                                                    corticosteroid

- medrysone: HMS Liquifilm

**MECHANISM OF ACTION**   • See entry for drug class (p. 598).
**INDICATIONS**   Ophthalmic conditions Medrysone is applied topically to the eye to control inflammation.
**CONTRAINDICATIONS**   • See entry for drug class (p. 603).
**DOSAGE**   Ophthalmic:   ADULTS: One drop in the conjunctival sac every 4 hours, or more often if required. *Special patient populations:*   CHILDREN: Pediatric doses have not been reported.   PREGNANCY: Safe use has not been established.
**PREPARATIONS**   *Ophthalmic suspension:* 0.1%.
**DRUG INTERACTIONS**   • See entry for drug class (p. 603).
**DIAGNOSTIC TEST INTERFERENCE**   • See entry for drug class (p. 603).
**FATE**   Little drug is expected to be absorbed when used as directed topically in the eye.
**❧ NURSING CONSIDERATIONS**

### Side effects, toxicities, and associated nursing actions   Few side effects are expected, other than occasional local reactions. For side effects of related drugs, see entry for drug class (p. 603).
### Nursing interventions related to drug administration
- See entry for drug class (p. 606).
### Patient and family education
- See entry for drug class (p. 606).

---

## methylprednisolone   (meth-ill-pred-NIS-oh-lone)                              corticosteroid

- methylprednisolone (methylprednisolone acetate, methylprednisolone sodium succinate): Medrol (also see Preparations)

**MECHANISM OF ACTION**   • See entry for drug class (p. 598).
**INDICATIONS**   Shock Methylprednisolone may be used in massive doses to aid in control of shock. • The immunosuppressive and anti-inflammatory effects of methylprednisolone may also be useful for the following conditions: • Cerebral edema • Collagen diseases • Dermatologic conditions • Rectal inflammation • Rheumatoid diseases. • For a full discussion, see entry for drug class (p. 602).
**CONTRAINDICATIONS**   • See entry for drug class (p. 603).
**DOSAGE**   PO:   ADULTS: Methylprednisolone, 2 to 60 mg daily divided into four doses, given with food to minimize irritation.   CHILDREN: Methylprednisolone, 0.117 to 1.66 mg/kg or 3.3 to 50 mg/M$^2$ daily, divided into three or four doses.   IV, IM:   ADULTS: Methylprednisolone sodium succinate, 10 mg to 1.5 g or higher, depending on the severity of the condition. Usual doses of 10 to 250 mg may be repeated up to six times daily.   CHILDREN: Methylprednisolone, 0.03 to 0.2 mg/kg or 1 to 6.25 mg/M$^2$ IM once or twice daily.   IA, IL, ST:   ADULTS: Methylprednisolone acetate, 4 to 80 mg depending on the site; repeat if necessary every 1 to 5 weeks. Methylprednisolone acetate is also administered IM at doses of 10 to 80 mg.   *Special patient populations:*   PREGNANCY: Use of this drug in pregnancy carries substantial risk to the fetus.

**PREPARATIONS**   Methylprednisolone *Tablets:* 2, 4, 8, 16, 24, and 32 mg (Medrol).   **Methylprednisolone acetate** *Suspension for IM, IA, IL, or ST injection:* 20, 40, or 80 mg/ml (Depo-Medrol, Depopred, Depo-Predate, Duralone, Rep-Pred); *topical ointment:* 0.25% or 1% (Medrol acetate); *rectal:* 40 mg powder for suspension (Medrol Enpak).   **Combinations products** *Topical ointment:* 0.25% or 1% methylprednisolone acetate with neomycin sulfate 0.5%.   **Methylprednisolone sodium succinate** *Powder for reconstitution for IM, IV injection:* 40 mg, 125 mg, 500 mg, 1 g or 2 g (A-MethaPred, Solu-Medrol).

**DRUG INTERACTIONS**   • See entry for drug class (p. 603).

**DIAGNOSTIC TEST INTERFERENCE**   • See entry for drug class (p. 603).

**FATE**   Methylprednisolone is adequately absorbed following oral administration. Methylprednisolone acetate is slowly absorbed from IM sites or from injections in joints. Methylprednisolone sodium succinate is rapidly absorbed from IM sites. Metabolism of the drug is primarily in liver, with metabolites being excreted in urine.

❦ **NURSING CONSIDERATIONS**

**Side effects, toxicities, and associated nursing actions**
  • See entry for drug class (p. 603).

**Nursing interventions related to drug administration**
  • Read orders and labels carefully to prepare dose for ordered route of administration.
  • Administer direct IV at a rate of 500 mg over at least 1 minute.
  • See entry for drug class (p. 606).

**Patient and family education**
  • See entry for drug class (p. 606).

---

# parametasone acetate   (pare-uh-METH-uh-zone)                    corticosteroid

  • parametasone acetate: Haldrone

**MECHANISM OF ACTION**   • See entry for drug class (p. 598).

**INDICATIONS**   The immunosuppresive and anti-inflammatory effects of parametasone acetate may be useful in oral therapy for the following conditions: • Allergic states • Collagen diseases • GI diseases • Hematologic disorders • Respiratory diseases • Rheumatoid diseases. • For a full discussion, see entry for drug class (p. 602).

**CONTRAINDICATIONS**   • See entry for drug class (p. 603).

**DOSAGE**   PO:   **ADULTS:** Initially 2 to 24 mg daily divided into three or four doses. Decrease dose to lowest level possible for control symptoms.   **CHILDREN:** Initially 0.058 to 0.8 mg/kg or 1.67 to 25 mg/M$^2$ divided into three or four doses. Decrease dose to lowest level possible for control of symptoms. *Special patient populations:*   **PREGNANCY:** Use of this drug in pregnancy carries substantial risk to the fetus.

**PREPARATIONS**   *Tablets:* 1 or 2 mg.

**DRUG INTERACTIONS**   • See entry for drug class (p. 603).

**DIAGNOSTIC TEST INTERFERENCE**   • See entry for drug class (p. 603).

**FATE**   Parametasone is well absorbed following oral administration. The drug is metabolized in the liver, and the metabolites are excreted in urine.

❦ **NURSING CONSIDERATIONS**

**Side effects, toxicities, and associated nursing actions**
  • See entry for drug class (p. 603).

**Nursing interventions related to drug administration**
  • See entry for drug class (p. 606).

**Patient and family education**
  • See entry for drug class (p. 606).

## prednisolone   (pred-NIS-oh-lone)                                    corticosteroid

- prednisolone (prednisolone acetate, prednisolone sodium phosphate, prednisolone tebutate): See Preparations

**MECHANISM OF ACTION** • See entry for drug class (p. 598).

**INDICATIONS**   The immunosuppressive and anti-inflammatory effects of prednisolone are useful for the following conditions: For a full discussion, see entry for drug class (p. 602). • Allergic states • Collagen disease • Dermatologic diseases • GI disease • Hepatic diseases • Ophthalmic conditions • Rheumatoid diseases. For a full discussion, see entry for drug class (p. 602).

**CONTRAINDICATIONS**   See entry for drug class (p. 603).

**DOSAGE**   PO:   **ADULTS:** Prednisolone, 5 to 60 mg daily, divided into two to four doses. Prednisolone sodium phosphate, 4 to 60 mg daily.   **CHILDREN:** Prednisolone, 0.14 to 2 mg/kg or 4 to 60 mg/M$^2$ daily, divided into four doses.   IV:   **ADULTS:** Prednisolone sodium phosphate, 4 to 60 mg daily.   **CHILDREN:** Prednisolone sodium phosphate, 0.04 to 0.25 mg/kg or 1.5 to 7.5 mg/M$^2$, daily as one dose or divided into two equal doses.   IM:   **ADULTS:** Prednisolone acetate, 4 to 60 mg daily, divided into two doses. Prednisolone sodium phosphate, 4 to 60 mg daily. Combined suspension prednisolone acetate and prednisolone sodium phosphate, 0.25 to 1 ml of suspension (20 to 80 mg acetate and 5 to 20 mg sodium phosphate forms).   **CHILDREN:** Prednisolone acetate, 0.04 to 0.25 mg/kg or 1.5 to 7.5 mg/M$^2$, daily as one dose or divided into two equal doses.   **ST, IA:**   **ADULTS:** Prednisolone acetate, 4 to 60 mg daily, divided into two doses. Prednisolone sodium phosphate, 2 to 30 mg, repeated every 3 days to 3 weeks, depending on the site and severity of the condition. Prednisolone tebutate, 4 to 40 mg, repeated at 2 to 3 week intervals. Combined suspension prednisolone acetate and prednisolone sodium phosphate, 0.25 to 1 ml of suspension (20 to 80 mg acetate and 5 to 20 mg sodium phosphate forms).   **CHILDREN:** Prednisolone acetate, 0.04 to 0.25 mg/kg or 1.5 to 7.5 mg/M$^2$ daily, as one dose or divided into two equal doses.   **Ophthalmic:**   **ADULTS OR CHILDREN:** Solution may be applied 1 or 2 drops as often as every hour for acute cases. Ointment is instilled into the conjunctival sac three or four times daily.   **Otic:**   **ADULTS OR CHILDREN:** Instill 3 or 4 drops into ear canal two or three times daily.   *Special patient populations:*   **PREGNANCY:** Use of this drug in pregnancy carries substantial risk to the fetus.

**PREPARATIONS**   Prednisolone *Tablets:* 5 mg (Cortalone, Delta-Cortef, Fernisolone-P); *oral solution:* 15 mg/5 ml (Prelone syrup).   **Prednisolone acetate** *Suspension for Im, IA, or ST use:* 25, 50 or 100 mg/ml (Articulose, Key-Pred, Predaject, Predate, Predcor); Ophthalmic suspension: 0.12%, 0.125%, or 1% (Enconopred, Ocu-Pred-A, Predair-A, Pred Forte).   **Prednisolone sodium phosphate** *Oral solution:* 5 mg/ 5 ml (Pediapred); *Solution for Im, IV, IA, IL, or St use:* 20 mg/ ml (Hydeltrasol, Key-Pred-Sp, Predate S); *Ophthalmic solution:* 0.125%, 0.5% or 1% (Ak-Pred, Inflamase, Ocu-Pred, Predair); *Otic solution:* 0.5% (Metreton).   **Prednisolone acetate with prednisolone sodium phosphate** *Suspension for Im, IA, IB, IS, or ST use:* 80 mg/ml prednisolone acetate and 20 mg/ml prednisolone sodium phosphate.   **Prednisolone tebutate** *Suspension for IA, IL, or St use:* 20 mg/ml (Hydeltra-TBA, Predate TBA, Predcor-TBA).   **Combination products** *Ophthalmic ointments:* 0.2%, 0.25%, or 0.5% prednisolone acetate with 10% sulfacetamide sodium (Blephamide SOP, Cetapred, Metimyd, Ocu-Lone-C, Predsulfair, Vasocidin);   *ophthalmic suspensions:* 0.2%, 0.25%, or 0.5% prednisolone acetate with 10% sulfacetamide sodium (Blephamide Liquifilm, Isopto Cetapred, Metimyd, Ocu-Lone-C, Ophtha P/S, Sulfamide, Sulphrin); 0.25% prednisolone acetate with 1% atropine sulfate (Mydrapred); 0.5% prednisolone acetate with neomycin sulfate 0.5% and 10,000 units/ml of polymyxin B sulfate; *ophthalmic solutions:* 0.2% or 0.5% prednisolone sodium phosphate with sulfacetamide sodium 10% (Vasocidin, Optimyd).

**DRUG INTERACTIONS** • See entry for drug class (p. 603).

**DIAGNOSTIC TEST INTERFERENCE** • See entry for drug class (p. 603).

**FATE**   Prednisolone and prednisolone sodium phosphate may be absorbed orally. Prednisolone acetate is slowly absorbed from IM or other sites of injection. Prednisolone sodium phosphate is rapidly absorbed from IM sites. is inactivated in the liver, and the metabolites are excreted in urine.

## ❦ NURSING CONSIDERATIONS
### Side effects, toxicities, and associated nursing actions
- See entry for drug class (p. 603).
### Nursing interventions related to drug administration
- Read orders and labels carefully to prepare doses for ordered routes of administration.
- Administer direct IV at a rate of 10 mg or less over 1 minute.
- See entry for drug class (p. 606).
### Patient and family education
- See entry for drug class (p. 606).

---

## prednisone    (PRED-ni-zone)                                    corticosteroid

- prednisone: Deltasone, Meticorten, Orasone

**MECHANISM OF ACTION**  • See entry for drug class (p. 598).

**INDICATIONS**   The immunosuppressive and anti-inflammatory effects of prednisone make this agent the drug of choice for oral therapy of the following conditions.  **Allergic states** Acute conditions may be treated with large doses gradually tapered off over several days and then stopped.  **Collagen disorders** Large doses may be required during acute episodes.  **Hematologic disorders** Prednisone may be used along with other appropriate therapy.  **Hepatic disease** Autoimmune chronic active hepatitis may respond.  **Renal disease** Nephrotic syndrome may respond to prednisone.  **Respiratory disorders** Sarcoidosis may respond.  **Rheumatoid diseases** Oral doses of prednisone may control symptoms of chronic arthritis.  **Neoplastic diseases** Lymphoid tumors such as leukemias and lymphomas are most sensitive. • For a full discussion, see entry for drug class (p. 602).

**CONTRAINDICATIONS**  • See entry for drug class (p. 603).

**DOSAGE   PO:   ADULTS:** Initially 5 to 60 mg daily divided into two or four doses after meals.  **CHILDREN:** 0.14 to 2 mg/kg or 4 to 60 mg/$M^2$ daily, divided into four doses.  *Special patient populations:* **PREGNANCY:** Use of this drug in pregnancy carries substantial risk to the fetus.

**PREPARATIONS**   *Tablets:* 1, 2.5, 5, 10, 20, 25, or 50 mg; *tablets, film-coated:* 5 or 50 mg; *oral solution:* 5 mg/ml concentrate or 5 mg/5 ml solution; *syrup:* 5 mg/5 ml.

**DRUG INTERACTIONS**  • See entry for drug class (p. 603).

**DIAGNOSTIC TEST INTERFERENCE**  • See entry for drug class (p. 603).

**FATE**   Prednisone is well absorbed following oral administration. The drug is activated by metabolism in the liver. The drug is ultimately eliminated by the action of different enzymes in the liver, which form inactive metabolites that are excreted in urine.

## ❦ NURSING CONSIDERATIONS
### Side effects, toxicities, and associated nursing actions
- See entry for drug class (p. 603).
### Nursing interventions related to drug administration
- See entry for drug class (p. 606).
### Patient and family education
- See entry for drug class (p. 606).

---

## triamcinolone    (tri-am-SIN-oh-lone)                           corticosteroid

- triamcinolone (triamcinolone acetonide, triamcinolone diacetate, triamcinolone hexaacetonide): Aristocrat (also see Preparations)

**MECHANISM OF ACTION**  • See entry for drug class (p. 598).

**INDICATIONS**    The immunosuppressive and anti-inflammatory effects of triamcinolone are useful for the following conditions: • Allergic states • Asthma • Dermatologic diseases • Rheumatoid diseases. • For a full discussion, see entry for drug class, (p. 602).

**CONTRAINDICATIONS**    • See entry for drug class (p. 603).

**DOSAGE    PO:    ADULTS:** Triamcinolone and triamcinolone diacetate, initially 4 to 48 mg daily, given as a single dose or divided into two to four equal doses.    **CHILDREN:** Triamcinolone and triamcinolone diacetate, 0.117 to 1.66 mg/kg or 3.3 to 50 mg/M$^2$ daily, divided into four equal doses.    **IM: ADULTS:** Triamcinolone diacetate, 40 mg once weekly. Triamcinolone acetonide, 60 mg once every 6 weeks, or when symptoms recur.    **CHILDREN OVER AGE 6:** Triamcinolone acetonide, 0.03 to 0.2 mg/kg or 1 to 6.25 mg/M$^2$ at 1 to 7 day intervals.    **IL:    ADULTS:** Triamcinolone diacetate—doses should not exceed 75 mg weekly. Triamcinolone acetonide—doses should not exceed 30 mg. Triamcinolone hexacetonide, 0.5 mg for each square inch of affected skin.    **IA, IS, ST:    ADULTS:** Triamcinolone diacetate, 2 to 40 mg, repeated at 1- to 8-week intervals. Triamcinolone acetonide, 2.5 to 40 mg to be repeated when symptoms recur. Triamcinolone hexacetonide, 2 to 20 mg to be repeated every 3 to 4 weeks.    **Inhalation:    ADULTS:** Triamcinolone acetonide, inhaler delivers 100 μg per spray. Initially two sprays three or four times daily may be used.    **CHILDREN OVER AGE 6:** Triamcinolone acetonide, inhaler delivers 100 μg per spray. Initially one or two sprays three or four times daily, not to exceed 120 μg daily.    **Topical:    ADULTS:** Triamcinolone acetonide—apply as thin film to affected area and rub in two to four times daily.    *Special patient populations:*    **CHILDREN:** Use in children under 6 years is to be avoided.    **PREGNANCY:** Use of this drug in pregnancy carries substantial risk to the fetus.

**PREPARATIONS**    **Triamcinolone** *Tablets:* 1, 2, 4, or 8 mg (Aristocort).    **Triamcinolone acetonide** *Oral inhalation:* 100 ug per metered spray of aerosol (Azmacort Oral Inhaler); *suspension for IM, IA, IS, IL, or ST use:* 10 or 40 mg/ml (Cenocort, Cinonide, Kenaject, Kenalog, Triam-A, Tiramonide, Trilog); *topical aerosol:* 0.2 mg per 2 second spray (Kenalog spray); *topical creams:* 0.025%, 0.1%, and 0.5% (Aristocort, Flutex, Kenalog, Triacet, Trymex); *topical lotions:* 0.025% or 0.1% (Kenalog); *topical ointments:* 0.025%, 0.1%, or 0.5% (Aristocort, Kenalog, Trymex); *topical paste:* 0.1% Kenalog in Orabase.    **Triamcinolone diacetate** *Oral solution:* 2 or 4 mg/5 ml (Aristocort, Kenacort); *suspension for IM, IA, IS, IL, or ST use:* 25 or 40 mg/ml (Amcort, Aristocort, Articulose LA, Cenocort, Cinalone, Triam-Forte, Triamolone, Trilone, Trisoject).    **Triamcinolone hexacetonide** *Suspension for IA or IL use:* 5 or 20 mg/ml (Aristospan).    **Combination products** *Topical cream:* 0.1% triamcinolone acetonide with nystatin 100,000 units/g (Mycobiotic II, Mycolog-II, Myco-Triacet II, Mytrex F, NGT, Nyst-olone II, Tri-Statin II); *topical ointment:* 0.1% triamcinolone acetonide with nystatin 100,000 units/g (Mycobiotic II, Mycolog II, Myco-Triacet II, Mytrex F, Nyst-olone II, Tri-Statin II).

**DRUG INTERACTIONS**    • See entry for drug class (p. 603).

**DIAGNOSTIC TEST INTERFERENCE**    • See entry for drug class (p. 603).

**FATE**    Triamcinolone or triamcinolone diacetate is adequately absorbed following oral administration. Other forms are slowly absorbed from various injection sites. The drug is metabolized in the liver and excreted in urine.

## ❦ NURSING CONSIDERATIONS

### Side effects, toxicities, and associated nursing actions
• See entry for drug class (p. 603).

### Nursing interventions related to drug administration
• Read orders and labels carefully to prepare doses for ordered routes of administration.
• See entry for drug class (p. 606).

### Patient and family education
• See entry for drug class (p. 606).

# Chapter Thirty-two

# Drugs affecting the female reproductive system

| | |
|---|---|
| **Estrogens** | **Progestins** |
| chlorotrianisene | ethynodiol diacetate (See Table 32-4, p. 640) |
| dienestrol | hydroxyprogesterone caproate |
| diethylstilbestrol | levonorgestrel (See Table 32-4, p. 640) |
| diethylstilbestrol diphosphate | medroxyprogesterone acetate |
| diethylstilbestrol diphosphate sodium | megestrol |
| esterified estrogens (see Estrone, p. 632) | norethindrone |
| estradiol | norethindrone acetate |
| estradiol cypionate | norethynodrel (See Table 32-4, p. 640) |
| estradiol valerate | norgestrel |
| estrogens, conjugated | progesterone |
| estrone | **Oral contraceptives** |
| estropipate (See Estrone, p. 632) | See Table 32-4, p. 640 |
| ethinyl estradiol (See Estradiol, p. 629) | |
| polyestradiol phosphate (See Estradiol, p. 629) | |

**INTRODUCTION**   Estrogens and progestins are potent hormones capable of widespread effects on the body. The ability of these compounds to modulate reproductive function allows their use in replacement therapy for a number of conditions caused by estrogen or progestin deficiency. Both classes of drugs are also used in palliative therapy of carcinomas of breast, prostate, kidney, and endometrium. The powerful actions of these drugs also create the potential for serious side effects, including cardiovascular, CNS, and reproductive reactions.

Estrogens and progestins are widely used in fixed combinations. Menopausal symptoms may occasionally be treated with combinations including estrogens with androgens (Chapter 33, Table 33-2, p. 650) or estrogens with meprobamate (see Conjugated Estrogens, p. 631). The most important combinations are those containing estrogens and progestins, which are used as oral contraceptives (Table 33-4, p. 640).

## Estrogens

chlorotrianisene ~ dienestrol ~ diethylstilbestrol ~ estradiol ~ estrogens, conjugated ~ esterified estrogens ~ estrone ~ estropipate

**OVERVIEW OF THE DRUG CLASS**   Estrogens include both natural steroids and synthetic compounds. Both types of compounds are used to replace natural estrogen function, to inhibit growth of certain tumors of reproductive tissues, or for contraception. Preparations differ mostly in oral bioavailability and duration of action.

**MECHANISM OF ACTION**   Estrogens interact with receptors within cells, eventually altering nucleic acid and protein synthesis by actions on the nucleus. The physiologic effects of estrogens include initiating development of female sex organs and maintaining secondary sex characteristics. Estrogens are required for development of breasts and adult female body contours. They promote bone growth and hasten closure of epiphyses. Estrogens also regulate onset of menstruation in mature women and influence secretion of gonadotropins.

**INDICATIONS**   **Estrogen deficiency** Primary ovarian failure, hypogonadism, or castration requires replacement of estrogens to relieve atrophic vaginitis, kraurosis valvae, or vasomotor symptoms of menopause. • Short-acting oral preparations may be appropriate.   **Carcinoma of the breast** Men or postmenopausal women with selected advanced tumors may receive relief of symptoms with estrogens. • Long-acting preparations may be appropriate.   **Prostatic carcinoma** Estrogens may be used along with chemotherapy and/or orchiectomy.

**CONTRAINDICATIONS**   **Asthma** These patients may be unable to tolerate fluid retention caused by estrogens. **Cardiovascular disease** These patients may be more sensitive to fluid retention and more at risk of thromboembolic complications.    **Hepatic insufficiency** These patients may be unable to tolerate fluid retention caused by estrogens.    **Hypercalcemia** Estrogens contribute to calcium retention, which may worsen hypercalcemia.    **Migraine** Fluid retention caused by estrogens may worsen episodes of migraine.    **Pregnancy** Estrogens administered to pregnant patients greatly increase risk of damage to the fetus.    **Renal insufficiency** These patients may be at increased risk of hypercalcemia.    **Seizure disorders** Fluid retention caused by estrogens may increase the likelihood of seizures.    **Thrombo-embolic diseases** Estrogens increase risk of thrombophlebitis and thromboembolic events; their use in patients with pre-existing related diseases constitutes unacceptable risk in most cases.

**DRUG INTERACTIONS**    **Anticoagulants** Oral anticoagulants may be less effective in patients also receiving estrogens. Doses of the anticoagulant may need to be increased.    **Barbiturates** Barbiturates induce liver microsomal enzymes that degrade estrogens, resulting in loss of estrogen effect. The combination should be avoided if possible.    **Carbamazepine** This drug may induce liver microsomal enzymes that degrade estrogens, resulting in loss of estrogen effect. The combination should be avoided if possible.    **Corticosteroids** Corticosteroids may be more effective in patients also receiving estrogens. Doses of the corticosteroid may need to be decreased.    **Phenylbutazone** This drug may induce liver microsomal enzymes that degrade estrogens, resulting in loss of estrogen effect. The combination should be avoided if possible.    **Phenytoin** This drug may induce liver microsomal enzymes that degrade estrogens, resulting in loss of estrogen effect. The combination should be avoided if possible. **Primidone** This drug may induce liver microsomal enzymes that degrade estrogens, resulting in loss of estrogen effect. The combination should be avoided if possible.

**DIAGNOSTIC TEST INTERFERENCE**    **Thyroid function tests** are altered by the estrogen-induced increase in thyroid-binding globulin. Total serum thyroxine is increased and triiodothyronine resin uptake is decreased without any evidence of actual changes in thyroid function.    **Metyrapone tests** may falsely suggest impaired adrenal function because corticosteroid-binding globulin concentrations are increased in serum.

**FATE**    Natural estrogens such as estradiol or estrone are inactivated by the GI tract and liver, which lowers oral absorption. Conjugated estrogens and nonsteroidal estrogens such as chlorotrianisene, dienestrol, and diethylstilbestrol are not inactivated in the same way and therefore are better absorbed orally. Absorption from IM sites may be delayed by forming esters or polymerizing the preparation. Metabolism is by the liver with excretion of metabolites principally in urine.

## 🐾 NURSING CONSIDERATIONS

### Side effects, toxicities, and associated nursing actions

**CNS** Depression, dizziness, changes in libido, migraine headache, or suicidal behavior may be precipitated by estrogen therapy.
- Assess for signs of depression: withdrawal, insomnia, anorexia, and lack of interest in personal appearance.
- Caution patients to avoid driving or operating hazardous equipment if dizziness occurs.
- Obtain a thorough health history before administering the drug. Consult with the physician before administering to patients with a history of depression, suicide attempts, or migraine headaches.
- Reinforce to patients the importance of notifying the physician if new signs or symptoms develop.
- Assess tactfully for changes in libido. Provide emotional support as needed.

**CV** Blood pressure may be elevated, becoming frankly hypertensive in some patients. Risk of thrombophlebitis, pulmonary embolism, stroke, myocardial infarction, subarachnoid hemorrhage, and other thromboembolitic disorders are elevated by estrogens. Fluid retention occurs in many patients.
- Obtain a history of any thromboembolitic problems before administering.
- Monitor blood pressure and pulse.
- Monitor weight and have patient monitor and record weight at home.
- Instruct patients to report leg pain, sudden onset of chest pain, shortness of breath, coughing up blood, dizziness, changes in vision or speech, or weakness or numbness of an arm or leg.

**Blood** Blood coagulation factors VII, VIII, IX, and X may increase, along with prothrombin.
- Monitor coagulation factors if indicated in specific patients.

**GI** Nausea is a common complaint. Abdominal cramps, bloating, changes in appetite, diarrhea,

vomiting, and weight change may occur.
- Instruct the patient to notify the physician if GI symptoms are severe or persistent.
- Instruct patients to take doses in the evening with a light, mild snack to decrease gastric irritation.

**Eye** Changes of corneal curvature may occur, making contact lenses difficult to wear.
- Warn patients about this potential problem, and instruct patients to consult with an ophthalmologist if trouble with contact lenses develops.

**Liver** Liver function tests may be altered. Hepatic porphyria may be exacerbated.
- Instruct patients to report the development of right upper quadrant abdominal pain, jaundice, fever, malaise, or change in the color or consistency of stools.
- Monitor liver function tests.

**Skin** Chloasma or melasma is the most common side effect. Hirsutism, alopecia, or erythema may occur.
- Instruct patients to report the development of skin changes. If the changes are severe, or intolerable to patient, the physician may change the drug or dose.

**Reproductive** Breakthrough bleeding, changes in menstrual flow, missed menses, or spotting may occur. Amenorrhea may follow use. Breast tenderness, enlargement, or secretions may occur.
- Assess for these problems.
- Instruct women to keep a record of menstrual periods and irregularities if they occur. Instruct the patient to notify the physician immediately if pregnancy is suspected.
- Teach the patient how to examine the breasts, and encourage patients to examine their breasts monthly.

**Metabolic** Glucose tolerance may be decreased. Serum triglycerides may increase.
- Instruct diabetic patients to monitor serum and urine glucose levels carefully, as an adjustment in insulin or diet may be necessary.
- Monitor serum glucose and triglyceride levels.

**Nursing interventions related to drug administration**
- Vaginal preparations should usually be applied at bedtime, if used once a day.
- Teach the patient to wear a sanitary napkin, rather than tampons, when vaginal medications are used.

**Patient and family education**
- Review anticipated benefits and possible drug side effects with patient.
- Instruct patients to report the development of any new sign or symptom.
- Remind patients to keep all health care providers informed of all medications being used.
- Note Drug Interactions. Caution patients to avoid the use of any medication that has not been first approved by the physician.
- Caution patients taking estrogens to stop smoking.
- Caution patients to take a missed dose as soon as remembered, unless it is almost time for the next scheduled dose, in which case the late dose should just be omitted. Patients should not double up to make up for missed doses.

## chlorotrianisene (kloh-ro-tri-AN-i-seen) estrogen

- chlorotrianisene: Tace

**MECHANISM OF ACTION** • See entry for drug class (p. 625).
**INDICATIONS** **Estrogen deficiency** Primary ovarian failure, hypogonadism, or castration requires replacement of estrogens to relieve atrophic vaginitis, kraurosis valvae, or vasomotor symptoms of menopause.
• Short-acting oral preparations may be appropriate. **Prostatic carcinoma** Estrogens may be used along with chemotherapy and/or orchiectomy.
**CONTRAINDICATIONS** • See entry for drug class (p. 625).
**DOSAGE** **PO:** **ADULTS:** 12 to 25 mg daily for 21 days, followed by 7 days without drug. Repeat as necessary, attempting at 3 to 6 month intervals to reduce or discontinue dosage. *Special patient populations:*

**CHILDREN:** Pediatric use has not been established.     **PREGNANCY:** FDA pregnancy category X.

**PREPARATIONS**     *Capsules:* 12, 25, or 72 mg (capsules contain tartrazine).

**DRUG INTERACTIONS**   • See entry for drug class (p. 626).

**DIAGNOSTIC TEST INTERFERENCE**   • See entry for drug class (p. 626).

**FATE**   • See entry for drug class (p. 626).

### ❦ NURSING CONSIDERATIONS

#### Side effects, toxicities, and associated nursing actions

**Allergy** Patients who are sensitive to aspirin may be more likely to suffer allergic reactions to the tartrazine contained in preparations of chlorotrianisene.

• For other side effects, see entry for drug class (p. 626).

#### Patient and family education

• See entry for drug class (p. 627).

---

## dienestrol   (dye-en-ES-trol)                                                      estrogen

• dienestrol: DV, Estraguard

**MECHANISM OF ACTION**   • See entry for drug class (p. 625).

**INDICATIONS**   **Atrophic vaginitis or kraurosis vulvae** These symptoms arising from estrogen deficiency may respond to topical estrogen.

**CONTRAINDICATIONS**   • See entry for drug class (p. 625).

**DOSAGE**   **Vaginally:**   **ADULTS:** 6 to 12 g of cream one or two full applicators daily for 1 to 2 weeks. Reduce by one-half and continue for 1 to 2 weeks. Maintenance doses are one full applicator one to three times weekly. Reduce dosage or discontinue when symptoms allow. *Special patient populations:* **CHILDREN:** Pediatric uses have not been established.   **PREGNANCY:** FDA pregnancy category X.

**PREPARATIONS**   *Vaginal cream:* 0.01%.

**DRUG INTERACTIONS**   • See entry for drug class (p. 626).

**DIAGNOSTIC TEST INTERFERENCE**   • See entry for drug class (p. 626).

**FATE**   Dienstrol can be absorbed through the vaginal mucosa, leading to systemic symptoms.

### ❦ NURSING CONSIDERATIONS

#### Side effects, toxicities, and associated nursing actions

• See entry for drug class (p. 626).

#### Nursing interventions related to drug administration

• Ascertain that patients can administer intravaginal doses correctly. Caution patients to use only in the amounts ordered. Caution patients not to use estrogen-containing creams as a lubricant during vaginal intercourse, as overdose may occur, and the male partner may suffer effects from the estrogen hormone.

#### Patient and family education

• See entry for drug class (p. 627).

---

## diethylstilbestrol   (dye-eth-ill-still-BES-trol)                                      estrogen

• diethylstilbestrol (diethylstilbestrol diphosphate, dethylstilbestrol diphosphate disodium): Stilphostrol

**MECHANISM OF ACTION**   • See entry for drug class (p. 625).

**INDICATIONS**   • See entry for drug class (p. 625).

**CONTRAINDICATIONS**   • See entry for drug class (p. 625).

**DOSAGE**   **PO:**   **ADULTS:** For estrogen replacement, 0.2 to 0.5 mg daily for 3 weeks, followed by 1 week without drug. Repeat cycles as necessary, making attempts every 3 to 6 months to reduce or discontinue therapy. For breast carcinoma, 15 mg daily for at least 3 months. For carcinoma of the prostate, 1 to 3 mg daily of diethylstilbestrol or 50 mg three times daily of diethylstilbestrol diphosphate. **IV: ADULTS:** For carcinoma of the prostate, diethylstilbestrol diphosphate disodium 0.5 g initially, then 1 g daily for 5 days. Maintenance is with 0.25 to 0.5 g by IV infusion once or twice weekly. *Special patient populations:* **CHILDREN:** Pediatric uses have not been established. **PREGNANCY:** FDA pregnancy category X.

**PREPARATIONS** Diethylstilbestrol *Tablets:* 1 to 5 mg; *tablets, enteric-coated:* 0.1, 1 or 5 mg. **Combinations with diethylstilbestrol** *Tablets:* 0.25 mg with methyltestosterone 5 mg. **Diethylstilbestrol diphosphate** *Tablets:* 50 mg. **Diethylstilbestrol diphosphate sodium** *Injection:* 50 mg/ml.

**DRUG INTERACTIONS** • See entry for drug class (p. 626).

**DIAGNOSTIC TEST INTERFERENCE** • See entry for drug class (p. 626).

**FATE** • See entry for drug class (p. 626).

## 🐾 NURSING CONSIDERATIONS

### Side effects, toxicities, and associated nursing actions

**Reproductive** Diethylstilbesterol has been associated with increased risk of cancers in reproductive tissues in offspring of women who received the drug during pregnancy. Thirty percent to 90% of female fetuses exposed in utero develop adenosis, and the risk of various cancers is increased. Risk of breast cancer is increased in adult females receiving the drug. Males exposed in utero have increased risk of genital abnormalities and low sperm counts.

• Caution women taking this drug to notify the physician immediately if pregnancy is suspected.

• See entry for drug class (p. 626).

### Nursing interventions related to drug administration

• For IV use, dilute dose in 300 ml of saline or dextrose for infusion. Infuse slowly for first few minutes (1 to 2 ml/min for 10 to 15 minutes) to monitor patient response, then increase rate to infuse ordered dose within 1 hour of starting infusion.

### Patient and family education

• See entry for drug class (p. 627).

---

## estradiol (es-tra-DYE-ol)                                   estrogen

• estradiol: estradiol cypionate, estradiol valerate, ethinyl estradiol, polyestradiol phosphate: Estrace (also see preparations)

**MECHANISM OF ACTION** • See entry for drug class (p. 625).

**INDICATIONS** • See Table 32-1; for a full discussion, see entry for drug class (p. 625).

**CONTRAINDICATIONS** • See entry for drug class (p. 625).

**DOSAGE** **PO:** **ADULTS:** *Estradiol:* For estrogen replacement, initial doses are 1 to 2 mg daily for 3 weeks followed by 1 week without drug. Repeat the cycle as necessary, attempting to reduce dosage or discontinue drug at 3 to 6 month intervals. For carcinoma of the breast, 10 mg three times daily for at least 3 months. For carcinoma of the prostate, 1 to 2 mg three times daily for at least 3 months. *Ethinyl estradiol:* For vasomotor symptoms of menopause 0.02 to 0.05 mg daily on a shedule alternating 3 weeks on and 1 week off drug; for estrogen replacement 0.05 one to three times daily for 2 weeks alternating with 2 weeks of progesterone therapy to attempt to induce menstruation; for breast carcinoma 1 mg three times daily for at least 3 months; for carcinoma of the prostate, 0.15 to 2 mg daily. **IM:** **ADULTS:** *Estradiol cypionate:* 1 to 5 mg once every 3 to 4 weeks for vasomotor symptoms of menopause; 1.5 to 2 mg once every month for replacement therapy. *Estradiol valerate:* 10 to 20 mg once every 4 weeks for vasomotor symptoms of menopause or estrogen replacement; 30 mg every 1 to 2 weeks for carcinoma of the prostate. *Polyestradiol phosphate:* 40 mg once every 2 to 4 weeks for carcinoma of the prostate. **Transdermal:** **ADULTS:** Estradiol, 0.05 mg daily in a transdermal sys-

| Table 32-1. | Summary of clinical uses of forms of estradiol | | | |
|---|---|---|---|---|
| Name | Estrogen replacement | Vasomotor symptoms of menopause | Breast carcinoma | Prostatic carcinoma |
| Estradiol | X | X | X | X |
| Estradiol cypionate | X | X | | |
| Estradiol valerate | X | X | | X |
| Ethinyl estradiol* | X | X | | X |
| Polyestradiol phosphate | | | | X |

*Ethinyl estradiol is also a component of oral contraceptives (Table 32-4, p. 640).

tem applied twice weekly on a schedule alternating 3 weeks on and 1 week off drug.   **Intravaginal:** ADULTS: Estradiol, 2 to 4 g of cream once daily for 1 to 2 weeks, then half the dose for an additional 1 to 2 weeks. Maintenance may be with 1 g one to three times weekly on a schedule alternating 3 weeks on and 1 week off drug.   *Special patient population:*   CHILDREN: Pediatric uses have not been established.   PREGNANCY: FDA pregnancy category X.

**PREPARATIONS**   **Estradiol** *Tablets:* 1 or 2 mg (Estrace); *topical transdermal system:* 0.05 mg/24 hours or 0.1 mg/24 hours (Estraderm); *vaginal cream:* 0.01% (Estrace).   **Estradiol cypionate** *Injection (in oil) for IM use:* 1 or 5 mg/ml (Depanate, depGynogen, Depo-Estradiol, Depogen, Dura-Estrin, E-Cypionate, Estro-Cyp, Estrofem, Estroject-LA, Estronol-LA, Hormogen Depot).   **Combination products with estradiol cypionate** *Injection (in oil) for IM use:* 2 mg/ml estradiol cypionate with 50 mg/ml testosterone cypionate (Andro/Fem, depAndrogyn, Depo-Testadiol, Depotestrogen, Duo-Cyp, Duratestrin, Menoject-LA).   **Estradiol valerate** *Injection (in oil) for IM use:* 10, 20, or 40 mg/ml (Delestrogen, Dioval, Duragen, Estradiol-LA, Estra-L, Feminate, Gynogen, Menaval, Valergen).   **Combination products with estradiol valerate** *Injection (in oil) for IM use:* 4 or 8 mg/ml estradiol valerate with 90 or 180 mg/ml testosterone enanthate (Androgyn-LA, Deladumone, Ditate, estra-Testrin, Teev, Testaval, Valertest).   **Ethinyl estradiol** *Tablets:* 0.02, 0.05, or 0.5 mg.   **Combination products with ethinyl estradiol** *Tablets:* 0.02 mg ethinyl estradiol with 1 mg fluoxymesterone • Also see listing for oral contraceptive agents in this chapter (Tablet 32-4, p. 640).   **Polyestradiol phosphate** Powder to be reconstituted for IM injection: 40 mg (Estradurin).

**DRUG INTERACTIONS**   • See entry for drug class (p. 626).

**DIAGNOSTIC TEST INTERFERENCE**   • See entry for drug class (p. 626).

**FATE**   Oral doses of estradiol are large to offset extensive metabolism in liver and the GI tract. Ethinyl estradiol is not readily metabolized and is used orally at smaller doses. Estradiol cypionate and estradiol valerate are esters designed to be slowly absorbed from IM sites, producing a long *duration* of action. Polyestradiol phosphate is a relatively insoluble form of estradiol that is also slowly absorbed from IM sites.

🦃 **NURSING CONSIDERATIONS**

**Side effects, toxicities, and associated nursing actions**

• See entry for drug class (p. 626).

**Nursing interventions related to drug administration**

• For IM administration of preparations in oil: Heat unopened vial in warm water for several minutes to decrease the viscosity of the oil. Vigorously agitate the ampule to resuspend the drug, which is usually an inconspicuous spot on the side of the vial. Resuspension is adequate when no particles of medication remain visible on the sides or bottom of the vial. Draw up the correct dose in a syringe fitted with a 19 to 21 gauge, 1½ inch needle. Administer immediately, before oil cools completely. Inject the medication2 inch needle. Administer immediately, before oil cools completely. Inject the medication with slow, even pressure. Attempts to inject too rapidly may cause the needle and syringe to separate, causing spilling of the medication and inaccurate dosage administration. Appropriate injection sites in adults include the buttocks, thigh, or ventrogluteal sites. Because the drug leaves palpable lumps at injection sites, avoid the deltoid muscles. Record and rotate injection sites. Oil-based preparations should never be given intravenously.

- Ascertain that patients can administer intravaginal doses correctly. Caution patients to use only in amounts ordered. Caution patients not to use estrogen-containing creams as a lubricant during vaginal intercourse, as overdose may occur and the male partner may suffer effects of the estrogen hormone.
- For transdermal administration, instruct the patient to apply a patch to a clean area, usually an inconspicuous place on the abdomen. Areas with excessive hair should be avoided. If the patch falls off, it should be replaced with a new one and the days of dosage administration readjusted. If severe skin irritation occurs, instruct the patient to notify the physician. Review with the patient the instruction leaflet supplied by the manufacturer.
- The following brands contain FD & C yellow dye number 5 (tartrazine) in the dosage listed. This dye may cause an allergic reaction in susceptible individuals. Although rare, this side effect is seen more commonly in persons with aspirin hypersensitivity: Estrace, 2 mg; Estinyl, 0.02 mg.

**Patient and family education**
- See entry for drug class (p. 627).

**Table 32-2.**

| Summary of clinical uses of estrogens | | | | | |
|---|---|---|---|---|---|
| Drug | Estrogen deficiency | Menopausal osteoporosis | Breast carcinoma | Prostatic carcinoma | Oral contraceptive |
| Chlorotrianisene | X | | | X | |
| Dienestrol | X | | | | |
| Diethylstilbestrol | X | | X | X | |
| Estradiol | X | | X | X | |
| Estradiol cypionate | X | | | | |
| Estradiol valerate | X | | | X | |
| Estrogens, conjugated | X | X | X | X | |
| Estrone | X | | | X | |
| Estropipate | X | | | | |
| Ethinyl estradiol | X | | X | X | X |
| Mestranol | | | | | |
| Polyestradiol | | | | X | |

## estrogens, conjugated (es-tro-jens KON-joo-ga-ted) estrogen

- estrogens, conjugated: Premarin, Progens

**MECHANISM OF ACTION**  Conjugated estrogens includes sodium salts of sulfate esters of estrone, equilin, or other estrogenic substances from pregnant mare's urine. The mechanism is as for other estrogens (see entry for drug class, p. 625).

**INDICATIONS**  **Uterine bleeding** When hormonal imbalance is involved, estrogen therapy may be a useful part of initial emergency treatment.  **Menopausal osteoporosis** Estrogens, along with proper diet, adequate calcium intake, and exercise, may slow bone loss in this age patient. Short-acting oral preparations may be appropriate. For other uses of conjugated estrogens, see entry for drug class (p. 625).

**CONTRAINDICATIONS**  • See entry for drug class (p. 625).

**DOSAGE**  **PO:**  **ADULTS:** For estrogen replacement, 0.3 to 1.25 mg daily usually on a schedule alternating 21 days with drug and 7 days without drug. For breast carcinoma, 10 mg three times daily for at least 3 months. For carcinoma of the prostate, 1.25 to 2.5 mg three times daily for at least 3 months.    **IM, IV:** **ADULTS:** For abnormal uterine bleeding, 25 mg as part of initial emergency treatment. Repeat at 6 to 12 hours if necessary.    **Intravaginal:**    **ADULTS:** For atrophic vaginitis or kraurosis vulvae, 2 to 4 g of vaginal cream applied once daily on a schedule alternating 21 days with drug and 7 days without drug. *Special patient populations:* **CHILDREN:** Pediatric uses have not been established. **PREGNANCY:** FDA pregnancy category X.

**PREPARATIONS**    *Tablets:* 0.3, 0.625, 0.9, 1.25, 2.5 mg; *powder for reconstitution:* 25 mg; *vaginal cream:* 0.0625%.    **Combination products with conjugated estrogens** 0.45 mg conjugated estrogens with 200 or 400 mg meprobamate (Milprem, PMB); 0.625 mg or 1.25 mg conjugated estrogens with 5 or 10 mg methyltestosterone (Premarin with methyltestosterone).

**DRUG INTERACTIONS** • See entry for drug class (p. 626).

**DIAGNOSTIC TEST INTERFERENCE** • See entry for drug class (p. 626).

   **FATE** • See entry for drug class (p. 626).

### ☙ NURSING CONSIDERATIONS

**Side effects, toxicities, and associated nursing actions**
- See entry for drug class (p. 626).

**Nursing interventions related to drug administration**
- Ascertain that patients can administer intravaginal doses correctly. Caution patients to use only in amounts ordered. Caution patients not to use estrogen-containing creams as a lubricant during vaginal intercourse, as overdose may occur, and the male partner may suffer effects of the estrogen hormone.
- For IV use, the drug may be given undiluted; administer slowly.

**Patient and family education**
- See entry for drug class (p. 627).

---

## estrone    (ES-trone)                      estrogen

- estrone, esterified estrogens, estropipate: Estratab, Menest, Ogen, Theelin

**MECHANISM OF ACTION** • See entry for drug class (p. 625).

**INDICATIONS** • See entry for drug class (p. 625).

**CONTRAINDICATIONS** • See entry for drug class (p. 625).

**DOSAGE**    **PO:**    **ADULTS:** For estrogen replacement with esterified estrogens, 0.3 to 7.5 mg daily, with dose depending on the severity of symptoms. The schedule usually alternates 21 days of therapy with 7 days off drug. For breast carcinoma, 10 mg three times daily for at least 3 months. For carincoma of the prostate, 1.25 to 2.5 mg one to three times daily for at least 3 months. For estrogen replacement with estropipate, 0.75 to 9 mg daily on a schedule that alternates 21 days with drug and 7 to 10 days without drug.    **IM:**    **ADULTS:** Estrone, for estrogen replacement, 0.1 to 1 mg two or three times weekly. For carcinoma of the prostate, 2 to 4 mg, two or three times weekly for at least 3 months. **Intravaginal:**    **ADULTS:** Estropipate, for atrophic vaginitis or kraurosis vulvae, 2 to 4 g of vaginal cream once daily on a schedule that alternates 21 days with drug and 7 days without drug.    *Special patient populations:*    **CHILDREN:** Pediatric uses have not been established.    **PREGNANCY:** FDA pregnancy category X.

**PREPARATIONS**    **Estrone** *Suspension for IM use:* 2 or 5 mg/ml (Estrogenic Substance, Estronol, Kestrone, Theelin Aqueous).    **Estropipate** *Tablets:* 0.75, 1.5, 3, or 6 mg (Ogen, Orapate); *vaginal cream:* 0.15%.    **Esterified estrogens** *Tablets:* 0.3, 0.625, 1.25, or 2.5 mg (Estratab, Menest).

**DRUG INTERACTIONS** • See entry for drug class (p. 626).

**DIAGNOSTIC TEST INTERFERENCE** • See entry for drug class (p. 626).

   **FATE**    See entry for drug class (p. 626).

### ☙ NURSING CONSIDERATIONS

**Side effects, toxicities, and associated nursing actions**
- See entry for drug class (p. 626).

**Nursing interventions related to drug administration**
- Ascertain that patients can administer intravaginal doses correctly. Caution patients to use only in amounts ordered. Caution patients not to use estrogen-containing creams as a lubricant during vaginal intercourse, as overdose may occur, and the male partner may suffer effects of the estrogen hormone.

**Patient and family education**
- See entry for drug class (p. 627).

# Progestins

ethynodiol diacetate (see Table 32-4) ~ hydroxyprogesterone caproate ~ levonorgestrel (see Table 32-4) ~ medroxyprogesterone acetate ~ megestrol ~ norethindrone ~ norethindrone acetate ~ norethynodrel (see Table 32-4) ~ norgestrel ~ progesterone

**OVERVIEW OF THE DRUG CLASS**    Progestins used in clinical situations include synthetic forms such as norethindrone and norgestrel, as well as the natural hormone, progesterone. Progestins are used alone for a variety of dysfunctions of reproductive tissues. Progestins are also used alone (Table 32-3, p. 638) or with estrogens as oral contraceptives (Table 32-4, p. 640).

**MECHANISM OF ACTION**    Progestins convert endometrium to the secretory phase, alter secretions in the vagina, and induce withdrawal bleeding in the presence of estrogen. These actions form the basis for the clinical uses of progestins. When used as contraceptives, progestins alter the endometrium to prevent normal implantation, alter the cervical mucus to lower the numbers of sperm entering the uterus, and may block ovulation in some patients. Other actions of progestins (relaxing uterine smooth muscle, stimulating growth of breast alveolar tissue, and increasing basal body temperature) may not be directly exploited in the clinical uses of these agents. The variable estrogenic, androgenic, or adrenocortical effects of progestins may contribute to side effects in certain patients.

**INDICATIONS**    **Amenorrhea** If the endometrium has been properly primed with estrogen, progestins may induce menstruation.    **Uterine bleeding** Hormonal imbalance may lead to a hyperplastic nonsecretory endometrium that bleeds abnormally; progestins may convert the endometrium to a more normal form and thus control bleeding.    **Carcinomas** Carcinomas of breast, prostate, kidney, or endometrium may respond to palliative therapy with progestins.    **Contraception** Alone or in combination with estrogens, progestins can prevent conception by a variety of mechanisms.

**CONTRAINDICATIONS**    **Asthma** These patients may be unable to tolerate fluid retention caused by progestins.    **Cardiovascular disease** These patients may be more sensitive to fluid retention and more at risk of thromboembolic complications.    **Hepatic insufficiency** These patients may be unable to metabolize progestins normally, and the drugs may accumulate.    **Migraine** Fluid retention caused by progestins may worsen episodes of migraine.    **Pregnancy** Progestins administered to pregnant patients greatly increase risk of damage to the fetus.    **Renal insufficiency** These patients may be unable to tolerate the fluid retention caused by progestins.    **Seizure disorders** Fluid retention caused by progestins may increase the likelihood of seizures.    **Thromboembolic diseases** Progestins increase risk of thrombophlebitis and thromboembolic events; their use in patients with pre-existing related diseases constitutes unacceptable risk in most cases.    **Undiagnosed vaginal bleeding** Progestins may worsen certain conditions leading to vaginal bleeding; they should be used only when hormonal imbalance is known to be the cause of symptoms.

**DRUG INTERACTIONS**    Most experience has been with oral contraceptives (p. 639).

**DIAGNOSTIC TEST INTERFERENCE**    Most experience has been with oral contraceptives (p. 642).

**FATE**    Oral absorption of synthetic progestins used in oral contraceptives is much higher than that of the natural hormone, progesterone. Bioavailability of these synthetic progestins ranges from 40% to 70% and is determined largely by rapid metabolism in the liver. Progestins may bind to plasma proteins. Free progestins distribute to many tissues and fluids, including bile and milk. Progestins are metabolized in the liver and excreted in urine and feces.

## ❦ NURSING CONSIDERATIONS

### Side effects, toxicities, and associated nursing actions

**CNS** Depression, dizziness, headache, nervousness, and fatigue may be observed.
- Assess for signs of depression: withdrawal, insomnia, anorexia, lack of interest in personal appearance.
- Caution patients to avoid driving or operating hazardous equipment if dizziness occurs.
- Obtain a thorough health history before administering the drug. Consult with the physician before administering to patients with a history of depression or suicide attempts.
- Reinforce to patients the importance of notifying the physician if new signs or symptoms develop.

**CV** Fluid retention may occur, leading to edema. Risk of thrombophlebitis and other embolic diseases is increased by progestins.
- Obtain history of any thromboembolitic problems before administering.
- Monitor blood pressure and pulse.
- Monitor weight, and have patient monitor and record weight at home.
- Instruct patients to report leg pain, sudden onset of chest pain, shortness of breath, coughing up blood, headache, dizziness, changes in vision or speech, or weakness or numbness of an arm or leg.

**Blood** Coagulation factors VII, VIII, IX, and X may be increased.
- Monitor coagulation factors if indicated in specific patients.

**GI** Weight gain, weight loss, or changes in appetite may occur.
- Monitor weight.
- Instruct patients to take doses in the evening with a light, mild snack to decrease gastric irritation.

**Eye** Optic neuritis, retinal thrombosis, and other eye changes have been reported.
- Instruct patients to notify the physician of any changes in eyes or vision.

**Allergic** Allergic rash or pruritis can occur.
- Instruct patients to report the development of any skin irritation or problem.

**Skin** Chloasma, melasma, baldness, hirsutism, erythema multiforme, erythema nodosum, hemorrhagic skin eruption, or itching may occur.
- Instruct patients to report the development of skin changes. If these changes are severe, or intolerable to patient, the physician may change drug or dose.

**Reproductive** Amenorrhea, breakthrough bleeding, cervical erosion, changes in secretions, changes in menstrual flow, and spotting have been reported.
- Assess for these problems.
- Instruct women to keep a record of menstrual periods and irregularities if they occur. Instruct the patient to notify the physician immediately if pregnancy is suspected.
- Teach the patient how to examine breasts, and encourage patients to perform self breast exam monthly.

### Patient and family education
- Review anticipated benefits and possible side effects of drug therapy.
- Instruct patients to report the development of any new sign or symptom.
- Remind patients to keep all health care providers informed of all medications being used.
- Note Drug Interactions. Caution patients to avoid the use of any medication that has not been first approved by the physician.
- Caution patients to avoid smoking.
- Caution patients to take a missed dose as soon as remembered, unless it is almost time for the next scheduled dose, in which case the late dose should be omitted. Patients should not double-up to make up for a missed dose.

---

## ethynodiol diacetate    (eh-thy-no-DYE-ol)                              progestin

- ethynodiol: Demulen, Ovulen (see Table 32-4)

**MECHANISM OF ACTION** • See Overview of Oral Contraceptives (p. 639).

**INDICATIONS** Oral contraception This progestin is used only as a component of oral contraceptives (Table 32-4, p. 640).

**CONTRAINDICATIONS** • See Overview of Oral Contraceptives (p. 639).

**DOSAGE** PO: ADULTS: See Table 32-4 (p. 640). *Special patient populations:* CHILDREN: Pediatric uses have not been established. PREGNANCY: FDA pregnancy category X.

**PREPARATIONS** • See Table 32-4 (p. 640). For other information on ethynodiol diacetate, see Overview of Oral Contraceptives (p. 639).

## hydroxyprogesterone caproate
(hy-drox-ee-pro-JES-ter-one KAP-ro-ate) progestin

• hydroxyprogesterone caproate: Duralutin, Gesterol, Hylutin, Hypogest

**MECHANISM OF ACTION** Hydroxyprogesterone caproate shares the action of other natural progestins but also possess estrogenic, androgenic, and adrenocorticoid activity. • See entry for drug class (p. 633).

**INDICATIONS** • See Table 32-3 (p. 638).

**CONTRAINDICATIONS** • See entry for drug class (p. 633).

**DOSAGE** IM: ADULTS: For amenorrhea and uterine bleeding, 375 mg as a single dose at 4 week intervals as necessary. For endometrial carcinoma, 1 g as a single dose once a week or more often; the maximum dose is 7 g weekly. Discontinue after 12 weeks if a response is not seen. *Special patient populations:* CHILDREN: Pediatric uses have not been established. PREGNANCY: FDA pregnancy category X.

**PREPARATIONS** Solution for IM injection: 125 or 250 mg/ml in castor oil with benzyl benzoate and benzyl alcohol.

**DRUG INTERACTIONS** • See entry for drug class (p. 639).

**DIAGNOSTIC TEST INTERFERENCE** • See entry for drug class (p. 642).

**FATE** Hydroxyprogesterone is a natural progestin from the adrenal glands. As the caproate ester, the compound is a more potent progestin than progesterone and has a longer *duration* of action. See entry for drug class (p. 633).

### ✿ NURSING CONSIDERATIONS

#### Side effects, toxicities, and associated nursing actions
• See entry for drug class (p. 634).

#### Nursing interventions related to drug administration
• See entry for drug class (p. 634).

#### Patient and family education
• See entry for drug class (p. 634).

## levonorgestrel (lee-vo-nor-JES-trel) progestin

• levonorgestrel: Leven, Nordette, Tri-leven, Triphasil (see Table 32-4)

**MECHANISM OF ACTION** • See Overview of Oral Contraceptives (p. 639).

**INDICATIONS** Oral contraception This progestin is used only as a component of oral contraceptives (Table 32-4).

**CONTRAINDICATIONS** • See Overview of Oral Contraceptives (p. 639).

**DOSAGE** PO: ADULTS: See Table 32-4 (p. 640). *Special patient populations:* CHILDREN: Pediatric uses have not been established. PREGNANCY: FDA pregnancy category X.

**PREPARATIONS**   • See Table 32-4 (p. 640).• For other information on levonorgestrel, see Overview of Oral Contraceptives (p. 640).

## medroxyprogesterone acetate   (meh-droxy-pro-JES-ter-one)                     progestin

- medroxyprogesterone acetate: Amen, Curretab, Provera

**MECHANISM OF ACTION**   Medroxyprogesterone acetate is a synthetic progestin with adrenocorticoid, androgenic, and anabolic activity but little estrogenic activity. See entry for drug class (p. 633).

**INDICATIONS**   **Amenorrhea or uterine bleeding** Medroxyprogesterone acetate is used as other progestins for these conditions. • See entry for drug class (p. 633).   **Renal or endometrial carcinoma** Medroxyprogesterone acetate may be used in palliative treatment of advanced disease.

**CONTRAINDICATIONS**   • See entry for drug class (p. 633).

**DOSAGE**   **PO:**   **ADULTS:** For amenorrhea or uterine bleeding, 5 to 10 mg for 5 to 10 days. Estrogen therapy may be needed to prepare the endometrium for a successful response to progestins.   **IM:**   **ADULTS:** For carcinoma, 400 to 1000 mg/week.   *Special patient populations:*   **CHILDREN:** Pediatric uses have not been established.   **PREGNANCY:** FDA pregnancy category X.

**PREPARATIONS**   *Tablets:* 2.5, 5, or 10 mg; *suspension for IM use: 100 or 400 mg/ml (Depo-Provera).*

**DRUG INTERACTIONS**   • See entry for drug class (p. 639).

**DIAGNOSTIC TEST INTERFERENCE**   • See entry for drug class (p. 642).

**FATE**   • See entry for drug class (p. 633).

### ☙ NURSING CONSIDERATIONS

#### Side effects, toxicities, and associated nursing actions
- See entry for drug class (p. 634).

#### Patient and family education
- See entry for drug class (p. 634).

## megestrol acetate   (meh-GES-trol)                     progestin

- megestrol acetate: Megace

**MECHANISM OF ACTION**   Megestrol acetate is a synthetic progestin used only for palliative management of advanced carcinoma of the breast. For a full discussion, see listing in Chapter 28 (p. 543).

## norethindrone   (nor-ETH-in-drone)                     progestin

- norethindrone (norethindrone acetate): Aygestin, Norlutate, Norlutin

**MECHANISM OF ACTION**   • See entry for drug class (p. 633).

**INDICATIONS**   • See Tables 32-3 (p. 638) and 32-4 (p. 640).

**CONTRAINDICATIONS**   • See entry for drug class (p. 633).

**DOSAGE**   **PO:**   **ADULTS:** *For amenorrhea or uterine bleeding,* 5 to 20 mg daily of norethindrone or 2.5 to 10 mg daily of norethindrone acetate administered from the fifth to the twenty-fifth day of the menstrual cycle. If estrogen priming is required, norethindrone acetate may be given for 5 to 10 days during the presumed last half of the menstrual cycle to induce menstruation. *For endometriosis,* initial doses are

10 mg daily for norethindrone or 5 mg daily for norethindrone acetate. These doses continue for 14 days and are then increased in 5 or 2.5 mg increments every 14 days up to maximal doses of 30 mg daily of norethindrone or 15 mg daily of norethindrone acetate. Therapy for this condition is continuous for 6 to 9 months. *As an oral contraceptive,* 0.35 mg daily continuously so long as contraception is desired (Table 32-4, p. 640). *Special patient populations:* CHILDREN: Pediatric uses have not been established. PREGNANCY: FDA pregnancy category X.

**PREPARATIONS** Norethindrone *Tablets:* 5 mg or 0.35 mg (for use as an oral contraceptive; see Table 32-4, p. 640). Norethindrone acetate *Tablets:* 5 mg.

**DRUG INTERACTIONS** • See entry for drug class (p. 639).

**DIAGNOSTIC TEST INTERFERENCE** • See entry for drug class (p. 642).

**FATE** Oral administration of norethindrone is adequate. Bioavailability is about 65% of an oral dose. Norethindrone acetate is more efficiently absorbed into the bloodstream and hence requires lower doses than does norethindrone. Norethindrone distributes well in many tissues and fluids. Concentrations in milk are about 10% of serum concentrations. Norethindrone acetate is rapidly converted to norethindrone in the body. Norethindrone is metabolized in the liver and excreted primarily in urine. The elimination *half-life* is 5 to 14 hours.

**✿ NURSING CONSIDERATIONS**

**Side effects, toxicities, and associated nursing actions**
• See entry for drug class (p. 642).

**Patient and family education**
• See entry for drug class (p. 643).

## norethynodrel (ner-eh-THIN-oh-drel) progestin

• norethynodrel: Enovid (see Table 32-4)

**MECHANISM OF ACTION** • See Overview of Oral Contraceptives (p. 639).

**INDICATIONS** Oral contraception This progestin is used only as a component of oral contraceptives (Table 32-4, p. 640).

**CONTRAINDICATIONS** • See Overview of Oral Contraceptives (p. 639).

**DOSAGE** PO: ADULTS: See Table 32-4 (p. 640). *Special patient populations:* CHILDREN: Pediatric uses have not been established. PREGNANCY: FDA pregnancy category X.

**PREPARATIONS** • See Table 32-4 (p. 640). • For other information on norethynodrel, see Overview of Oral Contraceptives (p. 639).

## norgestrel (nor-GES-trel) progestin

• norgestrel: Lo/Ovral, Ovral

**MECHANISM OF ACTION** Norgestrel is the progestin component in a number of oral contraceptive agents. For a full discussion, see Overview of Oral Contraceptives (p. 639).

**INDICATIONS** Contraception Norgestrel alone or in combination with estrogens may prevent conception (p. 639).

**CONTRAINDICATIONS** • See entry for drug class (p. 639).

**DOSAGE** PO: ADULTS: For norgestrel alone, 0.075 mg daily throughout the time protection from conception is required. For norgestrel in combinations with estrogens, see Oral Contraceptives (p. 640). *Special patient populations:* CHILDREN: Pediatric uses have not been established. PREGNANCY: FDA pregnancy category X.

**PREPARATIONS** *Tablets:* 0.075 mg. • For combinations with estrogens, see Table 32-4 (p. 640).

**DIAGNOSTIC TEST INTERFERENCE**   • See entry for drug class (p. 642).
> **FATE**   • See entry for drug class (p. 642).

☙ **NURSING CONSIDERATIONS**
> **Side effects, toxicities, and associated nursing actions**
>> • See entry for drug class (p. 642).
>
> **Patient and family education**
>> • See entry for drug class (p. 643).

---

## progesterone   (pro-JES-ter-one)                                    progestin

> • progesterone: Gesterol, Progestoject, Progestronaq-LA

**MECHANISM OF ACTION**   • See entry for drug class (p. 633).
**INDICATIONS**   **Amenorrhea** Amenorrhea caused by hormonal imbalance may respond to progestins.   **Uterine bleeding** Bleeding caused by hormonal imbalance may be halted by progestins.
**CONTRAINDICATIONS**   • See entry for drug class (p. 633).
**DOSAGE**   **IM:**   ADULTS: For amenorrhea, 5 to 10 mg daily for 6 to 8 days. Treatment usually starts 8 to 10 days before anticipated start of menstruation; withdrawal of progestin facilitates induction of menstruation. For uterine bleeding, 5 to 10 mg daily for 6 days. Estrogen therapy may precede progestin administration.   *Special patient populations:*   CHILDREN: Pediatric uses are not established.   PREGNANCY: FDA pregnancy category X.
**PREPARATIONS**   *Solution for IM use:* 50 mg/ml.
**DRUG INTERACTIONS**   • See entry for drug class (p. 639).
**DIAGNOSTIC TEST INTERFERENCE**   • See entry for drug class (p. 642).
> **FATE**   • See entry for drug class (p. 633).

☙ **NURSING CONSIDERATIONS**
> **Side effects, toxicities, and associated nursing actions**
>> • See entry for drug class (p. 634).
>
> **Patient and family education**
>> • See entry for drug class (p. 634).

---

**Table 32-3.**   **Summary of clinical uses of progestins**

| Drug | Amenor-rhea | Uterine bleeding | Oral contra-ceptive | Endo-metrial carcin-oma | Breast carcin-oma | Endo-metriosis |
|------|-------------|------------------|---------------------|-------------------------|-------------------|----------------|
| Ethynodiol diacetate | | | x | | | |
| Hydroxyprogesterone | x | x | | x | | |
| Levonorgestrel | | | x | | | |
| Medroxyprogesterone | x | x | | x | | |
| Megestrol | | | | | x | |
| Norethindrone | x | x | x | | | x |
| Norethynodrel | | | x | | | |
| Norgestrel | | | x | | | |
| Progesterone | x | x | | | | |

# Oral contraceptives

Brevicon ~ Demulen ~ Enovid ~ Genora ~ Leven ~ Loestrin ~ Lo/Ovral ~ Micronor ~ Modicon ~ Nordette ~ Norinyl ~ Norlestrin ~ Nor-Q.D. ~ Ortho-Novum ~ Ovcon ~ Ovral ~ Ovrette ~ Ovulen ~ Tri-Norinyl

**OVERVIEW OF THE DRUG CLASS**   Oral contraceptive agents include progestins alone and progestins in various combinations with estrogens. Progestins used alone for contraception are administered continuously. Combination products are administered on various schedules. Most combinations are administered on a schedule alternating 21 days on drug with 7 days off drug. Biphasic combinations use low-dose estrogen with low-dose progestin for 10 days, then higher-dose progestin for 11 days, followed by 7 days without drug. Triphasic combinations may vary the progestin dosage or both the estrogen and progestin dosage during the cycle (Table 32-4, p. 640).

**MECHANISM OF ACTION**   Oral contraceptives containing estrogens suppress the LH surge at midcycle, which is the primary trigger for ovulation. By these hormonal changes, ovulation is prevented. Progestins are less likely to prevent ovulation but have other actions that may prevent conception. Progestins change the endrometrium in ways that make implantation of an ovum unlikely. Progestins also alter cervical mucus, preventing normal entry of sperm into the uterus.

**INDICATIONS**   **Prevention of pregnancy** Women under age 40 who elect to use oral contraceptives should be made aware of the risks as well as the reliability of these agents.

**CONTRAINDICATIONS**   **Asthma** These patients may be unable to tolerate fluid retention caused by estrogens and progestins.   **Cardiovascular disease** These patients may be more sensitive to fluid retention and more at risk of thromboembolic complications.   **Cerebrovascular or coronary artery disease** These patients may be more at risk for strokes or myocardial infarction when receiving oral contraceptives.   **Hepatic disease** These patients may be unable to metabolize estrogens or progestins normally. Risk of liver tumor is increased in patients receiving oral contraceptives.   **Hypertension** Many patients receiving oral contraceptives experience an increase in blood pressure, which can be harmful in patients who are already hypertensive.   **Migraine** Fluid retention caused by oral contraceptives may worsen episodes of migraine.   **Ophthalmic vascular disease** Oral contraceptives may worsen this condition.   **Pregnancy** Oral contraceptives administered to pregnant patients greatly increase the risk of damage to the fetus.   **Renal insufficiency** These patients may be unable to tolerate fluid retention caused by oral contraceptives.   **Seizure disorders** Fluid retention caused by progestins and estrogens may increase the likelihood of seizures.   **Smoking** Heavy smoking greatly increases the risk of cardiovascular complications with oral contraceptives; patients should be counseled to stop smoking, at least while receiving these agents.   **Thromboembolic diseases** Oral contraceptives increase the risk of thrombophlebitis and thromboembolic events; their use in patients with pre-existing related diseases constitutes unacceptable risk in most cases.   **Undiagnosed vaginal bleeding** Oral contraceptives may worsen certain conditions, leading to vaginal bleeding.

**DRUG INTERACTIONS**   **Antibiotics** Several classes of antibiotics may disrupt GI flora and thereby inhibit bacterial release of active steroids from oral contraceptive preparations. Without the normal bacterial action to release active drug, oral contraceptive action may be reduced.   **Anticoagulants** Oral anticoagulants may be less effective in patients also receiving oral contraceptives; doses of the anticoagulant may need to be increased.   **Barbiturates** Barbiturates induce liver microsomal enzymes that degrade estrogens and progestins, resulting in loss of oral contraceptive effect; the combination should be avoided if possible.   **Benzodiazepines** Benzodiazepines are metabolized by the liver. Metabolism of individual members of this class may be inhibited or enhanced by oral contraceptive agents; dosage may have to be carefully monitored.   **Carbamazepine** This drug may induce liver microsomal enzymes that degrade estrogens and progestins, resulting in loss of oral contraceptive effect; the combination should be avoided if possible.   **Corticosteroids** Corticosteroids may be more effective in patients also receiving oral contraceptives; doses of the corticosteroid may need to be decreased.   **Metoprolol** Oral contraceptives may slow elimination of this beta-adrenergic receptor blocker; doses

Table 32-4.

## Clinical summary of oral contraceptive agents

| Progestin | Estrogen | Tablet content progestin/estrogen | Trade name | Monthly dosage |
|---|---|---|---|---|
| Ethynodiol diacetate | Ethinyl estradiol | 1 mg/35 µg | Demulen 1/35 | One tablet daily for 21 days, then 7 days with no drug |
| | | 1 mg/50 µg | Demulen 1/50 | One tablet daily for 21 days, then 7 days with no drug |
| Ethynodiol diacetate | Mestranol | 1 mg/100 µg | Ovulen | One tablet daily for 21 days, then 7 days with no drug |
| Levonorgestrel | Ethinyl estradiol | 0.15 mg/30 µg | Leven, Nordette | One tablet daily for 21 days, then 7 days with no drug |
| Levonorgestrel | Ethinyl estradiol | 0.05 mg/30 µg, 0.075 mg/40 µg, 0.125 mg/30 µg | Tri-leven, Triphasil | One tablet, 0.05 mg/30 µg, daily for 6 days then one tablet, 0.075 mg/40, µg daily for 5 days, followed by one tablet, 0.125 mg/30 µg, daily for 10 days; no drug for last 7 days |
| Norethindrone | — | 0.35 mg | Micronor, Nor-Q.D. | One tablet daily as long as contraception is desired |
| Norethindrone | Ethinyl estradiol | 0.4 mg/35 µg | Ovcon 35 | One tablet daily for 21 days, then 7 days with no drug |
| Norethindrone | Ethinyl estradiol | 0.5 mg/35 µg | Brevicon, Modicon | One tablet daily for 21 days, then 7 days with no drug. |
| Norethindrone | Ethinyl estradiol | 1 mg/35 µg | Genora 1/35, Norinyl 1 + 35, Ortho-Novum 1/35 | One tablet daily for 21 days, then 7 days with no drug |
| Norethindrone | Ethinyl estradiol | 1 mg/50 µg | Ovcon 50 | One tablet daily for 21 days, then 7 days with no drug |
| Norethindrone | Ethinyl estradiol | 0.5 mg/35 µg, 1 mg/35 µg | Ortho-Novum 10/11 | One 0.5 mg/35 µg tablet daily for 10 days, then one 1 mg/35 µg tablet daily for 11 days, followed by 7 days with no drug |
| Norethindrone | Ethinyl estradiol | 0.5 mg/35 µg, 0.75 mg/35 µg, 1 mg/35 µg | Ortho-Novum 7/7/7 | One 0.5 mg/35 µg tablet daily for 7 days, then one 0.75 mg/35 µg tablet daily for 7 days, then one 1 mg/35 µg tablet daily for 7 days followed by 7 days with no drug |

| Progestin | Estrogen | Amount | Trade name | Dosage schedule |
|---|---|---|---|---|
| Norethindrone | Ethinyl estradiol | 0.5 mg/35 µg, 1 mg/35 µg, 0.5 mg/35 µg | Tri-Norinyl | One 0.5 mg/35 µg tablet daily for 7 days, then one 1 mg/35 µg daily for 9 days, then one 0.5 mg/35 µg daily for 5 days followed by 7 days with no drug |
| Norethindrone | Mestranol | 1 mg/50 µg | Genora 1/50, Norinyl 1 + 50, Ortho-Novum 1/50 | One tablet daily for 21 days, then 7 days with no drug |
| Norethindrone | Mestranol | 1 mg/80 µg | Norinyl 1 + 80, Ortho-Novum 1/80 | One tablet daily for 21 days, then 7 days with no drug |
| Norethindrone | Mestranol | 2 mg/100 µg | Norinyl 2 mg, Ortho-Novum 2 mg | One tablet daily for 21 days, then 7 days with no drug |
| Norethindrone acetate | Ethinyl estradiol | 1 mg/20 µg | Loestrin 1/20 | One tablet daily for 21 days, then 7 days with no drug |
| Norethindrone acetate | Ethinyl estradiol | 1.5 mg/30 µg | Loestrin 1.5/30 | One tablet daily for 21 days, then 7 days with no drug |
| Norethindrone acetate | Ethinyl estradiol | 1 mg/50 µg | Norlestrin 1/50 | One tablet daily for 21 days, then 7 days with no drug |
| Norethindrone acetate | Ethinyl estradiol | 2.5 mg/50 µg | Norlestrin 2.5/50 | One tablet daily for 21 days, then 7 days with no drug |
| Norethynodrel | Mestranol | 5 mg/75 µg | Enovid 5 mg | One tablet daily for 21 days, then 7 days with no drug |
| Norethynodrel | Mestranol | 2.5 mg/100 µg | Enovid-E | One tablet daily for 21 days, then 7 days with no drug |
| Norethynodrel | Mestranol | 9.85 mg/150 µg | Enovid 10 mg | One tablet daily for 21 days, then 7 days with no drug |
| Norgestrel | — | 0.075 mg | Ovrette | One tablet daily for as long as contraception is desired |
| Norgestrel | Ethinyl estradiol | 0.3 mg/30 µg | Lo/Ovral | One tablet daily for 21 days, then 7 days with no drug |

may need to be reduced. **Phenylbutazone** This drug may induce liver microsomal enzymes that degrade estrogens and progestins, resulting in loss of oral contraceptive effect; the combination should be avoided if possible. **Phenytoin** This drug may induce liver microsomal enzymes that degrade estrogens and progestins, resulting in loss of oral contraceptive effect; the combination should be avoided if possible. **Primidone** This drug may induce liver microsomal enzymes that degrade estrogens and progestins, resulting in loss of oral contraceptive effect; the combination should be avoided if possible.

**DIAGNOSTIC TEST INTERFERENCE** **Thyroid function tests** are altered by the estrogen-induced increase in thyroid-binding globulin. Total serum thyroxine is increased and triiodothyronine resin uptake is decreased without any evidence of actual changes in thyroid function. **Metyrapone tests** may falsely suggest impaired adrenal function because corticosteroid-binding globulin concentrations are increased in serum.

**FATE** The active components of oral contraceptives are generally well absorbed, but bioavailability may vary considerably. Some of the agents are metabolized in the GI mucosa as well as on first pass through the liver. The drugs distribute into body fluids, including bile and milk. *Elimination* is primarily by metabolism in the liver. Some drugs undergo enterohepatic circulation. Excretion of intact drug and metabolites is in urine and feces.

---

## ❦ NURSING CONSIDERATIONS

### Side effects, toxicities, and associated nursing actions

**CNS** Aggressiveness, anxiety, depression, dizziness, headache, irritability, nervousness, and fatigue may be observed. Severe depression has led to suicide.

- Assess for signs of depression: withdrawal, insomnia, anorexia, and lack of interest in personal appearance.
- Caution patients to avoid driving or operating hazardous equipment if dizziness occurs.
- Obtain a thorough health history before administering the drug. Consult with the physician before administering to patients with a history of depression or suicide attempts.
- Reinforce to patients the importance of notifying the physician if new signs or symptoms develop.
- Obtain a careful baseline assessment of mental status and affect and repeat regularly.

**CV** Fluid retention may occur, leading to edema. Risk of thrombophlebitis and other embolic diseases is increased by progestins. Stroke and myocardial infarction are increased. Blood pressure is also increased in many patients.

- Obtain a history of any thromboembolic problems before administering.
- Monitor blood pressure and pulse. Inspect the patient for edema.
- Monitor weight and have the patient monitor and record weight at home.
- Instruct patients to report leg pain, sudden onset of chest pain, shortness of breath, coughing up blood, headache, dizziness, changes in vision or speech, or weakness or numbness of an arm or leg.

**Blood** Blood coagulation factors II, VII, VIII, IX, X, XII, and fibrinogen may be increased. Antithrombin III may fall.

- Monitor coagulation factors if indicated in specific patients.

**GI** Nausea is the most frequent side effect of oral contraceptives. Weight gain, weight loss, or changes in appetite may also occur. Oral absorption of folates may be reduced, creating the potential for folate deficiency.

- Instruct the patient to notify the physician if GI symptoms are severe or persistent.
- Instruct patients to take doses in the evening with a light, mild snack to decrease gastric irritation.
- Assess for folic acid deficiency: fatigue, pallor, nausea, anorexia, dyspnea, palpitations, and tachycardia.
- Monitor serum folate levels.
- Encourage a diet high in sources of folic acid: liver and lean meats, milk, eggs, leafy vegetables, bananas, oranges, beans, and whole wheat bread.

**Eye** Optic neuritis, retinal thrombosis, and other eye changes have been reported.

- Instruct patients to notify the physician about any eye problems or changes in vision.

**Liver** Liver function tests may be altered. Cholestatic jaundice may also occur. The risk of developing noncancerous hepatic adenomas is greatly increased in long-term users of oral contraceptives.

- Instruct patients to report the development of right upper quadrant abdominal pain, jaundice, fever, malaise, and change in the color or consistency of stools.
- Monitor liver function tests.

**Skin** Chloasma and melasma are the most common skin changes caused by oral contraceptives. Baldness, hirsutism, erythema multiforme, erythema nodosum, hemorrhagic skin eruption, or itching may also occur.

- Instruct patients to report the development of skin changes. If these changes are severe, or intolerable to patient, the physician may change the drug or dose.

**Reproductive** Amenorrhea, breakthrough bleeding, cervical erosion, changes in secretions, changes in menstrual flow, and spotting have all been reported. Breast tenderness may also occur.

- Assess for these problems.
- Instruct women to keep a record of menstrual periods and irregularities if they occur. Instruct the patient to notify the physician immediately if pregnancy is suspected.
- Teach the patient how to examine breasts, and encourage patients to examine their breasts monthly.

**Endocrine** Glucose tolerance may be decreased. Plasma triglyceride, low-density lipoprotein (LDL), and phospholipid levels may increase. Serum proteins such as albumin and thyroxine-binding globulin may be increased.

- Instruct diabetic patients to monitor blood and urine glucose frequently when initiating therapy or changing dose or brand; an adjustment in diet or insulin dose may be necessary.
- Monitor triglycerides and lipoproteins and other serum tests as needed.

**Other** Gallbladder disease is increased in young women using oral contraceptives. Systemic lupus erythematosus may be precipitated in some women, especially those with a history of this condition.

- Instruct patients to report the development of signs and symptoms that may indicate gallbladder disease: anorexia, vomiting, right upper quadrant abdominal pain, fever, and mild jaundice.

## Patient and family education

- Review anticipated benefits and possible side effects of drug therapy with patient.
- Instruct the patient to report the development of any new sign or symptom.
- Remind patients to keep all health care providers informed of all medications being used.
- Note Drug Interactions. Caution patients to avoid the use of any medication that has not been first approved by the physician.
- Caution patients to avoid smoking.
- Teach the patient to use a back-up form of birth control during the first week of the first cycle of therapy.
- Instruct the patient to take the pill at the same time each day.
- Instruct patients that missed dose should be taken as soon as she remembers it. If two consecutive pills are missed, the patient should double up on each of the next 2 days, then resume her regular schedule, but use additional contraceptive measures until she completes that cycle. If three or more consecutive tablets are missed, the patient should stop the pills for 7 days after the first missed tablet, then begin a new cycle of tablets. She should also use additional contraceptive measures from the time the missed tablets are noticed until 7 days after the new course of therapy is started.
- Caution patients that anovulation and amenorrhea may persist for as long as 6 months after oral contraceptive therapy has been discontinued.
- If a woman discontinues therapy in order to become pregnant, caution her to use alternate methods of birth control for at least 2 months to allow for more complete excretion of the hormones in the oral contraceptives.
- Remind patients to keep these and all medications out of the reach of children.

Chapter Thirty-three

# Drugs acting on the male reproductive system

**Androgens**
danazol
fluoxymesterone
methyltestosterone
testolactone (See Chapter 28)
testosterone
testosterone cypionate
testosterone enanthate
testosterone propionate

**Anabolic steroids**
dromostanolone propionate (See Chapter 28)
ethylestrenol
nandrolone decanoate
nandrolone phenpropionate
oxandrolone
oxymetholone
stanozolol

**INTRODUCTION**   The drugs covered in this chapter are all chemically related to the natural androgen, testosterone. Some of the drugs are used primarily for their androgenic effects, but others are used for their actions on blood factors or on pituitary gonadotropins. These drugs may also partially reverse certain types of growth retardation, but use in children exposes the child to premature closure of the epiphyses, which prevents attainment of full adult height. Anabolic steroids are widely used by athletes seeking to increase muscle mass and strength, but such use is against the precepts of the American College of Sports Medicine. Risks of dangerous, deforming, or even deadly side effects far outweigh potential benefits.

## Androgens

danazol ~ fluoxymesterone ~ methyltestosterone ~ testosterone ~ testosterone cypionate ~ testosterone enanthate ~ testosterone propionate

**OVERVIEW OF THE DRUG CLASS**   Androgens are responsible for proper development of primary and secondary sexual characteristics in males. The most important natural androgen is testosterone, which is produced in interstitial cells in the testes. Testosterone production is initiated by FSH and maintained by LH (p. 564). These gonadotropins are produced by the pituitary gland, rising when testosterone levels are low. When testosterone levels are high, gonadotropin production is suppressed.

Clinical uses of androgens include simple replacement therapy for certain conditions. Androgens are also used to block estrogens, to reverse catabolism, and to suppress gonadotropins.

**MECHANISM OF ACTION**   Androgens enter target cells, bind to specific receptors, and enter the nucleus, where transcription and translation of genes is regulated. Metabolic activity of the cell is changed by these events. Nitrogen, phosphorus, potassium, and sodium are retained, and protein synthesis increases. Urinary calcium losses decline.

The physiologic results of these molecular changes include growth and normal development of male sex organs, development of male hair distribution, thickening of vocal cords, bone growth, increase in body mass, and increased production of erythrocytes.

**INDICATIONS**   **Primary hypogonadism** Males without normal testicular production of androgens require replacement therapy with androgens to allow development and maintenance of male sexual characteristics.   **Carcinoma of the breast** Postmenopausal females may benefit from palliative therapy (See Chapter 28).   **Vasomotor symptoms of menopause** Women who fail to respond to estrogens alone may respond to androgens with estrogens. • The oral preparations contain fluoxymesterone or methyltestosterone. • Also See Table 33-1.

**CONTRAINDICATIONS**   **Severe renal, hepatic, or cardiac disease** Androgens cause sodium and fluid retention, which may increase risk of dangerous edema or congestive heart failure in these patients.   **Carcinoma of prostate or breast in males** These tumors may be stimulated by androgens.   **Hypercalcemia** Hypercalcemia may be worsened by the calcium-retaining effects of androgens.   **Pregnancy** Risk of fetal abnormalities exceeds potential benefits.

| Table 33-1. | Summary of clinical uses of androgens and anabolic steroids | | | | | | |
|---|---|---|---|---|---|---|---|
| **Drug** | **Male hypo-gonadism** | **Retarded growth** | **Anabolic** | **Anemias** | **Breast diseases** | **Endometri-osis** | **Angio-edema** |
| **Androgens** | | | | | | | |
| Danazol | | | | | + | + | + |
| Fluoxymesterone | + | + | | | + | | |
| Methyltestosterone | + | + | | | + | | |
| Testosterone | + | + | | | | | |
| **Anabolic steroids** | | | | | | | |
| Dromostanolone | | | + | | + | | |
| Ethylestrenol | | | + | + | | | |
| Nandrolone | | | + | + | + | | |
| Oxandrolone | | | + | | | | |
| Oxymetholone | | | + | + | | | |
| Stanozolol | | | + | | | | + |

**DRUG INTERACTIONS**    Oral anticoagulants may be potentiated by androgens, leading to bleeding episodes. Doses may require reduction.    **Insulin** requirements may be diminished by the hypoglycemic action of androgens.

**DIAGNOSTIC TEST INTERFERENCE**    Total serum thyroxine levels may be reduced because androgens lower levels of thyroxine-binding globulin. Thyroid function is unimpaired.

**FATE**    Testosterone is absorbed following oral administration but is rapidly metabolized in the GI mucosa and liver so that *bioavailability* is low. Testosterone esters are less water soluble and are slowly absorbed from IM depot sites. Fluoxymesterone and methyltestosterone are less well metabolized than testosterone and may be adequately absorbed orally. Conjugates of the drugs and metabolites are excreted in urine and, to a lesser degree, in feces.

## ☙ NURSING CONSIDERATIONS

### Side effects, toxicites, and associated nursing actions

**CNS** Anxiety, depression, excitation, headache, paresthesias, and sleeplessness may occur.
- Obtain baseline assessment of mental status and neurologic function, and repeat at regular intervals.
- Assess for signs of depression: insomnia, lack of appetite, loss of interest in personal appearance, and withdrawal.
- Assess for tingling of fingers and toes.

**CV** Retention of water and sodium may cause edema and contribute to congestive heart failure.
- Monitor weight, pulse, and blood pressure. Monitor serum electrolytes.
- Assess for development of edema. Auscultate lung and heart sounds. Watch for jugular venous distention.

**Blood** Androgens suppress clotting factors II, V, VII, and X. Polycythemia and leukopenia may occur.
- Instruct patients to report the development of bleeding or bruising, sore throat, or fever.
- Monitor complete blood count, and white blood cell differential.

**GI** Nausea is a common side effect.
- If nausea is severe or persistent, notify physician.
- Instruct patients to take doses with meals to lessen gastric irritation.

**Renal** Chloride, sodium, phosphates, potassium, and water may be retained. Bladder irritability has also occurred. Calcium excretion is diminished.
- Monitor weight, blood pressure, and pulse.

- Instruct patients to report bladder irritation.
- Instruct patients, if indicated by the medical condition, about calorie or sodium-restricted diets.
- Assess for hypercalcemia: thirst, polyuria, anorexia, nausea, vomiting, constipation, lethargy, and eventually coma. Review these symptoms with patients, and instruct patients to report the development of any new sign or symptom.
- Monitor serum electrolytes.

**Bone** Bone growth may be promoted, but in children the epiphyses may be induced to fuse prematurely, preventing the child from attaining full adult height.

- Review with children and families the proposed long-term treatment plan. Therapy for children is often intermittent, to allow drug-free periods to permit normal bone growth. The child's progress may be monitored with regular x-rays of wrists and hands to monitor bone maturation.
- Monitor weight and height.

**Liver** Abnormal liver function tests, cholestatic hepatitis, and jaundice may occur, especially with fluoxymesterone or methyltestosterone.

- Assess for signs of liver dysfunction: right upper quadrant abdominal pain, malaise, fever, jaundice, change in color or consistency of stools, and pruritis.
- Monitor liver function tests.

**Skin** Acne may occur. Flushing is also possible.

- Assess for skin changes. If acne is severe, consult physician about a change in drug or dose. Refer patients as indicated to a dermatologist.
- Reinforce to patients the importance of careful personal hygiene when acne is a problem.
- Warn patients about the possibility of flushing.

**Metabolic** Serum cholesterol may increase. Hypercalcemia may also occur, especially in cancer patients.

- Monitor serum cholesterol; if elevated, consult with physician about a change in dose. Refer patients to a dietitian for a low-cholesterol diet if indicated.
- Assess for hypercalcemia (see Renal, above).

**Allergic** Anaphylaxis is rare. Urticaria and inflammation at the injection site may occur with parenteral androgens.

- Assess injection sites carefully, and question patients about sites used previously. Consult physician about a change of drug form if inflammation is severe or persistent.

**Reproductive** Gynecomastia, oligospermia, decreased ejaculatory volume, and male-pattern baldness may be expected with long-term use or high doses. Priapism is especially likely with elderly males. Females suffer amenorrhea, menstrual irregularities, inhibition of gonadotropic secretion, virilization, hirsutism, and clitoral enlargement. Some of the virilizing side effects may not be reversed when treatment is stopped.

- Assess patients tactfully for these side effects. Some patients may not wish to discuss sexual problems, while children may be unable to describe some of the problems accurately. Provide emotional support as needed. Remind patients to take drugs as ordered for best effect, and not to stop taking the drug without notifying the physician.
- Instruct women to keep a record of menstrual periods. While pregnancy may be unlikely during drug therapy with androgens, instruct women to consult with the physician about the advisability of using birth control measures during the first few weeks of androgen therapy, and for the first several weeks after androgen therapy has stopped. Instruct women to notify the physician immediately if pregnancy is suspected.
- Instruct patients to report the development of any new sign or symptom. Some of the side effects may be lessened with a reduction in dose; consult the physician.

**Patient and family education**

- Review with patients and families the anticipated benefits and possible side effects of drug therapy.
- Caution diabetic patients to monitor blood glucose levels frequently for the first 2 weeks of therapy, and after androgen therapy is finished, as a change in insulin or dietary requirements may be necessary (see Drug interactions).
- Caution patients receiving oral anticoagulants to watch for any unexplained bruising or bleeding (see

Drug interactions). Encourage patients to have prothrombin time or other appropriate tests monitored for possible changes in dose of anticoagulant.

## danazol (DAN-a-zol)

• danazol: ✦Cyclomen, Danocrine

**MECHANISM OF ACTION**   Danazol has less androgenic activity than other members of this class. The actions sought with this drug are suppression of gonadotropin secretion, antiestrogen action, and inhibition of Cl esterase. See entry for drug class (p. 644).

**INDICATIONS**   **Endometriosis** Inhibition of gonadotropin and estrogen production causes relief of symptoms in up to 87% of patients. • The condition may return after therapy is halted.   **Hereditary angioedema** Androgenic effects of the drug limit use in children and pregnant women.   **Fibrocystic breast disease** Pain, tenderness, and nodularity may be relieved with therapy extending over several months, but the condition usually recurs when therapy is stopped.

**CONTRAINDICATIONS**   See entry for drug class (p. 644).

**DOSAGE**   **PO:**   **ADULTS:** For endometriosis, 200 to 800 mg daily divided into 2 equal doses. Therapy continues for up to 9 months. For fibrocystic breast disease, 100 to 400 mg daily divided into 2 equal doses. Therapy continues for up to 6 months. For hereditary angioedema, initially 400 to 600 mg daily divided into 2 or 3 equal doses. Reduce dosage by half after 3 months; maintenance should be with lowest dose that prevents recurrences.   *Special patient population:*   **ELDERLY:** Geriatric males are most at risk of priapism with androgen therapy.   **CHILDREN:** These drugs should be used short term at the lowest possible doses if used at all. Children are at risk of premature closure of the epiphyses, resulting in reduced adult height.   **PREGNANCY:** FDA pregnancy category X.

**PREPARATIONS**   *Capsules:* 50, 100, or 200 mg.

**DRUG INTERACTIONS**   See entry for drug class (p. 645).

**DIAGNOSTIC TEST INTERFERENCE**   See entry for drug class (p. 645).

**FATE**   See entry for drug class (p. 645).

### ☙ NURSING CONSIDERATIONS

#### Side effects, toxicities, and associated nursing actions

**Endocrine** The most common side effects are androgenic effects in females. Amenorrhea is reported by most women, but menstruation resumes within 2 or 3 months of discontinuing the drug in most women. For other possible side effects, see entry for drug class (p. 645).

#### Patient and family education

• See entry for drug class (p. 646).

## fluoxymesterone (floo-oxy-MES-ter-one)

• fluoxymesterone: Halotestin, Hysterone

**MECHANISM OF ACTION**   See entry for drug class (p. 644).

**INDICATIONS**   See entry for drug class (p. 644).

**CONTRAINDICATIONS**   See entry for drug class (p. 644).

**DOSAGE**   **PO:**   **ADULTS:** For hypogonadism in males, 5 to 20 mg daily as a single dose or divided into 3 or 4 doses. For carcinoma of the breast in females, 10 to 40 mg daily, divided into multiple doses. For vasomotor symptoms of menopause, 1 or 2 mg fluoxymesterone with 0.02 or 0.04 mg ethinyl estradiol for 21 days. After 7 days without drug, repeat the course as necessary.   *Special patient populations:*   **ELDERLY:** Geriatric males are most at risk of priapism with androgen therapy.   **CHILDREN:** These drugs should be used short term at the lowest possible doses if used at all. Children are at risk of premature closure of the epiphyses, resulting in reduced adult height.  **PREGNANCY:** FDA pregnancy category X.

**PREPARATIONS**  *Tablets:* 2, 5, OR 10 mg. Combination products include *tablets:* 1 mg fluoxymesterone with 0.02 mg ethinyl estradiol (Halodrin).

**DRUG INTERACTIONS**  See entry for drug class (p. 645).

**DIAGNOSTIC TEST INTERFERENCE**  See entry for drug class (p. 645).

**FATE**  See entry for drug class (p. 645).

### ❧ NURSING CONSIDERATIONS

#### Side effects, toxicities, and associated nursing actions
**Liver** Abnormal liver function tests, cholestatic hepatitis, and jaundice occur even at low doses. Peliosis of the liver, hepatic adenoma, and hepatic carcinoma are possible side effects of long-term therapy.
- For other side effects, see entry for drug class (p. 645).

#### Patient and family education
- See entry for drug class (p. 646).

---

## methyltestosterone  (meth-ill-tes-TOS-ter-one)  androgen

- methyltestosterone: Android, Metandren, Oreton, Testred, Virilon

**MECHANISM OF ACTION**  See entry for drug class (p. 644).

**INDICATIONS**  See entry for drug class (p. 644).

**CONTRAINDICATIONS**  See entry for drug class (p. 644).

**DOSAGE**  **PO:**  **ADULTS:** For male hypogonadism, 10 to 50 mg daily, in divided doses. For breast carcinoma in women, 50 to 200 mg daily. For vasomotor symptoms of menopause, use minimum doses of methyltestosterone with estrogen to control symptoms.  **Buccal:**  **ADULTS:** For male hypogonadism, 5 to 25 mg daily. For breast carcinoma in women, 25 to 100 mg daily.  *Special patient populations:*  **ELDERLY:** Geriatric males are most at risk of priapism with androgen therapy.  **CHILDREN:** These drugs should be used short term at the lowest possible doses if used at all. Children are at risk of premature closure of the epiphyses, resulting in reduced adult height.  **PREGNANCY:** FDA pregnancy category X.

**PREPARATIONS**  *Buccal tablets:* 5 or 10 mg. *Oral capsules:* 10 mg. *Oral tablets:* 10 or 25 mg. Combination products containing methyltestosterone include *oral tablets:* 1.25 mg with 0.625 mg esterified estrogens, or 2.5 mg with 1.25 esterified estrogens (Estratest). *Oral tablets:* 5 mg with 0.625 mg conjugated estrogens, or 10 mg with 1.25 mg conjugated estrogens (Premarin with Methyltestosterone). *Oral tablets:* 5 mg with 0.25 mg diethylstilbestrol (Tylosterone).

**DRUG INTERACTIONS**  See entry for drug class (p. 645).

**DIAGNOSTIC TEST INTERFERENCE**  See entry for drug class (p. 645).

**FATE**  See entry for drug class (p. 645).

### ❧ NURSING CONSIDERATIONS

#### Side effects, toxicities, and associated nursing actions
- See entry for drug class (p. 645).

#### Nursing interventions related to drug administration
- For buccal tablets: instruct patients to place tablet(s) in the mouth between the upper or lower gum and the cheek, and allow tablet to dissolve. While the tablet is in place, patients should refrain from eating, drinking, chewing, or smoking. Instruct patients to rotate sites with each administration. Remind patient to maintain a program of good, regular oral hygiene, and to report any oral irritation to the physician.

#### Patient and family education
- See entry for drug class (p. 646).

## testosterone   (tes-TOS-ter-one)                                    androgen

- testosterone: Andro, Androlan, Andronaq, Histerone, ♣Malogen, Testolin
- testosterone cypionate: Andro-cyp, Andronate, Depo-testosterone, Duratest
- testosterone enanthate: Android-T, Andro-L.A., Delatestryl, ♣Malogex
- testosterone propionate: Androlan, ♣Malogen

**MECHANISM OF ACTION**   See entry for drug class (p. 644).

**INDICATIONS**   See entry for drug class (p. 644).

**CONTRAINDICATIONS**   See entry for drug class (p. 644).

**DOSAGE**   **IM:**   **ADULTS:** For male hypogonadism, 10 to 25 mg testosterone or testosterone propionate two or three times weekly, or 50 to 400 mg testosterone cypionate or testosterone enanthate every 2 to 4 weeks. For carcinoma of the breast in women, 100 mg testosterone or 50 to 100 mg testosterone propionate three times weekly, or 200 to 400 mg testosterone cypionate or testosterone enanthate every 2 to 4 weeks.   **SC:**   **ADULTS:** For male hypogonadism, 2 to 6 pellets (150 to 450 mg) may be implanted after dosage is established by other routes.   *Special patient populations:*   **ELDERLY:** Geriatric males are most at risk of priapism with androgen therapy.   **CHILDREN:** These drugs should be used short term at the lowest possible doses if used at all. Children are at risk of premature closure of the epiphyses, resulting in reduced adult height.   **PREGNANCY:** FDA pregnancy category X.

**PREPARATIONS**   Testosterone, *pellets for SC implantation:* 75 mg. *Suspension:* 25, 50, or 100 mg/ml. Testosterone cypionate, *injection (in oil):* 50, 100, or 200 mg/ml. Combination products containing testosterone cypionate include *injection (in oil):* 50 mg/ml with estradiol cypionate 2 mg/ml; and testosterone enanthate, *injection (in oil):* 100 or 200 mg/ml. Combination products containing testosterone enanthate include *injection (in oil):* 90 mg/ml with estradiol valerate 4 mg/ml, or 180 mg with estradiol valerate 8 mg/ml; and testosterone propionate, *injection (in oil):* 25, 50, or 100 mg/ml.

**DRUG INTERACTIONS**   See entry for drug class (p. 645).

**DIAGNOSTIC TEST INTERFERENCE**   See entry for drug class (p. 645).

**FATE**   See entry for drug class (p. 645).

### ❦ NURSING CONSIDERATIONS

#### Side effects, toxicities, and associated nursing actions

- See entry for drug class (p. 645).

#### Nursing interventions related to drug administration

- Pellets for subcutaneous implantation can be inserted surgically or with a specially designed injector. Either procedure can be done easily in the physician's office; aseptic technique must be used. Usual sites of insertion are the infrascapular area or along the posterior axillary line. Two or more pellets may be inserted at one time, although not necessarily into the same subcutaneous pouch. The drug will be absorbed slowly from the pellets for up to 4 to 6 months. Sloughing of the pellets can occur; instruct patient to notify physician. Sloughing often indicates placement too superficially or lack of aseptic technique. Because the dose of subcutaneous pellets cannot be regulated easily, proper dosage for the patient is determined by oral medication before a switch is made to the subcutaneous route. For additional information, see the information supplied by the manufacturer.
- For IM oil-based suspensions: heat the unopened vial in warm water for several minutes to decrease the viscosity of the oil. Vigorously rotate the ampule/vial to resuspend the medication, which can often be seen as an inconspicuous film on the side of the vial. Resuspension is adequate when no particles of medication are visible on the side or bottom of the glass container. Insufficient resuspension will result in erratic absorption. Draw up the correct dose into a syringe fitted with a large-bore (19 to 21 gauge), 1 1/2 in needle, and administer using usual aseptic technique for IM administration. Administer as soon as possible after preparing to prevent oil from cooling completely. Inject the medication with slow, even pressure on the plunger. Attempts to inject too rapidly can increase pressure within the syringe, causing the needle and syringe to separate and the medication to spill. Appropriate injection sites include the buttocks, thigh, or ventrogluteal sites. The oil base, which allows slow absorption, can produce palpable lumps at injection sites; rotate injection sites, and avoid the deltoid muscle. Oil-based medications should never be given IV.

# Anabolic steroids

dromostanolone propionate (see Chapter 28) ~ ethylestrenol ~ nandrolone
~ oxandrolone ~ oxymetholone ~ stanozolol

**OVERVIEW OF THE DRUG CLASS**   Anabolic steroids are modified to reduce androgenic properties while retaining the anabolic effects of those compounds. Anabolic steroids nevertheless retain sufficient androgenic activity to limit their use in most patients. The drugs should be used only for the specific indications given below and should never be used for trivial purposes. The dangerous and deforming side effects of these agents preclude their use by healthy persons of any age seeking only to change body size or function for athletic purposes.

**MECHANISM OF ACTION**   Like androgens, the anabolic steroids favor protein synthesis, increase body mass, increase calcium retention, cause erythrocyte formation, alter blood factors, and function as antiestrogens.

**Table 33-2.**

## Summary of combinations including androgenic steroids

| Androgen | Other components | Trade names | Uses |
|---|---|---|---|
| Fluoxymesterone 1 mg | Ethinyl estradiol 0.02 mg | Halodrin | Vasomotor symptoms of menopause |
| Methyltestosterone 1.25 mg 2.5 mg | Esterified estrogens 0.625 mg 1.25 mg | Estratest Estratest | Vasomotor symptoms of menopause |
| Methyltestosterone 5 mg | Conjugated estrogens 0.625 mg | Premarin with Methyltestosterone | Vasomotor symptoms of menopause |
| 10 mg | 1.25 mg | Premarin with Methyltestosterone | |
| Methyltestosterone 5 mg | Diethylstilbestrol 0.25 mg | Tylosterone | Vasomotor symptoms of menopause |
| Testosterone cypionate 50 mg/ml | Estradiol cypionate 2 mg/ml | Andro/Fem, depAndrogyn, Depo-Testadiol, Depotestogen, Duo-Cyp, Duratestrin, Menoject-L.A., T-E Cypionate | Postpartum breast engorgement |
| Testosterone enanthate 90 mg/ml | Estradiol valerate 4 mg/ml | Androgyn L.A., Deladumone, Estra-Testrin, Teev, Testaval, Valertest | Postpartum breast engorgement |
| 180 mg/ml | 8 mg/ml | Deladumone OB, Ditate-DS, Valertest | |

**INDICATIONS**  **Tissue-depleting processes** Anabolic steroids may be used along with conventional therapy to reverse chronic catabolic processes in rare patients.  **Anemias** Anabolic steroids may be helpful along with conventional therapy for certain specific anemias.  **Carcinoma of breast** Dromostanolone is palliative therapy for advanced tumors in selected females (see Chapter 28).  **Hereditary angioedema** Stanozolol may be used prophylactically to reduce attacks.  **Arthritis** Ethylestrenol may be used as an adjunct to conventional therapy.

**CONTRAINDICATIONS**  **Severe renal or hepatic disease** Anabolic steroids cause sodium and fluid retention, which may increase risk of dangerous edema or congestive heart failure in these patients.  **Carcinoma of prostate or breast in males** These tumors may be stimulated by the androgenic action of anabolic steroids.  **Hypercalcemia** Hypercalcemia may be worsened by the calcium-retaining effects of anabolic steroids.  **Pregnancy** Risk of fetal abnormalities exceeds potential benefits.

**DRUG INTERACTIONS**  **Oral anticoagulants** may be potentiated by anabolic steroids, leading to bleeding episodes. Doses may require reduction.  **Insulin** requirements may be diminished by the hypoglycemic action of anabolic steroids.  **Corticosteroids** may increase the sodium-retaining properties of anabolic steroids and contribute to other side effects such as development of acne.

**FATE**  Ethylestrenol, oxandrolone, oxymetholone, and stanozolol are adequately absorbed orally, but other members of the class are used parenterally. Anabolic steroids, like the androgens, are metabolized by liver and excreted in urine and feces.

---

## ☙ NURSING CONSIDERATIONS

### Side effects, toxicities, and associated nursing actions

**CNS** Depression, headache, sleeplessness, or tiredness may occur. Rare cases of steroid-induced psychosis have been reported in healthy young athletes who took anabolic steroids for bodybuilding.
- Monitor mental status. Assess for signs of depression: lack of interest in personal appearance, insomnia, loss of appetite, and withdrawal.
- Caution patients to avoid driving or operating hazardous equipment if tiredness develops.
- If CNS symptoms are severe or persistent, instruct patient to notify physician.

**CV** Water retention and edema may occur.
- Monitor weight, blood pressure, and pulse. Assess for development of edema.

**Blood** Unusual bleeding may occur because clotting factors can be suppressed.
- Instruct patients to report the development of unexplained bruising or bleeding. Caution patients taking oral anticoagulants to be especially wary (see Drug interactions). Encourage patients on oral anticoagulants to have physician monitor prothrombin time or other tests to monitor anticoagulant dosage.

**GI** Abdominal discomfort, loss of appetite, altered appearance of stools, or vomiting may occur.

**Liver** Jaundice may occur. Long-term use of high doses increases the risk of peliosis hepatitis or hepatic neoplasms, causing weight loss, altered stools, and skin changes.
- Assess for signs of hepatic dysfunction and have patient report development of malaise, fever, jaundice, change in the color or consistency of stools, or right upper quadrant abdominal pain.
- Instruct patients to take doses with meals or snack to reduce gastric irritation.
- If GI symptoms are severe or persistent, have patient notify physician.

**Renal** Fluid retention is common. Bladder irritability may occur in adult males. Prostatic hypertrophy or carcinoma may interfere with urination in older males.
- Monitor weight and blood pressure.
- Warn patients about the possibility of difficulty with urination, and instruct them to report feelings of inability to empty the bladder. Monitor intake and output if indicated.

**Skin** Acne and oily skin are common. Hives or colored spots on skin or mucous membranes may be a sign of peliosis hepatitis.
- Assess for skin changes. If acne or oily skin is severe, consult physician about a change in drug or dose. Refer patients as indicated to a dermatologist.
- Review aspects of good personal hygiene with patients.
- Instruct patients to report the development of any unusual skin changes.

**Endocrine** Females may suffer virilization with enlarged clitoris, deepening of voice, and changes in hair growth. These changes may not be reversible. Males may suffer gynecomastia, increased erections, priapism, or decreased sexual activity.

- Assess tactfully for these changes. Provide emotional support as needed. Remind patients to take medications as ordered for best effects, and not to stop medications without notifying physician.
- Instruct patients to notify physician if priapism develops.

**Patient and family education**

- Review with patients the anticipated benefits and possible side effects of drug therapy.
- Caution diabetic patients to monitor blood glucose levels carefully when starting or ending therapy with steroids, as an adjustment in insulin dosage or diet may be necessary.
- Instruct patients that the effectiveness of anabolic steroids in burned, traumatized, or immobilized patients may be enhanced by the concomitant use of a diet high in calories, protein, vitamins, and minerals. Continue regular physical therapy to help reduce demineralization of bone.

---

## dromostanolone propionate  (dro-mo-STAN-oh-lone)    anabolic steroid

- dromostanolone propionate: Drolban

**MECHANISM OF ACTION**   See entry for drug class (p. 650) and complete listing in Chapter 28.

---

## ethylestrenol  (eth-ill-ES-tre-nol)    anabolic steroid

- ethylestrenol: Maxibolin

**MECHANISM OF ACTION**   See entry for drug class (p. 650).
**INDICATIONS**   See entry for drug class (p. 651) and Table 33-1.
**CONTRAINDICATIONS**   See entry for drug class (p. 651).
**DOSAGE**   **PO:**   **ADULTS:** 4 mg daily for 6 weeks. After a 4-week interval, the drug may be given for another 6 weeks.   **CHILDREN:** 1 to 3 mg daily.   *Special patient populations:*   **ELDERLY:** Older males may require lower doses to prevent excessive sexual stimulation or prostatic hypertrophy.   **CHILDREN:** These drugs should be used short term at the lowest possible doses if used at all. Children are at risk of premature closure of the epiphyses, resulting in reduced adult height.   **PREGNANCY:** FDA pregnancy category X.
**PREPARATIONS**   *Tablets:* 2 mg. *Oral elixir:* 2 mg/5 ml.
**DRUG INTERACTIONS**   See entry for drug class (p. 651).
   **FATE**   See entry for drug class (p. 651).
**☙ NURSING CONSIDERATIONS**
   **Side effects, toxicities, and associated nursing actions**
      - See entry for drug class (p. 651).
   **Patient and family education**
      - See entry for drug class (p. 652).

---

## nandrolone decanoate, nandrolone phenpropionate
(NAN-dro-lone)    anabolic steroid

- nandrolone decanoate, nandrolone phenpropionate: Anabolin, Androlone, Durabolin, Hybolin, Kabolin, Nandrobolic

**MECHANISM OF ACTION**   See entry for drug class (p. 650).
**INDICATIONS**   See entry for drug class (p. 651) and Table 33-1.

**CONTRAINDICATIONS**  See entry for drug class (p. 651).

**DOSAGE**  IM:  **ADULTS:** For nandrolone decanoate, 50 to 100 mg per week in females or 100 to 200 mg per week in males. For nandrolone phenpropionate, 50 to 100 mg weekly in males or females.  **CHIL-DREN OLDER THAN 2 YEARS:** For nandrolone decanoate, 25 to 50 mg every 3 to 4 weeks.  *Special patient populations:*  **ELDERLY:** Older males may require lower doses to prevent excessive sexual stimulation or prostatic hypertrophy.  **CHILDREN:** These drugs should be used short term at the lowest possible doses if used at all. Children are at risk of premature closure of the epiphyses, resulting in reduced adult height.  **PREGNANCY:** FDA pregnancy category X.

**PREPARATIONS**  Nandrolone decanoate, *solution for IM injection:* 50, 100, or 200 mg/ml. Nandrolone phenpropionate, *solution for IM injection:* 25 or 50 mg/ml.

**DRUG INTERACTIONS**  See entry for drug class (p. 651).

**FATE**  See entry for drug class (p. 651).

☙ **NURSING CONSIDERATIONS**

### Side effects, toxicities, and associated nursing actions
- See entry for drug class (p. 651).

### Patient and family education
- See entry for drug class (p. 652).

## oxandrolone  (ox-AN-dro-lone)  anabolic steroid

- oxandrolone: Anavar

**MECHANISM OF ACTION**  See entry for drug class (p. 650).

**INDICATIONS**  See entry for drug class (p. 651) and Table 33-1.

**CONTRAINDICATIONS**  See entry for drug class (p. 651).

**DOSAGE**  PO:  **ADULTS:** 2.5 mg two to four times daily.  **CHILDREN:** 0.25 mg/kg daily.  *Special patient populations:*  **ELDERLY:** Older males may require lower doses to prevent excessive sexual stimulation or prostatic hypertrophy.  **CHILDREN:** These drugs should be used short term at the lowest possible doses if used at all. Children are at risk of premature closure of the epiphyses, resulting in reduced adult height.  **PREGNANCY:** FDA pregnancy category X.

**PREPARATIONS**  *Tablets:* 2.5 mg.

**DRUG INTERACTIONS**  See entry for drug class (p. 651).

**FATE**  See entry for drug class (p. 651).

☙ **NURSING CONSIDERATIONS**

### Side effects, toxicities, and associated nursing actions
- See entry for drug class (p. 651).

### Patient and family education
- See entry for drug class (p. 651).

## oxymetholone  (oxy-METH-oh-lone)  anabolic steroid

- oxymetholone: Anadrol, Anapolon

**MECHANISM OF ACTION**  See entry for drug class (p. 650).

**INDICATIONS**  See entry for drug class (p. 651) and Table 33-1.

**CONTRAINDICATIONS**  See entry for drug class (p. 651).

**DOSAGE**  PO:  **ADULTS AND CHILDREN:** 1 to 5 mg/kg daily.  **NEONATES:** 0.175 mg/kg or 5 mg/$M^2$ each day in a single dose. *Special patient populations:*  **ELDERLY:** Older males may require lower doses to prevent excessive sexual stimulation or prostatic hypertrophy.  **CHILDREN:** These drugs should be used short term at the lowest possible doses if used at all. Children are at risk of premature closure of the epiphyses, resulting in reduced adult height. **PREGNANCY:** FDA pregnancy category X.

**PREPARATIONS** *Tablets:* 50 mg.
**DRUG INTERACTIONS** See entry for drug class (p. 651).
    **FATE** See entry for drug class (p. 651).

### 🐇 NURSING CONSIDERATIONS

#### Side effects, toxicities, and associated nursing actions
• See entry for drug class (p. 651).

#### Patient and family education
• See entry for drug class (p. 652).

---

## stanozolol (sta-NOZ-oh-lol) anabolic steroid

• stanozolol: Winstrol✤

**MECHANISM OF ACTION** See entry for drug class (p. 650).
**INDICATIONS** Stanozolol is used only for hereditary angioedema. • See entry for drug class (p. 651) and Table 33-1.
**CONTRAINDICATIONS** See entry for drug class (p. 651).
**DOSAGE** **PO:** **ADULTS:** 2 mg two or three times daily. **CHILDREN:** 1 to 2 mg daily, only during attacks of angioedema. *Special patient populations:* **ELDERLY:** Older males may require lower doses to prevent excessive sexual stimulation or prostatic hypertrophy. **CHILDREN:** These drugs should be used short term at the lowest possible doses if used at all. Children are at risk of premature closure of the epiphyses, resulting in reduced adult height. **PREGNANCY:** FDA pregnancy category X.
**PREPARATIONS** *Tablets:* 2 mg.
**DRUG INTERACTIONS** See entry for drug class (p. 651).
    **FATE** See entry for drug class (p. 651).

### 🐇 NURSING CONSIDERATIONS

#### Side effects, toxicities, and associated nursing actions
• See entry for drug class (p. 651).

#### Patient and family education
• See entry for drug class (p. 652).

# Chapter Thirty-four

# Drugs used to treat diabetes mellitus

| **Insulins** | **Sulfonylureas** |
|---|---|
| extended insulin zinc | acetohexamide |
| insulin zinc | chlorpropamide |
| isophane insulin | glipizide |
| prompt insulin zinc | glyburide |
| protamine zinc insulin | tolazamide |
| regular insulin | tolbutamide |

**Hyperglycemic agent**
glucagon

**INTRODUCTION**   Diabetes mellitus is a disease characterized by loss of insulin action. In one type of diabetes, insulin production is lost. This form of diabetes is now termed *insulin-dependent diabetes mellitus* (IDDM) but was once called juvenile-onset diabetes because many patients with this disorder are first diagnosed in childhood. In other diabetics, insulin production may be normal or even higher than normal, but the target tissues fail to respond appropriately. This type of diabetes, which is now called *non–insulin-dependent diabetes mellitus (NIDDM),* is much more common than IDDM. NIDDM is most often found in overweight people over the age of 40 and has been referred to as adult-onset diabetes or Type II diabetes.

Treatment of IDDM is by replacement therapy with a form of insulin, the hormone lacked by these patients. Treatment of NIDDM requires dietary manipulation and drug therapy to reverse the nonresponsiveness of target tissues.

## Insulins

extended insulin zinc  ~  insulin zinc  ~  isophane insulin  ~  prompt insulin zinc  ~  protamine zinc insulin  ~  regular insulin

**OVERVIEW OF THE DRUG CLASS**   Many insulin preparations used in humans are isolated and purified from porcine or bovine pancreas. Human insulin is prepared by recombinant DNA techniques or by chemical conversion of porcine insulin. Human insulin and pork insulin are less immunogenic than beef insulin.

Insulin from each of the three sources described above may be modified to alter the onset, peak, and duration of action (Table 34-1). Insulin preparations are summarized in Table 34-2.

**MECHANISM OF ACTION**   Insulin promotes glucose transport into muscle cells, making that carbohydrate available for use as an energy source. In addition, insulin stimulates the formation of lipids and inhibits the release of fatty acids from fat cells. Insulin also promotes protein synthesis. Without insulin, glucose accumulates in the blood because the sugar cannot be moved into cells to be metabolized. Ketone bodies may accumulate as fat metabolism becomes deranged. Protein is degraded faster than it is formed, and the muscles waste away.

**INDICATIONS**   **IDDM** Use in this disease constitutes replacement therapy.   **NIDDM** Patients with NIDDM may require insulin during a severe illness or surgery. • Insulin may also be used in patients with NIDDM who do not respond to diet, exercise, and other therapy for their disease.   **Gestational diabetes** This condition is often temporary and may respond to diet alone. • If these measures do not control hyperglycemia, insulin may be prescribed until the pregnancy ends.   **Total parenteral nutrition (TPN)** Regular insulin may be required for proper utilization of the high concentrations of glucose in some TPN formulations (see Chapter 10).   **Diagnosis of growth hormone deficiency** Regular insulin may be administered to test for the ability of the pituitary gland to release growth hormone.

**CONTRAINDICATIONS**   **Hypoglycemia** Patients who are hypoglycemic should not receive insulin. • Diabetics must learn to recognize the signs of a hypoglycemic reaction and distinguish that from hyperglycemia (Table 34-3). • Diabetic coma requires treatment with insulin, but stupor or coma from hypoglycemia requires treatment with glucose or glucagon (p. 672).

**DRUG INTERACTIONS**    **Corticosteroids** may antagonize the hypoglycemic action of insulin.    **Dextrothyroxine** sodium may antagonize the hypoglycemic action of insulin.    **Diazoxide** may inhibit insulin secretion from the patient's pancreas, resulting in hyperglycemia. The dose of insulin may need to be increased.    **Epinephrine** may antagonize the hypoglycemic action of insulin.    **Ethacrynic acid, furosemide, or thiazide diuretics** may elevate blood glucose levels and alter the dose of insulin.    **Oral contraceptives** may increase insulin requirements in diabetics.    **Phenytoin sodium** may inhibit insulin secretion from the patient's pancreas, resulting in hyperglycemia. The dose of insulin may need to be increased.    **Procarbazine** may potentiate the hypoglycemic effect of insulin.    **Propranolol** may alter insulin requirements.

**Table 34-1.    Properties of insulin preparations***

| Generic name | Classification | Description | Pharmacokinetic properties | | |
|---|---|---|---|---|---|
| | | | Onset of action | Peak action | Duration of action |
| Insulin injection | Rapid acting | Clear solution containing no zinc or modifying agents; intravenous or subcutaneous injection. | Within 1 hr | 2 to 4 hr | 6 to 8 hr |
| Prompt insulin zinc suspension | Rapid acting | Cloudy suspension of amorphous insulin precipitated with zinc to slow absorption; subcutaneous only. | 1½ to 2 hr | 4 to 7 hr | 12 to 16 hr |
| Isophane insulin suspension | Intermediate acting | Cloudy suspension of insulin complexed with protamine to slow absorption; subcutaneous only. | 1 to 2 hr | 10 to 16 hr | 18 to 30 hr |
| Insulin zinc suspension | Intermediate acting | Cloudy suspension containing 30% Semilente insulin and 70% Ultralente insulin; subcutaneous only. | 1 to 2 hr | 10 to 16 hr | 18 to 30 hr |
| Protamine zinc insulin | Long acting | Cloudy when well mixed; suspension of insulin complexed with more protamine than NPH insulin; subcutaneous only. | 6 to 8 hr | 14 to 24 hr | 24 to 36 hr or longer |
| Extended insulin zinc suspension | Long acting | Cloudy when well mixed; large complexes of insulin with zinc to slow absorption; no protein modifiers; subcutaneous only. | 5 to 8 hr | 16 to 18 hr | 24 to 36 hr or longer |

*From Clark JB, Queener SF, and Karb, VB: Pharmacological Basis of Nursing Practice, ed. 2, St. Louis, 1986, The C.V. Mosby Co.

**Table 34-2.**

## Summary of insulin preparations

| Generic name | Trade name | Source | Concentration |
|---|---|---|---|
| Insulin injection | Regular Iletin I | Beef/pork mixture | 40 or 100 units/ml |
| | Regular Insulin | Pork | 100 units/ml |
| | Regular Iletin II Purified Beef | Beef purified | 100 units/ml |
| | Regular Iletin II Purified Pork, Regular Insulin Purified Pork, Velosulin | Pork purified | 100 units/ml |
| | Regular Concentrated Iletin II Purified Pork | Pork purified | 500 units/ml |
| | Novolin R, Velosulin Human | Semisynthetic human from pork | 100 units/ml |
| | Humulin R, Humulin BR | Human from recombinant DNA | 100 units/ml |
| Prompt insulin zinc suspension | Semilente Iletin | Beef/pork mixture | 40 or 100 units/ml |
| | Semilente Insulin | Beef | 40 or 100 units/ml |
| | Semilente Purified Pork | Pork purified | 100 units/ml |
| Isophane insulin suspension (NPH) | Iletin I NPH | Beef/pork mixture | 40 or 100 units/ml |
| | Insulin NPH | Beef | 40 or 100 units/ml |
| | Iletin II NPH Purified Beef | Beef purified | 100 units/ml |
| | Iletin II NPH Purified Pork, Insulin NPH Purified Pork, Insulatard NPH | Pork purified | 100 units/ml |
| | Mixtard | Pork purified (70% NPH, 30% regular insulin) | 100 units/ml |
| | Insulatard NPH Human, Novolin N | Semisynthetic human from pork | 100 units/ml |
| | Novolin 70/30 | Semisynthetic human from pork (70% NPH, 30% regular insulin) | 100 units/ml |
| | Humulin N | Human from recombinant DNA | 100 units/ml |
| Insulin zinc suspension | Lente Iletin I | Beef/pork mixture | 40 or 100 units/ml |
| | Lente Insulin | Beef | 40 or 100 units/ml |
| | Lente Iletin II Purified Beef | Beef purified | 100 units/ml |
| | Lente Iletin II Purified Pork, Lente Insulin Purified Pork | Pork purified | 100 units/ml |
| | Novolin L | Semisynthetic human from pork | 100 units/ml |

*Continued.*

**Table 34-2.**

### Summary of insulin preparations—cont'd.

| Generic name | Trade name | Source | Concentration |
|---|---|---|---|
| | Humulin L | Human from recombinant DNA | 100 units/ml |
| Protamine zinc insulin suspension | Protamine Zinc Iletin I | Beef/pork mixture | 40 or 100 units/ml |
| | Protamine Zinc Iletin II Purified Beef | Beef purified | 100 units/ml |
| | Protamine Zinc Iletin II Purified Pork | Pork purified | 100 units/ml |
| Extended insulin | Ultralente Iletin I | Beef/pork mixture | 40 or 100 units/ml |
| | Ultralente Insulin | Beef | 100 units/ml |
| | Ultralente Insulin Purified Beef | Beef purified | 100 units/ml |

**Table 34-3.**

### Differential diagnosis of diabetic coma and hypoglycemic reactions*

| Clinical data | Diabetic coma | Hypoglycemic reactions |
|---|---|---|
| Symptoms | Thirst | Nervousness |
| | Abdominal pain | Hunger |
| | Nausea and vomiting | Sweating |
| | Headache | Weakness |
| | Constipation | Stupor |
| | Shortness of breath (Kussmaul breathing) | Convulsions |
| Signs | Facial flushing | Pallor |
| | Air hunger | Shallow respiration |
| | Soft eyeballs | Normal eyeballs |
| | Normal or absent reflexes | Babinski reflex may be seen |
| | Acetone breath | |
| Urine glucose | Positive | Negative or low |
| Urine acetone | Positive | Negative |
| Blood glucose | High (above 250 mg/dl) | Low (below 60 mg/dl |
| Blood $CO_2$ | Low | Normal |
| Precipitating factors | Untreated diabetes | Insulin overdosage |
| | Infection or disease appearing in a previously controlled diabetic patient | Skipping meals |
| | | Excessive exercise before meals |
| | High degree of emotional or psychological stress | |
| History | Onset of symptoms usually occurs over a period of days. | Onset of symptoms is somewhat related to the type of medication used; regular insulin overdose produces symptoms more rapidly than the longer-acting insulins or oral agents. |

*From Clark JB, Queener SF, and Karb, VB: Pharmacological Basis of Nursing Practice, ed. 2, St. Louis, 1986, The C.V. Mosby Co.

# NURSING CONSIDERATIONS

## Side effects, toxicities, and associated nursing actions

**Hypoglycemia** Insulin overdosage results in hypoglycemia, which can be life-threatening. Hypoglycemia must be distinguished from diabetic coma (Table 34-3).

- Review the signs and symptoms of hyperglycemia and hypoglycemia with the patient. The appearance of hypoglycemia may relate to the time of the last dose of insulin (Table 34-1). If possible, obtain blood for blood glucose. Whether blood is obtained or not, treat by administering a fast-acting carbohydrate. Example sources of glucose are ½ C fruit juice, ½ C sugar cola drink, ½ C regular gelatin dessert, 4 cubes or 2 packs of sugar, 2 squares of graham crackers, or 2 to 3 pieces of hard candy.
- Instruct patients to carry hard candy or other sources of carbohydrate with them at all times.
- Review signs and symptoms of hypoglycemia with family members, and discuss appropriate treatment.
- If hypoglycemia is severe, repeated, or occurring without explanation, have patient notify physician.

**Allergy** Local allergic reactions involving itching, redness, swelling, or stinging at the injection site are usually transient and are not uncommon. Anaphylaxis is very rare. Insulin resistance occasionally involves antibodies to insulin.

- It may not be possible to eliminate local allergic reactions. Supervise insulin administration technique, as scrupulous attention to technique may lessen local irritation. Record and rotate sites on a systematic basis so that accessible sites are not overused. (See p. 16 for a diagram of commonly used sites of subcutaneous injection.) Prepare dose of insulin as ordered, and let warm to room temperature. Cleanse injection site carefully, and allow skin surface to dry completely. Pinch skin between thumb and fingers of one hand, and insert needle into the "pocket" between the subcutaneous fat and muscle; a 45° to 90° angle can be used, depending on the amount of subcutaneous fat and the length of the needle. Aspirate for blood, then inject insulin and withdraw needle. Apply pressure to injection site, but do not rub the area. Disposable syringes can be safely reused by the patient for up to 3 days, but reused syringes may have duller needle tips; if irritation is a problem, the patient may want to use a new needle more often.
- If local irritation is severe or persistent, consult physician about a change in type of insulin.
- As noted, systemic reactions are rare and may be due to the animal source of the insulin: beef, pork, or mixed beef and pork. Treat symptomatically, and consult physician about changing source of insulin.

**Other** Atrophy or hypertrophy of subcutaneous fat may occur at the injection site. Rotation of injection sites minimizes this problem.

## Nursing interventions related to drug administration

- For IV use: only regular insulin can be used for IV use. Insulin may adsorb to the tubing and container, but the rate of adsorption is variable. Monitor patients receiving IV insulin carefully.
- Because most diabetics practice self-administration of insulin, other aspects of drug administration are discussed below.

## Patient and family education

- Review carefully and frequently the treatment of diabetes, including insulin administration, with patient and family. Caution patient to seek the advice of the nurse or physician when in doubt or when new signs and symptoms develop.
- The specific regimen prescribed for any patient is based on the age of the patient, severity of the diabetes, weight of the patient, philosophy of the health care team, and other medical problems or disabilities, etc. While general guidelines are noted in this monograph, more detailed information can be found in fundamental nursing texts and other printed resources.
- Caution patients to use only the insulin prescribed and to check carefully each time insulin is purchased that the correct form, brand, and strength of insulin have been supplied. Any change in insulin purity, strength, manufacturer, type, or source of insulin may result in a need to adjust dosage.

- Instruct patients to keep the vial of insulin currently in use at room temperature, but to store extra vials in the refrigerator; avoid freezing. Hospitals and pharmacies usually store insulin in the refrigerator, but this necessitates that insulin be warmed to room temperature before administering.
- Instruct patient to inspect vial of insulin before preparing ordered dose. Regular insulin should be crystal clear, while other forms of insulin will be cloudy.
- Rotate insulin vial between both hands before preparing dose to help resuspend modified insulin preparations and to warm refrigerated vials to room temperature. Avoid shaking vials and creating foam.
- Use only syringes designed for insulin administration. Check dosages carefully. In hospitals and other agencies, observe policies related to checking insulin dosages, such as having two nurses check that the correct dose of insulin has been prepared for administration.
- Two kinds of insulin can be mixed within the same syringe, within the following guidelines: regular insulin can be mixed with any other insulin. The lente forms can be mixed with other lente insulins but should not be mixed with any other kind of insulin except regular insulin. A single form of insulin in a syringe is stable for weeks to months. Mixtures of insulins are not stable and should be administered within 5 minutes of preparation. The exception to this is the commercially prepared combination insulins such as Mixtard or Novolin 70/30, which are also stable for long periods.
- When insulins are mixed, regular (unmodified) insulin should always be drawn into the syringe first. Instruct patients to always use the same procedure in drawing up two insulins to avoid inadvertant contamination of the two vials of insulin with each other.
- Insulin may be used in an insulin subcutaneous injection pump. See manufacturer's guidelines accompanying the infusion pump.
- Teach and/or refer patients as needed to a dietitian about appropriate dietary restrictions. Review foot care and other aspects of personal hygiene to prevent infections.
- Teach patients how to test blood glucose and/or urinary glucose. Review methods of testing and frequency, and supervise patient performing test activities for accuracy.
- Work with the patient and family to determine the best methods for insulin administration for that patient. Decisions to be made include whether to use disposable syringes, whether to reuse syringes, and whether patient has the facility and/or satisfactory vision for drawing up insulin doses, etc.
- Refer patients to the local health department for follow-up. Work with the public health nurse to address any problems in the home situation related to the management of diabetes.
- Refer patients to the American Diabetes Association or local support groups for additional information and resources; examples of such resources include syringes adapted for the visually impaired, information booklets, automatic insulin injectors, and so on.
- Review with diabetic patients what to do if the patient is ill or unable to eat. The patient should maintain hydration by drinking 8 oz of fluid per hour (of noncaloric beverages). Notify physician if illness is severe or persistent. Monitor blood glucose.
- Caution patients to keep track of amount of insulin and syringes on hand to avoid running out.
- Teach patients who travel to carry insulin and syringes in carry-on luggage.
- Encourage patients with diabetes to wear a medical identification tag or bracelet.
- Caution patients to avoid the use of alcohol.
- Caution patients to avoid taking any medications that have not been approved by the physician.

## extended insulin zinc   (IN-soo-lin)                                      hypoglycemic

- extended insulin zinc: Humulin ultralente, Ultralente Iletin I, Ultralente insulin, Ultralente Purified Beef

**MECHANISM OF ACTION**    See entry for drug class (p. 655).

**INDICATIONS**    As a slow-acting insulin, this preparation is not suitable for emergencies but is intended for routine use in stable diabetes. • See entry for drug class (p. 655).

**CONTRAINDICATIONS**    See entry for drug class (p. 655).

| Table 34-4. | Preparations of extended insulin zinc | | | |
|---|---|---|---|---|
| | Trade name | Source | Concentration | Purity |
| | Ultralente Humulin | Human recombi- nant DNA | 100 units/ml | No proinsulin |
| | Ultralente Iletin I | Beef and pork | 40 units/ml or 100 units/ml | <20 ppm proinsulin |
| | Ultralente insulin | Beef | 100 units/ml | <= 10 ppm proinsulin |
| | Ultralente Purified Beef Insulin | Beef | 100 units/ml | <=1 ppm proinsulin |

**DOSAGE**  All insulin dosage must be individualized based on careful monitoring of the patient. The doses listed below are guidelines only; doses for individual patients may vary from the ranges given. Doses for children are determined by the severity of disease, as well as body weight of the child.  **SC: ADULTS OR CHILDREN:** Initially, up to 26 units as a single dose 30 to 60 minutes before breakfast. May be combined with other forms such as regular insulin and administered two thirds before breakfast and one third before the evening meal.  *Special patient populations:*  **PREGNANCY:** Insulin is required for the diabetic mother. Uncontrolled diabetes is a risk factor for abnormal pregnancies.

**PREPARATIONS**  All preparations listed in Table 34-4 are suspensions.

**DRUG INTERACTIONS**  See entry for drug class (p. 656).

**FATE**  Insulin is a protein and is not stable in GI fluids. For this reason the hormone must be administered parenterally. Subcutaneous injections are preferred for routine use. Extended insulin zinc has been modified so that the suspension is slowly absorbed from the injection site, prolonging the duration of action (Table 34-1). Once absorbed, insulin is rapidly degraded by various tissues.

## ❦ NURSING CONSIDERATIONS

### Side effects, toxicities, and associated nursing actions
- See entry for drug class (p. 659).

### Nursing interventions related to drug administration
- See entry for drug class (p. 659).

### Patient and family education
- See entry for drug class (p. 659).

## insulin zinc  (IN-soo-lin)  hypoglycemic

- insulin zinc: Humulin L, Lente Iletin I, Lente Iletin II, Lente Insulin, Novolin L

**MECHANISM OF ACTIONS**  See entry for drug class (p. 655).

**INDICATIONS**  This intermediate-acting insulin preparation is used for routine management of diabetes but is not suitable for emergencies where rapid effect is required. • See entry for drug class (p. 655).

**CONTRAINDICATIONS**  See entry for drug class (p. 655).

**DOSAGE**  All insulin dosage must be individualized, based upon careful monitoring of the patient. The doses listed (Table 34-5) are guidelines only; doses for individual patients may vary from the ranges given. Doses for children are determined by the severity of disease, as well as body weight of the child.  **SC: ADULTS OR CHILDREN:** Initially up to 26 units as a single dose 30 to 60 minutes before breakfast. A second dose may be required before supper or at bedtime.  *Special patient populations:*  **PREG-**

**Table 34-5.**

### Preparations of insulin zinc*

| Trade name | Source | Concentration | Purity |
|---|---|---|---|
| Humulin L | Human, recombinant DNA | 100 units/ml | No proinsulin, <4 ppm contaminating polypeptides |
| Lente Iletin I | Beef and pork | 40 or 100 units/ml | <20 ppm proinsulin |
| Lente Iletin II Purified Beef | Beef | 100 units/ml | <1=10 ppm proinsulin |
| Lente Iletin II Purified Pork | Pork | 100 units/ml | <=10 ppm proinsulin |
| Lente Insulin | Beef | 100 units/ml | <10 ppm proinsulin |
| Lente Insulin Purified Pork | Pork | 100 units/ml | <=1 ppm proinsulin |
| Novolin L | Human, semisynthetic | 100 units/ml | Not reported |

*All preparations listed are suspensions. Preparations are not necessarily equivalent. When switching patients from one preparation to another, dosage adjustment may be necessary.

**NANCY:** Insulin is required for the diabetic mother. Uncontrolled diabetes is a risk factor for abnormal pregnancies.

**DRUG INTERACTIONS**   See entry for drug class (p. 656).

**FATE**   Insulin is a protein and is not stable in GI fluids. For this reason the hormone must be administered parenterally. Subcutaneous injections are preferred for routine use. Insulin zinc has been modified so that the suspension is more slowly absorbed from the injection site than regular insulin, prolonging the duration of action. Once absorbed, insulin is rapidly degraded by various tissues.

### ☙ NURSING CONSIDERATIONS
#### Side effects, toxicities, and associated nursing actions
   • See entry for drug class (p. 659).
#### Nursing interventions related to drug administration
   • See entry for drug class (p. 659).
#### Patient and family education
   • See entry for drug class (p. 659).

## isophane insulin   (EYE-so-fane)                          hypoglycemic

   • isophane insulin: Humulin N, Iletin I NPH, Insulin NPH, Insulatard, Insulatard NPH Human, Novolin N

**MECHANISM OF ACTION**   See entry for drug class (p. 655).

**INDICATIONS**   As a slow-acting insulin, this preparation is not suitable for emergencies when rapid action is critical, but is intended for routine use in stable diabetes. • See entry for drug class (p. 655).

**CONTRAINDICATIONS**   See entry for drug class (p. 655).

**DOSAGE**   All insulin dosage must be individualized, based on careful monitoring of the patient. The doses listed below are guidelines only; doses for individual patients may vary from the ranges given. Doses for children are determined by the severity of disease as well as body weight of the child.   **SC:**

| Table 34-6. | Preparations of isophane insulin* | | | |
|---|---|---|---|---|
| | **Trade name** | **Source** | **Concentration** | **Purity** |
| | Humulin N | Human, recombinant DNA | 100 units/ml | No proinsulin, <4 ppm contaminating polypeptides |
| | Iletin I NPH | Beef and pork | 40 or 100 units/ml | <20 ppm proinsulin |
| | Iletin II NPH Purified Beef | Beef | 100 units/ml | <=10 ppm proinsulin |
| | Iletin II NPH Purified Pork | Pork | 100 units/ml | <=10 ppm proinsulin |
| | Insulatard NPH | Pork | 100 units/ml | <=10 ppm proinsulin |
| | Insulatard NPH Human | Human, semisynthetic | 100 units/ml | Not reported |
| | Insulin NPH | Beef | 100 units/ml | <10 ppm proinsulin |
| | Insulin NPH Purified Pork | Pork | 100 units/ml | <=1 ppm proinsulin |
| | Mixtard | Pork | 70 units/ml of NPH insulin and 30 units/ml of regular insulin | <=10 ppm proinsulin |
| | Novolin N | Human, semisynthetic | 100 units/ml | <1 ppm proinsulin |
| | Novolin 70/30 | Human, semisynthetic | 70 units/ml NPH insulin and 30 units/ml of regular insulin | <1 ppm proinsulin |

*Preparations are not necessarily equivalent. When switching patients from one preparation to another, dosage adjustment may be necessary.

**ADULTS OR CHILDREN:** Initially up to 26 units as a single dose 30 to 60 minutes before breakfast. *Special patient populations:* **PREGNANCY:** Insulin is required for the diabetic mother. Uncontrolled diabetes is a risk factor for abnormal pregnancies.

**PREPARATIONS**    All preparations listed in the table above (Table 34-6) are suspensions.

**DRUG INTERACTIONS**    See entry for drug class (p. 656).

**FATE**    Insulin is a protein and is not stable in GI fluids. For this reason the hormone must be administered parenterally. Subcutaneous injections are preferred for routine use. Isophane insulin has been modified so that the suspension is slowly absorbed from the injection site, prolonging the duration of action. Once absorbed, insulin is rapidly degraded by various tissues.

❧ **NURSING CONSIDERATIONS**

**Side effects, toxicities, and associated nursing actions**
• See entry for drug class (p. 659).

**Nursing interventions related to drug administration**
• See entry for drug class (p. 659).

**Patient and family education**
• See entry for drug class (p. 659).

## prompt insulin zinc    (IN-soo-lin)                                        hypoglycemic

• prompt insulin zinc: Semilente Iletin I, Semilente Insulin

**MECHANISM OF ACTION**    See entry for drug class (p. 655).

| Table 34-7. | Preparations of prompt insulin zinc | | | |
|---|---|---|---|---|
| | Trade name | Source | Concentration | Purity |
| | Semilente Iletin I | Beef and pork | 40 or 100 units/ml | <20 ppm proinsulin |
| | Semilente Insulin | Beef | 100 units/ml | <10 ppm proinsulin |
| | Semilente Insulin Purified Pork | Pork | 100 units/ml | <=1 ppm proinsulin |

**INDICATIONS**  This rapidly acting preparation is usually combined with insulin zinc or with extended insulin zinc. • It is not suitable for use in emergencies; regular insulin IV is preferred. • See entry for drug class (p. 655).

**CONTRAINDICATIONS**  See entry for drug class (p. 655).

**DOSAGE**  All insulin dosage must be individualized based on careful monitoring of the patient. The doses listed below are guidelines only; doses for individual patients may vary from the ranges given. Doses for children are determined by the severity of disease as well as body weight of the child.  **SC: ADULTS OR CHILDREN:** Initially 10 to 20 units 30 minutes before breakfast, usually with one other dose during the day.  *Special patient populations:*  **PREGNANCY:** Insulin is required for the diabetic mother. Uncontrolled diabetes is a risk factor for abnormal pregnancies.

**PREPARATIONS**  The preparations listed in Table 34-7 are suspensions.

**DRUG INTERACTIONS**  See entry for drug class (p. 656).

**FATE**  Insulin is a protein and is not stable in GI fluids. For this reason the hormone must be administered parenterally. Subcutaneous injections are preferred for routine use. Prompt insulin zinc has been modified so that the preparation has a slightly longer duration of action than regular insulin. Once absorbed, insulin is rapidly degraded by various tissues.

## ☙ NURSING CONSIDERATIONS

### Side effects, toxicities, and associated nursing actions
• See entry for drug class (p. 659).

### Nursing interventions related to drug administration
• See entry for drug class (p. 659).

### Patient and family education
• See entry for drug class (p. 659).

## protamine zinc insulin  (PRO-ta-meen)  hypoglycemic

• protamine zinc insulin: Protamine zinc Iletin I, Protamine zinc Iletin II

**MECHANISM OF ACTION**  See entry for drug class (p. 655).

**INDICATIONS**  This long-acting preparation is intended for use primarily in stable diabetics and is not suitable for emergencies requiring rapid onset of action. • See entry for drug class (p. 655).

**CONTRAINDICATIONS**  See entry for drug class (p. 655).

**DOSAGE**  All insulin dosage must be individualized based on careful monitoring of the patient. The doses listed in Table 34-8 are guidelines only; doses for individual patients may vary from the ranges given. Doses for children are determined by the severity of disease as well as body weight of the child.  **SC: ADULTS OR CHILDREN:** Initially, up to 26 units in one dose 30 to 60 minutes before breakfast. *Special patient populations:*  **PREGNANCY:** Insulin is required for the diabetic mother. Uncontrolled diabetes is a risk factor for abnormal pregnancies.

| Table 34-8. | Preparations of protamine zinc insulin | | | |
|---|---|---|---|---|
| | **Trade Name** | **Source** | **Concentration** | **Purity** |
| | Protamine zinc Iletin I | Beef and pork | 40 or 100 units/ml | < 20 ppm proinsulin |
| | Protamine zinc Iletin II Purified Beef | Beef | 100 units/ml | < = 10 ppm proinsulin |
| | Protamine zinc Iletin II Purified Pork | Pork | 100 units/ml | < = 10 ppm proinsulin |

**PREPARATIONS**   All preparations listed in Table 34-8 are suspensions.

**DRUG INTERACTIONS**   See entry for drug class (p. 656).

  **FATE**   Insulin is a protein and is not stable in GI fluids. For this reason the hormone must be administered parenterally. Subcutaneous injections are preferred for routine use. Protamine zinc insulin has been modified so that the suspension is slowly absorbed from the injection site, prolonging the *duration of action*. Once absorbed, insulin is rapidly degraded by various tissues.

**❦ NURSING CONSIDERATIONS**

  **Side effects, toxicities, and associated nursing actions**

  • See entry for drug class (p. 659).

  **Nursing interventions related to drug administration**

  • See entry for drug class (p. 659).

  **Patient and family education**

  • See entry for drug class (p. 659).

## regular insulin   (IN-soo-lin)   hypoglycemic

  • regular insulin: Humulin BR, Humulin R, Iletin, Insulin, Novolin R, Velosulin, Velosulin R

**MECHANISM OF ACTION**   See entry for drug class (p. 655).

**INDICATIONS**   Regular insulin is the only preparation that is suitable for IV use when rapid action is necessary to control diabetic coma or diabetic ketoacidosis. • See entry for drug class (p. 655).

**CONTRAINDICATIONS**   See entry for drug class (p. 655).

**DOSAGE**   All insulin dosage must be individualized based on careful monitoring of the patient. The doses listed below are guidelines only; doses for individual patients may vary from the ranges given. Doses for children are determined by the severity of disease, as well as body weight of the child.   **IV: ADULTS:** For severe ketoacidosis and coma, 100 to 200 units total initial dose, with half given IV and half SC. Doses are repeated as necessary based on hourly glucose, acetone, or ketone measurements. Alternate therapy is with an IV loading dose of 2.4 to 7.2 units followed by an IV infusion of 2.4 to 7.2 units/hr.   **CHILDREN:** For severe ketoacidosis and coma, initially 1 to 2 units/kg total, with half given IV and half SC. Doses are repeated as necessary based on hourly glucose, acetone, or ketone measurements. Alternate therapy is with an IV loading dose of 0.1 units/kg followed by an IV infusion of 0.1 units/kg per hour. To test growth hormone secretion, 0.05 to 0.15 units/kg by rapid IV injection, with blood sampling before and 30, 45, and 60 minutes after the dose. Normal growth hormone responses are indicated by concentrations exceeding 10 mg/ml within 45 minutes of the injection.   **IM: ADULTS:** For ketoacidosis and coma, initially 0.22 units/kg, followed by 5 units every hour as necessary.   **CHILDREN:** For ketoacidosis and coma, initially 0.25 units/kg, followed by 0.1 units/kg per hour as necessary.   **SC: ADULTS:** For complicated, severe, or unstable diabe-

| Table 34-9. | Preparations of regular insulin* | | | |
|---|---|---|---|---|
| | **Trade name** | **Source** | **Concentration** | **Purity** |
| | Humulin BR | Human, recombinant DNA | 100 units/ml | For use in insulin pumps only |
| | Humulin R | Human, recombinant DNA | 100 units/ml | No proinsulin, <4 ppm contaminating polypeptides |
| | Novolin R | Human, semisynthetic | 100 units/ml | Not reported |
| | Regular Iletin I | Beef and Pork | 40 or 100 units/ml | <20 ppm proinsulin |
| | Regular Iletin II Purified Beef | Beef | 100 units/ml | <=10 ppm proinsulin |
| | Regular Iletin II Purified Pork | Pork | 100 or 500 units/ml | <=10 ppm proinsulin |
| | Regular Insulin | Pork | 100 units/ml | <10 ppm proinsulin |
| | Regular Insulin Purified Pork | Pork | 100 units/ml | <=1 ppm proinsulin |
| | Velosulin | Pork | 100 units/ml | <=10 ppm proinsulin |
| | Velosulin Human | Human, semisynthetic | 100 units/ml | Not reported |

*Preparations are not necessarily equivalent. When switching patients from one preparation to another, dosage adjustment may be necessary.

tes, 5 to 10 units 15 to 30 minutes before meals and at bedtime.   **CHILDREN:** For complicated, severe, or unstable diabetes, 2 to 4 units 15 to 30 minutes before meals and at bedtime.   *Special patient populations:*   **PREGNANCY:** Insulin is required for the diabetic mother. Uncontrolled diabetes is a risk factor for abnormal pregnancies.

**PREPARATIONS**   The preparations listed in Table 34-9 are the only insulin preparations that may be used IV or IM, as well as SC.

**DRUG INTERACTIONS**   See entry for drug class (p. 656).

**FATE**   Insulin is a protein and is not stable in GI fluids. For this reason the hormone must be administered parenterally. Subcutaneous injections are preferred for routine use, but regular insulin may be given IV for very rapid action. Absorbed insulin is rapidly degraded by various tissues. Doses of regular insulin must be repeated three or four times daily or combined with other forms of insulin for more prolonged action.

**☙ NURSING CONSIDERATIONS**
### Side effects, toxicities, and associated nursing actions
   • See entry for drug class (p. 659).
### Nursing interventions related to drug administration
   • See entry for drug class (p. 659).
### Patient and family education
   • See entry for drug class (p. 659).

# Sulfonylureas

acetohexamide ~ chlorpropamide ~ glipizide ~ glyburide ~ tolazamide ~ tolbutamide

**OVERVIEW OF THE DRUG CLASS**   Patients with NIDDM retain the ability to secrete insulin but resist the action of insulin in their tissues. For many of these patients, dietary restrictions may offer control of the disease. Others may require treatment with one of the sulfonylureas, along with dietary manipulations. Insulin is occasionally required in these patients when they are acutely stressed by illness or injury.

**MECHANISM OF ACTION**    Sulfonylureas have several effects that may contribute to the overall hypoglycemic action. The drugs stimulate release of insulin from the pancreas, at least during early phases of treatment. Sulfonylureas are not effective in patients lacking the ability to form insulin, e.g. patients with IDDM (type I or juvenile-onset). With long-term therapy the sulfonylureas may reduce the amount of glucose formed by the liver and may increase the sensitivity of peripheral tissues to insulin. These latter effects may be the most important for chronic control of NIDDM.

**INDICATIONS**    NIDDM NIDDM not adequately controlled by diet may be treated with oral doses of sulfonylureas.

**CONTRAINDICATIONS**    **IDDM** Patients must secrete some insulin in order to respond to sulfonylureas.    **Diabetic ketoacidosis, acidosis, or coma** Insulin is the appropriate therapy for these emergencies. **Pregnancy** Insulin is appropriate therapy for pregnant patients.    **Hepatic porphyria** Sulfonylureas may worsen this condition.    **Severe renal disease** Such patients may be more prone to side effects, including severe hypoglycemia.

**DRUG INTERACTIONS**    **Alcohol** with sulfonylureas may cause a disulfiram reaction in some patients (p. 715). **Beta adrenergic blocking agents** may block some signs of hypoglycemia and may worsen the patient's response to it. Patients may suffer more frequent and worse episodes of hypoglycemia.    **Calcium channel blocking agents** may decrease the hypoglycemic effect of sulfonylureas.    **Chloramphenicol** may enhance the hypoglycemic effect of sulfonylureas.    **Cimetidine** may enhance hypoglycemic action of sulfonylureas.    **Corticosteroids** may decrease the hypoglycemic effect of sulfonylureas. **Coumarin oral anticoagulants** may displace sulfonylureas from protein binding sites, increasing the hypoglycemic effect.    **Estrogens** may decrease the hypoglycemic effect of sulfonylureas.    **Furosemide** may decrease the hypoglycemic effect of sulfonylureas.    **Isoniazid** may decrease the hypoglycemic effect of sulfonylureas.    **Monoamine oxidase inhibitors** may enhance the hypoglycemic effect of sulfonylureas.    **Nicotinic acid** may decrease the hypoglycemic effect of sulfonylureas.    **Nonsteroidal antiinflammatory agents** may displace sulfonylureas from protein binding sites, increasing the hypoglycemic effect.    **Oral contraceptives** may decrease the hypoglycemic effect of sulfonylureas. **Phenothiazines** may decrease the hypoglycemic effect of sulfonylureas.    **Phenylbutazone** may displace sulfonylureas from protein binding sites or compete for urinary excretion, increasing the hypoglycemic effect.    **Phenytoin** may displace sulfonylureas from protein binding sites, increasing the hypoglycemic effect.    **Probenecid** may enhance the hypoglycemic effect of sulfonylureas.    **Rifampin** may decrease the hypoglycemic effect of sulfonylureas.    **Salicylates** may displace sulfonylureas from protein binding sites, increasing the hypoglycemic effect.    **Sulfonamides** may displace sulfonylureas from protein binding sites, increasing the hypoglycemic effect.    **Sympathomimetic agents** may decrease the hypoglycemic effect of sulfonylureas.    **Thiazide diuretics** may worsen diabetes and increase the dosage requirement for the sulfonylureas.    **Thyroid hormones** may decrease the hypoglycemic effect of sulfonylureas.

## ❦ NURSING CONSIDERATIONS

### Side effects, toxicities, and associated nursing actions

**Blood** Agranulocytosis, aplastic anemia, hemolytic anemia, leukopenia, pancytopenia, and thrombocytopenia are rare side effects of sulfonylureas.
- Assess patients for and ask them to report fever, sore throat, pallor, fatigue, malaise, and unexplained bruising or bleeding.
- Monitor complete blood count, white blood cell differential, and platelet count.

**GI** The most common side effects to several sulfonylureas are GI reactions, including anorexia, constipation, diarrhea, gastralgia, and vomiting.
- Monitor weight.
- Review possible GI side effects with patients. Caution patients to notify physician if side effects are severe or persistent, as a change in drug or dosage may be necessary.

- For constipatīon, instruct patients to increase fluid intake of noncaloric fluids to 2500 to 3000 ml per day, increase daily exercise, and increase amount of roughage in the diet.
- Caution patients to take ordered doses with meals.

**Metabolic** Hypoglycemia is a potentially life-threatening side effect of sulfonylurea therapy. Older patients or patients who are inadvertently overdosed are more susceptible to this reaction.

- Review signs and symptoms of hypoglycemia (see Table 34-2). Instruct patients to treat hypoglycemia by taking a fast-acting carbohydrate. Example sources of glucose are 1/2 C fruit juice, 1/2 C sugar cola drink, 1/2 C regular gelatin dessert, 4 cubes or 2 packs of sugar, 2 squares of graham crackers, or 2 to 3 pieces of hard candy.
- Instruct patients to carry hard candy or other sources of carbohydrates with them at all times.
- If hypoglycemia is severe, repeated, or occurring without explanation, have patient notify physician.

**Allergic** Reactions may include eczema, erythema, pruritis, skin eruptions, and urticaria.

- Caution patients to report the development of skin changes.

**Liver** Hepatic porphyria may be exacerbated. Jaundice is occasionally reported.

- Assess for signs of liver dysfunction: malaise, fever, jaundice, right upper quadrant abdominal pain, or change in color or consistency of stools.
- For specific side effects, see individual drug monographs.

**Patient and family education**

- Review carefully and frequently the treatment of diabetes with patient and family. Caution patient to seek the advice of the nurse or physician when in doubt, or when new signs and symptoms develop.
- The specific regimen prescribed for any patient will be based on the age of the patient, severity of the diabetes, weight of the patient, philosophy of the health care team, and other medical problems or disabilities, etc. While general guidelines are noted in this monograph, more detailed information can be found in nursing textbooks and other printed resources.
- Teach and/or refer patients as needed to a dietitian about appropriate dietary restrictions. Patients with NIDDM may find that adhering to the prescribed diet or losing weight to ideal body weight will be all that is necessary to maintain the blood glucose levels at the normal level. Reinforce to patients the importance of following dietary prescriptions.
- Teach patients how to test blood glucose and/or urinary glucose as prescribed. Review methods of testing, frequency, and supervise patient performing test activities for accuracy.
- Refer the patient to the health department for follow-up if indicated.
- Caution patients to take medication as prescribed, but if a dose is missed, not to "double-up" with 2 doses at the next dose time.
- Caution patients to keep track of the drug on hand to avoid running out.
- Encourage patients with diabetes to wear a medical identification tag or bracelet.
- Caution patients to avoid the use of alcohol.
- See Drug Interactions; caution patients to avoid all medications unless first approved by the physician. Remind patient to keep all health care providers informed of all drugs being used. Remind patients to keep these and all medications out of the reach of children.
- These agents are not to be used during pregnancy. Instruct women of childbearing age to notify physician immediately if pregnancy is suspected.

## acetohexamide    (a-see-to-HEX-uh-mide)                    oral hypoglycemic

- acetohexamide: Dymelor

**MECHANISM OF ACTION**   See entry for drug class (p. 667).
**INDICATIONS**   See entry for drug class (p. 667).
**CONTRAINDICATIONS**   See entry for drug class (p. 667).
**DOSAGE**   PO:   **ADULTS:** Doses range from 250 mg to 1.5 g daily, individualized according to patient need.
*Special patient populations:*   **ELDERLY:** Geriatric patients may be more sensitive to hypoglycemia

or other side effects of sulfonylureas. Geriatric patients should receive 250 mg as initial dosage and be carefully monitored before increasing dosage.   **CHILDREN:** Sulfonylureas are not indicated for sole therapy of IDDM.   **PREGNANCY:** Avoid use during pregnancy. Insulin may be substituted.

**PREPARATIONS**   *Tablets:* 250 or 500 mg.

**DRUG INTERACTIONS**   See entry for drug class (p. 667).

**FATE**   Acetohexamide is well absorbed following oral administration, producing *peak* serum concentrations of active forms of the drug within 4 hours. Acetohexamide is metabolized to active forms in the liver. The elimination *half-life* of the principal metabolite is 5 to 6 hours. Excretion is in urine.

### 🐾 NURSING CONSIDERATIONS

#### Side effects, toxicities, and associated nursing actions
- See entry for drug class (p. 667).

#### Patient and family education
- See entry for drug class (p. 668).

---

## chlorpropamide   (klor-PRO-pa-mide)                           oral hypoglycemic

- chlorpropamide: Diabinese, Glucamide

**MECHANISM OF ACTION**   See entry for drug class (p. 667).

**INDICATIONS**   See entry for drug class (p. 667).

**CONTRAINDICATIONS**   See entry for drug class (p. 667).

**DOSAGE**   PO:   **ADULTS:** Initially 250 mg at breakfast each day. Doses as low as 100 mg or as high as 500 mg may be required for individual patients. *Special patient populations:* **ELDERLY:** Geriatric patients may be more sensitive to hypoglycemia or other side effects of sulfonylureas. Geriatric patients should receive 100 to 125 mg as initial dosage and be carefully monitored before increasing or decreasing dosage.   **CHILDREN:** Sulfonylureas are not indicated for sole therapy of IDDM.   **PREGNANCY:** Avoid use during pregnancy. Insulin may be substituted.

**PREPARATIONS**   *Tablets:* 100 or 250 mg.

**DRUG INTERACTIONS**   See entry for drug class (p. 667).

**FATE**   Chlorpropamide is well absorbed following oral administration, producing *peak* plasma concentrations within 2 to 4 hours. Peak hypoglycemic effect is at 3 to 6 hours (see Table 32-10). The plasma *half-life* is about 36 hours. Chlorpropamide is partially metabolized in liver and excreted in urine.

### 🐾 NURSING CONSIDERATIONS

#### Side effects, toxicities, and associated nursing actions
**CNS** Headache, paresthesia, and weakness may occur as dose-related side effects.
- Assess patient for tingling of fingers, and toes.
- If CNS symptoms are severe or persistent, notify physician.

**Skin** Photosensitivity reactions can occur.
- Caution patients to avoid exposure to the sun or other sources of ultraviolet light, to wear a wide-brimmed hat, to keep extremities covered, and to wear a maximum-protection sunscreen on exposed skin surfaces.

**Endocrine** Inappropriate secretion of antidiuretic hormone (SIADH) may be induced, leading to water intoxication, with symptoms including confusion, dizziness, depression, nausea, decreased sodium concentration in serum, and increased urinary osmolality. Geriatric patients are more prone to this reaction than younger adults.
- Monitor weight and blood pressure; assess for the symptoms of SIADH.
- Monitor serum and urinary electrolytes and urine osmolality.
- For other reactions to chlorpropamide, see entry for drug class (p. 667).

#### Patient and family education
- See entry for drug class (p. 668).

| Table 34-10. | Summary of oral hypoglycemic agents | | | | |
|---|---|---|---|---|---|

| | | Hypoglycemic activity | | |
|---|---|---|---|---|
| Generic name | Trade name | Onset | Peak | Duration |
| Acetohexamide | Dymelor | <1 hr | 1 to 2 hr | 12 to 24 hr |
| Chlorpropamide | Diabenese | <1 hr | 3 to 6 hr | Up to 60 hr |
| Glipizide | Glucotrol | 15 to 30 min | 1 to 2 hr | 12 to 24 hr |
| Glyburide | Diabeta, Micronase | 45 to 60 min | 1.5 to 3 hr | 16 to 24 hr |
| Tolazamide | Tolinase | 4 to 6 hr | 10 hr | 12 to 16 hr |
| Tolbutamide | Orinase | <1 hr | 5 to 8 hr | 6 to 12 hr |

## glipizide    (GLIP-i-zide)                                    oral hypoglycemic

● glipizide: Glucotrol

**MECHANISM OF ACTION**    See entry for drug class (p. 667).

**INDICATIONS**    See entry for drug class (p. 667).

**CONTRAINDICATIONS**    See entry for drug class (p. 667).

**DOSAGE**    PO:    **ADULTS:** Initially 5 mg once daily. Maintenance doses may be as high as 30 mg daily, given in 2 divided doses, taken on empty stomach. *Special patient populations:* **ELDERLY:** Geriatric patients may be more sensitive to hypoglycemia or other side effects of sulfonylureas. Geriatric patients should receive 2.5 mg as initial dosage and be carefully monitored before increasing dosage. **CHILDREN:** Sulfonylureas are not indicated for sole therapy of IDDM. **PREGNANCY:** Avoid use during pregnancy. Insulin may be substituted.

**PREPARATIONS**    *Tablets:* 5 or 10 mg.

**DRUG INTERACTIONS**    **Cimetidine** may potentiate the hypoglycemic action of glipizide. Glipizide may potentially be involved in any interactions noted for other sulfonylureas (see entry for drug class p. 667).

**FATE**    Glipizide is completely absorbed following oral administration, producing *peak* serum concentrations within 1 to 3 hours (Table 34-10). Glipizide is less tightly bound to plasma proteins than the older sulfonylureas and therefore potentially less likely to be potentiated by drugs such as oral anticoagulants, nonsteroidal antiinflammatory agents, phenytoin, salicylates, or sulfonamides. Glipizide is completely metabolized by liver and excreted in urine.

## ☙ NURSING CONSIDERATIONS

### Side effects, toxicities, and associated nursing actions

**CNS** Up to 2% of patients report dizziness, drowsiness, or headache.

● Caution patients to avoid driving or operating hazardous equipment if dizziness or drowsiness occurs.

● Instruct patient to notify physician if CNS side effects are severe or persistent.

**GI** Up to 2% of patients suffer anorexia, constipation, diarrhea, gastralgia, nausea, pyrosis, and vomiting.

● Monitor weight. If GI symptoms are severe, monitor intake and output.

● Caution patients with diarrhea or vomiting to maintain fluid intake. If GI symptoms persist longer than 48 hours, instruct patients to notify physician.

**Allergic** About 1.5%of patients report allergic skin reactions or photosensitivity.

● Caution patients with photosensitivity to avoid exposure to the sun or other sources of ultraviolet light, to wear a wide-brimmed hat, to keep extremities covered, and to use a maximum-protection sunscreen.

- Instruct patients to report skin changes to the physician.
- For other side effects of glipizide, see entry for drug class (p. 667).

**Patient and family education**
- See entry for drug class (p. 668).

---

## glyburide   (GLY-byoo-ride)                                    oral hypoglycemic

- glyburide: DiaBeta, Micronase

**MECHANISM OF ACTION**   See entry for drug class (p. 667).
**INDICATIONS**   See entry for drug class (p. 667).
**CONTRAINDICATIONS**   See entry for drug class (p. 667).
**DOSAGE**   **PO:**   **ADULTS:** Initially 2.5 to 5 mg daily as a single dose. Maintenance doses may range up to 20 mg daily, given in 2 divided doses.   *Special patient populations:*   **ELDERLY:** Geriatric patients may be more sensitive to hypoglycemia or other side effects of sulfonylureas. Geriatric patients should receive 1.25 mg as initial dosage and be carefully monitored before increasing dosage.   **PATIENTS WITH IMPAIRED RENAL OR HEPATIC FUNCTION:** These patients should receive 1.25 mg as initial dosage and be carefully monitored before increasing dosage.   **CHILDRENS:** Sulfonylureas are not indicated for sole therapy of IDDM.   **PREGNANCY:** Avoid use during pregnancy. Insulin may be substituted.
**PREPARATIONS**   *Tablets:* 1.25, 2.5, or 5 mg.
**DRUG INTERACTIONS**   See entry for drug class (p. 667).
**FATE**   Glyburide is well absorbed following oral administration, producing *peak* serum concentrations within 1 to 2 hours (Table 34-10). The elimination *half-life* is 1.4 to 1.8 hours. The drug is completely metabolized in liver and excreted in equal proportions in feces and urine.

### ❦ NURSING CONSIDERATIONS
**Side effects, toxicities, and associated nursing actions**
**Allergic** About 1.5% of patients suffer allergic skin reactions. Rare patients may suffer generalized hypersensitivity reactions, which in one patient involved toxic erythema, cholestatic jaundice, eosinophilia, visceral arteritis, and death.
- Caution patients to notify physician of any unexpected sign or symptom.
- For other reactions to glyburide, see entry for drug class (p. 667).

**Patient and family education**
- See entry for drug class (p. 668).

---

## tolazamide   (tol-AZ-uh-mide)                                   oral hypoglycemic

- tolazamide: Ronase, Tolinase

**MECHANISM OF ACTION**   See entry for drug class (p. 667).
**INDICATIONS**   See entry for drug class (p. 667).
**CONTRAINDICATIONS**   See entry for drug class (p. 667).
**DOSAGE**   **PO:**   **ADULTS:** Initially 100 to 250 mg as a single dose at breakfast. Maintenance doses range up to 1 g daily.   *Special patient populations:*   **ELDERLY:** Geriatric patients may be more sensitive to hypoglycemia or other side effects of sulfonylureas. Geriatric patients should receive 100 mg as initial dosage and be carefully monitored before increasing dosage.   **CHILDREN:** Sulfonylureas are not

indicated for sole therapy of IDDM. **PREGNANCY:** Avoid use during pregnancy. Insulin may be substituted.

**PREPARATIONS** *Tablets:* 100, 250, or 500 mg.

**DRUG INTERACTIONS** See entry for drug class (p. 667).

**FATE** Oral doses of tolazamide are slowly absorbed, producing *peak* hypoglycemic effects within 4 to 6 hours. The *half-life* of the drug is about 7 hours. Tolazamide is extensively metabolized in liver, and some of the metabolites are active. Excretion is primarily in urine.

**❦ NURSING CONSIDERATIONS**

**Side effects, toxicities, and associated nursing actions**
- See entry for drug class (p. 667).

**Patient and family education**
- See entry for drug class (p. 668).

---

## tolbutamide (tol-BYOO-tuh-mide) oral hypoglycemic

- tolbutamide: Oramide, Orinase

**MECHANISM OF ACTION** See entry for drug class (p. 667).

**INDICATIONS** See entry for drug class (p. 667).

**CONTRAINDICATIONS** See entry for drug class (p. 667).

**DOSAGE** **PO:** **ADULTS:** Initially 1 to 2 g daily; maintenance doses range from 250 mg to 3 g daily. *Special patient populations:* **ELDERLY:** Geriatric patients may be more sensitive to hypoglycemia or other side effects of sulfonylureas. Geriatric patients should receive small initial doses and be carefully monitored before increasing dosage. **CHILDREN:** Sulfonylureas are not indicated for sole therapy of IDDM. **PREGNANCY:** Avoid use during pregnancy. Insulin may be substituted.

**PREPARATIONS** *Tablets:* 250 or 500 mg.

**DRUG INTERACTIONS** See entry for drug class (p. 667).

**DIAGNOSTIC TEST INTERFERENCE** **Uptake of radioactive iodine** may be falsely lowered in the presence of tolbutamide. **Urinary albumin tests** based on acetic acid or sulfosalicylic acid precipitation may be falsely positive because tolbutamide metabolites precipitate in the test.

**FATE** Tolbutamide is well absorbed following oral administration, producing *peak* plasma concentrations within 3 to 5 hours. Tolbutamide has the shortest *duration of action* of the sulfonylureas. The drug is metabolized in liver and excreted mostly in urine.

**❦ NURSING CONSIDERATIONS**

**Side effects, toxicities, and associated nursing actions**
- See entry for drug class (p. 667).

**Patient and family education**
- See entry for drug class (p. 668).

---

# Hyperglycemic agent

glucagon hydrochloride

---

## glucagon hydrochloride (GLOO-ka-gon) hyperglycemic agent

- hyperglycemic agent: Glucagon for Injection

**MECHANISM OF ACTION** Glucagon causes liberation of glucose from glycogen stored in the liver. This action may be of benefit in patients suffering acute hypoglycemic reactions.

**INDICATIONS**   **Hypoglycemia** Glucagon is ineffective in starvation or chronic hypoglycemia because in those situations glycogen stores in the liver are depleted; therefore no glucose is released by glucagon.

**CONTRAINDICATIONS**   **Insulinoma** Glucagon stimulates release of insulin, which may produce serious rebound hypoglycemia in these patients.   **Pheochromocytoma** Glucagon stimulates release of catecholamines, which may cause dangerous elevation of blood pressure in these patients.

**DOSAGE**   IV, IM, or SC:   ADULTS: 0.5 to 1 unit as a single dose, which may be repeated if the patient fails to regain consciousness within 20 minutes. Parenteral dextrose may be more reliable and safer.   CHILDREN: 0.025 mg/kg as a single dose, which may be repeated if the patient fails to regain consciousness within 20 minutes. Parenteral dextrose may be more reliable and safer.   *Special patient populations:*   ELDERLY: Special geriatric doses have not been established.   PREGNANCY: FDA pregnancy category B.

**PREPARATIONS**   *Powder for reconstitution:* 1 to 10 units of glucagon.

**DRUG INTERACTIONS**   **Anticoagulants** such as coumarins may be potentiated by massive doses of glucagon.

**FATE**   Glucagon is a polypeptide and cannot be administered orally. Parenteral administration results in hyperglycemic effects within 30 minutes; the effect is over within 1 to 2 hours. The plasma *half-life* of the drug is 3 to 10 minutes, with extensive degradation by liver and kidneys.

## 🐝 NURSING CONSIDERATIONS

### Side effects, toxicities, and associated nursing actions

**GI** Adverse effects of single dose therapy are limited to occasional nausea or vomiting.

- Monitor intake and output. If vomiting is severe, notify physician. Have suction machine available.
- Monitor blood glucose level.

### Nursing interventions related to drug administration

- For direct IV use, administer at a rate of 1 unit or less over 1 minute.

### Patient and family education

- Review with patient and family the patient's present condition. Obtain history of hypoglycemic event if appropriate, and review signs and symptoms of hypoglycemia with patient.
- Consult with physician, then teach family how to administer glucagon at home if patient's condition suggests this may be necessary in the future.

# DRUGS TO MODIFY MENTAL AND EMOTIONAL BEHAVIOR

**INTRODUCTION**   A variety of agents is available to alter functions of the CNS. Perhaps the most commonly prescribed are the sedative-hypnotic and antianxiety agents. A few barbiturates are widely used as sedative-hypnotic medications, however, the benzodizepines are the most rapidly expanding drug class for insomnia, sedation, or anxiety and the most commonly prescribed medications for these actions. Miscellaneous sedative-hypnotic drugs are also still used. The antialcohol drug, disulfiram is not a sedative-hypnotic drug. It is used selectively to produce alcohol aversion in recovering alcoholics.

Perhaps the most dramatic therapeutic effects are those seen with antipsychotic drugs. These are effective in controlling many psychoses and manifestations of schizophrenia. In addition, several antipsychotic drugs are used to curb nausea and vomiting, especially that of chemotherapy.

Many effective drugs are now available to treat the most common of the mental illnesses, depression. Many phobias also respond to therapy with antidepressant medication. The tricyclic antidepressants revolutionized the treatment of mental depression, but the newer antidepressants have fewer side effects than the older tricyclic antidepressants. Monoamine oxidase inhibitors have significant side effects and drug and food interactions. Nevertheless, they are useful in treating selected types of depression and phobias. Lithium has proven uniquely effective in controlling manic episodes and some types of depression as well.

Less widely used therapeutically are the CNS stimulants. Clinical use is made of selected CNS stimulants in controlling narcolepsy and hyperkinesis. CNS stimulants also have limited use in weight control.

**X**

# Chapter Thirty-five

# Sedative-hypnotic and antianxiety agents

**Barbiturates**
amobarbital
butabarbital
pentobarbital
phenobarbital
secobarbital

**Benzodiazepines**
alprazolam
♣bromazepam
clorazepate
chlordiazepoxide
diazepam
flurazepam
halazepam
♣ketazolam
lorazepam
♣nitrazepam
oxazepam
prazepam
quazepam
temazepam
triazolam

**Miscellaneous sedative-hypnotic drugs**
buspirone
chloral hydrate
chlormezanone
ethchlorvynol
ethinamate
glutethimide
hydroxyzine HCl/pamoate
meprobamate
methotrimeprazine HCl
methyprylon
paraldehyde
promethazine HCl
propiomazine HCl

**Antialcohol agent**
disulfiram

**INTRODUCTION**   The drugs prescribed for insomnia and anxiety are presented in three sections. The first section is the barbiturates, an old class of drugs, many of which are used as CNS depressants. The second section is the benzodiazepines, now the most popular drug class for treating insomnia and anxiety. The third section presents miscellaneous drugs occasionally prescribed for insomnia or anxiety.

The term *sedative-hypnotic* is used for the older drug classes, primarily the barbiturates. A small dose to calm an anxious patient is called a sedative. A larger dose to induce sleep is a hypnotic. These drugs act pharmacologically as general depressants of the central nervous system since they depress the reticular activating system of the brain stem. The reticular activating system determines the level of our awareness of the environment and therefore governs our reactions to it.

The newer antianxiety drugs of the benzodiazepine class can reduce anxiety with a far lesser degree of sedation than the barbiturates and other sedative-hypnotic drugs.

Recent research has demonstrated that hypnotic therapy is of limited value. Tolerance develops to hypnotic drugs in 3 days to a month or more, depending on the drug. Furthermore, hypnotic drugs, to a varying degree, supress REM (rapid eye movement) sleep, so that when the hypnotic drug is discontinued, there is a rebound in REM sleep with vivid dreams and increased awakening.

# Barbiturates

amobarbital (Schedule II [C-II],* ♣Schedule G) ~ butabarbital (Schedule II [C-II],* ♣Schedule G) ~ pentobarbital (Schedule II [C-II],* ♣Schedule G) ~ phenobarbital (Schedule IV [C-IV],* ♣Schedule G) ~ secobarbital (Schedule II [C-II],* ♣Schedule G)

**DRUG COMBINATIONS**   amobarbital sodium and secobarbital sodium: Tuinal • butabarbital sodium, phenobarbital, and secobarbital sodium: S.B.P.

**OVERVIEW OF THE DRUG CLASS**   More than 50 derivatives have been marketed for clinical use since the early 1900s, and 9 are still widely used. The barbiturates have been classified according to their

*Schedule III as a suppository.

676

duration of action and have been traditionally divided into four classes: ultra-short-acting, short-acting, intermediate-acting, and long-acting. However, the duration of action of barbiturates given orally for sedation tends to be similar. The ultra-short-acting barbiturates, thiamylal, thiopental, and methohexital, are administered intravenously for the induction and/or maintenance of anesthesia. These are discussed in Chapter 48. The five barbiturates widely used as sedative-hypnotic drugs are listed above and presented here.

**MECHANISM OF ACTION**    The barbiturates are general central nervous system depressants. The drugs act throughout the CNS and especially depress the reticular activating system of the brain stem, the system that determines the level of our awareness of the environment and therefore our reaction to the environment. The molecular mechanisms by which barbiturates act are not well described.

**INDICATIONS**    **Insomnia and anxiety** Barbiturates are useful only for short-term treatment of insomnia and should not be used for more than 2 weeks. Barbiturates are primarily used as preoperative sedatives. Since barbiturates have a high potential for tolerance and addiction, they are no longer widely used for outpatient sedation as single-entity drugs, although they are combined with other drugs.    **Convulsions** Phenobarbital and mephobarbital are used as prophylactic treatment for grand mal epilepsy (see Chapter 40). Barbiturates are occasionally used IV to control seizure episodes.

**CONTRAINDICATIONS**    • Activities requiring mental alertness. • History of drug abuse. • Depression. • Acute or chronic pain: paradoxical excitement may be experienced. • Hypersensitivity. • Bronchopneumonia or pulmonary insufficiency: respiration will be depressed. • Porphyria: patient or family history.

**DRUG INTERACTIONS**    **CNS depressants** Barbiturates potentiate other CNS depressants, including other sedatives and hypnotics, benzodiazepines, antihistamines, narcotic analgesics, antipsychotics, and alcohol.    **Oral anticoagulants, corticosteroids, doxycycline, oral contraceptives** Barbiturates may induce liver microsomal enzymes, increasing the metabolism of these drugs and thereby decreasing their action.    **Oral anticoagulants and griseofulvin** Barbiturates may acutely delay the absorption of these drugs.

**DIAGNOSTIC TEST INTERFERENCE**    The retention of sulfobromophthalein may increase, resulting in elevated readings. Barbiturates should not be administered within 24 hours of this test.

## 🕸 NURSING CONSIDERATIONS

### Side effects, toxicities, and associated nursing actions

**CNS** Drowsiness, lethargy, depression; pain in nerves, joints, or muscle. Increased dreaming or insomnia or nightmares may be experienced when hypnotic doses are discontinued. Prolonged therapy with sedative doses (600 to 800 mg daily) for 8 weeks or more will produce physical dependence.
- Caution patients to avoid driving or operating hazardous equipment until the effects of the medication can be evaluated. Supervise the play of children, especially when they are riding bicycles or engaging in other potentially dangerous activities.
- Supervise ambulation of hospitalized patients and discourage smoking.
- Keep side rails up.
- Keep a night light on.
- In the outpatient setting, be alert to patients who return for prescription refills on an increasingly frequent basis, as this may indicate improper use or physical dependence on the drug.
- Assess carefully for the development of suicidal tendencies in patients with symptoms of depression.

**CV** Hypotension may accompany a rapid IV injection.
- Monitor the vital signs and blood pressure.
- Maintain the patient in a recumbent position when administering parenterally.

**GI** Nausea, vomiting, diarrhea, or constipation are occasionally experienced.
- Monitor for development of GI side effects. If symptoms are persistent or severe, it may be necessary to discontinue the drug.
- Monitor intake and output.
- Taking the oral preparation with milk, crackers, or a small snack may decrease nausea.

**Hematologic** Rarely: agranulocytosis, thrombocytopenic purpura, or megaloblastic anemia.

- Monitor complete blood count (CBC) and differential and platelet count.
- Visually inspect the patient for appearance of bruising or petechiae. Instruct the patient to report the development of any unexplained bruising or bleeding, such as bleeding from gums or nose or heavy menses.
- Instruct the patient to report development of fever or sore throat or possible signs of a granulocytosis.

**Lung** Newborns are especially sensitive to respiratory depression caused by barbiturates. Toxic doses will depress respiration in children and adults.

- Monitor the respiratory rate.
- Symptoms of overdose include ataxia, decreased level of consciousness or mental dullness, nystagmus, and respiratory depression. Eventually coma will develop. Treatment should be supportive and should involve ventilatory support as needed, IV fluids, appropriate drugs to correct cardiovascular difficulties, and oxygen.

**Metabolic** Elevation in blood ammonia levels.

- Monitor blood ammonia levels if available. Elevated blood ammonia levels are most commonly associated with hepatic failure, but may be seen in other conditions.

**Allergic** Urticaria, angioedema, morbilliform or scarlatiniform rash, fever, serum sickness, erythema multiforme, or Stevens-Johnson syndrome.

- Monitor vital signs.
- Assess for these or other unexpected signs and symptoms.
- Have drugs, equipment, and personnel available to treat acute allergic reactions.

**Patient and family education**

- Review with the patient the expected benefits and possible side effects of therapy. Instruct the patient to report the development of any unexpected sign or symptom.
- Caution patients to avoid the use of any other medications, including over-the-counter preparations, without prior clearance with the physician. Review Drug Interactions in Overview of Drug Class.
- Caution the patient to avoid the use of alcohol.
- Remind patients to take the medication only as ordered. Patients should not double up if a dose is missed. Patients should not share medications with others.
- Instruct patients that the frequently encountered ''hangover effect'' in the morning following use of a sedative-hypnotic is a side effect of the medication and not a sign that the patient needs a larger dose that evening.
- For insomnia, instruct patients to take the prescribed dose about 30 minutes prior to bedtime.
- Caution patients taking medication as an anticonvulsant that drowsiness may continue for several days to weeks but should gradually diminish.
- Remind patients to keep these and all medications out of the reach of children. Child-proof caps should be used on medication vials.
- To avoid accidental overdose, caution patients to keep drugs in clearly marked containers, away from the bedside, so that the patient does not inadvertently repeat a dose if wakened during the night.

## amobarbital   (am-oh-BAR-bi-tal)                                                hypnotic*

- amobarbital (amobarbital sodium): Amytal, ✿Isobec (Schedule II, ✿Schedule G)

**MECHANISM OF ACTION**   Barbiturates depress the reticular activating system.

**INDICATIONS**   **Anxiety** For sedation, especially preoperatively.   **Insomnia** Should not be used for more than 2 weeks because tolerance develops.   **Seizures** For critical conditions, amobarbital may be administered IV or IM to control ongoing seizures.   **Narcoanalysis, narcotherapy** Patients are queried while under sedation.   **Schizophrenia** Diagnostic aid.

**CONTRAINDICATIONS**   • See entry for drug class (p. 677).

*Anticonvulsant.

**DOSAGE** **Sedation PO:** ADULTS: 30 to 50 mg two or three times daily. Range: 15 to 120 mg two to four times daily. CHILDREN: 2 mg/kg or 70 mg/M$^2$ daily, divided into four doses. **Preoperative sedation PO:** ADULTS: 200 mg 1 or 2 hours before surgery. **Hypnotic PO:** ADULTS: 65 to 200 mg at bedtime. Give for no longer than 2 weeks, preferably tapering the dose to avoid rebound insomnia. **IM:** ADULTS: 65 to 200 mg. CHILDREN: 2 to 3 mg/kg. **Anticonvulsant IV:** ADULTS AND CHILDREN OVER 6 YEARS: 65 to 500 mg. Rate should not exceed 100 mg/min for adults or 60 mg/M$^2$/min for children. *Special patient populations:* ELDERLY: Elderly patients are more likely to respond with paradoxical excitement. PREGNANCY: Barbiturates can cause fetal harm, including fetal abnormalities. Barbiturates can also cause postpartum hemorrhage and hemorrhagic disease in the newborn. Barbiturates are distributed to breast milk. For these reasons, barbiturates should be avoided by pregnant and nursing women.

**PREPARATIONS** *Amobarbital, Powder, tablets:* 30, 50, and 100 mg. *Amobarbital sodium, Powder, capsules:* 65 and 200 mg; parenteral: 250 and 500 mg. Dissolve in 2.5 or 5 ml, respectively, sterile water for a 10% (100 mg/ml) solution. Solutions should be used within 30 minutes. They should not be used if they contain a precipitate. *Combinations:* Amobarbital sodium, 25, 50, and 100 mg with equivalent weight of secobarbital sodium.

**DRUG INTERACTIONS** • See entry for drug class (p. 677).

**FATE** Amobarbital is well absorbed and has a plasma *half-life* of 14 to 42 hours. It is metabolized by the liver and excreted in the urine as the metabolite and its glucuronide.

### ☙ NURSING CONSIDERATIONS

**Side effects, toxicities, and associated nursing actions**
  • See entry for drug class (p. 677).

**Nursing interventions related to drug administration** After reconstituting the parenteral form, the solution should be used within 30 minutes.
  • Rate of IV administration should not exceed 100 mg/min for adults or 60 mg/m$^2$ of body surface per minute for children. Monitor respiratory rate. A suction machine should be readily available.
  • IV extravasation may cause tissue injury. Assess patency of IV infusion before administering.
  • Parenteral amobarbital is incompatible with most other drugs in a syringe.
  • IM injection should be made only into large muscles such as the gluteus maximus or vastus lateralis.
  • IM injection volume should not exceed 5 ml regardless of concentration.

**Patient and family education**
  • See entry for drug class (p. 678).

---

## butabarbital sodium   (byoo-ta-BAR-bi-tal)                                 sedative-hypnotic

  • butabarbital sodium: Butalan, Butatran, Buticaps, Butisol Sodium (Schedule II, ♣Schedule G)

**MECHANISM OF ACTION** Barbiturates depress the reticular activating system.

**INDICATIONS** **Insomina** Should not be used for more than 2 weeks because tolerance develops. **Anxiety** Common use is for preoperative sedation.

**CONTRAINDICATIONS** • See entry for drug class (p. 677).

**DOSAGE**

**Hypnotic PO:** ADULTS: 50 to 100 mg at bedtime. Give no more than 2 weeks, preferably tapering the dose to avoid rebound insomnia.

**Sedative PO:** ADULTS: 15 to 30 mg three or four times daily. Preoperatively, 50 to 100 mg 60 to 90 minutes before surgery. CHILDREN: 6 mg/kg or 180 mg/M$^2$ daily divided in three doses. Preoperatively, 2 to 6 mg/kg 60 to 90 minutes before surgery. *Special patient populations:* ELDERLY: Elderly patients are more likely to respond with paradoxical excitement. PREGNANCY: Barbiturates can cause fetal harm, including fetal abnormalities. Barbiturates can also cause postpartum hemorrhage and hemorrhagic disease in the newborn. Barbiturates are distributed to breast milk. For these reasons, barbiturates should be avoided by pregnant and nursing women.

**PREPARATIONS**    *Powder, capsules:* 15 and 30 mg; *elixir:* 30 mg/5 ml, 33.33 mg/5 ml; tablets: 15, 30, 50, and 100 mg. *Combination:* butabarbital sodium 30 mg with phenobarbital 15 mg and 50 mg secobarbital sodium.

**DRUG INTERACTIONS**    See entry for drug class (p. 677).

**FATE**    Butabarbital is well absorbed and *peak* plasma concentrations are seen in about 3 hours. The plasma *half-life* is 100 hours

❦ **NURSING CONSIDERATIONS**

**Side effects, toxicities, and associated nursing actions**
- See entry for drug class (p. 677).

**Patient and family education**
- See entry for drug class (p. 678).
- Butisol sodium brand 30 mg and 50 mg tablets and elixir contain FD & C yellow dye # 5 (tartrazine), which may cause an allergic-type reaction in some individuals. Although rare, this reaction is seen more often in persons with aspirin hypersensitivity.

---

## pentobarbital    (pen-toe-BAR-bi-tal)    sedative-hypnotic

- pentobarbital (pentobarbital sodium): Nembutal, Nembutal Sodium (Schedule II, ✤Schedule G)

**MECHANISM OF ACTION**    Barbiturates depress the reticular activating system.

**INDICATIONS**    **Insomnia** Should not be used for more than 2 weeks because tolerance develops.    **Anxiety** Common use is for preoperative sedation.    **Seizures** Pentobarbital may used to control status epilepticus or other seizures.    **Withdrawal** Pentobarbital may be substituted for other barbiturates or nonbarbiturate sedative-hypnotics or alcohol. Doses are then lowered 10% per day to achieve withdrawal without withdrawal symptoms.

**CONTRAINDICATIONS**    • See entry for drug class (p. 677).

**DOSAGE**

**Hypnotic    PO:    ADULTS:** 100 to 200 mg at bedtime. Give for no longer than 2 weeks, preferably tapering the dose to avoid rebound insomnia.    **CHILDREN:** 2 months to 1 year, 30 mg; 1 to 4 years, 30 to 60 mg; 5 to 12 years, 60 mg; 12 to 14 years, 60 or 120 mg.    **IM:    ADULTS:** 150 to 200 mg.    **CHILDREN:** 2 to 6 mg/kg or 125 mg/$M^2$, maximum, 100 mg.    **Sedative    PO:    ADULTS:** 20 to 40 mg two to four times daily.    **Preoperative sedation    ADULTS:** 150 to 200 mg 60 to 90 minutes before surgery.    **CHILDREN:** 5 mg/kg. Give rectally in children under 10 years old.

**Emergency anticonvulsant**

**IV:    ADULTS:** 100 mg is given initially. Additional smaller doses may be given if necessary, up to 200 to 500 mg.    **CHILDREN:** 50 mg is given initially. *Special patient populations:*    **ELDERLY:** Elderly patients are more likely to respond with paradoxical excitement.    **PREGNANCY:** Barbiturates can cause fetal harm, including fetal abnormalities. Barbiturates can also cause postpartum hemorrhage and hemorrhagic disease in the newborn. Barbiturates are distributed to breast milk. For these reasons, barbiturates should be avoided by pregnant and nursing women.

**PREPARATIONS**    *Pentobarbital, elixir:* 18.2 mg/5 ml. *Pentobarbital sodium, powder, capsules:* 50 and 100 mg; *injection:* 50 mg/ml; *suppositories:* 30, 60, 120, and 200 mg.

**DRUG INTERACTIONS**    • See entry for drug class (p. 677).

**FATE**    Pentobarbital is well absorbed. *Peak* plasma concentrations are reached in 30 to 60 minutes. Plasma *half-life* is 35 to 50 hours. Pentobarbital is metabolized by the liver and metabolites, and their glucuronides are excreted in the urine.

❦ **NURSING CONSIDERATIONS**

**Side effects, toxicities, and associated nursing actions**
- See entry for drug class (p. 677).

**Nursing interventions related to drug administration** IV dose may be given undiluted or further diluted with sterile water, sodium chloride for injection, or Ringer's lactate. Dilution of 9 ml diluent with 1 ml pentobarbital (50 mg/ml) equals 5 mg/ml. Use only clear solutions.
  * Rate of IV administration should not exceed 50 mg/min. Monitor respiratory rate. A suction machine should be readily available.
  * IV extravasation may cause tissue injury. Assess patency of IV infusion prior to administering. Intra-arterial injection may cause gangrene.
  * Parenteral pentobarbital is incompatible with most other drugs in a syringe.
  * IM injection should be made only into large muscles such as the gluteus maximus or vastus lateralis.
  * IM injection volume should not exceed 5 ml regardless of concentration.
  * Suppositories should not be divided, as doses may not be accurate. Obtain suppository of correct dosage.

**Patient and family education**
  * Nembutal sodium brand 100 mg capsules contain FD & C yellow dye # 5 (tartrazine), which may cause an allergic reaction in susceptible individuals. Although rare, this reaction is seen more commonly in individuals with aspirin hypersensitivity.
  * See entry for drug class (p. 678).

---

## phenobarbital (fen-noe-BAR-bi-tal) sedative, anticonvulsant

  * phenobarbital: Barbita, Solfoton (Schedule IV, ❦Schedule G) Luminal, ❦Eskabarb (Schedule IV, ❦Schedule G)

**MECHANISM OF ACTION** Barbiturates depress the reticular activating system.

**INDICATIONS** **Anxiety** As a routine antianxiety agent or as a preoperative sedative. **Anticonvulsant** Prophylaxis for the treatment of epilepsy (see Chapter 11). This is a major use of phenobarbital. **Withdrawal** Phenobarbital may be substituted for other barbiturates or nonbarbiturate sedative-hypnotics or alcohol. Doses are then lowered 10% per day to achieve withdrawal without withdrawal symptoms.

**CONTRAINDICATIONS** • See entry for drug class (p. 677).

**DOSAGE**

**Sedation** **PO:** **ADULTS:** 30 to 120 mg daily. Because of the long half-life of phenobarbital, this may be administered as a single dose. **CHILDREN:** 6 mg/kg or 180 mg/M$^2$ daily. This dose may also be administered rectally. **IM:** **ADULTS:** 100 to 200 mg 60 to 90 minutes before surgery. **CHILDREN:** 16 to 100 mg 60 to 90 minutes before surgery.

**Anticonvulsant** See Chapter 40. *Special patient populations:* **ELDERLY:** Elderly patients are more likely to respond with paradoxical excitement. **PREGNANCY:** Barbiturates can cause fetal harm, including fetal abnormalities. Barbiturates can also cause postpartum hemorrhage and hemorrhagic disease in the newborn. Barbiturates are distributed to breast milk. For these reasons, barbiturates should be avoided by pregnant and nursing women.

**PREPARATIONS** *Phenobarbital; powder; capsules:* 16, 65 (extended release) mg; elixir: 15 mg/5 ml; *tablets:* 8, 15, 16, 30, 32, 60, 65, and 100 mg. *Phenobarbital sodium; powder;* injection: 30, 60, 65, and 130 mg/ml.

**DRUG INTERACTIONS** • See entry for drug class (p. 677).

**FATE** Phenobarbital is the longest acting of the commonly used barbiturates. After oral administration, *peak* blood concentrations are reached in 10 to 15 hours, although the *onset of action* is generally 30 to 60 minutes. Plasma *half-life* is 2 to 6 days. Phenobarbital is metabolized by the liver, but slowly, and at least 25% of the drug is excreted in the urine unchanged. Phenobarbital is potent in inducing the liver metabolizing enzymes, accounting for the decreased effectiveness of many other drugs.

## ❦ NURSING CONSIDERATIONS
### Side effects, toxicities, and associated nursing actions
- See entry for drug class (p. 677).

### Nursing interventions related to drug administration
- Sterile powder must be diluted with sterile water for injection. Use at least 10 ml, regardless of prescribed dose. If using manufacturer-prepared sterile solution, it should also be diluted to make a volume of at least 10 ml. The sterile solution is compatible with most IV fluids, including 0.45% and 0.9% sodium chloride, 5% dextrose, Ringer's, or lactated Ringer's. Use only clear solutions. Solution should be used within 30 minutes.
- Rate of IV administration should not exceed 65 mg/min. Monitor respiratory rate. A suction machine should be readily available.
- IV extravasation may cause tissue injury. Assess patency of IV infusion prior to administering. Intra-arterial injection may cause gangrene.
- Parenteral phenobarbital is incompatible with most other drugs in a syringe.
- IM injection should be made only into large muscles such as the gluteus maximus or vastus lateralis.
- IM injection volume should not exceed 5 ml regardless of concentration.

### Patient and family education
- Phenobarbital may increase vitamin D requirements. The major sources of vitamin D are fortified milk products and exposure to sunshine. A vitamin supplement may be prescribed.
- See entry for drug class (p. 678).

---

## secobarbital sodium   (see-koe-BAR-bi-tal)                    sedative-hypnotic

- secobarbital sodium: Seconal, ♣Seral (Schedule II, ♣Schedule G)

**MECHANISM OF ACTION**   Barbiturates depress the reticular activating system.

**INDICATIONS**   **Insomnia** Should not be used for more than 2 weeks because tolerance develops.   **Anxiety** Preoperative sedation.

**CONTRAINDICATIONS**   • See entry for drug class (p. 677).

**DOSAGE**

**Hypnotic   PO or IM:   ADULTS:** 100 to 200 mg.   **IM:   CHILDREN:** 3 to 5 mg/kg or 125 mg/M$^2$, up to a maximum of 100 mg.

**Preoperative sedation   PO:   ADULTS:** 100 to 300 mg 60 to 90 minutes before surgery.   **CHILDREN:** 50 to 100 mg 60 to 90 minutes before surgery.   **Rectal:   CHILDREN:** 6 months to 3 years; 30 to 60 mg; over 3 years, 60 to 120 mg.   *Special patient populations:*   **ELDERLY:** Elderly patients are more likely to respond with paradoxical excitement.   **PREGNANCY:** Barbiturates can cause fetal harm, including fetal abnormalities. Barbiturates can also cause postpartum hemorrhage and hemorrhagic disease in the newborn. Barbiturates are distributed to breast milk. For these reasons, barbiturates should be avoided by pregnant and nursing women.

**PREPARATIONS**   *Powder, capsules:* 50 and 100 mg; *injection:* 50 mg/ml; *suppositories:* 120 mg. *Combinations:* secobarbital sodium, 25, 50, or 100 mg, with an equivalent weight of amobarbital sodium; secobarbital sodium, 50 mg, with butabarbital sodium, 30 mg, and phenobarbital, 15 mg.

**DRUG INTERACTIONS**   • See entry for drug class (p. 677).

**FATE**   Secobarbital is relatively short-acting. It is well absorbed orally, and *peak* plasma concentrations are achieved in 2 to 4 hours. Secobarbital is readily metabolized by the liver and excreted in the urine as metabolites. Plasma *half-life* is about 30 hours.

## ❦ NURSING CONSIDERATIONS
### Side effects, toxicities, and associated nursing actions
- See entry for drug class (p. 677).

### Nursing interventions related to drug administration
- For parenteral administration, dilute powder form as directed on vial with sterile water for injection. A commercially prepared injection form may be further diluted with sterile water for injection, 0.9% sodium chloride, or Ringer's injection. Lactated Ringer's should *not* be used. Administer only clear solutions.

- After reconstituting parenteral form, solution should be used within 30 minutes.
- Rate of IV administration should not exceed 50 mg/min. Monitor respiratory rate. A suction machine should be readily available.
- IV extravasation may cause tissue injury. Assess patency of IV infusion prior to administering. Intra-arterial injection may cause gangrene.
- Parenteral secobarbital is incompatible with most other drugs in a syringe.
- IM injection should be made only into large muscles such as the gluteus maximus or vastus lateralis.
- IM injection volume should not exceed 5 ml regardless of concentration.

### Patient and family education
- See entry for drug class (p. 678).

---

# Benzodiazepines

| | United States* | Canada* |
|---|---|---|
| alprazolam | Schedule IV | NC |
| ✽bromazepam | NA | NC |
| chlordiazepoxide | Schedule IV | NC |
| clonazepam (see Chapter 40) | Schedule IV | NC |
| clorazepate | Schedule IV | NC |
| diazepam | Schedule IV | NC |
| flurazepam | NC | NC |
| halazepam | Schedule IV | NC |
| ✽ketazolam | NA | NC |
| lorazepam | Schedule IV | NC |
| midazolam (see Chapter 48) | Schedule IV | NA |
| ✽nitrazepam | NA | NC |
| oxazepam | Schedule IV | NC |
| prazepam | Schedule IV | NA |
| quazepam | Schedule IV | NA |
| temazepam | Schedule IV | NC |
| triazolam | Schedule IV | NC |

*NA = not available; NC = not a controlled substance.

## DRUG COMBINATIONS
- chlordiazepoxide HC1 and clidinium Br: Chlordinium, Clindex, Clinoxide, Clipoxide, Librax, Lidox
- chlordiazepoxide and amitriptyline HC1: Limbitrol
- chlordiazepoxide with esterified estrogens: Menrium

**OVERVIEW OF THE DRUG CLASS**   Diazepam and chlordiazepoxide were introduced clinically in the 1960s as antianxiety drugs. The number of benzodiazepines in clinical use has increased dramatically, and this drug class is now widely used. Benzodiazepines have four actions: anxiety reducing (anxiolytic), sedative-hypnotic, muscle relaxing, and anticonvulsant. The popularity of the benzodiazepines rests in part on the very high therapeutic index. Overdoses of 1000 times the therapeutic dose have been reported not to result in death. However, benzodiazepines do have additive effects with other general central nervous system drugs. The combination of a benzodiazepine with alcohol can be deadly, although neither agent alone is likely to be.

All benzodiazepines are Schedule IV drugs in the United States and Schedule F drugs in Canada. The potential for abuse is mild. However, dependence occurs, particularly in patients with a history of drug and alcohol abuse.

The major difference among the benzodiazepines lies in their metabolism. The older benzodiazepines are metabolized to active compounds that are only slowly eliminated from the body, whereas

| Table 35-1. | Benzodiazepines classified by half-life* | | |
|---|---|---|---|
| | Generic name/trade name | Sedative-hypnotic use | Other uses |

**SHORT HALF-LIFE: 6–20 HOURS, NO METABOLITES, OR WEAK, INACTIVE, OR SHORT-LIVED METABOLITES**

| Generic name | Trade name | Sedative-hypnotic use | Other uses |
|---|---|---|---|
| Alprazolam | Xanax | Anxiety | |
| ✽Bromazepam | Lectopam | Anxiety | |
| Flunitrazepam | Rohypnol | Insomnia | Induction of anesthesia |
| Lorazepam | Ativan | Anxiety, insomnia | Preanesthetic |
| Midazolam | Versed | — | Induction of anesthesia |
| Oxazepam | Serax | Anxiety | Alcohol withdrawal |
| Temazepam | Restoril | Insomnia | |
| Triazolam | Halcion | Insomnia | Preanesthetic |

**INTERMEDIATE TO LONG HALF-LIFE (ACTIVE METABOLITES)**

| Generic name | Trade name | Sedative-hypnotic use | Other uses |
|---|---|---|---|
| Clorazepate | Tranxene | Anxiety | Alcohol withdrawal, anticonvulsant |
| Chlordiazepoxide | Librium | Anxiety | Preanesthetic, alcohol withdrawal |
| Clonazepam | Klonopin | — | Anticonvulsant |
| Diazepam | Valium | Anxiety | Preanesthetic, induction of anesthesia, alcohol withdrawal, Anticonvulsant, skeletal muscle hyperactivity |
| Flurazepam | Dalmane | Insomnia | |
| Halazepam | Paxipam | Anxiety | |
| ✽Ketazolam | Loftran | Anxiety | |
| ✽Nitrazepam | Mogadon | Insomnia | Anticonvulsants |
| Prazepam | Centrax | Anxiety | |
| Quazepam | Dormalin | Insomnia | |

*Benzodiazepines with intermediate to long half-lives (drugs with active metabolites) may not have a long duration of action from a single dose because of drug redistribution in the body. These drugs and their active metabolites will, however, tend to accumulate and thereby produce a level of sedation that may cause problems if these drugs are used continuously.

many of the newer benzodiazepines have weakly active or inactive metabolites. The advantage of these newer drugs is that they do not tend to cumulate and thereby cause problems with continued use. Table 35-1 classifies the benzodiazepines by their half-life and summarizes their clinical uses.

**MECHANISM OF ACTION**    Specific receptors for the benzodiazepines have been identified in the rat cerebral cortex and limbic system. Since the limbic system is a major integrating system governing emotional behavior associated with self-preservation, the presence of receptors for benzodiazepines in this system may account for their antianxiety action.

One action of benzodiazepines is to increase the action of the inhibitory neurotransmitter, gamma-aminobutyric acid (GABA). Both benzodiazepines and barbiturates help GABA open a chloride channel in the postsynaptic membrane of many neurons, which reduces the neuron's excitability. Many investigators believe that the receptors for benzodiazepines and barbiturates modulate this action.

**INDICATIONS**    Anxiety.    **Insomnia** Several benzodiazepines are effective as hypnotics: flurazepam, lorazepam, quazepam, nitrazepam, temazepam, and triazolam.    **Presurgical sedation** Diazepam, lorazepam, and triazolam are used.    **Alcohol withdrawal** Diazepam, chlordiazepoxide, chlorazepate, and oxazepam are used.    **Seizure disorders** Diazepam is most commonly used for terminating status epilepticus. Clorazepate and nitrazepam are also used. Clonazepam is used only as an anticonvulsant. **Skeletal muscle spasticity** Diazepam is most commonly used.

**CONTRAINDICATIONS** • Renal failure: active metabolites may not be excreted and may accumulate. • Depressed or psychotic patients in the absence of anxiety. • Pregnancy: fetal damage has been reported. Alprazolam, halazepam, and lorazepam are classified FDA pregnancy category D, whereas temazepam and triazolam are classified FDA pregnancy category X. • Breast-feeding: benzodiazepines are excreted into breast milk. • Acute angle-closure glaucoma. • Myasthenia gravis.

**DRUG INTERACTIONS** **CNS depressants** Benzodiazepines produce additive CNS depression. **Disulfiram and cimetidine** may inhibit the metabolism of benzodiazepines. **Levodopa** may be less effective if given concurrently with benzodiazepines. **Antacids** decrease the rate of absorption of benzodiazepines.

## ☙ NURSING CONSIDERATIONS

### Side effects, toxicities, and associated nursing actions

**CNS** Drowsiness, incoordination, fatigue, confusion, dizziness. Patients should not undertake activities requiring alertness. Paradoxical CNS stimulation may be seen.

**Eye** Double or blurred vision.

- Tell patients to avoid driving or operating hazardous equipment until the effects of the medication can be evaluated.
- Supervise ambulation of hospitalized patients and discourage smoking.
- Keep side rails up.
- Keep a night light on.
- Assess the patient for development of visual complaints.

**GI** Complaints include changes in appetite and weight (increased or decreased), dry mouth, increased salivation.

- Monitor weight.
- If significant weight changes occur (gain or loss of greater than 5 pounds), obtain a thorough diet history. Goals of diet modification vary with the patient. If excessive weight gain has occurred, instruct the patient about a low-calorie diet, and encourage increased exercise. If excessive weight loss has occurred, encourage intake of high-calorie foods. If weight gain or loss is excessive, it may be necessary to change drugs.
- For dry mouth, encourage patients to suck on sugerless hard candy or chew sugarless gum. Frequent oral hygiene may improve comfort. Avoid drying agents such as lemon-glycerin swabs. Some patients may wish to use a commercially available saliva substitute.
- If increased salivation is excessive, a change in dose or drug may be necessary.

**GU** Changes in libido; menstrual irregularities.

- Assess menstrual history. If menstrual irregularities are severe or troublesome to the patient, refer to a gynecologist. May require change in drug.
- Have the patient keep a record of menstrual periods. Instruct the patient to notify the physician immediately if pregnancy is suspected. Teach about birth control measures if appropriate or requested by patient.
- Assess for changes in libido. Treatment varies with the significance of the problem to the patient. May require a reduction in dosage or change in drug.

**Hematologic** Rarely, depression of blood elements.

**Metabolic** Changes in liver or renal function tests.

- Monitor complete blood cound (CBC) and platelets. AST (SGOT), ALT (SGPT), LDH, BUN, and creatinine.
- Assess for development of fever, petechiae, bruising, or unexplained bleeding. Caution the patient to report the development of any unexpected sign or symptom.
- Assess for the development of jaundice, right upper quadrant abdominal pain, malaise, or fever.

**Lung** Shortness of breath.

- Monitor respiratory rate.
- Assess breath sounds.

**Skin** Urticaria, rash, and photosensitivity.

**Allergic** Hypersensitivity reactions. See Skin.

- Inspect the patient for development of skin changes.
- Caution patients to avoid prolonged exposure to the sun, to wear a hat and long-sleeved clothing, and to use maximum-protection sunscreens.
- Be alert for acute allergic reactions. Know the location of drugs and equipment for treatment of allergic response.

**Other** Joint pain, muscle cramps, or tingling sensation.

- Question the patient about the appearance of any unusual sign or symptom.

**Patient and family education**

- Review with the patient expected benefits and possible side effects of therapy. Instruct the patient to report the development of any unexpected sign or symptom.
- Caution the patient to avoid the use of any other medications, including over-the-counter preparations, without prior clearance with the physician.
- Caution the patient to avoid the use of alcohol.
- Remind patients to take the medication only as ordered. Instruct patients that these drugs may be habit forming. Be alert in the outpatient setting for patients who return for prescription refills on an increasingly frequent basis, as this may indicate improper use or abuse of the drug.
- Caution patients not to discontinue the drug suddenly without consulting the physician.
- Patients should not double up if a dose is missed. Patients should not share medications with others.
- Remind patients to keep these and all medications out of the reach of children. Child-proof caps should be used.
- Smoking may decrease the sedative effects of the benzodiazepines. Ideally, patients should avoid smoking while taking benzodiazepines. Heavy smokers may need a larger dose.

## alprazolam    (al-PRAY-zoe-lam)    anxiolytic

- alprazolam: Xanax (Schedule IV)

**MECHANISM OF ACTION**    Alprazolam is a benzodiazepine. These drugs seem to depress the limbic system.

**INDICATIONS** • Anxiety.

**CONTRAINDICATIONS** • Depressed or psychotic patients in the absence of anxiety. • Pregnancy: fetal damage has been reported. • Breast-feeding: benzodiazepines are excreted into breast milk. • Acute angle-closure glaucoma. • Myasthenia gravis.

**DOSAGE**    PO:    ADULTS: 0.25 to 0.5 mg three times daily. Maximum dose is 4 mg daily.    *Special patient populations:*    ELDERLY: Doses for the elderly must be reduced. Initial dose is 0.25 mg two or three times daily. This may be increased if no adverse effects occur.    CHILDREN: Safety for children under 18 years old has not been established.    PREGNANCY: Benzodiazepines are not considered safe for use during pregnancy. Fetal abnormalities have been documented. FDA pregnancy category D.

**PREPARATIONS**    *Tablets:* 0.25, 0.5, and 1 mg.

**DRUG INTERACTIONS** • See entry for drug class (p. 685).

**FATE**    The *half-life* is 12 to 15 hours. Alprazolam does not have active metabolites.

**☙ NURSING CONSIDERATIONS**

**Side effects, toxicities, and associated nursing actions**

- See entry for drug class (p. 685).

**Patient and family education**

- See entry for drug class (p. 685).

## ✹bromazepam    (brome-AZ-e-pam)    anxiolytic

- bromazepam: ✹Lectopam

**MECHANISM OF ACTION**   Bromazepam is a benzodiazepine. These drugs seem to depress the limbic system.
**INDICATIONS**   • Anxiety.
**CONTRAINDICATIONS**   • Depressed or psychotic patients in the absence of anxiety. • Pregnancy: fetal damage has been reported. • Breast-feeding: benzodiazepines are excreted into breast milk. • Acute angle-closure glaucoma. • Myasthenia gravis.
**DOSAGE**   PO:   ADULTS: 6 to 18 mg daily in divided doses initially. The optimum dose can vary from 6 to 30 mg daily.   *Special patient populations:*   ELDERLY: Doses for the elderly must be reduced. Initial dose is 3 mg in divided doses. This may be increased if no adverse effects occur.   CHILDREN: Safety for children under 18 years old has not been established.   PREGNANCY: Benzodiazepines are not considered safe for use during pregnancy. Fetal abnormalities have been documented.
**PREPARATIONS**   *Tablets (scored):* 3 and 6 mg.
**DRUG INTERACTIONS**   See entry for drug class (p. 685).
**FATE**   *Peak* blood levels are achieved 1 to 4 hours after administration. The serum *half-life* of the drug is 8 to 19 hours. Metabolites are weakly active.

🦌 **NURSING CONSIDERATIONS**
  **Side effects, toxicities, and associated nursing actions**
    • See entry for drug class (p. 685).
  **Patient and family education**
    • See entry for drug class (p. 686).

## chlordiazepoxide   (klor-dye-az-e-POX-ide)   anxiolytic

  • chlordiazepoxide: Libritabs
  • chlordiazepoxide hydrochloride: Librium, Lipoxide, SK-Lygen, Reponans, ✦Relaxil, Sereen, ✦Trilium (Schedule IV)

**MECHANISM OF ACTION**   Chlordiazepoxide is a benzodiazepine. These drugs seem to depress the limbic system.
**INDICATIONS**   • Anxiety. • Preanesthetic. • Alcohol withdrawal.
**CONTRAINDICATIONS**   • Renal failure: active metabolites may not be excreted and may accumulate. • Depressed or psychotic patients in the absence of anxiety. • Pregnancy: fetal damage has been reported. • Breast-feeding: benzodiazepines are excreted into breast milk. • Acute angle-closure glaucoma. • Myasthenia gravis.
**DOSAGE**   PO:   ADULTS: *Anxiety:* 5 to 10 mg three or four times daily for mild anxiety. 20 to 25 mg three or four times daily for severe anxiety. *Alcohol withdrawal:* 50 to 100 mg initially to control agitation; additional doses may be given, up to 300 to 800 mg.   IV:   ADULTS: *Anxiety:* 50 to 100 mg initially with subsequent doses of 25 to 50 mg as required to manage acute or severe anxiety. IM:   ADULTS: *Preanesthetic medications:* 50 to 100 mg is given 1 hour before surgery.   *Special patient populations:*   ELDERLY: Doses for the elderly must be reduced. *PO:* Initial dose is 5 mg two to four times daily. This may be increased if no adverse effects occur. *IM:* 25 to 50 mg 1 hour before surgery.   CHILDREN: *PO:* Initial dose is 5 mg two to four times daily. This may be increased if no adverse effects occur. *IM:* 25 to 50 mg 1 hour before surgery for children over 12 years old.   PREGNANCY: Benzodiazepines are not considered safe for use during pregnancy. Fetal abnormalities have been documented.
**PREPARATIONS**   *Chlordiazepoxide, tablets:* 5, 10, and 25 mg. *Chlordiazepoxide* HCl, *capsules:* 5, 10, and 25 mg, *injection:* 100 mg. *Combinations:* chlordiazepoxide, 5 mg, with amitriptyline HCl, 12.5 mg; chlordiazepoxide, 10 mg, with amitriptyline HCl, 25 mg. Chlordiazepoxide, 5 mg, with 0.2 or 0.4 mg esterified estrogens; 10 mg with 0.4 esterified estrogens. Chlordiazepoxide HCl, 5 mg, with clidinium Br, 2.5 mg.
**DRUG INTERACTIONS**   • See entry for drug class (p. 685).
**DIAGNOSTIC TEST INTERFERENCE**   **Pregnancy test** Chlordiazepoxide may cause a false-positive reaction in the Gravindex pregnancy test.   **17-Ketosteroids** Chlordiazepoxide intereferes with the Zimmerman

reaction, resulting falsely high or low values.    **Urine alkaloids** Chlordiazepoxide may interefere with the Frings thin-layer chromatography procedure, resulting in falsely elevated readings.

**FATE**    The *half-life* of the parent drug is 5 to 30 hours. Chlordiazepoxide is metabolized to several long-lived active metabolites, including oxazepam.

## ❦ NURSING CONSIDERATIONS

### Side effects, toxicities, and associated nursing actions

- See entry for drug class (p. 685).

**CV** Parenteral administration may produce bradycardia or cardiac arrest. The elderly and debilitated are at most risk.

- Monitor vital signs and blood pressure.

### Nursing interventions related to drug administration

- The oral route is the preferred route of administration.
- For IM administration, dilute the drug powder with the diluent provided by the manufacturer. Administer via deep IM injection into a large muscle mass. Absorption via the IM route is erratic, so this route of administration is least acceptable.
- To administer IV, reconstitute 100 mg of sterile powder with 5 ml of 0.9% sodium chloride or sterile water for injection. This makes a concentration of 20 mg of chlordiazepoxide per milliliter. Gently rotate the vial to completely dissolve powder. Administer only freshly prepared solutions. Do not mix with infusion fluids. Administer direct IV push as close to IV insertion site as possible. Administer at a rate of 100 mg or less over at least 1 minute.
- Maintain the patient on bedrest for at least 3 hours following IV administration. Monitor vital signs and blood pressure. Have drugs and equipment available for resuscitation.

### Patient and family education

- See entry for drug class (p. 686).

---

## clorazepate dipotassium    (klor-AZ-e-pate)    anxiolytic

- clorazepate: Tranxene (Schedule IV)

**MECHANISM OF ACTION**    Clorazepate is a benzodiazepine. These drugs seem to depress the limbic system.

**INDICATIONS**    • Anxiety. • Acute alcohol withdrawal (to control agitation). • Partial seizures.

**CONTRAINDICATIONS**    **Renal failure** Active metabolites may not be excreted and may accumulate. **Depressed or psychotic patients in the absence of anxiety.**    **Pregnancy** Fetal damage has been reported.    **Breast-feeding** Benzodiazepines are excreted into breast milk.    **Acute angle-closure glaucoma.**    **Myasthenia gravis.**

**DOSAGE**    **PO:**    **ADULTS:** *Anxiety:* 30 mg daily in divided doses. May also be given as a single bedtime dose, but initial dose should not be greater than 15 mg. *Acute alcohol withdrawal:* first day, 30 mg initially, with 30 to 60 mg more. Second day, 45 to 90 mg in divided doses. Subsequent days the dose should be reduced 7.5 to 15 mg daily until the daily dose is 7.5 to 15 mg daily. *Partial seizures:* Initially, up to 7.5 mg three times daily. If needed, increase by 7.5 mg increments weekly. Maximum dose: 90 mg daily in divided doses.    **Special patient populations:**    **ELDERLY:** Doses for the elderly must be reduced. Initial dose is 7.5 mg in divided doses or as a single bedtime dose. This may be increased if no adverse effects occur.    **CHILDREN:** Not recommended for children under 9 years old. May be used as an adjuvent in the control of partial seizures. For children 9 to 12 years old: 7.5 mg two times a day. May increase the dose weekly if required in 7.5 mg increments. Maximum dose: 60 mg daily. **PREGNANCY:** Benzodiazepines are not considered safe for use during pregnancy. Fetal abnormalities have been documented.

**PREPARATIONS**    *Capsules:* 3.75, 7.5, and 15 mg; *tablets:* 3.75 7.5, 11.25, 15, and 22.5 mg.

**DRUG INTERACTIONS**    • See entry for drug class (p. 685).

**FATE**    Metabolities of clorazepate are active and have long plasma *half-lives.*

🐝 **NURSING CONSIDERATIONS**
### Side effects, toxicities, and associated nursing actions
- See entry for drug class (p. 685).
### Patient and family education
- See entry for drug class (p. 686).

## diazepam (dye-AZ-e-pam)         anxiolytic, anticonvulsant

- diazepam: Q-pam, Valium, Vazepam, ♣Vivol (Schedule IV)

**MECHANISM OF ACTION**   Diazepam is a benzodiazepine. These drugs seem to depress the limbic system.

**INDICATIONS**   • Anxiety. • Presurgical sedation: widely used for light anesthesia; anterograde amnesia for unpleasant procedures. • Acute and chronic relief of muscle spasms. • Status epilepticus: diazepam is the drug of choice for terminating these seizures. • Alcohol withdrawal.

**CONTRAINDICATIONS**   Renal failure: active metabolites may not be excreted and may accumulate. • Depressed or psychotic patients in the absence of anxiety. • Pregnancy: fetal damage has been reported. • Breast feeding: diazepam and its active metabolites are excreted in breast milk. • Acute angle-closure glaucoma. • Myasthenia gravis.

**DOSAGE**   **PO:**   **ADULTS:** *Anxiety, prophylaxis for epilepsy, relief of muscle spasticity:* 10 mg three or four times for the first day, then 5 mg three or four times daily. *Alcohol withdrawal:* 10 mg three or four times the first day, followed by 15 mg daily thereafter.   **IV:**   **ADULTS:** *Light anesthesia, anterograde amnesia:* 10 mg given slowly. *Anticonvulsant:* Initially, 5 to 10 mg, repeated at 10 to 15 minute intervals as necessary, for a total of not more than 30 mg. *Tetanus:* 5 to 10 mg initially, repeated in three to four hours. *Acute alcohol withdrawal:* 10 mg (up to 20 mg) initially, with additional doses of 5 to 10 mg every 3 to 4 hours. Some clinicians administer 10 mg at 20 to 30 minute intervals to severely agitated patients.   ***Special patient populations;***   **ELDERLY:** Doses for the elderly must be reduced. *PO;* 2.5 mg once or twice daily for anxiety. *IV;* 2 to 5 mg for anxiety.   **CHILDREN:** *PO:* 6 to 15 mg daily in divided doses for epilepsy. *IV for management of seizures:* 0.25 mg/kg, repeated at 15 to 30 minute intervals as needed, up to a cumulative dose of 0.75 mg/kg. for children ages 30 days to 5 years, 0.2 to 0.5 mg, repeated every 2 to 5 minutes, to a total cumulative dose of 5 mg.   **PREGNANCY:** Benzodiazepines are not considered safe for use during pregnancy. Fetal abnormalities have been documented.

**PREPARATIONS**   *Capsules, extended release:* 15 mg; tablets: 2, 5, and 10 mg; injection: 5 mg/ml.

**DRUG INTERACTIONS**   • See entry for drug class (p. 685).

**DIAGNOSTIC TEST INTERFERENCE**   **Urine alkaloids** Diazepam may cause falsely elevated readings in the Frings thin-layer chromatography procedure.   **Urinary glucose** False-negative reactions when the test is performed with Clinistix and Diastix but not with Testape.

**FATE**   Diazepam is metabolized to active metabolites with long plasma *half-lives*.

🐝 **NURSING CONSIDERATIONS**
### Side effects, toxicities, and associated nursing actions
- See entry for drug class (p. 685).

   **CV** Parenteral administration may produce bradycardia or cardiac arrest. The elderly and debilitated are at most risk.
- Monitor the vital signs and blood pressure.

### Nursing interventions related to drug administration
- For IV administration, do not dilute. Administer slowly, at a rate not exceeding 5 mg/min. Do not mix with other drugs or IV solutions; administer as close to the IV insertion site as possible. Monitor respirations, blood pressure, and level of consciousness. Suction equipment should be at the bedside.
- Maintain the patient on bedrest for at least 3 hours following IV administration.
- Keep drugs and equipment available for resuscitation.
- Diazepam may be given IM if it is not possible to administer IV.

**Patient and family education**
- See entry for drug class (p. 686).

## flurazepam hydrochloride    (flure-AZ-e-pam)    hypnotic

- flurazepam: Dalmane, Durapam

**MECHANISM OF ACTION**    Flurazepam is a benzodiazepine. These drugs seem to depress the limbic system.
**INDICATIONS**    • Insomnia.
**CONTRAINDICATIONS**    • Renal failure: active metabolites may not be excreted and may accumulate. • Depressed or psychotic patients in the absence of anxiety. • Pregnancy: fetal damage has been reported. • Breast-feeding. benzodiazepines are excreted in breast milk. • Acute angle-closure glaucoma. • Myasthenia gravis.
**DOSAGE    PO:    ADULTS:** 15 or 30 mg at bedtime.    *Special patient populations:*    **ELDERLY:** Doses for the elderly must be reduced. Usual dose is 15 mg at bedtime.    **CHILDREN:** Safety for children under 15 years old has not been established.    **PREGNANCY:** Benzodiazepines are not considered safe for use during pregnancy. Fetal abnormalities have been documented.
**PREPARATIONS**    *Capsules:* 15 and 30 mg.
**DRUG INTERACTIONS**    • See entry for drug class (p. 685).
**FATE**    Flurazepam is metabolized to active metabolites with long *half-lives.*
**❦ NURSING CONSIDERATIONS**
**Side effects, toxicities, and associated nursing actions**
- See entry for drug class (p. 685).
**Patient and family education**
- See entry for drug class (p. 686).

## halazepam    (hal-AZ-e-pam)    anxiolytic

- halazepam: Paxipam (Schedule IV)

**MECHANISM OF ACTION**    Halazepam is a benzodiazepine. These drugs seem to depress the limbic system.
**INDICATIONS**    • Anxiety.
**CONTRAINDICATIONS**    • Renal failure active metabolites may not be excreted and may accumulate. • Depressed or psychotic patients in the absence of anxiety. • Pregnancy: fetal damage has been reported. • Breast-feeding: benzodiazepines are excreted in breast milk. • Acute angle-closure glaucoma. • Myasthenia gravis.
**DOSAGE    PO:    ADULTS:** 20 to 40 mg three or four times daily.    *Special patient populations:*    **ELDERLY:** Doses for the elderly must be reduced. The initial dose is 20 mg one or two times daily. This may be increased if no adverse effects occur.    **CHILDREN:** Safety for children under 18 years old has not been established.    **PREGNANCY:** Benzodiazepines are not considered safe for use during pregnancy. Fetal abnormalities have been documented. FDA pregnancy category D.
**PREPARATIONS**    *Tablets:* 20 and 40 mg.
**DRUG INTERACTIONS**    • See entry for drug class (p. 685).
**FATE**    Halazepam has a plasma *half-life* of about 14 hours. It is metabolized to an active, long-lived metabolite.
**❦ NURSING CONSIDERATIONS**
**Side effects, toxicities, and associated nursing actions**
- See entry for drug class (p. 685).
**Patient and family education**
- See entry for drug class (p. 686).

## ✽ketazolam    (keet-AY-zoe-lam)                                    anxiolytic

- ketazolam: ✽Loftran

**MECHANISM OF ACTION**    Ketazolam is a benzodiazepine. These drugs seem to depress the limbic system.

**INDICATIONS**    • Anxiety.

**CONTRAINDICATIONS**    • Renal failure: active metabolites may not be excreted and may accumulate. • Depressed or psychotic patients in the absence of anxiety. • Pregnancy: fetal damage has been reported. • Breast-feeding: benzodiazepines are excreted in breast milk. • Acute angle-closure glaucoma. • Myasthenia gravis.

**DOSAGE**    **PO:**    **ADULTS:** 15 mg one or two times daily. Increments of 15 mg daily may be made. The largest dose should be at bedtime.    *Special patient populations:*    **ELDERLY:** Doses for the elderly must be reduced. The initial dose is half the regular adult dose. This may be increased if no adverse effects occur.    **CHILDREN:** Safety for children under 18 years old has not been established.    **PREGNANCY:** Benzodiazepines are not considered safe for use during pregnancy. Fetal abnormalities have been documented.

**PREPARATIONS**    *Capsules:* 15 and 30 mg.

**DRUG INTERACTIONS**    • See entry for drug class (p. 685).

**FATE**    *Peak* concentrations occur 3 hours after oral administration. The metabolites are active and have long *half-lives.*

## ❧ NURSING CONSIDERATIONS

### Side effects, toxicities, and associated nursing actions

- See entry for drug class (p. 685).

### Patient and family education

- See entry for drug class (p. 686).

## lorazepam    (lor-A-ze-pam)                                    anxiolytic

- lorazepam: Ativan (Schedule IV)

**MECHANISM OF ACTION**    Lorazepam is a benzodiazepine. These drugs seem to depress the limbic system.

**INDICATIONS**    • Anxiety. • Preoperative sedation. • Status epilepticus. • Insomnia.

**CONTRAINDICATIONS**    • Depressed or psychotic patients in the absence of anxiety. • Pregnancy: fetal damage has been reported. • Breast-feeding: benzodiazepines are excreted in breast milk. • Acute angle-closure glaucoma. • Myasthenia gravis.

**DOSAGE**    **PO, anxiety:**    **ADULTS:** 2 to 3 mg daily, divided in two or three doses.    **IM, preoperatively** 0.05 mg/kg, 2 hours before surgery.    **IV, preoperatively** 0.044 mg/kg, 15 to 20 mg before surgery. *Special patient populations:*    **ELDERLY:** Doses for the elderly must be reduced. This may be increased if no adverse effects occur.    **CHILDREN:** Safety for children under 18 years old has not been established.    **PREGNANCY:** Benzodiazepines are not considered safe for use during pregnancy. Fetal abnormalities have been documented.

**PREPARATIONS**    *Tablets:* 0.5, 1, and 2 mg; *injection;* 2 and 4 mg/ml.

**DRUG INTERACTIONS**    • See entry for drug class (p. 685).    **Scopolamine** There is an increased incidence of sedation, hallucinations, and irrational behavior when administered with lorazepam.

**FATE**    Lorazepam has a plasma *half-life* of 10 to 20 hours. There are no active metabolites.

## ❧ NURSING CONSIDERATIONS

### Side effects, toxicities, and associated nursing actions

- See entry for drug class (p. 685).

CV Parenteral administration may produce bradycardia or cardiac arrest. The elderly and debilitated are at most risk.

- Monitor the pulse and blood pressure.

### Nursing interventions related to drug administration
- For IV administration, dilute the ordered dose with equal amounts of sterile water, 5% dextrose, or 0.9% sodium chloride for injection. Administer as close to IV insertion site as possible. Avoid intra-arterial injection, as it may cause gangrene. Administer at a rate of 2 mg or less over 1 minute.
- Maintain the patient on bedrest for at least 3 hours following IV administration. Have a suction machine at the bedside and drugs and equipment for resuscitation nearby.
- Lorazepam may also be administered IM.

### Patient and family education
- See entry for drug class (p. 686).

---

## ✤nitrazepam  (nye-TRAY-ze-pam)  hypnotic, anticonvulsant

- nitrazepam: ✤Mogadon

**MECHANISM OF ACTION**  Nitrazepam is a benzodiazepine. These drugs seem to depress the limbic system.

**INDICATIONS**  • Insomnia. • Myoclonic seizures.

**CONTRAINDICATIONS**  • Depressed or psychotic patients in the absence of anxiety. • Pregnancy: fetal damage has been reported. • Breast-feeding benzodiazepines are excreted in breast milk. • Acute angle-closure glaucoma. • Myasthenia gravis.

**DOSAGE**  PO:  **ADULTS:** 5 to 10 mg before bedtime. *Special patient populations:*  **ELDERLY:** Doses for the elderly must be reduced. The initial does is 2.5 mg at bedtime. This may be increased if no adverse effects occur.  **CHILDREN:** Safety for children under 18 years old has not been established.  **PREGNANCY:** Benzodiazepines are not considered safe for use during pregnancy. Fetal abnormalities have been documented.

**PREPARATIONS**  *Tablets:* 5 and 10 mg.

**DRUG INTERACTIONS**  • See entry for drug class (p. 688).

**FATE**  Nitrazepam is rapidly absorbed, and *peak* blood levels are achieved in 3 hours. The plasma *half-life* is 16 to 48 hours. Metabolites are not active.

### ☙ NURSING CONSIDERATIONS
#### Side effects, toxicities, and associated nursing actions
- See entry for drug class (p. 685).
- Monitor respiratory rate.
- Assess breath sounds.

**Skin** Urticaria, rash, and photosensitivity.

**Allergic** Hypersensitivity reactions. See Skin.
- Inspect the patient for the development of skin changes.
- Caution patients to avoid prolonged exposure to the sun, to wear a hat and long-sleeved clothing, and to use maximum protection sunscreens.
- Be alert for acute allergic reactions. Know the location of drugs and equipment for the treatment of allergic response.

**Other** Joint pain, muscle cramps, and tingling sensation.
- Question the patient about the appearance of any unusual sign or symptom.

#### Patient and family education
- Review with the patient the expected benefits and possible side effects of therapy. Instruct the patient to report the development of any unexpected sign or symptom.
- Caution the patient to avoid the use of any other medications, including over-the-counter preparations, without prior clearance with the physician.
- Caution patient to avoid the use of alcohol.

- Remind patients to take the medication only as ordered. Instruct patients that these drugs may be habit forming. Be alert in the outpatient setting to patients who return for prescription refills on an increasingly frequent basis, as this may indicate improper use or abuse of the drug.
- Caution patients not to discontinue the drug suddenly without consultation with the physician.
- Patients should not double up if a dose is missed. Patients should not share medications with others.
- Remind patients to keep these and all medications out of the reach of children. Child-proof caps should be used.
- Smoking may decrease the sedative effects of the benzodiazepines. Ideally, patients should avoid smoking while taking benzodiazepines. Heavy smokers may need a larger dose.

## oxazepam   (ox-A-ze-pam)                                                         anxiolytic

- oxazepam: Serax (Schedule IV)

**MECHANISM OF ACTION**   Oxazepam is a benzodiazepine. These drugs seem to depress the limbic system.
**INDICATIONS**   • Anxiety. • Alcohol withdrawal.
**CONTRAINDICATIONS**   • Depressed or psychotic patients in the absence of anxiety. • Pregnancy: fetal damage has been reported. • Breast-feeding: benzodiazepines are excreted in breast milk. • Acute angle-closure glaucoma. • Myasthenia gravis.
**DOSAGE**   PO:   ADULTS: Anxiety: 10 to 15 mg three or four times daily. *Alcohol withdrawal:* 15 to 30 mg three or four times daily.   *Special patient populations:*   ELDERLY: Doses for the elderly are initially 10 mg three times daily. This may be increased to 15 mg three times daily if required and if no adverse effects occur.   CHILDREN: Safety for children under 18 years old has not been established.   PREGNANCY: Benzodiazepines are not considered safe for use during pregnancy. Fetal abnormalities have been documented.
**PREPARATIONS**   *Capsules:* 10, 15, and 30 mg; *tablets:* 15 mg (contain tartrazine).
**DRUG INTERACTIONS**   • See entry for drug class (p. 685).
**FATE**   Oxazepam has a plasma *half-life* of 3 to 21 hours. There are no active metabolites.
**🌺 NURSING CONSIDERATIONS**
### Side effects, toxicities, and associated nursing actions
- See entry for drug class (p. 685).
### Nursing interventions related to drug administration
- Serax, 15 mg, tablets contain FD & C yellow dye # 5 (tartrazine), which may cause an allergic reaction in susceptible individuals. Although rare, this reaction is seen more commonly in persons with aspirin hypersensitivity.
### Patient and family education
- See entry for drug class (p. 686).

## prazepam   (PRA-ze-pam)                                                         anxiolytic

- prazepam: Centrax (Schedule IV)

**MECHANISM OF ACTION**   Prazepam is a benzodiazepine. These drugs seem to depress the limbic system.
**INDICATIONS**   • Anxiety.
**CONTRAINDICATIONS**   • Renal failure: active metabolites may not be excreted and may accumulate. • Depressed or psychotic patients in the absence of anxiety. • Pregnancy: fetal damage has been reported. • Breast-feeding: benzodiazepines are excreted in breast milk. • Acute angle-closure glaucoma. • Myasthenia gravis.
**DOSAGE**   PO:   ADULTS: 30 mg daily in divided doses; range: 20 to 60 mg. Alternatively, give as a single bedtime dose. *Special patient populations:*   ELDERLY: Doses for the elderly must be reduced.

The initial dose is 10 to 15 mg daily in two or three doses. This may be increased if no adverse effects occur. **CHILDREN:** Safety for children under 18 years old has not been established. **PREGNANCY:** Benzodiazepines are not considered safe for use during pregnancy. Fetal abnormalities have been documented.

**PREPARATIONS** *Capsules:* 5, 10, and 20 mg; *tablets:* 10 mg.

**DRUG INTERACTIONS** • See entry for drug class (p. 685).

**FATE** Prazepam is metabolized to long-lived, active metabolites.

### ☙ NURSING CONSIDERATIONS

#### Side effects, toxicities, and associated nursing actions
• See entry for drug class (p. 685).

#### Patient and family education
• See entry for drug class (p. 686).

---

## quazepam (KWA-ze-pam) hypnotic

• quazepam: Dormalin (Schedule IV)

**MECHANISM OF ACTION** Quazepam is a benzodiazepine. These drugs seem to depress the limbic system.

**INDICATIONS** • Insomnia.

**CONTRAINDICATIONS** • Renal failure: quazepam and its active metabolites have long plasma half-lives and may accumulate. • Depressed or psychotic patients in the absence of anxiety. • Pregnancy: fetal damage has been reported. • Breast feeding: Benzodiazepines are excreted in breast milk. • Acute angle-closure glaucoma. • Myasthenia gravis.

**DOSAGE** **PO:** **ADULTS:** Initially, 15 mg. Some patients may require only 7.5 mg. *Special patient populations:* **ELDERLY:** Doses for the elderly must be reduced. The Initial dose should be 7.5 mg. This may be increased if adverse effects do not occur and the response is not sufficient. **CHILDREN:** Safety for children under 18 years old has not been established. **PREGNANCY:** Benzodiazepines are not considered safe for use during pregnancy. Fetal abnormalities have been documented.

**PREPARATIONS** *Tablets:* 15 mg.

**DRUG INTERACTIONS** See entry for drug class (p. 685).

**FATE** Quazepam is rapidly absorbed. The plasma *half-life* is 39 hours. Quazepam is metabolized in the liver and has at least two active metabolites with long half-lives. Quazepam may accumulate with repeated doses.

### ☙ NURSING CONSIDERATIONS

#### Side effects, toxicities, and associated nursing actions
• See entry for drug class (p. 685).

#### Patient and family education
• See entry for drug class (p. 686).

---

## temazepam (te-MAZ-e-pam) hypnotic

• temazepam: Restoril (Schedule IV)

**MECHANISM OF ACTION** Temazepam is a benzodiazepine. These drugs seem to depress the limbic system.

**INDICATIONS** • Insomnia.

**CONTRAINDICATIONS** • Depressed or psychotic patients in the absence of anxiety. • Pregnancy: fetal damage has been reported. FDA pregnancy category X. • Breast feeding: benzodiazepines are excreted in breast milk. • Acute angle-closure glaucoma. • Myasthenia gravis.

**DOSAGE** **PO:** **ADULTS:** 15 or 30 mg at bedtime. *Special patient populations:* **ELDERLY:** Dose for the elderly is 15 mg at bedtime. This may be increased if required and if there are no adverse effects.

**CHILDREN:** Safety for children under 18 years old has not been established. **PREGNANCY:** Benzodiazepines are not considered safe for use during pregnancy. Fetal abnormalities have been documented.

**PREPARATIONS** *Capsules:* 15 and 30 mg.

**DRUG INTERACTIONS** • See entry for drug class (p. 685).

**FATE** Temazepam has a plasma *half-life* of 10 to 20 hours. There are no active metabolites.

☙ **NURSING CONSIDERATIONS**

### Side effects, toxicities, and associated nursing actions
• See entry for drug class (p. 685).

### Patient and family education
• See entry for drug class (p. 686).

---

## triazolam (trye-AY-zoe-lam) anxiolytic

• triazolam: Halcion

**MECHANISM OF ACTION** Triazolam is a benzodiazepine. These drugs seem to depress the limbic system.

**INDICATIONS** • Insomnia.

**CONTRAINDICATIONS** • Depressed or psychotic patients in the absence of anxiety. • Pregnancy: fetal damage has been reported. • Breast-feeding: benzodiazepines are excreted in breast milk. • Acute angle-closure glaucoma. • Myasthenia gravis.

**DOSAGE** **PO:** **ADULTS:** 0.25 to 0.5 mg at bedtime. *Special patient populations:* **ELDERLY:** Doses for the elderly must be reduced. The initial dose is 0.125 mg at bedtime. This may be increased if necessary, and if there are no adverse effects. **CHILDREN:** Safety for children under 18 years old has not been established. **PREGNANCY:** Benzodiazepines are not considered safe for use during pregnancy. Fetal abnormalities have been documented. FDA pregnancy category X.

**PREPARATIONS** *Tablets:* 0.125, 0.25, and 0.5 mg.

**DRUG INTERACTIONS** • See entry for drug class (p. 685).

**FATE** Triazolam has a plasma *half-life* of 2 to 6 hours. There are no active metabolites.

☙ **NURSING CONSIDERATIONS**

### Side effects, toxicities, and associated nursing actions
• See entry for drug class (p. 685).

### Patient and family education
• See entry for drug class (p. 686).

---

# Miscellaneous sedative-hypnotic drugs*

| | United States | Canada |
|---|---|---|
| buspirone HCl | NC | NA |
| chloral hydrate | Schedule IV | NC |
| chlormezanone | NC | NC |
| ethchlorvynol | Schedule IV | NC |
| ethinamate | Schedule IV | NA |
| glutethimide | Schedule III | NC |
| hydroxyzine HCl/pamoate | NC | NC |
| meprobamate | Schedule IV | NC |
| methotrimeprazine HCl | NC | NC |
| methyprylon | Schedule III | NC |
| paraldehyde | Schedule IV | NC |
| promethazine HCl | NC | NC |
| propiomazine HCl | NC | NA |

*NA = not available; NC = not a controlled substance.

**DRUG COMBINATIONS**
- meprobamate and aspirin: Epromate, Equagesic, Equazine-M, Hepto-M, Mepro Compound, Meprogesic, Micrainin (Schedule IV)
- meprobamate and benactyzine HCl: Deprol (Schedule IV)
- meprobamate and conjugate estrogens: Milprem, PMB
- meprobamate and tridihexethyl Cl: Pathibamate
- promethazine HCl and meperidine HCl: Mepergan, Mepergan Fortis (Schedule II)
- promethazine HCl and phenylephrine HCl: Phenergan VC syrup, Promethazine HCl VC plain syrup

**OVERVIEW OF THE DRUG CLASS**    These drugs come from different chemical classes, but all are used for their sedative-hypnotic properties. Hydroxyzine is an antihistamine. Methotrimeprazine, promethazine, and propiomazine are phenothiazines. Chloral hydrate and paraldehyde are very old drugs. The remainder, ethchlorvynol, ethinamate, and methprylon, were introduced in the 1950s as improvements over the barbiturates. In fact, they are also readily abused and are used principally short-term as hypnotics.

**MECHANISM OF ACTION**    • See individual drugs.

**INDICATIONS**    • See individual drugs.

**CONTRAINDICATIONS**    • See individual drugs.

**DRUG INTERACTIONS**    **CNS depressants** Sedative-hypnotic drugs have an additive CNS depressant effect with other drugs having this property, including alcohol.

---

## buspirone hydrochloride    (BYOO-spi-rone)                    anxiolytic

- buspirone: BuSpar

**MECHANISM OF ACTION**    Buspirone is a new anxiolytic that alleviates anxiety without causing sedation or functional impairment. There seems to be a negligible potential for abuse or physical dependence. Buspirone appears to have a more selective CNS depressant activity through the dopaminergic system than do the benzodiazepines.

**INDICATIONS**    • Anxiety.

**CONTRAINDICATIONS**    • Not yet established.

**DOSAGE**    **PO:**    **ADULTS:** 5 to 10 mg three times daily.    *Special patient populations:*    **PREGNANCY:** Safe use has not been established.

**PREPARATIONS**    *Tablets:* 5 and 10 mg.

**DRUG INTERACTIONS**    Not yet established. Unlike other anxiolytics, CNS depression is not additive with alcohol.

**FATE**    Buspirone is well absorbed, especially in the presence of food. The drug is readily metabolized by the liver to metabolites that are inactive or weakly active. The plasma *half-life* is 2 to 11 hours and is increased in patients with liver disease.

### 🐾 NURSING CONSIDERATIONS

#### Side effects, toxicities, and associated nursing actions
**CNS** Nervousness, restlessness, headache, weakness, dizziness, and depression. These are infrequent.
- Tell patients to avoid driving or operating hazardous equipment if dizziness develops; notify the physician.

- Assess for signs of depression: withdrawal, lack of interest in personal appearance, insomnia, or weight change.

  **GI** Nausea is the most common side effect.
- Advise patients to take the drug with milk or a snack to lessen gastric side effects. If nausea is severe or persistent, notify the physician.

### Patient and family education

- Review with the patient the expected benefits and possible side effects of therapy. Instruct the patient to report the development of any unexpected sign or symptom.
- Caution the patient to avoid the use of any other medication, including over-the-counter preparations, without prior clearance with the physician.
- For insomnia, instruct patients to take the prescribed dose about 30 minutes prior to bedtime.
- Remind patients not to share medications with others.
- Remind the patient to keep these and all medications out of the reach of children. Child-proof caps should be used.
- To avoid accidental overdose, caution patient to keep drugs in clearly labeled containers, away from the bedside, so that the patient does not inadvertently repeat a dose if wakened during the night.
- Caution the patient to report excessive morning drowsiness to the physician. Excessive morning drowsiness represents a response to the medication or too high a prescribed dose; the patient should not increase the dose of medication to alleviate this ''fatigue.''
- Review with the patient other aids to sleep that might be effective, including drinking warm milk in the evening or taking a warm bath. Sedative-hypnotics should only be used for short-term treatment of insomnia.

---

## chloral hydrate    (KLOR-al HYE-drate)                                   sedative-hypnotic

- chloral hydrate: Aquachloral, Noctec (Schedule IV; ✤Novochlorhydrate ✤Schedule F)

**MECHANISM OF ACTION**   The mechanism of action is not well understood, but the CNS depressant effects are similar to those of the barbiturates.

**INDICATIONS**   **Insomnia** The drug is considered to cause less paradoxical excitement in children and the elderly than the barbiturates. Should not be used for more than 2 weeks because it loses its effectiveness. **Sedation** Especially preoperatively and postoperatively in children and the elderly.

**CONTRAINDICATIONS**   • Severe cardiac disease. • Depression: like other CNS depressants, chloral hydrate should be prescribed with caution. • Impaired renal or liver function: elimination of the drug will be markedly impaired. • Irritated GI system: esophagitis, gastritis, gastric or duodenal ulcers are contraindications.

**DOSAGE**   **PO or rectal:**   **ADULTS:** For hypnosis or presurgically, 500 mg to 1 g 15 to 30 minutes before bedtime or before surgery. In managing the symptoms of alcohol withdrawal, this dose may be given every 6 hours to control symptoms. The sedative dose is 250 mg three times daily after meals. **CHILDREN:** For hypnosis or presurgically, 50 mg/kg or 1.5 g/$M^2$; maximum, 1 g. As a sedative, 8.3 mg/kg or 250 mg/$M^2$ three times daily after meals.   *Special patient populations:*   **PREGNANCY:** Chloral hydrate crosses the placenta, but the effects on the fetus are unknown. Chloral hydrate should not be used by nursing mothers because it will distribute to breast milk and may sedate the infant.

**PREPARATIONS**   *Capsules:* 250 and 500 mg; *solution:* 250 mg/5 ml, 500 mg/5 ml, *suppository:* 325, 500, and 650 mg.

**DRUG INTERACTIONS**   **CNS depressants** Depression of the CNS is additive with other CNS depressants, including alcohol, paraldehyde, and barbiturates. Chloral hydrate may also induce a vasodilation reaction with alcohol that is characterized by palpitations, tachycardia, flushing, and a dysphoria. **Furosemide** Chloral hydrate in combination with furosemide may cause a variable blood pressure, an uneasy feeling, or flushing with perspiration.   **Oral anticoagulants** Chloral hydrate may potentiate the decrease in prothrombin levels, causing increased anticoagulant effects.

**DIAGNOSTIC TEST INTERFERENCE**   **Urine glucose** Chloral hydrate may produce a false-positive reaction in tests using cupric sulfate (Benedict's solution, Clinitest, Clinistix, Tes-Tape).   **Urine catecholamines** Chloral hydrate may interfere with fluorometric tests for 48 hours after administration.   **17-Hyroxysteroids** Chloral hydrate may interfere with the Reddy, Jenkins, and Thorn procedure.

**FATE**   Chloral hydrate is rapidly absorbed following oral or rectal administration and has a rapid *onset of action*. The drug is metabolized by the liver to an active product, trichloroethanol, by alcohol dehydrogenase, which has a *half-life* of 8 to 11 hours. Trichloroethanol is excreted in three forms: unchanged, as the glucuronide, and metabolized to trichloroacetic acid.

## ❦ NURSING CONSIDERATIONS

### Side effects, toxicities, and associated nursing actions

**CNS** Occasionally, disorientation and incoherence. Other CNS effects characteristic of depressants are rare.
- Caution patients to avoid driving or operating hazardous equipment after taking this medication.
- Supervise ambulation of hospitalized patients and discourage smoking.
- Keep side rails up.
- Keep a night light on.

**CV** Overdose can cause arrhythmias.
- If overdose is suspected, move the patient to an intensive care unit. Monitor electrocardiogram.

**GI** Gastric irritation with nausea, vomiting, and diarrhea is the most common side effect.
- Assess for presence of GI complaints.
- Taking the dose with a snack or milk may help reduce gastric irritation.
- If vomiting and diarrhea are severe or persistent, it may be necessary to discontinue the medication. Notify the physician.

**Skin** Rashes or urticaria are uncommon.
- Visually inspect the patient for the development of rashes or skin changes.

### Nursing interventions related to drug administration
- Capsules should not be chewed but administered with a glass of chilled fluids and swallowed whole.
- Dilute oral solutions or syrups in a half glass of chilled water, juice, or ginger ale.
- Lubricate a suppository for insertion with water only. Assess anal area for irritation.

### Patient and family education
- Review with the patient the expected benefits and possible side effects of therapy. Instruct the patient to report the development of any unexpected signs or symptom.
- Caution the patient to avoid the use of any other medications, including over-the-counter preparations, without prior clearance with the physician.
- Caution the patient to avoid the use of alcohol.
- For insomnia, instruct patients to take the prescribed dose about 30 minutes prior to bedtime.
- Remind patients that these drugs may be habit forming. Be alert in the outpatient setting for patients who return for prescription refills on an increasingly frequent basis, as this may indicate improper use or abuse of the drug.
- Remind patients not to share medications with others.
- Remind patients to keep these and all medications out of the reach of children. Child-proof caps should be used.
- To avoid accidental overdose, caution patient to keep drugs in clearly labeled containers, away from the bedside, so that the patient does not inadvertently repeat a dose if wakened during the night.
- Caution the patient to report excessive morning drowsiness to the physician. Excessive drowsiness in the morning represents a response to the medication, or too high a prescribed dose; the patient should not increase the dose of medication to alleviate this "fatigue."
- Review with the patient other aids to sleep that might be effective, including drinking warm milk in the evening or taking a warm bath. Sedative-hypnotics should only be used for short-term treatment of insomnia.

## chlormezanone (klor-MEZ-a-none)                    antianxiety

- chlormezanone: Trancopal (Schedule IV, ♣Schedule F)

**MECHANISM OF ACTION**   The mechanism of action is not well understood, but the CNS depressant effects are similar to those of the barbiturates.

**INDICATIONS**   **Anxiety** May not be as effective as benzodiazepines.

**CONTRAINDICATIONS**   • Hypersensitivity to the drug. • Hazardous activities: as with other CNS depressants, alertness and coordination will be compromised.

**DOSAGE**   **PO:**   **ADULTS:** 100 to 200 mg, three to four times daily. May give 400 mg at bedtime to promote sleep.   **CHILDREN:** 5 to 12 years, 50 to 100 mg three to four times daily. Not recommended for children under 5 years of age.   *Special patient populations:*   **PREGNANCY:** Safe use has not been established.

**PREPARATIONS**   *Tablets:* 100 and 200 mg.

**DRUG INTERACTIONS**   **CNS depressants** Additive CNS depression with other depressants, including alcohol.

**FATE**   Rapidly absorbed from the GI tract. *Onset* of action is 15 to 30 minutes. Plasma *half-life* is 24 hours. About half of the drug is bound to plasma albumin. Chlormezanone is metabolized in part by the liver, with the unchanged drug and metabolites excreted in the urine and feces.

### ☙ NURSING CONSIDERATIONS

#### Side effects, toxicities, and associated nursing actions

**CNS** Drowsiness is the most common side effect. Other CNS effects may include dizziness, slurred speech, headache, and ataxia.
- Caution patients to avoid driving or operating hazardous equipment after taking this medication. Supervise the play of children, especially when they are riding bicycles or engaging in other potentially dangerous activities.
- Supervise ambulation of hospitalized patients and discourage smoking.
- Keep side rails up.
- Keep a night light on.

**GI** Nausea, anorexia, and dry mouth.
- Assess for presence of GI complaints.
- Monitor weight.
- Taking the dose with snack or milk may help reduce gastric irritation.

**GU** Difficulty in voiding.
- Caution the patient about this side effect. Instruct the patient to report any difficulty in voiding.
- Suggest that the patient void before taking each dose.
- Monitor intake and output.

**Allergic** Rash.
- Visually inspect the patient for skin changes.

#### Patient and family education

- Review with the patient the expected benefits and possible side effects of therapy. Instruct the patient to report the development of any unexpected signs or symptom.
- Caution the patient to avoid the use of any other medications, including over-the-counter preparations, without prior clearance with the physician.
- Caution the patient to avoid the use of alcohol.
- For insomnia, instruct patients to take the prescribed dose about 30 minutes prior to bedtime.
- Remind patients that these drugs may be habit forming. Be alert in the outpatient setting to patients who return for prescription refills on an increasingly frequent basis, as this may indicate improper use or abuse of the drug.
- Remind patients not to share medications with others.
- Remind patients to keep these and all medications out of the reach of children. Child-proof caps should be used.

- To avoid accidental overdose, caution patient to keep drugs in clearly labeled containers, away from the bedside, so that the patient does not inadvertently repeat a dose if wakened during the night.
- Caution the patient to report excessive morning drowsiness to the physician. Excessive drowsiness in the morning represents a response to the medication or too high a prescribed dose; the patient should not increase the dose of medication to alleviate this "fatigue."
- Review with the patient other aids to sleep that might be effective, including drinking warm milk in the evening or taking a warm bath. Sedative-hypnotics should only be used for short-term treatment of insomnia.

## ethchlorvynol    (eth-klor-VI-nole)                                        hypnotic

- ethchlorvynol: Placidyl (Schedule IV; ✚Schedule F)

**MECHANISM OF ACTION**    The mechanism of action is not well understood, but the CNS depressant effects are similar to those of the barbiturates.

**INDICATIONS**    Insomnia Use short-term, no more than 1 week.

**CONTRAINDICATIONS**    • Impaired hepatic or renal function. • Hypersensitivity or porphyria.

**DOSAGE**    PO:   ADULTS: 500 mg at bedtime. Another 200 mg may be taken on early awakening.   *Special patient populations:*   PREGNANCY: Should not be used during pregnancy. May produce CNS depression and withdrawal symptoms in the neonate.

**PREPARATIONS**    *Capsules:* 200, 500, and 750 mg. The 750 mg capsule contains tartrazine.

**DRUG INTERACTIONS**    **CNS depressants** Ethchorvynol will enhance the CNS depressant effects of other drugs, including alcohol.   **MAO inhibitors** Enhances depression.   **Amitriptyline** Transient delirium.   **Oral anticoagulants** Decreases anticoagulant effects by enhancing metabolism. Ethchlorvynol appears to induce liver microsomal enzymes.

**FATE**    Rapidly absorbed with an *onset* of action in about 30 minutes. *Duration of action* is about 5 hours. Plasma *half-life* is 10 to 20 hours. Ethchlorvynol is metabolized by both the liver and kidney, and metabolites are excreted in the urine.

### ❧ NURSING CONSIDERATIONS
#### Side effects, toxicities, and associated nursing actions
**CNS** Occasionally, nightmares or hangover.

**Eye** Blurring of vision. Occasionally, amblyopia after long-term therapy.
- Caution patients to avoid driving or operating hazardous equipment after taking this medication.
- Supervise ambulation of hospitalized patients and discourage smoking.
- Keep side rails up.
- Keep a night light on.
- Caution patients to report the development of any visual changes.

**CV** Hypotension
- Monitor blood pressure, especially in the elderly.
- Supervise ambulation.

**GI** Gastric upset, nausea, and vomiting.
- Assess for presence of GI complaints.
- Monitor weight.
- Taking the dose with a snack or milk may help reduce gastric irritation.
- If vomiting is persistent or severe, it may be necessary to discontinue the medication. Notify the physician.

**Allergic** Rash; rarely, thrombocytopenia.
- Visually inspect the patient for skin changes.
- Monitor CBC and platelet count.
- Inspect the patient for the development of bruising, petechiae, or unexplained bleeding.

**Other** Unpleasant aftertaste.
- Caution the patient about this possible effect. If it develops, and is severe, it may be necessary to discontinue the medication.

- Instruct the patient to suck sugarless hard candy or chew sugarless gum to try to improve taste if it persists into the next day.

### Patient and family education

- Review with the patient the expected benefits and possible side effects of therapy. Instruct the patient to report the development of any unexpected signs or symptom.
- Caution the patient to avoid the use of any other medications, including over-the-counter preparations, without prior clearance with the physician.
- Caution the patient to avoid the use of alcohol.
- For insomnia, instruct patients to take prescribed dose about 30 minutes prior to bedtime.
- Remind patients that these drugs may be habit forming. Be alert in the outpatient setting for patients who return for prescription refills on an increasingly frequent basis, as this may indicate improper use or abuse of the drug.
- Remind patients not to share medications with others.
- Remind patients to keep these and all medications out of the reach of children. Child-proof caps should be used.
- To avoid accidental overdose, caution patient to keep drugs in clearly labeled containers, away from the bedside, so that the patient does not inadvertently repeat a dose if wakened during the night.
- Caution the patient to report excessive morning drowsiness to the physician. Excessive drowsiness in the morning represents a response to the medication or too high a prescribed dose; the patient should not increase the dose of medication to alleviate this "fatigue."
- Review with the patient other aids to sleep that might be effective, including drinking warm milk in the evening or taking a warm bath. Sedative-hypnotics should only be used for short-term treatment of insomnia.
- Placidyl brand 750 mg capsules contain FD & C dye # 5 (tartrazine), which may cause an allergic response in susceptible patients. Although rare, this response is seen more often in persons with aspirin hypersensitivity.

## ethinamate (e-THIN-a-mate) hypnotic

- ethinamate: Valmid (Schedule IV, ✿Schedule F)

**MECHANISM OF ACTION** The mechanism of action is not well understood, but the CNS depressant effects are similar to those of the barbiturates.

**INDICATIONS** Insomnia Not effective after 1 week.

**CONTRAINDICATIONS** Hazardous activities As with other CNS depressants, alertness and coordination will be compromised.

**DOSAGE** PO: ADULTS: 500 mg to 1 g 20 minutes before bedtime. *Special patient populations:* ELDERLY: Doses for the elderly should be kept at 500 mg. PREGNANCY: Safe use has not been established.

**PREPARATIONS** *Capsules:* 500 mg.

**DRUG INTERACTIONS** CNS depressants Additive CNS depression with other depressants, including alcohol.

**DIAGNOSTIC TEST INTERFERENCE** 17-Ketosteroids Values from the modified Zimmerman reaction or the Porter-Silber test may be falsely high.

**FATE** Ethinamate is rapidly absorbed from the GI tract. *Onset of action* is in about 20 minutes and the *duration of action* is 3 to 5 hours. Ethinamate is rapidly metabolized by the liver, and the metabolites are excreted in the urine.

### ❦ NURSING CONSIDERATIONS

#### Side effects, toxicities, and associated nursing actions

GI Rarely, mild GI upset.
- Assess for presence of GI complaints.
- Taking the dose with a snack or milk may help reduce gastric irritation.

Allergic Rarely, hypersensitivity reactions.
- Assess the patient for development of allergic reactions.
- Visually inspect the patient for skin rashes.

### Patient and family education

- Review with the patient the expected benefits and possible side effects of therapy. Instruct the patient to report the development of any unexpected signs or symptom.
- Caution the patient to avoid the use of any other medications, including over-the-counter preparations, without prior clearance with the physician.
- Caution the patient to avoid the use of alcohol.
- For insomnia, instruct patients to take prescribed dose about 30 minutes prior to bedtime.
- Remind patients that these drugs may be habit forming. Be alert in the outpatient setting to patients who return for prescription refills on an increasingly frequent basis, as this may indicate improper use or abuse of the drug.
- Remind patients not to share medications with others.
- Remind patients to keep these and all medications out of the reach of children. Child-proof caps should be used.
- To avoid accidental overdose, caution patient to keep drugs in clearly labeled containers, away from the bedside, so that the patient does not inadvertently repeat a dose if wakened during the night.
- Caution the patient to report excessive morning drowsiness to the physician. Excessive drowsiness in the morning represents a response to the medication or too high a prescribed dose; the patient should not increase the dose of medication to alleviate this ''fatigue.''
- Review with the patient other aids to sleep that might be effective, including drinking warm milk in the evening or taking a warm bath. Sedative-hypnotics should only be used for short-term treatment of insomnia.

## glutethimide   (gloo-TETH-i-mide)                                    hypnotic

- glutethimide: Doriden (Schedule III)

**MECHANISM OF ACTION**   The mechanism of action is not well understood, but the CNS depressant effects are similar to those of the barbiturates. In addition, gluthethimide has anticholinergic activity.

**INDICATIONS**   **Insomnia** Effective for no more than 1 week.

**CONTRAINDICATIONS**   **Conditions aggravated by anticholinergic activity** These include prostatic hypertrophy, stenosing peptic ulcer, pyloroduodenal obstruction, bladder neck obstruction, angle-closure glaucoma, and cardiac arrhythmias.

**DOSAGE**   PO:   ADULTS: 250 to 500 mg at bedtime.   *Special patient populations:*   ELDERLY: Doses for the elderly should not exceed 500 mg;   PREGNANCY: Safe use has not been established.

**PREPARATIONS**   *Capsules:* 500 mg; *tablets:* 250 and 500 mg.

**DRUG INTERACTIONS**   **CNS depressants** Additive CNS depression with other depressants, including alcohol.   **Tricyclic antidepressants** These have anticholinergic effects that are additive when combined with glutethimide.   **Oral anticoagulants** Gluthethimide will induce liver microsomal enzymes that increase the degradation of oral anticoagulants. A higher dose of anticoagulant may therefore be required.   **Anticholinergic drugs** Gluthethimide has weak anticholinergic effects and may potentiate those of other drugs with anticholinergic effects, especially the phenothiazines.

**DIAGNOSTIC TEST INTERFERENCE**   **17-Hydroxycorticosteroids** Glutethimide interferes with the Glenn-Nelson technique.

**FATE**   Glutethimide is irregularly absorbed. *Onset of action* is in about 30 minutes; *duration of action* is 4 to 6 hours. Elimination requires metabolism of glutethimide by the liver for subsequent excretion in the urine.

### ☙ NURSING CONSIDERATIONS

#### Side effects, toxicities, and associated nursing actions

**CNS** ''Hangover,'' paradoxical excitement, vertigo.

**Eye** Blurring of vision.

- Caution patients to avoid driving or operating hazardous equipment after taking this medication.
- Supervise ambulation of hospitalized patients and discourage smoking.
- Keep side rails up.

- Keep a night light on.
- If the patient displays paradoxical excitement, monitor carefully. Notify the physician.

**GI** Gastric irritation, nausea, dry mouth, hiccups, and diarrhea.

- Assess for the presence of GI complaints.
- Taking the dose with a snack or milk may help reduce gastric irritation.
- If vomiting, diarrhea, or hiccups are severe or persistent, it may be necessary to discontinue medication. Notify the physician.
- For dry mouth, encourage the patient to suck on sugarless hard candy or chew sugarless gum. Frequent oral hygiene may improve comfort. Avoid drying agents such as lemon-glycerin swabs. Some patients may wish to use a commercially available saliva substitute.

**Hematologic** Rarely, blood dyscrasias.

- Monitor CBC, differential, and platelets.
- Caution the patient to report the development of fever, sore throat, bruising, or unexplained bleeding.
- Visually inspect the patient for petechiae, and bruises.

### Patient and family education

- Review with the patient the expected benefits and possible side effects of therapy. Instruct the patient to report the development of any unexpected signs or symptoms.
- Caution the patient to avoid the use of any other medications, including over-the-counter preparations, without prior clearance with the physician.
- Caution the patient to avoid the use of alcohol.
- For insomnia, instruct patients to take prescribed dose about 30 minutes prior to bedtime.
- Remind patients that these drugs may be habit forming. Be alert in the outpatient setting for patients who return for prescription refills on an increasingly frequent basis, as this may indicate improper use or abuse of the drug.
- Remind patients not to share medications with others.
- Remind patients to keep these and all medications out of the reach of children. Child-proof caps should be used.
- To avoid accidental overdose, caution patient to keep drugs in clearly labeled containers, away from the bedside, so that the patient does not inadvertently repeat a dose if wakened during the night.
- Caution the patient to report excessive morning drowsiness to the physician. Excessive drowsiness in the morning represents a response to the medication or too high a prescribed dose; the patient should not increase the dose of medication to alleviate this ''fatigue.''
- Review with the patient other aids to sleep that might be effective, including drinking warm milk in the evening or taking a warm bath. Sedative-hypnotics should only be used for short-term treatment of insomnia.

---

## hydroxyzine HCl    (hye-DROX-i-zeen)                                    antianxiety

- hydroxyzine HCl: Atarax, Atozine, Durrax, ✱Mulipax, Vistacon, Vistaril
- hydroxyzine pamoate: Hy-Pam, Vamate, Vistaril Oral

**MECHANISM OF ACTION**   Hydroxyzine is an antihistamine with CNS depressant, anticholinergic, and antispasmodic activities.

**INDICATIONS**   • Anxiety. • Management of itching associated with allergic conditions. • Nausea and vomiting: hydroxyzine has antiemetic effects. • Alcohol withdrawal. • Preoperative medication.

**CONTRAINDICATIONS**   • Hypersensitivity. • Hazardous activities: as with other CNS depressants, alertness and coordination will be compromised.

**DOSAGE**   **PO:**   **ADULTS:** *Anxiety:* Agitation caused by alcohol withdrawal: 50 to 100 mg four times daily. *Management of itching caused by allergic conditions:* 25 mg three or four times daily.   **IM:** **ADULTS:** Sedation preoperatively and postoperatively; control of nausea and vomiting: 25 to 100 mg. *Special patient populations:*   **CHILDREN:** The pediatric dose if half the adult dose.   **PREGNANCY:**

Hydroxyzine has been shown to be teratogenic in animals and is not recommended for use during pregnancy.

**PREPARATIONS**    *Hydroxyzine HCl, tablets:* 10, 25, 50, and 100 mg; *tablets, film-coated:* 10, 25, 50, and 100 mg; *solution:* 10 mg/5 ml; *injection:* 25, 50 mg/ml. *Hydroxyzine pamoate, capsules:** 25, 50, 100 mg; *suspension*:* 25 mg/5 ml; ♣*Syrup:* 10 mg/ml.

**DRUG INTERACTIONS**    **CNS depressants** Additive CNS depression with other depressants, including alcohol. **Anticholinergic agents** Additive anticholinergic effects are seen with hydrolyzine.    **Epinephrine** Hydroxyzine can inhibit and reverse the vasopressor response.

**DIAGNOSTIC TEST INTERFERENCE**    **17-Hydroxycorticosteroids** Hydroxyzine can cause falsely high urinary values.

**FATE**    Hydroxyzine is rapidly absorbed with an *onset of action* in 15 to 30 minutes and a *duration of action* of 4 to 6 hours for the sedative action. The antihistaminic action may be effective for several days. Hydroxyzine is metabolized by the liver, and products are excreted through the bile in the feces.

## ❦ NURSING CONSIDERATIONS
### Side effects, toxicities, and associated nursing actions

**CNS** Sedative and antiemetic activity.

**Eye** Anticholinergic activity could cause blurring of vision.
* Caution patients to avoid driving or operating hazardous equipment until the effects of the medication can be evaluated. Supervise the play of children, especially when they are riding bicycles or engaging in other potentially dangerous activities.
* Supervise ambulation of hospitalized patients and discourage smoking.
* Keep side rails up.
* Keep a night light on.
* Antiemetic activity may be desirable effect for specific patients.
* Caution the patient to notify the physician if blurred vision occurs.

**CV** Rarely, cardiac arrhythmias. Overdose can cause hypotension.
* Monitor pulse and blood pressure, especially after parenteral injection.
* Assess for symptoms of hypotension: dizziness, visual changes, syncope, and light-headedness. Instruct the patient to notify the physician if these occur. Caution patients to move slowly from lying to sitting or standing positions to prevent falling from sudden hypotension.

**GI** Hydroxyzine has an antispasmodic effect.
* Monitor frequency of stools. If constipation occurs, encourage the patient to increase the fluid intake to at least 3000 ml/day and to add roughage and fiber and prune or other juices to the diet. Constipation is also more common in the immobilized patient; encourage the patient to increase the amount of daily exercise. In rare instances it may be necessary to add a laxative or stool softener to the drug regimen.
* For dry mouth, instruct the patient to chew sugarless gum or suck on sugarless hard candy. A dry mouth can often lead to a bad taste in the mouth, which may be partly relieved by frequent oral hygiene, including brushing the teeth and/or rinsing with a mouthwash or gargle. Avoid drying agents such as lemon-glycerin swabs. Increasing the fluid intake may also help to decrease the dry feeling. Some patients may wish to use a commercially available saliva substitute.

**Lung** Bronchodilation.
* Monitor vital signs.
* Assess breath sounds.

**Other** Anticholinergic effects.
* Urinary retention may occur, although this is more common in men with pre-existing prostatic hypertrophy. Instruct the patient to report inability to void, increasing difficulty in initiating urination, or a feeling of incomplete bladder emptying. Instruct patients to void prior to taking each dose of this drug.
* Monitor intake and output.
* Inability to perspire may occur. Caution patients about this possible hazard, and encourage them to take frequent rest periods to cool off if they are engaged in strenuous activities.

Weights are those equivalent to HCl form.

**Nursing interventions related to drug administration**

- The parenteral form is designed for IM administration. Inadvertent subcutaneous, intravenous, or intra-arterial administration may lead to gangrene or thrombosis. Aspirate carefully before injecting the solution to ascertain that the needle is not in a vein. Only large muscle masses should be used, including the dorsogluteal site or the vastus lateralis in young children.
- Tablets may be crushed and mixed with food or fluid for easier administration.
- Contents of capsules may be mixed with food or fluids for easier administration.

**Patient and family education**

- Review with the patient the expected benefits and possible side effects of therapy. Instruct the patient to report the development of any unexpected sign or symptom.
- Caution the patient to avoid the use of any other medication, including over-the-counter preparations, without prior clearance with the physician.
- Caution the patient to avoid the use of alcohol.
- For insomnia, instruct patients to take prescribed dose about 30 minutes prior to bedtime.
- For motion sickness, instruct patients to take the prescribed dose about 30 to 45 minutes prior to departing.
- Remind patients not to share medications with others.
- Remind the patient to keep these and all medications out of the reach of children. Child-proof caps should be used.
- To avoid accidental overdose, caution patient to keep drugs in clearly labeled containers, away from the bedside, so that the patient does not inadvertently repeat a dose if wakened during the night.
- Caution the patient to report excessive morning drowsiness to the physician. Excessive morning drowsiness represents a response to the medication or too high a prescribed dose; the patient should not increase the dose of medication to alleviate this ''fatigue.''
- Review with the patient other aids to sleep that might be effective, including drinking warm milk in the evening or taking a warm bath. Sedative-hypnotics should only be used for short-term treatment of insomnia.

---

## meprobamate    (me-proe-BA-mate)                                   antianxiety

- meprobamate: ♣Apo-Meprobamate, Equanil, ♣Meditran, Meprospan-400, Miltown, ♣Neotran, Neurate, ♣Novomepro, Sedabamate, Tranmep (Schedule IV, Schedule F)

**MECHANISM OF ACTION**    Meprobamate has CNS depressant actions similar to the barbiturates. The mechanism of action is not known.

**INDICATIONS**    • Anxiety. • Preoperative sedation.

**CONTRAINDICATIONS**    • Porphyria: meprobamate may exacerbate acute intermittent porphyria. • Hypersensitivity to meprobamate or the chemically related drugs such as carisoprodol, mebutamate, or carbromal.

**DOSAGE**    **PO:**    **ADULTS:** 1.2 to 1.6 g daily in three or four divided doses. *Extended-release capsules:* 400 to 800 mg in the morning and evening. Maximum daily dose is 2.4 g.    **CHILDREN 6 TO 12 YEARS OLD:** 100 to 200 mg two or three times daily. Alternatively, 25 mg/kg daily or 700 mg/m$^2$ daily in two or three divided doses. *Extended release capsules:* 200 mg in the morning and at bedtime.    *Special patient populations:*    **ELDERLY:** Administration should start with the smallest dose to avoid oversedation.    **PREGNANCY:** There appears to be an increased risk of congenital malformations during the first trimester. Avoidance of meprobamate by pregnant women is advised. Nursing mothers should also avoid meprobamate since it is excreted in breast milk.

**PREPARATIONS**    *Tablets:* 200, 400 and 600 mg; *tablets (film-covered):* 400 mg; *capsules (extended-release):* 200 and 400 mg *(Equanil brand tablets contain tartrazine). Combinations:* 200 mg with aspirin, 325 mg; 200, 400 mg with conjugated estrogens, 0.45 mg; 200, 400 mg with tridihexethyl chloride, 25 mg; 400 mg with benactyzine hydrochloride.

**DRUG INTERACTIONS**    **CNS depressants** Depression of the CNS is additive with other CNS depressants, including alcohol.

**DIAGNOSTIC TEST INTERFERENCE**   **17-ketosteroids and 17-ketogenicsteroids** Falsely high values with the Zimmerman reaction and in the modified Glenn-Nelson technique.

**FATE**   Meprobamate is well absorbed and has a *peak* plasma concentration is 1 to 3 hours. The *onset of action* is about 1 hour. The plasma *half-life* is 10 to 11 hours. Meprobamate is rapidly metabolized in the liver and can induce liver microsomal enzymes, although this does not appear to produce clinically significant drug interactions. Metabolites and the parent drug are excreted in the urine.

## ❦ NURSING CONSIDERATIONS

### Side effects, toxicities, and associated nursing actions

**CNS** Drowsiness and ataxia are the most frequent side effects. Others include dizziness, slurred speech, headache, vertigo, weakness, paresthesia, impaired visual accommodation, euphoria, and paradoxical CNS stimulation.
* Tell patients to avoid driving or operating hazardous equipment if dizziness, vertigo, or visual changes occur; notify the physician.
* Instruct patients to report the development of any new sign or symptom.
**CV** Palpitation, tachycardia, arrhythmias, transient ECG changes, syncope, and hypotension.
* Monitor blood pressure and pulse prior to administering and within 15 minutes of first few doses. Be alert to cardiovascular changes in patients with pre-existing heart problems.
* Instruct patients to report subjective changes in pulse, or development of palpitations or funny sensations in the chest. Discourage smoking and supervise ambulation of hospitalized patients, especially the elderly.
* Keep side rails up and a nightlight on. Keep call bell within easy reach.
**GI** Anorexia, nausea, vomiting, and diarrhea.
* Monitor weight weekly. If GI symptoms are present, monitor intake and output.
* Instruct patients to take doses with meals or snack to lessen GI side effects.
**Allergic** Mild to severe allergic reactions may occur. These are usually skin rashes but may affect blood cells.
* Inspect the patient for rashes, as well as for development of pallor, bruising, and petechiae.
* Monitor complete blood cell count and platelet count.

### Nursing interventions related to drug administration
* Equanil Wyseals brand film-coated tablets and Deprol brand combination product tablet contain FD & C yellow dye # 5 (tartrazine), which may cause an allergic response in susceptible individuals. Although rare, this side effect is seen more commonly in persons with aspirin hypersensitivity.

### Patient and family education
* Review with the patient the expected benefits and possible side effects of therapy. Instruct the patient to report the development of any unexpected sign or symptom.
* Caution the patient to avoid the use of any other medication, including over-the-counter preparations, without prior clearance with the physician.
* Caution the patient to avoid the use of alcohol.
* For insomnia, instruct patients to take prescribed dose about 30 minutes prior to bedtime.
* Remind patients not to share medications with others.
* Remind the patient to keep these and all medications out of the reach of children. Child-proof caps should be used.
* To avoid accidental overdose, caution patient to keep drugs in clearly labeled containers, away from the bedside, so that the patient does not inadvertently repeat a dose if wakened during the night.
* Caution the patient to report excessive morning drowsiness to the physician. Excessive morning drowsiness represents a response to the medication or too high a prescribed dose; the patient should not increase the dose of medication to alleviate this "fatigue."
* Review with the patient other aids to sleep that might be effective, including drinking warm milk in the evening or taking a warm bath. Sedative-hypnotics should only be used for short-term treatment of insomnia.

# methotrimeprazine HCL (meth-oh-trye-MEP-ra-zeen) sedative

- methotrimeprazine (✱levomepromazine): Levoprome, ✱Nozinan (✱Schedule F)

**MECHANISM OF ACTION** Methotrimeprazine is a phenothiazine derivative with pronounced tranquilization and sedative effects. Other activities include analgesic, antiemetic, and antihistaminic effects.

**INDICATIONS** **Anxiety** Methotrimeprazine is principally used for bed-fast patients experiencing pain. It is also used before delivery and preoperatively and postoperatively.

**CONTRAINDICATIONS** **Hazardous activities** As with other CNS depressants, alertness and coordination will be compromised.

**DOSAGE** **IM:** **ADULTS:** 10 to 20 mg every 4 to 6 hours for sedation with analgesia. Preoperatively, the dose is 2 to 20 mg 45 minutes to 3 hours before surgery. Postoperatively, only a low dose, 2.5 to 7.5 mg, should be given because of residual effects of other drugs. *Special patient populations:* **ELDERLY:** Initial doses are half the usual dose. Methotrimeprazine can produce a pronounced othostatic hypotensive response that is dangerous for patients unable to tolerate an abrupt drop in blood pressure. **CHILDREN:** Not recommended for children under 12 years old. **PREGNANCY:** Not recommended for use during pregnancy except during labor.

**PREPARATIONS** *Injection:* 20 mg/ml.

**DRUG INTERACTIONS** **CNS depressants** Methotrimeprazine is additive with other CNS depressants such as opiates, barbiturates, other sedatives, antihistamines, tranquilizers, and alcohol. **Anticholinergic agents** May potentiate the action of anticholinergic agents such as atropine and scopalamine and skeletal muscle relaxants such as succinylcholine that are frequently administered presurgically. **Antihypertensive agents** Methotrimeprazine causes hypotension that can be additive with other antihypertensive agents. **Epinephrine** Methotrimeprazine will reverse the vasopressor effect of epinephrine, so phenylephrine, methoxamine, or norepinephrine should be used if a vasopressor is needed.

**FATE** *Onset of action* is in 20 to 40 minutes, and the *duration of action* is about 4 hours. Methotrimeprazine is metabolized by the liver, and products are excreted in the urine and feces.

## ✿ NURSING CONSIDERATIONS
### Side effects, toxicities, and associated nursing actions

**CNS** Drowsiness, excessive sedation, and amnesia are frequent. Disorientation and euphoria are other common side effects.
- Caution patients to avoid driving or operating hazardous equipment until the effects of the medication can be evaluated.
- Supervise ambulation of hospitalized patients and discourage smoking.
- Keep side rails up.
- Keep a night light on.
- Antiemetic activity may be a desirable effect for specific patients.

**CV** Orthostatic hypotension.
- Monitor pulse and blood pressure. Be especially alert for hypotension in the elderly or those on other drugs causing hypotension such as antihypertensives.
- Assess for symptoms of hypotension: dizziness, visual changes, syncope, and light-headedness. Instruct the patient to notify the physician if these occur. Caution patients to move slowly from lying to sitting or standing positions to prevent falling from sudden hypotension.

**GI** Abdominal discomfort, nausea, and vomiting.
- Monitor intake and output.
- If nausea and vomiting are persistent or severe, it may be necessary to reduce the dosage or discontinue the medications.

**GU** Difficulty in urination secondary to the anticholinergic effect.
- Urinary retention may occur, although this is more common in men with pre-existing prostatic hypertrophy. Instruct the patient to report inability to void, increasing difficulty in initiating urination, or feeling of incomplete bladder emptying. Suggest that patients void prior to taking each dose.

- Monitor intake and output.

**Hematologic** Long-term use at high doses can cause jaundice and severe blood dyscrasias.
- Inspect the patient for jaundice.
- Monitor liver function studies, CBC, platelets, and differential.
- Assess the patient for development of petechiae, bruising, unexplained bleeding or bruising, fever, and sore throat.

**Other** Anticholinergic effects can manifest as nasal congestion, change in heart rate, or dry mouth. Extrapyramidal symptoms characteristic of phenothiazines are possible, particularly in patients with a history of convulsive disorders.
- Monitor pulse rate.
- Nasal congestion can be uncomfortable for the patient. Excessive blowing of the nose will not relieve the congestion and may irritate nasal passages. If nasal congestion is extreme, it may be necessary to discontinue the medication.
- For dry mouth, instruct the patient to chew sugarless gum or suck on sugarless hard candy. A dry mouth can often lead to a bad taste in the mouth, which may be partly relieved by frequent oral hygiene, including brushing the teeth and/or rinsing with a mouthwash or gargle. Avoid drying agents such as lemon-glycerin swabs. Increasing the fluid intake may also help to decrease the dry feeling. Some patients may wish to use a commercially available saliva substitute.
- Four major extrapyramidal syndromes are recognized: *Acute dystonia:* neck twisting, facial grimacing, abnormal eye movements, involuntary muscle movements. *Akathisia:* restlessness, difficulty in sitting still, strong urge to move about. *Parkinsonism:* motor retardation, masklike face, tremor, rigidity, salivation, shuffling gait. *Tardive dyskinesia:* protrusion of tongue, puffing of cheeks, chewing movements, involuntary movements of extremities, involuntary movements of trunk. A frequent diagnostic error is to attribute these reactions to psychiatric or other causes and to increase the dose of the causative medication, when in fact the medication should usually be discontinued. Notify the physician.

### Nursing interventions related to drug administration
- Administer this drug IM into a large muscle mass. Avoid accidental subcutaneous injection, as local tissue injury may occur.
- Because of frequent side effects of hypotension, patients should remain in bed for 3 to 6 hours following dose administration. Monitor carefully a patient's first attempts to sit or ambulate after a dose is administered.

### Patient and family education
- Review with the patient the expected benefits and possible side effects of therapy. Instruct the patient to report the development of any unexpected sign or symptom.
- Caution the patient to avoid the use of any other medication, including over-the-counter preparations, without prior clearance with the physician.
- Caution the patient to avoid the use of alcohol.
- For insomnia, administer prescribed dose about 30 minutes prior to bedtime.
- Caution the patient to report excessive morning drowsiness to the physician. Excessive morning drowsiness represents a response to the medication or too high a prescribed dose; the patient should not increase the dose of medication to alleviate this "fatigue."
- Review with the patient other aids to sleep that might be effective, including drinking warm milk in the evening or taking a warm bath. Sedative-hypnotics should only be used for short-term treatment of insomnia.

## methyprylon    (meth-i-PRYE-lon)                                          hypnotic

- methyprylon: Noludar (Schedule III, ✿Schedule F)

**MECHANISM OF ACTION**    The mechanism of action is not well understood, but the CNS depressant effects are similar to those of the barbiturates.

**INDICATIONS**    Insomnia For short-term treatment only.

**CONTRAINDICATIONS** • Hazardous activities: as with other CNS depressants, alertness and coordination will be compromised. • Renal or hepatic impairment.

**DOSAGE** PO: ADULTS: 200 to 400 mg 15 minutes before bedtime. Special patient populations: CHILDREN: Not for children under 12 years old. For children over 12 years old: 50 mg at bedtime initially; may give up to 200 mg. PREGNANCY: Safe use has not been established.

**PREPARATIONS** *Capsules:* 300 mg; *tablets:* 50 and 200 mg.

**DRUG INTERACTIONS** **CNS depressants** Additive CNS depression may occur with other CNS depressants, including alcohol.

**DIAGNOSTIC TEST INTERFERENCE** **17-Ketosteroids** Methyprylon interferes with the Holtorff Koch modification of the Zimmerman reaction. **17-Hydroxycorticosteroids** Methyprylon interferes with the modified Glenn-Nelson technique and the Porter-Silber reaction.

**FATE** *Onset of action* is within an hour, and *duration of action* is 5 to 8 hours. Methyprylon is metabolized in the liver to metabolites that are excreted in the urine. These metabolites enter the enterohepatic circulation.

## 🐾 NURSING CONSIDERATIONS

### Side effects, toxicities, and associated nursing actions

**CNS** Morning drowsiness, dizziness, vertigo, paradoxical excitation, anxiety, depression, nightmares, and dreaming.
* Caution patients to avoid driving or operating hazardous equipment until the effects of the medication can be evaluated. Supervise the play of children, especially when they are riding bicycles or performing other potentially dangerous activities.
* Supervise ambulation of hospitalized patients and discourage smoking.
* Keep side rails up.
* Keep a night light on.
* Assess for signs of depression: indifference, change in affect, insomnia, neglect of personal appearance, loss of appetite.

**Hematologic** May precipitate an attack of porphyria in patients prone to intermittent porphyria.
* Assess for patient history of intermittent prophyria prior to administering.
* Assess patient for symptoms of porphyria: moderate to severe abdominal pain, mild fever, vomiting, diarrhea, constipation, and sinus tachycardia. Monitor pulse.

**GI** Nausea, vomiting, diarrhea, constipation, and esophagitis.
* Monitor intake and output and question patients about GI symptoms.
* If constipation occurs, encourage the patient to increase the fluid intake to at least 3000 ml/day and to add roughage and fiber and prune or other juices to the diet. Constipation is also more common in the immobilized patient; encourage the patient to increase the amount of daily exercise. In rare instances it may be necessary to add a laxative or stool softener to the drug regimen.
* If GI symptoms persist or are severe, it may be necessary discontinuing the medication.

**Allergic** Generalized allergic reactions, itching, and rash.
* Assess the patient for allergic response.
* Have drugs and equipment available for acute allergic response.

### Patient and family education
* Review with the patient the expected benefits and possible side effects of therapy. Instruct the patient to report the development of any unexpected sign or symptom.
* Caution the patient to avoid the use of any other medication, including over-the-counter preparations, without prior clearance with the physician.
* Caution the patient to avoid the use of alcohol. Remind patients to take the medication only as ordered. Instruct patients that this drug may be habit forming. Be alert in the outpatient setting to patients who return for prescription refills on an increasingly frequent basis, as this may indicate improper use or abuse of the drug.
* For insomnia, instruct patients to take prescribed dose about 30 minutes prior to bedtime.
* Remind patients not to share medications with others.
* Remind the patient to keep these and all medications out of the reach of children. Child-proof caps should be used.

- To avoid accidental overdose, caution patient to keep drugs in clearly labeled containers, away from the bedside, so that the patient does not inadvertently repeat a dose if wakened during the night.
- Caution the patient to report excessive morning drowsiness to the physician. Excessive morning drowsiness represents a response to the medication or too high a prescribed dose; the patient should not increase the dose of medication to alleviate this ''fatigue.''
- Review with the patient other aids to sleep that might be effective, including drinking warm milk in the evening or taking a warm bath. Sedative-hypnotics should only be used for short-term treatment of insomnia.

## paraldehyde    (par-AL-de-hyde)                                    sedative, hypnotic

- paraldehyde: Paral (Schedule IV; Schedule F)

**MECHANISM OF ACTION**    The mechanism of action is not well understood, but the CNS depressant effects are similar to those of the barbiturates.

**INDICATIONS**    • Alcohol withdrawal: paraldehyde has been largely replaced by chlordiazepoxide and diazepam. • Seizures: paraldehyde can control seizures arising from tetanus, eclampsia, poisons, or status epilepticus. • Anxiety.

**CONTRAINDICATIONS**    • Hepatic insufficiency. • Hazardous activities: as with other CNS depressants, alertness and coordination will be compromised.

**DOSAGE**    **PO or rectal:**   **ADULTS:** 5 to 10 ml for sedation; 10 to 30 ml for hypnosis. For alcohol withdrawal, 5 to 10 mg every 4 to 6 hours the first day, then every 6 hours. Daily dose is decreased from 60 ml in 20 ml increments.   **CHILDREN:** 0.15 mg/kg or 6 ml/M$^2$ for sedation and double for hypnosis.   **IM, IV:** **ADULTS:** 5 ml for sedation, 10 ml for hypnosis; 4 to 5 ml IV or 5 to 10 ml IM to control seizures. For status epilepticus, may administer 0.2 to 0.4 ml/kg in 0.9% saline injection IV or 5 to 10 ml IM.   **CHILDREN:** 0.1 to 0.15 ml/kg in 0.9% saline injection.   *Special patient populations:*   **PREGNANCY:** Paraldehyde crosses the placenta and enters fetal circulation. Newborns of mothers given paraldehyde for sedation suffer respiratory depression.

**PREPARATIONS**    *Liquid, formulated for oral, parenteral or rectal administration:* 1 ml = 1 g.

**DRUG INTERACTIONS**    **CNS depressants** Depression of the CNS is additive with other CNS depressants. **Disulfiram** slows the metabolism of paraldehyde.

**FATE**    Paraldehyde is rapidly absorbed with an *onset of action* in 20 to 60 minutes. The *half-life* is 4 to 10 hours. Paraldehyde is largely metabolized by the liver, mainly by aldehyde dehydrogenase, the enzyme also important to the metabolism of alcohol. The metabolites are used by the body. Paraldehyde is also excreted unchanged through the lung, giving patients to whom paraldehyde has been given a characteristic odor.

## 🐦 NURSING CONSIDERATIONS

### Side effects, toxicities, and associated nursing actions

**CNS** CNS depression.
- Caution patients to avoid driving or operating hazardous equipment until the effects of the medication can be evaluated. Supervise the play of children, especially when they are riding bicycles or performing other potentially dangerous activities.
- Supervise ambulation of hospitalized patients and discourage smoking.
- Keep side rails up.
- Keep a night light on.

**GI** Gastric irritation is the most frequent side effect.
- Dilute the oral dose with chilled juice or milk to reduce gastric irritation.

**Lung** IV administration can cause pulmonary edema, leading to hemorrhage, respiratory distress, or cardiac collapse.
- Monitor vital signs and breath sounds.
- Have suction machine at the bedside during IV administration.

**Skin** Erythematous rash. IM administration is painful and can cause skin damage.
- Visually inspect the patient for development of rash.

- Administer IM doses into large muscle masses such as the dorsogluteal site or the vastus lateralis in children.

### Nursing interventions related to drug administration

- Paraldehyde has a characteristic odor. On exposure to air it oxidizes quickly. Use fresh solutions. Avoid exposure of the drug to the air. Discard solutions that smell like vinegar or that have been open over 24 hours.
- For IV administration, use only glass syringes. Dilute each 1 ml of medication with at least 2 ml of sodium chloride for injection. Administer diluted mixture at a rate of 1 ml/min. Position patients on their sides for IV administration. Have a suction machine available. In some agencies, only physicians may administer paraldehyde IV.
- For IM administration, use only large muscle masses (see skin).
- For oral administration, dilute the ordered dose in chilled juice or milk. Capsules are also available.
- For rectal instillation, mix dose with 120 ml olive oil and administer as a retention enema. It is difficult to control this route of administration, so this is the least accurate dosage route.
- Regardless of route of administration, the drug imparts a characteristic odor to the patient's breath.

### Patient and family education

- Review with the patient the expected benefits and possible side effects of therapy. Instruct the patient to report the development of any unexpected sign or symptom.
- Caution the patient to avoid the use of any other medication, including over-the-counter preparations, without prior clearance with the physician.
- Caution the patient to avoid the use of alcohol.
- Remind patients not to share medications with others.
- Remind the patient to keep these and all medications out of the reach of children. Child-proof caps should be used.
- To avoid accidental overdose, caution patient to keep drugs in clearly labeled containers, away from the bedside, so that the patient does not inadvertently repeat a dose if wakened during the night.
- Caution the patient to report excessive morning drowsiness to the physician. Excessive morning drowsiness represents a response to the medication or too high a prescribed dose; the patient should not increase the dose of medication to alleviate this "fatigue."
- Review with the patient other aids to sleep that might be effective, including drinking warm milk in the evening or taking a warm bath. Sedative-hypnotics should only be used for short-term treatment of insomnia.

---

## promethazine HCl   (proe-METH-a-zeen)                                      sedative

- promethazine HCl: Anergan, ✚Histanil, Phenergan, Quadnite, Remsed

**MECHANISM OF ACTION**   Promethazine is a phenothiazine derivative with pronounced tranquilization and sedative effects. Other activities include analgesic, antiemetic, and antihistaminic effects.

**INDICATIONS**   • Anxiety: promethazine is used as a sedative and antiemetic principally before surgery. May be used with a narcotic analgesic and an anticholinergic. • Motion sickness.

**CONTRAINDICATIONS**   Hazardous activities As with other CNS depressants, alertness and coordination will be compromised.   Respiratory impairment Particularly children and in patients with sleep apnea.

**DOSAGE**   PO, IM, IV, Rectal:   ADULTS: For preoperative or postoperative sedation: 25 to 50 mg. For prevention and management of nausea and vomiting: 12.5 to 25 mg.   CHILDREN: For preoperative or postoperative sedation: 12.5 to 25 mg or 0.5 to 1.1 mg/kg. For prevention and management of nausea and vomiting: 0.25 to 0.5 mg/kg or 7.5 to 15 mg/$M^2$ every 4 to 6 hours. Children who are acutely ill, dehydrated or showing symptoms of Reye's syndrome should not take promethazine because of the extrapyramidal side effects. Sleep apnea or respiratory depression is another contraindication of this drug, especially in young children. *Special patient populations:*   PREGNANCY: Safe use has not been established.

**PREPARATIONS** *Solution:* 6.25, ♣10, 25 mg/5 ml; *tablets:* ♣10, 12.5, 25, 50 mg; injection: 25, 50 mg/ml; rectal: 12.5, 25, 50 mg; ♣*cream:* 2%.

**DRUG INTERACTIONS** **CNS depressants** Promethazine is additive with other CNS depressants such as opiates, barbiturates, other sedatives, antihistamines, tranquilizers, and alcohol. **Epinephrine** Promethazine will reverse the vasopressor effect of epinephrine, so phenylephrine, methoxamine, or norepinephrine should be used if a vasopressor is needed. **Monoamine oxidase inhibitors** Promethazine will intensify the anticholinergic effects.

**DIAGNOSTIC TEST INTERFERENCE** **Pregnancy tests** May get a false-positive test with Gravindex brand test and false-negative with Prepurex and Dap brand tests. **ABO blood typing** Promethazine may interfere with typing. **Allergen tests** Promethazine alters the flare response to intradermal injections.

**FATE** Promethazine is well absorbed. The *onset of action* is about 20 minutes for oral and IM administration, and the *duration of action* is 2 to 8 hours. Promethazine is metabolized by the liver, and the inactive metabolites are excreted in the feces.

## ♥ NURSING CONSIDERATIONS

### Side effects, toxicities, and associated nursing actions

**CNS** Confusion and disorientation are the most frequent side effects. Extrapyramidal side effects may be seen at high doses.

**Eye** Blurring of the vision due to the anticholinergic effects.

- Caution patients to avoid driving or operating hazardous equipment until the effects of the medication can be evaluated. Supervise the play of children, especially when they are riding bicycles or performing other potentially dangerous activities.
- Supervise ambulation of hospitalized patients and discourage smoking.
- Keep side rails up.
- Keep a night light on.
- Antiemetic activity may be a desirable effect for specific patients.
- Instruct the patient to notify the physician if blurring of vision occurs.
- Four major extrapyramidal syndromes are recognized: *Acute dystonia:* neck twisting, facial grimacing, abnormal eye movements, involuntary muscle movements. *Akathisia:* restlessness, difficulty in sitting still, strong urge to move about. *Parkinsonism:* motor retardation, masklike face, tremor, rigidity, salivation, shuffling gait. *Tardive dyskinesia:* protrusion of tongue, puffing of cheeks, chewing movements, involuntary movements of extremities, involuntary movements of trunk. A frequent diagnostic error is to attribute these reactions to psychiatric or other causes and to increase the dose of the causative medication, when in fact the medication should usually be discontinued. Notify the physician.

**CV** Parenteral administration raises or lowers heart rate. Rapid IV administration may temporarily decrease blood pressure.

- Monitor pulse and blood pressure. Be especially alert for hypotension in the elderly or in those on other drugs causing hypotension such as antihypertensives.
- Assess for symptoms of hypotension: dizziness, visual changes, syncope, and light-headedness. Instruct the patient to notify the physician if these occur. Caution patients to move slowly from lying to sitting or standing to prevent falling from sudden hypotension.

**Hematologic** Leukopenia and agranulocytosis have been occasionally reported.

- Monitor CBC, platelets, and differential.
- Assess patients for development of petechiae, bruising, unexplained bleeding or bruising, fever, and sore throat.

**Skin** Photosensitivity.

- Alert patients to this possible side effect.
- Instruct patients to wear a hat and long-sleeved clothing, to avoid exposure to the sun, and to use maximum-protection sunscreens.

**Allergic** Itching, dermatitis, asthma, and angioedema have been reported.

- Assess the patient for allergic response.
- Have drugs and equipment available for acute allergic response.

**Other** Anticholinergic effects include dry mouth.

- Nasal congestion can be uncomfortable for the patient. Excessive blowing of the nose will not relieve the congestion and may irritate nasal passages. If nasal congestion is extreme, it may be necessary to discontinue the medication.
- For dry mouth, instruct the patient to chew sugarless gum or suck on sugarless hard candy. A dry mouth can often lead to a bad taste in the mouth, which may be partly relieved by frequent oral hygiene, including brushing the teeth and/or rinsing with a mouthwash or gargle. Avoid drying agents such as lemon-glycerin swabs. Increasing the fluid intake may also help to decrease the dry feeling. Some patients may wish to use a commercially available saliva substitute.
- Urinary retention may occur, although this is more common in men with pre-existing prostatic hypertrophy. Instruct the patient to report inability to void, increasing difficulty in initiating urination, or feeling of incomplete bladder emptying. Suggest that patients void prior to taking ordered dose.
- Monitor intake and output.

### Nursing interventions related to drug administration
- Promethazine hydrochloride may be given IM, IV, orally, or rectally. Avoid subcutaneous or intra-arterial injection.
- For IV administration, it is preferable to dilute the dose with up to 9 ml of normal saline. Final dilution should never exceed a concentration of 25 mg/ml. Administer at a rate not exceeding 25 mg over 1 minute.
- The parenteral form is sensitive to light. May be used if slightly discolored. Discard highly discolored solutions.
- Parenteral form may cause contact dermatitis. Exercise care in handling.
- After parenteral administration, maintain the patient in a recumbent position until effects of drug on blood pressure can be ascertained.
- Administration of oral doses with milk, meals, or snacks may reduce gastric irritation.
- Tablets may be crushed and mixed with food or fluids.

### Patient and family education
- Review with the patient the expected benefits and possible side effects of therapy. Instruct the patient to report the development of any unexpected sign or symptom.
- Caution the patient to avoid the use of any other medication, including over-the-counter preparations, without prior clearance with the physician.
- Caution the patient to avoid the use of alcohol.
- For insomnia, instruct patients to take the prescribed dose about 30 minutes prior to bedtime.
- For motion sickness, instruct patients to take prescribed dose about 30 to 45 minutes prior to departing.
- Remind patients not to share medications with others.
- Remind the patient to keep these and all medications out of the reach of children. Child-proof caps should be used.
- To avoid accidental overdose, caution patient to keep drugs in clearly labeled containers, away from the bedside, so that the patient does not inadvertently repeat a dose if wakened during the night.
- Caution the patient to report excessive morning drowsiness to the physician. Excessive morning drowsiness represents a response to the medication or too high a prescribed dose; the patient should not increase the dose of medication to alleviate this "fatigue."
- Review with the patient other aids to sleep that might be effective, including drinking warm milk in the evening or taking a warm bath. Sedative-hypnotics should only be used for short-term treatment of insomnia.

## propiomazine HCl   (proe-pee-OH-ma-zeen)                                    sedative
- propiomazine: Largon

**MECHANISM OF ACTION**   Propiomazine is a phenothiazine derivative with pronounced tranquilization and sedative effects. Other activities include analgesic, antiemetic, and antihistaminic effects.

**INDICATIONS**    **Anxiety** Promethahazine is used as a sedative and antiemetic principally before surgery. • May be used with a narcotic analgesic and an anticholinergic.

**CONTRAINDICATIONS**    **Hazardous activities** As with other CNS depressants, alertness and coordination will be compromised.

**DOSAGE**    **IM, IV:**   ADULTS: 20 to 40 mg. Repeat in 3 hours if necessary.   *Special patient populations:* CHILDREN: 2 to 4 years old: 10 mg; 4 to 6 years old: 15 mg; 6 to 12 years old: 25 mg.   PREGNANCY: Safe use has not been established.

**PREPARATIONS**    *Injection:* 20 mg/ml.

**DRUG INTERACTIONS**    **CNS depressants** Propiomazine is additive with other CNS depressants such as opiates, barbiturates, other sedatives, antihistamines, tranquilizers, and alcohol.   **Epinephrine** Propiomazine will reverse the vasopressor effect of epinephrine, so phenylephrine, methoxamine, or norepinephrine should be used if a vasopressor is needed.

**FATE**    *Onset of action* is 15 to 30 minutes (IV) and 40 to 60 minutes (IM); *duration of action* is 3 to 6 hours.

☙ **NURSING CONSIDERATIONS**

### Side effects, toxicities, and associated nursing actions

**CNS** Dizziness, confusion, and amnesia may be experienced.
* Caution patients to avoid driving or operating hazardous equipment until the effects of the medication can be evaluated. Supervise the play of children, especially when they are riding bicycles or performing other potentially dangerous activities.
* Supervise ambulation of hospitalized patients and discourage smoking.
* Keep side rails up.
* Keep a night light on.
* Antiemetic activity may be a desirable effect for specific patients.
* Instruct the patient to notify the physician if blurring of vision occurs.
* Four major extrapyramidal syndromes are recognized: *Acute dystonia:* neck twisting, facial grimacing, abnormal eye movements, involuntary muscle movements. *Akathisia:* restlessness, difficulty in sitting still, strong urge to move about. *Parkinsonism:* motor retardation, masklike face, tremor, rigidity, salivation, shuffling gait. *Tardive dyskinesia:* protrusion of tongue, puffing of cheeks, chewing movements, involuntary movements of extremities, involuntary movements of trunk. A frequent diagnostic error is to attribute these reactions to psychiatric or other causes and to increase the dose of the causative medication, when in fact the medication should usually be discontinued. Notify the physician.

**CV** Tachycardia.
* Monitor pulse and blood pressure. Be especially alert for hypotension in the elderly or in those on other drugs causing hypotension such as antihypertensives.
* Assess for symptoms of hypotension: dizziness, visual changes, syncope, and light-headedness. Instruct the patient to notify the physician if these occur. Caution patients to move slowly from lying to sitting or standing positions to prevent falling from sudden hypotension.

**GI** Gastrointestinal upset.
* Monitor intake and output.
* If GI symptoms are severe, it may be necessary to discontinue the medications.

**Lung** Respiration is depressed.
* Monitor respiratory rate.
* Assess breath sounds.

**Allergic** Rashes.
* Assess the patient for allergic response.
* Visually inspect the patient for development of skin manifestations.

**Other** Anticholinergic effects include dry mouth.
* Nasal congestion can be uncomfortable for the patient. Excessive blowing of the nose will not relieve the congestion and may irritate nasal passages. If nasal congestion is extreme, it may be necessary to discontinue the medication.

- For dry mouth, instruct the patient to chew sugarless gum or suck on sugarless hard candy. A dry mouth can often lead to a bad taste in the mouth, which may be partly relieved by frequent oral hygiene, including brushing the teeth and/or rinsing with a mouthwash or gargle. Avoid drying agents such as lemon-glycerin swabs. Increasing the fluid intake may also help to decrease the dry feeling. Some patients may wish to use a commercially available saliva substitute.
- Urinary retention may occur, although this is more common in men with pre-existing prostatic hypertrophy. Instruct the patient to report inability to void, increasing difficulty in initiating urination, or feeling of incomplete bladder emptying. Suggest that patient void prior to taking ordered dose.
- Monitor intake and output.

### Nursing interventions related to drug administration
- Propiomazine HCl may be given IM or IV. Avoid subcutaneous or intraarterial injection.
- For IV administration, dilute each milliliter (20 mg) with 9 ml of normal saline. Final dilution will be 1 ml equals 2 mg. Administer at a rate not exceeding 10 mg over 1 minute.
- Discard discolored solutions.
- After parenteral administration, maintain the patient in a recumbent position until effects of drug on blood pressure can be ascertained.

**Patient and family education**    Review with the patient the expected benefits and possible side effects of therapy. Instruct the patient to report the development of any unexpected sign or symptom.
- Caution the patient to avoid the use of any other medication, including over-the-counter preparations, without prior clearance with the physician.
- Caution the patient to avoid the use of alcohol.
- For insomnia, instruct patients to take prescribed dose about 30 minutes prior to bedtime.
- Remind patients not to share medications with others.
- Caution the patient to report excessive morning drowsiness to the physician. Excessive morning drowsiness represents a response to the medication or too high a prescribed dose; the patient should not increase the dose of medication to alleviate this "fatigue."
- Review with the patient other aids to sleep that might be effective, including drinking warm milk in the evening or taking a warm bath. Sedative-hypnotics should only be used for short-term treatment of insomnia.

---

# Antialcohol agent

disulfiram

**OVERVIEW OF THE DRUG CLASS**    Alcoholism is being treated as an addictive disease. Alcohol is a CNS depressant to which tolerance develops, so that the first step in the treatment of alcoholism is detoxification. Since withdrawal from alcohol is often accompanied by acute agitation, one of the benzodiazepines, usually chlordiazepoxide, chlorazepate, diazepam, or oxazepam, is frequently used to treat the symptoms of alcohol withdrawal. After the patient is free of alcohol, disulfiram is the only agent available to promote alcohol avoidance. The ingestion of alcohol by a person who has been taking disulfiram results in an unpleasant reaction that includes nausea, vomiting, flushing, light-headedness, abdominal pain, and tachycardia. The rationale of disulfiram therapy is that the highly unpleasant symptoms of the disulfiram-ethanol reaction will cause the person to avoid alcohol.

---

## disulfiram    (dye-SUL-fi-ram)    alcohol avoidance

- disulfiram: Antabuse

**MECHANISM OF ACTION**    Disulfiram blocks the metabolism of alcohol at an intermediate step. The metabolite that accumulates, acetaldehyde, probably causes the unpleasant symptoms associated with ingestion of alcohol in the presence of disulfiram. Disulfiram irreversibly inactivates the enzyme alcohol dehydrogenase, so the effects persist for 1 to 2 weeks.

**INDICATIONS** **Alcoholism** Disulfiram should be used only by those individuals desiring to avoid alcohol ingestion.

**CONTRAINDICATIONS** • Alcohol intoxication: disulfiram is indicated only for nondrinking alcoholics. • History of seizures: disulfiram may aggravate neurologic disorders and should also be avoided by those with an abnormal EEG or brain damage. • Diabetes mellitus, hypothyroidism: metabolic abnormalities may aggravate these conditions. • Cardiovascular disease. • Liver or kidney disease: disulfiram may damage the liver. • Multiple drug dependence or psychosis.

**DOSAGE** **PO:** **ADULTS:** Initially, 500 mg every morning for 1 to 2 weeks. Maintenance: 250 mg daily, range 125 to 500 mg. If drowsiness is a problem, the dose may be taken in the Evening. *Special patient populations:* **PREGNANCY:** Safety for use during pregnancy has not been established. Because disulfiram is an irreversible enzyme inhibitor, its use is not recommended during pregnancy.

**PREPARATIONS** *Tablets:* 250 and 500 mg.

**DRUG INTERACTIONS** **Alcohol** This is the reaction for which disulfiram is taken. **Barbiturates, coumarins, anticoagulants, paraldehyde, phenytoin** Disulfiram interferes with the metabolism of these drugs by the liver. **Isoniazid** Patients may experience incoordination, unsteady gain, or behavioral changes. **Metronidizole** Avoid combining with disulfiram. Patients may have an acute psychotic reaction or confusion. **Amitriptyline** Enhances the alcohol-disulfiram reaction.

**FATE** Disulfiram is readily absorbed but requires 3 to 12 hours to become effective. It is slowly metabolized by the liver with metabolites excreted in the urine. Some of the drug and metabolites may be expired from the lungs. Because disulfiram irreversibly inactivates aldehyde dehydrogenase, the effects persist for 1 to 2 weeks after the last dose.

### ❦ NURSING CONSIDERATIONS

#### Side effects, toxicities, and associated nursing actions in the absence of alcohol

**CNS** Drowsiness, fatigue, and headaches may be experienced, especially at the beginning of therapy. Vertigo, irritability, insomnia, disorientation, confusion, personality changes, abnormal gait, and slurred speech have also been reported. Occasionally there have been reports of seizures, peripheral neuropathy, polyneuritis, delirium, and psychoses.
* Tell patients to avoid driving or operating hazardous equipment if drowsiness, vertigo, disorientation, or confusion develop.
* Provide emotional support to the patient faced with significant CNS side effects, as the will to continue this drug may be lessened.
* Suggest that the patient take the daily dose in evening rather than the morning if drug side effects are interefering with the performance of daily activities.
* Remind patients that side effects may lessen with continued use of the drug.

**Eye** Optic neuritis (rare).
* Assess the patient for changes in vision, both subjective and objective.

**GU** Impotence, occasional and transient.
* Question the patient tactfully about the development of this side effect. Provide emotional support as needed. Remind the patient that impotence is usually transient. Remind the patient not to discontinue medication without discussing it with physician.

**Allergic** Acne-like or allergic dermatitis. May be controlled with antihistamines.
* Inspect the patient for development of dermatitis. Refer patient to dermatologist if dermatitis cannot be controlled or is intolerable to patient.

**Other** Metallic or garlic aftertaste. Forewarn patients about this side effect. If aftertaste is contributing to anorexia or weight loss, consult with the physician about a possible reduction in dosage.
* Monitor weight.
* Review aspects of good oral hygiene with patients. Suggest that patients suck on sugarless hard candy or chew sugarless gum to lessen unpleasant taste.

#### Side effects, toxicities, and associated nursing actions in the presence of alcohol

**CNS** Anxiety, weakness, vertigo, and confusion.

**CV** Palpitations, flushing, throbbing headache, chest pain, tachycardia, hypotension, and fainting.

**Eye** Blurred vision.
**GI** Nausea, copious vomiting.
**Lung** Dyspnea.
**Skin** Sweating.

* Review these side effects with the patient, as they will develop if patient consumes any products containing alcohol while also taking disulfiram. Tell patients that these symptoms may last for a short period (from 30 minutes to several hours). If they are severe, the patient should go to the emergency room.
* Discuss with patients the many potential sources of alcohol that the patient must be alert to: alcohol-containing foods or sauces, liquid medicines, elixirs, tonics, vinegars, cough syrups, mouth washes, gargles. Tell the patient not to apply to the skin any alcohol-containing products such as rubbing alcohol, after-shave lotions, cologne, perfume, toilet water.

### Nursing interventions related to drug administration

* Do not administer this drug if the patient has consumed any alcohol-containing product within the last 12 hours.
* Do not administer this drug to any patient without the patient's knowledge.

### Patient and family education

* Review the anticipated benefits and possible side effects of drug therapy with patient and family. Review carefully the side effects that can occur when alcohol is consumed (see preceding discussion).
* Administration of this drug is usually limited to patients who have been carefully evaluated for probable success, and the drug should be used in conjunction with other forms of supportive therapy for the patient.
* Instruct patients to wear a medical identification tag or bracelet or to carry a card in the wallet indicating that disulfiram is being used.
* Teach patients to discuss all medications with the pharmacist prior to using to ascertain if they contain alcohol.
* Teach the patient to read the labels of food items prior to consuming them to determine if they contain alcohol.
* Tell patients that the effects of disulfiram may persist in the blood for up to 14 days after the last dose of the drug is taken.
* Instruct patients to keep all health care providers aware of all drugs being used.

# Chapter Thirty-six

# Antipsychotic drugs

| | |
|---|---|
| acetophenazine | molindone |
| chlorpromazine | perphenazine |
| chlorprothixene | prochlorperazine |
| droperidol | promazine |
| fluphenazine | thioridazine |
| haloperidol | thiothixene |
| loxapine | trifluperazine |
| mesoridazine | triflupromazine |

**DRUG COMBINATIONS**
- perphenazine and amitriptyline hydrochloride: Etrafon, Triavil
- droperidol and pentanyl citrate: Innovar

**INTRODUCTION**     There are five chemical classes of antipsychotic drugs in clinical use. These drug classes have an identical mechanism of action; they are dopamine antagonists and block CNS dopamine receptors. The drug classes differ in their potency and incidence of side effects. These differences are compared in Table 36-1.

Although the antipsychotic drugs are unique in allowing symptomatic treatment of psychoses, several of these drugs are commonly used as antiemetics or to potentiate other CNS drugs, mainly anesthetics and analgesics. Chlorpromazine, the first antipsychotic drug introduced in the United States, originally was licensed as an antiemetic drug, later as a drug to potentiate anesthesia, and finally as an antipsychotic drug.

The phenothiazines are the largest class of antipsychotic drugs. There are three chemical subdivisions of the phenothiazines: aliphatic, piperidine, and piperazine. These subclasses differ in the incidence of side effects. The other chemical classes of antipsychotic drugs include the thioxanthene, butyrophenone, dibenzoxazepine, and dihydroindolone classes. Although it is common to see these chemical classes listed, as they are in Table 36-1, the major emphasis will be placed on the similarities of actions of the antipsychotic drugs. The specific chemical classes will not be separately discussed because of the high degree of overlap in uses and actions.

**OVERVIEW OF THE DRUG CLASS**     Psychoses account for most of the patients hospitalized for mental illness and disable as many Americans as heart disease and cancer combined.

The antipsychotic drugs are unique in allowing symptomatic treatment of psychoses. A psychosis is a major emotional disorder with an impairment of mental function great enough to prevent the individual from participating in everyday life. The hallmark of a psychosis is the loss of contact with reality. There is no one symptom of a psychosis. The symptoms may include agitation, hostility, combativeness, hyperactivity, as well as delusions, hallucinations, disordered thought and perception, emotional and social withdrawal, paranoid symptoms, and personal neglect. Antipsychotic drugs specifically decrease at least some of these symptoms so the patient can think and function more coherently.

**MECHANISM OF ACTION**     **Antipsychotic drugs as dopamine antagonists** The antipsychotic drugs block dopamine receptors in various parts of the brain. The antipsychotic effect arises from receptor blockade in the limbic system. The limbic system is the area of the brain that regulates emotional behavior. The antiemetic effect comes from receptor blockade in the chemoreceptor trigger zone. Extensive therapeutic use is made of several of the antipsychotic drugs for their potent antiemetic effect, particularly as an adjunct to chemotherapy and to surgery.

Undesired actions arising from dopamine receptor blockade include the extrapyramidal and endocrine side effects. Extrapyramidal reactions arise from the blockade of dopamine receptors in certain nuclei of the basal ganglia of the brain. This area of the brain is responsible for the coordination of movement. Extrapyramidal actions are described in detail under Nursing Considerations below. Dopamine inhibits the release of the hormone prolactin by the pituitary gland. Blockade of dopamine leads to the hypersecretion of prolactin and secondarily to endocrine disturbances of the reproductive system by mechanisms not yet understood.     **Anticholinergic actions of antipsychotic drugs** All

Table
36-1.

## Antipsychotic drugs listed according to drug class, potency, and major side effects*

| Drug | Equipotent dose† | Relative incidence of side effects | | | |
|---|---|---|---|---|---|
| | | Sedative effect | Orthostatic hypotension | Anticholinergic effects | Extrapyramidal symptoms |
| **Phenothiazines** | | | | | |
| Aliphatic | | | | | |
|   Chlorpromazine | 100 | High | Moderate | Moderate/high | Moderate |
|   Promazine | 200 | Moderate | Moderate | High | Moderate |
|   Triflupromazine | 25 | High | Moderate | Moderate/high | Moderate/high |
| Piperidine | | | | | |
|   Mesoridazine | 50 | High | Moderate | Moderate | Low |
|   Thioridazine | 100 | High | Moderate | Moderate/high | Low |
| Piperazine | | | | | |
|   Acetophenazine | 20 | Moderate | Low | Low | High |
|   Fluphenazine | 2 | Low/moderate | Low | Low | High |
|   Perphenazine | 8 | Low/moderate | Low | Low | High |
|   Prochlorperazine | 10 | Moderate | Low | Low | High |
|   Trifluoperazine | 4 | Moderate | Low | Low | High |
| **Thioxanthenes** | | | | | |
|   Chlorprothixene | 100 | High | Moderate/high | Moderate/high | Low/moderate |
|   Thiothixene | 4 | Low | Low/moderate | Low | Moderate/high |
| **Butyrophenone** | | | | | |
|   Haloperidol | 2 | Low | Low | Low | High |
| **Dibenzoxazepine** | | | | | |
|   Loxapine | 10 | Moderate | Low/moderate | Low/moderate | Moderate/high |
| **Dihydroindolone** | | | | | |
|   Molindone | 10 | Moderate | Low/moderate | Moderate | Moderate |

*From Clark JB, Queener SF, Karb, VB: Pharmacological Basis of Nursing Practice, ed. 2, St. Louis, 1986,
The C.V. Mosby Co.
†Compared to 100 mg chlorpromazine.

antipsychotic drugs have some anticholinergic action. The atropine-like effects include dry mouth, blurred vision, difficulty in urination, and constipation. **Actions from adrenergic blockade** The phenothiazines and thioxanthenes also block alpha adrenergic receptors for norepinephrine in the brain. Neurons containing norepinephrine in the reticular activating system of the brain are associated with alertness. The sedative effect of the phenothiazines and the thioxanthenes is believed to result from their blockade of these receptors for norepinephrine. The blockade of adrenergic receptors in the vasomotor center inhibits peripheral sympathetic tone and causes orthostatic hypotension. **Antihistaminergic action** The antipsychotic drugs block histamine receptors in the CNS. This activity causes drowsiness and sedation.

**INDICATIONS** **Psychosis** Antipsychotic drugs are effective for functional psychoses, especially those caused by a major traumatic event • Schizophrenia, a chronic illness with psychotic episodes, can often be effectively treated. Organic psychoses, those secondary to physical damage from disease, trauma, poisoning, etc., are not as successfully treated. • Toxic psychoses from alcohol or drug withdrawal are treated with diazepam. • Amphetamine psychosis is specifically treated with antipsychotic drugs. **Emesis** Antipsychotic drugs are very effective antiemetics. • Because of the numerous side effects of the antipsychotic drugs, their use is restricted to the management of postoperative nausea and vomiting, radiation and chemotherapy sickness, nausea and vomiting caused by toxins, and intractable vomiting. **Potentiation of narcotic analgesics** This is a useful combination in treating pain in terminal cancer patients.

**CONTRAINDICATIONS** **History of seizures** Use antipsychotic drugs with caution, as they may lower the seizure threshold. **Elderly or debilitated patients** Use antipsychotic drugs with caution, as antipsychotic drugs may blunt mental acuity. **Renal or liver disease** Degradation and elimination of antipsychotic drugs requires hepatic and renal mechanisms. **Respiratory disorder** Supression of coughing heightens the danger of aspiration of secretions or vomitus. **Glaucoma, prostatic hypertrophy** These conditions may be exacerbated by the anticholinergic effects of antipsychotic drugs.

**DRUG INTERACTIONS** **CNS depressants** Antipsychotic drugs are additive or potentiate the action of other CNS depressants. This includes opiates, barbiturates, general anesthetics, and alcohol. **Anticonvulsants** Antipsychotic drugs lower the seizure threshold, so adjustments of anticonvulsant medications may be needed. Chlorpromazine has been reported to decrease the metabolism of phenytoin, which may lead to phenytoin toxicity. Phenobarbital may increase the metabolism of chlorpromazine so that increased doses of chlorpromazine may be required. **Lithium** In the presence of high lithium concentrations, antipsychotic drugs may cause an acute encephalopathic syndrome. **Metrizamide** Antipsychotic drugs should be discontinued 48 hours before and after the administration of metrizamide. This recommendation is based on animal studies that indicate an increased risk of seizures.

**DIAGNOSTIC TEST INTERFERENCE** **Urinary false-positive results** The incidence of false-positive measurements is increased in tests for urobilinogen, amylase, uroporphrins, porphobilinogens, and 5-hydroxyindolacetic acid by urinary metabolites of phenothiazines. Some pregnancy tests (Gravindex, HCG test, Pregnosticon, UCG test) have an increase in false-positive results when patients are receiving antipsychotic drugs. This is secondary to the endocrine effects of antipsychotic drugs.

## ❦ NURSING CONSIDERATIONS

### Side effects, toxicities, and associated nursing actions

A number of side effects are characteristic of the antipsychotic drugs.

**Extrapyramidal reactions** These are most important side effects. The origin of the extrapyramidal reactions is the dopamine blockade in areas of the brain governing motor coordination and movement. Four extrapyramidal syndromes are associated with antipsychotic drugs: acute dystonia, akathisia, pseudoparkinsonism, and tardive dyskinesia.

**ACUTE DYSTONIA** is a spasm of muscles of the tongue, face, neck, or back and may mimic seizures. Dystonia is usually seen in the first 5 days of antipsychotic therapy. It may be treated with an antihistaminic or anticholinergic antiparkinsoian drug. Dystonia reactions are most common in patients under 25 years of age and rarely persist after treatment of the acute reaction. Some of the classic reactions seen in dystonia include torticollis (neck twisting), an oculogyric crisis (upward gaze paralysis), stereotyped motions of the jaw, and opisthotonus (a spasm in which the head and feet go back to make an inverted U-shape of the body).

**AKATHISIA** is motor restlessness and may be mistaken for psychotic restlessness or agitation. Akathisia commonly appears after the first few days of therapy, and if not recognized, the antipsychotic drug dosage may again be mistakenly increased to relieve the agitation. Patients experiencing akathisia will have difficulty in sitting still and may pace about, fidget, or constantly move their legs. Anticholinergic drugs or a muscle relaxant such as diazepam may be effective in treating these symptoms. If these treatments are not effective, a different antipsychotic drug may have to be tried. Tolerance does not quickly develop to akathisia, but akathisia disappears when the drug is discontinued.

**PSEUDOPARKINSONISM** is marked by motor retardation and rigidity. The patient finds it difficult to initiate or to carry out movements. The face even resembles a mask because emotions do not register on the face. The patient has a shuffling gait and hypersalivates. A tremor is seen in the hands and legs. These parkinsonian symptoms commonly appear after a week of therapy and are treated with antiparkinsonian drugs. Tolerance does not develop to the parkinsonian symptoms. If they cannot be controlled with drug therapy, the antipsychotic drug has to be changed.

**TARDIVE DYSKINESIA** is classically associated with long term, high-dose antipsychotic therapy. It is most common in elderly women and in patients who have had a cerebrovascular accident (stroke). Tardive dyskinesia is the worst of the extrapyramidal reactions, since it cannot be readily treated, is persistent, and may not altogether disappear when drug therapy is discontinued. Tardive dyskinesia usually appears some months after therapy has been started, when the drug dosage is reduced or discontinued. Tardive dyskinesia is believed to represent the development of receptors that are supersensitive to dopamine after prolonged blockade by the antipsychotic drugs. Removing the antipsychotic drug worsens the condition, since dopamine then has ready access to these supersensitive receptors. Antiparkinsonian drugs also worsen tardive dyskinesia, since they either increase dopamine or block the acetylcholine opposing the effects of dopamine. Some common symptoms of tardive dyskinesia are protrusion of the tongue (fly-catcher sign), puffing of the cheeks or the tongue in a cheek (bonbon sign), chewing movements, and involuntary movements of the extremities and trunk (choreoid or athetoid movements). The recognition that tardive dyskinesia is a common reaction (up to 50%) in patients treated for a long time with high doses of antipsychotic drugs has prompted reevaluation of long-term therapy with these drugs. The current choice is to use as low a dose as possible and to put the patient on a ''drug holiday'' during periods of remission.

- Assess carefully and systematically for development of extrapyramidal side effects. Errors in diagnosis may lead to inadvertently increasing the dose of medication when the correct choice should be to decrease the dose of medication. In addition, once additional medications to treat side effects are added to the treatment regimen, the assessment of the patient becomes even more difficult.
- Review the extrapyramidal side effects with patients and families. Instruct patients and families to notify the physician if any unusual signs or symptoms develop.

**Sedation and postural hypotension** Sedation and postural hypotension are most often seen early in treatment with the aliphatic phenothiazines, the class of phenothiazines with the most prominent adrenergic blocking activity. These side effects are most likely to be prominent in elderly or debilitated patients. If sedation and hypotension are not severe, the dosage can be reduced and then gradually increased to produce tolerance.

- Caution patients to avoid driving and operating hazardous equipment until sedation diminishes.
- Instruct patients to move slowly from lying to sitting or standing positions.
- Supervise ambulation of hospitalized patients until the degree of hypotension can be determined. Keep siderails up at night.
- Monitor the blood pressure. These medications may take several weeks to achieve the desired blood levels, and patients may be at risk for hypotension for weeks to a couple of months.
- Instruct patients to remain recumbent for at least 30 to 60 minutes following parenteral administration.
- For treatment of severe hypotension, norepinephrine or phenylephrine should be used.

**Electrocardiographic changes** The aliphatic phenothiazines are also the most likely to produce nonspecific changes in the T wave of the ECG. This change has no particular meaning but is undesirable for a patient with concurrent heart disease who is being monitored for ECG changes.

- Obtain a baseline ECG prior to initiating therapy with phenothiazines, and at regular intervals.
- Monitor the pulse.

**Seizure potential** The antipsychotic drugs must be used with caution in patients with epilepsy, since convulsions can be precipitated by these drugs. This lowering of the convulsion threshold makes antipsychotic drugs unsuitable for the treatment of drug withdrawal.

- Use cautiously in patients with a history of seizures. Pad siderails. Have a suction machine at hand.

**Endocrine disturbances** The endocrine impairment that results in sexual dysfunction in men and women derives from the dopaminergic blocking action. Women may experience delayed ovulation and menstruation, lack of menstruation (amenorrhea), milk production (galactorrhea), or weight gain. Men may experience impotence, decreased libido, retrograde ejaculation, or moderate breast growth (gynecomastia).

- If appropriate, caution patient about these possible side effects.
- Assess patients carefully for these endocrine problems. Patients may be reluctant to discuss these problems. Other patients may not be troubled by these side effects. Still other patients will find these side effects so distressing that they refuse to take the medication or discontinue the drugs after discharge from the acute care facility.
- Be supportive of patients experiencing endocrine side effects, and their spouses or sexual partners. In some patients, changing the drug or lowering the dose may be helpful.
- Monitor weight.
- Keep a record of menstrual periods, especially for institutionalized women.
- If weight gain is significant, instruct patients in a low calorie diet. Suggest patients initiate a regular program of physical exercise.
- Note that antipsychotics may produce false-positive pregnancy test results. The safe use of these drugs during pregnancy has not been established. Advise women who may suspect they are pregnant to notify the physician. Women of childbearing age may wish to use birth control measures while taking antipsychotics.

**Allergic reactions** Photosensitivity and cholestatic hepatitis are allergic reactions that occasionally develop during therapy with antipsychotic drugs.

**PHOTOSENSITIVITY** is fairly common and represents an allergic reaction to a metabolite produced by sunlight. Since antipsychotic drugs have metabolites with long half-lives and these metabolites accumulate in the skin, photosensitivity can result. Patients taking antipsychotic drugs should not sunbathe.

- Caution patients to avoid exposure to the sun. If they must go out, advise patients to wear a hat, long-sleeve shirt and long pants, and to use maximum-protection sunscreens.

**CHOLESTATIC HEPATITIS** can develop when an allergic inflammation arises in the bile duct. The allergy is to metabolites that are excreted in the bile. Jaundice can result if the bile duct is blocked. This condition is reversible when the drug is stopped.

- Assess for malaise, fever, nausea, jaundice, right upper quadrant abdominal pain, and change in the color or consistency of stools.
- Monitor liver function tests.

**Anticholinergic effects** All the antipsychotic drugs have some anticholinergic action, producing dry mouth, blurred vision, delayed micturition, and constipation most frequently.

- Monitor intake and output, and record frequency of stools.
- If constipation develops, advise patients to increase fluid intake to 2500 to 3000 ml per day, increase intake of fruits, juices, and fiber, and increase daily exercise. For some patients, it may be necessary for the physician to prescribe a stool softener.
- For xerostomia (dry mouth), advise patients to suck on hard candies or chew gum (sugarless, to avoid dental caries and weight gain), drink frequent sips of water, avoid lemon-glycerin swabs or other rinses that are drying or irritating, but perform regular oral hygiene. Some patients may wish to use a commercially available saliva substitute.
- If blurred vision occurs, caution patients to avoid driving or operating hazardous equipment until the effects of the medication lessen. Notify the physician.

- Urinary retention is more common in the elderly, the immobilized, and in men with preexisting prostatic hypertrophy.

### Nursing interventions related to drug administration

- Supervise the patient carefully to ascertain that the medication is swallowed and not hidden in the mouth to be discarded later or stored by the patient. Some antipsychotic drugs are available in syrup, injection, or depot injection forms to help ensure that the patient receives the prescribed dose.
- Because antipsychotic drugs may suppress the cough reflex, administer them cautiously to patients with chronic obstructive lung disease, emphysema, or asthma; the elderly; postoperative patients; the immobilized; or anyone with a decreased level of consciousness.
- Prior to beginning antipsychotic therapy, monitor the vital signs and blood pressure. Check blood pressure with the patient in lying, sitting, and standing positions.
- Concentrated oral forms of most antipsychotics are available for institutional use. The dose should be diluted in at least 60 ml of one of the diluents suggested by the manufacturer.
- Contact dermatitis with the phenothiazines has been reported. Personnel preparing and administering these drugs should avoid direct contact with the drug on the skin, or should wear gloves while working with these drugs.
- Be alert to potentiation of hypotension and depression of the CNS if other CNS depressants are added to the drug regimen. Examples include narcotic analgesics and antihypertensives.

### Patient and family education

- Review with patients and families the expected benefits and possible side effects of therapy. Caution patients and families to report the development of any new sign or symptom.
- Remind patients and families that it may be weeks to months before the full benefits and effects of the medication can be seen.
- Instruct patients to avoid the use of alcohol while taking antipsychotics.
- Advise patients on long-term therapy to have periodic ophthalmic examinations.
- Antipsychotics may interfere with the body's ability to regulate temperature. Caution patients to avoid prolonged exposure to extremes of temperature, to allow for frequent cooling-off periods when exercising or in extremely hot situations, and to dress warmly for exposure to the cold.
- Instruct patients to report the symptoms of blood dyscrasias: fever, sore throat, and weakness.
- These drugs are excreted in breast milk. Warn lactating women to consult the physician prior to beginning drug therapy.
- Caution patients to avoid the use of over-the-counter preparations without first checking with the physician, to avoid potentiation of side effects. Remind patients to keep all health care providers informed of all medications being taken.
- Caution patients on long-term therapy with antipsychotics to avoid suddenly discontinuing the medication.
- Remind patients to keep these and all medications out of the reach of children.

---

## acetophenazine maleate    (a-set-oh-FEN-a-zeen)    antipsychotic

- acetophenazine maleate: Tindal

**MECHANISM OF ACTION**    The major actions are characteristic of dopamine receptor antagonists.

**INDICATIONS**    • Psychosis.

**CONTRAINDICATIONS**    • History of seizures. • Renal or liver disease. • Respiratory disorder. • Glaucoma, prostatic hypertrophy. • For more complete information, see entry for drug class (p. 720).

**DOSAGE**    PO:    **ADULTS:** Initially, 20 mg three times daily: range, 40 to 80 mg total in divided doses. For hospitalized patients, the dose may be increased to 80 to 120 mg daily. Occasionally, doses of 400 to 600 mg daily are required. *Special patient populations:*    **ELDERLY:** Elderly or debilitated patients may require a lower dose.    **PREGNANCY:** Safe use has not been established.

**PREPARATIONS**    Tablets: 20 mg.

**DRUG INTERACTIONS**    CNS depressants including opiates, barbiturates, general anesthetics, and alcohol are potentiated by antipsychotic drugs. **Anticonvulsants** Increased doses may be required. **Lithium** CNS toxicity is potentiated by antipsychotic drugs. **Mitrizamide** should not be administered concurrently with antipsychotic drugs. See entry for drug class (p. 720) for more complete information.

**FATE** Acetophenazine is a piperazine phenothiazine. The fate of this compound has not been well characterized.

### ☙ NURSING CONSIDERATIONS

#### Side effects, toxicities, and associated nursing actions
- See entry for drug class (p. 720).

#### Nursing interventions related to drug administration
- See entry for drug class (p. 723).

#### Patient and family education
- See entry for drug class (p. 723).

---

## chlorpromazine, chlorpromazine hydrochloride
(klor-PROE-ma-zeen)                                    antipsychotic, antiemetic, tranquilizer

- chlorpromazine, chlorpromozine hydrochloride: ✿Apo-Chlorpromazine, ✿Chlor-Promanl, ✿Largactil, ✿Novochlorpromazine, Thorazine, Promapar, Thor-Prom, Chlorazine, Ormazine, Promaz

**MECHANISM OF ACTION**   The major actions are characteristic of dopamine receptor antagonists.

**INDICATIONS** **Psychosis.** **Excessive anxiety, tension, agitation** Severe behavioral problems in children, especially of a combative or hyperexcitable nature, are treated with chlorpromazine. **Nausea and vomiting** Mainly that associated with surgery, chemotherapy, or radiation therapy. **Intermittent porphyria.** **Intractable hiccups.** **Tetanus** Chlorpromazine is adjunctive therapy. **Surgery** To control restlessness and apprehension before surgery or acute nausea and vomiting during surgery.

**CONTRAINDICATIONS**   • History of seizures. • Renal or liver disease • Respiratory disorder. • Glaucoma, prostatic hypertrophy. • For more complete information, see entry for drug class (p. 720).

**DOSAGE** **Psychotic disorders: excessive tension, anxiety, agitation:** *PO:* **ADULTS:** 30 to 75 mg daily divided into 2 to 4 doses. Dosage may be gradually increased every 3 days by 20 to 50 mg to control symptoms. Maintain for at least 2 weeks, then gradually reduce to the lowest effective dose, generally around 200 mg daily. *IM:* **ADULTS:** Intial doses may be given IM rather than PO. Generally, 25 mg is given, and repeated in an hour if necessary. In severely agitated, hospitalized patients, the daily dose is increased to a maximum of 400 mg every 4 to 6 hours over the first few days. Administration is switched to PO after several days or when the patient becomes calm. **CHILDREN 6 MONTHS OR OLDER:** 0.55 mg/kg every 4 to 6 hours. The initial dose is usually twice this. In children under 5 years, the maximum daily dose is 40 mg; 5 to 12 years old, 75 mg daily. **Nausea and vomiting:** *PO:* **ADULTS:** 10 to 25 mg every 4 to 6 hours. **CHILDREN 6 MONTHS OR OLDER:** 0.55 mg/kg every 4 to 6 hours. *IM:* **ADULTS:** 25 mg initially and 25 to 50 mg every 3 to 4 hours as necessary. **CHILDREN:** Same as PO. *Rectal:* **ADULTS:** 100 mg every 6 to 8 hours. **CHILDREN:** 1.1 mg/kg every 6 to 8 hours. **Intermittent porphyria:** *PO or IM:* **ADULTS:** 25 to 50 mg three or four times daily for the acute phase. **Intractable hiccups:** **ADULTS:** PO dose is 25 to 50 mg three or four times daily; if no relief in 2 to 3 days, the dose is given in IM. If still no relief, the dose is given by slow IV infusion with the patient lying down and with the blood pressure monitored. **Tetanus:** *IM or IV:* **ADULTS:** 25 to 50 mg three or four times daily. **CHILDREN 6 MONTHS OR OLDER:** 0.55 mg/kg three or four times daily. **Surgery:** **ADULTS:** 25 to 50 mg is given PO 2 to 3 hours before surgery or half that dose is given IM 1 to 2 hours before surgery. *PO or IM:* **CHILDREN 6 MONTHS OR OLDER:** 0.55 mg/kg 2 to 3 or 1 to 2 hours before surgery, respectively. *Special patient populations:* **ELDERLY:** Elderly or debilitated patients may require a lower dose. **PREGNANCY:** Safe use has not been established. Chlorpromazine and its metabolites cross the placenta and are distributed into milk.

**PREPARATIONS**   Chlorpromazine *suppositories:* 25, 100 mg. Chlorpromazine hydrochloride, *tablets:* 10, 25, 50, 100, 200 mg; *capsules, extended-release:* 30, 75, 150, 200, 300 mg; *solution (oral):* 10 mg/5 ml, 30 mg/ml, 100 mg/ml; *injection:* 25 mg/ml.

**DRUG INTERACTIONS**   **CNS depressants** including opiates, barbiturates, general anesthetics, and alcohol are potentiated by antipsychotic drugs.   **Anticonvulsants** Increased doses may be required.   **Lithium** CNS toxicity is potentiated by antipsychotic drugs.   **Mitrizamide** Should not be administered concurrently with antipsychotic drugs. See entry for drug class (p. 720) for more complete information.

**FATE**   Chlorpromazine is well absorbed from the GI tract but is metabolized by the intestinal mucosa and the liver. The *onset* for tranquilizing effect is 30 to 60 minutes, with a *duration of action* of 4 to 6 hours. Many metabolites are formed and are probably largely excreted in the urine.

## ☙ NURSING CONSIDERATIONS

### Side effects, toxicities, and associated nursing actions
- See entry for drug class (p. 720).

### Nursing interventions related to drug administration
- See entry for drug class (p. 723).
- Slight discoloration of injection or oral solution will not affect drug action. Discard solutions that are markedly discolored.
- For IM injection, choose a large, well-developed muscle mass such as the dorsogluteal site or rectus femoris muscle in adults, or the vastus lateralis in children. Aspirate before injecting to avoid inadvertent IV administration. Rotate and record sites.
- To avoid irritation at the IM injection site, dilute ordered dose in 0.9% sodium chloride or 2% procaine hydrochloride (check with physician).
- For direct IV push, dilute chlorpromazine hydrochloride in 0.9% sodium chloride to make a dilution of 1 mg/ml. Administer at a rate of 1.0 mg/min in adults and 0.5 mg/min in children.
- For IV infusion, dilute ordered dose in 500 to 1000 ml of 0.9% sodium chloride and infuse slowly.
- Side effects such as extrapyramidal reactions and blood dyscrasias are rare with short-term administration, as when chlorpromazine is used as an antiemetic. On the other hand, any side effect mentioned here can occur in that rare individual who is extremely sensitive to the drug. Be alert for the development of side effects.

### Patient and family education
- See entry for drug class (p. 723).

---

# chlorprothixene, chlorprothixene hydrochloride, chlorprothixene lactate   (klor-proe-THIX-een)   antipsychotic

- chlorprothixene, chlorprothixene hydrochloride, chlorprothixene lactate: ✦Tarasan, Taractan

**MECHANISM OF ACTION**   The major actions are characteristic of dopamine receptor antagonists.

**INDICATIONS**   • Psychosis.

**CONTRAINDICATIONS**   • History of seizures. • Renal or liver disease. • Respiratory disorder. • Glaucoma, prostatic hypertrophy. • For more complete information, see entry for drug class (p. 720).

**DOSAGE**   PO:   **ADULTS:** Initially, 25 to 50 mg three or four times daily. The dosage may be gradually increased if needed, but should not exceed 600 mg daily.   **CHILDREN OVER 6 YEARS:** 10 to 25 mg three or four times daily. Dose is adjusted as needed.   IM:   **ADULTS AND CHILDREN OVER 12 YEARS OLD:** 25 to 50 mg, repeated three or four times daily. Usually IM therapy is used only initially; when the patient is under control, PO therapy is used.   *Special patient populations:*   **ELDERLY:** Elderly or debilitated patients may require a lower dose.   **CHILDREN:** Safety has not been established for oral therapy in children under 6 years old or for parenteral therapy for children under 12 years old.    **PREGNANCY:** Safe use has not been established.

**PREPARATIONS**    Chlorprothixene, *tablets:* 10, 25, 50, 100 mg. Chlorprothixene hydrochloride, *injection:* 12.5 mg/ml. Chlorprothixene hydrochloride and lactate, *solution:* 100 mg/5 ml.

**DRUG INTERACTIONS**    **CNS depressants** including opiates, barbiturates, general anesthetics, and alcohol are potentiated by antipsychotic drugs.    **Anticonvulsants** Increased doses may be required.    **Lithium** CNS toxicity is potentiated by antipsychotic drugs.    **Mitrizamide** should not be administered concurrently with antipsychotic drugs. See entry for drug class (p. 720) for more complete information.

**FATE**    Chlorprothixene is erratically absorbed. The *onset of action* for the tranquilizing effect is 10 to 30 minutes, depending on the route of administration. The metabolic fate of chlorprothixene has not been well characterized. The unchanged drug and metabolites have been found in the urine and feces.

## 🦢 NURSING CONSIDERATIONS

### Side effects, toxicities, and associated nursing actions
- See entry for drug class (p. 720).

### Nursing interventions related to drug administration
- See entry for drug class (p. 723).
- For IM injection, choose a large, well-developed muscle mass such as the dorsogluteal site or rectus femoris muscle in adults, or the vastus lateralis in children. Aspirate before injecting to avoid inadvertent IV administration. Rotate and record sites.
- Taractan brand tablets contain FD & C coloring number 5 (tartrazine), which may cause an allergic reaction in susceptible individuals. While rare, this side effect is more common in persons with aspirin hypersensitivity.

### Patient and family education
- See entry for drug class (p. 723).

---

# droperidol    (droe-PER-i-dole)                                                    tranquilizer

- droperidol: Inapsine

**MECHANISM OF ACTION**    The major actions are characteristic of dopamine receptor antagonists. Droperidol also has pronounced activity as an alpha adrenergic receptor blocker.

**INDICATIONS**    **Surgery** Droperidol is used to produce tranquilization and to reduce nausea and vomiting. Droperidol is also used with opiate analgesics to produce anesthesia for surgery.

**CONTRAINDICATIONS**    • History of seizures. • Renal or liver disease. • Respiratory disorder. • Glaucoma, prostatic hypertrophy. • For more complete information, see entry for drug class (p. 720).

**DOSAGE**    **IM, IV:    ADULTS:** For premedication, 2.5 to 10 mg 30 to 60 minutes before induction of general anesthesia. As an adjunct for induction of anesthesia, 0.22 to 0.275 mg/kg. For tranquilization for diagnostic procedures (with topical anesthetics), 2.5 to 10 mg 30 to 60 minutes before the procedure. As an adjunct to regional anesthesia, 2.5 to 5 mg.    **CHILDREN 2 TO 12 YEARS:** For premedication or induction of anesthesia, 0.088 to 0.165 mg/kg.    *Special patient populations:*    **ELDERLY:** Elderly or debilitated patients may require a lower dose, and smaller doses are administered initially.    **PREGNANCY:** Safe use has not been established.

**PREPARATIONS**    *Injection:* 2.5 mg/ml.

**DRUG INTERACTIONS**    **CNS depressants** including opiates, barbiturates, general anesthetics, and alcohol are potentiated by antipsychotic drugs.    **Anticonvulsants** Increased doses may be required.    **Lithium** CNS toxicity is potentiated by antipsychotic drugs.    **Mitrizamide** should not be administered concurrently with antipsychotic drugs. See entry for drug class (p. 720) for more complete information.

**FATE**    *Onset of action* is 3 to 10 minutes, with full effects in 30 minutes. The *duration of action* is 2 to 4 hours for the sedative-tranquilization effects. An altered consciousness may be experienced for up to 12 hours.

## ❦ NURSING CONSIDERATIONS

### Side effects, toxicities, and associated nursing actions
- See entry for drug class (p. 720).

### Nursing interventions related to drug administration
- See entry for drug class (p. 723).
- For IV administration, may be given undiluted. Administer each 10 mg or less over 1 minute. Dose frequently titrated by patient response.
- Dose may be diluted in 5% dextrose or Ringer's lactate, and infused slowly.
- For IM injection, choose a large, well-developed muscle mass such as the dorsogluteal site or rectus femoris muscle in adults, or the vastus lateralis in children. Aspirate before injecting to avoid inadvertent IV administration. Rotate and record sites.
- Monitor blood pressure. While hypotension may occur, hypertension has also been reported.

### Patient and family education
- See entry for drug class (p. 723).
- Because this drug is only available in parenteral form, its use outside of the hospital setting is rare.

---

## fluphenazine   (floo-FEN-a-zeen)                                    antipsychotic

- fluphenazine decanoate: ❧Modecate, Prolixin Decanoate
- fluphenazine enanthate: ❧Moditen Enanthate, Prolixin Enanthate
- fluphenazine hydrochloride: ❧Apo-Fluphenazine, ❧Moditen Hydrochloride, Permitil, Prolixin

**MECHANISM OF ACTION**    The major actions are characteristic of dopamine receptor antagonists.

**INDICATIONS**    • Psychosis.

**CONTRAINDICATIONS**    • History of seizures. • Renal or liver disease. • Respiratory disorder. • Glaucoma, prostatic hypertrophy. • For more complete information, see entry for drug class (p. 720).

**DOSAGE**    **PO hydrochloride form:**   **ADULTS:** 0.5 to 10 mg daily divided into 3 or 4 doses initially. Dosage may be increased gradually to optimize response. Optimum dose is usually under 20 mg. Dosages up to 40 mg daily may be required for severely disturbed patients. After control of symptoms is achieved, the dosage is gradually decreased to a maintenance dose that is usually 1 to 5 mg daily.   **IM:** **ADULTS:** 1/2 to 1/3 the oral dose. The usual initial dose is 1.25 mg.   **IM decanoate or enanthate form:**   **ADULTS:** These are long-acting depot forms of the drug and should only be used for a patient who is stabilized on the daily hydrochloride form and shows no signs of side effects. The conversion factor is 25 mg fluphenazine decanoate every 3 weeks for every 20 mg daily of fluphenazine hydrochloride. The usual initial dose of fluphenazine enanthate is 25 mg every 2 weeks.   *Special patient populations:*   **ELDERLY:** Elderly or debilitated patients are begun at the lowest dose and the dose is increased gradually if necessary   **PREGNANCY:** Safe use has not been established.

**PREPARATIONS**    Hydrochloride, *elixir:* 2.5 mg/5 ml; *solution,* 5 mg/ml; *tablets,* 1, 2.5, 5, 10 mg; *IM injection,* 2.5 mg/ml. Decanoate form, *injection:* 25 mg/ml. Enanthate form, *injection:* 25 mg/ml.

**DRUG INTERACTIONS**    **CNS depressants** including opiates, barbiturates, general anesthetics, and alcohol are potentiated by antipsychotic drugs.   **Anticonvulsants** Increased doses may be required.   **Lithium** CNS toxicity is potentiated by antipsychotic drugs.   **Mitrizamide** should not be administered concurrently with antipsychotic drugs. See entry for drug class (p. 720) for more complete information.

**FATE**    The hydrochloride form is rapidly absorbed, with an *onset of action* within 60 minutes and a *duration of action* of 6 to 8 hours. The decanoate or enanthate forms have an *onset of action* of 2 to 3 days and a *duration of action* of 1 to 6 weeks, with an average of 2 weeks for the enanthate form and 3 weeks for the decanoate form.

## ❦ NURSING CONSIDERATIONS

### Side effects, toxicities, and associated nursing actions
- See entry for drug class (p. 720).

### Nursing interventions related to drug administration
- See entry for drug class (p. 723).
- Read orders carefully: decanoate and enanthate forms are long-acting depot forms.
- For decanoate and enanthate forms, use a dry needle and syringe. A wet needle or syringe will cause drug to turn cloudy. A large-bore needle should be used, such as a 21 gauge needle.
- For IM injection, choose a large, well-developed muscle mass such as the dorsogluteal site or rectus femoris muscle in adults, or the vastus lateralis in children. Aspirate before injecting to avoid inadvertent IV administration. Rotate and record sites.

### Patient and family education
- See entry for drug class (p. 723).

---

## haloperidol   (ha-loe-PER-i-dole)                              antipsychotic, antiemetic

- haloperidol, haloperidol lactate: ✚Apo-Haloperidol, Haldol, ✚Peridol

**MECHANISM OF ACTION**   The major actions are characteristic of dopamine receptor antagonists.

**INDICATIONS**   • Psychosis. • Gilles de la Tourette syndrome. • Nausea and vomiting: for that associated with chemotherapy.

**CONTRAINDICATIONS**   • History of seizures. • Renal or liver disease. • Respiratory disorder. • Glaucoma, prostatic hypertrophy. • For more complete information, see Overview of Drug Class (p. 720).

**DOSAGE**   PO:   **ADULTS:** Psychosis or Tourette's syndrome, initial dose of 0.5 to 2 mg two or three times daily, then adjusted for therapeutic response. For severe psychosis, initial dose is 3 to 5 mg two or three times daily. Daily doses up to 100 mg or more may be required in resistant cases.   **CHILDREN, 3 TO 12 YEARS:** Tourette's syndrome or severe hyperactive behavior problems, 0.05 to 0.075 mg/kg daily, divided into 2 or 3 doses. Psychoses, 0.5 mg daily or 0.05 to 0.15 mg/kg daily, divided into 2 or 3 doses.   IM:   **ADULTS:** Psychosis, initially, 2 to 5 mg, repeated every 1 to 8 hours to control symptoms, then switch to oral dose.   *Special patient populations:*   **ELDERLY:** Elderly or debilitated patients may require a lower dose.   **CHILDREN:** Safety or effectiveness for children under 3 years old has not been established.   **PREGNANCY:** Limb abnormalities have been reported in two infants whose mothers had taken haldoperidol early in pregnancy. Animal studies report teratogenicity. Haldoperidol is found in breast milk.

**PREPARATIONS**   *Tablets:* 0.5, 1, 2, 5, 10, 20 mg. Hydrochloride, *solution:* 2 mg/ml; *IM injection,* 5 mg/ml.

**DRUG INTERACTIONS**   **CNS depressants** including opiates, barbiturates, general anesthetics, and alcohol are potentiated by antipsychotic drugs.   **Anticonvulsants** Increased doses may be required.   **Lithium** CNS toxicity is potentiated by antipsychotic drugs.   **Mitrizamide** should not be administered concurrently with antipsychotic drugs. See entry for drug class (p. 720) for more complete information.

**FATE**   Haloperidol is well absorbed, with *peak* levels seen 10 minutes after IM or 2 to 6 hours after oral administration. The metabolic fate of haloperidol has not been well characterized. Haloperidol is metabolized by the liver and metabolites excreted in the urine and feces.

## ❦ NURSING CONSIDERATIONS

### Side effects, toxicities, and associated nursing actions
- See entry for drug class (p. 720).

### Nursing interventions related to drug administration
- See entry for drug class (p. 720).
- For IM injection, choose a large, well-developed muscle mass such as the dorsogluteal site or rectus femoris muscle in adults, or the vastus lateralis in children. Aspirate before injecting to avoid inadvertent IV administration. Rotate and record sites.
- The IM route of administration is not recommended for children.
- Haldol brand tablets in 1, 5, and 10 mg doses contain FD & C coloring # 5 (tartrazine), which may cause an allergic response in susceptible individuals. While rare, this response is seen more often in persons with aspirin hypersensitivity.

  - See entry for drug class (p. 720).

## loxapine hydrochloride, loxapine succinate  (LOX-a-peen)   antipsychotic

  - loxapine hydrochloride, loxapine succinate: Loxitane

**MECHANISM OF ACTION**   The major actions are characteristic of dopamine receptor antagonists.

**INDICATIONS**   • Psychosis.

**CONTRAINDICATIONS**   • History of seizures. • Renal or liver disease. • Respiratory disorder. • Glaucoma, prostatic hypertrophy. • For more complete information, See Overview of Drug Class (p. 720).

**DOSAGE**   PO:   **ADULTS:** Initially, 10 mg twice daily. Dosage may be increased rapidly to improve response if no side effects appear. For severe schizophrenic states, initial dose may be 50 mg daily. Maintenance dose is usually 60 to 100 mg, given in 2 to 4 doses. Doses should not exceed 250 mg daily.
IM:   **ADULTS:** 12.5 to 50 mg every 4 to 6 hours for prompt control of acutely agitated patients. *Special patient populations:*   **ELDERLY:** Elderly or debilitated patients may require a lower dose.   **CHILDREN:** Not recommended for children under 16 years of age.   **PREGNANCY:** Safe use has not been established.

**PREPARATIONS**   Hydrochloride, *solution (oral):* 25 mg/ml. *Injection (IM):* 50 mg/ml. Succinate, *capsules:* 5, 10, 25, 50 mg.

**DRUG INTERACTIONS**   **CNS depressants** including opiates, barbiturates, general anesthetics, and alcohol are potentiated by antipsychotic drugs.   **Anticonvulsants** Increased doses may be required.   **Lithium** CNS toxicity is potentiated by antipsychotic drugs.   **Mitrizamide** should not be administered concurrently with antipsychotic drugs. See entry for drug class (p. 720) for more complete information.

**FATE**   Loxapine is well absorbed. *Peak* serum concentrations appear in about 2 hours. *Onset* of sedative effect is 20 to 30 minutes. *Peak* effect is in 1.5 to 3 hours. *Duration* of sedative action is 12 hours. Loxapine is metabolized by the liver. Metabolites are excreted in the feces and urine.

**NURSING CONSIDERATIONS**

Side effects, toxicities, and associated nursing actions
  - See entry for drug class (p. 720).

Nursing interventions related to drug administration
  - See entry for drug class (p. 723).
  - For IM injection, choose a large, well-developed muscle mass such as the dorsogluteal site or rectus femoris muscle in adults, or the vastus lateralis in children. Aspirate before injecting to avoid inadvertent IV administration. Rotate and record sites.
  - Loxapine hydrochloride should not be given IV.

Patient and family education
  - See entry for drug class (p. 723).

## mesoridazine besylate   (mez-oh-RID-a-zeen)        antipsychotic, tranquilizer

  - mesoridazine besylate: Serentil

**MECHANISM OF ACTION**   The major actions are characteristic of dopamine receptor antagonists.

**INDICATIONS**   Psychosis.   **Tranquilizer** Used in reducing the anxiety, tension, depression, and nausea and vomiting of alcohol dependence. Also used in reducing the anxiety and tension of neuroses.

**CONTRAINDICATIONS**   • History of seizures. • Renal or liver disease. • Respiratory disorder. • Glaucoma, prostatic hypertrophy. • For more complete information, see entry for drug class (p. 720).

**DOSAGE** **PO:** **ADULTS:** *Psychosis,* initially, 50 mg three times daily, then adjusted as needed. Usual therapeutic dosage is 100 to 400 mg daily. ***Special patient populations:*** *Hyperactive* associated with mental deficiency or chronic brain syndrome: 25 mg three times daily, up to maximum daily dose of 300 mg. *Adjunctive therapy of alcohol dependence:*25 mg two times daily, up to a maximum daily dose of 200 mg. *Anxiety and tension associated with neuroses:* 10 mg three times daily, up to a maximum daily dose of 150 mg. **IM:** **ADULTS:** 25 mg, repeated in 30 to 60 minutes if needed. Maximum daily dose is 200 mg. **ELDERLY:** Elderly or debilitated patients should be started at a lower dose. **CHILDREN:** Not recommended for children under 12 years. **PREGNANCY:** Safe use has not been established.

**PREPARATIONS** *Solution (oral):* 25 mg/ml. *Tablets:* 10, 25, 50, 100 mg. *Injection:* 25 mg/ml.

**DRUG INTERACTIONS** **CNS depressants** including opiates, barbiturates, general anesthetics, and alcohol are potentiated by antipsychotic drugs. **Anticonvulsants** Increased doses may be required. **Lithium** CNS toxicity is potentiated by antipsychotic drugs. **Mitrizamide** should not be administered concurrently with antipsychotic drugs. See entry for drug class (p. 720) for more complete information.

**FATE** Mesoridazine is well absorbed. The metabolism of mesoridazine has not been well characterized.

❦ **NURSING CONSIDERATIONS**

**Side effects, toxicities, and associated nursing actions**
- See entry for drug class (p. 720).

**Nursing interventions related to drug administration**
- See entry for drug class (p. 723).
- For IM injection, choose a large, well-developed muscle mass such as the dorsogluteal site or rectus femoris muscle in adults, or the vastus lateralis in children. Aspirate before injecting to avoid inadvertent IV administration. Rotate and record sites.
- Serentil brand tablets contain FD & C brand coloring (tartrazine), which may cause an allergic response in some individuals. While rare, this side effect is seen more commonly in persons with aspirin hypersensitivity.

**Patient and family education**
- See entry for drug class (p. 723).

---

## molindone hydrochloride  (moe-LIN-done)                              antipsychotic

- molindone hydrochloride: Moban

**MECHANISM OF ACTION** The major actions are characteristic of dopamine receptor antagonists.

**INDICATIONS** • Psychosis, used primarily in treating schizophrenia.

**CONTRAINDICATIONS** • History of seizures. • Renal or liver disease. • Respiratory disorder. • Glaucoma, prostatic hypertrophy. • For more complete information, see entry for drug class (p. 720).

**DOSAGE** **PO:** **ADULTS:** *Mild symptoms,* 5 to 15 mg three or four times daily. *Moderately severe symptoms,* 10 to 25 mg daily. Doses larger than 150 mg daily are seldom beneficial. **CHILDREN:** *Mentally retarded, schizophrenic children 3 to 5 years old,* single daily dose of 1.5 to 2.5 mg. ***Special patient populations:*** **ELDERLY:** Elderly or debilitated patients should be started at a lower dose. **CHILDREN:** In general, not recommended for children under 12 years old. **PREGNANCY:** Safe use has not been established.

**PREPARATIONS** *Solution (oral):* 20 mg/ml. *Tablets:* 5, 10, 25, 50, 100 mg.

**DRUG INTERACTIONS** **CNS depressants** including opiates, barbiturates, general anesthetics, and alcohol are potentiated by antipsychotic drugs. **Anticonvulsants** Increased doses may be required. **Lithium** CNS toxicity is potentiated by antipsychotic drugs. **Mitrizamide** should not be administered concurrently with antipsychotic drugs. See entry for drug class (p. 720) for more complete information.

**FATE** Molindone is well absorbed, and *peak* effects occur in about 1 hour. *Duration of action* is about 36 hours. Molindone is metabolized in the liver and products are excreted in the feces and urine.

## ❦ NURSING CONSIDERATIONS

### Side effects, toxicities, and associated nursing actions
- See entry for drug class (p. 720).

### Nursing interventions related to drug administration
- See entry for drug class (p. 723).

### Patient and family education
- See entry for drug class (p. 723).

---

## perphenazine    (per-FEN-a-zeen)                     antipsychotic, antiemetic

- perphenazine: ♣Apo-Perphenazine, ♣Phenazine, ♣PMS Levazine, Trilafon

**MECHANISM OF ACTION**    The major actions are characteristic of dopamine receptor antagonists.

**INDICATIONS**    • Psychosis. • Antiemetic.

**CONTRAINDICATIONS**    • History of seizures. • Renal or liver disease. • Respiratory disorder. • Glaucoma, prostatic hypertrophy. • For more complete information, see Overview of Drug Class (p. 720).

**DOSAGE**    **PO:**    **ADULTS:** *Psychosis, outpatient,* 4 to 8 mg three times daily or 1 extended-release tablet, 8 or 16 mg, twice daily. *Psychosis, hospitalized patient,* 8 to 16 mg two to four times daily, or 8 to 32 mg in extended-release tablets, twice daily. *Severe nausea and vomiting,* 8 to 16 mg daily in divided doses. **IM:**    **ADULTS:** *Psychosis,* for prompt control of severe symptoms, 5 mg, repeated every 6 hours as needed. IM therapy is continued only until oral therapy can be startd, generally within 2 days. *Severe nausea and vomiting,* 5 mg.    **IV:**    **ADULTS:** 5 mg, given 1 mg at a time. Each mg is given by slow IV infusion over a 1- to 2-minute interval. Give only to control severe vomiting, retching during surgery, or to stop intractable hiccups.    ***Special patient populations:***    **ELDERLY:** Elderly or debilitated patients should be started at the lower dose.    **CHILDREN:** Not recommended for children under 12 years old. Older children are given the same doses as adults.    **PREGNANCY:** Safe use has not been established.

**PREPARATIONS**    *Solution (oral):* 16 mg/5 ml. *Tablets:* 2, 4, 8, 16 mg. *Tablet, extended-release:* 8 mg. *Injection:* 5 mg/ml.

**DRUG INTERACTIONS**    **CNS depressants** including opiates, barbiturates, general anesthetics, and alcohol are potentiated by antipsychotic drugs.    **Anticonvulsants** Increased doses may be required.    **Lithium** CNS toxicity is potentiated by antipsychotic drugs.    **Mitrizamide** should not be administered concurrently with antipsychotic drugs. See entry for drug class (p. 720) for more complete information.

**FATE**    The metabolic fate of perphenazine is not well characterized.

## ❦ NURSING CONSIDERATIONS

### Side effects, toxicities and associated nursing actions
- See entry for drug class (p. 720).

### Nursing interventions related to drug administration
- See entry for drug class (p. 723).
- For IM injection, choose a large, well-developed muscle mass such as the dorsogluteal site or rectus femoris muscle in adults, or the vastus lateralis in children. Aspirate before injecting to avoid inadvertent IV administration. Rotate and record sites.
- For direct IV push, dilute with 0.9% normal saline to a dilution of 0.5 mg/ml. Infuse at a rate of 0.5 mg/min.
- For intermittent infusion, further dilute dose in 0.9% normal saline and infuse slowly (use infusion pump, microdip infusion set).

### Patient and family education
- See entry for drug class (p. 723).

## prochlorperazine, prochlorperazine edisylate, prochlorperazine maleate (proe-klor-PER-a-zeen)

antipsychotic, tranquilizer, antiemetic

- prochlorperazine, prochlorperazine edisylate, prochlorperazine maleate: Compazine, ✽Stemetil

**MECHANISM OF ACTION**    The major actions are characteristic of dopamine receptor antagonists.

**INDICATIONS**    **Psychosis.**    **Neurosis** Prochlorperazine is effective in relieving moderate to severe anxiety and tension.    **Emesis** To control nausea and vomiting associated with surgery, chemotherapy, or radiation therapy.

**CONTRAINDICATIONS**    • History of seizures. • Renal or liver disease. • Respiratory disorder. • Glaucoma, prostatic hypertrophy. • For more complete information, see entry for drug class (p. 720).

**DOSAGE**    **PO:**    **ADULTS:** *Psychosis, outpatients,* 5 or 10 mg three or four times daily. *Psychosis, hospitalized patients,* 10 mg three or four times daily. Dosage may be increased every 2 or 3 days to control symptoms. *Excessive anxiety of neurosis,* 5 or 10 mg three or four times daily. A single 15 mg extended-release capsule may be taken. *Severe nausea and vomiting,* 5 or 10 mg three or four times daily or a 15 mg extended-release capsule in the morning, or a 10 mg extended-release capsule twice daily.    **CHILDREN:** *Psychosis,* 2 to 12 years old, 2.5 mg two or three times daily initially. Dosage may be gradually adjusted up if necessary to a maximum of 20 mg for children 2 to 5 years old and 25 mg for children 6 to 12 years old.    **IM:**    **ADULTS:** *Psychosis,* 10 to 20 mg. *Neurotic anxiety,* 5 to 10 mg. *Severe nausea and vomiting,* 5 to 10 mg. Prior to surgery, 5 or 10 mg may be given 1 to 2 hours before the induction of anesthesia. During or after surgery, 5 or 10 mg may be given, repeated once in 30 minutes if necessary.    **CHILDREN:** *Psychosis,* 0.13 mg/kg. *Severe nausea and vomiting,* children over 2 years old, 0.4 mg/kg or 10 mg/M$^2$ daily in 3 or 4 divided doses. Alternatively, the following doses may be used: 20 to 30 lb, 2.5 mg two or three times daily; 30 to 40 lb, 2.5 mg, two to four times daily; 40 to 85 lb, 2.5 mg three times daily or 5 mg twice daily, maximum 15 mg. Children should not be given prochlorperazine for more than 24 hours.    **Rectal:**    **ADULTS:** *Excessive anxiety,* 25 mg twice daily.    **CHILDREN:** *Severe nausea and vomiting,* children over 2 years old, 0.4 mg/kg or 10 mg/M$^2$ daily in 3 or 4 divided doses. Alternatively, the following doses may be used: 20 to 30 lb, 2.5 mg two or three times daily; 30 to 40 lb, 2.5 mg, two to four times daily; 40 to 85 lb, 2.5 mg three times daily or 5 mg twice daily, maximum 15 mg. Children should not be given prochlorperazine for more than 24 hours.    **IV:**    **ADULTS:** *For control of severe nausea or vomiting prior to surgery,* an infusion of 20 mg/L is begun 15 to 30 minutes before the induction of anesthesia.    ***Special patient populations:***    **ELDERLY:** Elderly or debilitated patients should be started at a lower dose.    **CHILDREN:** Pediatric doses are given above.    **PREGNANCY:** Safe use has not been established.

**PREPARATIONS**    Prochlorperazine, *suppositories:* 2.5, 5, 25 mg. Edisylate form, *solution (oral):* 5 mg/5 ml. *Injection:* 5 mg/ml. Maleate form, *capsules, extended-release:* 10, 15, 30 mg. *Tablets:* 5, 10, 25 mg.

**DRUG INTERACTIONS**    **CNS depressants** including opiates, barbiturates, general anesthetics, and alcohol are potentiated by antipsychotic drugs.    **Anticonvulsants** Increased doses may be required.    **Lithium** CNS toxicity is potentiated by antipsychotic drugs.    **Mitrizamide** should not be administered concurrently with antipsychotic drugs. See entry for drug class (p. 720) for more complete information.

**FATE**    The metabolic fate of prochlorperazine is not well characterized.

### ☙ NURSING CONSIDERATIONS
#### Side effects, toxicities, and associated nursing actions
- See entry for drug class (p. 720).

#### Nursing interventions related to drug administration
- See entry for drug class (p. 723).
- Slight discoloration of injection or oral solution will not affect drug action. Discard solutions that are markedly discolored.
- For IM injection, choose a large, well-developed muscle mass such as the dorsogluteal site or rectus

femoris muscle in adults, or the vastus lateralis in children. Aspirate before injecting to avoid inadvertent IV administration. Rotate and record sites.
- For IV use, dilute prochlorperazine with 0.9% sodium chloride to make a dilution of 0.5 mg/ml. Further dilute 10 to 20 mg with 1000 ml of isotonic IV solution.
- For IV push, may be given undiluted. A single dose should not exceed 10 mg. Rate of administration should not exceed 5 mg/ml/min.
- Side effects such as extrapyramidal reactions and blood dyscrasias are rare with short-term administration, as when chlorpromazine is used as an antiemetic. On the other hand, any side effect mentioned here can occur in that rare individual who is extremely sensitive to the drug. Be alert for the development of side effects.

**Patient and family education**
- See entry for drug class (p. 723).

---

## promazine hydrochloride    (PROE-ma-zeen)                        antipsychotic

- promazine hydrochloride: ✿Promanyl, Sparine

**MECHANISM OF ACTION**    The major actions are characteristic of dopamine receptor antagonists.

**INDICATIONS**    • Psychosis.

**CONTRAINDICATIONS**    • History of seizures. • Renal or liver disease. • Respiratory disorder. • Glaucoma, prostatic hypertrophy. • For more complete information, see entry for drug class (p. 720).

**DOSAGE**    PO, IM:    **ADULTS:** 10 to 200 mg every 4 to 6 hours. Dosage is individualized. Single doses of up to 500 mg may be tolerated as may daily doses of 800 mg. Total daily dose should not exceed 1 g. **CHILDREN OVER 12 YEARS OLD:** 10 to 25 mg every 4 to 6 hours.    **IM, IV:**    **ADULTS:** 50 to 150 mg for severely agitated patients. If response is not sufficient in 30 minutes, an additional dose of up to 300 mg may be given. *Special patient populations:*    **ELDERLY:** Elderly or debilitated patients may require a lower dose.    **CHILDREN:** Not recommended for children under 12 years old.    **PREGNANCY:** Safe use has not been established.

**PREPARATIONS**    *Solution (oral):* 10 mg/5 ml. *Tablets:* 25, 50, 100 mg. *Injection:* 25, 50 mg/ml.

**DRUG INTERACTIONS**    **CNS depressants** including opiates, barbiturates, general anesthetics, and alcohol are potentiated by antipsychotic drugs.    **Anticonvulsants** Increased doses may be required    **Lithium** CNS toxicity is potentiated by antipsychotic drugs.    **Mitrizamide** should not be administered concurrently with antipsychotic drugs. See entry for drug class (p. 720.) for more complete information.

**FATE**    The metabolic fate of promazine has not been well characterized.

☙ **NURSING CONSIDERATIONS**

**Side effects, toxicities, and associated nursing actions**
- See entry for drug class (p. 720).

**Nursing interventions related to drug administration**
- See entry for drug class (p. 723).
- For IM injection, choose a large, well-developed muscle mass such as the dorsogluteal site or rectus femoris muscle in adults, or the vastus lateralis in children. Aspirate before injecting to avoid inadvertent IV administration. Rotate and record sites.
- For IV use, may be given undiluted, but concentration should not exceed 25 mg/ml. May be further diluted with 9 ml of 0.9% sodium chloride to make a dilute of 2.5 to 5 mg/ml. Administer at a rate of 25 mg or less over 1 minute.
- Sparine brand 25 mg tablets and Sparine brand syrup contain FD & C coloring # 5 (tartrazine), which may cause an allergic reaction is susceptible individuals. While rare, this side effect is found more frequently in persons with aspirin hypersensitivity.

**Patient and family education**
- See entry for drug class (p. 723).

# thioridazine, thioridazine hydrochloride
(thye-or-RID-a-zeen)                                   antipsychotic, tranquilizer

- thioridazine, thioridazine hydrochloride: ♣Apo-Thioridazine, Mellaril, Millazine, ♣Novorida-zine, ♣PMS Thioridazine

**MECHANISM OF ACTION**   The major actions are characteristic of dopamine receptor antagonists.

**INDICATIONS**   Psychosis.   **Behavioral problems in children** Thioridazine is used to control severe behavioral problems marked by combativeness, explosive hyperexcitability, or hyperactivity marked by excessive motor activity.

**CONTRAINDICATIONS**   • History of seizures. • Renal or liver disease. • Respiratory disorder. • Glaucoma, prostatic hypertrophy. • For more complete information, see entry for drug class (p. 720).

**DOSAGE**   PO:   **ADULTS:** *Psychosis,* 50 to 100 mg three times daily initially. Dosages may be adjusted if necessary. Patients requiring more than 300 mg daily should be hospitalized. *Depression with anxiety or agitiation, anxiety, tension, sleep disturbances, fears in the elderly,* 25 mg three times daily initially. Range for the total dose is 20 to 200 mg. Treatment should be only short-term.   **CHILDREN 2 TO 12 YEARS OLD:** 0.5 to 3 mg/kg daily. Initial dose is usually 10 mg two or three times daily for children with moderate behavioral problems; the dose is 25 mg two or three times daily for children hospitalized with severe disturbances or psychosis.   *Special patient populations:*   **CHILDREN:** Not recommended for children less than 2 years old.   **PREGNANCY:** Safe use has not been established.

**PREPARATIONS**   Thioridazine, *suspension (oral):* 25, 100 mg/5 ml. Hydrochloride form, *solution (oral):* 30, 100 mg/ml. *Tablets:* 10, 15, 25, 50, 100, 150, 200 mg. *Tablets, film-coated:* 10, 15, 25, 50, 100, 200 mg.

**DRUG INTERACTIONS**   **CNS depressants** including opiates, barbiturates, general anesthetics, and alcohol are potentiated by antipsychotic drugs.   **Anticonvulsants** Increased doses may be required.   **Lithium** CNS toxicity is potentiated by antipsychotic drugs.   **Mitrizamide** should not be administered concurrently with antipsychotic drugs. See entry for drug class (p. 720) for more complete information.

**FATE**   The metabolic fate of thioridazine has not been well characterized.

❦ **NURSING CONSIDERATIONS**

**Side effects, toxicities, and associated nursing actions**
- See entry for drug class (p. 720).

**Nursing interventions related to drug administration**
- See entry for drug class (p. 723).

**Patient and family education**
- See entry for drug class (p. 723).

# thiothixene, thiothixene hydrochloride
(thye-oh-THIX-een)                                   antipsychotic, antidepressant

- thiothixene, thiothixene hydrochloride: Navane

**MECHANISM OF ACTION**   The major actions are characteristic of dopamine receptor antagonists.

**INDICATIONS**   Psychosis.   **Depression** May be useful in treating depression associated with neurosis.

**CONTRAINDICATIONS**   • History of seizures. • Renal or liver disease. • Respiratory disorder. • Glaucoma, prostatic hypertrophy. • For more complete information, see entry for drug class (p. 720).

**DOSAGE**   PO:   **ADULTS:** *For mild to moderate psychosis,* 2 mg three times daily. This may be increased up to 15 mg daily. *For severe psychosis,* 5 mg twice daily initially, increase to 60 mg daily if necessary.   IM:   **ADULTS:** *For acutely agitated patients,* 4 mg two to four times daily.   *Special patient pop-*

*ulations:*   **ELDERLY:** Elderly or debilitated patients may require a lower dose.   **CHILDREN:** Not recommended for children under 12 years old.   **PREGNANCY:** Safe use has not been established.

**PREPARATIONS**   *Capsules:* 1, 2, 5, 10, 20 mg. Hydrochloride form, *solution (oral):* 5 mg/ml. *Injection:* 2 mg/ml, 10 mg.

**DRUG INTERACTIONS**   **CNS depressants** including opiates, barbiturates, general anesthetics, and alcohol are potentiated by antipsychotic drugs.   **Anticonvulsants** Increased doses may be required.   **Lithium** CNS toxicity is potentiated by antipsychotic drugs.   **Mitrizamide** should not be administered concurrently with antipsychotic drugs. See entry for drug class (p. 720) for more complete information.

**FATE**   Thiothixene is well absorbed. Therapeutic response is seen in 1 to 6 hours after IM injection, several days after oral administration. Thiothixene is metabolized in the liver and excreted mainly in the feces.

### ❦ NURSING CONSIDERATIONS

#### Side effects, toxicities, and associated nursing actions
- See entry for drug class (p. 720).

#### Nursing interventions related to drug administration
- See entry for drug class (p. 723).
- For IM injection, choose a large, well-developed muscle mass such as the dorsogluteal site or rectus femoris muscle in adults, or the vastus lateralis in children. Aspirate before injecting to avoid inadvertent IV administration. Rotate and record sites.

#### Patient and family education
- See entry for drug class (p. 723).

---

## trifluoperazine hydrochloride   (trye-floo-PROE-ma-zeen)    antipsychotic

- trifluoperazine hydrochloride: ✽Apo-Trifluoperazine, Stelazine, Suprazine

**MECHANISM OF ACTION**   The major actions are characteristic of dopamine receptor antagonists.

**INDICATIONS**   Psychosis.   Anxiety Trifluoperazine may be used short term for nonpsychotic anxiety.

**CONTRAINDICATIONS**   • History of seizures. • Renal or liver disease. • Respiratory disorder. • Glaucoma, prostatic hypertrophy. • For more complete information, see entry for drug class (p. 720).

**DOSAGE**   PO:   **ADULTS:** *Outpatients,* 1 to 2 mg twice daily is usually sufficient. *Hospitalized patients,* 2 to 5 mg twice daily initially. Dose may be increased. Optimum dose is usually found to be 15 to 20 mg daily. *For nonpsychotic anxiety,* 2 to 6 mg daily. Duration should not be more than 12 weeks because of the potential for persistent tardive dyskinesia.   **CHILDREN 6 TO 12 YEARS OLD:** 1 mg one or two times daily, increased gradually to control symptoms. Daily doses rarely exceed 15 mg.   **IM: ADULTS:** *To control severe psychotic symptoms,* 1 to 2 mg every 4 to 6 hours as necessary, not exceeding 10 mg in 24 hours.   *Special patient populations:*   **ELDERLY:** Elderly or debilitated patients may require a lower dose.   **CHILDREN:** Not recommended for children under 6 years old. **PREGNANCY:** Safe use has not been established.

**PREPARATIONS**   *Solution (oral):* 10 mg/ml. *Tablets:* 1, 2, 5, 10 mg. *Injection:* 2 mg/ml.

**DRUG INTERACTIONS**   **CNS depressants** including opiates, barbiturates, general anesthetics, and alcohol are potentiated by antipsychotic drugs.   **Anticonvulsants** Increased doses may be required.   **Lithium** CNS toxicity is potentiated by antipsychotic drugs.   **Mitrizamide** should not be administered concurrently with antipsychotic drugs. See entry for drug class (p. 720) for more complete information.

**FATE**   The metabolic fate of trifluoperazine has not been well characterized.

### ❦ NURSING CONSIDERATIONS

#### Side effects, toxicities, and associated nursing actions
- See entry for drug class (p. 720).

#### Nursing interventions related to drug administration
- See entry for drug class (p. 723).

- For IM injection, choose a large, well-developed muscle mass such as the dorsogluteal site or rectus femoris muscle in adults, or the vastus lateralis in children. Aspirate before injecting to avoid inadvertent IV administration. Rotate and record sites.

**Patient and family education**
- See entry for drug class (p. 723).

---

# triflupromazine hydrochloride

antipsychotic, antiemetic

- triflupromazine hydrochloride: Vesprin

**MECHANISM OF ACTION**   The major actions are characteristic of dopamine receptor antagonists.

**INDICATIONS**   • Psychosis. • Severe nausea and vomiting.

**CONTRAINDICATIONS**   • History of seizures. • Renal or liver disease. • Respiratory disorder. • Glaucoma, prostatic hypertrophy. • For more complete information, see Overview of Drug Class (p. 720).

**DOSAGE**   IM:   ADULTS: *For control of psychotic disorder,* 60 mg daily in divided doses. Maximum dose is 150 mg daily. *Nausea and vomiting,* 5 to 15 mg. Repeat every 4 hours if necessary, maximum 60 mg daily.   CHILDREN: *For control of psychotic disorder,* or *for control of nausea and vomiting,* 0.2 to 0.25 mg/kg daily. Maximum dose is 10 mg daily.   IV:   ADULTS: *For the control of nausea and vomiting,* 1 mg. This may be repeated to a maximum total dose of 3 mg daily.   *Special patient populations:* ELDERLY: Elderly or debilitated patients require a lower dose. Initial dose is 2.5 mg. Maximum daily dose is 15 mg.   CHILDREN: Not recommended for children younger than 2 1/2 years old.   PREGNANCY: Safe use has not been established.

**PREPARATIONS**   *Injection:* 10, 20 mg/ml.

**DRUG INTERACTIONS**   **CNS depressants** including opiates, barbiturates, general anesthetics, and alcohol are potentiated by antipsychotic drugs.   **Anticonvulsants** Increased doses may be required.   **Lithium** CNS toxicity is potentiated by antipsychotic drugs.   **Mitrizamide** should not be administered concurrently with antipsychotic drugs. See entry for drug class (p. 720) for more complete information.

**FATE**   The metabolic fate of triflupromazine has not been well characterized.

## ❧ NURSING CONSIDERATIONS

**Side effects, toxicities, and associated nursing actions**
- See entry for drug class (p. 720).

**Nursing interventions related to drug administration**
- See entry for drug class (p. 723).
- For IM injection, choose a large, well-developed muscle mass such as the dorsogluteal site or rectus femoris muscle in adults, or the vastus lateralis in children. Aspirate before injecting to avoid inadvertent IV administration. Rotate and record sites.
- For IV use, dilute each 10 mg with 9 ml of 0.9% normal saline to make a dilution of 1 mg/ml. Rate of administration should not exceed 8 mg/min.

**Patient and family education**
- See entry for drug class (p. 723).

# Chapter Thirty-seven

# Antidepressant drugs

**Tricyclic antidepressants**
amitriptyline
desipramine
doxepine
imipramine
nortriptyline
protriptyline
trimipramine

**Second-generation antidepressants**
amoxapine
bupropion
maprotiline
trazodone

**Monamine oxidase (MAO) inhibitors**
isocarboxazid
phenelzine
tranylcypromine

**Antimanic drug**
lithium

**INTRODUCTION** Depression is a disorder of mood (affect) that occurs in an estimated 15% to 30% of all adults at some time during their lives. Depression is not a single entity; rather it is a syndrome that can include various symptoms. These symptoms can include:

1. A general mood that has been low for more than a week
2. A change in appetite and/or weight
3. A change in sleep pattern, particularly early morning awakening
4. Loss of energy
5. Loss of interest in activities and/or sex
6. Feelings of guilt or self-reproach
7. Inability to concentrate
8. Thoughts of suicide

Depression becomes a medical problem when normal functioning is significantly hampered. Three major categories of depression are recognized: reactive depression, endogenous depression, and manic-depressive disorder.

*Reactive depression* is experienced after some significant loss in life. This depression is usually acute for a couple of weeks and resolves within 3 months. Therapy for reactive depression is to provide emotional support. One of the benzodiazepines, the antianxiety drugs, may be prescribed to relieve anxiety or insomnia if required. An antidepressant drug typically is not needed.

*Endogenous depression* is depression with no apparent cause. The current view is that endogenous depression is a neurochemical disorder treatable with appropriate drug therapy. This concept arose from the observation in the 1950s that reserpine caused depression in patients treated for hypertension. Reserpine was found to deplete the neurotransmitter norepinephrine. About the same time, isoproniazid, a drug then used to treat tuberculosis, was found to relieve depression in patients. Isoproniazid inhibited the degradation of norepinephrine by inhibiting the enyzme monoamine oxidase. These two observations suggested that a deficiency in the brain neurotransmitter norepinephrine is associated with depression. Current evidence favors a biogenic amine theory of depression, in which a deficiency either in brain norepinephrine or in another amine neurotransmitter, serotonin, is associated with depression. Two drug classes currently used to treat depression, tricyclic antidepressants and the monoamine oxidase inhibitors, have pharmacologic mechanisms that restore norepinephrine and serotonin in the brain.

*Manic-depressive* is the third major type of depressive disorder. The classic manic-depressive patient has a manic period characterized by excessive euphoria, overactivity, a flow of ideas, extreme self-confidence, and little need for sleep, alternating with a period of depression. Lithium is the specific drug treatment for mania.

Depression is also the side effect of some drugs, especially the antihypertensive drugs reserpine, methyldopa, guanethidine, and propranolol. Alcohol and antianxiety drugs often unmask depression by alleviating the anxiety that frequently accompanies depression. Steroids, particularly glucocorticoids and oral contraceptives, can cause depression. Drug-induced depression mimics endogenous depression but is treated by removing the drug or lowering the dose.

# Tricylic antidepressants

amitriptyline ~ desipramine ~ doxepine ~ imipramine ~ nortriptyline ~ protriptyline ~ trimipramine

**DRUG COMBINATIONS**    amitriptyline hydrochloride and perphenazine: Etrafon, Triavil

**OVERVIEW OF THE DRUG CLASS**    The tricyclic antidepressants derive their name from their basic three-ring chemical structure. The pharmacology of these drugs is complex and in many ways resembles that of the phenothiazines with the sedative and anticholinergic side effects. The tricyclic antidepressants vary in the degree of sedation and anticholinergic side effects they produce.

**MECHANISM OF ACTION**    The tricyclic antidepressants block the reuptake of norepinephrine and/or serotonin into their presynaptic neurons. This action causes an increase in the synaptic concentration of these neurotransmitters, which is an early effect of the drug. However, clinically no antidepressant response is seen for 2 weeks. Recent research suggests that the tricyclic antidepressants also alter the sensitivity of brain tissue to the action of norepinephrine and serotonin. Since this effect takes 2 weeks to become established, this action more closely correlates with the onset of the clinical antidepressant action.

**INDICATIONS**    Depression.

**CONTRAINDICATIONS**    **Recent myocardial infarction or cardiac disease** The anticholinergic, adrenolytic, and quinidine-like actions of the tricyclic antidepressants can compromise cardiac function.    **Hyperthyroidism** These patients are at risk for developing cardiac arrhythmias.

**DRUG INTERACTIONS**    **Monoamine oxidase inhibitors** May cause a hypertensive crisis and/or a high fever if combined with tricyclic antidepressants.    **Guanethidine, clonidine** The antihypertensive effects with these drugs may be blocked by tricyclic antidepressants.    **Anticholinergics** The anticholinergic effects are potentiated by tricyclic antidepressants.    **Sympathomimetics** Sympathomimetic effects are potentiated by tricyclic antidepressants.    **Alcohol, barbiturates, benzodiazepines** The CNS depressant effect of these drugs is potentiated by the tricyclic antidepressants.    **Methylphenidate** decreases the metabolism of the tricyclic antidepressants.

---

## ☙ NURSING CONSIDERATIONS

### Side effects, toxicities, and associated nursing actions

**CNS** Drowsiness is the most common; fatigue, lethargy, weakness or agitation, excitement, restlessness, and insomnia may occur.

- Assess for the development of these side effects.
- If drowsiness occurs, caution patients to avoid driving or operating hazardous equipment until the effects of the medication wear off. Tolerance to this side effect usually develops, but if severe or persistent, it may be necessary to lower the dose of drug. Notify the physician.
- Extrapyramidal side effects have been reported, and these are described in the Overview of Drug Class (p. 720) for antipsychotic drugs.
- Notify the physician if agitation, unusual behavior, anxiety, or extrapyramidal symptoms occur.

**CV** Postural hypotension, conduction arrhythmias, alterations in ECG pattern.

- Prior to beginning therapy, obtain baseline vital signs, blood pressure, and ECG rhythm strip.
- Monitor blood pressure every 4 to 8 hours when initiating therapy.
- Caution patients to move slowly from lying to sitting or standing. Supervise ambulation, especially of the elderly, if hypotension is present.
- Keep siderails up at night.

**Hematologic** Rarely, hypersensitivity reactions causing alteration in white blood cell counts. Monitor complete blood cell counts.

- Monitor complete blood count and white blood cell differential.
- Assess for agranulocytosis: fever, chills, malaise, sore throat.
- Assess for thrombocytopenia: unexplained bleeding or bruising, or development of petechiae.

**Anticholinergic** Anticholinergic side effects may include dry mouth, blurred vision, constipation, and

urinary retention.
- Monitor intake and output, and record frequency of stools. Auscultate bowel sounds.
- If constipation develops, advise patients to increase fluid intake to 2500 to 3000 ml per day, increase intake of fruits, juices, and fiber, and increase daily exercise. For some patients, it may be necessary for the physician to prescribe a stool softener.
- For xerostomia (dry mouth), advise patients to suck on hard candies or chew gum (sugarless, to avoid dental caries and weight gain), drink frequent sips of water, avoid lemon-glycerin swabs or other rinses that are drying or irritating, but perform regular oral hygiene. Some patients may wish to use a commercially available saliva substitute.
- If blurred vision occurs, caution patient to avoid driving or operating hazardous equipment until the effects of the medication lessen. Notify the physician.
- Urinary retention is more common in the elderly, the immobilized, and in men with preexisting prostatic hypertrophy.

**Allergic** Rash, edema, drug fever, photosensitivity.
- Assess for manifestations of allergic response.
- Caution patients to avoid prolonged exposure to the sun. If photosensitivity appears to be developing, caution patients to wear a hat, long-sleeve shirt, and long pants while in the sun, and to use a maximum-protection sunscreen.

**Other** Changes in transaminase or alkaline phosphatase levels may be seen.
- Monitor liver function tests.
- Assess for development of jaundice, right upper quadrant abdominal pain, change in color or consistency of stools.

## Nursing interventions related to drug administration
- Concentrated solutions are available for some of the antidepressants; consult manufacturer's literature for appropriate diluents.
- Supervise the patient carefully to ascertain that the medication is swallowed and not hidden in the mouth to be discarded or stored by the patient.
- The risk of suicide is present in seriously depressed patients and may persist for several weeks after the patient begins antidepressant therapy. Be alert to patient comments and behavior. Use institutional guidelines for initiation of suicide precautions.

## Patient and family education
- Review the expected benefits and possible side effects of therapy with the patient and/or family.
- Reassure patients that several weeks of drug therapy are needed to produce a significant change in the patient's condition.
- Review with patients that need to continue taking the medication as ordered, even if the patient begins to feel subjective improvement. It is the continued therapeutic blood levels of the drugs that help maintain subjective feelings of improvement.
- Caution patients to avoid taking over-the-counter medications without prior approval from the physician and to keep all health care providers informed of all medications being taken.
- As the patient's mood improves, appetite may improve, and some patients will find weight gain to be a problem. If weight gain is significant, a change in drug or dosage may be indicated, or the patient may need to be instructed in a calorie-restricted diet.
- Safe use in pregnancy has not been established for many of these drugs. Advise women who think they may be pregnant to consult their physicians. Women of childbearing age may wish to use some form of birth control. Lactating women who are prescribed antidepressants should consult their physicians before breastfeeding.
- Caution patients to avoid stopping these medications suddenly.
- Caution patients to keep these and all medications out of the reach of children.
- Tricyclic antidepressants may elevate or lower blood glucose levels. Caution diabetic patients about this. Diabetic patients may need to monitor blood glucose levels more often, and may need a change in diet or dose of insulin.
- Instruct patients to avoid the use of alcohol.
- Instruct patients to take these drugs with meals or snack to lessen gastric irritation.

## amitriptyline hydrochloride    (a-mee-TRIP-ti-leen)    antidepressant

- amitriptyline hydrochloride: Amitril, ✤Apo-Amitriptyline, Elavil, Emitrip, Endep, ✤Levate, ✤Meravil, ✤Novotriptyn, SK-Amitriptyline

**MECHANISM OF ACTION**    The tricyclic antidepressants all block the reuptake of norepinephrine and/or serotonin into their presynaptic neurons.

**INDICATIONS**    Depression.

**CONTRAINDICATIONS**    **Recent myocardial infarction or cardiac disease** The anticholinergic, adrenolytic, and quinidine-like actions of the tricyclic antidepressants can compromise cardiac function.    **Hyperthyroidism** These patients are at risk for developing cardiac arrhythmias.

**DOSAGE**    **PO:**    **ADULTS:** Initial doses are 75 to 100 mg daily. Hospitalized patients may be started at a higher dose. Dosage is gradually adjusted to produce maximum therapeutic effect with minimum toxicity. Maximum antidepressant effects may take 2 weeks or more and may require up to 300 mg daily. When symptoms are controlled, the dose should be gradually lowered to a maintenance therapeutic range of 25 to 100 mg daily.    **IM:**    **ADULTS:** 20 to 30 mg 4 times daily.    *Special patient populations:* **ELDERLY:** Geriatric patients should be started with 10 mg three times daily with 20 mg at bedtime. **CHILDREN:** Adolescent patients should be started with 10 mg three times daily with 20 mg at bedtime. Not recommended for children under 12 years old.    **PREGNANCY:** Safe use has not been established. Amitriptyline and its metabolite appear in breast milk, but the concentrations are not large enough to be detected in the serum of a nursing infant.

**PREPARATIONS**    *Tablets, film-coated:* 10, 25, 50, 75, 100, 150 mg. *Injection:* 10 mg/ml. ✤*Syrup:* 10 mg/5 ml.

**DRUG INTERACTIONS**    **Monoamine oxidase inhibitors** May cause a hypertensive crisis and/or a high fever if combined with tricyclic antidepressants.    **Guanethidine clonidine** The antihypertensive effects with these drugs may be blocked by tricyclic antidepressants.    **Anticholinergics** The anticholinergic effects are potentiated by tricyclic antidepressants.    **Sympathomimetics** Sympathomimetic effects are potentiated by tricyclic antidepressants.    **Alcohol, barbiturates, benzodiazepines** The CNS depressant effect of these drugs is potentiated by the tricyclic antidepressants.    **Methylphenidate** decreases the metabolism of the tricyclic antidepressants.

**FATE**    Amitriptyline is rapidly absorbed. It is metabolized to nortriptyline, which is also active. The plasma *half-life* is 10 to 50 hours. Metabolites are excreted in the urine.

### ☙ NURSING CONSIDERATIONS

#### Side effects, toxicities, and associated nursing actions
- See entry for drug class (p. 738).

#### Nursing interventions related to drug administration
- See entry for drug class (p. 739).
- For IM injection, choose a large, well-developed muscle mass such as the dorsogluteal site or rectus femoris muscle in adults, or the vastus lateralis in children. Aspirate before injecting to avoid inadvertent IV administration. Rotate and record sites.
- While this drug is often administered in divided doses, it is long acting and may usually be administered once a day with satisfactory results.
- Administration of a daily single dose, or of any increases in dosage, at bedtime, may lessen daytime sedation. Patients who experience insomnia or stimulation may benefit from taking the single dose in the morning.

#### Patient and family education
- See entry for drug class (p. 739).

## desipramine hydrochloride    (dess-IP-ra-meen)    antidepressant

- desipramine hydrochloride: Norpramin, Pertofrane

**MECHANISM OF ACTION**    The tricyclic antidepressants all block the reuptake of norepinephrine and/or serotonin into their presynaptic neurons.

**INDICATIONS**    Depression.

**CONTRAINDICATIONS**   **Recent myocardial infarction or cardiac disease** The anticholinergic, adrenolytic, and quinidine-like actions of the tricyclic antidepressants can compromise cardiac function.   **Hyperthyroidism** These patients are at risk for developing cardiac arrhythmias.

**DOSAGE**   **PO:**   **ADULTS:** Initial doses are 75 to 150 mg daily. Hospitalized patients may be started at a higher dose. Dosage is gradually adjusted to produce maximum therapeutic effect with minimum toxicity. Maximum antidepressant effects may take 2 weeks or more and may require up to 300 mg daily. When symptoms are controlled, the dose should be gradually lowered to a maintenance therapeutic range of 25 to 100 mg daily.   *Special patient populations:*   **ELDERLY:** Geriatric patients should be started with 25 to 50 mg daily. Doses greater than 100 mg are seldom needed.   **CHILDREN:** Adolescent patients should be started with 25 to 50 mg daily. Doses greater than 100 mg are seldom needed. Not recommended for children under 12 years old.   **PREGNANCY:** Safe use has not been established.

**PREPARATIONS**   *Capsules:* 25, 50 mg. *Tablets:* 10, 25, 50, 75, 100, 150 mg. Tablets contain tartrazine.

**DRUG INTERACTIONS**   **Monoamine oxidase inhibitors** may cause a hypertensive crisis and/or a high fever if combined with tricyclic antidepressants.   **Guanethidine, clonidine** The antihypertensive effects with these drugs may be blocked by tricyclic antidepressants.   **Anticholinergics** The anticholinergic effects are potentiated by tricyclic antidepressants.   **Sympathomimetics** Sympathomimetic effects are potentiated by tricyclic antidepressants.   **Alcohol, barbiturates, benzodiazepines** The CNS depressant effect of these drugs is potentiated by the tricyclic antidepressants.   **Methylphenidate** decreases the metabolism of the tricyclic antidepressants.

**FATE**   Desipramine is well absorbed. The plasma *half life* ranges from 7 to 60 hours. Desipramine is metabolized by the liver and metabolites are excreted in the urine.

☙ **NURSING CONSIDERATIONS**

**Side effects, toxicities, and associated nursing actions**
- See entry for drug class (p. 738).

**Nursing interventions related to drug administration**
- See entry for drug class (p. 739).
- While this drug is often administered in divided doses, it is long-acting and may usually be administered once a day with satisfactory results.
- Administration of a daily single dose, or of any increases in dosage, at bedtime, may lessen daytime sedation. Patients who experience insomnia or stimulation may benefit from taking the single dose in the morning.
- Normpramin brand tablets in 25, 50, 75, and 100 mg strengths contain FD & C coloring # 5 (tartrazine), which may cause an allergic reaction in susceptible individuals. While rare, this side effect is seen more often in persons with aspirin hypersensitivity.

**Patient and family education**
- See entry for drug class (p. 739).

---

## doxepin hydrochloride   (DOX-e-pin)                                        antidepressant

- doxepin hydrochloride: Adapin, Sinequan, ✽Triadapin

**MECHANISM OF ACTION**   The tricyclic antidepressants all block the reuptake of norepinephrine and/or serotonin into their presynaptic neurons.

**INDICATIONS**   Depression.

**CONTRAINDICATIONS**   **Recent myocardial infarction or cardiac disease** The anticholinergic, adrenolytic, and quinidine-like actions of the tricyclic antidepressants can compromise cardiac function.   **Hyperthyroidism** These patients are at risk for developing cardiac arrhythmias.

**DOSAGE**   **PO:**   **ADULTS:** Initial doses are 30 to 150 mg daily. Dosage is gradually adjusted for therapeutic effect with minimum toxicity and seldom exceeds 300 mg daily. A single dose should not exceed 150 mg. After the therapeutic effect is established, the dosage may be gradually reduced to a level that still maintains relief of symptoms.   *Special patient populations:*   **ELDERLY:** Altered doses for the elderly have not been specifically established. In general, geriatric patients require a lower dose.

**CHILDREN:** Not recommended for children under 12 years old.    **PREGNANCY:** Safe use has not been established. Doxepin is excreted in breast milk and has been reported to cause sedation and respiratory depression in a nursing infant whose mother was taking doxepin. For this reason, doxepin should not be taken by nursing mothers.

**PREPARATIONS**    *Capsules:* 10, 25, 50, 75, 100, 150 mg. *Solution (oral):* 10 mg/ml.

**DRUG INTERACTIONS**    **Monoamine oxidase inhibitors** may cause a hypertensive crisis and/or a high fever if combined with tricyclic antidepressants.    **Guanethidine, clonidine** The antihypertensive effects with these drugs may be blocked by tricyclic antidepressants.    **Anticholinergics** The anticholinergic effects are potentiated by tricyclic antidepressants.    **Sympathomimetics** Sympathomimetic effects are potentiated by tricyclic antidepressants.    **Alcohol, barbiturates, benzodiazepines** The CNS depressant effect of these drugs is potentiated by the tricyclic antidepressants.    **Methylphenidate** decreases the metabolism of the tricyclic antidepressants.

**FATE**    Doxepin is well absorbed. The plasma *half-life* is 6 to 8 hours. Doxepin is metabolized by the liver, and at least one metabolite is active. Excretion is in the urine.

**☙ NURSING CONSIDERATIONS**

**Side effects, toxicities, and associated nursing actions**
- See entry for drug class (p. 738).

**Nursing interventions related to drug administration**
- See entry for drug class (p. 739).
- The oral concentrate should be diluted with 120 ml of compatible diluent. Consult manufacturer's literature. Grape juice should not be used as a diluent for patients also on methadone therapy, and many carbonated beverages are incompatible.
- While this drug is often administered in divided doses, it is long-acting and may usually be administered once a day with satisfactory results.
- Administration of a daily single dose, or of any increases in dosage, at bedtime, may lessen daytime sedation. Patients who experience insomnia or stimulation may benefit from taking the single dose in the morning.

**Patient and family education**
- See entry for drug class (p. 739).

---

# imipramine hydrochloride, imipramine pamoate
(im-IP-ra-meen)                                                                                antidepressant

- imipramine hydrochloride, imipramine pamoate: ♣Apo-Imipramine, Janimine Filmtab, ♣Novopramine, SK-Pramine, Tipramine, Tofranil

**MECHANISM OF ACTION**    The tricyclic antidepressants all block the reuptake of norepinephrine and/or serotonin into their presynaptic neurons.

**INDICATIONS**    Depression. **Enuresis** Imipramine can help control function enuresis in children.

**CONTRAINDICATION**    **Recent myocardial infarction or cardiac disease** The anticholinergic, adrenolytic, and quinidine-like actions of the tricyclic antidepressants can compromise cardiac function.    **Hyperthyroidism** These patients are at risk for developing cardiac arrhythmias.

**DOSAGE**    **PO:**    **ADULTS:** Initial dose is 75 to 100 mg daily. Dosage may be increased gradually up to 200 mg but no more than 300 mg if needed. Hospitalized patients may be started at higher doses. When symptoms have been controlled, dosage may be decreased gradually to maintain relief with minimum side effects. Maintenance dose is generally 50 to 150 mg daily.    **CHILDREN:** *For depression, children over 12 years old,* 30 to 40 mg daily initially. Dosage may be increased gradually to 100 mg if necessary. *Children under 12 years old:* 1.5 mg/kg daily initially, increased every 3 to 4 days by 1 mg/kg daily to a maximum of 5 mg/kg daily if required. *For enuresis, children over 6 years old only:* 25 mg daily initially, 1 hour before bedtime. If response is not satisfactory after 1 week, increase to 50 mg nightly for children under 12 years old; 75 mg is the maximum dose for children over 12 years old.

**IM:**    **ADULTS:** 100 mg daily in divided doses.    *Special patient populations:*    **ELDERLY:** Geriatric patients are given 30 to 40 mg daily initially. Dosage may be increased gradually to 100 mg if necessary.    **CHILDREN:** Pediatric doses are given above.    **PREGNANCY:** Safe use has not been established.

**PREPARATIONS**    Hydrochloride form, *tablets:* 10, 25, 50 mg. *Tablets, film-coated:* 10, 25, 50 mg. *Injection:* 12.5 mg/ml. Pamoate form, *capsules:* 75, 100, 125, 150 mg.

**DRUG INTERACTIONS**    **Monoamine oxidase inhibitors** may cause a hypertensive crisis and/or a high fever if combined with tricyclic antidepressants.    **Guanethidine, clonidine** The antihypertensive effects with these drugs may be blocked by tricyclic antidepressants.    **Anticholinergics** The anticholinergic effects are potentiated by tricyclic antidepressants.    **Sympathomimetics** Sympathomimetic effects are potentiated by tricyclic antidepressants.    **Alcohol, barbiturates, benzodiazepines** The CNS depressant effect of these drugs is potentiated by the tricyclic antidepressants.    **Methylphenidate** decreases the metabolism of the tricyclic antidepressants.

**FATE**    Imipramine is well absorbed and metabolized by the liver to desipramine, which is also active, and other compounds. The plasma *half-life* of imipramine is 8 to 16 hours. Metabolites are excreted in the urine.

## ☙ NURSING CONSIDERATIONS

### Side effects, toxicities, and associated nursing actions
- See entry for drug class (p. 738).

### Nursing interventions related to drug administration
- See entry for drug class (p. 739).
- For IM injection, choose a large, well-developed muscle mass such as the dorsogluteal site or rectus femoris muscle in adults, or the vastus lateralis in children. Aspirate before injecting to avoid inadvertent IV administration. Rotate and record sites.
- While this drug is often administered in divided doses, it is long-acting and may usually be administered once a day with satisfactory results.
- Administration of a daily single dose, or of any increases in dosage, at bedtime, may lessen daytime sedation. Patients who experience insomnia or stimulation may benefit from taking the single dose in the morning.
- For enuresis, the prescribed daily dose is usually administered 1 hour before bedtime. For early night bedwetters, it may be better to administer the dose in the late afternoon. Consult the physician.
- Tofranil brand tablets, Janimine Filmtab brand in 10 and 25 mg dose tablets, and Tofranil-PM brand 100 and 125 mg capsules contain FD & C coloring number 5 (tartrazine), which may cause an allergic response in susceptible individuals. While rare, this reaction is seen more often in persons with aspirin hypersensitivity.

### Patient and family education
- See entry for drug class (p. 739).

## nortriptyline hydrochloride    (nor-TRIP-ti-leen)    antidepressant

- nortriptyline hydrochloride: Aventyl, Pamelor

**MECHANISM OF ACTION**    The tricyclic antidepressants all block the reuptake of norepinephrine and/or serotonin into their presynaptic neurons.

**INDICATIONS**    • Depression.

**CONTRAINDICATIONS**    **Recent myocardial infarction or cardiac disease** The anticholinergic, adrenolytic, and quinidine-like actions of the tricyclic antidepressants can compromise cardiac function.    **Hyperthyroidism** These patients are at risk for developing cardiac arrhythmias.

**DOSAGE**    **PO:**    **ADULTS:** Initial doses are 75 to 100 mg daily. Hospitalized patients may be started at a higher dose. Dosage is gradually adjusted to produce maximum therapeutic effect with minimum toxicity. Maximum antidepressant effects may take 2 weeks or more and may require up to 300 mg daily. When symptoms are controlled, the dose may be gradually lowered. *Special patient populations:* **ELDERLY:** Geriatric patients should be started with 30 to 50 mg daily. Doses greater than 100 mg are seldom needed.    **CHILDREN:** Adolescent patients should be started with 30 to 50 mg daily. Doses greater than 100 mg are seldom needed. Not recommended for children under 12 years old.    **PREGNANCY:** Safe use has not been established.

**PREPARATIONS**    *Capsules:* 10, 25, 75 mg. *Solution (oral):* 10 mg/5 ml.

**DRUG INTERACTIONS**    **Monoamine oxidase inhibitors** may cause a hypertensive crisis and/or a high fever if combined with tricyclic antidepressants.    **Guanethidine, clonidine** The antihypertensive effects with these drugs may be blocked by tricyclic antidepressants.    **Anticholinergics** The anticholinergic effects are potentiated by tricyclic antidepressants.    **Sympathomimetics** Sympathomimetic effects are potentiated by tricyclic antidepressants.    **Alcohol, barbiturates, benzodiazepines** The CNS depressant effect of these drugs is potentiated by the tricyclic antidepressants.    **Methylphenidate** decreases the metabolism of the tricyclic antidepressants.

**FATE**    Nortriptyline has a plasma *half-life* of 16 to 90 hours. Nortriptyline is metabolized by the liver and metabolites are excreted in the urine.

## ❦ NURSING CONSIDERATIONS

### Side effects, toxicities, and associated nursing actions
- See entry for drug class (p. 738).

### Nursing interventions related to drug administration
- See entry for drug class (p. 739).
- While this drug is often administered in divided doses, it is long-acting and may usually be administered once a day with satisfactory results.
- Administration of a daily single dose, or of any increases in dosage, at bedtime, may lessen daytime sedation. Patients who experience insomnia or stimulation may benefit from taking the single dose in the morning.

### Patient and family education
- See entry for drug class (p. 739).

---

## protriptyline hydrochloride    (pro-TRIP-ti-leen)    antidepressant

- protriptyline hydrochloride: ✸Triptil, Vivactil

**MECHANISM OF ACTION**    The tricyclic antidepressants all block the reuptake of norepinephrine and/or serotonin into their presynaptic neurons.

**INDICATIONS**    • Depression.

**CONTRAINDICATIONS**    **Recent myocardial infarction or cardiac disease** The anticholinergic, adrenolytic, and quinidine-like actions of the tricyclic antidepressants can compromise cardiac function.    **Hyperthyroidism** These patients are at risk for developing cardiac arrhythmias.

**DOSAGE**    **PO:**    **ADULTS:** Initial doses are 15 to 40 mg daily. Hospitalized patients may be started at a higher dose. Dosage is gradually adjusted to produce maximum therapeutic effect with minimum toxicity. Maximum antidepressant effects may take 2 weeks or more and may require up to 60 mg daily. When symptoms are controlled, the dose may be gradually lowered. *Special patient populations:* **ELDERLY:** Geriatric patients should be started with 5 mg three times daily. Doses greater than 20 mg are seldom needed.    **CHILDREN:** Adolescent patients should be started with 5 mg three times daily. Doses greater than 20 mg are seldom needed. Not recommended for children under 12 years old.    **PREGNANCY:** Safe use has not been established.

**PREPARATIONS**    *Tablets (film-coated):* 5, 10 mg.

**DRUG INTERACTIONS**    **Monoamine oxidase inhibitors** May cause a hypertensive crisis and/or a high fever if combined with tricyclic antidepressants.    **Guanethidine, clonidine** The antihypertensive effects with these drugs may be blocked by tricyclic antidepressants.    **Antichlolinergics** The anticholinergic effects are poteniated by tricyclic antidepressants.    **Sympathomimetics** Sympathomimetic effects are potentiated by tricyclic antidepressants.    **Alcohol, barbiturates, benzodiazepines** The CNS depressant effect of these drugs is potentiated by the tricyclic antidepressants.    **Methylphenidate** Decreases the metabolism of the tricyclic antidepressants.

**FATE**    Protriptyline is well absorbed. Metabolism and excretion are slow. Only 50% of the drug is excreted in 16 days.

## ☙ NURSING CONSIDERATIONS

### Side effects, toxicities, and associated nursing actions
- See entry for drug class (p. 738).

### Nursing interventions related to drug administration
- See entry for drug class (p. 739).
- While this drug is often administered in divided doses, it is long-acting and may usually be administered once a day with satisfactory results.
- Administration of a daily single dose, or of any increases in dosage, at bedtime, may lessen daytime sedation. Patients who experience insomnia or stimultion may benefit from taking the single dose in the morning.

### Patient and family education
- See entry for drug class (p. 739).

---

## trimipramine maleate    (trye-MIP-ra-meen)    antidepressant

- trimipramine maleate: Surmontil

**MECHANISM OF ACTION**    The tricyclic antidepressants all block the reuptake of norepinephrine and/or serotonin into their presynaptic neurons.

**INDICATIONS**    • Depression.

**CONTRAINDICATIONS**    **Recent myocardial infarction or cardiac disease** The anticholinergic, adrenolytic, and quinidine-like actions of the tricyclic antidepressants can compromise cardiac function.    **Hyperthyroidism** These patients are at risk for developing cardiac arrhythmias.

**DOSAGE**    **PO:**    **ADULTS:** Initial doses are 75 to 100 mg daily. Hospitalized patients may be started at a higher dose. Dosage is gradually adjusted to produce maximum therapeutic effect with minimum toxicity. Maximum antidepressant effects may take 2 weeks or more and may require up to 300 mg daily. When symptoms are controlled, the dose may be gradually lowered. *Special patient populations:* **ELDERLY:** Geriatric patients should be started with 50 mg daily. Doses greater than 150 mg are seldom needed.    **CHILDREN:** Adolescent patients should be started with 50 mg daily. Doses greater than 300 mg are seldom needed. Not recommended for children under 12 years old.    **PREGNANCY:** Safe use has not been established.

**PREPARATIONS**    *Capsules*: 25, 50, 100 mg.

**DRUG INTERACTIONS**    **Monoamine oxidase inhibitors** may cause a hypertensive crisis and/or a high fever if combined with tricyclic antidepressants.    **Guanethidine, clonidine** The antihypertensive effects with these drugs may be blocked by tricyclic antidepressants.    **Anticholinergics** The anticholinergic effects are potentiated by tricyclic antidepressants.    **Sympathomimetics** Sympathomimetic effects are potentiated by tricyclic antidepressants.    **Alcohol, barbiturates, benzodiazepines** The CNS depressant effect of these drugs is potentiated by the tricyclic antidepressants.    **Methylphenidate** Decreases the metabolism of the tricyclic antidepressants.

**FATE**    Trimipramine is well absorbed and metabolized by the liver. The plasma *half-life* is 9 hours. Metabolites are excreted in the urine.

## ☙ NURSING CONSIDERATIONS

### Side effects, toxicities, and associated nursing actions
- See entry for drug class (p. 738).

### Nursing interventions related to drug administration
- See entry for drug class (p. 739).

- While this drug is often administered in divided doses, it is long-acting. If the daily dose does not exceed 200 mg, it may usually be administered once a day with satisfactory results.
- Administration of a daily single dose, or of any increases in dosage, at bedtime, may lessen daytime sedation. Patients who experience insomnia or stimulation may benefit from taking the single dose in the morning.

**Patient and family education**
- See entry for drug class (p. 739).

# Second-generation antidepressants

amoxapine ~ bupropion ~ maprotiline ~ trazodone

**OVERVIEW OF THE DRUG CLASS**    New antidepressant drugs have been introduced that are neither tricyclics nor monoamine oxidase inhibitors. They are regarded as alternatives to tricyclic antidepressants, although their action on norepinephrine and serotonin uptake is not necessarily similar to that of the tricyclics. The new antidepressant drugs have, to a varying degree, a lesser incidence of anticholinergic side effects, less cardiotoxicity, and a faster onset of action than the tricyclics.

**MECHANISM OF ACTION**    These compounds tend to have a selective effect on norepinephrine or serotonin uptake. See the individual drug.

**INDICATIONS**    • Depression.

**CONTRAINDICATIONS**    • See the individual drug.

**DRUG INTERACTIONS**    In general, the drug interactions for these newer drugs are not well characterized. Until experience is gathered, the drug interactions characteristic of the tricyclic antidepressants should be assumed.

## amoxapine    (a-mox-a-peen)                                                                                     antidepressant

- amoxapine: Asendin

**MECHANISM OF ACTION**    Amoxapine inhibits monoamine uptake. Amoxapine is a more potent inhibitor of norepinephrine uptake than of serotonin uptake. Amoxapine also blocks dopamine receptors. This action makes amoxapine effective in relieving anxiety and agitation.

**INDICATIONS**    Depression Amoxapine is also effective in relieving anxiety and agitation associated with depression.

**CONTRAINDICATIONS**    • Hypersensitivity to the drug. • Myocardial infarction, immediate recovery period. • Acute congestive heart failure.

**DOSAGE**    PO:    ADULTS: Initially, 150 mg daily. This is usually given as 1 dose at bedtime. The dose is raised gradually. The effective dose is usually 200 to 300 mg daily. Hospitalized patients may be started at higher doses. The therapeutic effect is generally evident in 2 weeks or less.    *Special patient populations:*    ELDERLY: Geriatric patients should be started at lower doses, usually 75 mg daily, increasing to 150 mg after 3 days if the drug is tolerated.    CHILDREN: Not currently recommended for children under 16 years of age.    PREGNANCY: Safe use has not been established. FDA pregnancy category C.

**PREPARATIONS**    *Tablets:* 25, 50, 100, 150 mg.

**DRUG INTERACTIONS**    **Monoamine oxidase inhibitors** At least 2 weeks should elapse between the time an MAO inhibitor is discontinued and bupropion is started.    **CNS depressants** Amoxapine potentiates the CNS depression of other drugs, including opiates, barbiturates, and alcohol.    **Anticholinergic drugs** Amoxapine potentiates anticholinergic effects.    **Sympathomimetic drugs** Amoxapine potentiates sympathomimetic effects.    **Cimetidine** Inhibits the metabolism of amoxapine.

**FATE**    Amoxapine is well absorbed and has a plasma *half-life* of 8 hours. Amoxapine is metabolized in the liver to active metabolites which are excreted principally in the urine, but also in the feces.

## ❦ NURSING CONSIDERATIONS

### Side effects, toxicities, and associated nursing actions

- See entry for drug class (p. 738). The following are unique to amoxapine:

**CNS** Sedation is minimum compared to traditional tricyclic antidepressants. Infrequently, extrapyramidal side effects.

**CV** Tachycardia and arrhythmias are less frequent than with the traditional tricyclic antidepressants.

**GI** Constipation.

**GU** Sexual disturbances have been reported occasionally.

- Assess patients tactfully for sexual disturbances; many patients are unwilling to discuss sexual problems. Provide emotional support as needed. Caution patients to avoid stopping medications without notifying the physician. Caution patients to take medications as ordered for best effect. Consult with physician about changes in drug or dosage.

**Other** Anticholinergic effects are minimum. Serum prolactin may be elevated and galactorrhea has been reported.

### Nursing interventions related to drug administration

- See entry for drug class (p. 739).
- While this drug is often administered in divided doses, it is long-acting and may usually be administered once a day with satisfactory results.
- Administration of a daily single dose, or of any increases in dosage, at bedtime, may lessen daytime sedation. Patients who experience insomnia or stimulation may benefit from taking the single dose in the morning.

### Patient and family education

- See entry for drug class (p. 739).

---

## bupropion hydrochloride   (byoo-PROE-pee-on)                                antidepressant

- bupropion hydrochloride: Wellbutrin

**MECHANISM OF ACTION**   Bupropion is unique in that no marked effect on norepinephrine or serotonin uptake has been demonstrated. Bupropion does block the reuptake of dopamine.

**INDICATIONS**   • Depression.

**CONTRAINDICATIONS**   • History of seizures.

**DOSAGE**   PO:   **ADULTS:** The recommended daily dose is 75 to 600 mg.   *Special patient populations:* **PREGNANCY:** Safe use has not been established. FDA pregnancy category C.

**PREPARATIONS**   *Tablets:* 75 mg.

**DRUG INTERACTIONS**   **Monoamine oxidase inhibitors** At least 2 weeks should elapse between the time an MAO inhibitor is discontinued and bupropion is started.   **Anticonvulsants** Higher doses may be required. In general, bupropion appears to carry a higher risk of seizure than other antidepressants, especially at doses exceeding 450 mg/day.

**FATE**   Bupropion is well absorbed but is readily metabolized by the liver. The *half-life* is about 12 hours.

## ❦ NURSING CONSIDERATIONS

### Side effects, toxicities, and associated nursing actions

- See entry for drug class (p. 738). The following are unique to bupropion:

**CNS** Agitation, insomnia, tremor, dizziness; headache or migraine; weight loss.

**Other** Dry mouth is the most common side effect. Other anticholinergic side effects include nausea or vomiting, excessive sweating. Bupropion increases the concentration of serum prolactin.

### Nursing interventions related to drug administration

- See entry for drug class (p. 739).
- While this drug is often administered in divided doses, it is long-acting and may usually be administered once a day with satisfactory results.

- Administration of a daily single dose, or of any increases in dosage, at bedtime, may lessen daytime sedation. Patients who experience insomnia or stimulation may benefit from taking the single dose in the morning.

**Patient and family education**
- See entry for drug class (p. 739).

---

## maprotiline hydrochloride  (ma-PROE-ti-leen)  antidepressant

- maprotiline hydrochloride: Ludiomil

**MECHANISM OF ACTION**  Maprotiline is a tetracyclic antidepressant that inhibits norepinephrine but not serotonin uptake.

**INDICATIONS**  • Depression.

**CONTRAINDICATIONS**  • Hypersensitivity to the drug. • Acute (closed-angle) glaucoma. • Recent myocardial infarction. • Acute congestive heart failure. • History of seizures.

**DOSAGE**  **PO:**  **ADULTS:** Initially, 75 mg daily. May be given in 3 divided doses or, more commonly, 1 dose. If no improvement in 2 weeks, gradually increase daily dose by 25 mg increments. A dose of 150 mg is usually effective for most outpatients. Hospitalized patients can be started at a 150 mg daily dose. Antidepressant effects should occur within 2 to 3 weeks.  *Special patient populations:*  **ELDERLY:** Geriatric patients should be started at lower doses, generally 10 mg three times daily. Maximum range for maintenance is 50 to 75 mg daily.  **CHILDREN:** Not recommended for children.  **PREGNANCY:** Safe use has not been established. FDA pregnancy category B.

**PREPARATIONS**  *Tablets (film-coated):* 25, 50, 75 mg.

**DRUG INTERACTIONS**  **Monoamine oxidase inhibitors** Maprotiline should not be taken concurrently with an MAO inhibitor. The MAO inhibitor should be discontinued for at least 14 days before maprotiline is administered.

**FATE**  Maprotiline is slowly absorbed, and *peak* plasma concentrations are reached only 8 to 24 hours after administration. The plasma *half-life* is about 51 hours. Maprotiline is metabolized in the liver to active metabolites. These are excreted primarily in the urine but also in the feces.

**☙ NURSING CONSIDERATIONS**

**Side effects, toxicities, and associated nursing actions**
- See entry for drug class (p. 738). The following are unique to maprotiline:
  **CNS** Drowsiness is the most common; fatigue, lethargy, weakness or agitation, excitement, restlessness, and insomnia may occur.
  **CV** Postural hypotension, conduction arrhythmias, alteration in ECG pattern.

**Nursing interventions related to drug administration**
- See entry for drug class (p. 739).
- While this drug is often administered in divided doses, it is long-acting and may usually be administered once a day with satisfactory results.
- Administration of a daily single dose, or of any increases in dosage, at bedtime, may lessen daytime sedation. Patients who experience insomnia or stimulation may benefit from taking the single dose in the morning.

**Patient and family education**
- See entry for drug class (p. 739).

---

## trazodone hydrochloride  (TRAY-zoe-done)  antidepressant

- trazodone hydrochloride: Desyrel

**MECHANISM OF ACTION**  Trazodone is chemically unrelated to other antidepressant drugs. Trazodone is on inhibitor of serotonin uptake.

**INDICATIONS**    • Depression. • Alcohol dependence.

**CONTRAINDICATIONS**    • Hypersensitivity to the drug. • Recent myocardial infarction.

**DOSAGE**    PO:    **ADULTS:** Initially, 150 mg daily in divided doses. Hospital patients can be started at higher doses. The dosage may be increased every 3 or 4 days if necessary. The maximum dosage is 400 mg daily for outpatients, 600 mg for hospitalized patients.    *Special patient populations:*    **ELDERLY:** Geriatric patients should be started at lower doses, 25 to 50 mg daily. May increase gradually to 100 to 150 mg daily if required.    **CHILDREN:** Not recommended for children under 18 years of age.    **PREGNANCY:** Safe use has not been established. FDA pregnancy category C.

**PREPARATIONS**    *Tablets:* 150 mg. *Tablets (film-coated):* 50, 100 mg.

**DRUG INTERACTIONS**    **MAO inhibitors** Trazodone should not be taken concurrently.    **Antihypertensive medications** Trazodone may lower the dose required since it has hypotensive effects.

**FATE**    Trazodone is rapidly absorbed, and absorption is aided when the drug is taken after a meal. Trazodone is metabolized by the liver and is eliminated principally in the urine within 72 hours. Trazodone disappears from the plasma in two phases. The first phase has a *half-life* of 3 to 6 hours, and the second phase is 5 to 9 hours.

### ❦ NURSING CONSIDERATIONS

#### Side effects, toxicities, and associated nursing actions

• See entry for drug class (p. 738). The following are unique to trazodone:
**CNS** Drowsiness is the most common; fatigue, lethargy, weakness.    **CV** Postural hypotension, conduction arrhythmias, or alteration in ECG pattern are not common for trazodone compared to traditional tricyclic antidepressants.

#### Nursing interventions related to drug administration

• See entry for drug class (p. 739).
• Trazodone should be taken shortly after a meal or light snack to decrease the incidence of dizziness or lightheadedness. Absorption of trazodone is affected by food, but with chronic therapy, the effect of food on effectiveness of the drug is not clinically important.
• Administration of any increases in dosage at bedtime may lessen daytime sedation. Patients who experience insomnia or stimulation may benefit from taking the single dose in the morning.

#### Patient and family education

• See entry for drug class (p. 739).

---

# Monoamine oxidase (MAO) inhibitors

isocarboxazid ~ phenelzine ~ tranylcypromine

**OVERVIEW OF THE DRUG CLASS**    The monoamine oxidase (MAO) inhibitors were in use before the tricyclic antidepressants were discovered. The MAO inhibitors are not as effective as the tricyclic antidepressants in treating common endogenous depression, but the MAO inhibitors are more effective in treating depression exhibited as phobias.

**MECHANISM OF ACTION**    The MAO inhibitors irreversibly inhibit the enzyme monoamine oxidase. According to the biogenic amine hypothesis of depression, the MAO inhibitors are effective because they prevent the degradation of norepinephrine and serotonin, so that the concentration of these central nervous system neurotransmitters is increased.

**INDICATIONS**    **Depression,** mainly atypical depression, agoraphobia (fear of open spaces), or hypochondriasis (anxiety about one's health). MAO inhibitors seem especially effective in reducing psychomotor retardation and morbid preoccupation of patients who are resistant to tricyclic antidepressants.

**CONTRAINDICATIONS**    **Noncompliance** MAO inhibitors are characterized by a number of food (Patient populations) and drug interactions that the patient must respect.

**DRUG INTERACTIONS**    **Sympathomimetic drugs, tricyclic antidepressants** These can cause a hypertensive crisis if given concurrently with an MAO inhibitor. Two weeks should be allowed between discontinuing a tricyclic antidepressant and starting a sympathomimetic drug.    **Alcohol, meperidine, sedatives, antihistamines** These are CNS depressants that have a synergistic depression with the MAO inhibitors.    **Antihypertensive drugs, diuretics** These act synergistically with MAO inhibitors to these drugs is exaggerated by an MAO inhibitor.

## ❧ NURSING CONSIDERATIONS

### Side effects, toxicities, and associated nursing actions

**CNS** Effects can be excitatory or inhibitory: restlessness, insomnia/drowsiness, anorexia/increased appetite, dizziness, weakness, headache. At high doses: variable effects on seizure threshold, activation of latent schizophrenia, hypomania, mania.

**Eye** Blurred vision, amblyopia.

- Assess for the development of these side effects.
- If drowsiness, dizziness, or visual disturbances occur, caution patients to avoid driving or operating hazardous equipment until the effects of the medication wear off or are evaluated. Notify the physician.
- Monitor weight. It may be necessary to monitor mealtimes or measure intake and output.
- Notify physician if agitation, anxiety, mania, or any marked changes in behavior occur.
- Be alert to alterations in seizure threshold. In patients with a history of seizures, pad siderails, and supervise patients carefully until the effects of the medication can be evaluated.

**CV** Orthostatic hypotension, suppression of anginal pain.

- Prior to beginning therapy, obtain baseline vital signs, blood pressure, ECG rhythm strip.
- Monitor blood pressure every 4 to 8 hours when initiating therapy or changing dosages.
- Caution patients to move slowly from lying to sitting or standing. Supervise ambulation, especially of the elderly, if hypotension is present.
- Keep siderails up at night.
- Caution patients with a history of heart disease or angina to avoid situations requiring exertion.

**GI** Constipation.

- Record frequency of stools.
- If constipation develops, advise patients to increase fluid intake to 2500 to 3000 ml per day, increase intake of fruits, juices, and fiber, and increase daily exercise. For some patients, it may be necessary for the physician to prescribe a stool softener.

**GU** Urinary retention.

- Urinary retention is more common in the elderly, the immobilized, and in men with preexisting prostatic hypertrophy.
- Monitor intake and output. Notify the physician if retention is suspected.

**Other** MAO inhibitors may lead to a hypertensive crisis if tyramine-containing foods or beverages are ingested.

- *Tyramine-containing foods* include avocados; bananas; beer; bologna; canned figs; chocolate; cheese (except cottage cheese); cheese-containing food such as pizza or macaroni and cheese; liver; meat extracts such as Marmite, Bovril; offal, papaya products, including meat tenderizers; paté; pickled and kippered herring; pepperoni; pods of broad beans (fava beans); raisins; raw yeast or yeast extracts; salami; sausage; sour cream; soy sauce; wine; chianti; yogurt.
- Review in detail with patient and household cook the sources of tyramine. Take diet history, and caution patients about food preferences or habits that may lead to tyramine ingestion.
- Caution patients to avoid excessive amounts of caffeine, although small amounts are acceptable. Review sources of caffeine: coffee, tea, many soft drinks, some over-the-counter medications.
- Symptoms of hypertensive crisis that might occur after ingestion of tyramine-rich foods include headache, palpitations, visual changes, neck stiffness or soreness, nausea, vomiting, sweating, photophobia, pupillary changes, and bradycardia or tachycardia. Hypertensive crisis is an emergency. Instruct the patient to seek medical attention if these symptoms occur.
- Instruct patients taking MAO inhibitors to wear a medical identification tag or bracelet.
- Instruct patients to avoid tyramine-containing foods for at least 3 weeks following cessation of therapy with MAO inhibitors.
- Phentolamine, the alpha receptor antagonist, is used to reduce the blood pressure in hypertensive crisis.

### Nursing interventions related to drug administration

- Supervise the patient carefully to ascertain that the medication is swallowed and not hidden in the mouth to be discarded or stored by the patient.

- The risk of suicide is present in seriously depressed patients and may persist for several weeks after the patient begins drug therapy. Be alert to patient comments and behavior. Use institutional guidelines for initiation of suicide precautions.

### Patient and family education

- Review the expected benefits and possible side effects of therapy with the patient and/or family.
- Review dietary restrictions with patient and family (see above).
- Reassure patients that several weeks of drug therapy are needed to produce significant changes in the patient's condition.
- Review with patients the need to continue taking the medication as ordered, even if the patient begins to feel subjective improvement. It is the continued therapeutic blood levels of the drugs that help maintain subjective feelings of improvement.
- Caution the patient to avoid taking over-the-counter medications without prior approval of the physician. Note the Drug interactions (p. 749). Caution patients to keep all health care providers informed of all medications being taken.
- If weight gain is significant, a change in drug or dosage may be indicated, or the patient may need to be instructed in a calorie-restricted diet.
- Safe use in pregnancy has not been established. Advise women who think they may be pregnant to consult their physicians. Women of childbearing age may wish to use some form of birth control. Lactating women who are prescribed MAO inhibitors should consult their physicians before breast-feeding.
- Caution patients to avoid the use of alcohol.
- MAO inhibitors may interact with insulin or oral hypoglycemic agents. Caution diabetic patients about this. Diabetic patients may need to monitor blood glucose levels more often and may need a change in diet or dose of insulin or hypoglycemic agent.
- Caution patients to report the development of jaundice, malaise, right upper quadrant abdominal pain, or change in the color or consistency of stools, as these may indicate liver involvement.
- Caution patients not to discontinue the medication without discussion with the physician.

---

## isocarboxazid (eye-so-kar-BOX-a-zid) antidepressant

- isocarboxazid: Marplan

**MECHANISM OF ACTION** The MAO inhibitors irreversibly inhibit the enzyme monoamine oxidase. According to the biogenic amine hypothesis of depression, the MAO inhibitors are effective because they prevent the degradation of norepinephrine and serotonin, so that the concentration of these central nervous system neurotransmitters is increased.

**INDICATIONS** • Depression.

**CONTRAINDICATIONS** Noncompliance MAO inhibitors are characterized by a number of food (see Patient populations) and drug interactions that the patient must respect.

**DOSAGE** PO: ADULTS: Initially, 30 mg daily, in single or divided doses. When the patient is improved, the dosage should be lowered, generally to a maintenance dose of 10 to 20 mg. *Special patient populations:* ELDERLY: Elderly patients are more prone to the side effects of MAO inhibitors, so these drugs should be used especially cautiously with geriatric patients. CHILDREN: MAO inhibitors are not recommended for children. PREGNANCY: Safe use has not been established.

**PREPARATIONS** *Tablets:* 10 mg.

**DRUG INTERACTIONS** Sympathomimetic drugs, tricyclic antidepressants These can cause a hypertensive crisis if given concurrently with an MAO inhibitor. Two weeks should be allowed between discontinuing a tricyclic antidepressant and starting a sympathomimetic drug. Alcohol, meperidine, sedatives, antihistamines These are CNS depressants that have a synergistic depression with the MAO inhibitors. Antihypertensive drugs, diuretics These act synergistically with MAO inhibitors to cause orthostatic hypotension. Insulin, oral hypoglycemic agents The hypoglycemic response to these drugs is exaggerated by an MAO inhibitor.

**FATE** The metabolic fate of MAO inhibitors is not well characterized. These drugs are cumulative. The *onset of action* may take several days or weeks. The effects persist for up to 3 weeks after the drug is discontinued.

### ❦ NURSING CONSIDERATIONS

#### Side effects, toxicities, and associated nursing actions
- See entry for drug class (p. 750).

#### Nursing interventions related to drug administration
- See entry for drug class (p. 750).
- Administration of a single daily dose, or of any increases in dosage, at bedtime, may lessen daytime sedation. Patients who experience insomnia or stimulation may benefit from taking the single dose in the morning.

#### Patient and family education
- See entry for drug class (p. 751).

---

## phenelzine sulfate  (FEN-el-zeen)  antidepressant

- phenelzine sulfate: Nardil

**MECHANSIM OF ACTION** The MAO inhibitors irreversibly inhibit the enzyme monoamine oxidase. According to the biogenic amine hypothesis of depression, the MAO inhibitors are effective because they prevent the degradation of norepinephrine and serotonin, so that the concentration of these central nervous system neurotransmitters is increased.

**INDICATIONS** • Depression.

**CONTRAINDICATIONS** **Noncompliance** MAO inhibitors are characterized by a number of food (see Patient populations) and drug interactions that the patient must respect.

**DOSAGE** **PO:** **ADULTS:** Initially, 15 mg three times daily. May be increased to 60 mg daily if tolerated. Maximum effect is seen in 2 to 6 weeks. Thereafter, the dose should be lowered slowly. The maintenance dose may be as low as 15 mg daily or every other day. *Special patient populations:* **ELDERLY:** Elderly patients are more prone to the side effects of MAO inhibitors, so these drugs should be used especially cautiously for geriatric patients. **CHILDREN:** MAO inhibitors are not recommended for children. **PREGNANCY:** Safe use has not been established.

**PREPARATIONS** *Tablets:* 15 mg.

**DRUG INTERACTIONS** **Sympathomimetic drugs, tricyclic antidepressants** These can cause a hypertensive crisis if given concurrently with an MAO inhibitor. Two weeks should be allowed between discontinuing a tricyclic antidepressant and starting a sympathomimetic drug. **Alcohol, meperidine, sedatives, antihistamines** These are CNS depressants that have a synergistic depression with the MAO inhibitors. **Antihypertensive drugs, diuretics** These act synergistically with MAO inhibitors to cause orthostatic hypotension. **Insulin, oral hypoglycemic agents** The hypoglycemic response to these drugs is exaggerated by an MAO inhibitor.

**FATE** The metabolic fate of MAO inhibitors is not well characterized. These drugs are cumulative. The *onset of action* may take several days or week. The effects persist for up to 3 weeks after the drug is discontinued.

### ❦ NURSING CONSIDERATIONS

#### Side effects, toxicities, and associated nursing actions
- See entry for drug class (p. 750).

#### Nursing interventions related to drug administration
- See entry for drug class (p. 750).
- Administration of a single daily dose, or of any increases in dosage, at bedtime, may lessen daytime sedation. Patients who experience insomnia or stimulation may benefit from taking the single dose in the morning.

- See entry for drug class (p. 751).

---

## tranylcypromine sulfate    (tran-ill-SIP-roe-meen)    antidepressant

- tranylcypromine sulfate: Parnate

**MECHANISM OF ACTION**    The MAO inhibitors irreversibly inhibit the enzyme monoamine oxidase. According to the biogenic amine hypothesis of depression, the MAO inhibitors are effective because they prevent the degradation of norepinephrine and serotonin, so that the concentration of these central nervous system neurotransmitters is increased.

**INDICATIONS**  • Depression.

**CONTRAINDICATIONS**    Noncompliance MAO inhibitors are characterized by a number of food (see Patient populations) and drug interactions that the patient must respect.

**DOSAGE**    **PO:**    **ADULTS:** Initially, 20 mg daily in 2 doses, 10 mg in the morning and 10 mg in the afternoon. If no response after 2 to 3 weeks, increase the morning dose to 20 mg for a total of 30 mg daily. After a response is established, the dosage may be gradually lowered to a daily dose of 10 to 20 mg.    *Special patient populations:*    **ELDERLY:** Elderly patients are more prone to the side effects of MAO inhibitors, so these drugs should be used especially cautiously for geriatric patients.    **CHILDREN:** MAO inhibitors are not recommended for children.    **PREGNANCY:** Safe use has not been established.

**PREPARATIONS**    *Tablets:* 10 mg.

**DRUG INTERACTIONS**    **Sympathomimetic drugs, tricyclic antidepressants** These can cause a hypertensive crisis if given concurrently with an MAO inhibitor. Two weeks should be allowed between discontinuing a tricyclic antidepressant and starting a sympathomimetic drug.    **Alcohol, meperidine, sedatives, antihistamines** These are CNS depressants that have a synergistic depression with the MAO inhibitors.    **Antihypertensive drugs, diuretics** These act synergistically with MAO inhibitors to cause orthostatic hypotension.    **Insulin, oral hypoglycemic agents** The hypoglycemic response to these drugs is exaggerated by an MAO inhibitor.

**FATE**    The metabolic fate of MAO inhibitors is not well characterized. These drugs are cumulative. The *onset of action* may take several days or week. The effects persist for up to 3 weeks after the drug is discontinued.

### ❦ NURSING CONSIDERATIONS

#### Side effects, toxicities, and associated nursing actions
- See entry for drug class (p. 750).

#### Nursing interventions related to drug administration
- See entry for drug class (p. 750).
- Administration of a single daily dose, or of any increases in dosage, at bedtime, may lessen daytime sedation. Patients who experience insomnia or stimulation may benefit from taking the single dose in the morning.

#### Patient and family education
- See entry for drug class (p. 751).

---

# Antimanic drug

lithium

**OVERVIEW OF THE DRUG CLASS**    The classic manic-depressive patient has a manic period characterized by excessive euphoria, overactivity, a flow of ideas, extreme self-confidence, and little need for sleep, alternating with a period of severe depression. Lithium is the drug of choice for treating the manic phase of a manic-depressive disorder. If the patient is severely manic, an antipsychotic drug or electroconvulsive shock therapy may be used initially to subdue behavior. Lithium may also be effective in treating the depression of the manic-depressive disorder and even endogenous depression per se.

## lithium carbonate, lithium citrate (LI-thee-um) antimanic, antidepressant

- lithium carbonate, lithium citrate: ✤Carbolith, Cibalith-S, ✤Duralith, Eskalith, ✤Lithane, Lithium Carbonate Capsules, ✤Lithizine, Lithonate, Lithobid, Lithotabs

**MECHANISM OF ACTION** Lithium acts to lower concentrations of norepinephrine and serotonin by inhibiting their release from and enhancing their reuptake by neurons. These effects, along with the side effects and toxic effect of lithium, are believed to be related to the partial replacement of sodium by lithium in membrane reactions.

**INDICATIONS** • Mania. • Major depression.

**CONTRAINDICATIONS** **Early pregnancy** Congenital malformations in infants of mothers on lithium therapy have been documented.

**DOSAGE** Serum lithium concentrations must be monitered during therapy and doses adjusted accordingly. The therapeutic range is very narrow: 1 to 1.4 mEq/L (mmolar) for acute therapy, 0.5 to 1.3 mEq/L (mmolar) for maintenance therapy. Side effects are common at higher doses. **PO:** **ADULTS:** *For acute manic episode,* initially 1.8 g of the carbonate or 30 ml of the citrate form daily divided into 2 or 3 doses. On a weight basis, 20 to 30 mg/kg daily. *Maintenance,* 900 to 1200 mg of the carbonate form or 15 to 20 ml of the citrate form daily, divided into 2 to 4 doses. *Special patient populations:* **ELDERLY:** Doses for geriatric patients are reduced to 600 to 900 mg daily of the carbonate form or 15 to 20 ml of the citrate form divided into 2 or 3 doses. Geriatric patients require doses to produce low serum concentrations (about .5 mEq/L [mmolar]) for maintenance therapy. This must be individually determined. **CHILDREN:** Lithium is not labeled for pediatric use. However, pediatric doses are 15 to 60 mg/kg or 0.5 to 1.5 $g/M^2$ to achieve serum concentrations of 0.5 to 1.3 mEq/ml. **PREGNANCY:** Lithium is considered teratogenic in early pregnancy. Lithium is distributed into breast milk and nursing should be avoided by mothers maintained on lithium.

**PREPARATIONS** Carbonate, *capsules:* 300 mg. *Tablets:* 300 mg. *Tablets, film-coated:* 300 mg. *Tablets, extended-release:* 450 mg. *Tablets, extended-release, film-coated:* 300 mg. Citrate, *solution:* 8 mEq/5 ml.

**DRUG INTERACTIONS** **Thiazide diuretics** These reduce the clearance of lithium and can cause lithium intoxication. Usually, the dose of lithium must be reduced about 50%. **Antipsychotic drugs** Lithium may decrease serum concentrations and phenothiazines may increase renal clearance of lithium. The result of these interactions is unpredictable. Extrapyramidal reactions may be more common. The nausea and vomiting of lithium intoxication may be masked by the antipsychotic drug. **Nonsteroidal antiinflammatory agents** These increase the serum concentration of lithium by 30% to 60%, making lithium toxicity more common. The NSAIAs decrease the renal excretion of lithium. **Anticonvulsants** Various neurologic side effects have been reported for patients taking carbamazepine or phenytoin and lithium. **Neuromuscular blocking agents** Lithium prolongs the action of succinylcholine or pancuonium. **Iodides** The combination of lithium and iodides may give an additive or synergic hypothyroid effect. **Sodium** Lithium clearance is altered by sodium in that increased sodium increases lithium clearance and vice versa.

**FATE** Lithium is readily absorbed and *peak* concentrations are found in 30 minutes to 3 hours. In general, in adults, a 300 mg dose of lithium carbonate gives a serum concentration of about 0.5 mEa/L (mmolar). Lithium is widely distributed in the body. Red blood cells only take in lithium gradually due to an electrochemical gradiant that opposes the chemical gradient. Red blood cell concentrations can therefore be used to determine whether a patient has been noncompliant and has taken only the most recent dosage to produce acceptable serum concentrations. Lithium is excreted by the kidney by the same processes that control sodium excretion. Of the lithium filtered in the kidney, 80% is reabsorbed in the proximal tubule and 20% is excreted in the urine. The *half-life* of lithium in the plasma is 24 hours, and this is increased to 36 hours in the elderly.    **Side effects** Side effects are related to the blood level of lithium as follows:

### Below 1.5 mEq/L*
Fine tremor of hands
Dry mouth
Increased thirst
Increased urination
Nausea
### 1.5 to 2.0 mEq/L
Vomiting
Diarrhea
Muscle weakness
Incoordination (ataxia)
Dizziness
Confusion
Slurred speech
### 2.0 to 2.5 mEq/L
Persistent nausea and vomiting.
Blurred vision
Muscle twitching (fasciculations)
Hyperactive deep tendon reflexes
### 2.5 to 3.0 mEq/L
Myoclonic twitches or movements of an entire limb
Choreathetoid movements
Urinary and fecal incontinence
### Above 3.0 mEq/L
Seizures
Cardiac arrhythmias
Hypotension
Peripheral vascular collapse
Death

## ❧ NURSING CONSIDERATIONS
### Side effects, toxicities, and associated nursing actions
- See above for side effects.
- Note the side effects seen at increasing serum drug levels, above.
- Review the side effects with patient and family, and the need to seek medical attention if the side effects occur.
- For *fine tremor*, provide reassurance and support. This effect may lessen in time. The patient may have to learn to tolerate it.
- For *dry mouth* or *increased thirst*, suggest that the patient increase intake of fluids, take frequent sips of water, chew sugarless gum or suck on sugarless hard candy, and perform regular oral hygiene. Avoid the use of drying mouthwashes. Some patients may wish to use a commercially available saliva substitute.
- For *increased urination*, suggest the patient try to limit fluid intake after 8 PM, to avoid having to get up at night to void. Monitor intake and output. If urinary output is excessive, assess for development of diabetes insipidus: excessive dilute urine, of low specific gravity, 1.000 to 1.003.
- For *nausea*, suggest the patient take ordered doses with meals.

### Nursing interventions related to drug administration
- Caution patients on extended-release preparations to swallow these whole, not to chew or suck on them.

*NOTE: 1 mEq/L = 1 mmolar.

- Lithane brand tablets contain FD & C coloring number 5 (tartrazine), which may cause an allergic response in susceptible individuals. While rare, this side effect is seen more often in persons with aspirin hypersensitivity.
- Monitoring serum drug levels is important in assessing patient response to lithium but does not diminish the need for careful, systematic nursing assessment.
- Supervise the patient carefully to ascertain that the medication is swallowed and not hidden in the mouth to be discarded or stored by the patient.
- The risk of suicide is present in seriously depressed patients and may persist for several weeks after the patient begins drug therapy. Be alert to patient comments and behavior. Use institutional guidelines for initiation of suicide precautions.

## Patient and family education

- Review with patients and/or families the expected benefits and possible side effects of therapy.
- Reassure patients that several weeks of drug therapy are needed to produce a significant change.
- Caution patients taking lithium to return for blood work as directed, so dosage can be adjusted according to patient response.
- Caution patients to report the development of any unexpected sign or symptom.
- Review with patients the need to continue taking the medication as ordered, even if the patient begins to feel subjective improvement. It is the continued therapeutic blood levels of the drug that help maintain subjective feelings of improvement.
- Caution patients to avoid taking over-the-counter medications without prior approval of the physician. Caution patients to keep all health care providers informed of all medications being taken.
- As the patient's mood improves, appetite may improve, and some patients will find weight gain to be a problem. If weight gain is significant, the patient may need to be instructed in a calorie-restricted diet.
- Instruct patients to monitor weight on a weekly basis. Excessive weight gain (greater than 2 to 5 lb/week) should be reported to the physician.
- Safe use in pregnancy has not been established. Advise women who think they may be pregnant to consult their physicians. Women of childbearing age may wish to use some form of birth control. Lactating women who are prescribed lithium should consult their physicians before breastfeeding.
- Caution patients to avoid stopping this medication suddenly.
- Caution patients to keep these and all medications out of the reach of children.
- Caution patients to avoid the use of alcohol.
- Caution patients to avoid significant changes in sodium intake (see Drug interactions, above). Review with patients and household cook the common sources of dietary sodium.
- Patients requiring restricted fluid intake or low sodium intake for treatment of other health conditions may be unable to take lithium. Be supportive of patients and families.
- Caution patients to notify the physician if fever or severe or persistent vomiting or diarrhea occurs, as resulting electrolyte depletion may contribute to lithium toxicity.
- If a metallic taste in the mouth occurs, it will probably persist throughout therapy. While not medically significant, it may be annoying to the patient.

# Chapter Thirty-eight
# Central nervous system stimulants

amphetamine sulfate
benzphetamine hydrochloride
caffeine
dextroamphetamine sulfate
diethylpropion hydrochloride
doxapram hydrochloride
fenfluramine hydrochloride
mazindol

methamphetamine hydrochloride
methylphenidate hydrochloride
pemoline
phendimetrazine tartrate
phenmetrazine hydrochloride
phentermine hydrochloride
phenylpropanolamine hydrochloride

**OVERVIEW OF THE DRUG CLASS**   Drugs that stimulate the central nervous system (CNS) have few clinical uses. Narcolepsy, a sleep disorder, may respond to CNS stimulants; paradoxically, hyperactivity in children may also respond to CNS stimulants. The other clinical uses of these compounds are to stimulate respiration and to suppress appetite (Table 38-1). When these compounds must be used, care must always be taken to avoid abuse and to avoid excessive stimulation of the CNS by overdose with the agents. Many of these drugs are schedule II agents with very high abuse potentials.

**MECHANISM OF ACTION**   Amphetamines and related drugs increase the release and effectiveness of norepinephrine and dopamine. These compounds are catecholamines that serve as neurotransmitters in the brain. The level of arousal is increased by action on the reticular activating system; amphetamines also stimulate the medial forebrain bundle, or reward center, creating a perception of pleasure unrelated to external stimuli. Analeptic drugs (used to stimulate respiration) have a variety of effects on several systems, including the CNS.

**INDICATIONS**   **Narcolepsy** CNS stimulants used during the daytime can help control narcolepsy, a condition in which patients abruptly fall asleep during normal daytime activities.   **Hyperkinesis** Children displaying overactivity and associated symptoms may receive CNS stimulants to control the condition. These drugs, which cause agitation and activity in adults, may have a calming effect in children. Hyperkinesis is also referred to as attention deficit disorder.   **Obesity** Appetite suppression is a side effect of CNS stimulants, which may be used as a temporary aid in weight reduction programs.   **Respiratory depression** CNS stimulants are occasionally used to stimulate respiration, most often in newborns.

**Table 38-1.**

**Clinical indications for CNS stimulants**

| | Narcolepsy | Hyperkinesis | Obesity | Respiratory depression |
|---|---|---|---|---|
| Amphetamine | + | + | + | |
| Benzphetamine | | | + | |
| Caffeine* | | | | + |
| Dextroamphetamine | + | + | + | |
| Diethylpropion | | | + | |
| Doxapram | | | | + |
| Fenfluramine | | | + | |
| Mazindol | | | + | |
| Methamphetamine | | + | + | |
| Methylphenidate | + | + | | |
| Pemoline | | + | | |
| Phendimetrazine | | | + | |
| Phenmetrazine | | | + | |
| Phentermine | | | + | |
| Phenylpropanolamine* | | | + | |

*For additional uses, see the drug monograph.

**CONTRAINDICATIONS**    **Convulsive disorders** Convulsions may be triggered by these stimulatory agents. **Cardiovascular disease** Blood pressure may be elevated and arrhythmias may be induced.    **History of drug abuse** Because of their high abuse potential, many of these agents are unsuitable for unsupervised use in patients with a history of drug abuse. • For other specific contraindications, see specific drugs.

**DRUG INTERACTIONS**    **Antihypertensive agents** may be less effective when given with certain CNS stimulants.    **CNS stimulants** should never be combined with each other because of the danger of excessive CNS stimulation. • For specific interactions, see specific drug listing.

## ☙ NURSING CONSIDERATIONS

### Side effects, toxicities, and associated nursing actions

**CNS** Nervousness, agitation, sleeplessness, tremor, or seizures can result from excessive stimulation.
- If CNS side effects are severe, it may be necessary to reduce drug dosage; notify the physician.
- In the hospital setting, pad side rails and keep them up, and have a suction machine at the bedside.
- To prevent insomnia, take the last dose of the day at least 6 hours before bedtime.

**CV** Tachycardia, arrhythmias, hypertension, and other signs of cardiovascular stimulation can arise from direct or secondary actions of CNS stimulants.
- Monitor vital signs and blood pressure.
- Caution patients to avoid ingestion of other drugs or food that also contribute to cardiovascular side effects, such as caffeine and caffeine-containing beverages and over-the-counter cold preparations containing phenylpropanolamine.

### Patient and family education

- Review the anticipated benefits and possible side effects of drug therapy with patients and families.
- Forewarn patients that several days to weeks of therapy may be necessary before the full effect of drug therapy can be evaluated.
- Impress upon patients the importance of returning for regular medical follow-up.
- Remind patients that the use of these drugs to treat general fatigue is inappropriate. Rebound exhaustion may be severe.
- Teach patients taking CNS stimulants for appetite suppression that the use of the drug should be combined with a total treatment program, which may include dietary counseling, exercise, and behavior modification.
- Teach patients to take the medications only as ordered. Patients should not double up if a dose is missed.
- Remind patients to keep these and all drugs out of the reach of children. Parents should supervise medication administration in children with hyperkinesis.
- Warn patients to avoid discontinuing the medication suddenly, as abrupt withdrawal may precipitate psychiatric manifestations and lethargy.
- Remind patients to keep all health care providers informed of all medications being taken.
- Because of the effect on appetite and weight, teach diabetic patients to monitor blood sugar closely. A change in the dose of insulin, oral hypoglycemic agent, or diet may be necessary.

## amphetamine, amphetamine sulfate    (am-FET-uh-meen)    anorexiant*

- sold under generic name (CII)

**MECHANISM OF ACTION**    Amphetamines increase the release and effectiveness of norepinephrine and dopamine in the central nervous system. The catecholamines norepinephrine and dopamine act as neurotransmitters in the CNS, in addition to serving as neurotransmitters in the peripheral autonomic nervous system. Amphetamines increase the level of arousal by action on the reticular activating

*CNS stimulant.

system. Amphetamine action on the medial forebrain bundle, or reward center, creates a perception of pleasure that is unrelated to external stimuli.

**INDICATIONS**  **Narcolepsy** Amphetamines used during the daytime can help control narcolepsy, a condition in which patients abruptly fall asleep during normal daytime activities.  **Hyperkinesis** Children displaying overactivity and associated symptoms may receive amphetamines to control the condition. These drugs, which cause agitation and activity in adults, may have a calming effect in children.  **Obesity** Appetite suppression is a side effect of amphetamine, which may be used as a temporary aid in weight reduction programs.

**CONTRAINDICATIONS**  **Advanced arteriosclerosis** Amphetamines may cause vasoconstriction or sudden elevations in blood pressure.  **Hypertension** Amphetamines may elevate blood pressure.  **Hyperthyroidism** Amphetamines may dangerously increase the symptoms of agitation and cardiovascular overstimulation in hyperthyroidism.  **Cardiovascular disease** Amphetamines may elevate blood pressure or induce arrhythmias.  **Glaucoma (narrow angle)** Amphetamines may increase intraocular pressure. **Mental instability or history of drug abuse** The mood-altering effects of amphetamines and the strong potential for abuse make them especially dangerous for patients with a history of susceptibility. **Hypersensitivity to sympathomimetic amines** The catecholamines released by amphetamines can trigger dangerous reactions in sensitive individuals.

**DOSAGE**  **For narcolepsy:** *PO:*  **ADULTS:** Dosage should be individualized, starting with smaller doses and increasing until therapeutic effect is achieved or toxicity supervenes. Daily doses normally range between 5 and 60 mg in single or multiple doses. Doses should not be given within 6 hours of bedtime to avoid insomnia.  **For hyperkinesis:** *PO:*  **CHILDREN OVER 6 YEARS:** Initially, 5 mg once or twice daily. Increase weekly by 5 mg increments until desired effect is achieved. Daily doses should not exceed 40 mg.  **CHILDREN 3 TO 5 YEARS:** Initial dose is 2.5 mg, increased as necessary by 2.5 mg at weekly intervals.  **For obesity:** *PO:*  **ADULTS:** 5 to 30 mg daily, given in divided doses 30 to 60 minutes before meals. Therapy should not be continued beyond a few weeks because tolerance develops to the anorexiant effects, whereas the abuse potential remains.  *Special patient populations:*  **PREGNANCY:** Amphetamine should not be used in pregnancy.  **CHILDREN:** Avoid in children under age 3.

**PREPARATIONS**  *Tablets:* 5 or 10 mg, scored. Not available in Canada.

**DRUG INTERACTIONS**  **Monoamine oxidase (MAO) inhibitors** block normal pathways for destruction of sympathomimetic amines; therefore, the catecholamines released by amphetamines may not be efficiently metabolized and can accumulate to dangerous levels. Fatalities have resulted.  **Halothane and cyclopropane** used as general anesthetics may sensitize the heart to the catecholamines released by amphetamines. The result may be dangerous or fatal arrhythmias.

**FATE**  Amphetamine is readily absorbed orally and distributed to many tissues, especially the central nervous system. *Peak* effects are observed 2 to 3 hours after ingestion; the *duration* of effect ranges from 4 to 24 hours. The primary route of elimination of amphetamine is through the kidneys, with excretion enhanced in an acidic urine. Some metabolism of amphetamine also occurs.

### ☙ NURSING CONSIDERATIONS

#### Side effects, toxicities, and associated nursing actions

**CNS** Acute effects of amphetamine include nervousness, increased motor activity, talkativeness, irritability, insomnia, increased libido, dizziness, headaches, hyperexcitability, tremors, twitching, and changes in vision. Pupils may be dilated. Chronic use may cause habituation or addiction. Chronic users often show emotional lability, loss of appetite, and impaired mental processes. Chronic use of high doses can cause a reaction resembling paranoid schizophrenia, with auditory and visual hallucinations.
* Obtain a thorough baseline assessment before starting therapy.
* Instruct the patient and family to report changes in mood or affect.
* Caution patients to avoid driving or operating hazardous equipment until the effects of medication can be evaluated.
* Monitor weight.
* In the hospital setting, pad side rails and keep them up. Have a suction machine at the bedside.

**CV** Tachycardia, palpitation, hypertension or hypotension, cardiac arrhythmias, flushing, or pallor can occur.

- Monitor pulse and blood pressure.
- Obtain a baseline ECG, and monitor ECG at regular intervals throughout therapy.
- Caution patients to avoid the use of over-the-counter medications without first clearing them with the physician. Medications containing phenylpropanolamine, caffeine, and other substances that also have cardiovascular effects are readily available to the consumer and may contribute to excessive cardiovascular stimulation.

**GI** Nausea, vomiting, anorexia, dryness of the mouth, intestinal cramps, and diarrhea or constipation have been reported.

- If vomiting or diarrhea is severe or persistent, notify the physician.
- Monitor weight. Instruct patients to record weight at least twice a week.
- If constipation occurs, increase fluid intake to 2500 ml/day, increase dietary intake of fruits, fruit juices, and fiber, and increase the level of exercise.
- For dry mouth, instruct the patient to chew sugarless gum, suck on sugarless candy, and rinse the mouth frequently. Avoid drying mouthwashes. Encourage good oral hygiene (brushing and flossing), which will improve patient comfort and lessen the chance of tooth decay. Some patients may wish to use commercially available saliva substitutes.

**Metabolic** Children receiving amphetamine for hyperkinesis may suffer growth retardation. For this reason, children should have the drug discontinued periodically to assess whether the drug must be continued for control of the condition and to allow growth to proceed normally.

- Instruct parents to measure and record height and weight of children taking this drug for hyperkinesis at least weekly.

**Peripheral nerves** Motor and vocal tics and Tourette's disorder may be worsened by amphetamine.

- Monitor patients for development of or worsening of tics.

### Nursing interventions related to drug administration
- When used for appetite suppression, the drug should be given 30 to 60 minutes prior to a meal.

### Patient and family education
- Review the anticipated benefits and possible side effects of drug therapy with patients and families.
- See entry for drug class (p. 758).

---

## benzphetamine hydrochloride (benz-FET-uh-meen) anorexiant

- benzphetamine hydrochloride: Didrex (CIII)

**MECHANISM OF ACTION** Benzphetamine is similar to amphetamine in its mechanism of action and anorexiant action.

**INDICATIONS** Obesity Appetite suppression is a side effect of CNS stimulants such as benzphetamine. This action may be temporarily helpful in weight control programs including caloric restriction and dietary retraining.

**CONTRAINDICATIONS** Advanced arteriosclerosis Benzphetamine may cause vasoconstriction or sudden elevations in blood pressure. Hypertension Benzphetamine may elevate blood pressure. Hyperthyroidism Benzphetamine may dangerously increase the symptoms of agitation and cardiovascular overstimulation in hyperthyroidism. Cardiovascular disease Benzphetamine may elevate blood pressure or induce arrhythmias. Glaucoma Benzphetamine may increase intraocular pressure. Mental instability or history of drug abuse Benzphetamine has a potential for abuse; its use may be inappropriate for patients with a history of susceptibility. Hypersensitivity to sympathomimetic amines The catecholamines released by benzphetamine can trigger dangerous reactions in sensitive individuals.

**DOSAGE** PO: ADULTS: Initially 25 to 50 mg once daily, usually in midmorning. Dosage may be increased as needed and tolerated to 50 mg three times daily. *Special patient populations:* CHILDREN: Children under 12 years should not receive benzphetamine.    **PREGNANCY:** Benzphetamine is toxic to fetuses and should not be given to pregnant patients, nor to nursing mothers.

**PREPARATIONS**    *Tablets:* 25 mg (with tartrazine) and 50 mg, scored.

**DRUG INTERACTIONS    Monoamine oxidase (MAO) inhibitors** block normal destruction of catecholamines that may be released by benzphetamine. The result may be a dangerous overstimulation caused by the accumulated catecholamines.

**FATE**    Benzphetamine is orally absorbed to produce anorexiant effects within 1 to 2 hours. The *duration* of action is about 4 hours.

## ❦ NURSING CONSIDERATIONS

### Side effects, toxicities, and associated nursing actions

**CNS** Overstimulation of the CNS may produce restlessness, tremor, dizziness, headache, insomnia, changes in libido, and impaired coordination. Occasionally, patients suffer psychotic episodes. Seizures have occured. Habituation is possible.

* Obtain a thorough baseline assessment before starting therapy.
* Instruct the patient and family to report changes in mood or affect.
* Caution patients to avoid driving or operating hazardous equipment until the effects of medication can be evaluated.
* Monitor weight.
* In the hospital setting, pad side rails and keep them up. Have a suction machine at the bedside.

**CV** Tachycardia, palpitations, and increased blood pressure are common effects.

* Monitor pulse and blood pressure.
* Obtain a baseline ECG, and monitor ECG at regular intervals throughout therapy.
* Caution patients to avoid the use of over-the-counter medications without first clearing them with the physician. Medications containing phenylpropanolamine, caffeine, and other substances that also have cardiovascular effects are readily available to the consumer and may contribute to excessive cardiovascular stimulation.

**GI** Nausea, vomiting, dryness of the mouth, and an unpleasant taste can occur.

* If vomiting or diarrhea are severe or persistent, notify the physician.
* Monitor weight. Instruct patients to record weight at least twice a week.
* If constipation occurs, increase fluid intake to 2500 ml/day, increase dietary intake of fruits, fruit juices, and fiber, and increase level of exercise.
* For dry mouth, instruct the patient to chew sugarless gum, suck on sugarless candy, and rinse the mouth frequently. Avoid drying mouthwashes. Encourage good oral hygiene (brushing and flossing), which will improve patient comfort and lessen the chance of tooth decay. Some patients may wish to use commercially available saliva substitutes.

**Allergic** Allergic skin reactions and urticaria occur rarely.

* Monitor patients for rashes and skin changes.

### Nursing interventions related to drug administration

* Didrex brand, 25 mg, tablets contain FD & C yellow dye #5 (tartrazine), which may cause an allergic reaction in susceptible individuals. Although rare, this response is seen more commonly in persons with aspirin hypersensitivity.

### Patient and family education

* Review the anticipated benefits and possible side effects of drug therapy with patients and families.
* See entry for drug class (p. 758).

---

## caffeine    (ka-FEEN)                                                          CNS stimulant

* caffeine: Caffedrine, Caffeine and Sodium Benzoate, Citrated Caffeine, Dexitac, NōDōz, Stimtabs, Tirend, Vivarin

**MECHANISM OF ACTION**    Caffeine inhibits phosphodiesterase, the enzyme that normally destroys the intracellular second messenger cyclic AMP. As a result of the increased concentrations of cyclic AMP and its longer persistence, the function of many cells and tissues are altered. Caffeine is especially effective at altering function of cells in the CNS; the mild stimulatory effects on the CNS are the primary reason for using caffeine. In addition to CNS effects, caffeine causes vasoconstriction, mild diuresis, cardiac stimulation, increased gastric acidity, and increased strength of contraction in skeletal muscle.

**INDICATIONS**   **CNS stimulation** Caffeine is widely used to improve mental alertness, primarily in the form of oral OTC preparations.   **Respiratory depression** Although parenteral forms of caffeine have been used to stimulate respiration following overdose with CNS depressant drugs, other forms of therapy are more specific and probably more efficacious. Caffeine was specifically employed to combat neonatal apnea in low-birth-weight infants, but this is not an approved indication for the drug at present.   **Headache** Caffeine causes vasoconstriction of cerebral blood vessels and can therefore relieve symptoms of migraine or cluster headaches in selected patients, especially when given with ergotamine. For simple tension headaches, caffeine is often combined with analgesics such as aspirin or acetaminophen; no carefully controlled trials clearly show benefits from such combinations. Caffeine and sodium benzoate injection may be used to relieve headache following spinal puncture.   **Fluid retention** Caffeine has mild diuretic action and has been used to counteract the fluid retention preceding menstruation.

**CONTRAINDICATIONS**   **Peptic ulcers** Caffeine promotes acid secretion in the stomach and may exacerbate ulcers.   **Cardiac arrhythmias** Caffeine causes palpitations and may worsen arrhythmias of many kinds. The drug is usually avoided for a few weeks after myocardial infarction.   **Neonates with high bilirubin levels** Caffeine may uncouple bilirubin from albumin, causing kernicterus in these infants already at risk.

**DOSAGE**   **For alerting effects:** *PO:*   ADULT: Doses of 100 to 200 mg of anhydrous caffeine are usually sufficient; citrated caffeine at 65 to 325 mg three times daily (equivalent to 32 to 162 mg anhydrous caffeine) have also been used. Oral doses of 18 to 50 g (18,000 to 50,000 mg) have proven fatal in adults.   **For respiratory stimulation:** *IM, IV:*   ADULT: Doses of 500 mg to 1 g of caffeine and sodium benzoate injection have been used in emergency respiratory failure caused by CNS depressants or electric shock.   CHILDREN: Caffeine is not approved to treat neonatal apnea. The drug was used in the past as caffeine and sodium benzoate injection in doses equivalent to 20 mg/kg caffeine as a loading dose, followed in 2 or 3 days by 5 to 10 mg/kg twice or three times daily.   *Special patient populations:*   CHILDREN: Children may be more prone to adverse CNS effects of caffeine than are adults. Infants who receive caffeine and sodium benzoate injection are at increased risk of kernicterus. PREGNANCY: Caffeine is mutagenic in animals and in laboratory tests but has not clearly been associated with such effects in humans. Caffeine intake is usually discouraged in pregnancy because the drug crosses the placenta.

**PREPARATIONS**   *Caffeine, anhydrous, tablets:* 75, 100, and 200 mg; *capsules, extended release:* 200 and 250 mg. *Citrated caffeine, tablets:* 65 mg (equivalent to 32 mg anhydrous caffeine). *Caffeine and sodium benzoate, solution for injection:* 250 mg/l, which is equivalent to 125 mg/l of anhydrous caffeine and 125 mg/l sodium benzoate.

**DRUG INTERACTIONS**   **Beta-adrenergic stimulating agents** may have increased inotropic effects when given with caffeine.

**DIAGNOSTIC TEST INTERFERENCES**   **Serum urate** may be falsely increased by caffeine when the Bittner method of assay is used.   **Urinary catecholamines, vanillylmandelic acid (VMA), and 5-hydroxyindoleacetic levels acid** may be increased by caffeine, possibly leading to false diagnoses of pheochromocytoma or neuroblastoma.

**FATE**   Caffeine is well absorbed orally, producing *peak* blood concentrations within 50 to 75 minutes. The drug is well distributed, crossing freely into amniotic fluid and into the brain. Caffeine is metabolized by the liver, and metabolites and unaltered drug are eliminated in urine. The elimination *half-life* is 3 to 4 hours.

## ☙ NURSING CONSIDERATIONS
### Side effects, toxicities, and associated nursing actions
**CNS** Irritability, insomnia, anxiety, nervousness may occur with overuse of caffeine. Acute toxicity

resulting from very high doses may cause stomach pain, delirium, fever, or clonic-tonic seizures. Chronic ingestion of high doses can produce tolerance and psychologic dependence.

- Obtain a thorough baseline assessment before starting therapy.
- Instruct the patient and family to report changes in mood or affect.
- In the hospital setting, pad side rails and keep them up. Have a suction machine at the bedside.

**CV** Cardiac arrhythmias may follow large doses.

- Monitor pulse and blood pressure.
- Obtain a baseline ECG, and monitor ECG at regular intervals throughout therapy.
- Caution patients with a known history of cardiac disease to limit caffeine intake unless specifically approved by the physician.

**Renal** Diuresis and dehydration may occur.

- Monitor intake, output, weight, and blood pressure. Assess skin turgor.

### Nursing interventions related to drug administration

- IM injection is preferred over IV use. Use anatomic landmarks to identify injection sites. Record sites and rotate sites.
- For IV use, caffeine may be given undiluted. Administer at a rate of 250 mg or less over 1 minute.

### Patient and family education

- Review the anticipated benefits and possible side effects of drug therapy with patients and families.
- See entry for drug class (p. 758).

---

# dextroamphetamine, dextroamphetamine sulfate
(dex-troh-am-FET-uh-meen)                                                                    anorexiant*

- dextroamphetamine: Biphetamine (with amphetamine), Dexampex, Dexedrine, Fernex, Oxydess (CII)

**MECHANISM OF ACTION** Amphetamine is a mixture of two isomers: levamphetamine (the levorotatory isomer) and dextroamphetamine (or dexamphetamine; the dextrorotatory isomer). Of the two isomers, dextroamphetamine has the stronger effect on the CNS. Amphetamines increase the release and effectiveness of norepinephrine and dopamine in the central nervous system. The catecholamines norepinephrine and dopamine act as neurotransmitters in the CNS, in addition to serving as neurotransmitters in the peripheral autonomic nervous system. Amphetamines increase the level of arousal by action on the reticular activating system. Amphetamine action on the medial forebrain bundle, or reward center, creates a perception of pleasure that is unrelated to external stimuli.

**INDICATIONS** **Narcolepsy** Dextroamphetamine is used during the daytime to help control narcolepsy, a condition in which patients abruptly fall asleep during normal daytime activities. **Hyperkinesis** Children displaying overactivity and associated symptoms may receive dextroamphetamine to control the condition. These drugs, which cause agitation and activity in adults, may have a calming effect in children. **Obesity** Appetite suppression is a side effect of dextroamphetamine, which may be used as a temporary aid in weight reduction programs.

**CONTRAINDICATIONS** **Advanced arteriosclerosis** Dextroamphetamine may cause vasoconstriction or sudden elevations in blood pressure. **Hypertension** Dextroamphetamine may elevate blood pressure. **Hyperthyroidism** Dextroamphetamine may dangerously increase the symptoms of agitation and cardiovascular overstimulation in hyperthyroidism. **Cardiovascular disease** Dextroamphetamine may elevate blood pressure or induce arrhythmias. **Glaucoma** Dextroamphetamine may increase intraocular pressure. **Mental instability or history of drug abuse** The mood-altering effects of dextroamphetamine and the strong potential for abuse make the drug especially dangerous for patients with a history of susceptibility. **Hypersensitivity to sympathomimetic amines** The catecholamines released by dextroamphetamine can trigger dangerous reactions in sensitive individuals.

*CNS stimulant.

**DOSAGE**    For narcolepsy: *PO:*    ADULTS: Dosage should be individualized, starting with smaller doses and increasing until therapeutic effect is achieved or toxicity supervenes. Daily doses normally range between 5 and 60 mg in single or multiple doses. Doses should not be given within 6 hours of bedtime to avoid insomnia.    **For hyperkinesis:** *PO:*    CHILDREN OVER 6 YEARS: Initially, 5 mg once or twice daily. Increase weekly by 5 mg increments until desired effect is achieved. Daily doses should not exceed 40 mg.    CHILDREN 3 TO 5 YEARS: Initial dose is 2.5 mg, increased as necessary by 2.5 mg at weekly intervals.    **For obesity:** *PO:*    ADULTS: 5 to 30 mg daily, given in divided doses 30 to 60 minutes before meals. Therapy should not be continued beyond a few weeks because tolerance develops to the anorexiant effects, while the abuse potential remains. Extended-release preparations may be given as a single morning dose.    *Special patient populations:*    PREGNANCY: Dextroamphetamine should not be administered to pregnant women.    CHILDREN: Avoid in children under 3 years of age.

**PREPARATIONS**    *Dextroamphetamine sulfate, tablets:* 5, 10, or 15 mg, scored; *capsules:* 15 mg; *capsules, extended release:* 5, 10, or 15 mg; *elixir:* 5 mg/ml. *Dextroamphetamine (as a resin complex) with amphetamine, capsules:* 6.25 or 10 mg each of dextroamphetamine and amphetamine. *Mixtures containing dextroamphetamine* are available as tablets and capsules (see Table 38-1, p. 757).

**DRUG INTERACTIONS**    **Monoamine oxidase (MAO) inhibitors**    block normal pathways for destruction of sympathomimetic amines; therefore, the catecholamines released by dextroamphetamine may not be efficiently metabolized and can accumulate to dangerous levels. Fatalities have resulted. At least 14 days should elapse between end of therapy with MAO inhibitors and start of dextroamphetamine. **Halothane and cyclopropane** used as general anesthetics may sensitize the heart to the catecholamines released by dextroamphetamine. The result may be dangerous or fatal arrhythmias.

**FATE**    Dextroamphetamine is readily absorbed orally and distributed to many tissues, especially the central nervous system. *Peak* effects are observed 2 to 3 hours after ingestion; the *duration* of effect ranges from 4 to 24 hours. The primary route of elimination is through the kidneys, with excretion enhanced in an acidic urine. Some metabolism of dextroamphetamine also occurs.

## 🐾 NURSING CONSIDERATIONS

### Side effects, toxicities, and associated nursing actions
- See Amphetamine (p. 758).

### Nursing interventions related to drug administration
- When used for appetite suppression, the drug should be given 30 to 60 minutes prior to a meal.
- Dexedrine brand extended-release capsules in 5, 10, and 15 mg dosages and Dexedrine brand, 5 mg, tablets contain FD & C yellow dye # 5 (tartrazine), which may cause an allergic reaction in susceptible individuals. Although rare, this reaction is seen more commonly in persons with aspirin hypersensitivity.

### Patient and family education
- Review the anticipated benefits and possible side effects of drug therapy with patients and families.
- See entry for drug class (p. 758).

---

## diethylpropion hydrochloride, amfepramone
(dye-eth-ill-PRO-pee-ahn)                                                                anorexiant

---

- diethylpropion hydrochloride: Depletite, Dietic, Tenuate, Tepanil (CIV), ♣Nobesine, ♣Propion, ♣Regibon

**MECHANISM OF ACTION**    Diethylpropion is similar to amphetamine in its mechanism of action and anorexiant action.

**INDICATIONS**    **Obesity** Appetite suppression is a side effect of CNS stimulants such as diethylpropion. This action may be temporarily helpful in weight control programs that include caloric restriction and dietary retraining.

**CONTRAINDICATIONS**    **Advanced arteriosclerosis** Diethylpropion may cause vasoconstriction or sudden elevations in blood pressure.    **Hypertension** Diethylpropion may elevate blood pressure.    **Hyperthyroidism** Diethylpropion may dangerously increase the symptoms of agitation and cardiovascular overstimulation in hyperthyroidism.    **Cardiovascular disease** Diethylpropion may elevate blood pressure or induce arrhythmias.    **Glaucoma** Diethylpropion may increase intraocular pressure.    **Mental instability or history of drug abuse** Diethylpropion has a potential for abuse; its use may be inappropriate for patients with a history of susceptibility.    **Hypersensitivity to sympathomimetic amines** The catecholamines released by diethylpropion can trigger dangerous reactions in sensitive individuals.

**DOSAGE**    **PO:**    ADULTS: 25 mg three times daily, usually 1 hour before meals. An extended-release preparation, 75 mg, may be taken once daily at midmorning.    *Special patient populations:*    CHILDREN: Children should not receive diethylpropion.    PREGNANCY: Diethylpropion should be avoided by pregnant patients and nursing mothers.

**PREPARATIONS**    *Tablets:* 25 mg; *tablets, extended release:* 75 mg.

**DRUG INTERACTIONS**    **Monoamine oxidase (MAO) inhibitors** block normal destruction of catecholamines that may be released by diethylpropion. The result may be a dangerous overstimulation caused by the accumulated catecholamines.    **Guanethidine** effects may be diminished by diethylpropion, resulting in loss of control of hypertension.

**FATE**    Diethylpropion hydrochloride is orally absorbed to produce anorexiant effects within 1 to 2 hours. The *duration of action* is about 4 hours.

## ❦ NURSING CONSIDERATIONS

### Side effects, toxicities, and associated nursing actions

**CV** Tachycardia, palpitations, and increased blood pressure are common effects. Bone marrow depression and blood dyscrasias have rarely occurred.
- See benzamphetamine (p. 760).

### Nursing interventions related to drug administration
- Read labels carefully; extended-release formulations are available.

### Patient and family education
- Review the anticipated benefits and possible side effects of drug therapy with patients and families.
- See entry for drug class (p. 758).

---

# doxapram hydrochloride    (DOX-uh-pram)    CNS stimulant*

- doxapram hydrochloride: Dopram

**MECHANISM OF ACTION**    Doxapram stimulates the CNS at all levels, but the action usually sought is stimulation of respiration. Doxapram directly stimulates the respiratory centers in the medulla, resulting in variable and transient increases in the depth and rate of respiration. Doses in excess of those required to stimulate respiration induce tonic-clonic seizures. Cardiovascular effects of doxapram are secondary, resulting from actions on the CNS.

**INDICATIONS**    **Respiratory depression following anesthesia** Doxapram can increase respiration in these patients, but therapy must include other measures as well. The action of doxapram is transient, and the drug has a high potential for toxicity.    **Drug-induced respiratory depression** Doxapram can stimulate respiration in patients overdosed with CNS depressants, but other more specific measures are usually more beneficial.    **Acute respiratory failure caused by chronic obstructive pulmonary disease (COPD)** If used at all, doxapram must be used for 2 hours or less. Because doxapram increases the work of respiration, the extra oxygen demand may offset any benefit of increased respiration.

**CONTRAINDICATIONS**    **Epilepsy, seizures, or head injury** Doxapram increases the likelihood of seizure activity.    **Cardiovascular disease** Doxapram may increase blood pressure and heart rate, which may be

*Respiratory stimulant.

dangerous in persons predisposed to stroke, coronary artery disease, heart failure, or hypertension. **Acute bronchial asthma** Doxapram does not improve this condition. **Respiratory failure caused by neuromuscular blockade, airway obstruction, pulmonary embolism, pneumothorax, or pulmonary fibrosis** Doxapram does not improve these conditions. **Mechanical ventilation** Doxapram adds unnecessary risk.

**DOSAGE** **IV:** ADULT: Doses may vary slightly, depending on the specific condition being treated. In general, single doses of doxapram should not exceed 1.5 mg/kg; patients should not receive the drug for longer than 2 hours. The maximum daily dose is 3 g (4 mg/kg). *Special patient populations:* ELDERLY: Elderly, debilitated patients may not be able to tolerate the increased work load caused by respiratory stimulation with doxapram. The drug should be avoided if possible. CHILDREN: Children under 12 should not receive doxapram. PREGNANCY: Pregnant or lactating patients should not receive doxapram.

**PREPARATIONS** *Solution for injection:* 20 mg/ml with benzyl alcohol.

**DRUG INTERACTIONS** **Sympathomimetic amines** may add to the increases in blood pressure caused by doxapram. **Monoamine oxidase inhibitors** used as antidepressants or antihypertensives may add to the increases in blood pressure caused by doxapram. **Halothane and cyclopropane** used as general anesthetics may sensitize the heart to catecholamines, which increases the risk of arrhythmias. Doxapram may add to that risk. **Muscle relaxants** may have a longer duration of action than doxapram, therefore, muscle relaxation may recur after the effects of doxapram have disappeared.

**FATE** The *onset* of respiratory stimulation with IV injection of doxapram is 2 minutes; the *duration of action* is 5 minutes. Continuous infusion is required to maintain effects. Doxapram is well distributed to tissues and is metabolized in the liver. Metabolites are excreted by the kidneys.

## ☙ NURSING CONSIDERATIONS

### Side effects, toxicities, and associated nursing actions

**CNS** Headache, dizziness, disorientation, apprehension, pupillary dilation, paresthesias, sweating, flushing, and hyperpyrexia may occur. Positive bilateral Babinski signs may be noted. Tonic-clonic seizures may be induced, which require treatment with IV diazepam or a short-acting barbiturate.

- Obtain a thorough baseline assessment before starting therapy. Monitor temperature.
- Instruct the patient and family to report changes in mood or affect.
- Monitor deep tendon reflexes and Babinski reflexes. Provide a calm, reassuring attitude. Do not leave the patient unattended.
- In the hospital setting, pad side rails and keep them up. Have a suction machine at the bedside.

**CV** Increased blood pressure, tachycardia, ECG changes, and chest pain occur frequently.

- Monitor pulse and blood pressure.
- Obtain continuous ECG tracing throughout therapy.

**Blood** Doxapram causes hemolysis. This and other local reactions can be minimized by using dilute solutions infused slowly.

- May be given undiluted or diluted with equal parts of sterile water for injection, or dilute 250 mg in 250 ml 5% or 10% dextrose in water or normal saline, and administer as an infusion. Verify that infusion is patent before administering. Administer slowly to reduce hemolysis and thrombophlebitis. An undiluted dose may be given over 1 minute. The diluted dose is titrated to patient response, beginning with a rate of 5 mg/min, decreasing to 1 to 3 mg/min. The use of an infusion control device and microdrip tubing will help in titration.

**GI** Nausea, vomiting, diarrhea, and an urge to defecate may be caused by doxapram.

- Monitor intake and output.
- If diarrhea or vomiting is severe or persistent, notify the physician.

**GU** Spontaneous voiding or urinary retention may occur.

- Monitor intake and output. If the patient has not voided in 2 to 4 hours, palpate bladder and assess for retention. In the acutely ill patient, it may be appropriate to insert a urinary catheter.

**Lung** Bronchospasm, laryngospasm, coughing, and gagging may occur. Hypoventilation and even apnea may arise because doxapram causes constriction of cerebral blood vessels and respiratory alkalosis.

- Monitor respiratory rate, and auscultate breath sounds at regular intervals.

- If the patient is not already intubated, have a laryngoscope and airway at the bedside, as well as oxygen and a suction machine.
- Do not leave the patient unattended.
- Monitor arterial blood gases.

**Nursing interventions related to drug administration**
- For IV use, see Blood.

**Patient and family education**
- Review with patients and families the anticipated benefits and possible side effects of drug therapy.

---

## fenfluramine hydrochloride   (fen-FLOOR-uh-meen)                    anorexiant

- fenfluramine: Ponderal, ✿Ponderax, Pondimin (CIV)

**MECHANISM OF ACTION**   Fenfluramine is chemically related to amphetamine, but unlike amphetamine, fenfluramine depresses the CNS. The anorexiant action of fenfluramine may be related to CNS actions and/or metabolic effects of the drug.

**INDICATIONS**   **Obesity** The anorexiant action of fenfluramine may be temporarily helpful in weight control programs that include caloric restriction and dietary retraining.

**CONTRAINDICATIONS**   **Hypertension** Fenfluramine may elevate or lower blood pressure.   **Cardiovascular disease** Fenfluramine may alter blood pressure or induce arrhythmias.   **Glaucoma** Fenfluramine may increase intraocular pressure.   **Mental instability or history of drug abuse** Fenfluramine has a potential for abuse; its use may be inappropriate for patients with a history of susceptibility.   **Alcoholism** Fenfluramine may cause psychotic reactions in alcoholics.   **Hypersensitivity to sympathomimetic amines** The catecholamines released by fenfluramine can trigger dangerous reactions in sensitive individuals.

**DOSAGE**   **PO:**   **ADULTS:** 20 mg three times daily, usually 1 hour before meals. Dosage may be increased weekly by 20 mg unless adverse reactions occur. The maximum dose is 40 mg three times daily. *Special patient populations:* **CHILDREN:** Children should not receive fenfluramine.   **PREGNANCY:** Fenfluramine should be avoided by pregnant patients and nursing mothers.

**PREPARATIONS**   *Tablets:* 20 mg, scored.

**DRUG INTERACTIONS**   **Monoamine oxidase (MAO) inhibitors** block normal destruction of catecholamines that may be released by fenfluramine. The result may be a dangerous overstimulation caused by the accumulated catecholamines.   **CNS depressants** can have additive effects with fenfluramine, leading to excessive depression.   **General anesthetics** can be dangerous to patients who have received fenfluramine for prolonged periods because such patients may have been depleted of the catecholamines required to handle the stress of anesthesia and surgery. The result can be cardiac arrest.

**FATE**   Fenfluramine hydrochloride is orally absorbed to produce anorexiant effects within 1 to 2 hours. The *duration of action* is 4 to 6 hours. Fenfluramine is metabolized extensively; metabolites are excreted in urine. The elimination *half-life* of the drug is about 20 hours. Acidifying the urine speeds excretion.

### ❦ NURSING CONSIDERATIONS
#### Side effects, toxicities, and associated nursing actions

**CNS** Drowsiness is common. Some patients report dizziness, headache, insomnia, depression, lethargy, anxiety, and impaired coordination. Occasionally, patients suffer psychotic episodes; alcoholic patients are more prone to this reaction.
- Obtain a thorough baseline assessment before starting therapy.
- Instruct the patient and family to report changes in mood or affect.
- Caution patients to avoid driving or operating hazardous equipment until the effects of medication can be evaluated.
- Monitor weight.

**CV** Palpitation, changes in blood pressure, and fainting have occurred. Cardiac arrest under general anesthesia is possible.

- Monitor pulse and blood pressure.
- Obtain a baseline ECG, and monitor ECG at regular intervals throughout therapy.
- Caution patients to avoid the use of over-the-counter medications without first clearing them with the physician. Medications containing phenylpropanolamine, caffeine, and other substances that also have cardiovascular effects are readily available to the consumer and may contribute to excessive cardiovascular stimulation.

**Renal** Increased urinary frequency, dysuria, and impotence have occurred.
- Caution patients to report the development of these symptoms. If they are severe or persistent, it may be necessary to change drugs; notify the physician.

**GU** Dryness of the mouth and diarrhea are common reactions.
- If diarrhea is severe or persistent, notify the physician.
- For dry mouth, instruct the patient to chew sugarless gum, suck on sugarless candy, and rinse the mouth frequently. Avoid drying mouthwashes. Encourage good oral hygiene (brushing and flossing), which will improve patient comfort and lessen the chance of tooth decay. Some patients may wish to use commercially available saliva substitutes.

### Patient and family education
- Review the anticipated benefits and possible side effects of drug therapy with patients and families.
- See entry for drug class (p. 758).

## mazindol   (MAZ-in-dol)                                                                anorexiant

- mazindol: Mazanor, Sanorex (CIV)

**MECHANISM OF ACTION**   Mazindol is similar to amphetamine in its anorexiant effect. CNS effects of mazindol may differ from those of amphetamine, although both drugs stimulate various processes.

**INDICATIONS**   **Obesity** Appetite suppression is a side effect of CNS stimulants such as mazindol. This action may be temporarily helpful in weight control programs that include caloric restriction and dietary retraining.

**CONTRAINDICATIONS**   **Advanced arteriosclerosis** Mazindol may cause vasoconstriction or sudden alterations in blood pressure.   **Hypertension** Mazindol may alter blood pressure.   **Cardiovascular disease** Mazindol may alter blood pressure or induce arrhythmias.   **Glaucoma** Mazindol may increase intraocular pressure.   **Mental instability or history of drug abuse** Mazindol has a potential for abuse; its use may be inappropriate for patients with a history of susceptibility.

**DOSAGE**   **PO:**   ADULTS: 1 mg three times daily, usually 1 hour before meals. Alternatively, 2 mg may be taken once daily (1 hour before lunch). *Special patient populations:*   CHILDREN: Children under age 12 should not receive mazindol.   PREGNANCY: Mazindol should be avoided by pregnant patients and nursing mothers.

**PREPARATIONS**   *Tablets:* 1 or 2 mg, scored.

**DRUG INTERACTIONS**   **Monoamine oxidase (MAO) inhibitors** block normal destruction of catecholamines that may be released by mazindol. The result may be a dangerous overstimulation caused by the accumulated catecholamines.   **Guanethidine** effects may be diminished by mazindol, resulting in loss of control of hypertension.   **Pressor agents** such as norepinephrine or isoproterenol may have excessive pressor effects in patients receiving mazindol.   **Insulin** requirements in diabetes mellitus may be altered.

**FATE**   Mazindol is orally absorbed to produce anorexiant effects within 1 hour. The *duration of action* is 8 to 15 hours. Mazindol is incompletely metabolized; both unchanged drug and conjugated metabolites are excreted in the urine.

### ❧ NURSING CONSIDERATIONS
#### Side effects, toxicities, and associated nursing actions
**CNS** Overstimulation of the CNS may produce restlessness, tremor, dizziness, headache, insomnia,

and shivering. Chronic schizophrenics suffer an increase in schizophrenic behavior. Habituation is possible, and abrupt withdrawal may result in depression, fatigue and other symptoms.
- See benzamphetamine (p. 760).

**Patient and family education**
- Review the anticipated benefits and possible side effects of drug therapy with patients and families.
- See entry for drug class (p. 758).

---

## methamphetamine hydrochloride   (meth-am-FET-uh-meen)   anorexiant*

- methamphetamine hydrochloride: Desoxyn, Methampex, Methedrine (CII)

**MECHANISM OF ACTION**   Methamphetamine, like other amphetamines, increases the release and effectiveness of norepinephrine and dopamine in the central nervous system. The catecholamines norepinephrine and dopamine act as neurotransmitters in the CNS, in addition to serving as neurotransmitters in the peripheral autonomic nervous system. Amphetamines increase the level of arousal by action on the reticular activating system. Amphetamine action on the medial forebrain bundle, or reward center, creates a perception of pleasure that is unrelated to external stimuli. Methamphetamine has a potency between that of dextroamphetamine and amphetamine for stimulating the CNS.

**INDICATIONS**   **Hyperkinesis** Children displaying overactivity and associated symptoms may receive methamphetamine to control the condition. Methamphetamine, which causes agitation and activity in adults, may have a calming effect in children.   **Obesity** Appetite suppression is a side effect of methamphetamine, which may be used as a temporary aid in weight reduction programs.

**CONTRAINDICATIONS**   **Advanced arteriosclerosis** Methamphetamine may cause vasoconstriction or sudden elevations in blood pressure. **Hypertension** Methamphetamine may elevate blood pressure. **Hyperthyroidism** Methamphetamine may dangerously increase the symptoms of agitation and cardiovascular overstimulation in hyperthyroidism.   **Cardiovascular disease** Methamphetamine may elevate blood pressure or induce arrhythmias.   **Glaucoma** Methamphetamine may increase intraocular pressure.   **Mental instability or history of drug abuse** The mood-altering effects of methamphetamine and the strong potential for abuse make this drug especially dangerous for patients with a history of susceptibility.   **Hypersensitivity to sympathomimetic amines** The catecholamines released by methamphetamine can trigger dangerous reactions in sensitive individuals.

**DOSAGE**   **For hyperkinesis:** *PO:*   CHILDREN OVER 6 YEARS: Initially, 2.5 to 5 mg once or twice daily. Increase weekly by 5 mg increments until desired effect is achieved, which normally requires 20 to 25 mg daily.   **For obesity:** *PO:*   ADULTS: 5 to 15 mg daily, given in divided doses 30 to 60 minutes before meals. Sustained-release preparations are administered before breakfast and contain either 10 or 15 mg of drug. Therapy should not be continued beyond a few weeks because tolerance develops to the anorexiant effects, while the abuse potential remains. *Special patient populations:* CHILDREN: Avoid in children under age 6.   PREGNANCY: Methamphetamine should not be administered to pregnant women.

**PREPARATIONS**   *Tablets:* 5 or 10 mg, scored; *tablets, extended release:* 5, 10, or 15 mg. The 15 mg extended-release tablets sold under the trade name of Desoxyn contain tartrazine, which may cause allergic reactions in susceptible patients.

**DRUG INTERACTIONS**   **Monoamine oxidase (MAO) inhibitors** block normal pathways for destruction of sympathomimetic amines; therefore, the catecholamines released by methamphetamine may not be efficiently metabolized and can accumulate to dangerous levels. Fatalities have resulted.   **Halothane and cyclopropane** used as general anesthetics may sensitize the heart to the catecholamines released by methamphetamine. The result may be dangerous or fatal arrhythmias.

**FATE**   Methamphetamine is readily absorbed orally and distributed to many tissues, especially the central nervous system. The *duration of effect* ranges from 4 to 24 hours. The primary route of elimination of amphetamine is through the kidneys, with excretion enhanced in an acidic urine.

*CNS stimulant.

### ❦ NURSING CONSIDERATIONS

#### Side effects, toxicities, and associated nursing actions
- See amphetamine (p. 758).

#### Nursing interventions related to drug administration
- When used for appetite suppression, the drug should be given 30 to 60 minutes prior to a meal. The extended-release tablet should be given before breakfast.
- Desoxyn brand extended-release tablets in 15 mg dosages contain FD & C yellow dye number 5 (tartrazine), which may cause an allergic reaction in susceptible individuals. While rare, this reaction is seen more commonly in persons with aspirin hypersensitivity.

#### Patient and family education
- Review the anticipated benefits and possible side effects of drug therapy with patients and families.
- See entry for drug class (p. 758).

---

## methylphenidate hydrochloride (meth-ill-FEN-i-date)    CNS stimulant

- methylphenidate hydrochloride: ✦Centedrin Ritalin (CII)

**MECHANISM OF ACTION**   Methylphenidate produces CNS stimulation that resembles the stimulation caused by amphetamines. The mechanism by which methylphenidate stimulates the CNS is not understood in detail and may differ from that of amphetamines.

**INDICATIONS**   **Narcolepsy** Methylphenidate used during the daytime can help control narcolepsy, a condition in which patients abruptly fall asleep during normal daytime activities.   **Hyperkinesis** Children displaying overactivity and associated symptoms may receive methylphenidate to control the condition.

**CONTRAINDICATIONS**   **Seizures** Methylphenidate may increase the likelihood of seizures in predisposed patients.   **Hypertension** Methylphenidate may increase hypertension.   **Agitation, anxiety, or tension** Methylphenidate may worsen these conditions.   **Tourette's disorder or motor tics** Methylphenidate may worsen these conditions.   **Glaucoma** Methylphenidate may increase intraocular pressure.

**DOSAGE**   **For narcolepsy:** *PO:*   **ADULTS:** 10 mg two or three times daily, given 30 to 45 minutes before meals. Dosage is individualized for control of symptoms with minimum doses.   **For hyperkinesis:** *PO:* **CHILDREN OLDER THAN 6 YEARS:** Initially, 5 mg before breakfast and lunch, increasing by 5 or 10 mg increments weekly until response is satisfactory. Alternatively, initial doses may be 0.25 mg/kg, doubling the dose weekly to until 2 mg/kg is achieved. Daily doses should not exceed 60 mg, nor should the drug be continued longer than 1 month if responses are not satisfactory. Children who do respond should have therapy interupted every few months to assess whether drug therapy is still required.   *Special patient populations:*   **CHILDREN:** Children younger than 6 should not receive methylphenidate.   **PREGNANCY:** Methylphenidate should not be used in pregnant or lactating patients.

**PREPARATIONS**   *Tablets:* 5, 10 or 20 mg; *tablets, extended release:* 20 mg.

**DRUG INTERACTIONS**   **Monoamine oxidase (MAO) inhibitors** may cause dangerous increases in blood pressure when combined with methylphenidate.   **Guanethidine or bretylium** have less hypotensive activity when given with methylphenidate.   **Coumarin anticoagulants** are metabolized less efficiently in patients also receiving methylphenidate; dangerous accumulation of the anticoagulants may occur. **Phenylbutazone,** an anti-inflammatory drug, is less efficiently metabolized in patients also receiving methylphenidate; dangerous toxic reactions to phenylbutazone may therefore occur.   **Phenobarbital, phenytoin, and primidone** agents used as anticonvulsants, are less efficiently metabolized in patients also receiving methylphenidate; dangerous accumulation of the drugs may occur.   **Tricyclic antidepressants (imipramine, desipramine)** are less efficiently metabolized in patients also receiving methylphenidate; dangerous toxic reactions to the antidepressants may therefore occur.

**FATE** Methylphenidate hydrochloride is well absorbed orally, and the *duration of action* is 3 to 6 hours. Methylphenidate is metabolized, and the metabolites are excreted in urine.

## NURSING CONSIDERATIONS

### Side effects, toxicities, and associated nursing actions

**CNS** Confusion, delirium, euphoria, hallucinations, and toxic psychosis may occur with overdosage; the reactions resemble those to amphetamine. Agitation, headache, confusion, mydriasis, hyperpyrexia, tremors, sweating, twitching, hyperreflexia, and seizures may also occur in response to overdoses. At normal therapeutic doses, nervousness, insomnia, anorexia, dizziness, headache, akathisia, dyskinesia, or drowsiness may occur.

* Obtain a thorough baseline assessment before starting therapy.
* Instruct the patient and family to report changes in mood or affect.
* Caution patients to avoid driving or operating hazardous equipment until the effects of medication can be evaluated.
* Monitor weight.
* In the hospital setting, pad side rails and keep them up. Have a suction machine at the bedside.

**CV** Cardiac arrythmias, hypertension, and tachycardia may occur at toxic doses. At normal therapeutic doses, blood pressure and heart rate may change, and angina or cardiac arrhythmias may occur.

* Monitor pulse and blood pressure.
* Obtain a baseline ECG, and monitor ECG at regular intervals throughout therapy.
* Caution patients to avoid the use of over-the-counter medications without first clearing them with the physician. Medications containing phenylpropanolamine, caffeine, and other substances that also have cardiovascular effects are readily available to the consumer and may contribute to excessive cardiovascular stimulation.

**GI** Nausea, vomiting, and dry mouth occur at toxic doses. Anorexia, abdominal pain, and weight loss may occur at normal therapeutic doses in children.

* If vomiting or diarrhea is severe or persistent, notify physician.
* Monitor weight. Instruct patients to record weight at least twice a week.
* If constipation occurs, increase fluid intake to 2500 ml/day, increase dietary intake of fruits, fruit juices, and fiber, and increase level of exercise.
* For dry mouth, instruct the patient to chew sugarless gum, suck on sugarless candy, and rinse the mouth frequently. Avoid drying mouthwashes. Encourage good oral hygiene (brushing and flossing), which will improve patient comfort and lessen the chance of tooth decay. Some patients may wish to use commercially available saliva substitutes.

**Metabolic** Children receiving methylphenidate for hyperkinesis may suffer growth retardation. For this reason, children should have the drug discontinued periodically to assess whether the drug must be continued for control of the condition and to allow growth to proceed normally.

* Instruct parents to measure and record height and weight of children taking this drug for hyperkinesis at least weekly.

**Allergic** Rash, urticaria, fever, pain in the joints (arthralgia), exfoliative dermatitis, or erythema multiforme may occur. Stevens-Johnson syndrome is a possible reaction.

* Monitor patients for rashes and skin changes. Instruct patients to report the development of high fever, headache, stomatitis, conjunctivitis, rhinitis, urethritis, and balanitis (inflammation of the glans penis), as these may signal the development of Stevens-Johnson syndrome.

### Nursing interventions related to drug administration

* Read labels carefully; the drug is available in a regular tablet form and an extended-release formulation.

### Patient and family education

* Review the anticipated benefits and possible side effects of drug therapy with patients and families.
* See entry for drug class (p. 758).

## pemoline (PEM-oh-lin) CNS stimulant

- pemoline: Cylert (CIV)

**MECHANISM OF ACTION** Pemoline produces CNS stimulation that resembles the stimulation caused by amphetamines or methylphenidate. The mechanism by which pemoline stimulates the CNS is not understood in detail and may differ from that of the other two drugs.

**INDICATIONS** **Hyperkinesis** Children displaying overactivity and associated symptoms may receive pemoline to control the condition.

**CONTRAINDICATIONS** **Hepatic dysfunction** Pemoline causes reversible hepatic damage in many patients. Persons with pre-existing hepatic impairment may be at greater risk of serious or life-threatening complications. **Tourett disorder or motor tics** Pemoline may worsen these conditions. **Renal impairment** Pemoline and its metabolites are excreted in the urine; the drug may accumulate if renal function is impaired. **Psychoses** Pemoline can cause signs and symptoms that complicate diagnosis and evaluation of therapy in psychotic patients.

**DOSAGE** **PO:** **CHILDREN OLDER THAN 6 YEARS:** Initially, 37.5 mg before breakfast, increasing by 18.75 mg increments weekly until response is satisfactory. Daily doses should not exceed 112.5 mg. Full beneficial effects may take as long as a month to become evident. Children who do respond should have therapy interupted every few months to assess whether drug therapy is still required. *Special patient populations:* **CHILDREN:** Children younger than 6 should not receive pemoline. **PREGNANCY:** Pemoline should not be used in pregnant or lactating patients.

**PREPARATIONS** *Tablets:* 18.75, 37.5, or 75 mg; *tablets, chewable:* 37.5 mg.

**DRUG INTERACTIONS** Specific interactions have not been reported.

**FATE** Pemoline is well absorbed orally, leading to *peak* serum concentrations within 2 to 4 hours. The *duration* of CNS stimulation is up to 8 hours. The therapeutic effects of pemoline on hyperkinetic children may take weeks to develop. The elimination *half-life* of pemoline in children is extremely variable, ranging from 2 to 12 hours. This value may increase when the drug is used for long periods.

## 🦃 NURSING CONSIDERATIONS

### Side effects, toxicities, and associated nursing actions

**CNS** Confusion, delirium, euphoria, hallucinations, and toxic psychosis may occur with overdosage; the reactions resemble those to amphetamine. At normal therapeutic doses, nervousness, insomnia, anorexia, dizziness, headache, akathisia, dyskineisa, or drowsiness may occur. In children, insomnia is the most common early side effect.

- Obtain a thorough baseline assessment before starting therapy.
- Instruct the patient and family to report changes in mood or affect.
- Caution patients to avoid driving or operating hazardous equipment until the effects of medication can be evaluated.
- Monitor weight.
- In the hospital setting, pad side rails and keep them up. Have a suction machine at the bedside.

**CV** Tachycardia may occur at toxic doses. At normal therapeutic doses, cardiovascular changes usually do not occur.

- Monitor pulse and blood pressure.
- Obtain a baseline ECG, and monitor ECG at regular intervals throughout therapy.
- Caution patients to avoid the use of over-the-counter medications without first clearing them with the physician. Medications containing phenylpropanolamine, caffeine, and other substances that also have cardiovascular effects are readily available to the consumer and may contribute to excessive cardiovascular stimulation.

**GI** Nausea, anorexia, abdominal pain, and weight loss may occur at normal therapeutic doses in children.

- If vomiting or diarrhea is severe or persistent, notify the physician.
- Monitor weight. Instruct patients to record weight at least twice a week.
- If constipation occurs, increase fluid intake to 2500 ml/day, increase dietary intake of fruits, fruit juices, and fiber, and increase level of exercise.

- For dry mouth, instruct the patient to chew sugarless gum, suck on sugarless candy, and rinse the mouth frequently. Avoid drying mouthwashes. Encourage good oral hygiene (brushing and flossing), which will improve patient comfort and lessen the chance of tooth decay. Some patients may wish to use commercially available saliva substitutes.

**Metabolic** Children receiving pemoline for hyperkinesis may suffer growth retardation. For this reason, children should have the drug discontinued periodically to assess whether the drug must be continued for control of the condition and to allow growth to proceed normally.

- Instruct parents to measure and record height and weight of children taking this drug for hyperkinesis at least weekly.

**Liver** Elevated serum AST (SGOT), ALT (SGPT), and alkaline phosphatase may indicate liver damage, with or without other symptoms. Rarely, jaundice or hepatitis occur. Elderly patients may show more severe signs.

- Monitor liver function tests.
- Instruct patients to report the development of jaundice, malaise, fever, right upper quadrant abdominal pain, or change in the color or consistency of stools.

**Allergic** Rash may occur. Liver damage may be an allergic reaction.

- Monitor patients for rashes and skin changes.

### Nursing interventions related to drug administration
- Chewable tablets should be chewed for several minutes prior to swallowing.

### Patient and family education
- Review the anticipated benefits and possible side effects of drug therapy with patients and families.
- See entry for drug class (p. 758).

---

## phendimetrazine tartrate   (fen-dye-ME-tra-zeen)    anorexiant

- phendimetrazine tartrate: Adipost, Bacarate, Bontril, Dyrexan-OD, Hyrex, Melfiat, Obalan, Obezine, Plegine, Prelu-2, SPRX-105, Statobex, Trimcaps, Trimstat, Trimtabs, Wehless, Weightrol (CIII)

**MECHANISM OF ACTION**   Phendimetrazine is similar to amphetamine in its mechanism of action and anorexiant effects.

**INDICATIONS**   **Obesity** Appetite suppression is a side effect of CNS stimulants such as phendimetrazine. This action may be temporarily helpful in weight control programs that include caloric restriction and dietary retraining.

**CONTRAINDICATIONS**   **Advanced arteriosclerosis** Phendimetrazine may cause vasoconstriction or sudden elevations in blood pressure.   **Hypertension** Phendimetrazine may elevate blood pressure.   **Hyperthyroidism** Phendimetrazine may dangerously increase the symptoms of agitation and cardiovascular overstimulation in hyperthyroidism.   **Cardiovascular disease** Phendimetrazine may elevate blood pressure or induce arrhythmias.   **Glaucoma** Phendimetrazine may increase intraocular pressure. **Mental instability or history of drug abuse** Phendimetrazine has a potential for abuse; its use may be inappropriate for patients with a history of susceptibility.   **Hypersensitivity to sympathomimetic amines** The catecholamines released by phendimetrazine can trigger dangerous reactions in sensitive individuals.

**DOSAGE**   **PO:**   **ADULTS:** 35 mg two or three times daily, usually 1 hour before meals. Although the dose may be cautiously increased if tolerated, the maximum dose is 70 mg three times daily. An extended-release preparation containing 105 mg may be taken once daily at midmorning.   *Special patient populations:*   **CHILDREN:** Children should not receive phendimetrazine.   **PREGNANCY:** Phendimetrazine should be avoided by pregnant patients and nursing mothers.

**PREPARATIONS**   *Capsules and tablets:* 35 mg. The capsules and tablets sold under the trade name Statobex contain tartrazine (FD & C yellow # 5), which may cause allergic reactions in susceptible individuals. *Capsules and tablets, extended release:* 105 mg.

**DRUG INTERACTIONS**   **Monoamine oxidase (MAO) inhibitors** block normal destruction of catecholamines that may be released by phendimetrazine. The result may be a dangerous overstimulation caused by the accumulated catecholamines.   **Guanethidine** effects may be diminished by phendimetrazine, resulting in loss of control of hypertension.

**FATE**   Phendimetrazine tartrate is well absorbed orally. The *duration of action* is about 4 hours.

## ☙ NURSING CONSIDERATIONS

### Side effects, toxicities, and associated nursing actions
- See benzphetamine (p. 760).

### Nursing interventions related to drug administration
- See Preparations. Statobex brand contains tartrazine.

### Patient and family education
- Review the anticipated benefits and possible side effects of drug therapy with patients and families.
- See entry for drug class (p. 758).

---

## phenmetrazine hydrochloride   (fen-MET-rah-zeen)   anorexiant

- phenmetrazine hydrochloride: Preludin (CII)

**MECHANISM OF ACTION**   Phenmetrazine is similar to amphetamine in its mechanism of action and anorexiant effects.

**INDICATIONS**   **Obesity** Appetite suppression is a side effect of CNS stimulants such as phenmetrazine. This action may be temporarily helpful in weight control programs that include caloric restriction and dietary retraining.

**CONTRAINDICATIONS**   **Advanced arteriosclerosis** Phenmetrazine may cause vasoconstriction or sudden elevations in blood pressure.   **Hypertension** Phenmetrazine may elevate blood pressure.   **Hyperthyroidism** Phenmetrazine may dangerously increase the symptoms of agitation and cardiovascular overstimulation in hyperthyroidism.   **Cardiovascular disease** Phenmetrazine may elevate blood pressure or induce arrhythmias.   **Glaucoma** Phenmetrazine may increase intraocular pressure.   **Mental instability or history of drug abuse** Phenmetrazine has a potential for abuse; its use may be inappropriate for patients with a history of susceptibility.   **Hypersensitivity to sympathomimetic amines** The catecholamines released by phenmetrazine can trigger dangerous reactions in sensitive individuals.

**DOSAGE**   **PO:**   **ADULTS:** 25 mg two or three times daily, usually 1 hour before meals. Although the dose may be cautiously increased if tolerated, the maximum dose is 25 mg three times daily. An extended-release preparation containing 75 mg may be taken once daily at midmorning. *Special patient populations:*   **CHILDREN:** Children should not receive phenmetrazine.   **PREGNANCY:** Phenmetrazine should be avoided by pregnant patients and nursing mothers.

**PREPARATIONS**   *Tablets:* 25 mg., *tablets, extended release:* 75 mg. The extended-release tablets contain tartrazine (FD & C yellow # 5), which may cause allergic reactions in susceptible individuals.

**DRUG INTERACTIONS**   **Monoamine oxidase (MAO) inhibitors** block normal destruction of catecholamines that may be released by phenmetrazine. The result may be a dangerous overstimulation caused by the accumulated catecholamines.   **Guanethidine** effects may be diminished by phenmetrazine, resulting in loss of control of hypertension.

**FATE**   Phenmetrazine hydrochloride is well absorbed orally. The *duration of action* is about 4 hours with the regular formulation.

## ☙ NURSING CONSIDERATIONS

### Side effects, toxicities, and associated nursing actions
- See benzphetamine (p. 760).

### Nursing interventions related to drug administration
- See Preparations. Extended-release tablets contain tartrazine.

**Patient and family education**
- Review the anticipated benefits and possible side effects of drug therapy with patients and families.
- See entry for drug class (p. 758).

## phentermine hydrochloride, phentermine (FEN-ter-meen) anorexiant

- phentermine hydrochloride: Adipex-P, Appi-Plex, Dapex, Fastin, Ionamin, Obephen, Obermine, Obestin, Paramine, Phentride, Phentrol, Tora, Unifast, Wilpowr (CIV)

**MECHANISM OF ACTION** Phentermine is similar to amphetamine in its mechanism of action and anorexiant effect.

**INDICATIONS** **Obesity** Appetite suppression is a side effect of CNS stimulants such as phentermine. This action may be temporarily helpful in weight control programs that include caloric restriction and dietary retraining.

**CONTRAINDICATIONS** **Advanced arteriosclerosis** Phentermine may cause vasoconstriction or sudden elevations in blood pressure. **Hypertension** Phentermine may elevate blood pressure. **Hyperthyroidism** Phentermine may dangerously increase the symptoms of agitation and cardiovascular overstimulation in hyperthyroidism. **Cardiovascular disease** Phentermine may elevate blood pressure or induce arrhythmias. **Glaucoma** Phentermine may increase intraocular pressure. **Mental instability or history of drug abuse** Phentermine has a potential for abuse; its use may be inappropriate for patients with a history of susceptibility. **Hypersensitivity to sympathomimetic amines** The catecholamines released by phentermine can trigger dangerous reactions in sensitive individuals.

**DOSAGE** **PO:** **ADULTS:** 8 mg three times daily, usually 30 minutes before meals. Alternate dosing schedules include 15 to 30 mg of phentermine resin complex or 15 to 37.5 mg phentermine hydrochloride once daily at midmorning. *Special patient populations:* **CHILDREN:** Children should not receive phentermine. **PREGNANCY:** Phentermine should be avoided by pregnant patients and nursing mothers.

**PREPARATIONS** *Phentermine hydrochloride, tablets:* 8 (scored) or 37.5 mg; capsules: 8, 15, 18.75, 30, or 37.5 mg. *Phentermine as resin complex, capsules:* 15 or 30 mg.

**DRUG INTERACTIONS** **Monoamine oxidase (MAO) inhibitors** block normal destruction of catecholamines that may be released by phentermine. The result may be a dangerous overstimulation caused by the accumulated catecholamines. **Guanethidine** effects may be diminished by phentermine, resulting in loss of control of hypertension.

**FATE** Phentermine is bioavailable following oral administration of phentermine hydrochloride or of the insoluble phentermine resin complex. The pharmacokinetics are similar to other appetite suppressants, with doses often being required three times daily for best effect.

## ☙ NURSING CONSIDERATIONS

**Side effects, toxicities, and associated nursing actions**
- See benzphetamine (p. 760).

**Patient and family education**
- Review the anticipated benefits and possible side effects of drug therapy with patients and families.
- See entry for drug class (p. 758).

## phenylpropanolamine hydrochloride
(fen-ill-pro-pan-OHL-uh-meen) decongestant*

- phenylpropanolamine hydrochloride: Appedrine, Control, Dexatrim, Dietac, Propadrine

**MECHANISM OF ACTION** Phenylpropanolamine is a sympathomimetic with central and peripheral action. Phenylpropanolamine constricts blood vessels, making the drug useful orally or topically as a decon-

*Anorexiant.

gestant. The CNS effects of phenylpropanolamine include mild, temporary appetite suppression much like that produced by the amphetamines and related CNS stimulants. The generally milder CNS effects of phenylpropanolamine enable the drug to be used without prescription.

**INDICATIONS**  **Nasal congestion** Phenylpropanolamine constricts the vessels in mucous membranes, reducing swelling and improving air flow (see Chapter 53).  **Obesity** Phenylpropanolamine may be used as a temporary aid in weight reduction programs.

**CONTRAINDICATIONS**  **Hypertension** Phenylpropanolamine may elevate blood pressure, complicating therapy of hypertension.  **Cardiovascular disease** Phenylpropanolamine may elevate blood pressure or induce arrhythmias that could be dangerous to patients with pre-existing cardiovascular disease. **Hyperthyroidism** Phenylpropanolamine may increase the symptoms of agitation and cardiovascular overstimulation in hyperthyroidism.  **Glaucoma** Phenylpropanolamine may increase intraocular pressure.

**DOSAGE**  **For nasal congestion:** *PO:*  ADULTS: 25 mg every 4 hours or 50 mg repeated no more frequently than 6 or 8 hours. Maximum total daily dosage is 150 mg. Sustained-release forms contain 75 mg and are taken twice daily.  CHILDREN: Ages 6 to 12, 12.5 mg every 4 hours or 25 mg every 8 hours. **For obesity** *PO:*  ADULTS: 25 mg three times daily; maximum daily dose is 75 mg. Dosage with sustained-release forms is 50 to 75 mg daily.  *Special patient populations:*  CHILDREN: Avoid in children under age 6.  PREGNANCY: Phenylpropanolamine should not be used by pregnant or lactating patients.

**PREPARATIONS**  *Tablets:* 25, 50, or 100 mg; *capsules:* 25 or 50 mg; *capsules, timed release:* 37.5 or 75 mg; *oral solution (drops):* 25 mg/4 drops. Phenylpropanolamine is included in several OTC preparations that also include caffeine, vitamins, mild diuretics, and other ingredients.

**DRUG INTERACTIONS**  **Monoamine oxidase (MAO) inhibitors** block normal pathways for destruction of sympathomimetic amines. Phenylpropanolamine may cause dangerous symptoms in these patients because of overstimulation of the sympathetic nervous system.  **Sympathomimetic amines** such as those found in OTC decongestants should not be used along with phenylpropanolamine. The combination may cause dangerous overstimulation of the sympathetic nervous system.

**FATE**  Phenylpropanolamine is readily absorbed orally. The *half-life* is 3 to 4 hours. Most of the drug is excreted by the kidneys, with the remainder being metabolized by the liver.

### ❦ NURSING CONSIDERATIONS

#### Side effects, toxicities, and associated nursing actions

**CNS** Nervousness, restlessness, dizziness, headache, tinnitus can occur at any dose but are more likely with excessive doses.

- Obtain a thorough baseline assessment before starting therapy.
- Instruct the patient and family to report changes in mood or affect.
- Instruct patients to report the development of tinnitus or hearing changes.
- Caution patients to avoid driving or operating hazardous equipment until the effects of medication can be evaluated.
- Monitor weight.

**CV** Tachycardia, palpitations, and excessive increases in blood pressure are possible.

- Monitor pulse and blood pressure.
- Obtain a baseline ECG, and monitor ECG at regular intervals throughout therapy.
- Caution patients to avoid the use of over-the-counter medications without first clearing them with the physician. Medications containing phenylpropanolamine, caffeine, and other substances that also have cardiovascular effects are readily available to the consumer and may contribute to excessive cardiovascular stimulation.

**Renal** Exceedingly high doses of phenylpropanolamine were reported as the possible cause of renal failure in two patients.

- Caution patients to report the development of edema or fluid retention.
- Monitor weight. Instruct patients to record weight at least twice a week.
- If renal failure is suspected, monitor serum creatinine and BUN. Monitor intake and output.

**Metabolic** Phenylpropanolamine may increase blood glucose.

- Caution diabetic patients to monitor blood glucose levels more frequently. A change in the dose of insulin and/or diet requirements may be necessary.

### Patient and family education

- Review the anticipated benefits and possible side effects of drug therapy with patients and families.
- See entry for drug class (p. 758).

# ANTICONVULSANTS AND DRUGS INFLUENCING MOTOR CONTROL

**INTRODUCTION**  This unit is divided into six chapters based on the five types of muscle disorders for which there are pharmacologic interventions: seizure disorders, spasticity, muscle spasms, myasthenia gravis, and parkinsonism. The sixth chapter reviews the neuromuscular blocking agents used to promote musculoskeletal relaxation during anesthesia.

Anticonvulsant drugs are used acutely and chronically to control a variety of seizure conditions. The severity of exaggerated reflexes (spinal spasticity) or inappropriate posture (cerebral spasticity) can sometimes be relieved by one of the antispastic drugs. When muscle spasms are not adequately controlled by analgesics and antiinflammatory drugs, one of the centrally acting skeletal muscle relaxants presented may be added. The drugs used to treat the disease myasthenia gravis are acetylcholinesterase inhibitors. Drugs for treating parkinsonism include anticholinergic drugs, antihistaminic drugs, amantadine, and levodopamine. All act to restore a balance of neurotransmitters in the basal ganglia controlling muscle tone. Neuromuscular blocking agents produce muscular relaxation to facilitate procedures and surgery on anesthetized patients.

**XI**

# Chapter Thirty-nine

# Anticonvulsant drugs

acetazolamide (see Chapter 9)
carbamazepine
clonazepam
diazepam (see Chapter 35)
ethosuximide
magnesium sulfate (see Chapter 62)
methsuximide

paraldehyde (see Chapter 35)
phenobarbital
phensuximide
phenytoin
primidone
valproic acid

**DRUG COMBINATIONS**

- phenobarbital and phenytoin: Dilantin with Phenobarbital, Kapseals

**OVERVIEW OF THE DRUG CLASS**  Epilepsy is a neurologic disorder characterized by a recurrent pattern of abnormal neuron discharges within the brain, resulting in a sudden loss or disturbance of consciousness, sometimes in association with motor activity (clonic or tonic seizures), sensory phenomena (aura and characteristic sensations), or inappropriate behavior. Between 1% and 2% of the population is estimated to have epilepsy. The cause of epilepsy may be unknown (idiopathic) or may be traced to a known brain lesion. In general, epilepsy appearing in childhood or adolescence is likely to be idiopathic, whereas epilepsy appearing in adulthood is likely to relate to a definable cause, such as a head injury, cerebrovascular accident (stroke), or brain tumor.

An appropriate choice of drugs taken on a long-term basis, can control the seizures of epilepsy in about 80% of patients. The choice of drugs depends on a careful diagnosis of the seizure pattern, which ideally is made from the observation of a seizure and the recording of the brain wave pattern with an electroencephalogram (EEG) during the seizure. The diagnosis is critical to the selection of a drug or drugs, since different seizure patterns are controlled by different drugs. The drug choice by seizure type is listed in Table 39-1. Only first and second-choice drugs are covered in this section.

**MECHANISM OF ACTION**  The molecular basis of anticonvulsant action is not known. These drugs depress the excitability of neurons, particularly those that fire inappropriately to initiate the seizure, and thus prevent the spread of seizure discharges. Presumably the mechanisms will be found to modify the ionic movements of sodium, potassium, or calcium across the nerve membrane associated with the action potential or to modify the release or uptake of neurotransmitters.

**INDICATIONS**  • Recurrent seizures.

**CONTRAINDICATIONS**  **Hepatic or renal disease** Several anticonvulsants can cause hepatic or renal damage.

**DRUG INTERACTIONS**  See the individual drug.

## carbamazepine  (kar-ba-MAZ-e-peen)                    anticonvulsant

- carbamazepine: ♣Apo-Carbamazepine, ♣Marzepine, Tegretol

**MECHANISM OF ACTION**  Limits seizure propagation by acting at the level of synaptic transmission. Carbamazepine is chemically related to the tricyclic antidepressants.

**INDICATIONS**  **Partial seizure disorders** Used prophylactically for psychomotor or temporal lobe seizures. **Grand mal seizures** For prophylactic management.  **Trigeminal neuralgia** For the symptomatic treatment of pain.

**CONTRAINDICATIONS**  **Cardiac damage** Carbamazepine can cause serious cardiovascular effects itself and should not be administered to a patient who already suffers cardiac damage.  **Liver disease** Carbamazepine can cause liver damage, and liver function studies are monitored in patients taking the drug. Pre-existing liver disease interferes with this necesasry monitoring.  **Bone marrow depression** Carbamazepine can cause aplastic anemia and should not be used by anyone with a history of bone marrow depression.

**Table 39-1.**

## Drug choice by seizure type

| Seizure type | First-choice drugs* | Additional drugs for second-choice drugs† |
|---|---|---|
| General: tonic-clonic (grand mal)<br><br>Partial: cortical focal (including jacksonian) | Alone or in combination:<br>1. Phenytoin (Dilantin)—adults<br>2. Phenobarbital (Luminal)—children<br>3. Carbamazepine (Tegratal) | 1. Other barbiturates: primidone (Mysoline) or mephobarbital (Mebaral)<br>2. Valproic acid (Depakene) |
| General: absence (petit mal) | Alone<br>1. Ethosuximide (Zarontin)<br>2. Valproic acid (Depakene) | 1. Other succinimides: methsuximide (Celontin) or phensuximide (Milontin)<br>2. Benzodiazepines: diazepam (Valium) or clonazepam (Clonopin) |
| General: myoclonus (Intentional of progressive) | 1. Valproic acid (Depakene) | 1. Chonazepam (Clonopin)<br>2. 1,5,-Hydroxytyptophan and carbidopa (experimental) |
| General: infantile spasms | 1. Adrenocorticotropic hormone (ACTH) | 1. Clonazepam (Clonopin) |
| Partial: complex (temporal lobe, psychomotor) | 1. Carbamazepine (Tegretol) | 1. Primidone (Mysoline)<br>2. Phenytoin (Dilantin) |
| Status epilepticus: continuous tonic-clonic | 1. Intravenous diazepam (Valium)<br>2. Intravenous phenytoin sodium (Dilantin)<br>3. Intravenous phenobarbital sodium (Luminal Sodium) | 1. Rectal paraldehyde<br>2. Intravenous amobarbital sodium (Amytal Sodium) |

*First-choice drugs are those generally effective for most patients with the least of toxic effects.

†Second-choice drugs are those sometimes effective when the first-choice drugs are not effective alone or those associated with a higher incidence of side effects.

From Clark JB, Queener SF, Karb, VB: Pharmacological Basis of Nursing Practice, ed. 2, St. Louis, 1986, The C.V. Mosby Co.

**DOSAGE**    For seizures:   *PO:*   ADULTS AND CHILDREN OVER 12 YEARS OLD: 200 mg two times daily initially, increasing by up to 200 mg daily to achieve control. Dosages over 400 mg daily are divided into 3 or 4 doses. Maximum dose is 1 g daily for children 13 to 15 years old, 1.2 g daily for those older.   CHILDREN 6 TO 12 YEARS OLD: 100 mg two times the first day, then increase by 100 mg daily to achieve control and divide into 3 or 4 doses. Maximum dose is 1 gm daily.   CHILDREN UNDER 6 YEARS OLD: 5 mg/kg daily. Dosage can be increased every week by 5 mg/kg if needed, up to 20 mg/kg.   Trigeminal neuralgia:   *PO:* 100 mg twice daily the first day. Then increase dose by 100 mg every 12 hours until pain is relieved. Maximum dose is 1.2 g. Pain relief is usually obtained at doses of 200 mg to 1.2 g daily. A maintenance dose is generally 400 to 800 mg daily. At least every 3 months the dosage should be reduced to see if the maintenance dose can be lowered or discontinued. *Special patient populations:*   PREGNANCY: Safe use during pregnancy has not been established. Nursing mothers should not take carbamazepine.

**PREPARATIONS**    *Tablets:* 200 mg. *Tablets (chewable):* 200 mg.

**DRUG INTERACTIONS**    **Phenytoin, phenobarbital, primidone** Carbamazepine decreases the half-life of these anticonvulsants, probably by increasing their metabolism.

**FATE**    Carbamazepine is only slowly absorbed from the GI tract. Two to four days may be required to achieve steady-state plasma levels. The *half-life* is 8 to 72 hours. Carbamazepine is metabolized by the liver and can induce liver microsomal enzymes, thereby increasing the rate of degradation of other drugs.

## ☙ NURSING CONSIDERATIONS

### Side effects, toxicities, and associated nursing actions

**CNS** Ataxia, dizziness, and anorexia are early signs of toxic levels. Other side effects include vertigo, drowsiness, fatigue and confusion.

- Obtain baseline neurologic and mental status examination prior to administering first dose. Monitor patient at regular intervals.
- Caution patients to avoid driving or operating hazardous equipment if ataxia, vertigo, or drowsiness occur.
- Instruct patient and family to notify physician if CNS side effects develop.
- Monitor serum drug levels.

**CV** Severe reactions include congestive heart failure, worsening of hypertension, hypotension, edema, and thrombophlebitis.

- Monitor blood pressure and weight.
- Instruct patients to monitor and record weight at home. Weight gain in excess of 2 to 5 lb in 1 week should be reported to the physician.

**Eye** Nystagmus is characteristic of early toxicity. Other effects include blurred vision, transient diplopia, and visual hallucinations.

- Caution patients to avoid driving or operating hazardous equipment if visual changes occur; notify physician.

**GI** Nausea, vomiting, gastric distress, diarrhea, constipation, dryness of the mouth, pharngitis, glossitis, and stomatitis.

- Inform patient about the possibility of these side effects. If vomiting or diarrhea is severe, monitor intake and output and weight.
- For dry mouth, instruct patient to rinse mouth frequently with water, suck sugarless hard candy or chew sugarless gum, and continue a regular program of oral hygiene (brushing and flossing), although drying mouthwashes should be avoided. Some patients may wish to use commercially available saliva substitutes.
- Encourage patients to have regular dental care.
- For constipation, keep a record of bowel movements. Increase fluid intake to 2500 to 3000 ml per day, increase amount of fruits, fruit juices, and bran, and increase daily exercise.
- Instruct patient to notify physician if any GI side effect is severe or persistent.

**GU** Urinary frequency and urinary retention are both reported.

- Inform patients about these side effects. Instruct patients to notify the physician if urinary symptoms occur.
- In hospitalized patients, it may be appropriate to monitor intake and output.

**Hematologic** Aplastic anemia, causing death, occasionally occurs. Patients must be carefully monitored for hematologic toxicity.
* Monitor complete blood count, white blood cell differential, and platelets.
* Instruct patients to report the development of pallor, fatigue, sore throat, fever, unexplained bleeding or bruising, nosebleeds, and bleeding gums.

**Skin** Rashes.
* Visually inspect patient for development of rashes.
* If photosensitivity develops, instruct patients to avoid exposure to the sun and other sources of ultraviolet light, keep extremeties well covered, wear a hat, and use maximum-protection sunscreen on exposed skin surfaces.
* Instruct patient to report to the physician the development of any skin changes.

**Allergic** Cholestatic hepatitis.
* Monitor liver function tests.
* Instruct the patient to report the development of right upper quadrant abdominal pain, malaise, change in the color or consistency of stools, and jaundice.

**Other** Alterations in liver function studies, aching joints and muscles, leg cramps.
* Instruct patients to report the development of any unexpected sign or symptom.

### Nursing interventions related to drug administration

* Question patient about allergy to other medications prior to administering. Patients allergic to tricyclic antidepressants may also be allergic to carbamazepine.
* Instruct patients to take doses with meals or a snack to lessen gastric irritation.

### Patient and family education

* Review with patients the anticipated benefits and possible side effects of drug therapy.
* Reinforce to patients the importance of continuing prescribed medications even if they have been seizure-free for an extended period of time. Reinforce the need to take drugs as ordered and to avoid suddenly discontinuing prescribed medications, as this may precipitate seizures.
* Counsel patients to find out from physician what actions to take in the event of a missed dose of drug.
* Female patients taking oral contraceptives may wish to consider alternative measures for birth control. Instruct patient to consult with physician.
* Women of childbearing age may wish to use birth control while taking this medication. If women wish to conceive, counsel them to keep physicians informed so that patient can be given most current information about drug effects during pregnancy.
* Encourage patients on long-term anticonvulsant therapy to wear a medical identification tag or bracelet. In addition, suggest that they carry in their wallets a card listing current drugs and dosages.
* Remind patients to keep all health care providers informed of all medications being taken.
* Refer patients as needed to local or national agencies, including the local visiting nurse agency, vocational rehabilitation, or Epilepsy Foundation of America.
* Instruct patients to avoid the use of alcohol unless permitted in small amounts by the physician.
* Instruct diabetic patients who are to receive carbamazepine to monitor blood glucose levels carefully until dosage is established, as adjustments in insulin or diet may be necessary.

---

## ethosuximide (eth-oh-SUX-i-mide)    anticonvulsant

* ethosuximide: Zarontin

**MECHANISM OF ACTION** Ethosuximide is chemically a succinimide. Ethosuximide elevates the seizure threshold in the cortex and basal ganglia and reduces the synaptic response to low-frequency, repetitive stimulation.

**INDICATIONS** **Absence (petit mal) seizures** Ethosuximide is a drug of choice.

**CONTRAINDICATIONS** • Known hepatic or renal disease.

**DOSAGE**    PO:    **CHILDREN:** Initially, for children 3 to 6 years old, 250 mg daily in a single dose; for children 6 years and older, 500 mg daily in divided doses. The daily dose is then increased by 250 mg every 4 to 7 days until the seizures are controlled. Maintenance is usually 20 mg/kg or 1.2 $g/M^2$ daily. Dose should not exceed 1.5 daily.    *Special patient populations:*    **PREGNANCY:** Safe use during pregnancy has not been established.

**PREPARATIONS**    *Capsules:* 250 mg. *Solution (oral):* 250 mg/5 ml.

**DRUG INTERACTIONS**    **Phenytoin** Serum concentration is increased if given concurrently with ethosuximide.

**FATE**    Ethosuximide is absorbed from the GI tract to reach *peak* level in about 4 hours. Four to seven days of therapy are required to reach steady-state plasma levels. The plasma *half-life* is 30 hours in children, 60 hours in adults. Ethosuximide is metabolized and excreted in the urine.

## ❧ NURSING CONSIDERATIONS

### Side effects, toxicities, and associated nursing actions

**CNS** Drowsiness, ataxia, irritability, and restlessness.
- Obtain baseline neurologic and mental status examination prior to administering first dose. Monitor patient at regular intervals.
- Tell patients to avoid driving or operating hazardous equipment if ataxia, vertigo, or drowsiness occur.
- Instruct patient and family to notify physician if CNS side effects occur.
- Monitor serum drug levels.

**Eye** Blurred vision, diplopia.
- Tell patients to avoid driving or operating hazardous equipment if visual changes occur; notify physician.

**GI** Gastrointestinal upset, hiccups.
- Inform patient about the possibility of GI upset. If GI symptoms are severe or persistent, notify physician.

**Hematologic** Agranulocytosis.
- Monitor complete blood count, white blood cell differential, and platelet count.
- Instruct patients to report the development of pallor, fatigue, sore throat, fever, unexplained bleeding or bruising, nosebleeds, and bleeding gums.

**Skin** Rashes.
- Visually inspect patient for development of rashes.
- Instruct patient to report to the physician the development of any skin changes.

**Allergic** Hepatic reactions, including hepatitis and jaundice.
- Monitor liver function tests.
- Instruct the patient to report the development of right upper quadrant abdominal pain, malaise, change in the color or consistency of stools, or jaundice.

### Nursing interventions related to drug administration
- Question patient about allergy to other medications prior to administering. Patients allergic to any of the succinimides may also be allergic to this one.
- Instruct patients to take doses with meals or a snack to lessen gastric irritation.

### Patient and family education
- Review with patients the anticipated benefits and possible side effects of drug therapy.
- Reinforce to patients taking anticonvulsants the importance of continuing prescribed medications even if they have been seizure-free for an extended period of time. Reinforce to patients taking anticonvulsants the need to take drugs as ordered and to avoid suddenly discontinuing prescribed medications, as this may precipitate seizures.
- Counsel patients to find out from physician what actions to take in the event of a missed dose of drug. Usually, if a missed dose is remembered within 4 hours, it should be taken, and the usual dosing schedule resumed. Tell patients not to double-up to make up for missed doses.
- Women of childbearing age may wish to use birth control while taking this medication. If women wish to conceive, counsel them to keep physicians informed so the patient can be given most current information about drug effects during pregnancy.

- Encourage patients on long-term anticonvulsant therapy to wear a medical identification tag or bracelet. In addition, suggest that they carry in their wallets a card listing current drugs and dosages.
- Remind patients to keep all health care providers informed of all medications being taken.
- Refer patients as needed to local or national agencies, including the local visiting nurse agency, vocational rehabilitation, or Epilepsy Foundation of America.
- Instruct patients to avoid the use of alcohol unless permitted in small amounts by the physician.

## methsuximide (meth-SUX-i-mide)

anticonvulsant

- methsuximide: Celontin Kapseals

**MECHANISM OF ACTION** Methsuximide is chemically a succinimide. Methsuximide elevates the seizure threshold in the cortex and basal ganglia and reduces the synaptic response to low-frequency, repetitive stimulation. Methsuximide is chemically related to ethosuximide.

**INDICATIONS** **Absence (petit mal) seizures** Methsuximide is a second-line drug.

**CONTRAINDICATIONS** • Known hepatic or renal disease.

**DOSAGE** **PO:** **ADULTS AND CHILDREN:** Initially, 300 mg daily. After 1 week, the dosage may be increased weekly by 300 mg daily if necessary to control seizures. Maximum daily dose, 1.2g. Administer in divided doses. *Special patient populations:* **PREGNANCY:** Safe use during pregnancy has not been established.

**PREPARATIONS** *Capsules:* 150, 300 mg.

**DRUG INTERACTIONS** **Phenytoin** Serum concentration may be increased if given concurrently with methsuximide.

**FATE** Methsuximide is absorbed from the gastrointestinal tract to give *peak* plasma levels in 1 to 3 hours. The plasma *half-life* is 3 hours. Methsuximide is metabolized in the liver and metabolites are excreted in the urine.

## ☙ NURSING CONSIDERATIONS

### Side effects, toxicities, and associated nursing actions

**CNS** Drowsiness, ataxia, irritability, and restlessness.
- Obtain baseline neurologic and mental status examination prior to administering first dose. Monitor patient at regular intervals.
- Tell patients to avoid driving or operating hazardous equipment if ataxia, vertigo, or drowsiness occur.
- Instruct patient and family to notify physician if CNS side effects occur.
- Monitor serum drug levels.

**Eye** Blurred vision, diplopia.
- Tell patients to avoid driving or operating hazardous equipment if visual changes occur; notify physician.

**GI** Gastrointestinal upset, hiccups.
- Inform patient about the possibility of GI upset. If GI symptoms are severe or persistent, notify physician.

**Hematologic** Agranulocytosis.
- Monitor complete blood count, white blood cell differential, and platelet count.
- Instruct patients to report the development of pallor, fatigue, sore throat, fever, unexplained bleeding or bruising, nosebleeds, or bleeding gums.

**Skin** Rashes.
- Visually inspect patient for development of rashes.
- Instruct patient to report to the physician the development of any skin changes.

**Allergic** Hepatic reactions, including hepatitis and jaundice.
- Monitor liver function tests.
- Instruct the patient to report the development of right upper quadrant abdominal pain, malaise, change in the color or consistency of stools, or jaundice.

### Nursing interventions related to drug administration

- Question patient about allergy to other medications prior to administering. Patients allergic to any of the succinimides may also be allergic to this one.
- Instruct patients to take doses with meals or a snack to lessen gastric irritation.

### Patient and family education

- Review with patients the anticipated benefits and possible side effects of drug therapy.
- Reinforce to patients taking anticonvulsants the importance of continuing prescribed medications even if they have been seizure-free for an extended period of time. Reinforce to patients taking anticonvulsants the need to take drugs as ordered and to avoid suddenly discontinuing prescribed medications, as this may precipitate seizures.
- Tell patients not to take any capsules that are not full or in which the contents have melted, as they may not be effective.
- Counsel patients to find out from physician what actions to take in the event of a missed dose of drug. Usually, if a missed dose is remembered within 4 hours, it should be taken, and the usual dosing schedule resumed. Tell patients not to double-up to make up for missed doses.
- Women of childbearing age may wish to use birth control while taking this medication. If women wish to conceive, counsel them to keep physicians informed so that the patient can be given the most current information about drug effects during pregnancy.
- Encourage patients on long-term anticonvulsant therapy to wear a medical identification tag or bracelet. In addition, suggest that they carry in their wallets a card listing current drugs and dosages.
- Remind patients to keep all health care providers informed of all medications being taken.
- Refer patients as needed to local or national agencies, including the local visiting nurse agency, vocational rehabilitation, or Epilepsy Foundation of America.
- Instruct patients to avoid the use of alcohol unless permitted in small amounts by the physician.

---

# phenobarbital, phenobarbital sodium
(fee-noe-BAR-bi-tal)

sedative
anticonvulsant

- phenobarbital, phenobarbital sodium: ♣Gardenal, Luminal, Solfoton, PBR/12 Schedule IV

**MECHANISM OF ACTION**    Barbiturates depress monosynaptic and polysynaptic transmission and thereby decrease the excitability of nerve cells.

**INDICATIONS**    **Anticonvulsant** Prophylaxis for the treatment of epilepsy. This is a major use of phenobarbital. Grand-mal epilepsy (clonic-tonic seizures) and partial seizures are the principal types effectively controlled by phenobarbital.    **Anxiety** As a routine antianxiety agent or as a preoperative sedative. **Withdrawal** Phenobarbital may be substituted for other barbiturates or nonbarbiturate sedative-hypnotics or alcohol. Doses are then lowered 10% per day to achieve withdrawal without withdrawal symptoms.

**CONTRAINDICATIONS**    **History of drug abuse.**    **Hypersensitivity.**    **Porphyria** Patient or family history. **Pulmonary insufficiency** Respiration will be depressed.

**DOSAGE**    Epilepsy: *PO:*    **ADULTS:** 100 to 300 mg daily. Because of the long half-life of phenobarbital, this may be administered as a single dose.    **CHILDREN:** 3 to 5 mg/kg or 125 mg/M$^2$ daily.    **For terminating status epilepticus and other acute seizure states:** *IM:*    **ADULTS:** 200 to 600 mg.    **CHILDREN:** 100 to 400 mg. Up to 30 minutes may be required to terminate the attack.    *IV:* See IM doses. Discontinue when seizures stop.    **Sedation** See Chapter 39.    *Special patient populations:* **ELDERLY:** Elderly patients are more likely to respond with paradoxical excitement.    **PREGNANCY:** Barbiturates can cause fetal harm, including fetal abnormalities. Barbiturates can also cause postpartum hemorrhage and hemorrhagic disease in the newborn. Barbiturates are distributed to breast milk. For these reasons, barbiturates should be avoided by pregnant and nursing women.

**PREPARATIONS**   Phenobarbital, *powder, capsules:* 16, 65 mg; *elixir:* 15 mg/5 ml: *tablets:* 8, 15, 16, 30, 32, 60, 65, 100 mg. Phenobarbital sodium, *powder, injection:* 30, 60, 65, 130 mg/ml.

**DRUG INTERACTIONS**   **CNS depressants** Barbiturates potentiate other CNS depressants, including other sedatives and hypnotics, benzodiazepines, antihistamines, narcotic analgesics, antipsychotics, and alcohol.   **Oral anticoagulants, corticosteroids, doxycycline, oral contraceptives** Barbiturates may induce liver microsomal enzymes, increasing the metabolism of these drugs and thereby decreasing their action.

**FATE**   Phenobarbital is the longest-acting of the commonly used barbiturates. After oral administration, *peak blood concentrations* are reached in 10 to 15 hours, although the *onset of action* is generally 30 to 60 minutes. Plasma *half-life* is 2 to 6 days. Phenobarbital is metabolized by the liver, but slowly, and at least 25% of the drug is excreted in the urine unchanged. Phenobarbital is potent in inducing the liver metabolizing enzymes, accounting for the decreased effectiveness of many other drugs.

## ☙ NURSING CONSIDERATIONS

### Side effects, toxicities, and associated nursing actions

**CNS** Drowsiness, lethargy, depression; pain in nerves, joints, or muscle. Increased dreaming or insomnia or nightmares may be experienced when hypnotic doses are discontinued. Prolonged therapy with sedative doses (600 to 800 mg daily) for 8 weeks or more will produce physical dependence.
* Reassure patients that CNS effects will often lessen with continued therapy.
* Tell patients to avoid driving or operating hazardous equipment until drowsiness wears off.
* Children occasionally manifest a paradoxical reaction, displaying hyperactivity and excitement. If this occurs, notify physician.

**CV** Hypotension may accompany a rapid IV injection.
* Monitor blood pressure before and at 5- to 15-minute intervals until stable during IV administration.
* Dilute ordered dose to at least 10 ml.
* Administer at a rate of 1 grain (60 to 65 mg) over 1 minute.

**GI** Nausea, vomiting, diarrhea, or constipation are occasionally experienced.
* Forewarn patient about GI side effects. If these side effects are severe or persistent, notify physician.
* For constipation, increase fluid intake to 2500 to 3000 ml per day, increase dietary intake of fruit, fruit juices, and fiber, and increase level of exercise.
* If vomiting or diarrhea occur, monitor intake, output, and weight.

**Hematologic** Rarely, agranulocytosis, thrombocytopenic purpura, and megaloblastic anemia.
* Instruct patients to report the development of pallor, fatigue, sore throat, fever, unexplained bleeding or bruising, nosebleeds, or bleeding gums.
* Monitor complete blood count, white blood cell differential, and platelets.

**Lung** Newborns are especially sensitive to respiratory depression caused by barbiturates. Toxic doses will depress respiration in children and adults.
* Monitor respiratory rate hourly when initiating therapy with this drug, when increasing the dose, or when patients are receiving other central nervous system depressants.
* Check dosage calculation and preparation of prescribed dose carefully for infants and children.

**Metabolic** Elevation in blood ammonia.
* Assess ammonia level prior to the start of therapy and again at regular intervals.

**Allergic** Urticaria, angioedema, morbilliform or scarlatiniform rash, fever, serum sickness, erythema multiforme, or Stevens-Johnson syndrome.
* Instruct patients to report immediately the appearance of any skin changes, fever, or malaise.
* Have available in settings where phenobarbital is administered drugs, equipment, and personnel for treatment of acute allergic reactions.

### Nursing interventions related to drug administration
* For IV use, dilute powder as directed on vial. Further dilute ordered dose to at least 10 ml, with sterile water for injection. Administer at a rate of 65 mg or less per minute. Doses prepared from powder must be used within 30 minutes of preparation. Ascertain patency of vein before adminis-

tering; intravenous administration may cause thrombosis, while intraarterial administration may cause gangrene. Have a suction machine at the bedside, and have readily available equipment for intubation.
- Oral or IM administration is preferred.
- Avoid dividing suppositories, as this may contribute to inaccurate dosage.

### Patient and family education
- Review with patients the anticipated benefits and possible side effects of drug therapy.
- Reinforce to patients taking anticonvulsants the importance of continuing prescribed medications even if they have been seizure-free for an extended period of time. Reinforce the need to take drugs as ordered and to avoid suddenly discontinuing prescribed medications, as this may precipitate seizures.
- Instruct patients to find out from the physician what actions to take in the event of a missed dose of drug. Usual instructions are to take the missed dose as soon as remembered, unless it is almost time for the next dose. Tell patients not to double-up for missed doses.
- Women of childbearing age may wish to use birth control measures while taking this medication. If women wish to conceive, counsel them to keep physicians informed so that the patients can be given the most current information about drug effects during pregnancy.
- Encourage patients on long-term anticonvulsant therapy to wear a medical identification tag or bracelet. In addition, suggest that they carry in their wallets a card listing current drugs and dosages.
- Remind patients to keep all health care providers informed of all medications being taken.
- Refer patients as needed to local or national agencies, including the local visiting nurse agency, vocational rehabilitation, or Epilepsy Foundation of America.
- Instruct patients to avoid the use of alcohol unless permitted in small amounts by the physician.

---

## phensuximide   (fen-SUX-i-mide)       anticonvulsant

- phensuximide: Milontin Kapseals

**MECHANISM OF ACTION**   Phensuximide is chemically a succinimide and chemically related to ethosuximide. Phensuximide elevates the seizure threshold in the cortex and basal ganglia and reduces the synaptic response to low-frequency, repetitive stimulation.

**INDICATIONS**   **Absence (petit mal) seizures** Phensuximide is a second-line drug.

**CONTRAINDICATIONS**   • Known hepatic or renal disease.

**DOSAGE**   PO:   ADULTS AND CHILDREN: 500 mg to 1 g two or three times daily.   *Special patient populations:*   PREGNANCY: Safe use during pregnancy has not been established.

**PREPARATIONS**   *Capsules:* 500 mg.

**DRUG INTERACTIONS**   **Phenytoin** Serum concentration may be increased if given concurrently with phensuximide.

**FATE**   Phensuximide is absorbed from the gastrointestinal tract to give *peak* plasma concentrations in 1 to 4 hours. The plasma *half-life* is 4 hours. Metabolites of phensuximide are excreted in the urine.

### ☙ NURSING CONSIDERATIONS
#### Side effects, toxicities, and associated nursing actions
**CNS** Drowsiness, ataxia, irritability, and restlessness.
- Obtain baseline neurologic and mental status examination prior to administering first dose. Monitor patient at regular intervals.
- Tell patients to avoid driving or operating hazardous equipment if ataxia, vertigo, or drowsiness occur.
- Instruct patient and family to notify physician if CNS side effects occur.
- Monitor serum drug levels.

**Eye** Blurred vision, diplopia.
- Tell patients to avoid driving or operating hazardous equipment if visual changes occur; notify physician.

**GI** Gastrointestinal upset, hiccups.
- Inform patient about the possibility of GI upset. If GI symptoms are severe or persistent, notify physician.

**Hematologic** Agranulocytosis.
- Monitor complete blood count, white blood cell differential, and platelet count.
- Instruct patients to report the development of pallor, fatigue, sore throat, fever, unexplained bleeding or bruising, nosebleeds, or bleeding gums.

**Skin** Rashes.
- Visually inspect patient for development of rashes.
- Instruct patient to report to the physician the development of any skin changes.

**Allergic** Hepatic reactions, including hepatitis and jaundice.
- Monitor liver function tests.
- Instruct the patient to report the development of right upper quadrant abdominal pain, malaise, change in the color or consistency of stools, or jaundice.

### Nursing interventions related to drug administration
- Question patient about allergy to other medications prior to administering. Patients allergic to any of the succinimides may also be allergic to this one.
- Instruct patients to take doses with meals or a snack to lessen gastric irritation.

### Patient and family education
- Review with patients the anticipated benefits and possible side effects of drug therapy.
- Reinforce to patients taking anticonvulsants the importance of continuing prescribed medications even if they have been seizure-free for an extended period of time. Reinforce to patients taking anticonvulsants the need to take drugs as ordered and to avoid suddenly discontinuing prescribed medications, as this may precipitate seizures.
- Counsel patients to find out from physician what actions to take in the event of a missed dose of drug.
- Women of childbearing age may wish to use birth control while taking this medication. If women wish to conceive, counsel them to keep physicians informed so that the patient can be given most current information about drug effects during pregnancy.
- Encourage patients on long-term anticonvulsant therapy to wear a medical identification tag or bracelet. In addition, suggest that they carry in their wallets a card listing current drugs and dosages.
- Remind patients to keep all health care providers informed of all medications being taken.
- Refer patients as needed to local or national agencies, including the local visiting nurse agency, vocational rehabilitation, or Epilepsy Foundation of America.
- Warn patients that phensuximide may discolor urine, turning it pink, red, or red-brown. The discoloration is harmless.
- Instruct patients to avoid the use of alcohol unless permitted in small amounts by the physician.

## phenytoin, phenytoin sodium  (FEN-i-toy-in)  anticonvulsant

- phenytoin, phenytoin sodium: Dilantin, Diphenylan Sodium

**MECHANISM OF ACTION**  Phenytoin is chemically a hydantoin. The anticonvulsant action of the hydantoins appears to be a limitation of seizure propagation by reduction of the post-tetanic potential. This may involve an effect on the sodium pump.

**INDICATIONS**  **Grand mal epilepsy** Phenytoin is the drug of choice for prophylactic treatment in adults.  **Partial seizure epilepsy** Phenytoin is the drug of choice for prophylactic treatment in adults.  **Cardiac arrhythmias** See Chapter 6.

**CONTRAINDICATIONS**  **Lymphadenopathy** This can be a side effect of phenytoin. Preexistence of the condition will make monitoring difficult.

**DOSAGE**   **PO:**   **ADULTS:** 100 mg three times daily. Seizure control may take 5 to 10 days. If necessary, dosage should be increased cautiously in increments of 100 mg every 2 to 4 weeks. Usual maintenance dose is 300 to 600 mg daily.   **CHILDREN:** 5 mg/kg or 250 mg/M$^2$ daily in 2 or 3 doses. Adjust dosage only gradually if necessary. Usual maintenance dose is 4 to 8 mg/kg daily.   **PO:**   **Loading dose:** In hospitalized patients, the first day therapy may be started as a loading dose.   **ADULTS:** 1 g total, divided into 3 doses given at 2-hour intervals.   **CHILDREN:** 500 to 600 mg total, divided into 3 doses given at 2-hour intervals. Effective serum concentrations of phenytoin are 10 to 20 µg/ml.   *Special patient populations:*   **PREGNANCY:** Safe use has not been established.

**PREPARATIONS**   Phenytoin, *suspension (oral):* 20, 125 mg/5 ml; *tablets (chewable):* 50 mg. Sodium salt, *injection:* 50 mg/ml; *capsules (extended-release):* 30, 100 mg; *capsules (prompt):* 30, 100 mg.

**DRUG INTERACTIONS**   **Phenobarbital** The interaction with phenytoin is variable. In some patients, phenytoin concentrations increase because phenobarbital competes for the degrading enzymes. In other patients, phenobarbital increases the amount of degrading enzymes to decrease the serum concentration of phenytoin.   **Oral anticoagulants, carbamazepine** These decrease the metabolism of phenytoin by competing for the degrading enzymes. The serum concentration of phenytoin is increased.   **Valproic acid** displaces phenytoin bound to protein to increase the effective concentration of phenytoin.   **Estrogen** The metabolism of estrogen is increased by phenytoin, so the effective concentration of estrogen is decreased.

**DIAGNOSTIC TEST INTERFERENCE**   **Thyroid tests** Protein-bound iodide (PBI) values are lowered.   **Steroids** Urinary 17 hydroxylcorticosteroids and 17 ketosteroids are decreased, while 6 beta hydroxycortisol is increased. The normal values for the dexamethasone and metyrapone tests are decreased.   **Serum enzymes** Alkaline phosphatase and gamma glutamyl transpeptidase concentrations may be increased.

**FATE**   Phenytoin is irregularly absorbed from the gastrointestinal tract. Phenytoin has a plasma *half-life* of 24 hours. The capacity of the liver to metabolize phenytoin is limited at serum concentrations much above therapeutic levels (10 to 20 µg/ml).

## ❧ NURSING CONSIDERATIONS

### Side effects, toxicities, and associated nursing actions

**CNS** Incoordination and slurred speech are symptoms when the serum concentration of phenytoin is above 30 µg/ml. At higher serum concentrations, tremors, nervousness or drowsiness, and fatigue may be seen.

**Eye** Nystagmus is a common symptom of elevated serum concentration.

* Review with patients and families these symptoms of overdose, and instruct patients to notify physician if symptoms occur.
* Review with patients or families administering drug suspension form to shake bottle vigorously before pouring ordered dose. Overdose occasionally occurs when suspension forms have not been shaken well, with the result that much of the drug has settled to the bottom of the bottle. As the bottle is used up, the concentration of drug per milliliter increases, and accidental overdose may occur.
* Monitor serum drug levels, and encourage patients to keep regular follow-up appointments with physician.

**CV** With IV use, hypotension and cardiovascular collapse may be produced.

* Oral administration is the preferred route of administration.
* Administer IV doses via direct intravenous administration. Prepare dose with diluent supplied by manufacturer; doses should not be further diluted. Slightly yellow solutions may be used; discard solutions that are not clear. Do not mix with other drugs or many IV solutions, as precipitation may occur. Flush tubing before and after administration with 0.9% sodium chloride. Administer at a rate of 50 mg or less per minute. Monitor blood pressure, and if possible have patient connected to ECG monitor to monitor cardiac rhythm during and immediately after IV administration.
* Remember that even if used as an anticonvulsant, phenytoin also has cardiovascular effects. See Chapter 6.

**GI** Gastrointestinal distress.

* Instruct patients to take dose with snack or meals to lessen gastric irritation. If GI symptoms are severe or persistent, notify physician.

**Hematologic** Depression of various white cells is not uncommon. Hematologic monitor should be part of therapy.
* Monitor complete blood cell count and white blood cell differential.
* Assess patient for signs of folic acid deficiency: easy fatigability, weakness, fainting, or headache.

**Skin** Rashes, hypertrichosis (overgrowth of a coarse hair), acne. Gingival hyperplasia occurs in about 20% of patients, especially in children. This is the limiting factor for use in children.
* Review with patients these possible side effects. Instruct patients to report the development of skin changes.
* Provide emotional support to patients who develop hypertrichosis, acne, or other skin changes, as patients may wish to discontinue the medication because of these side effects.
* Instruct patients to consult a dermatologist for severe acne or hypertrichosis.
* Encourage regular preventive dental care, careful toothbrushing, and flossing.

**Metabolic** Altered vitamin D metabolism sometimes leading to osteomalacia.
* Recommend foods high in vitamin D, such as fortified milk, herring, sardines, liver, and egg yolk, and encourage increased exposure to the sun.
* Monitor serum calcium, serum phosphorus, and alkaline phosphatase levels.

**Allergic** Rashes.
* Instruct patients to report the development of any skin changes.

### Nursing interventions related to drug administration
* For IV administration, see CV, above.
* Avoid switching brands or dosage forms without consultation with the physician.
* IM use produces erratic absorption and should be avoided.

### Patient and family education
* Review with patients the anticipated benefits and possible side effects of drug therapy.
* Reinforce to patients taking anticonvulsants the importance of continuing prescribed medications even if they have been seizure-free for an extended period of time. Reinforce the need to take drugs as ordered and to avoid suddenly discontinuing prescribed medications, as this may precipitate seizures.
* Instruct patients to use only the brand and dosage form prescribed by the physician. Different brands may vary in bioavailability, while prompt and extended-release forms cannot be substituted for each other without adjustment of dosage frequency.
* Instruct patients to find out from the physician what actions to take in the event of a missed dose of drug. Usual instructions are: if dose is taken once a day, take the missed dose as soon as remembered, unless it is the next day; resume the usual dosing schedule; do not double-up to make up for missed doses. If the doses are taken throughout the day: take the missed dose as soon as remembered, unless within 4 hours of the next dose, in which case the patient should omit the missed dose; do not double-up doses.
* Encourage diabetic patients to monitor blood glucose levels frequently when initiating drug therapy or adjusting dosage of phenytoin, as an adjustment in insulin or diet may also be necessary.
* Inform patients that phenytoin may produce a brownish or pinkish discoloration of urine.
* Women of childbearing age may wish to use birth control measures while taking this medication. If women wish to conceive, counsel them to keep physicians informed so that the patients can be given the most current information about drug effects during pregnancy.
* Encourage patients on long-term anticonvulsant therapy to wear a medical identification tag or bracelet. In addition, suggest that they carry in their wallets a card listing current drugs and dosages.
* Remind patients to keep all health care providers informed of all medications being taken.
* Refer patients as needed to local or national agencies, including the local visiting nurse agency, vocational rehabilitation, or Epilepsy Foundation of America.
* Instruct patients to avoid the use of alcohol unless permitted in small amounts by the physician.

# primidone (PRI-mi-done)

- primidone: ✹Apo-Primidone, Mysoline, ✹Sertan

**MECHANISM OF ACTION** Primidone is a structural analog of phenobarbital.

**INDICATIONS** **Grand mal epilepsy** Primidone is a second-choice drug. **Partial seizure epilepsy** Primidone is a second-choice drug.

**CONTRAINDICATIONS** **History of drug abuse. Hypersensitivity. Porphyria** Patient or family history. **Pulmonary insufficiency** Respiration will be depressed.

**DOSAGE** **PO:** **ADULTS AND CHILDREN OVER 8 YEARS OLD:** 100 to 125 mg at bedtime for the first 3 days, then the same dose is given twice a day for days 4 through 6, then three times a day for days 7 to 9, then 250 mg three times a day. The maintenance dose is usually 250 mg three or four times daily. The maximum daily dose is 2 g daily in divided doses. **CHILDREN UNDER 8 YEARS OLD:** 50 mg once a day for days 1 to 3; twice a day for days 4 to 6; 100 mg twice a day for days 7 to 9; then a maintenance dose of 125 to 250 mg three times a day. *Special patient populations:* **PREGNANCY:** Safe use has not been established.

**PREPARATIONS** *Suspension (oral):* 250 mg/5 ml. *Tablets:* 50, 250 mg.

**DRUG INTERACTIONS** Specific drug interactions have not been reported. However, the following interactions characteristic of barbiturates should be considered. **CNS depressants** Barbiturates potentiate other CNS depressants, including other sedatives and hypnotics, benzodiazepines, antihistamines, narcotic analgesics, antipsychotics, and alcohol. **Oral anticoagulants, corticosteroids, doxycycline, oral contraceptives** Barbiturates may induce liver microsomal enzymes, increasing the metabolism of these drugs and thereby decreasing their action. **Oral anticoagulants, griseofulvin** Barbiturates may acutely delay the absorption of these drugs.

**FATE** Primidone is incompletely absorbed from the gastrointestinal tract. *Peak* serum concentrations are measured in about 4 hours. The therapeutic serum concentration is 5 to 12 µ/ml. The plasma *half-life* is 10 to 20 hours. Primidone is metabolized by the liver, partly into active metabolites, including phenobarbital.

## ☙ NURSING CONSIDERATIONS

### Side effects, toxicities, and associated nursing actions

**CNS** Drowsiness, incoordination, vertigo, lethargy, loss of appetite. In children hyperexcitability may be seen.
- Caution patients and families about these possible side effects. Instruct patients to report the development of these side effects to the physician.
- If drowsiness, vertigo, or incoordination occur, caution patients to avoid driving or operating hazardous equipment.
- Monitor the weight of children.
- Monitor serum drug levels if available.

**Eye** Nystagmus, diplopia.
- Assess patients for these eye changes at regular intervals.
- Instruct patients to report the development of eye changes to the physician and to avoid driving or operating hazardous equipment if diplopia occurs.

**GI** Nausea and vomiting.
- If nausea and vomiting are severe or persistent, notify physician. These symptoms may lessen with continued use.
- Instruct patients to take doses with meals or snack to lessen gastric distress.

**Hematologic** Rarely, megaloblastic anemia that can be treated with folic acid.
- Monitor complete blood cell count and white blood cell differential.
- Monitor patients for signs of folic acid deficiency: easy fatigability, weakness, fainting, and headache.

**Skin** Rash.

**Allergic** Rarely, syndrome resembling lupus erythematosus.
- Instruct patients to report the development of any skin changes or any unexpected sign or symptom.

**Other** Loss of hair, edema of the eyelids and/or legs.
- Warn patients about these unusual side effects.
- Monitor patient's weight at regular intervals.

### Nursing interventions related to drug administration
- Tablets may be crushed and mixed with small amounts of food or fluid.

### Patient and family education
- Review with patients the anticipated benefits and possible side effects of drug therapy.
- Reinforce to patients taking anticonvulsants the importance of continuing prescribed medications even if they have been seizure-free for an extended period of time. Reinforce the need to take drugs as ordered and to avoid suddenly discontinuing prescribed medications, as this may precipitate seizures.
- Instruct patients to find out from the physician what actions to take in the event of a missed dose of drug. Usual instructions are to take the missed dose as soon as remembered, unless within 4 hours of the next dose, in which case the missed dose should be omitted. Patients should not double-up doses.
- Women of childbearing age may wish to use birth control measures while taking this medication. If women wish to conceive, counsel them to keep physicians informed so that the patients can be given the most current information about drug effects during pregnancy.
- Encourage patients on long-term anticonvulsant therapy to wear a medical identification tag or bracelet. In addition, suggest that they carry in their wallets a card listing current drugs and dosages.
- Remind patients to keep all health care providers informed of all medications being taken.
- Refer patients as needed to local or national agencies, including the local visiting nurse agency, vocational rehabilitation, or Epilepsy Foundation of America.
- Instruct patients to avoid the use of alcohol unless permitted in small amounts by the physician.

# valproic acid, valproate sodium, divalproex sodium
(val-PROE-ic)                                                              anticonvulsant

- valproic acid, valproate sodium, divalproex sodium: Depakene, Depakote

**MECHANISM OF ACTION**   The anticonvulsant action of valproic acid is not known but may be related to its ability to increase brain concentrations of the inhibitory neurotransmitter, gamma-aminobutyric acid (GABA).

**INDICATIONS**   **Myoclonic seizures** Valproic acid is the drug of choice.   **Petit mal epilepsy** Valproic acid is a second-choice drug.

**CONTRAINDICATIONS**   **Liver disease** Valproic acid can cause serious damage to the liver. • It is essential to monitor for liver damage, which is not possible with preexisting liver disease.

**DOSAGE**   **PO:**   **ADULTS AND CHILDREN:** 15 mg/kg daily. This may be increased by 5 to 10 mg/kg daily at weekly intervals to control seizures if necessary. Maximum dose 60 mg/kg daily.   *Special patient populations:* **PREGNANCY:** There seems to be an increase in neural tube defects in infants of mothers taking valproic acid. However, valproic acid should not be discontinued because of the risk of precipitating status epilepticus.

**PREPARATIONS**   Valproate sodium; *solution (oral):* 150 mg/5ml. Valproic acid; *capsules:* 250 mg. Divalproex sodium; *tablets (enteric-coated):* 125, 250, 500 mg.

**DRUG INTERACTIONS**   **CNS depressants** Additive depression, especially with phenobarbital, primidone, and alcohol.   **Phenobarbital, primidone** Valproic acid can cause increased plasma concentrations of phenobarbital.   **Clonazepam** The combination of clonazepam and valproic acid may cause an absence status.   **Phenytoin** Valproic acid can lead to decreased phenytoin concentrations.   **Monoamine oxidase inhibitors** Valproic acid can potentiate the effects of MAO inhibitors.   **Aspirin, oral anticoagulants** Valproic acid can increase bleeding time.

**DIAGNOSTIC TEST INTERFERENCE** **Urinary ketones** Valproic acid can lead to false-positive values. **Thyroid function tests** Valproic acid alters values, but the clinical effect is not known.

**FATE** *Peak* plasma concentrations are seen in 1 to 4 hours with valproic acid or its sodium salt and in 3 to 5 hours with the divalproex form. Valproate is highly (80% to 95%) bound to plasma protein. The plasma *half-life* is 5 to 20 hours. Valproic acid is metabolized by the liver and metabolites are excreted in the urine.

## ❦ NURSING CONSIDERATIONS

### Side effects, toxicities, and associated nursing actions

**CNS** Sedation and drowsiness, especially when taking other anticonvulsants. Rarely, anxiety, depression, confusion, and hallucinations. Rarely, in chidren, hyperactivity, aggressiveness, and behavioral disturbances.

**Eye** Nystagmus, diplopia, "spots."

- Caution patients about these side effects, and instruct patients to report their development to the physican.
- Caution patients to avoid driving if sedation, drowsiness, diplopia, or "spots" occur.
- Monitor serum drug levels if available.

**GI** Nausea, vomiting, and indigestion are the most frequent side effects. Other side effects include hypersalivation, abdominal cramps, diarrhea, or constipation.

- If GI symptoms are severe or persistent, notify physician.
- If vomiting or diarrhea occur, monitor intake, output, and weight.
- If constipation occurs, instruct patients to increase fluid intake to 2500 to 3000 ml per day, increase daily intake of fruits, fruits juices, and fiber, and increase level of exercise.
- Instruct patients to take ordered dose with meals or snack to lessen gastric irritation. Have patient switch to enteric-coated drug form to lessen gastric irritation; consult physician.

**Hematologic** Prolongation of bleeding.

- Instruct patients to report the development of unexplained bleeding or bruising, nosebleed, or bleeding gums.
- Monitor platelet count.

**Skin** Rashes.

- Instruct patient to report the development of any rashes or skin changes.

**Metabolic** Hyperammonemia.

**Other** Elevations in hepatic function tests, damage to the liver that may be serious; changes in hair texture or amount.

- Monitor liver function tests, serum ammonia level.
- Instruct patients to report the development of jaundice, right upper quadrant abdominal pain, change in color or consistency of stools, or malaise.

### Nursing interventions related to drug administration

- Capsules should not be opened, and enteric-coated tablets should not be crushed. For patients who may have difficulty swallowing capsules, suggest switching to oral solution.

### Patient and family education

- Review with patients the anticipated benefits and possible side effects of drug therapy.
- Reinforce to patients taking anticonvulsants the importance of continuing prescribed medications even if they have been seizure-free for an extended period of time. Reinforce the need to take drugs as ordered and to avoid suddenly discontinuing prescribed medications, as this may precipitate seizures.
- Instruct patients to find out from the physician what actions to take in the event of a missed dose of drug. Usual instructions are, for once a day dosing: take missed dose as soon as remembered, unless it is the next day. Do not double-up doses. Go back to the regular dosing schedule. If usual dosing is two or more times per day: take missed dose as soon as remembered, if within 6 hours of the missed dose. Take the rest of the day's doses in even-spaced intervals. Do not double-up doses.
- Women of childbearing age may wish to use birth control measures while taking this medication. If women wish to conceive, counsel them to keep physicians informed so that the patients can be given the most current information about drug effects during pregnancy.

- Encourage patients on long-term anticonvulsant therapy to wear a medical identification tag or bracelet. In addition, suggest that they carry in their wallets a card listing current drugs and dosages.
- Remind patients to keep all health care providers informed of all medications being taken.
- Refer patients as needed to local or national agencies, including the local visiting nurse agency, vocational rehabilitation, or Epilepsy Foundation of America.
- Instruct patients to avoid the use of alcohol unless permitted in small amounts by the physician.
- Remind patients to keep all medications out of the reach of children. The oral solution of valproate sodium is eye catching and pleasant tasting; small children may be tempted to drink it.

# Chapter Forty
# Drugs to control spasticity

baclofen
dantrolene
diazepam (see Chapter 35)

**INTRODUCTION**    Spasticity is the lack of fine control of motor activity resulting from the loss of inhibitory tone in the polysynaptic pathways in the spinal cord. Since the inhibitory tone is controlled largely by neural pathways from the brain, spasticity is seen in patients in whom these inhibitory pathways have been disrupted through spinal cord injury, cerebrovascular accidents (strokes), multiple sclerosis, or cerebral palsy. The patient with spasticity has exaggerated reflexes (spinal spasticity) or inappropriate posture (cerebral spasticity).

Three drugs have been found effective in relieving some cases of spasticity: baclofen, dantrolene, and diazepam. Diazepam is a benzodiazepine discussed in Chapter 40 as an antianxiety drug.

---

## baclofen    (BAK-loe-fen)                                                        antispasticity

- baclofen: Lioresal

**MECHANISM OF ACTION**    Baclofen is a derivative of gamma-aminobutyric acid (GABA). Baclofen decreases the frequency and amplitude of muscle spasms through an action in the spinal cord.

**INDICATIONS**    **Spasticity Choreiform movements** Arising from Huntington's chorea.

**CONTRAINDICATIONS**    **Epilepsy** Baclofen may deteriorate seizure control.

**DOSAGE**    PO:    **ADULTS AND CHILREN OVER 12 YEARS OF AGE:** 5 mg, three times daily. May increase dose 15 mg daily every 3 days if necessary. Maintenance doses are usually 40 to 80 mg daily. Allow at least 2 months to evaluate treatment.    *Special patient populations:*    **CHILDREN:** Not recommended for children under 12 years of age.    **PREGNANCY:** Safe use has not been established.

**PREPARATIONS**    *Tablets:* 10, 20 mg.

**DRUG INTERACTIONS**    **CNS depressants** Additive depression.

**FATE**    Baclofen is rapidly absorbed. *Peak* serum concentrations are reached in 2 to 3 hours. The plasma *half-life* is 2.5 to 4 hours. Baclofen is excreted largely in the urine, about 15% as metabolites.

## ☙ NURSING CONSIDERATIONS

### Side effects, toxicities, and associated nursing actions

**CNS** Most common, drowsiness. Occasionally, fatigue, dizziness, muscle weakness, hypotonia, depression, and headache.

**Eye** Miosis or mydriasis, diplopia, and nystagmus.

- Warn patients about these side effects.
- Obtain careful baseline mental status examination and repeat at regular intervals to monitor for depression.
- Caution patient to avoid driving or operating hazardous equipment if drowsiness, dizziness, or changes in vision due to mydriasis, miosis, or diplopia occur.
- Instruct patient to avoid bright lights and wear sunglasses when outside if mydriasis occurs.

**CV** Hypotension.

- Monitor blood pressure every 4 hours in hospital setting.
- Be alert to hypotension when ambulating patients, especially if patients have been immobilized or primarily sedentary prior to the start of drug therapy with baclofen.

**GI** Nausea, constipation. Rarely, dry mouth, anorexia, and alteration of taste perception.

- If GI symptoms are severe or persistent, notify physician.
- If constipation occurs, instruct patient to increase fluid intake to 2500 to 3000 ml per day, increase dietary intake of fruit, fruit juices, and fiber, and increase level of exercise if possible.

- If dry mouth occurs, instruct patient to try sucking on sugarless hard candies or chewing sugarless gum, performing frequent oral hygiene, but avoiding drying mouthwashes. Some patients may wish to consider the use of commerically available saliva substitutes.
- Tell patients that drug may be taken with meals or snack to lessen gastric irritation.
- Monitor weight at regular intervals. If patient is losing weight, monitor intake and output.

**GU** Urinary frequency, or rarely, retention, dysuria, nocturia, hematuria; impotence.
- Warn patients about these side effects and ask patients to report their development.
- Monitor intake and output, and keep a record of frequency of voidings.
- Monitor urinalysis, or test urine for presence of blood.
- Assess tactfully for the development of impotence. Caution patients not to discontinue taking medications without consulting the physician. Provide emotional support as indicated. Consult with physician about changing drugs or dosages if appropriate.

**Lung** Rarely, dyspnea.
- Monitor respiratory rate. Question patient about subjective assessment of breathing.

**Skin** Rashes, pruritis.
- Visually inspect patient for development of skin changes.
- Instruct patients to report the development of any rashes or skin changes.

**Metabolic** Rarely, edema.
- Monitor weight.

### Patient and family education
- Review with patients anticipated benefits and possible side effects of drug therapy.
- Reassure patients that several days to weeks of therapy may be necessary before improvement is seen. On the other hand, if improvement is not seen in 6 to 8 weeks, the drug is usually withdrawn.
- Caution diabetic patients to monitor blood glucose levels carefully when starting, stopping, or changing the dose of this medication, as an adjustment in diet or insulin dose may be necessary.
- Instruct patients to avoid the use of alcohol unless permitted in small amounts by the physician.
- Remind patients to keep all health care providers informed of all medications being taken.

## dantrolene sodium   (DAN-troe-leen)                          antispastic

- dantrolene sodium: Dantrium

**MECHANISM OF ACTION**   Dantrolene affects the muscle directly by interfering with the intracellular release of calcium necessary to initiate contraction.

**INDICATIONS**   **Spasticity** Especially when the spasticity causes pain, discomfort, or limits functional rehabilitation.   **Malignant hyperthermia** IV dantrolene is given immediately with other supportive measures.

**CONTRAINDICATIONS**   **Liver disease** Dantrolene can cause severe liver damage. Baseline functional studies are made before therapy is started. Ongoing liver disease would limit the ability to monitor for drug-induced damage.

**DOSAGE**   **Spasticity:** *PO:*   **ADULTS:** Initially, 25 mg daily. Dosage may be increased gradually to 25 mg two, three, and four times daily if necessary at 4- to 7-day intervals. Further increments are made by increasing the amount per dose in 25 mg increments. Doses rarely exceed 400 mg daily.   **CHILDREN OVER 5 YEARS OF AGE:** Initially, 0.5 mg/kg, two times daily. If necessary, dosage is increased first by increasing the number of doses to 3 and 4 per day, then by increasing the amount per dose in 0.5 mg/kg amounts.   **Malignant hyperthermia:** *IV:*   **ADULTS AND CHILDREN:** 1 mg/kg by rapid IV. Repeat if necessary. The total dose should not exceed 10 mg/kg. Oral doses of 4 to 8 mg/kg daily, divided into 4 doses, for 3 days, are given to prevent recurrence.   *Special patient populations:* **PREGNANCY:** Safe use has not been established.

**PREPARATIONS**   *Capsules:* 25, 50, 100 mg. *Injection:* 20 mg.

**DRUG INTERACTIONS**   **Estrogen** Hepatotoxicity is more common in women over 35 years old receiving concomitant estrogen therapy.

**FATE** Dantolene is poorly absorbed, and *peak* serum concentrations are measured about 5 hours after oral administration. Therapeutic blood concentrations are 100 to 600 ng/ml. The *half-life* is about 8 hours. Dantrolene is metabolized in the liver and excreted in the urine.

## ☙ NURSING CONSIDERATIONS

### Side effects, toxicities, and associated nursing actions

**CNS** Drowsiness, weakness, general malaise, and fatigue are the most frequent side effects. Speech disturbance, headache, and alteration of taste are rarely seen. Also rare are depression and confusion.

**Eye** Diplopia.

• Review side effects with patients and families; instruct them to report the development of these side effects.

• Caution patients to avoid driving or operating hazardous equipment if drowsiness, confusion, or diplopia occur.

• Obtain careful baseline mental status examination, and monitor for depression at regular intervals. Assess for withdrawal, lack of interest in personal appearance, insomnia, anorexia, and weight loss.

• Reassure patients that many of these side effects may lessen with continued use of the drug.

**CV** Tachycardia, erratic blood pressure.

• Monitor blood pressure and pulse at regular intervals. For treatment of malignant hyperthermia, patient should be attached to cardiac monitor.

• Be alert to hypotension when assisting patients to ambulate, especially if patient has been immobilized or primarily sedentary prior to drug therapy.

**GI** Constipation, GI bleeding, anorexia, and cramps.

• Keep a record of bowel movements. If constipation occurs, instruct patient to increase daily fluid intake to 2500 to 3000 ml per day, increase dietary intake of fruits, fruit juices, and fiber, and increase level of exercise, if possible.

• Monitor stools for presence of blood, and instruct patient to do the same.

• If GI symptoms are severe or persistent, notify physician.

**GU** Increased urinary frequency, hematuria, incontinence, nocturia; also difficulty in urination, retention. Difficulty in erection.

• Advise patients about these possible side effects and instruct them to report their development.

• Monitor intake and output and keep a record of frequency of voidings.

• Monitor urinalysis or check urine for blood.

• Assess tactfully for difficulty in erection. Provide emotional support as appropriate. Caution patient not to discontinue medications without consulting physician.

**Lung** Pleural effusion with carditis.

• Auscultate lung and heart sounds at regular intervals. Assess chest pain and difficulty in breathing.

**Skin** Abnormal hair growth, acne-like rash, urticaria, and sweating.

• Visually inspect patient for skin changes; report changes to the physician.

• Provide emotional support if skin changes occur; referral to a dermatologist may be appropriate for some patients.

**Liver** Hepatotoxicity. Baseline liver function studies are made before therapy starts and regularly during therapy.

• Monitor liver function tests.

• Instruct patients to report the development of jaundice, malaise, right upper quadrant abdominal pain, and change in the color or consistency of stools.

**Other** Myalgia, backache; chills and fever; feeling of suffocation; excessive tearing.

• Assess patients for these side effects. Caution patients to report the development of any unexpected sign or symptom.

### Nursing interventions related to drug administration

• For IV administration, dilute each 20 mg of drug with 60 ml of sterile water for injection that does not contain a bacteriostatic agent. Shake solution until clear. Administer as rapid IV push. Once reconstituted and diluted, solution must be protected from light and used within 6 hours.

**Patient and family education**

- Review with patients anticipated benefits and possible side effects of drug therapy.
- Reassure patients that several days to weeks of therapy may be necessary before improvement is seen. On the other hand, if improvement is not seen in 6 to 8 weeks, the drug is usually withdrawn.
- Instruct patients to avoid the use of alcohol unless permitted in small amounts by the physician.
- Remind patients to keep all health care providers informed of all medications being taken.
- Instruct patients who develop malignant hyperthermia to wear a medical identification tag or bracelet indicating this fact.
- If a patient develops photosensitivity, instruct patient to avoid exposure to the sun or other sources of ultraviolet light, wear a hat and long-sleeve clothing, and use maximum-protection sunscreen on exposed skin surfaces.

# Chapter Forty-one

# Drugs to relieve muscle spasms

| | |
|---|---|
| carisoprodol | cyclobenzaptrine |
| chlorphenesin | methocarbamol |
| chlorzoxazone | orphenadrine (see Chapter 43) |

**DRUG COMBINATIONS**
- carisoprodol and aspirin: Carisoprodol Compound, Sodol Compound, Soma Compound
- carisoprodol and aspirin and codeine phosphate: CIII—Soma Compound with Codeine
- chlorzoxazone and acetaminophen: Clorofon-F, Parafon Forte, Zoxaphen
- methocarbamol and aspirin: Robaxisal

**OVERVIEW OF THE DRUG CLASS**  Muscle spasms are local muscle contractions initiated by muscle or tendon injury and inflammation. Muscle spasms occur in conditions such as sprains, bursitis, arthritis, and lower back pain. The primary treatment of muscle spasms includes analgesics, antiinflammatory drugs, immobilization of the affected part, if possible, heat, and physical therapy. If relief is not achieved through these means, a centrally acting skeletal muscle relaxant may be added.

**MECHANISM OF ACTION**  The mechanism of action for the centrally acting skeletal muscle relaxants is not well understood. Muscle tone is in part modulated through complex pathways in the spinal cord, and these drugs seem to depress these spinal cord pathways. In addition, the centrally acting skeletal muscle relaxants are related to various antianxiety drugs. Since anxiety itself will make a muscle spasm worse, treatment of the anxiety that accompanies a muscle spasm may be a major mechanism of action.

**INDICATIONS**  • Muscle spasms not relieved by other therapy.

**CONTRAINDICATIONS**  • See individual drug.

**DRUG INTERACTIONS**  **CNS depressants** Additive depression with other CNS depressants, including alcohol.

---

## carisoprodol  (kar-eye-soe-PROE-dole)                central muscle relaxant

- carisoprodol: Rela, Sodol, Soma, Soprodol, Soridol

**MECHANISM OF ACTION**  Centrally acting skeletal muscle relaxants depress muscle tone through an action in the spinal cord. In addition, these drugs relieve anxiety, an effect that may contribute to their effectiveness.

**INDICATIONS**  • Muscle spasms not relieved by other therapy.

**CONTRAINDICATIONS**  • Impaired hepatic or renal function.

**DOSAGE**  PO:  **ADULTS AND CHILDREN OVER 12 YEARS OF AGE:** 350 mg four times daily.  **CHILDREN 5 TO 12 YEARS OF AGE:** 25 mg/kg or 750 mg/M$^2$ in 4 divided doses.  *Special patient populations:* **CHILDREN:** Not recommended for children under 5 years of age.  **PREGNANCY:** Safe use has not been established. Carisoprodol does concentrate in milk and should not be used by nursing mothers.

**PREPARATIONS**  *Tablets:* 350 mg.

**DRUG INTERACTIONS**  **CNS depressants** Additive depression with other CNS depressants, including alcohol.

**FATE**  The *onset of action* is 30 minutes and the *duration of action* is 4 to 6 hours. The plasma *half-life* is 8 hours. Carisoprodol is metabolized in the liver and excreted in the urine.

**☙ NURSING CONSIDERATIONS**
### Side effects, toxicities, and associated nursing actions
**CNS** Drowsiness, dizziness, ataxia, vertigo, incoordination, tremor, agitation, irritability, headache, fainting, and insomnia.
- Review with patients these side effects. If drowsiness, ataxia, incoordination, or vertigo occurs, instruct patient to avoid driving or operating hazardous equipment.

- Reassure patients that many of these side effects may diminish with continued therapy.

**CV** Fast heart rate, postural hypotension, and flushing.
- Monitor vital signs and blood pressure.
- Instruct patients to move slowly from lying to sitting or standing positions. Supervise ambulation of hospitalized patients. Keep siderails up. Keep a nightlight on.

**Eye** Idiosyncratic reactions include a temporary loss of vision, diplopia, and mydriasis, symptoms that usually disappear a few hours after carisoprodol is discontinued.
- Warn patients that eye problems may occur, and if they do, patients should notify the physician.

**GI** Nausea, vomiting, hiccups, and distress.
- Instruct patients that taking prescribed doses with meals or snack may lessen gastric irritation.
- If GI symptoms are severe or persistent, notify physician.

**Lung** Asthmatic episodes in susceptible individuals.

**Allergic** Hypersensitivity reactions, including anaphylactoid response.
- Check patients again within a few minutes of administering doses.
- Monitor vital signs.
- Have available drugs, equipment, and personnel for resuscitation in setting where muscle relaxants are used.

**Skin** Rashes, urticaria.
- Visually inspect patient for skin changes.
- Instruct patients to report skin changes to the physician.

### Nursing interventions related to drug administration
- Rela brand tablets contain FD & C yellow dye # 5, tartrazine, which may cause allergic reactions in susceptible individuals. While rare, this reaction is seen more commonly in persons with aspirin hypersensitivity.
- The final dose of the day should be taken at bedtime.

### Patient and family education
- Review with patients the anticipated benefits and possible side effects of therapy.
- Instruct patients to avoid the use of alcohol unless permitted in small amounts by the physician.
- Remind patients to keep all health care providers informed of all medications being used.

---

## chlorphenesin carbamate    (klor-FEN-e-sin)    central muscle relaxant

- chlorphenesin carbamate: Maolate, ✦Mycil

**MECHANISM OF ACTION**    Centrally acting skeletal muscle relaxants depress muscle tone through an action in the spinal cord. In addition, these drugs relieve anxiety, an effect that may contribute to their effectiveness.

**INDICATIONS**    • Muscle spasms not relieved by other therapy.

**CONTRAINDICATIONS**    **Hepatic disease** Use with caution.

**DOSAGE**    **PO:**    **ADULTS:** Initially, 800 mg three times daily, then adjust dose. Usual dose is 400 mg four times daily. Do not use longer than 8 weeks. *Special patient populations:* **CHILDREN:** Not recommended for children under 12 years of age. **PREGNANCY:** Safe use has not been established.

**PREPARATIONS**    *Tablets:* 400 mg.

**DRUG INTERACTIONS**    **CNS depressants** Additive depression with other CNS depressants, including alcohol.

**FATE**    Chlorphenesin is well absorbed. The plasma *half-life* is 2 to 5 hours. Chlorphenesin is metabolized in the liver and excreted in the urine.

### ❧ NURSING CONSIDERATIONS

#### Side effects, toxicities, and associated nursing actions
**CNS** Drowsiness, dizziness, confusion, headache, weakness; rarely, paradoxical stimulation, agitation, nervousness, insomnia.

- Review these side effects with patients. Tell patients to avoid driving or operating hazardous equipment if drowsiness, dizziness, or confusion occur, and to notify physician.
- Reassure patients that many of these side effects diminish with continued use of the medication.

**GI** Nausea, epigastric distress.

- Instruct patient that taking ordered doses with meals or snack may lessen gastric irritation.
- If GI symptoms are severe or persistent, notify physician.

**Hematologic** Rarely, leukopenia, thrombocytopenia, agranulocytosis, pancytopenia.

- Instruct patients to report the development of fever, sore throat, malaise, unexplained bruising or bleeding, nosebleed, bleeding gums.
- Monitor complete blood count, white blood cell differential, and platelet count.

**Allergic** Rash pruritis, anaphylactoid reaction.

- Visually inspect patient for development of rashes.
- Check patients within a few minutes of administering doses.
- Have available drugs, equipment, and personnel for resuscitation in settings where muscle relaxants are used.

### Nursing interventions related to drug administration

- Maolate brand tablets contain FD & C yellow dye # 5, tartrazine, which may cause allergic reactions in susceptible individuals. While rare, this reaction is seen more commonly in persons with aspirin hypersensitivity.
- The final dose of the day should be taken at bedtime.

### Patient and family education

- Review with patients the anticipated benefits and possible side effects of therapy.
- Instruct patients to avoid the use of alcohol unless permitted in small amounts by physician.
- Remind patients to keep all health care providers informed of all medications being used.

---

## chlorzoxazone    (klor-ZOX-a-zone)       central muscle relaxant

- chlorzoxazone: Paraflex

**MECHANISM OF ACTION**    Centrally acting skeletal muscle relaxants depress muscle tone through an action in the spinal cord. In addition, these drugs relieve anxiety, an effect that may contribute to their effectiveness.

**INDICATIONS**    • Muscle spasms not relieved by other therapy.

**CONTRAINDICATIONS**    • Hypersensitivity to the drug.

**DOSAGE**    **PO:**   **ADULTS:** 250 mg three or four times daily. Severe cases may require two or three times that dose initially.   **CHILDREN:** 20 mg/kg daily or 600 mg/M$^2$ in 3 or 4 divided doses.   *Special patient populations:*   **PREGNANCY:** Safe use has not been established.

**PREPARATIONS**    *Tablets:* 250 mg.

**DRUG INTERACTIONS**    **CNS depressants** Additive depression with other CNS depressants, including alcohol.

**FATE**    Chlorzoxazone is well absorbed. The *onset of action* is about 1 hour, and the *duration of action* is 3 to 4 hours. Chlorzoxazone is metabolized in part by the liver and excreted in the urine as glucuronides.

### ☙ NURSING CONSIDERATIONS

#### Side effects, toxicities, and associated nursing actions

**CNS** Drowsiness, dizziness, lightheadedness, malaise, headache, paradoxical overstimulation.

- Review these side effects with patients. Caution patients to avoid driving or operating hazardous equipment if drowsiness occurs.
- Reassure patients that these side effects may diminish with continued use of the drug.

**GI** Anorexia, nausea, vomiting, heartburn, constipation, or diarrhea.

- Inform patient that taking ordered doses with meals or snack may lessen gastric irritation.
- If GI symptoms are severe or persistent, notify physician.

- If constipation occurs, encourage patients to increase fluid intake to 2500 to 3000 ml per day, increase dietary intake of fruit, fruit juices, or fiber, and increase level of exercise if possible.
- If diarrhea or vomiting occur, monitor intake, output, and weight.

**GU** A metabolite of chlorzoxazone may color the urine orange or purple-red.
- Warn patients about this change in urine color.

**Hematologic** Rarely, anemia, granulocytopenia.
- Instruct patients to report the development of fatigue, malaise, sore throat, fever.
- Monitor complete blood cell count and white blood cell differential.

**Allergic** Rash, petechiae, urticaria, pruritis; rarely, angioedema, anaphylactic reactions.
- Inspect patients for development of skin changes.
- Check patients within a few minutes of administering dose to monitor for allergic reactions.
- Have available drugs, equipment, and personnel for resuscitation in settings where muscle relaxants are administered.

**Other** Rarely, hepatotoxicity with abnormalities in liver function tests.
- Instruct patients to report the development of jaundice, right upper quadrant abdominal pain, malaise, change in the color or consistency of stools.
- Monitor liver function tests.

### Nursing interventions related to drug administration
- Parafon Forte brand combination product containing chlorzoxazone with acetaminophen contains FD & C yellow dye # 5, tartrazine, which may cause allergic reactions in susceptible individuals. While rare, this reaction is seen more commonly in persons with aspirin hypersensitivity.
- Tablets may be crushed and mixed with a small amount of food or fluid for ease in taking ordered doses.

### Patient and family education
- Review with patients the anticipated benefits and possible side effects of therapy.
- Instruct patients to avoid the use of alcohol unless permitted in small amounts by the physician.
- Remind patients to keep all health care providers informed of all medications being used.

---

# cyclobenzaprine hydrochloride
(sye-kloe-BEN-za-preen)                                                    central muscle relaxant

- cyclobenzaprine hydrochloride: Flexeril

**MECHANISM OF ACTION**  Centrally acting skeletal muscle relaxants depress muscle tone through an action in the spinal cord. Cyclobenzaprine is related to the tricylic antidepressants and has sedative effects, potentiates norepinephrine, and has anticholinergic activity.

**INDICATIONS**  • Muscle spasms not relieved by other therapy.

**CONTRAINDICATIONS**  Urinary retention, glaucoma Cyclobenzaprine has anticholinergic activity that will worsen these conditions.

**DOSAGE**  PO:  ADULTS: 20 to 40 mg daily in 2 to 4 divided doses, maximum, 60 mg daily. Administer for no more than 3 weeks. *Special patient populations:*  CHILDREN: Not recommended for children. PREGNANCY: Safe use has not been established, although animal tests have not revealed harm to the fetus or impaired fertility.

**PREPARATIONS**  *Tablets (film-coated):* 10 mg.

**DRUG INTERACTIONS**  CNS depressants Additive depression with other CNS depressants, including alcohol.

**FATE**  Cyclobenzaprine is well absorbed and extensively metabolized by the liver. The *onset of action* is 1 hour and the *duration of action* is 12 to 24 hours. Metabolites are excreted in the urine. Unchanged drug is eliminated in the feces via biliary excretion.

## NURSING CONSIDERATIONS
### Side effects, toxicities, and associated nursing actions
**CNS** Drowsiness, dizziness, fatigue, headache, nervousness, confusion; rarely, stimulation, insomnia, nightmares, hallucinations.

- Review these side effects with patients. Tell patients that if drowsiness or dizziness occur to avoid driving or operating hazardous equipment.
- Reassure patients that side effects may diminish with continued use of the drug.

**CV** Rarely, fast heart rate, hypotension, fainting, palpitations.

- Monitor blood pressure and pulse.
- Instruct patients to move slowly from lying to sitting or standing. Keep siderails up. Keep a night-light on. Supervise ambulation, especially if patients are elderly or have been primarily immobilized or sedentary prior to use of this drug.

**GI** Dry mouth, nausea, unpleasant taste, constipation.

- If dry mouth occurs, instruct patients to take frequent sips of water, suck on sugarless hard candies or chew sugarless gum, perform regular oral hygiene, but avoid drying mouthwashes. Some patients may wish to try commercially available saliva substitutes.
- If constipation occurs, instruct patients to increase fluid intake to 2500 to 3000 ml per day, increase dietary intake of fruit, fruit juices, or fiber, and increase level of exercise, if possible.
- If GI symptoms are severe or persistent, notify physician.
- Instruct patients to try taking ordered doses with meals or snack to lessen gastric irritation.

**Allergic** Rash, urticaria, edema of face and tongue.

- Inspect patient at regular intervals for skin changes.
- Check patients within a few minutes of administering doses to ascertain development of allergic responses.

### Patient and family education

- Review with patients the anticipated benefits and possible side effects of therapy.
- Instruct patients to avoid the use of alcohol unless permitted in small amounts by the physician.
- Remind patients to keep all health care providers informed of all medications being used.

---

## methocarbamol    (meth-oh-KAR-ba-mole)                    central muscle relaxant

- methocarbamol: Delaxin, Robomol, Robaxin

**MECHANISM OF ACTION**    Centrally acting skeletal muscle relaxants depress muscle tone through an action in the spinal cord. In addition, these drugs relieve anxiety, an effect that may contribute to their effectiveness.

**INDICATIONS**    **Muscle spasms** not relieved by other therapy.    **Tetanus** Methocarbamol may be used, although other drugs are preferred.

**CONTRAINDICATIONS**    **Epilepsy, impaired renal function** Methocarbamol injection should not be used.

**DOSAGE**    **Skeletal muscle relaxation:** *PO:*    **ADULTS:** Initially, 6 to 8 g daily in 4 divided doses. Maintenance is 4 to 4.5 g daily in 3 to 6 divided doses.    *IM or IV:*    **ADULTS:** 1 g initially, not to exceed 3 g per day, and no longer than 3 days. Usually, after the initial dose, oral doses are begun.    **Tetanus:** *IV:* **ADULTS:** 1 to 2 g at 300 mg/min. May give additional doses, up to 3 g total. Repeat with 1 to 2 g every 6 hours. Switch to an oral dose when possible. Up to 24 g daily may be required for an oral dose. **CHILDREN:** 15 mg/kg or 500 mg/M$^2$ initially at 180 mg/M$^2$/min. Do not exceed 1.8 g/M$^2$/day nor for more than 3 days.    *Special patient populations:*    **CHILDREN:** Pediatric doses have been established for treating tetanus.    **PREGNANCY:** Safe use has not been established.

**PREPARATIONS**    *Tablets:* 500, 750 mg. *Tablets (film-coated):* 500, 750 mg. *Injection:* 100 mg/ml.

**DRUG INTERACTIONS**    **CNS depressants** Additive depression with other CNS depressants, including alcohol.    **Anticholinesterase inhibitors** Methocarbamol may make patients with myasthenia gravis weaker.

**DIAGNOSTIC TEST INTERFERENCE**    **Colored urine** Urine of patients taking methocarbamol may turn brown, black, blue, or green on standing.    **5-HIAA & VMA** Methocarbamol can give false-positive results for urine 5-hydroxyindolacetic acid (5-HIAA) and for vanilmandelic acid (VMA) in some procedures.

**FATE**    Methocarbamol is well absorbed. The *onset of action* is 30 minutes after an oral dose. The plasma *half-life* is 1 to 2 hours. Methocarbamol is metabolized by the liver and excreted in the urine.

## ❦ NURSING CONSIDERATIONS

### Side effects, toxicities, and associated nursing actions

**CNS** Drowsiness, dizziness, incoordination, headache, fever.

**Eye** Blurred vision, nystagmus.

* Review these side effects with patients. Tell patients to avoid driving or operating hazardous equipment if drowsiness, dizziness, incoordination, or diplopia occur.
* Reassure patients that many of these side effects will diminish with continued use of the medication.

**CV** Slow heart rate, fainting.

* Monitor heart rate and blood pressure. If heart rate drops below 60, notify physician.
* Instruct patients to move slowly from lying to sitting or standing. Keep siderails up and a nightlight on. Supervise ambulation, especially of the elderly and individuals who have been immobilized or primarily sedentary prior to drug administration.

**GI** Nausea, anorexia, metallic taste.

* Instruct patients to take oral doses with meals or snacks to lessen gastric irritation.
* If GI symptoms are severe or persistent, notify physician.

**Allergic** Urticaria, rash, pruritis, skin eruptions, nasal congestion.

* Visually inspect patient for skin changes.

### Nursing interventions related to drug administration

* For IV use, may be given undiluted at a rate of 300 mg or less over 1 minute. May also be diluted in up to 250 ml of isotonic sodium chloride or 5% dextrose solution, and administered as an infusion. Avoid extravasation, which may lead to thrombophlebitis or sloughing.
* Keep patients recumbent for at least 15 minutes following intravenous administration. Keep siderails up. Monitor blood pressure and pulse.
* Administer IM doses into large muscle masses such as the dorsogluteal site in adults or vastus lateralis in small children. Use anatomical landmarks to choose sites. Aspirate prior to injecting medication to avoid inadvertent intravenous administration. Record and rotate injection sites.

### Patient and family education

* Review with patients the anticipated benefits and possible side effects of drug therapy.
* Tell patients that their urine may turn black, brown, or green while on this drug. This side effect is harmless and will disappear when the drug is discontinued.
* Instruct the patient to avoid the use of alcohol unless permitted in small amounts by the physician.
* Remind patients to keep all health care providers informed of all medications being used.

Chapter Forty-two

# Drugs to treat myasthenia gravis

ambenonium          neostigmine
edrophonium          pyridostigmine

**OVERVIEW OF THE DRUG CLASS**   Myasthenia gravis is a disease in which the skeletal muscles quickly weaken and become fatigued. The muscles most commonly involved are those controlling facial movements. One early sign of myasthenia gravis is drooping eyelids (ptosis). As the disease progresses, chewing and swallowing become increasingly difficult, and the voice becomes less distinct. Death can result if the intercostal muscles and the diaphragm, muscles essential for breathing, become affected.

The basic defect in myasthenia gravis is that there are not enough receptors for acetylcholine at the neuromuscular junction. This reduction in the number of available receptors appears to be caused by an autoimmune disease in which antibodies block the active site for acetylcholine on the muscle (nicotinic) receptor and also increase the rate at which the receptors are degraded by the cell.

Drugs that inhibit the degradation of acetylcholine, acetylcholinesterase inhibitors, are the first-line treatment for myasthenia gravis.

**MECHANISM OF ACTION**   Acetylcholinesterase inhibitors allow the accumulation of acetylcholine at the neuromuscular junction, and this increase in the concentration of acetylcholine at the neuromuscular junction ensures that available receptors are activated.

**INDICATIONS**   • Myasthenia gravis.

**CONTRAINDICATIONS**   • Obstruction of the intestinal or urinary tracts.

**DRUG INTERACTIONS**   Many drugs block the neuromuscular receptor to a degree that it is not noticeable in a normal person, but can dangerously weaken the patient with myasthenia gravis. These drugs should either not be used or use cautiously, with appropriate adjustment of medication:

ACTH and glucocorticoids
**Anesthetics**
halothane (Fluothane)
lidocain IV (Xylocaine)
**Antiarrhythmics**
procainamide (Pronestyl)
propranolol (Inderal)
quinidine
**Antibiotics**
bacitracin (Bacitracin)
colistimethate (Coly-Mycin M)
colistin (Coly-Mycin S)
gentamicin (Garamycin)
kanamycin (Kantrex)
lincomycin (Lincocin)
neomycin (Mycifradin, Neobiotic)
paromomycin (Humatin)
polymyxin B (Aerosporin, Polymyxin B)
streptomycin (Streptomycin)
viomycin (Viocin)
**Anticonvulsants**
magnesium sulfate
**Antimalarials**
quinine
**Diuretics and other drugs or circumstances promoting low blood potassium concentration**
**Muscle relaxants**
gallamine (Flaxedil)
metocurine (Metubine)
pancuronium (Pavulon)

succinylcholine (Anectine)
tubocurarine

**Sedatives, especially those with respiratory depressant effects, such as barbiturates, narcotics, and tranquilizers.**

**Thyroid compound**

## ☙ NURSING CONSIDERATIONS

### Side effects, toxicities, and associated nursing actions

**CNS** Agitation and restlessness at toxic doses.

**CV** Slow heart rate (bradycardia), hypotension.

**Eye** Miosis.

**GI** Nausea, vomiting, diarrhea, abdominal cramps.

**Lung** Bronchospasm.

**Skin** Sweating.

**Other** The side effects are those characteristic of parasympathetic stimulation.

- All of these symptoms indicate cholinergic crisis, due to too high a dose of acetylcholinesterase inhibitor, or too short a period of time between doses.
- In attempting to regulate the dose of acetylcholinesterase inhibitors, monitor vital signs and blood pressure. Have a suction machine at the bedside. Remain calm and reassuring to the patient. Have available equipment for intubation in the event that the patient displays myasthenic crisis.
- Keep handy or at the bedside of patients with myasthenia gravis syringes, a tourniquet, and vials of atropine (antidote of acetylcholinesterase inhibitors) and an intravenous acetycholinesterase inhibitor such as edrophonium or neostigmine, to allow for rapid assessment or treatment of myasthenic or cholinergic crisis.

### Nursing interventions related to drug administration

- Assess the ability of the myasthenic patient to swallow before preparing an ordered dose of oral acetylcholinesterase inhibitor. If the ability to swallow is deteriorating, it may be necessary to administer a parenteral dose of medication rather than an oral dose. Ideally, the physician will have written orders for both oral and parenteral doses of acetycholinesterase inhibitors so that valuable time is not lost in trying to call the physician for a medication order if the patient is slipping into a myasthenic crisis.
- Administer doses of acetylcholinesterase inhibitors as close as possible to the time ordered, even if it requires leaving the patient care unit to find the patient in x-ray or therapy departments. Many myasthenics are very sensitive to changes in dosing frequency and will slip into myasthenic crisis if doses are late.
- Work with the patient to determine the best dosing schedule for medications. For example, patients may find it helpful to schedule doses of acetylcholinesterase inhibitors for 30 to 60 minutes before meals to have maximum strength for eating and swallowing.
- Instruct patients to take doses with snack or meals to lessen gastric irritation.

### Patient and family education

- Review with patients and families the anticipated benefits and possible side effects of drug therapy.
- Teach patients and families about, and give a list of, drugs known to cause weakness in patients taking acetylcholinesterase inhibitors.
- Emphasize to patients the importance of consulting with the physician before taking any medication, whether prescribed or over the counter. Remind patients to keep all health care providers informed of all medications being used.
- Instruct patients with myasthenia gravis to wear a medical identification tag or bracelet, and to carry with them the names and doses of medications being taken.
- Teach family members about the disease and signs and symptoms of myasthenic and cholinergic crisis. Instruct the family to bring the patient to an emergency care setting any time they feel the patient is not responding appropriately.
- Reinforce to patients the importance of taking acetylcholinesterase inhibitors exactly as ordered. In all but the mildest cases of the disease, forgetting a dose of medication, taking a dose too early or too

late, or omitting an inconvenient dose may cause the disease to go out of control. If the patient is required to take a nighttime dose at home, instruct the patient to obtain a reliable, nonelectric alarm clock to awaken the patient.
- Remind patients to keep careful watch on the supply of medication, and to refill prescriptions before the supply on hand has completely run out.
- Refer patients as needed to local visiting nurse agencies, and local, state, or national myasthenia gravis support groups.
- Remind patients to keep these and all medications out of the reach of children.

## ambenonium chloride (am-be-NOE-nee-um) acetylcholinesterase inhibitor

- ambenonium chloride: Mytelase

**MECHANISM OF ACTION** Inhibits the degradation of acetylcholine. The increase in acetylcholine at the neuromuscular junction increases muscle strength.

**INDICATIONS** Myasthenia gravis Symptomatic treatment to improve muscle strength.

**CONTRAINDICATIONS** • Obstruction of the intestinal or urinary tracts.

**DOSAGE** PO: **ADULTS:** Initially, 5 mg daily. The dosage is adjusted upward in 5 mg daily increments every 1 to 2 days until the desired response is obtained. The usual maintenance dose is highly variable, generally in the range of 5 to 25 mg three or four times a day. **CHILDREN:** Initially, 0.3 mg/kg or 10 mg/$M^2$ daily, divided into 3 to 4 doses. Dosage is gradually adjusted up to achieve desired response. Maintenance dosages may be 1.5 mg/kg or 50 mg/$M^2$ daily. *Special patient populations:* **PREGNANCY:** Safe use has not been established. Newborns may show transient weakness.

**PREPARATIONS** *Tablets:* 10 mg.

**DRUG INTERACTIONS** Many drugs block the neuromuscular receptor to a degree that is not noticeable in a normal person, but can dangerously weaken the patient with myasthenia gravis. These drugs should either not be used or used cautiously, with appropriate adjustment of medication. See entry for drug class (p. 806) for a complete listing.

**FATE** Ambenonium is poorly absorbed and has a variable duration of action. In general the *duration of action* is 4 to 8 hours. The metabolic fate of ambenonium has not been well characterized.

### ☙ NURSING CONSIDERATIONS

#### Side effects, toxicities, and associated nursing actions
- See entry for drug class (p. 807).

#### Nursing interventions related to drug administration
- See entry for drug class (p. 807).

#### Patient and family education
- See entry for drug class (p. 807).

## edrophonium chloride (ed-roe-FOE-nee-um) acetylcholinesterase inhibitor

- edrophonium chloride: Tensilon

**MECHANISM OF ACTION** Inhibits the degradation of acetylcholine. The increase in acetylcholine at the neuromuscular junction increases muscle strength.

**INDICATIONS** Myasthenia gravis Edrophonium has a very short duration of action and is used as a diagnostic agent. **Differential diagnosis** Edrophonium is used to differentiate whether muscle weakness is due to too much or too little anticholinesterase medication. If the muscle weakness is from too little medication, muscle strength will briefly improve after edrophonium is administered. If muscle strength decreases, there is an overdose of medication.

**CONTRAINDICATIONS** • Obstruction of the intestinal or urinary tracts.

**DOSAGE**   Differential diagnosis of myasthenia gravis: *IV or IM:*   ADULTS: 10 mg. If IV, 2 mg is first injected and the patient evaluated after 30 seconds. If no reaction, the remaining 8 mg is injected. If IM, inject 10 mg.   IV:   CHILDREN: 1 mg if under 75 lb (34 kg), 2 mg if over 75 lb. If no response in 45 seconds, inject an additional 1 mg and repeat every 30 seconds to a maximum dose of 5 mg (under 75 lb) or 10 mg (over 75 lb).   *IM:*   CHILDREN: 2 mg for children under 75 lb (34 kg), 5 mg for those over 75 lb. Reaction should appear in 2 to 10 minutes.   *Special patient populations:*   PREGNANCY: Safe use has not been established. Newborns may show transient weakness.

**PREPARATIONS**   *Injection:* 10 mg/ml.

**DRUG INTERACTIONS**   Many drugs block the neuromuscular receptor to a degree that is not noticeable in a normal person, but can dangerously weaken the patient with myasthenia gravis. These drugs should either not be used or used cautiously, with appropriate adjustment of medication. See entry for drug class (p. 806) for a complete listing.

**FATE**   The metabolic fate of edrophonium has not been well characterized. Edrophonium is short-acting.

☙ **NURSING CONSIDERATIONS**

**Side effects, toxicities, and associated nursing actions**
- See entry for drug class (p. 807).

**Patient and family education**
- See entry for drug class (p. 807).

---

# neostigmine bromide, neostigmine methylsulfate
(nee-oh-STIG-meen)                                            acetylcholinesterase inhibitor

- neostigmine bromide, neostigmine methylsulfate: Prostigmin Bromide, Prostigmin Methylsulfate

**MECHANISM OF ACTION**   Inhibits the degradation of acetylcholine. The increase in acetylcholine at the neuromuscular junction increases muscle strength.

**INDICATIONS**   Myasthenia gravis Diagnosis and symptomatic treatment to improve muscle strength.

**CONTRAINDICATIONS**   • Obstruction of the intestinal or urinary tracts.

**DOSAGE**   Diagnosis of myasthenia gravis:   ADULTS: Anticholinesterase medications are discontinued for at least 8 hours. Atropine, 0.011 mg/kg is given IM 30 minutes before neostigmine, and a muscle strength test is made. Alternatively, the same dose of atropine can be given IV at the same time as neostigmine. Atropine prevents adverse muscarinic effects (nausea, bronchospasm, hypotension, sweating). Neostigmine methylsulfate, 0.22 mg/kg, is given IM. More atropine can be administered if needed (0.4 to 0.6 mg IV).   CHILDREN: The same dose of atropine is given. The IM dose of neostigmine methylsulfate is 0.025 to 0.04 mg/kg.   **Treatment of myasthenia gravis:** *PO:* ADULTS: Initially, 15 mg three times daily of neostigmine, then gradually increase the dosage for optimum muscle strength. The maintenance dose is highly individualized, varying from 15 to 375 mg daily.   CHILDREN: 7.5 to 15 mg three to four times daily initially, then increase gradually. An alternate dosage regimen is 0.333 mg/kg or 10 mg/M$^2$ six times daily.   **Postoperative distention and urinary retention:** *IM or SC:*   ADULTS: 0.25 mg neostigmine methylsulfate every 4 to 6 hours for 2 to 3 days.   *Special patient populations:*   PREGNANCY: Safe use has not been established. Newborns may show transient weakness.

**PREPARATIONS**   Bromide, *tablets:* 15 mg. Methylsulfate, *injection:* 0.25, 0.5, 1 mg/ml.

**DRUG INTERACTIONS**   Many drugs block the neuromuscular receptor to a degree that is not noticeable in a normal person but can dangerously weaken the patient with myasthenia gravis. These drugs should either not be used or used cautiously, with appropriate adjustment of medication. See entry for drug class (p. 806) for a complete listing.

**FATE**   Neostigmine is poorly absorbed from the gastrointestinal tract, in part accounting for variation in dose requirements. The *onset of action* is 20 to 30 minutes after parenteral administration, 2.5 to 4 hours after oral administration. Neostigmine is hydrolyzed and metabolized. Neostigmine and its metabolites are excreted in the urine.

### ☙ NURSING CONSIDERATIONS
#### Side effects, toxicities, and associated nursing actions
- See entry for drug class (p. 807).

#### Nursing interventions related to drug administration
- See entry for drug class (p. 807).

#### Patient and family education
- See entry for drug class (p. 807).

---

## pyridostigmine bromide    (peer-id-oh-STIG-meen)    acetylcholinesterase inhibitor

- pyridostigmine bromide: Mestinon, Regonal

**MECHANISM OF ACTION**    Inhibits the degradation of acetylcholine. The increase in acetylcholine at the neuromuscular junction increases muscle strength.

**INDICATIONS**    *Myasthenia gravis* Symptomatic treatment to improve muscle strength.

**CONTRAINDICATIONS**    • Obstruction of the intestinal or urinary tracts.

**DOSAGE**    PO:    ADULTS: Initially, 60 mb, three times daily, adjusted every 2 days if necessary. The maintenance dose is highly individualized and varies from 60 to 1.5 g daily.    CHILDREN: Initially, 7 mg/kg or 200 mg/$M^2$ daily, divided into 5 or 6 doses. Adjust every few days as necessary.    IM or very slow IV:    ADULTS: 2 mg (1/30 the oral dose) every 2 to 3 hours.    *Special patient populations:*    PREGNANCY: Safe use has not been established. Newborns may show transient weakness.

**PREPARATIONS**    *Solution (oral):* 60 mg/5 ml. *Tablets:* 60 mg. *Tablets (extended-release):* 180 mg. *Injection:* 5 mg/ml.

**DRUG INTERACTIONS**    Many drugs block the neuromuscular receptor to a degree that is not noticeable in a normal person, but can dangerously weaken the patient with myasthenia gravis. These drugs should either not be used or used cautiously, with appropriate adjustment of medication. See entry for drug class (p. 806) for a complete listing.

**FATE**    Pyridostigmine is poorly absorbed. The *onset of action* is 30 to 45 minutes after oral administration, with a *duration of action* of 3 to 6 hours. After IM administration, the *onset of action* is 15 minutes and 2 to 5 minutes IV administration. Pyridostigmine is hydrolyzed and metabolized. Pyridostigmine and its metabolites are excreted in the urine.

### ☙ NURSING CONSIDERATIONS
#### Side effects, toxicities, and associated nursing actions
- See entry for drug class (p. 807).

#### Nursing interventions related to drug administration
- See entry for drug class (p. 807).
- For IV use, may be given undiluted at a rate of 0.5 mg per minute for treatment of myasthenia gravis. For use as a muscle relaxant antagonist, rate may be 5 mg per minute.

#### Patient and family education
- See entry for drug class (p. 807).

# Chapter Forty-three

# Drugs to treat parkinsonism

amantadine
benztropine
biperiden
bromocriptine (see Chapter 29)
carbidopa
diphenhydramine (see Chapter 53)

ethopropazine
levodopa
orphenadrine
procyclidine
trihexyphenidyl

**DRUG COMBINATIONS**
- carbidopa and levodopa: Sinemet
- orphenadrine and aspirin and caffeine: Norgesic

**INTRODUCTION** Parkinsonism is a movement disorder characterized by rigidity, akinesia, and tremor. *Rigidity* means that the muscle tone is greatly increased but reflex activity is not. When a limb is passively forced through flexor or extensor movements, the muscular resistance alternately increases and decreases to give a cogwheel effect. *Akinesia* (no motion) refers to the difficulty the patient has in initiating any movement. Early in the course of parkinsonism, the difficulty in initiating movement is not as marked and is termed *bradykinesia* (slow motion). The *tremor* of parkinsonism is seen mostly in the limbs at rest and decreases with movement of the limbs.

The present understanding of parkinsonism is that it represents a deficiency in the neurotransmitter dopamine in certain basal ganglia. Dopamine from these neuronal tracts is believed to exert an inhibitory influence on cholinergic neurons of the extrapyramidal system controlling muscle tone. When dopamine is lacking, muscle tone increases because of the unopposed action of acetylcholine, resulting in muscular rigidity, inhibition of spontaneous movements, and tremor. The lack of dopamine is secondary to a progressive degeneration of specific dopominergic neurons. This degeneration cannot be arrested. Drugs only alleviate the symptoms for a few years.

Drugs used early in the course of parkinsonism include anticholinergic drugs, antihistaminic drugs given for their anticholinergic activity, and amantidine. The *anticholinergic drugs* include benztropine, biperiden, ethopropazine, procyclidine, and trihexyphenidyl. The *antihistaminic drugs* include diphenhydramine and orphenadrine. *Amantadine* is an antiviral agent that also promotes the release of dopamine from central neurons.

Drugs used late in the course of parkinsonism include levodopa (which is metabolized to dopamine) and bromocriptine, a dopamine agonist. Carbidopa is an agent that inhibits the peripheral conversion of levodopa to dopamine.

Certain drugs can cause symptoms of parkinsonism, specifically reserpine and the antipsychotic drugs. Lowering the dose or discontinuing the drug eliminates the symptoms.

## amantadine hydrochloride (a-MAN-ta-deen) antiparkinson, antiviral

- amantadine hydrochloride: Symmetrel

**MECHANISM OF ACTION** Amantadine promotes the release of dopamine from the central neurons, an action unrelated to its antiviral effects. This promotion of dopamine release partially overcomes its deficiency.

**INDICATIONS** **Parkinsonism** Amantadine may be given alone or with an anticholinergic drug. **Influenza A virus respiratory tract illness** See Chapter 23.

**CONTRAINDICATIONS** **Epilepsy** Seizure activity may be increased. **Congestive heart failure or peripheral edema** may be worsened by amantadine.

**DOSAGE** **PO:** **ADULTS:** 100 mg two times daily. If given with other antiparkinson drugs, 100 mg once daily initially, then increased to 100 mg twice daily after a week or more. Up to 400 mg daily may be given if necessary. *Special patient populations:* **CHILDREN:** Pediatric doses are only for the antiviral action (see Chapter 23). **PREGNANCY:** Safe use has not been established.

**PREPARATIONS** *Capsules:* 100 mg. *Solution (oral):* 50 mg/5 ml.

**DRUG INTERACTIONS**    **Anticholinergic drugs** Dosage will have to be decreased when amantadine is added.

**FATE**    Amantadine is readily absorbed. The plasma *half-life* is about 24 hours; this is increased up to 8 days in patients with renal disease. Amantidine is excreted unchanged in the urine.

## ☙ NURSING CONSIDERATIONS

### Side effects, toxicities, and associated nursing actions

**CNS** Depression, psychosis; hallucinations, confusion, anxiety, irritability.
- Obtain careful baseline mental status examination prior to start of therapy, and evaluate at regular intervals.
- Tell patients to avoid driving or operating hazardous equipment if CNS side effects are prominent.
- Be alert to signs of increasing depression: lethargy, apathy, decreased appetite, loss of interest in personal appearance. Be alert to suicidal tendencies.
- If insomnia occurs, suggest patient take the last dose of the day several hours before bedtime.

**CV** Congestive heart failure, orthostatic hypotension.
- Monitor intake, output, daily weight, blood pressure, pulse. Auscultate lung sounds.
- Instruct patients to report the development of swelling of the lower extremeties.
- Instruct patients to move slowly from lying to sitting or standing. Supervise ambulation. Keep siderails up. Keep a nightlight on.

**GI** Nausea, constipation.
- If constipation occurs, encourage patients to increase fluid intake to 2500 to 3000 ml per day, increase dietary intake of fruit, fruit juices, and fiber, and increase level of exercise, if possible.
- If side effects are severe, consult with physician about the possibility of rearranging dosing schedule to have more frequent, but lower, doses during the day.
- If nausea is severe or persistent, notify physician.

**GU** Urinary retention.
- Instruct patient to report sensation of inadequate bladder emptying.
- Instruct patient to urinate prior to each dose.

**Hematologic** Rarely, leukopenia, neutropenia.
- Instruct patient to report the development of fever, sore throat, malaise, fatigue.
- Monitor white blood cell differential.

**Skin** Livedo reticularis (bluish or purplish mottling of the skin) generally appears during the first year of therapy and may take several weeks to subside when therapy is discontinued.

**Allergic** Skin rash.
- Visually inspect patients for skin changes.
- Instruct patients to report the development of any skin changes.

### Nursing interventions related to drug administration
- Capsules may be opened and content mixed with a small amount of food or fluid for ease in taking dose, although a liquid preparation is also available.

### Patient and family education
- Review with patients the anticipated benefits and possible side effects of drug therapy.
- Remind patients to take this drug only as directed.
- Caution patients to avoid the use of alcohol unless permitted in small amounts by the physician.

---

## benztropine mesylate    (BENZ-troe-peen)                    antiparkinson

- benztropine mesylate: ✿Apo-Bentropin, ✿Bensylate, ✿PMS Benztropine, Cogentin

**MECHANISM OF ACTION**    Benztropine is an anticholinergic agent. Anticholinergic agents are useful in treating parkinsonism because they help correct the relative cholinergic excess in the substantia nigra responsible for the parkinsonian symptoms.

**INDICATIONS** **Parkinsonism** Akinesia and rigidity are usually reduced by anticholinergic agents. • The parkinsonian tremor is not as effectively decreased.

**CONTRAINDICATIONS** • Acute glaucoma. • Pyloric or duodenal obstruction, peptic ulcers, prostatic hypertrophy, bladder obstruction. • Myasthenia gravis.

**DOSAGE** **PO:** **ADULTS:** 1 to 2 mg daily. May be increased gradually by 0.5 mg every 5 to 6 days if necessary. Maximum daily dose is 6 mg. Smaller doses are usually given at bedtime. If the dosage is larger than 2 mg daily, the dosage is divided, up to 4 times daily. *Special patient populations:* **ELDERLY:** Patients over 60 years old are usually more sensitive to anticholinergic drugs and a lower dose can be used. **CHILDREN:** Parkinsonism is not a pediatric disorder. Benztropine is contraindicated in children under 3 years old and used with caution in older children. **PREGNANCY:** Safe use has not been established.

**PREPARATIONS** *Tablets:* 0.5, 1, 2 mg. *Injection:* 1 mg/ml.

**DRUG INTERACTIONS** **Phenothiazines and tricyclic antidepressants** These drugs have anticholinergic effects. Paralytic ileus has been reported when one of these drugs is taken with an anticholinergic drug. **Orphenadrine and propoxyphene** Either of these, taken with an anticholinergic, may produce mental confusion, anxiety, and tremors. **Levodopa** Anticholinergics will delay gastric emptying, decreasing the amount of levodopa absorbed.

**FATE** The effects of benztropine are cumulative and may not be evident for 2 or 3 days after therapy is started. The metabolic fate of benztropine is not well characterized.

## ✿ NURSING CONSIDERATIONS

### Side effects, toxicities, and associated nursing actions

**CNS** Drowsiness, dizziness.

**Eye** Blurred vision.

• Tell patients to avoid driving or operating hazardous equipment if these side effects occur.
• Reassure patients that these side effects may diminish with continued use of the drug.
• Supervise ambulation of elderly clients. Keep siderails up. Keep a nightlight on. Keep call bell within easy reach.

**GI** Dry mouth, nausea, constipation.

• Keep a record of stools. If constipation occurs, encourage the patient to increase fluid intake to 2500 to 3000 ml per day, increase dietary intake of fruits, fruit juices, and fiber, and increase level of exercise if possible. Auscultate bowel sounds, especially in immobilized patients.
• For dry mouth, encourage patients to take frequent sips of water, suck on sugarless hard candy or chew sugarless gum, perform regular oral hygiene, but avoid drying mouthwashes (usually, ones containing alcohol). Some patients may wish to try commercially available saliva substitutes.
• To lessen nausea, suggest taking doses before or after meals.

**GU** Difficulty in urination.

• Monitor intake and output.
• Instruct patients to report any difficulty in voiding, or apparent sensation of inadequate bladder emptying.

**Skin** Rash.

• Inspect patients at regular intervals for skin changes.

### Nursing interventions related to drug administration

• Tablets may be crushed and mixed with a small amount of food or fluid for patients who have difficulty swallowing tablets.
• For IV use, may be given undiluted at a rate of 1 mg or less pre minute.

### Patient and family education

• Review anticipated benefits and possible side effects of drug therapy.
• Tell patients that ability to sweat may be diminished, so tolerance of heat may be reduced. Patients in hot environments should plan periods of rest in the shade during the course of the day.
• Inform patients that several days of therapy may be necessary before the full effects of therapy are seen.
• Tell patients to keep all health care providers informed of all medications being used.
• Instruct patients to consult with the physician prior to using any medication, whether prescribed or over the counter.

# biperiden hydrochloride, biperiden lactate (bye-PER-i-den) antiparkinson

● biperiden hydrochloride, biperiden lactate: Akineton

**MECHANISM OF ACTION**  Biperiden is an anticholinergic agent. Anticholinergic agents are useful in treating parkinsonism because they help correct the relative cholinergic excess in the substantia nigra responsible for the parkinsonian symptoms.

**INDICATIONS**  **Parkinsonism** Akinesia and rigidity are usually reduced by anticholinergic agents. ● The parkinsonian tremor is not as effectively decreased.

**CONTRAINDICATIONS**  ● Acute glaucoma. ● Pyloric or duodenal obstruction, peptic ulcers, prostatic hypertrophy, bladder obstruction. ● Myasthenia gravis.

**DOSAGE**  **PO:**  **ADULTS:** 2 mg three or four times daily. If tolerance develops after prolonged therapy, the dosage may be increased. If biperiden is to be discontinued, it should be reduced gradually while the new drug is started.  **IM or slow IV:**  **ADULTS:** 2 mg to treat acute, drug-induced extrapyramidal symptoms. May repeat every 30 minutes if necessary, up to 8 mg total in 24 hours.  *Special patient populations:*  **ELDERLY:** Patients over 60 years old are usually more sensitive to anticholinergic drugs and a lower dose can be used.  **PREGNANCY:** Safe use has not been established.

**PREPARATIONS**  Hydrochloride, *tablets:* 2 mg. Lactate, *injection:* 5 mg/ml.

**DRUG INTERACTIONS**  **Phenothiazines and tricyclic antidepressants** These drugs have anticholinergic effects. Paralytic ileus has been reported when one of these drugs is taken with an anticholinergic drug.  **Orphenadrine and propoxyphene** Either of these, taken with an anticholinergic, may produce mental confusion, anxiety, and tremors.  **Levodopa** Anticholinergics will delay gastric emptying, decreasing the amount of levodopa absorbed.

**FATE**  The metabolic fate of biperiden has not been well characterized.

**☙ NURSING CONSIDERATIONS**

### Side effects, toxicities, and associated nursing actions

**CNS** Drowsiness, dizziness.

**Eye** Blurred vision.

● Tell patients to avoid driving or operating hazardous equipment if this side effect occurs.

● Reassure patients that this side effect may diminish with continued use of the drug.

● Supervise ambulation of elderly clients. Keep siderails up. Keep a nightlight on. Keep call bell within easy reach.

**GI** Dry mouth; nausea, constipation.

● Keep a record of stools. If constipation occurs, encourage the patient to increase fluid intake to 2500 to 3000 ml per day, increase dietary intake of fruits, fruit juices, and fiber, and increase level of exercise if possible. Auscultate bowel sounds, especially in immobilized patients.

● For dry mouth, encourage patients to take frequent sips of water, suck on sugarless hard candy or chew sugarless gum, perform regular oral hygiene but avoid drying mouthwashes (usually, ones containing alcohol). Some patients may wish to try commercially available saliva substitutes.

● To lessen nausea, suggest taking doses before or after meals.

**GU** Difficulty in urination.

● Monitor intake and output.

● Instruct patients to report any difficulty in voiding or apparent sensation of inadequate bladder emptying.

**Skin** Rash.

● Inspect patients at regular intervals for skin changes.

### Nursing interventions related to drug administration

● Tablets may be crushed and mixed with a small amount of food or fluid for patients who have difficulty swallowing tablets.

● For IV use, may be given undiluted at a rate of 2 mg or less per minute. Patient should remain recumbent for at least 15 minutes following drug administration. Monitor vital signs.

### Patient and family education

● Review anticipated benefits and possible side effects of drug therapy.

- Tell patients that ability to sweat may be diminished, so tolerance of heat may be reduced. Patients in hot environments should plan periods of rest in the shade during the course of the day.
- Inform patients that several days of therapy may be necessary before the full effects of therapy are seen.
- Tell patients to keep all health care providers informed of all medications being used.
- Instruct patients to consult with the physician prior to using any medication, whether prescribed or over the counter.

## carbidopa    (kar-bi-DOE-pa)    antiparkinson

- carbidopa: Lodosyn

**MECHANISM OF ACTION**    Carbidopa is a decarboxylase inhibitor that does not cross the blood-brain barrier. Carbidopa is given with levodopa to inhibit the peripheral conversion of levodopa to dopamine. This means that levodopa is converted to dopamine primarily in the CNS. Plasma concentrations of dopamine are much lower than when levodopa is administered alone, and the incidence of side effects, particularly nausea and vomiting, is markedly decreased. The dose of levodopa required for therapeutic effectiveness is also decreased.

**INDICATIONS**    *Parkinsonism* Carbidopa decreases the dosage of levodopa required to control symptoms.

**CONTRAINDICATIONS**    Hypersensitivity.

**DOSAGE**    **PO:**    **ADULTS:** Dosage must be individually adjusted. Carbidopa is not effective alone. If the patient is not currently receiving levodopa, a starting dosage is 100 mg of levodopa and 25 mg of carbidopa, three times daily. This is increased every 2 to 3 days if necessary by 100 mg levodopa and 25 mg carbidopa to a maximum daily dose of 600 mg levodopa, 150 mg carbidopa. For patients currently receiving levodopa, levodopa is withheld for at least 8 hours, and a daily dose of levodopa-carbidopa is begun at 20% to 25% of the former levodopa dose.    *Special patient populations:*    **ELDERLY:** Geriatric patients are started at lower initial doses.    **PREGNANCY:** Safe use has not been established.

**PREPARATIONS**    *Tablets:* 25 mg. *Combination tablets:* 100 mg levodopa, 10 mg carbidopa; 100 mg levodopa, 25 mg carbidopa; 250 mg levodopa, 25 mg carbidopa.

**DRUG INTERACTIONS**    See those for levodopa.

**FATE**    About 50% of carbidopa is absorbed. Carbidopa does not cross the blood-brain barrier. The plasma *half-life* is 1 to 2 hours. The metabolic fate of carbidopa is not well characterized.

### 🐦 NURSING CONSIDERATIONS

#### Side effects, toxicities, and associated nursing actions

- No specific side effects have been attributed to carbidopa.

#### Nursing interventions related to drug administration

- See entry for levodopa (p. 817).

#### Patient and family education

- Review with patients the anticipated benefits of therapy. Point out the interaction between levodopa and carbidopa.
- Point out to patients just being started on carbidopa, or on carbidopa-levodopa combinations, that side effects due to levodopa may be troublesome until dosage adjustment is complete. Review with patients the information about levodopa.

## ethopropazine hydrochloride    (eth-oh-PROE-pa-zeen)    antiparkinson

- ethopropazine hydrochloride: Parsidol, ✤Parsitan

**MECHANISM OF ACTION**    Ethopropazine is an anticholinergic agent chemically related to the phenothiazines, an antipsychotic drug class with anticholinergic activity. Anticholinergic agents are useful in treating parkinsonism because they help correct the relative cholinergic excess in the substantia nigra responsible for the parkinsonian symptoms.

**INDICATIONS**  **Parkinsonism** Akinesia and rigidity are usually reduced by anticholinergic agents.
* The parkinsonian tremor is not as effectively decreased.

**CONTRAINDICATIONS**  • Acute glaucoma. • Pyloric or duodenal obstruction, peptic ulcers, prostatic hypertrophy, bladder obstruction. • Myasthenia gravis.

**DOSAGE**  **PO:**  **ADULTS:** 50 mg one or two times daily. If necessary, gradually increase dose. The usual therapeutic dose for mild to moderate symptoms is 100 to 400 mg daily; for severe symptoms, 500 to 600 mg daily. *Special patient populations:*  **ELDERLY:** Patients over 60 years old are usually more sensitive to anticholinergic drugs and a lower dose can be used.  **CHILDREN:** Parkinsonism is not a pediatric disorder. Benztropin is contraindicated in children under 3 years old and used with caution in older children.  **PREGNANCY:** Safe use has not been established.

**PREPARATIONS**  *Tablets:* 10, 50 mg.

**DRUG INTERACTIONS**  **Phenothiazines and tricyclic antidepressants** These drugs have anticholinergic effects. Paralytic ileus has been reported when one of these drugs is taken with an anticholinergic drug.  **Orphenadrine and propoxyphene** Either of these, taken with an anticholinergic, may produce mental confusion, anxiety, and tremors.  **Levodopa** Anticholinergics will delay gastric emptying, decreasing the amount of levodopa absorbed.

**FATE**  The *onset of action* is about 30 minutes. The *duration of action* is 4 hours. The metabolic fate of ethopropazine is not well characterized.

## ☙ NURSING CONSIDERATIONS

### Side effects, toxicities, and associated nursing actions

**CNS** Drowsiness, dizziness.

**Eye** Blurred vision.
* Tell patients to avoid driving or operating hazardous equipment if this side effect occurs.
* Reassure patients that this side effect may diminish with continued use of the drug.
* Supervise ambulation of elderly clients. Keep siderails up. Keep a nightlight on. Keep call bell within easy reach.

**GI** Dry mouth; nausea, constipation.
* Keep a record of stools. If constipation occurs, encourage the patient to increase fluid intake to 2500 to 3000 ml per day, increase dietary intake of fruits, fruit juices, and fiber, and increase level of exercise if possible. Auscultate bowel sounds, especially in immobilized patients.
* For dry mouth, encourage patients to take frequent sips of water, suck on sugarless hard candy or chew sugarless gum, perform regular oral hygiene but avoid drying mouthwashes (usually, ones containing alcohol). Some patients may wish to try commercially available saliva substitutes.
* To lessen nausea, suggest taking doses before or after meals.

**GU** Difficulty in urination.
* Monitor intake and output.
* Instruct patients to report any difficulty in voiding or apparent sensation of inadequate bladder emptying.
* Suggest that patients void prior to taking each ordered dose.

**Skin** Rash.
* Inspect patients at regular intervals for skin changes.

### Patient and family education
* Review anticipated benefits and possible side effects of drug therapy.
* Tell patients that ability to sweat may be diminished, so tolerance of heat may be reduced. Patients in hot environments should plan periods of rest in the shade during the course of the day.
* Inform patients that serveral days of therapy may be necessary before the full effects of therapy are seen.
* Tell patients to keep all health care providers informed of all medications being used.
* Instruct patients to consult with the physician prior to using any medication, whether prescribed or over the counter.

## levodopa    (lee-voe-DOE-pa)    antiparkinson

- levodopa: Dopar, Larodopa

**MECHANISM OF ACTION**    Levodopa is the chemical precursor of dopamine, and unlike dopamine, levodopa readily crosses the blood-brain barrier. Levodopa is converted to dopamine by the enzyme dopa decarboxylase. This dopamine can overcome the deficiency in the substantia nigra.

**INDICATIONS**    **Parkinsonism** Because of the side effects, levodopa is used when amantidine and the anticholinergics are no longer effective.

**CONTRAINDICATIONS**    **Acute glaucoma. Severe cardiovascular or pulmonary disease, bronchial asthma** Use only cautiously.    **Renal or hepatic disease** Use only cautiously.    **Endocrine disease** Use only cautiously.

**DOSAGE**    **PO:**    **ADULTS:** Initially, 500 mg to 1 g daily in 2 or more doses. Daily dosage is increased every 3 to 7 days by 100 to 750 mg until the desired response is achieved. Maximum dosage should not exceed 8 g daily. The usual dose is 3 to 6 g daily in 3 or more doses. Optimum therapy may require 3 to 6 months to achieve.    *Special patient populations:*    **ELDERLY:** Geriatric patients are started with lower doses.    **PREGNANCY:** Safe use has not been established.

**PREPARATIONS**    *Capsules:* 100, 250, 500 mg. *Tablets:* 100, 250 500 mg.

**DRUG INTERACTIONS**    **Monoamine oxidase inhibitors** Patients being treated with one of these antidepressants cannot readily metabolize dopamine and are at risk for a hypertensive crisis. Therapy with an MAO inhibitor should be discontinued at least 2 weeks before levodopa therapy is begun.    **Pyridoxine** can reverse the therapeutic effects of levodopa.    **Anticholinergic agents** These act synergistically with levodopa, especially to reduce the tremor. Also, anticholinergic drugs slow gastric emptying and thereby diminish the activity of levodopa by delaying its absorption.    **Hypotensive agents** Such as methyldopa or guanethidine may act synergistically with levodopa.    **Inhalation anesthetics** Levodopa can precipitate cardiac arrhythmias.    **Phenytoin** interferes with the therapeutic effects of levodopa.

**DIAGNOSTIC TEST INTERFERENCE**    **Urinary glucose** False-positive reactions in tests based on cupric sulfate reagent (Benedict's reagent, Clinitest tablets) and false-negative reactions in tests using glucose oxidase (Clinistix, TesTape).    **Urinary ketones** False-positive with sodium nitroprusside reagent (Acetest, Ketostix, Labstix).    **Phenylketonuria** Levodopa causes the urine to turn black-brown, interfering with the color change when the ferric chloride reagent is added.

**FATE**    Levodopa is well absorbed. The plasma *half-life* is about 1 hour. Levodopa is metabolized to dopamine in the digestive tract as well as by the liver. Since about 75% of levodopa is converted in the periphery, high plasma concentrations of levodopa result. These high concentrations are responsible for the side effects. Metabolites of dopamine are excreted in the urine.

### ☙ NURSING CONSIDERATIONS
#### Side effects, toxicities, and associated nursing actions

**CNS** Ataxia, increased hand tremor, dizziness, numbness, weakness and faintness, confusion, insomnia, nightmares, hallucinations and delusions, agitation and anxiety, fatigue, euphoria. Choreiform and/or dystonic movements, rarely, convulsions. Mental changes including paranoia, psychosis, depression, dementia.

**Eye** Diplopia, blurred vision.

- Obtain careful baseline assessment of function and mental status, and monitor patient at regular intervals. Caution patient about the numerous side effects, and instruct patients and families to report the development of any new sign or symptom. Some symptoms may indicate a need to lower dosage, while others may indicate a need to change the dosing frequency.
- Caution patients to avoid driving or operating hazardous equipment if CNS effects are prominent or eye problems occur.

**CV** Flushing, cardiac irregularities, palpitations, orthostatic hypotensive episodes, episodes of slow hear rate (bradycardia).

- Monitor blood pressure and pulse, especially during periods of dosage adjustment.
- Instruct patients to move slowly from lying to sitting or standing. Supervise ambulation, keep siderails up, keep a nightlight on.

- If appropriate, instruct patients of family members to take and record pulse at regular intervals at home. Consult with physician to determine guidelines for specific patients.

**GI** Anorexia, nausea and vomiting, abdominal pain, flatulence, diarrhea or constipation, dry mouth, bleeding, ulcer.

- Monitor intake, output, and weight.
- For constipation, encourage patients to increase intake of fluids to 2500 to 3000 ml per day, increase dietary intake of fruit, fruit juices, or bran, and increase level of exercise, if possible.
- For dry mouth, encourage patients to rinse their mouths frequently with water, suck on sugarless hard candy or chew sugarless gum, perform regular oral hygiene, but avoid drying mouthwashes. Some patients may wish to use commercially available saliva substitutes.
- Monitor stools for occult blood, and monitor hemoglobin and hematocrit.

**GU** Incontinence, dark urine, priapism.

- Warn patients that urine may be dark in color, especially if left standing.
- Caution male patients about the possibility of priapism, and instruct patients to notify the physician if it occurs.
- If incontinence is severe or disabling, work with the physician and patient to help determine a solution that is satisfactory to both.

**Hematologic** Agranulocytosis, hemolytic anemia, leukopenia.

- Instruct patients to report the development of sore throat, pallor, fever, malaise.
- Monitor complete blood cell count, white blood cell differential.

**Skin** Rashes, increased sweating, dark sweat.

- Visually inspect patient for skin changes.
- Forewarn patients that sweat may be dark.

**Metabolic** Elevations of BUN, SGOT, SGPT, LDH, bilirubin, alkaline phosphatase, protein bound iodine.

- Obtain baseline bloodwork prior to initiating drug therapy, and monitor at regular intervals. Remind patients to keep all health care providers informed of all medications being used.

### Nursing interventions related to drug administration

- Instruct patients to take levodopa or levodopa-carbidopa combinations with meals or snack to reduce gastric irritation.
- If patients have difficulty swallowing levodopa capsules or tablets, consult the pharmacist about preparing a liquid form.
- Dopar brand capsules in 100, 250, and 500 mg doses contain FD & C yellow dye #5 (tartrazine), which may cause an allergic reaction in susceptible individuals. While rare, this side effect is seen more commonly in persons with aspirin hypersensitivity.

### Patient and family education

- Review with patients the anticipated benefits and possible side effects of drug therapy.
- Instruct diabetic patients to monitor blood glucose levels carefully while taking levodopa, as urinary glucose and ketone measurements may be inaccurate (see Diagnostic test interference).
- Caution patients to avoid the use of any medications without first clearing their use with the physician. Point out specifically the need to avoid vitamin preparations containing pyridoxine (vitamin $B_6$).
- Reassure patients that several weeks or months of therapy may be needed before improvement is seen.
- Remind patients to keep all health care providers informed of all medications being used.
- Remind patients to use this medication only as directed.

## orphenadrine citrate, orphenadrine hydrochloride
(or-FEN-a-dreen)

antiparkinson

- orphenadrine citrate, orphenadrine hydrochloride: Banflex, ✤Disipa, Flexoject, Flexon, Marflex, Myolin, Neocyten, Noradex, Norflex, Orfenate, Orflagen, X-Otag,

**MECHANISM OF ACTION**    Orphenadrine is an antihistaminic with anticholinergic properties. Anticholinergic agents are useful in treating parkinsonism because they help correct the relative cholinergic excess in the substantia nigra responsible for the parkinsonian symptoms.

**INDICATIONS**    Parkinsonism Akinesia and rigidity are usually reduced by anticholinergic agents. The parkinsonian tremor is not as effectively decreased.

**CONTRAINDICATIONS**    • Acute glaucoma. • Pyloric or duodenal obstruction, peptic ulcers, prostatic hypertrophy, bladder obstruction. • Myasthenia gravis.

**DOSAGE**    PO:   **ADULTS:** 50 mg, three times daily. The dosage may be gradually increased if necessary. Usually, up to 250 mg daily is well tolerated.   *Special patient populations:*   **ELDERLY:** Patients over 60 years old are usually more sensitive to anticholinergic drugs and a lower dose can be used. **PREGNANCY:** Safe use has not been established.

**PREPARATIONS**    Citrate, *tablets:* 100 mg. *Tablets (extended-release):* 100 mg. *Injection:* 30 mg/ml. Hydrochloride, *tablets:* 50 mg.

**DRUG INTERACTIONS**    **Phenothiazines and tricyclic antidepressants** These drugs have anticholinergic effects. Paralytic ileus has been reported when one of these drugs is taken with an anticholinergic drug.   **Propoxyphene** taken with an orphenadrine may produce mental confusion, anxiety, and tremors.   **Levodopa** Anticholinergics will delay gastric emptying, decreasing the amount of levodopa absorbed.

**FATE**    Orphenadrine is well absorbed. The *onset of action* is about 1 hour and the *duration of action* is 4 to 6 hours. The plasma *half-life* is 14 hours. Orphenadrine is extensively metabolized and the metabolites are excreted in the urine.

## ❦ NURSING CONSIDERATIONS

### Side effects, toxicities, and associated nursing actions
**CNS** Stimulation, insomnia, restlessness, hallucinations, confusion.
**Eye** Blurred vision.
- Caution patients to avoid driving or operating hazardous equipment if confusion or hallucinations occur; notify physician.
- Reassure patients that these side effects may diminish with continued use of the drug.
- Supervise ambulation of elderly clients. Keep siderails up. Keep a nightlight on.
**GI** Dry mouth; nausea, constipation.
- Keep a record of stools. If constipation occurs, encourage the patient to increase fluid intake to 2500 to 3000 ml per day, increase dietary intake of fruits, fruit juices, and fiber, and increase level of exercise if possible. Auscultate bowel sounds, especially in immobilized patients.
- For dry mouth, encourage patients to take frequent sips of water, suck on sugarless hard candy or chew sugarless gum, perform regular oral hygiene but avoid drying mouthwashes. Some patients may wish to try commercially available saliva substitutes.
- For nausea, suggest taking doses before or after meals.
**GU** Difficulty in urination.
- Monitor intake and output.
- Instruct patients to report any difficulty in voiding or apparent sensation of inadequate bladder emptying.
- Suggest patients void prior to taking each ordered dose.
**Skin** Rash.
- Visually inspect patients at regular intervals for skin changes.

### Nursing interventions related to drug administration
- For IV use, may be given undiluted, or diluted in 5 to 10 ml of sterile water for injection. Administer at a rate of 30 mg or less over 1 minute. Monitor vital signs. Keep patient recumbent for 15 to 30 minutes. Assist patients to get up when ready.

### Patient and family education
- Review with patients the anticipated benefits and possible side effects of drug therapy.
- Caution patients that ability to sweat may be diminished, so tolerance of heat may be reduced. Patients in hot environments should plan into their day periods of rest in shade.

- Inform patients that several days of therapy may be necessary before the full effects of therapy are seen.
- Caution patients to keep all health care providers informed of all medications being used.
- Instruct patients to clear the use of any medication, prescribed or over the counter, with the physician prior to use.
- Caution the patient to avoid the use of alcohol unless permitted in small amounts by the physician.

---

## procyclidine hydrochloride    (proe-SYE-kli-deen)      antiparkinson

- procyclidine hydrochloride: Kemadrin

**MECHANISM OF ACTION**    Procyclidine is an anticholinergic agent. Anticholinergic agents are useful in treating parkinsonism because they help correct the relative cholinergic excess in the substantia nigra responsible for the parkinsonian symptoms.

**INDICATIONS**    **Parkinsonism** Akinesia and rigidity are usually reduced by anticholinergic agents. The parkinsonian tremor is not as effectively decreased.

**CONTRAINDICATIONS**    • Acute glaucoma. • Pyloric or duodenal obstruction, peptic ulcers, prostatic hypertrophy, bladder obstruction. • Myasthenia gravis.

**DOSAGE**    **PO:**    **ADULTS:** 2.5 mg, three times a day. The dose may be increased to 5 mg three times a day, and then in 5 mg increments as necessary to control symptoms. Severe cases may require 45 to 60 mg daily. *Special patient populations:*    **ELDERLY:** Patients over 60 years old are usually more sensitive to anticholinergic drugs and a lower dose can be used.    **PREGNANCY:** Safe use has not been established.

**PREPARATIONS**    *Tablets:* 5 mg.

**DRUG INTERACTIONS**    **Phenothiazines and tricyclic antidepressants** These drugs have anticholinergic effects. Paralytic ileus has been reported when one of these drugs is taken with an anticholinergic drug.    **Orphenadrine and propoxyphene** Either of these, taken with an anticholinergic, may produce mental confusion, anxiety, and tremors.    **Levodopa** Anticholinergics will delay gastric emptying, decreasing the amount of levodopa absorbed.

**FATE**    The metabolic fate of procyclidine is not well characterized.

### ☙ NURSING CONSIDERATIONS

#### Side effects, toxicities, and associated nursing actions

**CNS** Drowsiness, dizziness.

**Eye** Blurred vision.

- Tell patients to avoid driving or operating hazardous equipment if these side effects occur.
- Reassure patients that these side effects may diminish with continued use of the drug.
- Supervise ambulation of elderly clients. Keep siderails up. Keep a nightlight on. Keep call bell within easy reach.

**GI** Dry mouth; nausea, constipation.

- Keep a record of stools. If constipation occurs, encourage the patient to increase fluid intake to 2500 to 3000 ml per day, increase dietary intake of fruits, fruit juices, and fiber, and increase level of exercise if possible. Auscultate bowel sounds, especially in immobilized patients.
- For dry mouth, encourage patients to take frequent sips of water, suck on sugarless hard candy or chew sugarless gum, perform regular oral hygiene but avoid drying mouthwashes (usually, ones containing alcohol). Some patients may wish to try commercially available saliva substitutes.
- To lessen nausea, suggest taking doses before or after meals.

**GU** Difficulty in urination.

- Monitor intake and output.
- Instruct patients to report any difficulty in voiding or apparent sensation of inadequate bladder emptying.
- Suggest that patients void prior to taking each ordered dose.

**Skin** Rash.
- Inspect patients at regular intervals for skin changes.

**Patient and family education**
- Review anticipated benefits and possible side effects of drug therapy.
- Tell patients that ability to sweat may be diminished, so tolerance of heat may be reduced. Patients in hot environments should plan periods of rest in the shade during the course of the day.
- Inform patients that several days of therapy may be necessary before the full effects of therapy are seen.
- Tell patients to keep all health care providers informed of all medications being used.
- Instruct patients to consult with the physician prior to using any medication, whether prescribed or over the counter.

## trihexyphenidyl hydrochloride (trye-hex-ee-FEN-i-dill) antiparkinson

- trihexyphenidyl hydrochloride: Aphen, Artane, Tihexane

**MECHANISM OF ACTION** Trihexyphenidyl is an anticholinergic agent. Anticholinergic agents are useful in treating parkinsonism because they help correct the relative cholinergic excess in the substantia nigra responsible for the parkinsonian symptoms.

**INDICATIONS** **Parkinsonism** Akinesia and rigidity are usually reduced by anticholinergic agents. • The parkinsonian tremor is not as effectively decreased.

**CONTRAINDICATIONS** • Acute glaucoma. • Pyloric or duodenal obstruction, peptic ulcers, prostatic hypertrophy, bladder obstruction. • Myasthenia gravis.

**DOSAGE** **PO:** **ADULTS:** First day, 1 mg, then increase by 2 mg increments at 3- to 5-day intervals. Effective dose is usually 6 to 10 mg daily. *Special patient populations:* **ELDERLY:** Patients over 60 years old are usually more sensitive to anticholinergic drugs and a lower dose can be used. **PREGNANCY:** Safe use has not been established.

**PREPARATIONS** *Capsules (extended-release):* 5 mg. *Elixir:* 2 mg/5 ml. *Tablets:* 2, 5 mg.

**DRUG INTERACTIONS** **Phenothiazines and tricyclic antidepressants** These drugs have anticholinergic effects. Paralytic ileus has been reported when one of these drugs is taken with an anticholinergic drug. **Orphenadrine and propoxyphene** Either of these, taken with an anticholinergic, may produce mental confusion, anxiety, and tremors. **Levodopa** Anticholinergics will delay gastric emptying, decreasing the amount of levodopa absorbed.

**FATE** Trihexyphenidyl is rapidly absorbed from the gastrointestinal tract. The *onset of action* is about 1 hour, and the *duration of action* is 6 to 12 hours. The metabolic fate of trihexyphenidyl has not been well characterized, but it is believed to be excreted unchanged in the urine.

## 🦉 NURSING CONSIDERATIONS

**Side effects, toxicities, and associated nursing actions**

**CNS** Drowsiness, dizziness.

**Eye** Blurred vision.
- Tell patients to avoid driving or operating hazardous equipment if these side effects occur.
- Reassure patients that these side effects may diminish with continued use of the drug.
- Supervise ambulation of elderly patients. Keep siderails up. Keep a nightlight on. Keep call bell within easy reach.

**GI** Dry mouth; nausea, constipation
- Keep a record of stools. If constipation occurs, encourage the patient to increase fluid intake to 2500 to 3000 ml per day, increase dietary intake of fruits, fruit juices, and fiber, and increase level of exercise if possible. Auscultate bowel sounds, especially in immobilized patients.
- For dry mouth, encourage patients to take frequent sips of water, suck on sugarless hard candy or chew sugarless gum, perform regular oral hygiene, but avoid drying mouthwashes (usually, ones containing alcohol). Some patients may wish to try commercially available saliva substitutes.

- To lessen nausea, suggest taking doses before or after meals.

**GU** Difficulty in urination

- Monitor intake and output.
- Instruct patients to report any difficulty in voiding or apparent sensation of inadequate bladder emptying.
- Suggest that patients void prior to taking each ordered dose.

**Skin** Rash.

- Inspect patients at regular intervals for skin changes.

### Nursing interventions related to drug administration

- Read labels carefully; 5 mg doses are available in tablets and extended-release capsules.

### Patient and family education

- Review anticipated benefits and possible side effects of drug therapy.
- Tell patients that ability to sweat may be diminished, so tolerance of heat may be reduced. Patients in hot environments should plan periods of rest in the shade during the course of the day.
- Inform patients that several days of therapy may be necessary before the full effects of therapy are seen.
- Tell patients to keep all health care providers informed of all medications being used.
- Instruct patients to consult with the physician prior to using any medication, whether prescribed or over the counter.

# Chapter Forty-four

# Neuromuscular blockers

**Nondepolarizing (competitive) blocking drugs**
atracurium
gallamine
metocurine
pancuronium
tubocurarine
vecuronium

**Depolarizing drug**
succinylcholine

**INTRODUCTION**   Neuromuscular blocking drugs are used to provide skeletal muscle relaxation during diagnostic and surgical procedures. Patients receiving neuromuscular blocking drugs will be those undergoing anesthesia, patients having certain diagnostic studies in which brief muscle relaxation is necessary for the completing of the study, some patients who are ''bucking'' ventilators, and patients undergoing electroconvulsive therapy.

**OVERVIEW OF THE DRUG CLASS**   The neuromuscular blocking agents all act at the neuromuscular junction. Of the neuromuscular blockers in clinical use, only succinylcholine is a depolaring blocker. The other neuromuscular blockers are nondepolarizing agents.

   The neuromuscular blockers are distinguished by their duration of action and route of excretion. The route of excretion is the key factor in determining which patient populations experience prolonged neuromuscular blockade. Table 44-1 compares the duration of action and the sensitive patient populations.

**MECHANISM OF ACTION**   Neuromuscular blocking drugs produce complete muscle relaxation by binding to the receptor for acetylcholine at the neuromuscular junction. The nondepolarizing or competitive blockers bind to the receptor without initiating depolarization of the muscle membrane. The depolarizing drug also binds to the receptor for acetylcholine but does cause depolarization of the muscle membrane. Both types of blockade, nondepolarizing and depolarizing, result in muscle paralysis.

**INDICATIONS**   **Skeletal muscle relaxation during surgery** This action is particularly important for abdominal surgery. • Neuromuscular blockers should never be administered to a conscious patient but only to a patient after general anesthesia has been induced. • This is because the conscious patient would be distressed by the complete paralysis induced and be aware of all procedures and associated pain.

| Table 44-1. | Comparision of the neuromuscular blockers | | |
|---|---|---|---|
| | Drug | Duration of action (min) | Patient populations with risk for prolonged blockade |
| | **Non-depolarizing neuromuscular blockers** | | |
| | Atracurium | 20 - 35 | None |
| | Gallamine | 15 - 30 | Biliary obstruction |
| | | | Renal failure |
| | Metocurine | 35 - 60 | Elderly |
| | | | Renal failure |
| | Pancuronium | 35 - 75 | Elderly |
| | Tubocurarine | 20 - 40 | Elderly |
| | | | Renal failure |
| | Vecuronium | 25 - 30 | Biliary obstruction |
| | **Depolarizing neuromuscular blocker** | | |
| | Succinylcholine | 4 - 10 | Decreased plasma pseudo-cholinesterase |

**Endotracheal intubation** This is facilitated when the patient is pretreated with a neuromuscular blocker. **Laryngospasm** This is relieved with a neuromuscular blocker. **Electroconvulsive shock therapy.** Administration of a neuromuscular blocker will prevent dislocations and fractures.

**CONTRAINDICATIONS** **Pulmonary impairment or respiratory depression** This is not an absolute contraindication, but extreme care is required. **Myasthenia gravis** These patients already have severely compromised neuromuscular transmission.

**DRUG INTERACTIONS** **Aminoglycoside antibiotics** Kanamycin, neomycin, and streptomycin in particular increase or prolong skeletal muscle relaxation when administered with a neuromuscular blocker. **Other antibiotics** The polymyxin antibiotics, polymxin B sulfate, colistin, colistimethate sodium; the polypeptide antibiotic capreomycin sulfate; and clindamycin and lincomycin increase or prolong skeletal muscle relaxation when administered with a neuromuscular blocker. **Beta adrenergic drugs** potentiate the effect of neuromuscular blockers and can cause apnea when given to patients coming off neuromuscular blockers. **General anesthetics** Methoxyflurane, enflurane, and isoflurane in particular can cause a neuromuscular blockade that can add to or potentiate the effects of the nondepolarizing blockers. **Lidocaine** in high IV doses, potentiates the effect of neuromuscular blockers and can cause apnea when given to patients coming off neuromuscular blockers. **Opioids** Opiate analgesics add to the respiratory depression caused by the neuromuscular lockers. **Quinidine** potentiates the effect of neuromuscular blockers and can cause apnea when given to patients coming off neuromuscular blockers. **Edrophonium** This cholinomimetic may be used to reverse the neuromuscular blockade of the nondepolarizing neuromuscular blockers.

## ☙ NURSING CONSIDERATIONS

### Side effects, toxicities, and associated nursing actions

**CV** Changes in heart rate, blood pressure, and cardiac output may occur.
- Monitor the blood pressure, pulse, respirations, and respiratory status at frequent, regular intervals.
- Monitor electrocardiogram.

### Nursing interventions related to drug administration

- Neuromuscular blocking agents should only be used in settings where personnel and equipment are available to provide immediate endotracheal intubation of the patient. Have available a suction machine, oxygen, a mechanical ventilator or resuscitation bag, and resuscitation equipment and drugs.
- Note the many drug interactions for the class as a whole and for individual drugs. Patients receiving neuromuscular blocking drugs are often receiving a variety of other drugs and so may have a prolonged response to the neuromuscular blockade agent.
- Administer analgesics at regular intervals if the patient is thought to be in pain, as the patient cannot indicate a need for analgesics. Neuromuscular blocking agents are not anesthetics. Unless patients are also anesthetized, patients can still hear, feel, and, if the eyelids are open, see. Hospital personnel should avoid inappropriate talking within patient earshot and should take care to avoid carelessness in bumping the bed, placing equipment on or near patients in a painful way, or placing bed linens too tight or with wrinkles under the patient. Use radios and televisions judiciously, and not too loud.
- Keep readily available the reversing agent or antagonist for the neuromuscular blocking agent.
- When discontinuing therapy with a neuromuscular blocking agent, do not leave the patient unattended until sufficient muscle tone has returned so that the patient can breathe, handle secretions, and, if not intubated, call for assistance if needed. In infants, assess for the ability to hold the eyelids open or to hold up the legs.
- When administering these drugs via constant infusion, a microdrip tubing set and an infusion controlling device should be used.
- Consult the manufacturer's literature for specific guidelines regarding calculation of dosage. In many institutions, induction with a neuromuscular blocking agent must be done by the anesthesiologist or nurse anesthetist; consult agency policies for guidance.
- A peripheral nerve stimulator may be used to monitor the patient's response to the neuromuscular

blocking drug.
**Patient and family education**
- Review with patients and families the anticipated benefits and possible side effects of drug therapy. These drugs are used only in the acute care setting.
- Keep family members and patients informed of changes in the patient's condition and treatment plan.

## atracurium besylate   (a-tra-KYOOR-ee-um)                    neuromuscular blocker

- atracurium besylate: Tracrium

**MECHANISM OF ACTION**   Atracurium is a nondepolarizing neuromuscular blocker. For further information, see the entry for the drug class (p. 823).

**INDICATIONS**   **Skeletal muscle relaxation** Atracurium is used principally during surgery. • Pulmonary compliance for assisted respiration is also enhanced. • See the entry for the drug class (p. 823) for a fuller explanation of indications for neuromuscular blockers.

**CONTRAINDICATIONS**   • See the entry for the drug class (p. 824) for contraindications of neuromuscular blockers.

**DOSAGE**   **IV:**   **ADULTS:** 0.4 to 0.5 mg/kg initially. Endotracheal intubation can be performed in 2 to 2.5 minutes after administration; maximum relaxation occurs within 5 minutes. Atracurium is administered initially only by rapid IV injection and never by IV infusion or IM. The initial dose is decreased to 0.25 to 0.35 mg/kg if enflurane or isoflurane is to be used. The initial dose is reduced to 0.3 to 0.4 mg/kg if the initial dose of atracurium follows the use of succinylcholine. The maintenance dose during surgery is 0.08 to 0.1 mg/kg, generally given 20 to 45 minutes after the initial dose.   **IV:** **CHILDREN 1 MONTH TO 2 YEARS OF AGE:** 0.3 to 0.4 mg/kg. The adult dosage is used for children older than 2 years of age. More frequent administration of the maintenance dose may be required in children.   *Special patient populations:*   PREGNANCY: Safe use has not been established. Toxicity tests in rabbits established potential teratogenic effects in early pregnancy. FDA pregnancy category C.

**PREPARATIONS**   *Injection (parenteral):* 10 mg/ml in 5 and 10 ml containers. Atracurium besylate should not be mixed in the same syringe nor administered simultaneously through the same needle as an alkaline solution such as bicarbonate.

**DRUG INTERACTIONS**   See the entry for the drug class (p. 824) for drug interactions characteristic of neuromuscular blockers.   **Enflurane and isoflurane** These general anesthetics increase the potency and prolong the duration of neuromuscular blockade by about 35% to 50%.   **Succinylcholine** Prior use of succinylcholine, the depolarizing neuromuscular blocker, reduces the dose of atracurium needed.

**FATE**   The *peak* action is seen 3 to 5 minutes after IV administration. The *duration of action* depends on the dose and the type of anesthesia used, but is generally 20 to 35 minutes. Atracurium is about 80% bound to plasma protein, but the plasma *half-life* is only about 20 minutes. Atracurium is rapidly hydrolyzed by esterases to inactive metabolites that are excreted primarily in the urine. Renal and liver disease have little effect on the fate of atracurium.

## ❦ NURSING CONSIDERATIONS

### Side effects, toxicities, and associated nursing actions
- Clinically important side effects occur in less than 15% of patients.
  **CV** Changes in heart rate, blood pressure, and cardiac output occur occasionally but are minimum and transient.
- See entry for drug class (p. 824).
  **Other** The most frequent side effect (5%) of atracurium is cutaneous histamine release. This usually appears as a skin flush and less frequently as erythema, pruritis, or urticaria
- Be alert to this side effect; it usually requires no treatment.

### Nursing interventions related to drug administration
- See entry for drug class (p. 824).
- The neuromuscular blocking effects of this drug can be reversed with neostigmine, pyridostigmine, or edrophonium, usually given in conjunction with atropine or glycopyrrolate.

**Patient and family education**
- See entry for drug class (p. 825).

---

## gallamine triethiodide    (GAL-a-meen)                    neuromuscular blocker

- gallamine triethiodide: Flaxedil

**MECHANISM OF ACTION**    Gallamine is a nondepolarizing neuromuscular blocker. For further information, see the entry for the drug class (p. 823).

**INDICATIONS**    **Skeletal muscle relaxation** Gallamine is used during surgery. • Pulmonary compliance for assisted respiration is also enhanced. • See the entry for the drug class (p. 823) for more complete information on indications for neuromuscular blockers.

**CONTRAINDICATIONS**    • See the entry for the drug class (p. 824).    **Sensitivity to sulfites** Commercially available formulations of gallamine contain sulfites and may produce adverse reactions in individuals sensitive to sulfites.    **Renal impairment** Since gallamine is excreted unchanged in the urine, patients with significantly impaired renal function cannot excrete the drug and thereby terminate the neuromuscular blockade.    **Shock** Patients in shock have poor circulation and hence poor kidney function. • The remarks for renal impairment above therefore apply.

**DOSAGE**    IV:    ADULTS: Initially, 1 mg/kg is administered as an adjunct to general anesthesia. The total dose administered at one time should not exceed 100 mg. Additional doses of 0.5 to 1.0 mg/kg may be administered at 40-minute intervals as needed. When methoxyflurane is the anesthetic, the doses can be decreased by a third.    IV:    CHILDREN: Infants over 1 month of age and children receive the same dose as adults. Infants under 1 month of age, 0.25 to 0.75 mg/kg initially, then 0.1 to 0.5 mg/kg as needed.    *Special patient populations:* PREGNANCY: Safe use has not been established. FDA pregnancy category C.

**PREPARATIONS**    *Injection (IV use only):* 20 mg/ml. The solution contains sulfite and should not be used for individuals sensitive to sulfites.

**DRUG INTERACTIONS**    See the entry for the drug class (p. 824) for drug interactions characteristic of neuromuscular blockers.    **Enflurane and isoflurane** These general anesthetics increase the potency and prolong the duration of neuromuscular blockade by about 35% to 50%.    **Diazepam** IV diazepam may increase the intensity and duration of the neuromuscular blockade produced by gallamine.

**FATE**    The *peak* effect of gallamine is 3 minutes after administration. The *duration of action* is dose dependent, but is generally 15 to 20 minutes. Gallamine binds to serum albumin, and patients deficient in albumin require lower doses. Gallamine is excreted unchanged in the urine.

### ☙ NURSING CONSIDERATIONS
**Side effects, toxicities, and associated nursing actions**
- See entry for drug class (p. 824).

**Nursing interventions related to drug administration**
- See entry for drug class (p. 824).
- The neuromuscular blocking effects of this drug can be reversed with neostigmine, pyridostigmine, or edrophonium, usually given in conjunction with atropine or glycopyrrolate.

**Patient and family education**
- See entry for drug class (p. 825).

---

## metocurine iodide    (met-oh-KYOO-reen)                    neuromuscular blocker

- metocurine iodide: Metubine Iodide

**MECHANISM OF ACTION**    Metocurine is a nondepolarizing neuromuscular blocker. For further information, see entry for drug class (p. 823).

**INDICATIONS**  **Skeletal muscle relaxation** Metocurine is used during surgery. • Pulmonary compliance for assisted respiration is also enhanced. • For further information, see the entry for the drug class (p. 823) on indications for neuromuscular blockers.

**CONTRAINDICATIONS**  • See the entry for the drug class (p. 824) on contraindications of neuromuscular blockers.   **Renal impairment** Because metocurine is excreted mainly in the urine, patients with poor renal function or in shock should not receive metocurine.

**DOSAGE**  **IV injection over 30 to 60 seconds:**   ADULTS: For endotracheal intubation, 0.2 to 0.4 mg/kg; as an adjunct to general anesthesia, 0.1 to 0.3 mg/kg. Additional doses are generally 0.5 to 1 mg every 30 to 90 minutes as required. When methoxyflurane or fluroxene is the anesthesia, the doses are reduced 33% to 50%. *Special patient populations:* CHILDREN: Metocurine is not used in children. PREGNANCY: Safe use has not been established. FDA pregnancy category C.

**PREPARATIONS**  *Injection (IV):* 2 mg/ml in 20 ml container.

**DRUG INTERACTIONS**  See the entry for the drug class (p. 824) for drug interactions characteristic of neuromuscular blockers.   **Enflurane and isoflurane** These general anesthetics increase the potency and prolong the duration of neuromuscular blockade.

**FATE**  The *onset of action* is achieved in 1 to 4 minutes after IV injection and the *peak* effect 1.5 to 10 minutes. The *duration of action* is 15 to 90 minutes, depending on the dose and general anesthetic used. The plasma *half-life* of the drug is about 3.5 hours. Metocurine is excreted mainly unchanged in the urine.

## ☙ NURSING CONSIDERATIONS

### Side effects, toxicities, and associated nursing actions

**CV** Hypotension secondary to histamine release and ganglionic blockade.

**Other** Histamine release that can cause hypotension or even shock.

• Monitor the blood pressure.

• See entry for drug class (p. 824).

### Nursing interventions related to drug administration

• See entry for drug class (p. 824).

• The neuromuscular blocking effects of this drug can be reversed with neostigmine, pyridostigmine, or edrophonium, usually given in conjunction with atropine or glycopyrrolate.

### Patient and family education

• See entry for drug class (p. 825).

---

## pancuronium bromide   (pan-kyoo-ROE-nee-um)   neuromuscular blocker

• pancuronium bromide: Pavulon

**MECHANISM OF ACTION**  Pancuronium is a nondepolarizing neuromuscular blocker. For further information, see the entry for the drug class (p. 823).

**INDICATIONS**  **Skeletal muscle relaxation** Pancuronium is used during surgery. • Pulmonary compliance for assisted respiration is also enhanced. • See the entry for the drug class (p. 823) on indications for neuromuscular blockers.

**CONTRAINDICATIONS**  • See entry for drug class (p. 824).   **Renal impairment** Because pancuronium is excreted mainly in the urine, patients with poor renal function or in shock should not receive pancuronium.

**DOSAGE**  ADULTS AND CHILDREN OVER 1 MONTH OF AGE: For endotracheal intubation: 0.06 to 0.1 mg/kg; for adjunct to general surgery: 0.04 to 0.1 mg/kg initially, with additional doses of 0.01 mg/kg at 25- to 60-minute intervals. *Special patient populations:* PREGNANCY: Safe use has not been established, but pancuronium may be used during cesarean delivery.

**PREPARATIONS**  *Injection (IV):* 1 mg/ml in a 10 ml container, 2 mg/ml in a 2 or 5 ml container.

**DRUG INTERACTIONS**  See the entry for the drug class (p. 824) for drug interactions characteristic of neuromuscular blockers.   **Enflurane and isoflurane** Use of these anesthetics may decrease the dose of pancuronium needed.    **Succinylcholine** Prior use of succinylcholine, the depolarizing neuromuscular blocker, reduces the dose of pancuronium needed.

**FATE**    The *onset of action* is within 3 minutes, and the *duration of action* is 35 to 45 minutes. The plasma *half-life* is about 2 hours, and the drug is eliminated mainly unchanged by the kidneys.

## ❦ NURSING CONSIDERATIONS

### Side effects, toxicities, and associated nursing actions

**CV** Slight increase in heart rate and blood pressure.
• Monitor blood pressure and pulse.
• See entry for drug class (p. 824).

**Other** Excessive salivation may occur, especially in children, if an anticholinergic drug has not been given.
• Assess airway frequently and carefully.
• Have a suction machine at the bedside.

### Nursing interventions related to drug administration

• See entry for drug class (p. 824).
• The neuromuscular blocking effects of this drug can be reversed with neostigmine, pyridostigmine, or edrophonium, usually given in conjunction with atropine or glycopyrrolate.

### Patient and family education

• See entry for drug class (p. 825).

---

## succinylcholine chloride    (suk-sin-ill-KOE-leen)    neuromuscular blocker

• succinylcholine chloride: Anectine, Quelicin

**MECHANISM OF ACTION**    Succinylcholine is the only clinically used depolarizing neuromuscular blocker. For further information, see the entry for the drug class (p. 823).

**INDICATIONS    Skeletal muscle relaxation of short duration** Succinylcholine is the drug of choice for procedures of short duration (less than 3 minutes) such as endotracheal intubation, endoscopic examinations, electroconvulsive shock therapy, and orthopedic manipulations.

**CONTRAINDICATIONS**    • See entry for drug class (p. 824).    **Electrolyte disturbances** Patients with hyperkalemia or who are digitalized are sensitive to the release of intracelluar potassium characteristic of succinylcholine.    **Fractures or muscle spasms** Because succinylcholine is depolarizing, there is an initial period of muscular contraction and muscle fasciculations before relaxation is achieved. • These may be dangerous in patients with bone fractures.    **Denervated muscles** Denervated muscle is supersensitive to succinylcholine and releases large amounts of potassium that can cause ventricular arrhythmias and/or cardiac arrest. • Patients with denervated muscle include those with recent severe burns, major crush injuries, upper motor neuron lesions from stroke, tumor, spinal cord injury, multiple sclerosis (recent onset), tetanus, or diffuse lower motor neuron disease.

**DOSAGE**    **IV:**    ADULTS: 0.6 mg/kg (range 0.3 to 1.1 mg/kg) is given for short procedures. Administration should take 10 to 30 seconds. A test dose of 0.1 mg/kg may be administered first to the anesthetized patient who is breathing spontaneously. This dose should either not depress respiration or should depress respiration for less than 5 minutes. Individuals who do not metabolize succinylcholine will develop paralysis that persists for up to 60 minutes.    **IV infusion** When prolonged procedures are anticipated, infusion is preferred to intermittent injections, which more readily cause tachyphylaxsis and prolonged apnea. Succinylcholine is compatible with 5% dextrose, 5% dextrose and 0.9% sodium chloride, 0.9% sodium chloride, or 1/6 M sodium lactate. The concentration of succinylcholine for IV infusion is 1 or 2 mg/ml administered at a rate of 2.5 to 7.5 mg/min.    **IV:**    **CHILDREN:** 1 to 2 mg/kg. Neonates generally require 2 mg/kg.    **IM** 2.5 to 4 mg/kg. This route is preferred to continuous IV infusion for prolonged administration of succinylcholine to children. Malignant hyperthermia is a major risk of continuous IV infusion of this drug in children. *Special patient populations:*    **PREG-**

**NANCY:** Safe use has not been established. When succinylcholine must be used, a reduced adult dose is used. FDA pregnancy category C.

**PREPARATIONS**    *Injection (IV):* 20, 50, 100 mg/ml. *Powder (for IV infusion):* 100, 500, 1000 mg.

**DRUG INTERACTIONS**    See the entry for the drug class (p. 824) for drug interactions characteristic of neuromuscular blockers.    **Cholinesterase inhibitors** These inactivate plasma pseudocholinesterase, the enzyme that rapidly degrades succinylcholine. Cholinesterase inhibitors therefore can greatly prolong the action of succinylcholine. This action has even been noted when the irreversible cholinesterase inhibitor was one of the ophthalmic products: echothiophate, isofluorophate, demecarium. Many insecticides are organophosphate cholinesterase inhibitors.    **Procaine** in high concentrations can inhibit the hydrolysis of succinylcholine.

**FATE**    The *onset of action* is within 1 minute, and the *duration of action* is generally less than 10 minutes following administration of usual doses. Succinylcholine is rapidly hydrolyzed to an inactive form by a pseudocholinesterase in the plasma.

### 🐦 NURSING CONSIDERATIONS

#### Side effects, toxicities, and associated nursing actions

**CV** Bradycardia with hypotension and cardiac arrhythmias may result from vagal stimulation after administration of succinylcholine.

- Monitor blood pressure and pulse.
- See entry for drug class (p. 824).

**Eye** Transient increase in intraocular pressure that is too transient to be dangerous in the intact eye.
**Respiratory** Transient apnea is common. Oxygen should always be available for controlled respiration.
**Other** Muscle fasciculations may leave the patient sore on recovery.

- Reassure patients after procedures that this soreness is probably due to the drug.
- See entry for drug class (p. 824).

#### Nursing interventions related to drug administration

- See entry for drug class (p. 824).
- The neuromuscular blocking effects of this drug can be reversed with neostigmine, pyridostigmine, or edrophonium, usually given in conjuction with atropine or glycopyrrolate.

#### Patient and family education

- See entry for drug class (p. 824).

---

## tubocurarine chloride (curare)    (too-boe-kyoo-RAR-een) neuromuscular blocker

- tubocurarine chloride (curare): Tubocurarine Chloride, ♣Tubarine

**MECHANISM OF ACTION**    Tubocurarine is a nondepolarizing neuromuscular blocker. For further information, see the entry for the drug class (p. 808).

**INDICATIONS**    **Skeletal muscle relaxation** Tubocurarine is used during surgery of moderate or long duration.    • Pulmonary compliance for assisted respiration is also enhanced. • See the entry for the drug class (p. 823) on indications for neuromuscular blockers.    **Tetanus** Tubocurarine can reduce the muscle spasms of severe tetanus.    **Myasthenia gravis** Tubocurarine is sometimes used as a diagnostic tool.

**CONTRAINDICATIONS**    • See entry for drug class (p. 824).    **Histamine release** Since tubocurarine may cause histamine release, patients for whom histamine release is hazardous should not receive tubocurarine.

**DOSAGE**    **IV:    ADULTS AND CHILDREN:** As an adjunct to anesthesia, the initial dose is 0.2 to 0.5 mg/kg; supplemental doses are 0.04 to 0.1 mg/kg.    **IV:    INFANTS TO 1 MONTH OF AGE:** 0.3 mg/kg initially, with subsequent doses of 0.1 mg/kg.    *Special patient populations:*    **PREGNANCY:** Tubocurarine does not readily cross the placenta and may be used for obstetrical surgery. Large, continuous doses may paralyze a fetus. FDA pregancy category C.

**PREPARATIONS**    *Injection (IV):* 3 mg/ml. Do not use if the solution is discolored. Tubocurarine chloride injection should not be mixed with a barbiturate injection because the barbiturate may precipitate.

**DRUG INTERACTIONS**    See the entry for the drug class (p. 824) for drug interactions characteristic of neuro-muscular blocker.    **Enflurane and isoflurane** Use of these anesthetics will decrease the dose of tubocurarine needed by 33% to 50%.

**FATE**    The *peak* action is seen 2 to 5 minutes after IV administration and persists for 25 to 90 minutes. Tubocurarine is excreted unchanged in the urine.

### ☙ NURSING CONSIDERATIONS

#### Side effects, toxicities, and associated nursing actions

**CV** Hypotension, secondary to histamine release and ganglionic blockade.
- Monitor the blood pressure
- See entry for drug class (p. 824).

#### Nursing interventions related to drug administration
- See entry for drug class (p. 824).
- The neuromuscular blocking effects of this drug can be reversed with neostigmine, pyridostigmine, or edrophonium, usually given in conjunction with atropine or glycopyrrolate.

#### Patient and family education
- See entry for drug class (p. 824).

---

# vecuronium bromide    (vek-yoo-ROE-nee-um)    neuromuscular blocker

- vecuronium bromide: Norcuron

**MECHANISM OF ACTION**    Vecuronium is a nondepolarizing neuromuscular blocker. This new agent does not produce significant ganglionic or vagal blockade nor interfere with the uptake of norepinephrine nor cause histamine release as do older agents. For further information, see the entry for the drug class (p. 823).

**INDICATIONS**    **Skeletal muscle relaxation** Vecuronium may used for endotracheal intubation and during surgery. Pulmonary compliance for assisted respiration is also enhanced. See the entry for the drug class (p. 823) on indications for neuromuscular blockers.

**CONTRAINDICATIONS**    • See entry for drug class (p. 824).

**DOSAGE**    **IV:**    **ADULTS:** Initial intubating dose: 0.08 to 0.1 mg/kg; subsequent doses are 0.01 to 0.015 mg/kg as needed. If succinylcholine is used first, the subsequent doses of vecuronium are 0.04 to 0.06 mg/kg.    **IV:**    **CHILDREN (1 TO 10 YEARS OF AGE):** Slightly higher initial doses are used than for adults.    **IV:**    **CHILDREN (7 WEEKS TO 1 YEAR OF AGE):** Children in this age goup are more sensitive to vecuronium than adults and have a recovery time up to 50% longer.    *Special patient populations:*    **PREGNANCY:** Safe use has not been established. FDA pregnancy category C.

**PREPARATIONS**    *Powder:* 10 mg for dilution to 5 ml.

**DRUG INTERACTIONS**    See the entry for the drug class (p. 824) for drug interactions characteristic of neuro-muscular blockers.    **Enflurane and isoflurane** Use of these anesthetics will decrease the dose of vecuronium needed by 33% to 50%.    **Succinylcholine** Prior use increases the potency and prolongs the duration of neuromuscular blockade.

**FATE**    The *onset of action* is generally about 1 minute and maximum at 3 to 5 minutes. The *duration of action* is 20 to 40 minutes depending on the anesthetic used and whether succinylcholine was administered. Vecuronium is excreted mainly in the bile and appears in the feces, so vecuronium can be used for patients with impaired kidney function.

### ☙ NURSING CONSIDERATIONS

#### Side effects, toxicities, and associated nursing actions

These are infrequent with vecuronium as compared to other neuromuscular blockers. This new agent does not produce significant ganglionic or vagal blockade nor interfere with the uptake of norepinephrine nor cause histamine release as do older agents.

**Nursing interventions related to drug administration**
- See entry for drug class (p. 824).
- The neuromuscular blocking effects of this drug can be reversed with neostigmine, pyridostigmine, or edrophonium, usually given in conjunction with atropine or glycopyrrolate.

**Patient and family education**
- See entry for drug class (p. 825).

# DRUGS FOR SEVERE PAIN AND ANESTHESIA

**INTRODUCTION**   This unit presents drugs that block the patient's perception of severe pain. Narcotic analgesics have the ability to render the individual unreactive to pain even though the individual is conscious and the source of pain has not been removed. The antagonists block the actions of the narcotic analgesics.

Anesthetic agents may have systemic or local action. The general anesthetics render the patient unconscious and allow modern surgical procedures to be carried out. The intravenous anesthetic agents are used in the induction of anesthesia or sometimes alone for short procedures. The local anesthetics are used for topical anesthesia or infiltrated around nerves to provide regional anesthesia.

XII

# Chapter Forty-five

# Narcotic analgesics and antagonists

| Narcotic analgesics | methadone |
| --- | --- |
| alfentanil | morphine |
| alphaprodine | nalbuphine |
| buprenorphine | oxycodone |
| butorphanol | oxymorphone |
| codeine | pentazocine |
| fentanyl | propoxyphene |
| hydrocodone | sufentanil |
| hydromorphone | |
| levorphanol | **Narcotic antagonists** |
| meperidine (❋petnidine) | naloxone |
| | naltrexone |

**INTRODUCTION**   Opium has been used to produce analgesia and euphoria throughout the history of human-kind. Opium is the sticky brown gum collected from a type of poppy, and about 10% of the gum is morphine. Even today morphine remains the prototype of the narcotic analgesics. Chemically, drugs produced by modification of morphine or synthetic drugs with morphinelike activity are called *opioids*. More familiarly, the opioids are called narcotic analgesics. The term *narcotic* is derived from the Greek word meaning stupor or insensibility. The chief characteristic of the opioids is their ability to render the individual unreactive to pain even though the individual is conscious and the source of pain has not been removed.

All opioids have abuse potential to a greater or lesser degree and most are covered by the Controlled Substance Act.

## Narcotic analgesics

alfentanil ~ alphaprodine ~ buprenorphine ~ butorphanol ~ codeine ~ pentanyl ~ hydrocodone ~ hydromorphone ~ levorphanol ~ meperidine ~ methadone ~ morphine ~ nalbuphine ~ oxycodone ~ oxymorphone ~ pentazocine ~ propoxyphene ~ sufentanil

**DRUG COMBINATIONS**   Narcotic analgesics (opioids) are commonly combined with nonnarcotic analgesics, especially aspirin and acetaminophen. These combinations are listed in Table 47-1 (p. 867).

**OVERVIEW OF THE DRUG CLASS**   The pharmacology of morphine provides the standard for comparing the actions of opioids. Three will be summarized: actions in the CNS, actions in the periphery, and drug tolerance and dependence.   **Actions in the central nervous system**   ANALGESIA: The analgesia produced by morphine has three characteristics. First, morphine raises the threshold for pain perception at the level of the spinal cord and higher CNS centers, making the individual less aware of pain. Second, morphine reduces anxiety and fear, which are the emotional reactions to pain. Third, morphine induces sleep even in the presence of severe pain.   **MEDULLARY ACTIONS:** Morphine makes the respiratory center less sensitive to carbon dioxide, so that death from overdose of morphine is frequently respiratory arrest. Secondly, morphine depresses the cough center, and several cough suppressants are opioid derivatives. Third, morphine stimulates the chemoreceptor trigger zone, resulting in nausea and vomiting.   **BEHAVIOR:** The effect of morphine depends on the mental state of the individual. The person who has experienced pain, fear, or anxiety may experience euphoria. Larger doses can cause drowsiness or sleep. A few individuals become excited.   **Actions in the periphery:**   GASTROINTESTINAL TRACT: Morphine has a profound depressant effect on the gastrointestinal tract. Constipation is a common side effect. Some related opioids are used to treat nonspecific diarrhea.   SECRETIONS: Gastric, biliary, and pancreatic secretions are inhibited by morphine.   URINARY RETENTION: Morphine stimulates the release of vasopression (antidiuretic hormone), so that more water is absorbed in the kidney tubules, decreasing urine volume. Morphine also reduces perception of the need for voiding.   CARDIOVASCULAR EFFECTS: Morphine commonly causes hypotension. Morphine causes histamine release, and histamine is a potent vasodilator. In high doses, morphine slows the heart rate. **OCULAR EFFECT**: A classic effect of morphine is to reduce pupillary size. A pinpoint pupil is one characteristic of a narcotic overdose, however, if the victim is near death, hypoxia causes the release of epinephrine, which dilates the pupil. **Tolerance and dependence** **TOLERANCE**: Tolerance develops morphine's euphoric and respiratory depression effects. Daily use of one of the opioids can produce drug dependence in 3 weeks. Little or no tolerance develops to the pupillary constriction or to the constipating effect of the opioids. **DEPENDENCE**: A drug-dependent person will experience distinct physical reactions if the drug is suddenly discontinued; these reactions make up the abstinence syndrome. The opiate abstinence syndrome consists of a runny nose, goose flesh, tearing, sweating, and yawning 16 hours after the last dose. The pupils do not react readily to light. Over the next 20 hours, the individual becomes restless, cannot sleep, and experiences muscle twitching. Hot and cold flashes and abdominal cramping occur. By 36 hours, the individual feels nauseous, vomits, and has diarrhea. These reactions are generally the reverse of the drug effects. The body overcompensates when the drug is removed.

**MECHANISM OF ACTION** In the 1970s specific receptors for morphinelike drugs were identified. This finding led to the discovery of *endorphins,* named for endogenous morphinelike substances. All endorphins are polypeptides and are found in those specific locations long associated with the action of morphine and in which opiate receptors can be identified: the brain, spinal cord, and gut.

The smallest of the endorphins are the enkephalins. The enkephalins consist of five amino acids and seem to be neurotransmitters associated with (1) the mediation of pain and analgesia; (2) the release of growth hormone, prolactin, and vasopressin from the pituitary; (3) the modulation of locomotor activity; (4) the regulation of mood; and (5) the regulation of gut motility.

The actions of opioid drugs have been associated with three types of opiate receptors. The mu receptor mediates central analgesia, euphoria, respiratory depression, and physical dependence. These are the classic morphine effects. The kappa receptor mediates spinal analgesia, miosis, sedation, and appetite regulation. The receptor appears sensitive to opioids with mixed agonist-antagonist receptors. The sigma receptor mediates the dysphoric, hallucinogenic, and cardiac stimulant effects. The receptor appears sensitive to opioid antagonist activity. The opioid drugs vary in their spectrum of activity at these three types of sites. Morphinelike opioids are agonists for the mu and kappa receptors. Other opioids have only partial agonist activity at the mu and kappa receptors, and some are antagonists of the mu receptor. The complex spectrum of receptor activities therefore determines the characteristic action of each opioid.

**INDICATIONS** **Analgesia** Opioids vary in the degree of pain relieved. Table 45-1 summarizes the opioids used for analgesia with respect to the degree of pain for which they are prescribed, the equivalent analgesic dose, the time for peak effect, the duration of analgesia, and the U. S. schedule classification (C) under which each falls as a controlled substance. In Canada, opioids are Schedule G drugs (controlled).

**CONTRAINDICATIONS** **Pulmonary edema** caused by a chemical irritant (because of the respiratory depression.) Opiates, however, cause pooling of blood in the extremities by decreasing peripheral resistance, and this can relieve pulmonary edema secondary to acute left ventricular heart failure.

**DRUG INTERACTIONS** **CNS depressants** Opioids potentiate the effects of other CNS depressants, including other opioids, general anesthetics, tranquilizers, sedatives and hypnotics, alcohol, tricyclic antidepressants, and monoamine oxidase inhibitors. **Phenothiazines** may antagonize the analgesic effect of opioids. **Skeletal muscle relaxants** Opioids may enhance the neuromuscular blocking action.

## ☙ NURSING CONSIDERATIONS
### Side effects, toxicities, and associated nursing actions

**CNS** Respiratory depression; dizziness, mental clouding, sedation; rarely, agitation, restlessness, delirium, and insomnia.

- Monitor respiratory rate as an indicator of CNS depression. If the rate is less than 12 per minute in an adult, withhold additional doses unless ventilatory support is being provided.
- Auscultate breath sounds every 2 to 4 hours. Since narcotic analgesics suppress the cough reflex, it is especially important to have patients turn, cough, and breathe deeply every 2 hours.
- Narcotic antagonists, oxygen, and resuscitation equipment should be readily available in settings

| Table 45-1. | Comparison of the narcotic analgesics | | | | |
|---|---|---|---|---|---|
| **Level of pain** | **Drug** | **Equivalent analgesic dose (mg) given IM or SC** | **Time for peak effect (min)** | **Duration (hr)** | **Schedule\*** |
| Severe | Morphine | 10 | 30 to 90 | 3 to 7 | II |
| | Buprenorphine (Buprenex) | 0.5 | 45 | 4 to 6 | V |
| | Hydromorphone hydrochloride (Dilaudid) | 1.5 | 30 to 90 | 4 to 5 | II |
| | Levorphanol tartrate (Levo-Dromoran) | 2 to 3 | 60 to 90 | 5 to 8 | II |
| | Methadone (Dolophine) | 7.5 to 10 | 60 to 120 | 3 to 6 | II |
| | Oxymorphone (Numorphan) | 1 to 1.5 | 30 to 90 | 3 to 6 | II |
| Moderate to severe | Alphaprodine (Nisentil) | 40 to 60 | 30 | 1 to 2 | II |
| | Butorphanol (Stadol) | 1.5 to 3.5 | 30 | 3 to 4 | N.S. |
| | Meperidine (Demerol) | 75 to 100 | 30 to 60 | 2 to 4 | II |
| | Nalbuphine (Nubain) | 10 | 30 | 3 to 6 | N.S. |
| | Pentazocine (Talwin) | 40 to 60 | 30 to 60 | 2 to 3 | IV |
| Mild to moderate | Codeine phosphate | 120 | 60 to 90 | 4 to 6 | II |
| | Propoxyphene (Darvon) | 180 to 240 | 60 | 4 to 6 | IV |

*These are the U. S. schedules. In Canada, narcotic analgesics are Schedule G (controlled drugs).

where narcotic analgesics are administered.
- Monitor level of consciousness and mental status. Evaluate findings carefully. For example, restlessness may be due to pain, hypoxia, shock, or an unusual reaction to the analgesic.
- Keep side rails up, keep a nightlight on, supervise ambulation, and discourage smoking.
- If insomnia is present, a switch to another analgesic agent may be advised; consult with the physician.

**CV** Flushing, bradycardia.
- Monitor pulse. If bradycardia develops (pulse below 60 in adults or 110 in infants), withhold the dose and notify the physician.
- Monitor blood pressure. Hypotension is more common in the elderly, the immobilized, and in patients receiving other medications that have hypotension as a side effect. It may also be a sign of sepsis or shock.

**Eye** Visual disturbances, miosis.
- Monitor pupillary response to light. The presence of pupillary constriction may indicate narcotic use, when the patient is unable or unwilling to discuss drug use.
- Caution patients to report to the physician the development of visual changes.

**GI** Nausea, vomiting, and constipation.
- Monitor intake, output, and weight.
- If nausea and vomiting occur, a switch to another analgesic may be appropriate; consult with the physician.
- If nausea occurs, it may be appropriate to administer an antiemetic concomitantly with the narcotic. Note that the peak effect of many antiemetics occurs at a different time than that of the narcotic, so often the drugs should be on a different dosing schedule. Also, antiemetics may potentiate central nervous system depression but do not potentiate analgesic effects. Sedation and hypotension may be pronounced.
- Constipation may be severe. Increase fluid intake to 2500 to 3000 ml/day; increase dietary intake of fruit, fruit juices, and fiber; increase level of exercise. The use of stool softeners may be necessary.

**GU** Urinary retention.
- Monitor intake and output.
- Have the patient void before administering the next dose.
- Urinary retention may be more pronounced in the elderly, the immobilized, and men with preexisting prostatic hypertrophy. Question patients about difficulty in voiding, pain in the bladder area, or sensations of inadequate bladder emptying when narcotic analgesics are being used. Palpate bladder for distention.
- If urinary retention is a problem, have patients void prior to receiving dose of analgesic.

### Nursing interventions related to drug administration

- Analgesics, especially narcotic analgesics, constitute one of the most useful classes of medications, as they permit individuals to tolerate short-and-long-term pain, and thus tolerate surgery and trauma and perhaps to face death more peacefully. Failure of health care team members to be knowledgeable about adequate drug doses, frequency of drug administration, and choice of appropriate medication, as well as fear of causing addiction result in patients receiving inadequate pharmacologic treatment of pain. Thoughtful, individualized patient assessment should always be done prior to administering pain medication. If the decision is made to administer a medication, adequate doses should be used, and the medication or medications should be administered frequently enough to maintain a therapeutic blood level of the medication. Finally, the use of a narcotic is often enhanced by the concomitant use of aspirin or acetaminophen; consult the physician.
- Nursing measures that may help relieve pain should be included in the plan of care. These include massage, distraction, deep breathing or relaxation exercises, application of heat or cold, or just being there to provide care and comfort to the patient.
- Check the physician's orders carefully. Observe agency policy regarding the expiration date of narcotic medication orders.
- Record the patient's response to pain and the response to narcotic administration.
- Taking oral doses with a snack or milk may lessen gastric irritation.
- Use anatomic landmarks to choose injection sites. Aspirate prior to injecting dose to avoid inadvertent intravenous administration. Record injection sites and rotate sites.
- For constant infusion, microdrip tubing and an infusion monitoring device should be used.

### Patient and family education

- Review the anticipated benefits and possible side effects of therapy with patients and families. Caution patients to report the development of any unexpected sign or symptom.
- Teaching the patient about narcotic analgesics in preparation for discharge to home must be individualized. Review with patient or family the dose, frequency of administration, route of administration, and under what circumstances the physician should be contacted.
- If a combination drug product has been prescribed, review with patients the side effects associated with each of the drugs in the combined product.
- Caution patients to avoid the use of alcohol.
- Caution patients to avoid the use of other medications that also may cause central nervous system depression, such as barbiturates, antiemetics, antihistamines, or tranquilizers, unless first approved by the physician.
- Caution patients to keep these and all medications out of the reach of children. Accidental overdose with narcotic analgesics in a child may quickly lead to death.

---

## alfentanil hydrochloride   (al-FEN-ta-nil)                narcotic analgesic

- alfentanil hydrochloride: Alfenta (C-II)

**MECHANISM OF ACTION**   Alfentanil is a narcotic analgesic with opiate agonist activity. See entry for drug class for more complete information (p. 835).

**INDICATIONS**   **Analgesia** Used as an adjunct for anesthesia to induce and maintain general analgesia.

**CONTRAINDICATIONS**   • Hypersensitivity. • Head injury.

**DOSAGE** IV: ADULTS: For induction of anesthesia, the dose is 130 μg/mg. Administer as a bolus infusion over a 3 minute period if procedure is to last under 30 minutes. Administer as a continuous infusion if the procedure is to last more than 45 minutes. *Special patient populations;* ELDERLY: Dose should be decreased by 40% CHILDREN: Not tested in children under 12 years old. PREGNANCY: Safe use has not been established. FDA pregnancy category C.

**PREPARATIONS** *Injections:* 500 μg/ml.

**DRUG INTERACTIONS** **CNS depressants** CNS depressants (barbiturates, benzodiazepines, opioids, general anesthetics) give additive CNS depression. The dose of an inhalation anesthetic should be reduce 30% to 50%.

**FATE** Rapid *onset of action*. Respiratory depression action outlasts the analgesic action.

### ☙ NURSING CONSIDERATIONS

#### Side effects, toxicities, and associated nursing actions

**CV** Bradycardia or tachycardia; hypotension or hypertension.
- Monitor blood pressure and pulse.
- Supervise ambulation; keep side rails up. Instruct patients to move slowly from lying to sitting or standing positions if hypotension develops.
- If bradycardia develops (pulse below 60 beats per minute in adults or 110 in infants), withhold the dose and notify the physician.

**GI** Nausea and vomiting.
- Monitor intake, output, and weight.
- If nausea and vomiting occur, switching to another analgesic may be appropriate; consult with the physician.
- If nausea occurs, it may be appropriate to administer an antiemetic concomitantly with the narcotic. Note that the peak effect of many antiemetics occurs at a different time than that of the narcotic, so often the two drugs should be on different dosing schedules. Also, antiemetics may potentiate central nervous system depression but do not potentiate analgesic effects. Sedation and hypotension may be pronounced.

**Respiratory** Apnea.
- Monitor the respiratory rate. If the rate is less than 12 in an adult, withhold additional doses unless ventilatory support is being provided.
- Auscultate breath sounds every 2 to 4 hours. Since narcotic analgesics suppress the cough reflex, it is especially important to have patients turn, cough, and breathe deeply every 2 hours.

**Other** Muscular rigidity is common.
- Assess range of motion. If muscular rigidity is developing, notify the physician.

#### Nursing interventions related to drug administration
- See entry for drug class (p. 837).

#### Patient and family education
- See entry for drug class (p. 837).

---

## alphaprodine hydrochloride   (al-fa-PROE-deen)   narcotic analgesic

- alphaprodine hydrochloride: Nisentil (C-II)

**MECHANISM OF ACTION** Alphaprodine is a narcotic analgesic with opiate agonist activity. See the entry for drug class for more complete information (p. 835).

**INDICATIONS** **Analgesia** For moderate to severe acute pain. Uses include alleviation of pain and anxiety as preoperative medication, for urologic examination, labor, and dental procedures.

**CONTRAINDICATIONS** • Respiratory depression.

**DOSAGE** IV: ADULTS: 0.4 to 0.6 mg/kg. For urologic procedures, 20 to 30 mg. Prior to major surgery, 10 to 20 mg; minor surgery, 20 mg. SC: ADULTS: 0.4 to 1.2 mg/kg. Prior to major surgery, 20 to 40 mg; minor surgery, 40 mg; labor, 40 to 60 mg after cervical dilation has begun. Repeat as necessary at 2 hour intervals.    **Submucosal:**    CHILDREN: For dental procedures: 0.3 to 0.6 mg/kg.    *Special patient populations:*    CHILDREN: Not recommended for children under 12 years old except for dental procedures.    PREGNANCY: Used during labor after cervical dilation has begun. Safety for other use during pregnancy has not been established.

**PREPARATIONS**    *Injection:* 40 or 60 mg/ml.

**DRUG INTERACTIONS**    **CNS depressants** Opioids potentiate the effects of other CNS depressants, including other opioids, general anesthetics, tranquilizers, sedatives and hypnotics, alcohol, tricyclic antidepressants, and monoamine oxidase inhibitors.    **Phenothiazines** may antagonize the analgesic effect of opioids.    **Skeletal muscle relaxants** Opioids may enhance neuromuscular blocking action.

**FATE**    Alphaprodine has a more rapid onset and a shorter duration of action than meperidine. *Onset of action* is 5 to 10 minutes after SC and 1 to 2 minutes after IV administration. *Duration of action* is 1 to 2 hours after SC and 0.5 to 1.5 hours after IV administration. Alphaprodine is metabolized in the liver and excreted in the urine.

### ☙ NURSING CONSIDERATIONS

#### Side effects, toxicities, and associated nursing actions
- See entry for drug class (p. 835)

#### Nursing interventions related to drug administration
- Alphaprodine should *not* be administered via the IM route.
- For direct IV infusion, dilute dose with 5 to 10 ml of sterile water for injection. Administer at a rate of 20 mg or less over 1 minute.
- See entry for drug class (p. 837).

#### Patient and family education
- See entry for drug class (p. 837).

---

## buprenorphine hydrochloride    (byoo-pren-OR-feen)    narcotic analgesic

- buprenorphine hydrochloride: Buprenex (C-V)

**MECHANISM OF ACTION**    Buprenorphine is a narcotic analgesic with mixed agonist-antagonist activity. See entry for drug class for more complete information (p. 835).

**INDICATIONS**    **Analgesia** Buprenorphine is a new drug in the United States. Effective for moderate to severe pain associated with surgery, cancer, neuralgias, labor, renal colic, or myocardial infarction.

**CONTRAINDICATIONS**    • Respiratory depression.

**DOSAGE**    IM    ADULTS: 0.3 to 0.6 mg, every 6 to 8 hours as needed.    *Special patient populations:*    PREGNANCY: Safe use has not been established (FDA pregnancy category C).

**PREPARATIONS**    *Injection:* 0.3 mg/ml.

**DRUG INTERACTIONS**    **CNS depressants** Opioids potentiate the effects of other CNS depressants, including other opioids, general anesthetics, tranquilizers, sedatives and hypnotics, alcohol, tricyclic antidepressants, and monoamine oxidase inhibitors.    **Phenothiazines** may antagonize the analgesic effect of opioids.    **Skeletal muscle relaxants** Opioids may enhance the neuromuscular blocking action.

**FATE**    *Onset of action* is 15 to 45 minutes; *duration of action* is 6 to 8 hours. Buprenophine is excreted unchanged in the feces.

### ☙ NURSING CONSIDERATIONS

#### Side effects, toxicities, and associated nursing actions
- See entry for drug class (p. 834).

#### Nursing interventions related to drug administration
- See entry for drug class (p. 836).

#### Patient and family education
- See entry for drug class (p. 836).

## butorphanol tartrate (byoo-TOR-fa-nole) narcotic analgesic

- butorphanol tartrate: Stadol

**MECHANISM OF ACTION** Butorphanol is a narcotic analgesic with opiate agonist activity. See entry for drug class for more complete information (p. 835).

**INDICATIONS** **Analgesia** For moderate to severe pain, including cancer, neuropathic, spastic conditions, opthopedic, burns, surgery, and renal colic. Butorphanol is a new drug that has not been placed on the Controlled Substances Schedule.

**CONTRAINDICATIONS** • Respiratory depression.

**DOSAGE** IM: ADULTS: 1 to 4 mg every 3 to 4 hours as needed. The usual initial dose is 2 mg. IV: ADULTS: 0.5 to 2 mg every 3 to 4 hours as needed. The usual initial dose is 1 mg. *Special patient populations:* CHILDREN: Not recommended for children under 18 years old. PREGNANCY: Safe use has not been established. Animal tests have not shown adverse effects on the fetus.

**PREPARATIONS** *Injection:* 1 or 2 mg/ml.

**DRUG INTERACTIONS** **CNS Depressants** Opioids potentiate the effects of other CNS depressants, including other opioids, general anesthetics, tranquilizers, sedatives and hypnotics, alcohol, tricyclic antidepressants, and monoamine oxidase inhibitors. **Phenothiazines** may antagonize the analgesic effect of opioids. **Skeletal muscle relaxants** Opioids may enhance the neuromuscular blocking action.

**FATE** The onset and duration of action depend on the route of administration. After IM administration, the *onset of action* is 10 t0 30 minutes, and the *duration of action* is 3 to 4 hours. Maximum analgesia occurs after 30 to 60 minutes. After IV administration, the *onset of action* is 1 minute, and the *duration of action* is 2 to 4 hours. *Peak* analgesia occurs within 5 minutes. Butorphanol is metabolized in the liver and excreted in the urine.

### NURSING CONSIDERATIONS

**Side effects, toxicities, and associated nursing actions** Respiratory depression is not as common with butorphanol as with morphine.

- See entry for drug class (p. 835).

**Nursing interventions related to drug administration**

- For direct IV infusion, the drug may be given undiluted. Administer at a rate of 2 mg or less over 3 to 5 minutes.
- See entry for drug class (p. 837).

**Patient and family education**

- See entry for drug class (p. 837).

## codeine (KOE-deen) narcotic analgesic

- codeine (codeine phosphate, codeine sulfate): Generic, ♣Paveral (C-II)

**MECHANISM OF ACTION** Codeine is a narcotic analgesic with opiate agonist activity. See entry for drug class for more complete information (p. 835).

**INDICATIONS** **Analgesia** Codeine is used for mild to moderate pain. Codeine is commonly combined with aspirin or acetaminophen (see drug list). **Coughing** Codeine is a good antitussive.

**CONTRAINDICATIONS** • Respiratory depression.

**DOSAGE** PO, SC, IM: ADULTS: 30 mg every 4 hours as needed. Dose can range from 15 to 60 mg. CHILDREN: 3 mg/kg or 100 mg/$M^2$ daily in six divided doses. *Special patient populations:* PREGNANCY: Safe use has not been established (FDA pregnancy category C).

**PREPARATIONS** *Codeine phosphate, solution (oral):* 15 mg/5 ml, *tablets:* 15, 30, or 60 mg; *injection:* 15, 30, or 60 mg/ml. *Codeine sulfate, tablets:* 15, 30, or 60 mg.

**DRUG INTERACTIONS** **CNS depressants** Opioids potentiate the effects of other CNS depressants, including other opioids, general anesthetics, tranquilizers, sedatives and hypnotics, alcohol, tricyclic antidepressants, and monoamine oxidase inhibitors. **Phenothiazines** may antagonize the analgesic effect of opioids. **Skeletal muscle relaxants** Opioids may enhance neuromuscular blocking action.

**FATE**  Codeine is well absorbed orally. The *onset of action* is 15 to 30 minutes, and the *duration of action* is 4 to 6 hours. Codeine is metabolized in the liver and excreted in the urine.

## 🦫 NURSING CONSIDERATIONS

### Side effects, toxicities, and associated nursing actions
- See entry for drug class (p. 835).

### Nursing interventions related to drug administration
- Codeine is not administered intravenously.
- See entry for drug class (p. 837).

### Patient and family education
- See entry for drug class (p. 837).

---

## fentanyl citrate   (FEN-ta-nil)                    narcotic analgesic

- fentanyl citrate: Sublimaze (C-II)

**MECHANISM OF ACTION**  Fentanyl is a narcotic analgesic with opiate agonist activity. See entry for drug class for more complete information (p. 835).

**INDICATIONS**  **Analgesia** Used before, during, and after surgery. Supplements general or regional anesthesia. **Neuroleptanalgesia** The combination of fentanyl and droperidol is administered to provide anesthesia.

**CONTRAINDICATIONS**  • Myasthenia gravis. • Patients who have received MAO (monoamine oxidase) inhibitors within the previous 14 days.

**DOSAGE**  **IM:** **ADULTS:** Preoperatively, 50 to 100 μg 30 to 60 minutes before surgery. As an adjunct to regional anesthesia; 50 to 100 μg. Postoperative pain, 50 to 100 μg every 1 to 2 hours as needed.  **IV:** **ADULTS:** Adjunct to general surgery. Low dose (minor surgical procedures), 2 μg/kg; moderate dose (major surgical procedures), 2 to 20 μg/kg; high dose (open heart, neurologic, orthopedic surgery), 20 to 50 μg/kg.  **CHILDREN 2 TO 12 YEARS OLD:** 1.7 to 3.3 μg/kg as an adjunct to general surgery. *Special patient populations:*  **ELDERLY:** Reduced doses are required for geriatric patients.  **CHILDREN:** Not recommended for children under 2 years old.  **PREGNANCY:** Safe use has not been established.

**PREPARATIONS**  *Injection:* 50 μg/ml.

**DRUG INTERACTIONS**  **CNS depressants** Opioids potentiate the effects of other CNS depressants, including other opioids, general anesthetics, tranquilizers, sedatives and hypnotics, alcohol, tricyclic antidepressants, and monoamine oxidase inhibitors.  **Phenothiazines** may antagonize the analgesic effect of opioids.  **Skeletal muscle relaxants** Opioids may enhance neuromuscular blocking action.

**FATE**  After IV injection, the *onset of action* is a few minutes; the *duration of action* is 30 to 60 minutes. After IM injection, the *onset of action* is within 15 minutes; the *duration of action* is 1 to 2 hours. Fentanyl is metabolized in the liver and excreted in the urine.

## 🦫 NURSING CONSIDERATIONS

### Side effects, toxicities, and associated nursing actions
- See entry for drug class (p. 835).

### Nursing interventions related to drug administration
- For direct IV infusion, may be given undiluted. Administer dose over 2 to 3 minutes.
- See entry for drug class (p. 837).

### Patient and family education
- See entry for drug class (p. 837).

---

## hydrocodone bitartrate   (hye-droe-KOE-done)                    narcotic analgesic

- hydrocodone bitartrate: ✣Hycodan, ✣Robidone (C-III)

**MECHANISM OF ACTION**  Hydrocodone is a narcotic analgesic with opiate agonist activity. See entry for drug class for more complete information (p. 835).

**INDICATIONS** **Analgesia** Moderate to moderately severe pain. Hydrocodone is marketed only in combination with the nonnarcotic analgesics, aspirin, or acetaminophen (see drug list). **Coughing** Hydrocodone is an effective antitussive agent.

**CONTRAINDICATIONS** • Respiratory depression.

**DOSAGE** **PO:** **ADULTS:** Fixed combination with aspirin or acetaminophen only. The usual dose contains 5 to 10 mg hydrocodone and is administered every 4 to 6 hours as needed. *Special patient populations:* **CHILDREN:** Not recommended for children. **PREGNANCY:** Safe use has not been established (FDA pregnancy category C).

**PREPARATIONS** See drug list for combinations (Table 47-1, p. 867). These combinations contain 5 mg of hydrocodone bitartrate.

**DRUG INTERACTIONS** **CNS depressants** Opioids potentiate the effects of other CNS depressants, including other opioids, general anesthetics, tranquilizers, sedatives and hypnotics, alcohol, tricyclic antidepressants, and monoamine oxidase inhibitors. **Phenothiazines** may antagonize the analgesic effect of opioids. **Skeletal muscle relaxants** Opioids may enhance neuromuscular blocking action.

**FATE** Hydrocodone is metabolized in the liver and excreted in the urine. The *duration of action* is 4 to 8 hours.

**🐝 NURSING CONSIDERATIONS**

**Side effects, toxicities, and associated nursing actions**
• See entry for drug class (p. 835).

**Nursing interventions related to drug administration** Anodynos-DHC brand tablets containing hydrocodone 5 mg, acetaminophen 150 mg, aspirin 230 mg, and caffeine 30 mg contain FD & C yellow dye # 5 (tartrazine), which may cause an allergic reaction in susceptible individuals. Although rare, this response is seen more frequently in persons with aspirin hypersensitivity.
• See entry for drug class (p. 837).

**Patient and family education**
• See entry for drug class (p. 837).

---

# hydromorphone hydrochloride   (hye-droe-MOR-fone)    narcotic analgesic

• hydromorphone hydrochloride: Dilaudid (C-II)

**MECHANISM OF ACTION** Hydromorphone is a narcotic analgesic with opiate agonist activity. See entry for drug class for more complete information (p. 835).

**INDICATIONS** **Analgesia** Moderate to serve pain.

**CONTRAINDICATIONS** • Respiratory depression. • Intracranial lesion with intracranial pressure. • Status asthmaticus. • Pulmonary edema.

**DOSAGE** **PO:** **ADULTS:** 2 mg every 4 to 6 hours as needed. Severe pain may require 4 mg. As an antitussive, 1 mg every 3 to 4 hours. **CHILDREN:** As an antitussive agent for children 6 to 12 years old, 0.5 mg every 3 to 4 hours. **SC or IM:** **ADULTS:** 2 mg every 4 to 6 hours as needed. Severe pain may require 3 to 4 mg. **Rectal:** **ADULTS:** 3 mg every 6 to 8 hours, as needed. *Special patient populations:* **CHILDREN:** Not recommended for children under 6 years old. Pediatric doses for children 6 to 12 years old are for the antitussive action only. **PREGNANCY:** Safe use has not been established.

**PREPARATIONS** *Tablets:* 1, 2, 3, or 4 mg; *injection:* 1,2, 3, 4, or 10 mg/ml; *suppositories:* 3 mg.

**DRUG INTERACTIONS** **CNS depressants** Opioids potentiate the effects of other CNS depressants, including other opioids, general anesthetics, tranquilizers, sedatives and hypnotics, alcohol, tricyclic antidepressants, and monoamine oxidase inhibitors. **Phenothiazines** May antagonize the analgesic effect of opioids. **Skeletal muscle relaxants** Opioids may enhance neuromuscular blocking action.

**FATE** Hydromorphone is well absorbed. The *onset of action* is 15 to 30 minutes; the *duration of action* is 4 to 5 hours. Hydromorphone is metabolized in the liver and excreted in the urine.

## 🐾 NURSING CONSIDERATIONS

### Side effects, toxicities, and associated nursing actions
• See entry for drug class (p. 835).

### Nursing interventions related to drug administration
• For IV administration, dilute dose with 5 ml of sterile water or normal saline for injection. Administer at a rate of 2 mg or less over 3 to 5 minutes.
• Dilaudid brand tablets in 1, 2, and 4 mg dosages and Dilaudid brand cough syrup contain FD & C yellow dye # 5 (tartrazine), which may cause an allergic reaction in susceptible individuals. Although rare, this response is seen more frequently in persons with aspirin hypersensitivity.
• See entry for drug class (p. 837).

### Patient and family education
• See entry for drug class (p. 837).

---

## levorphanol tartrate   (lee-VOR-fa-nole)                    narcotic analgesic

• levorphanol tartrate: Levo-Dromoran, Dromoran, (C-III)

**MECHANISM OF ACTION**   Levorphanol is a narcotic analgesic with opiate agonist activity. See entry for drug class for more complete information (p. 835).

**INDICATIONS**   **Analgesia** Moderate to severe pain, preoperative sedation, adjunct to nitrous oxide/oxygen anesthesia.

**CONTRAINDICATIONS**   • Respiratory depression and anoxia. • Acute alcoholism. • Broncial asthma. • Intracranial pressure.

**DOSAGE**   **PO or SC:**   **ADULTS:** 2 mg or 3 mg if necessary.   *Special patient populations:*   **PREGNANCY:** Safe use has not been established.

**PREPARATIONS**   *Tablets:* 2 mg; *injection:* 2 mg/ml.

**DRUG INTERACTIONS**   **CNS depressants** Opioids potentiate the effects of other CNS depressants, including other opioids, general anesthetics, tranquilizers, sedatives and hypnotics, alcohol, tricyclic antidepressants, and monoamine oxidase inhibitors.   **Phenothiazines** may antagonize the analgesic effect of opioids.   **Skeletal muscle relaxants** Opioids may enhance neuromuscular blocking action.

**FATE**   Levorphanol is well absorbed. The *onset of action* is 60 to 90 minutes; the *duration of action* is 6 to 8 hours. Levorphanol is metabolized in the liver and excreted in the urine.

## 🐾 NURSING CONSIDERATIONS

### Side effects, toxicities, and associated nursing actions
• See entry for drug class (p. 835).

### Nursing interventions related to drug administration
• For IV administration of levorphanol, dilute dose with 5 ml of sterile water or normal saline for injection. Administer at a rate of 3 mg or less over 3 to 5 minutes.
• See entry for drug class (p. 837).

### Patient and family education
• See entry for drug class (p. 837)

---

## meperidine hydrochloride   (me-PER-i-deen)

## ✤pethidine hydrochloride   (PETH-i-deen)                    narcotic analgesic

• meperidine hydrochloride: Demerol (C-II)

**MECHANISM OF ACTION**   Meperidine is a narcotic analgesic with opiate agonist activity. See entry for drug class for more complete information (p. 835).

**INDICATIONS**    **Analgesia** Moderate to severe pain, as with myocardial infarction or labor. Also used for preoperative sedation and as a supplement to anesthesia.

**CONTRAINDICATIONS**    • Head injury with increased intracranial pressure. • Hypersensitivy. • Use of MAO (monoamine oxidase) inhibitors within 14 days. • Asthma and other conditions associated with compromised respiration. • Acute abdominal conditions.

**DOSAGE**    **PO, IM, SC:**    ADULTS: 50 to 150 mg every 3 to 4 hours as needed. For labor, 50 to 100 mg is given when labor pains become regular. May repeat at 1 to 3 hour intervals if necessary.    CHILDREN: 1.1 to 1.8 mg/kg every 3 to 4 hours as needed.    **IV:**    ADULTS: 15 to 35 mg/hr by slow, continuous infusion.    *Special patient populations:*    PREGNANCY: Safe use has not been established. Meperidine is excreted in breast milk.

**PREPARATIONS**    *Solution (oral):* 50 mg/5 ml; *tablets:* 50 or 100 mg; *injection:* 25, 50, 75, or 100 mg/ml; *injection for IV infusion:* 10 mg/ml.

**DRUG INTERACTIONS**    **CNS depressants** Opioids potentiate the effects of other CNS depressants, including other opioids, general anesthetics, tranquilizers, sedatives and hypnotics, alcohol, tricyclic antidepressants, and monoamine oxidase inhibitors.    **Phenothiazines** may antagonize analgesic effect of opioids.    **Skeletal muscle relaxants** Opioids may enhance neuromuscular blocking action.

**FATE**    Meperidine has a rapid *onset of action,* generally within 15 minutes. The *duration of action* is 2 to 4 hours. Meperidine is metabolized in the liver and excreted in the urine.

## ☙ NURSING CONSIDERATIONS

### Side effects, toxicities, and associated nursing actions
- See entry for drug class (p. 835).

### Nursing interventions related to drug administration
- For IV administration of meperidine, dilute dose with 5 ml of sterile water or normal saline for injection. Administer at a rate of 25 mg or less over 1 minute.
- Dilute dose of meperidine syrup in at least a half-glass of water. When taken undiluted, it may cause temporary mucous membrane anesthesia.
- See entry for drug class (p. 837).

### Patient and family education
- See entry for drug class (p. 837).

---

## methadone hydrochloride    (METH-a-done)    narcotic analgesic

- methadone hydrochloride: Dolophine (C-II)

**MECHANISM OF ACTION**    Methadone is a narcotic analgesic with opiate agonist activity. See entry for drug class for more complete information (p. 835).

**INDICATIONS**    **Analgesia** Severe pain. May be used for severe or chronic pain in terminally ill patients. **Detoxification and maintenance** Methadone is used as an oral substitute for other opioids. Methadone does not give the euphoria characteristic of shorter-acting opioids and blocks these drugs.

**CONTRAINDICATIONS**    • Pulmonary edema.

**DOSAGE**    **For pain:** *PO, IM, SC:*    ADULTS: 2.5 to 10 mg every 3 to 4 hours as needed. If used for chronic pain, 5 to 20 mg every 6 to 8 hours PO.    **For detoxification and maintenance:**    *PO:*    ADULTS: Initial dose is 15 to 20 mg to suppress withdrawal symptoms. Repeat as withdrawal symptoms appear. Usual daily dose is 40 mg the first 2 to 3 days. Dosage is then decreased every 1 to 2 days. If methadone is not discontinued after 3 weeks, the patient is considered to be on a maintenance program. In a methadone maintenance program, the patient does not give up the addiction but substitutes methadone for other opioids. Methadone is orally effective, does not cause euphoria, and blocks the euphoric action of other opioids. The patient is stabilized on a daily methadone dose that may range from 40 to 100 mg. Federal law prohibits daily doses higher than 120 mg without special authority. *Special patient populations:*    CHILDREN: Methadone is not recommended for children under 16 years of age.   **PREGNANCY:** Safe use has not been established. Infants born of methadone-maintained mothers may have a higher incidence of sudden infant death.

**PREPARATIONS**   *Solution (oral):* 5 or 10 mg/5 ml, 10 mg/ml; *tablets:* 5, 10, or 40 mg; *injection:* 10 mg/ml.

**DRUG INTERACTIONS**   **CNS depressants** Opioids potentiate the effects of other CNS depressants, including other opioids, general anesthetics, tranquilizers, sedatives and hypnotics, alcohol, tricyclic antidepressants, and monoamine oxidase inhibitors.   **Phenothiazines** may antagonize the analgesic effect of opioids.   **Skeletal muscle relaxants** Opioids may enhance neuromuscular blocking action.

**FATE**   Methadone is well absorbed. The *onset of action* is 10 to 15 minutes; the *duration of action* is 4 to 6 hours. Methadone is metabolized in the liver and excreted in the urine and feces.

☙ **NURSING CONSIDERATIONS**
### Side effects, toxicities and associated nursing actions
- See entry for drug class (p. 835).
### Nursing interventions related to drug administration
- When the oral concentrate solution is used, dilute dose with water to at least 90 ml prior to administration.
- Dispersible tablets should be diluted in at least 120 ml of water, orange juice, citrus flavor Tang brand drink, or other acidic fruit beverage. Complete dispersion occurs in about 1 minute.
- See entry for drug class (p. 837).
### Patient and family education
- See entry for drug class (p. 837).

---

## morphine sulfate   (MOR-feen)                                        narcotic analgesic

- morphine sulfate: Generic, Roxanol, MS Contin, ✾Epimorph, ✾Morphitec, ✾M.O.S., ✾Statex (C-II)

**MECHANISM OF ACTION**   Morphine is a narcotic analgesic with opiate agonist activity. See entry for drug class for more complete information.

**INDICATIONS**   **Analgesia** Severe pain.

**CONTRAINDICATIONS**   • Head injuries with increased intracanial pressure. • Acute asthma. • Pregnancy (prior to labor).

**DOSAGE**   **SC or IM:**   **ADULTS:** 10 mg every 4 hours as needed. For myocardial infarction: 8 to 15 mg. **CHILDREN:** 0.1 to 0.2 mg/kg every 4 hours as needed; maximum dose is 15 mg. Generally, children 1 to 3 years old receive 1 mg; 4 to 6 years old, 1.5 mg 7 to 9 years old, 2 mg; 10 to 12 years old, 4 mg. **IV:**   **ADULTS:** 2.5 to 15 mg is diluted in 5 ml and administered slowly over 4 to 5 minutes. Dosage is individualized for severe, chronic pain of cancer. Initially, 1 to 10 mg/hr, then increase to an effective maintenance dose, generally 20 to 150 mg/hr. These patients may be given a patient-controlled infusion device that allows the patient to self-administer morphine as needed.   **PO:**   **ADULTS:** 10 to 30 mg every 4 hours as needed. Alternatively, 30 mg extended-release tablet every 12 hours.   **Rectal:** **ADULTS:** 10 to 20 mg every 4 hours as needed.   **Epidural:**   **ADULTS:** For relief of severe pain, 5 mg initially, then add 1 to 2 mg increments after 1 hour if needed. Maximum daily dose, 10 mg. **Intrathecal:**   **ADULTS:** Use 1/10 the epidural dose. *Special patient populations:* **ELDERLY:** Generally, reduced doses are required, especially for the epidural and intrathecal routes. **PREGNANCY:** Safe use has not been established. Morphine is used during labor but should be avoided if a premature infant is to be delivered because of the possible respiratory depression (FDA pregnancy category C).

**PREPARATIONS**   *Solution (oral):* 10 or 20 mg/5 ml, 20 mg/ml; *tablets:* 10, 15, or 30 mg; *tablets (extended release):* 30 mg; *injection (IM, IV, SC):* 2, 4, 8, 10, or 15 mg/ml; *injection (epidural, intrathecal, IV):* 0.5 or 1 mg/ml; *suppositories:* 5, 10, or 20 mg.

**DRUG INTERACTIONS**   **CNS depressants** Opioids potentiate the effects of other CNS depressants, including other opioids, general anesthetics, tranquilizers, sedatives and hypnotics, alcohol, tricyclic antidepressants, and monoamine oxidase inhibitors.   **Phenothiazines** may antagonize analgesic effect of opioids.   **Skeletal muscle relaxants** Opioids may enhance neuromuscular blocking action.

**FATE**   Morphine is incompletely absorbed for the gastrointestinal tract. The *peak* analgesic effect varies with the route of administration: 60 minutes after oral administration, 20 to 60 minutes after rectal administration, 50 to 90 minutes after subcutaneous administration, 30 to 60 minutes after intramuscular administration, and 20 minutes after IV injection. Respiratory depression may precede the maximal analgesic effect. Morphine is metabolized in the liver and excreted in the urine.

### ☙ NURSING CONSIDERATIONS
#### Side effects, toxicities, and associated nursing actions
- See entry for drug class (p. 835).
#### Nursing interventions related to drug administration
- For IV administration, dilute ordered dose with at least 5 ml of normal saline or sterile water for injection. Administer diluted dose over 3 to 5 minutes.
- For intrathecal or epidural administration, the preservative-free solution for injection should be used.
- See entry for drug class (p. 837).
#### Patient and family education
- See entry for drug class (p. 837).

---

## nalbuphine hydrochloride   (NAL-byoo-feen)                        narcotic analgesic

- nalbuphine hydrochloride: Nubain (C-V)

**MECHANISM OF ACTION**   Nalbupine is a narcotic analgesic with mixed agonist-antagonist activity. See entry for drug class for more complete information (p. 835).

**INDICATIONS**   **Analgesia** Moderate to severe pain.

**CONTRAINDICATIONS**   **Patients dependent on opiate drugs.** Nalbuphine may induce withdrawal symptoms.

**DOSAGE**   **SC, IM, IV:**   ADULTS: 10 mg/70 kg, repeated every 3 to 6 hours as needed. Maximum daily dose: 160 mg.   *Special patient populations:* PREGNANCY: Safe use has not been established (FDA pregnancy category C).

**PREPARATIONS**   *Solution:* 10 mg/ml.

**DRUG INTERACTIONS**   **CNS depressants** Opioids potentiate the effects of other CNS depressants, including other opioids, general anesthetics, tranquilizers, sedatives and hypnotics, alcohol, tricyclic antidepressants, and monoamine oxidase inhibitors.   **Phenothiazines** may antagonize the analgesic effect of opioids.   **Skeletal muscle relaxants** Opioids may enhance neuromuscular blocking action.

**FATE**   The *onset of action* is 2 minutes after IV and 15 minutes after IM or SC administration. The *duration of action* is 3 to 6 hours.

### ☙ NURSING CONSIDERATIONS
#### Side effects, toxicities, and associated nursing actions
- See entry for drug class (p. 835).
#### Nursing interventions related to drug administration
- For IV administration nalbuphine may be administered undiluted. Administer each 10 mg or less over 3 to 5 minutes.
- See entry for drug class (p. 837).
#### Patient and family education
- See entry for drug class (p. 837).

---

## oxycodone                                                         narcotic analgesic

- oxycodone: Generic, ✿Supeudol, ✿Eudol, ✿Mictoben, ✿Proladone (C-II)

**MECHANISM OF ACTION**   Oxycodone is a narcotic analgesic with opiate agonist activity. See entry for drug class for more complete information (p. 835).

**INDICATIONS**    **Analgesia** Moderate to moderately severe pain, such as that associated with bursitis, injuries, dislocations, simple fractures, or neuralgia. Also used for postoperative, postextraction, and postpartum pain.

**CONTRAINDICATIONS**    • Decreased respiratory reserve, as in emphysema, asthma. • Elevated spinal fluid pressure.

**DOSAGE**    **PO:**   **ADULTS:** 5 mg every 6 hours.   **CHILDREN:** One-fourth the adult dose for children 6 to 12 years old; one-half the adult dose for children over 12 years old.   **Rectal:**   **ADULTS:** 10 or 20 mg (one or two suppositories) three to four times daily.   *Special patient populations:*   **PREGNANCY:** Safe use has not been established.

**PREPARATIONS**    *Solution (oral):* 5 mg/5ml; *tablets:* 5 mg. Oxycodone is administered mainly combined with aspirin or acetaminophen.

**DRUG INTERACTIONS**    **CNS depressants** Opioids potentiate the effects of other CNS depressants, including other opioids, general anesthetics, tranquilizers, sedatives and hypnotics, alcohol, tricyclic antidepressants, and monoamine oxidase inhibitors.   **Phenothiazines** may antagonize the analgesic effect of opioids.   **Skeletal muscle relaxants** Opioids may enhance neuromuscular blocking action.

**FATE**    The *onset of action* is 10 to 15 minutes, with a *peak effect* in 30 to 60 minutes. The *duration of action* is 3 to 6 hours. Oxycodone is metabolized in the liver and excreted in the urine.

**❦ NURSING CONSIDERATIONS**

**Side effects, toxicities, and associated nursing actions**

• See entry for drug class (p. 835).

**Nursing interventions related to drug administration**

• See entry for drug class (p. 837).

**Patient and family education**

• See entry for drug class (p. 837).

## oxymorphone hydrochloride   (ox-i-MOR-fone)    narcotic analgesic

• oxymorphone hydrochloride: Numorphan (C-II)

**MECHANISM OF ACTION**    Oxymorphone is a narcotic analgesic with opiate agonist activity. See entry for drug class for more complete information (p. 835).

**INDICATIONS**    **Analgesia** Moderate to severe pain. Also for preoperative sedation, a supplement to anesthesia, and labor.

**CONTRAINDICATIONS**    • Hypersensitivity to morphine analogs. • Respiratory depression. • Convulsive states.

**DOSAGE**    **SC, IM:**   **ADULTS:** 1 to 1.5 mg every 4 to 6 hours as needed. For labor, 0.5 to 1 mg.   **IV:** **ADULTS:** 0.5 mg.   **Rectal:**   **ADULTS:** 5 mg (one suppository) every 4 to 6 hours.   *Special patient populations:*   **ELDERLY:** Reduced doses are recommended.   **CHILDREN:** Not recommended for children under 12 years old.   **PREGNANCY:** Safe use has not been established except during labor.

**PREPARATIONS**    *Injection:* 1 or 1.5 mg/ml; *suppositories:* 5 mg.

**DRUG INTERACTIONS**    **CNS depressants** Opioids potentiate the effects of other CNS depressants, including other opioids, general anesthetics, tranquilizers, sedatives and hypnotics, alcohol, tricyclic antidepressants, and monoamine oxidase inhibitors.   **Phenothiazines** may antagonize the analgesic effect of opioids.   **Skeletal muscle relaxants** Opioids may enhance neuromuscular blocking action.

**FATE**    The *onset of action* is 5 to 10 minutes after IV administration, 10 to 15 minutes after SC or IM administration, and 15 to 30 minutes after rectal administration. The *duration of action* is 3 to 6 hours. Oxymorphone is metabolized in the liver and excreted in the urine.

**❦ NURSING CONSIDERATIONS**

**Side effects, toxicities, and associated nursing actions**

• See entry for drug class (p. 835).

### Nursing interventions related to drug administration
- For IV administration, dilute the ordered dose in 5 ml of sterile water or normal saline for injection. Administer the diluted dose over 3 to 5 minutes.
- See entry for drug class (p. 837).

### Patient and family education
- See entry for drug class (p. 837).

---

# pentazocine hydrochloride,
# pentazocine lactate    (pen-TAZ-oh-seen)                    narcotic analgesic

- pentazocine hydrochloride: Talwin (C-IV)

**MECHANISM OF ACTION**    Pentazocine is a narcotic analgesic with mixed agonist-antagonist activity. See entry for drug class for more complete information.

**INDICATIONS**    **Analgesia** Moderate to severe pain.

**CONTRAINDICATIONS**    • Renal or hepatic impairment: caution is required. • Acute myocardial infarction accompanied by hypertension or left ventricular failure.

**DOSAGE**    **PO:    ADULTS:** 50 mg every 3 to 4 hours as needed.    **IM, SC, IV:    ADULTS:** 30 mg every 3 to 4 hours. IM is preferred to the SC route. Total daily dose should not exceed 360 mg.    *Special patient populations:*    **PREGNANCY:** Safe use has not been established, except during labor (FDA pregnancy category C).

**PREPARATIONS**    *Pentazocine hydrochloride; tablets:* 50 mg (with 0.5 mg naloxone). The naloxone is added to negate the euphoric effect sought in illegal drug use. *Pentazocine lactate; injection:* 30 mg/ml.

**DRUG INTERACTIONS**    **CNS depressants** Opioids potentiate the effects of other CNS depressants, including other opioids, general anesthetics, tranquilizers, sedatives and hypnotics, alcohol, tricyclic antidepressants, and monoamine oxidase inhibitors.    **Phenothiazines** may antagonize the analgesic effect of opioids.    **Skeletal muscle relaxants** Opioids may enhance neuromuscular blocking action.

**FATE**    Pentazocine is well absorbed from all sites. The *onset of action* is 2 minutes after IV administration and 15 to 20 minutes after IM, SC, or oral administration. The *duration of action* is about 1 hour after IV administration and 2 to 3 hours after administration by other routes. Pentazocine is metabolized in the liver and excreted in the urine.

### ❦ NURSING CONSIDERATIONS
#### Side effects, toxicities, and associated nursing actions
- See entry for drug class (p. 835).

#### Nursing interventions related to drug administration
- For IV administration pentazocine may be administered undiluted, although diluting the dose is preferable. Dilute each 5 mg in 5 ml of sterile water for injection. Administer each 5 mg or less over 1 minute.
- This drug is incompatible in a syringe with many other drugs, including the barbiturates. Check with the pharmacist if in doubt.
- See entry for drug class (p. 837).

#### Patient and family education
- See entry for drug class (p. 837).

---

# propoxyphene hydrochloride,
# propoxyphene napsylate    (proe-POX-i-feen)                  narcotic analgesic

- propoxyphene hydrochloride: Darvon, ✿Novopropoxyn, ✿642 (C-IV)

**MECHANISM OF ACTION**    Propoxyphene is a narcotic analgesic with mixed agonist-antagonist activity. See entry for drug class for more complete information.

**INDICATIONS**   **Analgesia** Mild to moderate pain. Propoxyphene is commonly combined with aspirin or acet-aminophen.

**CONTRAINDICATIONS**   • Suicidal or addiction-prone patients. • Alcoholism; patients taking tranquilizers or antidepressants.

**DOSAGE**   **PO:**   **ADULTS:** 65 mg of the hydrochloride form, 100 mg of the Napsylate form, every 4 hours as needed. *Special patient populations:* **CHILDREN:** Not recommended for pediatric patients. **PREGNANCY:** Safe use has not been established (FDA pregnancy category C).

**PREPARATIONS**   *Propoxyphene hydrochloride; capsules:* 32 or 65 mg. *Propoxyphene napsylate; suspension:* 50 mg/ 5 ml; *tablets (film coated):* 100 mg.

**DRUG INTERACTIONS**   **CNS depressants** Opioids potentiate the effects of other CNS depressants, including other opioids, general anesthetics, tranquilizers, sedatives and hypnotics, alcohol, tricyclic antidepressants, and monoamine oxidase inhibitors.   **Phenothiazines** may antagonize the analgesic effect of opioids.   **Skeletal muscle relaxants** Opioids may enhance neuromuscular blocking action.

**FATE**   The *onset of action* is 15 to 60 minutes, and the *duration of action* is 4 to 6 hours. Propoxyphene is metabolized in the liver and excreted in the urine.

### ❦ NURSING CONSIDERATIONS

**Side effects, toxicities, and associated nursing actions**
  • See entry for drug class (p. 835).

**Nursing interventions related to drug administration**
  • See entry for drug class (p. 837).

**Patient and family education**
  • See entry for drug class (p. 837).

---

## sufentanil citrate   (soo-FEN-ta-nil)   narcotic analgesic

  • sufentanil citrate: Sufenta (C-II)

**MECHANISM OF ACTION**   Sufentanil is a narcotic analgesic with opiate agonist activity. See entry for drug class for more complete information.

**INDICATIONS**   **Analgesia** Used as the narcotic component in balanced anesthesia that also includes nitrous oxide and a skeletal muscle relaxant.

**CONTRAINDICATIONS**   • Hypersensitivity.

**DOSAGE**   **IV:**   **ADULTS:** Doses must be individualized according to the patient and the surgery involved. The dosage ranges from 1 to 2 µg/kg for surgical induction to 25 to 50 µg/kg for maintenance during major surgery.   **CHILDREN:** Doses must be individualized according to the patient and the surgery involved. The dosage ranges from 10 to 25 µg/kg initially, with supplements of 25 to 50 µg as required. Not recommended for children under 2 years old. *Special patient populations:* **ELDERLY:** In general, lower doses are required by elderly patients. **PREGNANCY:** Safe use has not been established.

**PREPARATIONS**   *Injection:* 50 µg/ml.

**DRUG INTERACTIONS**   **CNS depressants** Opioids potentiate the effects of other CNS depressants, including other opioids, general anesthetics, tranquilizers, sedatives and hypnotics, alcohol, tricyclic antidepressants, and monoamine oxidase inhibitors.   **Phenothiazines** may antagonize the analgesic effect of opioids.   **Skeletal muscle relaxants** Opioids may enhance neuromuscular blocking action.

**FATE**   Consciousness is generally lost within 3 minutes after IV administration. Time to regain consciousness depends on the total dose administered and can be 30 minutes to 6 hours. Sufentanil is metabolized in the liver and excreted in the urine and feces.

### ❦ NURSING CONSIDERATIONS

**Side effects, toxicities, and associated nursing actions**   Sufentanil tends not to cause the histamine release characteristic of other opioids.
  • See entry for drug class (p. 835).

**Nursing interventions related to drug administration**   For IV administration sufentanil may be administered slowly, undiluted.
- See entry for drug class (p. 837).

**Patient and family education**
- See entry for drug class (p. 837).

# Narcotic antagonists

naloxone ~ naltrexone

**OVERVIEW OF THE DRUG CLASS**   Two pure narcotic antagonists are in clinicial use. Naloxone is a short-acting drug used to reverse respiratory depression in narcotic overdosed individuals. Naltrexone is a long-acting drug used in adjunctive therapy for drug rehabilitation from narcotic addiction.

**MECHANISM OF ACTION**   Narcotic antagonists are opiate receptor antagonists. These drugs bind to the opiate receptor. They are used not to block the body's endorphins but to block the action in ingested opioids by addicted individuals.

**INDICATIONS**   • See individual drug.

**CONTRAINDICATIONS**   • See individual drug.

**DRUG INTERACTIONS**   See individual drug.

## naloxone hydrochloride   (nal-OX-one)        narcotic antagonist

- naloxone hydrochloride: Narcan

**MECHANISM OF ACTION**   Naloxone is an opioid antagonist. It has little pharmacologic activity of its own but will reverse the activity of an opioid. When administered to an individual who has overdosed on an opioid, naloxone will reverse the respiratory depression. When given to an addicted individual, naloxone will precipitate withdrawal symptoms.

**INDICATIONS**   **Respiratory depression** Naloxone will reverse the respiratory depression caused by an acute overdose of an opioid but not of other CNS depressants such as barbiturates or alcohol. Naloxone causes no respiratory depression of its own. Therefore, naloxone can be administered to a comatose individual regardless of the cause of the respiratory depression without making the patient's condition worse.

**CONTRAINDICATIONS**   **Addiction to opioids** Naloxone will precipitate withdrawal symptoms. This has been used as a test for opioid addiction.

**DOSAGE**   **Known or suspected opiate overdosage:** *IV:*  **ADULTS:** 0.2 to 4 mg initially, repeated at 2 to 3 minute intervals if necessary. If no response after 10 mg has been administed, the depression is probably not due to opiate overdosage.  **CHILDREN:** 0.01 mg/kg initially, then 0.1 mg/kg if needed. The duration of action of the opiate is often greater than that of naloxone. The patient must therefore be carefully observed. Continuous IV administration may be required.  **Postoperative opiate depression:** *IV:*  **ADULTS:** 0.1 to 0.2 mg, given at 2 minute intervals to achieve the desired response. May repeat at 1 to 2 hour intervals. Alternatively, 0.005 mg/kg, repeated after 15 minutes.  **CHILDREN:** 0.005 to 0.01 mg at 2 minute intervals to achieve the desired response. May repeat at 1 to 2 hour intervals.  **Neonatal opiate depression** 0.01 mg/kg into the umbilical vein at 2 minute intervals to achieve the desired response. *Special patient populations:*  **PREGNANCY:** Safe use has not been established.

**PREPARATIONS**   *Injection:* 0.02, 0.4, or 1 mg/ml.

**DRUG INTERACTIONS**   **Opioids** Naloxone reverses opiate effects.

**FATE**   Naloxone is effective within 2 minutes after IV administration. The *duration of action* is about 45 minutes. Naloxone is rapidly metabolized by the liver and excreted in the urine.

## ☙ NURSING CONSIDERATIONS

**Side effects, toxicities, and associated nursing actions**   Effects specifically attributable to naloxone have not been established.

**Nursing interventions related to drug administration**

- Monitor blood pressure, pulse, and respiratory rate every 5 minutes initially, tapering to every 15 minutes, then every 30 minutes when stable. In the acutely ill or comatose patient, attach patient to ECG monitor. Have a suction machine available.
- Have drugs, equipment, and personnel available for resuscitation if needed. Do not leave patient unattended until patient is stable.
- Continue to monitor the patient closely for several hours after naloxone administration, as the effects of naloxone may wear off, causing the patient to again display signs of narcotic overdose.
- For IV administration naloxone may be given undiluted at a rate of 0.4 mg or less over 15 seconds. Dose may be titrated to patient response.
- If desired, dilute with sterile water for injection. May be further diluted with normal saline or 5% dextrose solution and administered as an infusion.

**Patient and family education**   This drug is rarely administered outside of an acute care situation.

---

## naltrexone hydrochloride   (nal-TREX-one)                    narcotic antagonist

- naltrexone hydrochloride: Trexan

**MECHANISM OF ACTION**   Naltrexone is an opioid antagonist. It has little pharmacologic activity of its own but will reverse the activity of an opioid.

**INDICATIONS**   **Opiate dependence** Naltrexone is orally effective and long-acting. It is prescribed for individuals detoxified of opioids. Since naltrexone blocks the effects of opioids, it is used with behavioral therapy to discourage resumption of opioid use.

**CONTRAINDICATIONS**   **Individuals addicted to opioids** Naltrexone will precipitate withdrawal symptoms.

**DOSAGE**   PO:   **ADULTS:** Initially, 25 mg. If there are no withdrawal reactions, another 25 mg is administered. Thereafter, 50 mg daily is given as maintenance therapy. Doses of 100 to 150 mg may be administered every other day for outpatient therapy.   *Special patient populations:*   **CHILDREN:** Not recommended for children under 18 years old.   **PREGNANCY:** Safe use has not been established.

**PREPARATIONS**   *Tablets:* 50 mg.

**DRUG INTERACTIONS**   **Opioids** Naltrexone reverses opiate effects.

**FATE**   The *onset of action* is about 1 hour. The *duration of action* is 24 hours for a 50 mg dose and proportionately longer for doses up to 150 mg. Naltrexone is slowly metabolized in the liver and excreted in the urine.

## ☙ NURSING CONSIDERATIONS

**Side effects, toxicities, and associated nursing actions**

**CNS** Headache, nervousness, difficulty in sleeping, anxiety, irritability, and depression.

- Assess for CNS effects. It may be difficult to differentiate between effects due to naltrexone and those due to the emotional effect of narcotic withdrawal.
- Administering dose in the morning may help reduce insomnia.

**CV** Rare, increased blood pressure, nonspecific ECG changes.

- Obtain baseline measurements of blood pressure, pulse, and ECG tracing prior to initiating drug therapy.
- Monitor blood pressure and pulse daily initially, then taper to monthly measurements if no abnormalities are noted.

**GI** Abdominal pain and cramps.

- Monitor bowel sounds, keep record of bowel movements.
- If abdominal discomfort is persistent or severe, notify the physician; it may be necessary to reduce drug dose.

**Lung** Nasal congestion, sneezing, sinus, coughing, difficulty in breathing.
- Monitor respiratory rate, and auscultate breath sounds.
- If respiratory symptoms are severe or persistent, notify the physician.

**Skin** Rash.
- Inspect the patient for development of rash.

**Metabolic** Liver abnormalities occur mainly in individuals receiving large (300 mg) daily doses.
- Obtain baseline liver function test results before initiating therapy, and monitor these tests on a regular basis.
- Monitor for right upper quadrant abdominal pain, appreance of jaundice, change in the color or consistency of stools.

**Other** Joint and muscle pain; tremors.
- Monitor for other subjective and objective changes.

### Nursing interventions related to drug administration
- Naltrexone therapy should not be initiated until the patient has completed detoxification and been free of opiate drugs for 7 to 10 days.
- Prior to induction with oral naltrexone, the patient may be given a naloxone challenge test (see Naloxone). In this test, a subcutaneous or IV dose of naloxone is administered to the patient, then the patient is observed for signs of opiate withdrawal. The signs include nasal stuffiness, rhinorrhea, tearing, sweating, tremor, abdominal cramps, vomiting, goose flesh, and myalgia. If symptoms of withdrawal appear, the patient is not sufficiently drug free to begin naltrexone therapy. The naloxone challenge test may be repeated daily until the patient is opiate free.
- Monitor the patient carefully for a least 1 hour after the first dose for the appearance of withdrawal symptoms.
- Naltrexone therapy should be used only as a component of a medically supervised behavioral modification program designed to help the patient maintain an opiate-free state.
- Taking oral doses with meals or a snack may lessen gastric irritation.

### Patient and family education
- Review with patients the anticipated benefits and possible side effects of therapy. Instruct the patient to report the development of any unexpected sign or symptom.
- Review with patients the need to avoid ingestion of opiates via any route of aministration while patient is receiving naltrexone.
- Encourage patients in their efforts to remain opiate free and to return for maintenance doses of naltrexone.
- Remind the patient to keep all health care providers informed of all medications patient is taking.
- Instruct the patient to avoid the use of over-the-counter preparations unless first cleared by the physician, as some may contain opioids.
- Instruct the patient to wear a medical identification tag or bracelet indicating the patient is receiving naltrexone.

# Chapter Forty-six

# Anesthetics

| Inhalation anesthetics | Local anesthetics |
|---|---|
| cyclopropane | benoxinate |
| diethyl ether | benzocaine |
| enflurane | bupivacaine |
| halothane | butamben |
| isoflurane | chloroprocaine |
| methoxyflurane | cocaine |
| nitrous oxide | cyclomethycaine |
| | dibucaine |
| **Intravenous anesthetics** | dyclonine |
| diazepam | etidocaine |
| droperidol and fentanyl | lidocaine |
| etomidate | mepivacaine |
| fentanyl | pramoxine |
| flunitrazepam | prilocaine |
| ketamine | procaine |
| methohexital | proparacaine |
| midazolam | propoxycaine |
| sufentanil | tetracaine |
| thiamylal | |
| thiopental | |

**INTRODUCTION**   Modern surgery did not really begin until the introduction of nitrous oxide, ether, and chloroform as general anesthetics in the late 1800s. The agents commonly used today in developed countries include gases (nitrous oxide), volatile liquids (halothane, methoxyflurane, enflurane, isoflurane), and intravenous agents (ketamine, narcotic analgesics). The ultra-short-acting barbiturates, benzodiazepines, and etomidate are used intravenously for anesthesia induction. Local anesthetics directly block nerve conduction. These agents are useful for many topical applications, but several are also injected to infiltrate a major nerve branch, producing regional anesthesia.

# Inhalation anesthetics

cyclopropane ~ diethyl ether ~ enflurane ~ halothane ~ isoflurane ~ methoxyflurane ~ nitrous oxide

**OVERVIEW OF THE DRUG CLASS**   The inhalation anesthetics are gases or volatile liquids administered as gases. The effective concentration of an inhalation anesthetic in the brain does not depend on the solubility of the anesthetic in blood or tissue, but on its partial pressure, the effective pressure of the gas in the atmosphere. The potency of an inhalation anesthetic is determined by the minimum alveolar concentration (MAC) that will produce anesthesia, defined as insensitivity to a skin incision in 50% of the patients.

Since inhalation anesthetics are administered by highly trained personnel, only the general features of these agents will be summarized. This summary is presented in Table 46-1. Halothane and nitrous oxide are the most widely used inhalation anesthetics, whereas cyclopropane and diethyl ether are seldom used in modern hospitals because of their flammability.

**MECHANISM OF ACTION**   The general anesthetics are unusual in their mechanism of action because they do not appear to act by a receptor mechanism. Instead, general anesthetics are believed to alter the lipid structure of cell membranes so that physiologic functions are impaired. The network of neurons making up the CNS is especially vulnerable because alteration of the membrane structure interrupts the complex intercommunication necessary for function.

**INDICATIONS**   **Major surgery** The ideal anesthetic would produce analgesia, unconsciousness, muscle relaxation, and reduction of reflex activity. Because none of the anesthetics have all these properties, other drugs are commonly administered as well, especially analgesics and muscle relaxants.

**Table 46-1.**

## Properties of inhalation anesthetics

| Drug | Physical properties | Onset | MAC (%) | Cardiovascular effects | Muscle relaxation | Elimination | Other properties |
|---|---|---|---|---|---|---|---|
| Cyclopropane | Flammable gas | Very rapid | 9.2 | Sensitizes heart to catecholamines | Good | Lungs | Good analgesia Nausea, vomiting. headache, delirium on emergence |
| Diethyl ether | Flammable liquid | Slow | 1.92 | Minimum | Excellent | Lungs | Excellent analgesia Nausea, vomiting on emergence Secretions stimulated |
| Enflurane (Ethrane) | Nonflammable liquid | Rapid | 1.68 | Decreased blood pressure May sensitize heart to catecholamines | Good | Lungs 2% to 5% metabolized by liver | Causes low body temperature, hypothermia, shivering |
| Halothane (Fluothane) | Nonflammable liquid | Rapid | 0.77 | Decreased blood pressure Sensitizes heart to catecholamines | Fair | Lungs 20% metabolized by liver | Poor analgesia |
| Isoflurane (Forane) | Nonflammable liquid | Rapid | 1.3 | Minimum | Good | Lungs Little metabolism by liver | |
| Methoxyflurane (Penthrane) | Nonflammable liquid | Slow | 0.16 | Decreased blood pressure | Good | Lungs 70% metabolized by liver | Excellent analgesia |
| Nitrous oxide | Nonflammable gas | Very rapid | 101 | Minimum | — | Lungs | Widely used with other drugs for anesthesia Good analgesia |

**CONTRAINDICATIONS**    • Insufficient cardiovascular reserve.

**DRUG INTERACTIONS**    **CNS depressants** With the exception of enflurane, the inhalation anesthetics are CNS depressants that will act additively with other CNS depressants. In particular, nitrous oxide is used for major surgery only with a narcotic analgesic to provide analgesia and to potentiate the depressant effect of the nitrous oxide. By itself, nitrous oxide provides analgesia but not a deep anesthesia. Balanced anesthesia refers to the combination of nitrous oxide, a narcotic analgesic, and a skeletal muscle relaxant to produce surgical anesthesia.    **Catecholamines** Cyclopropane, enflurane, and halothane sensitize the heart to catecholamine stimulation. Arrhythmias may result.

## 🐾 NURSING CONSIDERATIONS

### Nursing interventions related to drug administration

- Administration of preoperative medications is an important part of the planned anesthesia for the patient. Take care to administer these medications as ordered.
- In caring for postoperative patients, note which anesthetic agents have been used (see Table 46-1). Note that agents vary in their likelihood to produce nausea, vomiting, and other effects that may be prominent in the immediate postoperative period.
- Drugs, equipment, and personnel should be readily available for patient resuscitation if needed.
- In the immediate postoperative period, monitor the vital signs every 5 minutes, tapering to every 15, then 30, then 60 minutes as the patient stabilizes. Have a suction machine at the bedside. Keep side rails up.

### Patient and family education

- Review with patients the anticipated benefits and possible side effects associated with anesthesia.
- Instruct patients and families prior to surgery about activities that will be required of patients after surgery, including the need to turn, cough, and breath deeply, ambulate, and so on. Patients should be assisted to practice these activities if appropriate.
- Obtain a thorough medication history prior to surgery. Many anesthetics may produce exaggerated responses in the presence of other drugs.
- Caution patients who exhibit a severe reaction or response to any anesthetic to carry with them the name of the anesthetic and to inform any health care providers about this response before having surgery again.

## Intravenous anesthetics

diazepam (see also Chapter 35) ~ droperidol and fentanyl ~ etomidate ~ fentanyl (see also Chapter 45) ~ flunitrazepam ~ ketamine ~ methohexital ~ midazolam ~ sufentanil (see also Chapter 45) ~ thiamylal ~ thiopental

**OVERVIEW OF THE DRUG CLASS**    The intravenous (IV) anesthetics include the ultra-short-acting barbiturates: thiopental, methohexital, and thiamytal; three benzodiazepines, diazepam, flunitrazepam, and midazolam; ketamine and etomidate. Only ketamine is a true anesthetic, abolishing the perception of and reaction to pain. The barbiturates and benzodiazepines are used primarily as induction agents or to allay anxiety for diagnostic and dental procedures. The advantage of the IV agents is that they are effective seconds after administration.

Since IV anesthetics are administered by highly trained personnel, only the general features of these agents will be summarized. This summary is presented in Table 46-2.

**MECHANISM OF ACTION**    The IV anesthetics are generally very lipid soluble, the exception being midazolam. They are initially distributed to the brain, liver, and kidneys, the organs with the largest blood flow, but later the drug is redistributed to body fat and skeletal muscle, which are less well perfused. This redistribution lowers the circulating concentration to one that no longer maintains anesthesia. This redistribution is responsible for the short duration of action. Metabolism of the drug proceeds as the drug passes through the liver.

**INDICATIONS**    • Induction for general anesthesia. • Basal sedation and amnesia.

**CONTRAINDICATIONS**    • Severe cardiovascular disease, hypotension, or shock.

**Table 46-2.** Injectable drugs for anesthesia

| Generic name | Trade name | Administration/dosage | Comments |
|---|---|---|---|
| **BARBITURATES** | | | |
| Methohexital sodium | Brevital Sodium ✦Brietal Sodium | IV: *Adults*—for induction, 5 to 12 ml of 1% solution no faster than 1 ml every 5 sec. Maintenance, 2 to 4 ml of 1% solution as required. | Has the shortest duration of action (5 to 7 min) of the barbiturates. Some patients develop hiccups after rapid injection. Schedule IV substance. |
| Thiamylal sodium | Surital | IV: *Adults*—for induction, 2 to 4 ml of 2.5% solution every 30 to 40 sec, with maximum dose 3 to 5 mg/kg body weight. Maintenance, 2 to 4 ml of 2.5% solution as required. | Duration of action about 15 min. Schedule III substance. |
| Thiopental sodium | Pentothal | IV: *Adults*—for induction, 50 to 100 mg (2 to 4 ml) in 2.5% solution every 30 to 40 sec or 3 to 5 mg/kg body weight. Maintenance, 2 to 4 ml of 2.5% solution as required. *Children*—3 to 5 mg/kg as described for adults | Duration of action about 15 min. May cause yawning, coughing, or laryngospasm Schedule III substance. |
| **BENZODIAZEPINES** | | | |
| Diazepam | Valium | IV: *Adults*—0.1 to 0.2 mg/kg body weight to induce sleep, maximum dose 10 to 20 mg. Basal sedation requires only 5 to 30 mg, so 2.5 to 5 mg is injected every 30 sec until light sleep or slurred speech is produced. | Do not mix with other liquids. A local anesthetic may be required for intravenous injection. |
| Flunitrazepam | Rohypnol | IV: *Adults*—for induction, 36 to 50 μg/kg body weight over 20 to 40 sec. Maintenance, 10 μg/kg as needed. | Used for induction of anesthesia. Also used to produce sedation, sleep, and amnesia for procedures such as endoscopy. |

| | | |
|---|---|---|
| Midazolam hydrochloride | Versed | For conscious sedation:<br>IV: *Adults*: (unpremedicated) 0.075 to 0.15 mg/kg body weight, administered slowly in 1 to 2 mg increments immediately prior to the procedure. Up to 0.2 mg/kg may be given and an additional maintenance dose of 25% of initial dose may be given. Patients over 60 yr or patients premedicated with a narcotic require an initial dose 25% to 30% less than for the unpremedicated patient. For presurgical sedation and amnesia:<br>IM: *Adults*: 0.07 to 0.08 mg/kg body weight 30 to 60 min before surgery.<br>Adjunct to general anesthesia:<br>IV: *Adults*: (unpremedicated) 0.2 to 0.4 mg/kg body weight initially, administered over 5 to 30 sec. Maximum dose: 0.6 mg/kg body weight. Premedicated adults should receive an initial dose of 0.15 to 0.25 mg/kg body weight. Dosage should be at the low range when the patient is over 55 yr old and debilitated. | A new agent for preoperative sedation; for conscious sedation with or without a narcotic for endoscopic procedures and dentistry; for induction of general anesthesia. Schedule IV substance. |
| **MISCELLANEOUS** | | |
| Droperidol | Inapsine | IV: *Adults and children over 2 yr*—0.15 mg/kg body weight. Onset: 10 to 15 min. Duration: 3 to 6 hr. | An antipsychotic drug. Used with fentanyl citrate and nitrous oxide to produce neuroleptanestresia. May cause extrapyramidal symptoms. |
| Etomidate | Amidate<br>Hypnomidate | IV: *Adults and children over 10 yr*—for induction, 0.3 mg/kg body weight injected over 30 to 60 sec, may vary between 0.2 and 0.6 mg/kg. | A new, nonbarbiturate agent used for induction and sometimes maintenance of anesthesia. |

*Continued.*

**Table 46-2.** **Injectable drugs for anesthesia—cont'd.**

| Generic name | Trade name | Administration/dosage | Comments |
|---|---|---|---|
| Fentanyl citrate | Sublimaze | IV: *Adults and children over 2 yr*—0.002 to 0.003 mg/kg body weight in divided doses over 6 to 8 min. Maintenance, 0.05 to 0.1 mg every 30 to 60 min. Onset: 1 to 2 min. | A potent, short-acting narcotic analgesic. Used with droperidol and nitrous oxide for neuroleptic anesthesia and with nitrous oxide for balanced anesthesia. |
| Ketamine | Ketaject Ketalar | IV: *Adults and children*—1 to 4.5 mg/kg body weight over 60 sec, ½ of initial dose used for maintenance as needed. IM: *Adults and children*—6.5 to 13 mg/kg body weight, ½ of initial dose for maintenance as needed. | Produces a cataleptic anesthesia with good analgesia. Not a scheduled drug. |
| Sufentanil citrate | Sufenta | IV: *Adults*—initial dose is 1 to 8 μg/kg with nitrous oxide and oxygen. Additional doses are 10 to 25 μ/kg. Doses depend on the severity of pain associated with the surgery. *Children over 2 yr*—for cardiovascular surgery: 10 to 25 μg/kg with oxygen and a muscular relaxant. Additional doses are 25 to 50 μg (1 to 2 μg/kg). | A potent, short-acting narcotic analgesic used with nitrous oxide for balanced anesthesia or alone with oxygen and a muscle relaxant. |

**DRUG INTERACTIONS** **CNS depressants** Except for ketamine, the IV anesthetics are CNS depressants that produce additive effects with other CNS depressants. **Droperidol and fentanyl citrate** This combination of an antipsychotic drug and a short-acting narcotic analgesic is marketed as Innovar and used to produce a neuroleptic anesthesia.

### ☙ NURSING CONSIDERATIONS

#### Nursing interventions related to drug administration

- Administration of preoperative medications is an important part of the planned anesthesia for the patient. Take care to administer these medications as ordered.
- In caring for postoperative patients, note which anesthetic agents have been used (see Table 46-1). Note that agents vary in their likelihood to produce amnesia, sedation, and other effects that may be prominent in the immediate postoperative period.
- In the immediate postoperative period, monitor vital signs every 5 minutes, tapering to every 15, then 30, then 60 minutes as the patient stabilizes. Have a suction machine available. Keep side rails up.
- Drugs, equipment, and personnel should be readily available if needed for resuscitation.
- Many of the agents are used alone for outpatient procedures and surgeries. Usually, the patient should not be permitted to drive home alone after receiving an injectable anesthetic.
- When ketamine is used, psychic disturbances are relatively common and include unpleasant dreams, emergence delirium, irrational behavior, disorientation, and hallucinations. The occurrence of these side effects may be lessened by providing the patient with a quiet wake-up period, perhaps in the quietest corner of the recovery room. Excessive stimulation should be avoided, although vital signs must still be monitored. If psychic side effects occur, provide calm reassurance and reorientation to the patient. Do not leave patient unattended. Once patient is returned to hospital room, keep room dimly lit, and keep noise and stimulation to a minimum. Inform family members of probable cause of behavior and enlist their aid in patient reorientation and reassurance.

#### Patient and family education

- Review with patients the anticipated benefits and possible side effects associated with anesthesia.
- Instruct patients and families prior to surgery about activities that will be required of patients after surgery, including the need to turn, cough, and breath deeply, ambulate, and so on. Patients should be assisted to practice these activities if appropriate.
- Obtain a thorough medication history prior to surgery. Many anesthetics may produce exaggerated responses in the presence of other drugs.
- Caution patients who exhibit a severe reaction or response to any anesthetic to carry with them the name of the anesthetic and to inform any health care providers about this response before having surgery again.

# Local anesthetics

benoxinate ~ benzocaine ~ bupivacaine ~ butamben ~ chloroprocaine ~ cocaine ~ cyclomethycaine ~ dibucaine ~ dyclonine ~ .etidocaine ~ lidocaine ~ mepivacaine ~ pramoxine ~ prilocaine ~ procaine ~ proparacaine ~ propoxycaine ~ tetracaine

**OVERVIEW OF THE DRUG CLASS** Local anesthetics can be divided into those applied topically to provide surface anesthesia and those injected into an area to produce local anesthesia. Only lidocaine (Xylocaine), dibucaine (Nupercaine), and tetracaine (Pontocaine) are used both topically and by injection. **Surface anesthesia** Those local anesthetics applied as drops, sprays, lotions, creams, or ointments are listed in Table 46-3. Distinction is made between those drugs safely applied to the eyes, those applied to the skin, and those applied to mucosal areas. Only tetracaine (Pontocaine) is suitable for application to all three sites. Systemic absorption is generally not a problem with those local anesthetics applied to the skin; however, those applied to the mucosal membranes of the nose, mouth, throat, urethra, rectum, and vagina may be readily absorbed. The lowest concentration should be used to avoid

| | Table 46-3 | Local anesthetics for surface anesthesia | | | | |

| Generic name | Trade name | Eye* | Mucous membranes† | Skin | Comments |
|---|---|---|---|---|---|
| Benoxinate hydrochloride | Dorsacaine | + | 0 | 0 | Applied topically to eye to anesthetize cornea and conjunctiva. |
| Benzocaine | Americaine | 0 | 0 | + | Widely used. Included in many nonprescription preparations for the relief of sunburn, itching, and mild burns. Long acting and poorly absorbed |
| Butamben picrate | Butesin Picrate | 0 | 0 | + | Nonprescription ointment for relief of itching and burning. |
| Cocaine hydrochloride | | + | + | 0 | Scheduled II drug. Medically used in ear, nose, and throat procedures when vasoconstriction and shrinking of mucous membranes are desired. Ophthalmic preparations anesthetize cornea and conjunctiva. |
| Cyclomethycaine sulfate | Surfacaine | 0 | +‡ | + | Nonprescription drug used as a cream, ointment, or jelly on skin. Prescription drug for use on genitourinary areas. |
| Dibucaine hydrochloride | Nupercaine Hydrochloride | 0 | 0 | + | Nonprescription skin ointment or cream |
| Dyclonine hydrochloride | Dyclone | 0 | + | + | Used to suppress the gag reflex and to lessen the discomfort of genitourinal endoscopy. Precipitated by the iodine of contrast media used in pyelography and should not be used. |
| Lidocaine | Xylocaine | 0 | + | + | Widely used for topical anesthesia in ear, nose, and throat procedures; upper digestive tract procedures; and genitourinary procedures. Rapid onset and intermediate duration. Not irritating and low incidence of hypersensitivity. |
| Lidocaine hydrochloride | Xylocaine hydrochloride | | | | |
| Pramoxine hydrochloride | Tronothane Hydrochloride | 0 | +‡ | + | Nonprescription cream or ointment primarily used to relieve pain of itching, burns and hemorrhoids. |
| Proparacaine hydrochloride | Ophthaine Hydrochloride | + | 0 | 0 | Applied topically to the eye to anesthetize the cornea and conjunctiva. |
| Tetracaine hydrochloride | Pontocaine Hydrochloride | + | + | + | Topically, the onset is 5 min and duration is 45 min. Usual topical dose is 20 mg; maximum, 50 mg because of toxicity and slow degradation. Ophthalmic preparations are dilute solutions for instillation |

*+indicates suitable site for application; 0 indicates site not suitable for application.
†Mucous membranes include the bronchotracheal mucosa and the mucosa of the urethra, rectum, and vagina.
‡Not for application to the bronchotracheal mucosa.

systemic toxicity.    **Injection anesthesia** The local anesthetics used by injection are listed in Table 46-4. The area affected by a local anesthetic depends on how and where it is injected. The anesthesia produced is described by the technique of injection: infiltration, nerve block, epidural, and spinal anesthesia. *Infiltration anesthesia* refers to the superficial application of a local anesthetic, as for a dental procedure or to suture a cut. *Nerve block anesthesia* refers to the injection of a local anesthetic along a nerve before it reaches the surgical site. The most extensive field of local anesthesia is achieved by applying the drug around the nerve roots near the spinal cords to produce *epidural* or *spinal* anesthesia. For epidural anesthesia, the local anesthetic is administered outside the dura mater. For spinal anesthesia, the local anesthetic is injected into the subarachnoid space between the arachnoid and pia mater membranes in the lumbar area.

**MECHANISM OF ACTION**    Local anesthetics reversibly inhibit nerve conduction by inhibiting the influx of sodium ions into the nerve. The resting potential of the neurons is not affected, but the action potential is depressed. All neurons in the area of administration, whether pain, motor, or autonomic neurons, are affected, so in addition to the loss of pain, loss of sensory, motor, and autonomic activities occurs. The size of the nerve fiber determines its sensitivity to local anesthetics, with the smaller fibers being the most sensitive. Since sensory fibers are smaller than motor activity and, conversely, motor activity is regained before sensory function.

**INDICATIONS**    Relief of itching and burning. Requirement for surface anesthesia. Examinations of the eye, bronchoscopy, endotracheal intubation, gastroscopy, genitourinary procedures.    **Surgery** When a nerve block or spinal block suffices to anesthetize the surgical area.    **Childbirth** Epidural anesthesia is common for vaginal births; spinal anesthesia for Cesarean births.

**CONTRAINDICATIONS**    • Hypersensitivity.

**DRUG INTERACTIONS**    There are no pronounced drug interactions with the local anesthetic agents per se, but the vasoconstriction often accompanying the injected local anesthetic has the following drug interactions.    **MAO inhibitors, tricylic antidepressants, antispychotic drugs** Hypotensive or hypertensive episodes.    **Oxytocic drugs** Hypertensive response.    **Halothane** Increased risk of cardiac arrhythmias.

## ❧ NURSING CONSIDERATIONS

### Nursing interventions related to drug administration

- Administration of preoperative medications are an important part of the planned anesthesia for the patient. Take care to administer these medications as ordered.
- In caring for postoperative patients, note which anesthetic agents have been used (see Table 46-1). Note that agents vary in their likelihood to produce amnesia, effects on the fetus after delivery, or other effects that may be prominent in the immediate postoperative period.
- Have drugs, equipment, and personnel available for resuscitation in any setting where local anesthetics are used.
- Question the patient carefully about allergic response to previous local anesthetics prior to use of these drugs. Note that to many patients the term Novocain means any local anesthetic, regardless of the actual preparation.
- As with inhalation or intravenous anesthetics, careful monitoring of vital signs and respirations should be done during and after surgery or procedures.
- Following spinal anesthesia, patients are usually kept flat for up to 12 hours.
- Following spinal or epidural anesthesia, the patient may be unaware of the need to void. Monitor intake and output, and palpate bladder for distention. Notify the physician if the patient has not voided in 8 hours.
- Supervise ambulation of patients getting up the first time after spinal or epidural anesthesia. Keep side rails up. Avoid tight sheets or irritations to the lower extremities, as the patient cannot identify irritants until sensation returns.
- Apply heat or cold with extreme caution to areas numb from anesthesia, since the patient will be unable to indicate if skin irritation or burning is occurring.

### Patient and family education

- Review with patients the anticipated benefits and possible side effects associated with anesthesia.

**Table 46-4.** **Local anesthetics for injection**

| Generic name | Trade name | Local infiltration or nerve block or epidural block* | Spinal block (subarachnoid) | Duration† | Comments |
|---|---|---|---|---|---|
| Bupivacaine hydrochloride | Marcaine | + | Investigational | Long‡ | Provides long-acting epidural anesthesia in labor with no reported effects on fetus. Maximum dose, 200 mg. |
| Chloroprocaine hydrochloride | Nesacaine | + | Investigational | Short | Little systemic toxicity because of rapid hydrolysis in the plasma. No effects reported on fetus after epidural anesthesia in mother. Maximum dose, 800 mg. |
| Dibucaine | Nupercaine Hydrochloride | 0 | + | Long | The most potent and toxic of the local anesthetics. Onset can take 15 min. Available in hyperbaric (heavy), isobaric, and hypobaric (light) solutions. Total dose, 2.5 to 10 mg, depending on use. |
| Etidocaine hydrochloride | Duranest | + | 0 | Long | Highly lipid soluble. Onset for epidural block, 5 min. Profound muscle relaxation is desirable for abdominal surgery but not for labor. |
| Lidocaine | Xylocaine Hydrochloride | + | + | Intermediate | Widely used local anesthetic. Maximum dose, 300 mg (4.5 mg/kg body weight). Can cause drowsiness, fatigue, and amnesia. |
| Mepivacaine | Carbocaine | + | 0 | Intermediate | Chemically related to lidocaine. Maximum dose, 400 mg (7 mg/kg body weight). |
| Prilocaine | Citanest Hydrochloride | + | 0 | Intermediate | Maximum dose, 600 mg (8 mg/kg body weight). Useful for outpatient surgery because of the low incidence of drowsiness of fatigue as side effects. Metabolites can cause methemoglobinemia. |
| Procaine hydrochloride | Novocain | + | + | Short | Noted for its safety because of its rapid hydrolysis in the plasma. Maximum dose, 600 mg (10 mg/kg body weight). Duration of epidural block is unreliable. |
| Propoxycaine hydrochloride | Ravocaine Hydrochloride | + | + | Intermediate | Available only in a combination product containing procaine and levonordefrin. Used for dental surgery, onset; 2-3 min. |
| Tetracaine | Pontocaine Hydrochloride | 0 | + | Long | The most widely used drug for spinal anesthesia. Onset, 5 min. Dose for spinal anesthesia, 2 to 15 mg. Available in hyperbaric (heavy), isobaric, and hypobaric (light) solutions. |

*+ indicates suitable use; 0 indicates use not suitable.

† Duration without epinephrine: short, 1 hr, intermediate, 2 hr; long, 3 hr (approximations).

‡ Duration of bupivacaine in nerve block is 6 to 13 hr.

- Instruct patients and families prior to surgery about activities that will be required of patients after surgery, including the need to turn, cough and breath deeply, ambulate, and so on. Patients should be assisted to practice these activities if appropriate.
- Obtain a thorough medication history prior to surgery. Many anesthetics may produce exaggerated responses in the presence of other drugs.
- Caution patients who exhibit a severe reaction or response to any anesthetic to carry with them the name of the anesthetic and to inform any health care providers about this response before having surgery again.
- If a local (surface) anesthetic has been prescribed for self-medication, review with the patient the frequency and route of administration. Caution the patient to use the medication only as directed and to take care to avoid inadvertent injury to anesthetized areas.

# DRUGS TO REDUCE SWELLING AND FEVER

**INTRODUCTION**   Pain, fever, and inflammation are common to many conditions. Analgesic-antipyretic drugs are the first-line drugs for treating these symptoms. Aspirin and acetaminophen are widely used over-the-counter analgesic-antipyretic agents. Aspirin not only relieves fever and mild pain, but its antiinflammatory action makes it the first-line drug in treating arthritis. Other salicylates are available as analgesic, antipyretic, and/or antiinflammatory agents. Nonsteroidal antiinflammatory drugs (NSAIDs) are also used to treat pain and inflammation. Many of these drugs have been introduced within the past 10 years. Ibuprofen has become available over-the-counter.

Rheumatoid arthritis is a progressive autoimmune disease affecting joints. In the early stages, aspirin and nonsteroidal antiinflammatory drugs can control the pain and swelling. In advanced cases, more potent drugs have been developed to treat rheumatoid arthritis resistant to control with aspirin and NSAIDs. Another joint disease is gout. Gout is a type of arthritis whose origin has been well characterized. Drugs can selectively control the causes of gout.

**XIII**

# Chapter Forty-seven

# Analgesic-antipyretic drugs

| | |
|---|---|
| acetaminophen | magnesium salicylate |
| **Salicylates** | salicylamide |
| aspirin | salsalate |
| choline salicylate | sodium salicylate |
| diflunisal | sodium thiosalicylate |

**COMBINATION DRUGS**    The analgesic-antipyretic drugs, especially aspirin and acetaminophen, are commonly combined with other drugs, especially the narcotic analgesics. These drug combinations of nonnarcotic and narcotic analgesics are listed in Table 47-1.

**INTRODUCTION**    Aspirin and acetaminophen are two widely used over-the-counter drugs, effective in relieving minor aches and pains (analgesia) and in lowering fever (antipyretic). Aspirin is chemically a salicylate, and other drugs of this class are also available. Acetaminophen is a paraaminophenol and unrelated chemically to the salicylates. Acetaminophen is an effective analgesic-antipyretic drug that has become an espically popular OTC drug in recent years because of minimal gastrointestinal bleeding, noninterference with blood clotting, few drug interactions, and a lack of association with Reye's syndrome in children.    **Analgesia** The analgesic effect of the analgesic-antipyretic drugs is due to a peripheral mechanism rather then the central effect characteristic of the narcotic analgesics. Analgesic-antipyretic drugs interfere with local mediators released in damaged tissue to stimulate nerve endings. In the presence of these drugs, the nerves are not stimulated. Objective pain, the component of pain that arises from stimulation of peripheral nerve endings, is therefore not felt. This mechanism is in contrast to that of the narcotic analgesics, which interfere with subjective pain at the level of the central nervous system.    **Antipyresis** An antipyretic drug is one that reduces a fever. Normally the balance between heat production and heat dissipation is carefully balanced by the brain. An area of the preoptic anterior hypothalamus is considered the thermostat of the body. Fever results from an increase in the ''set point'' of this hypothalamic center for body temperature. An endogenous fever-producing agent (pyrogen) is released by white cells engulfing foreign matter (phagocytic leukocytes). this endogenous pyrogen is the major, if not the only, final product that acts on the hypothalamic center to produce fever in response to infections, hypersensitivity, or inflammation. Even though it is clear that fever is produced by a protein synthesized by the body as part of an immunologic reaction, it is not clear how fever is a beneficial response, although phagocytosis, a process that inactivates virsues and bacteria, is enhanced by a higher body temperature. The nonnarcotic analgesics act as antipyretics by reversing the effect of the endogenous pyrogen on the hypothalamus so that the ''thermostat'' is returned to normal.

---

## acetaminophen    (a-seat-a-MEE-noe-fen)    analgesic, antipyretic

- acetaminophen: Anacin-3, Datril, Liquiprin, ♣Panadol, Phenaphen, Tylenol, Tempra, others

**MECHANISM OF ACTION**    Acetaminophen acts at peripheral nerve endings to relieve mild pain and at the hypothalamus to lower a fever. See Introduction for a more complete discussion.

**INDICATIONS**    Pain Acetaminophen is effective for mild to moderate pain. It is also commonly combined with aspirin, caffeine, or opioids (see Table 47-1)    **Fever** Acetaminophen is preferred for children because there is no association between acetaminophen and Reye's syndrome. Also, acetaminophen is available in flavored liquid forms for infants and young children.

**CONTRAINDICATIONS**    Anemia Acetaminophen decreases the oxygen capacity of blood because it leads to the formation of methemoglobin.    **Hypersensitivity** is rare but is marked by rash and urticaria.

**DOSAGE**    PO:    ADULTS AND CHILDREN OVER 11 YEARS OLD: 325 to 650 mg every 4 to 6 hours.    **PO or Rectal:**    CHILDREN 4 to 12 months old, 4 to 80 mg; 1 to 2 years old, 120 mg; 2 to 3 years old, 160 mg; 4 to 5 years old, 240 mg; 6 to 8 years old, 325 mg; 9 to 10 years old, 400 mg; 11 years old, 480

**Table 47-1.**

## Prescription combination products of nonnarcotic and narcotic analgesics

| Trade name | Analgesic 1 | Analgesic 2 | Other ingredients* | Prescription |
|---|---|---|---|---|
| Aceta with Codeine | Acetaminophen | Codeine | | C-III |
| Amaphen with Codeine | Acetaminophen | Codeine | BB, CF | C-III |
| Anexsia with Codeine | Aspirin | Codeine | CF | C-III |
| Anodynos-DHC | Acetaminophen | Aspirin hydrocodone | CF | C-III |
| APC with Codeine | Aspirin | Codeine | CF, PH | C-III |
| ASA and Codeine | Aspirin | Codeine | CF | C-III |
| ASA and Codeine Compound | Aspirin | Codeine | CF | C-III |
| Ascriptin with Codeine | Aspirin | Codeine | OT | C-III |
| Axotal | Aspirin | | BB | |
| B-A-C | Aspirin | Codeine | BB, CF | C-III |
| Bancap | Acetaminophen | | BB | |
| Bancap HC | Acetaminophen | Hydrocodone | BB | C-III |
| Bancap with Codeine | Acetaminophen | Codeine | BB | C-III |
| Co-Gesic | Acetaminophen | Hydrocodone | | C-III |
| Codalan | Acetaminophen | Codeine | CF | C-III |
| Codoxy | Aspirin | Oxycodone | | C-II |
| Darmacet-P | Acetaminophen | Hydrocodone | | C-III |
| Darvocet-N | Acetaminophen | Propoxyphene | | C-IV |
| Darvon Compound | Aspirin | Propoxyphene | CF | C-IV |
| Darvon with ASA | Aspirin | Propoxyphene | | C-IV |
| Demerol APAP | Acetaminophen | Meperidine | | C-II |
| Dia-Gesic | Acetaminophen | Aspirin/hydrocodone | CF | C-III |
| Dolacet | Acetaminophen | Hydrocodone | | C-III |
| Dolene | Acetaminophen | Propoxyphene | | C-IV |
| Doxapap | Acetaminophen | Propoxyphene | | C-V |
| Duradyne DHC | Acetaminophen | Hydrocodone | | C-III |
| Empirin with Codeine | Aspirin | Codeine | | C-III |
| Empracet with Codeine | Acetaminophen | Codeine | | C-III |
| Endolor | Acetaminophen | | BB, CF | |
| Equagesic | Aspirin | | MB | C-IV |
| Equazine-M | Aspirin | | MB | C-IV |
| Esgic | Acetaminophen | | BB, CF | |
| Fioricet | Acetaminophen | | BB, CF | |
| Fiorinal | Aspirin | | BB, CF | C-III |
| Fiorinal with Codeine | Aspirin | Codeine | BB, CF | C-III |
| G-2, G-3 | Acetaminophen | Codeine | BB | C-III |
| G-1 | Acetaminophen | | BB, CF | C-III |
| Hydrocet | Acetaminophen | Hydrocodone | | C-III |
| Mepro Compound | Aspirin | | MB | C-IV |
| Mepro-Analgesic | Aspirin | | MB | C-IV |
| Micrainin | Aspirin | | MB | C-IV |
| Norcet | Acetaminophen | Hydrocodone | | C-III |
| Oxycet | Acetaminophen | Oxycodone | | C-II |
| Oxycodone with Aspirin | Aspirin | Oxycodone | | C-II |
| Pabalate | Sodium salicylate | | OT | |
| Percocet | Acetaminophen | Oxycodone | | C-II |
| Percodan | Aspirin | Oxycodone | | C-II |
| Persistin | Salsalate | Aspirin | | |
| Phenaphen with Codeine | Acetaminophen | Codeine | | C-III |

*BB = butabarbital; CF = caffeine; MB = meprobamate; PH = phenacetin; OT = other.          *Continued.*

| Table 47-1. | Prescription combination products of nonnarcotic and narcotic analgesics—cont'd. | | | | |
|---|---|---|---|---|---|
| **Trade name** | **Analgesic 1** | **Analgesic 2** | **Other ingredients*** | **Prescription** | |
| Phrenilin | Acetaminophen | | BB | | |
| Phrenilin with Codeine | Acetaminophen | Codeine | BB | C-III | |
| Propacet | Acetaminophen | Propoxyphene | | C-V | |
| Proval #3 | Acetaminophen | Codeine | | C-III | |
| Roxicet | Acetaminophen | Oxycodone | | C-II | |
| Roxiprin | Aspirin | Oxycodone | | C-III | |
| S-A-C | Salicylamide | Acetaminophen | CF | | |
| Salimeth | Salicylamide | Acetaminophen | | | |
| SK-Oxycodone | Aspirin | Oxycodone | | C-III | |
| Synglos-DC | Aspirin | Dihydrocodeine | CF | C-III | |
| Talwin Compound | Aspirin | Pentazocine | CF | C-IV | |
| Trilisate Liquid | Choline salicylate | Magnesium salicylate | | | |
| Two-Dyne | Acetaminophen | | BB, CF | | |
| Tylenol with Codeine | Acetaminophen | Codeine | | C-III | |
| Tylox | Acetaminophen | Oxycodone | | C-III | |
| Vicodin | Acetaminophen | Hydrocodone | | C-II | |
| Wygesic | Acetaminophen | Propoxyphene | | C-V | |
| Zydone | Acetaminophen | Hydrocodone | | C-III | |

*BB = butabarbital; CF = caffeine; MB = meprobamate; PH = phenacetin; OT = other.

mg.    **INFANTS:** 1 to 3 months, 40 mg; 4 to 11 months, 80 mg. No more than five doses in any 24 hour period. *Special patient populations:* **PREGNANCY** No special problems have been identified affecting safety for use during pregnancy.

**PREPARATIONS**    *Capsules:* 325 or 500 mg; *elixir:* 120, 160, or 325 mg/5 ml; *solution:* 160 or 167 mg/5 ml; 48 or 100 mg/ml; *tablets:* 120, 325, 500, or 650 mg; *tablets (chewable):* 80 mg; *tablets (film-coated):* 160, 325, or 500 mg; *rectal:* 120, 125, 325, or 650 mg. Multiple combination products are available for analgesia and relief from colds and hayfever. See Tables 47-1 and 53-1.

**DRUG INTERACTIONS**    **Phenothiazines** Hypothermia is a possibility for patients taking phenothiazines and an antipyretic drug.

**FATE**    Acetaminophen is well absorbed and not highly bound to plasma protein. The *onset of action* is 10 to 60 minutes, and the *duration of action* is 4 to 6 hours. Acetaminophen is metabolized in the liver and the metabolite conjugated to glucuronic and sulfuric acid. These steps require glutathione and, in high doses, the liver is depleted of glutathione by the metabolism of acetaminophen. Toxic levels of a metabolite then accumulate that cause hepatic damage. Overdose of acetaminophen can cause death due to liver failure.

**☙ NURSING CONSIDERATIONS**

**Side effects, toxicities, and associated nursing actions**    Normal use of acetaminophen is not associated with many side effects. A few individuals may have a sensitivity reaction.

**Allergic** Rash, itching; rarely, laryngeal edema, angioedema, anaphylactoid reactions.

• Observe for allergic response. If severe, notify the physician.

• Tell patients with allergy to acetaminophen to wear a medical identification tag or bracelet noting the allergy.

**Nursing interventions related to drug administration**

• Remind patients to chew the chewable tablet form for several minutes before swallowing.

• Anodynos-DHC brand combination tablet containing acetaminophen 150 mg, aspirin 320 mg, caffeine 30 mg, and hydrocodone bitartrate 5 mg contains FD & C yellow dye #5 (tartrazine), which may cause an allergic reaction in susceptible individuals. Although rare, this reaction is seen more commonly in persons with aspirin hypersensitivity.

### Patient and family education

- Review the anticipated benefits and possible side effects of drug therapy with patients.
- Caution patients to keep these and all medications out of the reach of children. Children should never be encouraged to take medications by being told they are candy. Caution patients to seek medical help immediately if overdose is suspected.
- Tell patients to be alert to signs of acute toxicity: nausea, vomiting, abdominal pain. Severe poisoning may result in CNS stimulation, excitement, delirium, followed by CNS depression, stupor, hypothermia, rapid, shallow breathing, tachycardia, hypotension, and circulatory failure.
- Review with patients signs indicating possible chronic overdose: unexplained bleeding, bruising, fever, sore throat, malaise. Remind patients to report any unexpected sign or symptom to the physician.
- Caution patients to read labels of all medications carefully. Many over-the-counter products for pain and for treatment of sinus problems or cold contain acetaminophen alone or in combination with other drugs. Caution patients to avoid taking several drugs simultaneously unless absolutely necessary.
- Review with parents the dosages appropriate for children of various sizes and ages. Assist parents in finding a drug form that is easy to administer. Note that absorption from a rectal suppository is variable, and there may be rectal irritation. This route of administration may be the least desirable.
- Remind patients to take this drug only as directed.
- Pain or fever that persists beyond 3 to 5 days may signal a more serious health problem. Instruct patients to seek medical help rather than to self-medicate indefinitely.
- Remind patients to keep all health providers informed of all medications being taken.

# Salicylates

aspirin ~ choline salicylate ~ diflunisal ~ magnesium salicylate ~ salicylamide ~ salsalate ~ sodium salicylate ~ sodium thiosalicylate

**DRUG COMBINATIONS**  • See Table 47-1 for common prescription analgesic combination products.

**OVERVIEW OF THE DRUG CLASS**  The salicylates include aspirin and several other OTC drugs. These are popularly used for self-treatment of fever and minor aches and pains. In larger doses, aspirin and some of the salicylates are first-line treatment for arthritis. The salicylates are nonsteroidal antiinflammatory drugs (NSAIDs) and share the tendency of the other NSAIDs to reduce blood clotting and to cause gastrointestinal bleeding.

**MECHANISM OF ACTION**  Aspirin and the other salicylates, like other NSAIDs, are inhibitors of prostaglandin synthesis. Prostaglandins are discussed as examples of the nonsteroidal antiinflammatory drugs in Chapter 48.

**INDICATIONS**  **Pain** Especially mild pain, as minor headaches, muscle headaches, muscle aches.  **Fever. Inflammation** Especially that of muscle or joint pain. In large doses, aspirin in the drug-of-choice for treating arthritis.

**CONTRAINDICATIONS**  **Bleeding ulcers** In addition, caution should be used when patients have gastritis or peptic ulcers.  **Hemorrhagic disorders, hemophilia** In addition, caution should be used when patients are anemic, have impaired liver fucntion, hypoprothrombinemia, or other conditions that compromise blood clotting.  **Severe renal function impairment** Salicylates are excreted via the kidney. In addition, caution should be used with patients prone to fluid retention, as in hypertension and congestive heart failure.  **Hypersensitivity. Varicella infections or influenzalike symptoms in children** There seems to be an increased risk for the development of Reye's syndrome in children treated with aspirin, although a causal relationship has not been established. Acetaminophen appears to be safe to use. **Gastrointestinal bleeding or disturbance** can be made worse by salicylates.

**DRUG INTERACTIONS** **Protein-bound drugs** Salicylates are highly bound to plasma protein and can displace other drugs, including oral anticoagulants, sulfonylureas, hydantoins, penicillins, and sulfonamides. **Anticoagulants** Salicylates have an anti-vitamin K effect, inhibiting the vitamin K–dependent synthesis of clotting factors, including prothrombin. **Uricosuric drugs** Salicylates interfere with probenecid and sulfinpyrazone. **Oral hypoglycemic drugs** Salicylates enhance the hypoglycemic effect of these drugs. **Corticosteroids** Salicylate concentrations decrease when corticosteroids are given and increase when they are discontinued. **Methotrexate** Salicylates can increase the plasma concentration of methotrexate by displacing it from protein binding and by inhibiting its excretion. **Acidifying and alkalizing agents** The renal excretion of salicylates is enhanced by those agents promoting an alkaline urine (antacids, carbonic anhydrase inhibitors), thereby lowering plasma concentrations of the salicylate. Urine acidifying agents such as ammonium chloride decrease the renal excretion of salicylates, resulting in higher plasma concentrations of the salicylate. **Anticonvulsants** Salicylates can displace phenytoin and valproic acid from protein-binding sites. This seems to promote the metabolism of phenytoin, leading to lower effective concentrations. However, the effective concentrations of valproic acid, and hence the side effects, seem to increase. **Diuretics** Salicylates may slightly reduce the effectiveness of spironolactone and furosemide. **Vitamin C** Vitamin C in large doses can acidify the urine. In an acid urine, salicylate is reabsorbed from the renal tubule and therefore not readily excreted. Patients on high-dose aspirin or salicylate therapy can accumulate high plasma levels of salicylate when they ingest large amounts of vitamin C.

**DIAGNOSTIC TEST INTERFERENCE** **Urinary glucose** At doses higher than 2.4 g daily, salicylates may give false-positive results in glucose determinations using cupric sulfate (Benedict's solution, Clinitest) and false-negative results in glucose determinations using glucose-oxidase determinations (Clinistix, TesTape). **Acetoacetate** Salicylates react with the ferric chloride to produce a persistent color. **Vanillylmandelic acid** Salicylates can lead to false-positive or false-negative results, depending on the determination. **Phenolsulfonphthalein** Salicylates can decrease the urinary excretion of this test compound. **Thyroid tests** Salicylates in high concentrations can alter tyroxine-binding. **Theophylline** Salicylates may interfere with determinations of plasma theophylline determined by the Schack and Waxler method. **Uric acid** Salicylates can falsely increase serum uric acid determinations.

---

## aspirin (AS-pir-in) analgesic*
## ❧acetylsalicylic acid (a-SEAT-il-sal-i-SIL-ik)

---

- aspirin: Generic, ❧Aspirin, ❧Astrin, ❧Ecotrin, ❧Entrophen

**MECHANISM OF ACTION** Aspirin is an inhibitor of prostaglandin synthesis, as are other NSAIDs (see Chapter 48). In addition, aspirin has the unique capability among the salicylates or irreversibly inhibiting the enzyme cyclooxygenase by acetylating it. On a clinical level, this makes aspirin an effective antiplatelet drug. Aspirin acetylates the cyclooxygenase of platelets, thereby inhibiting the production of the prostaglandin, thromboxane $A_2$. Thromboxane $A_2$ is the prostaglandin promoting the aggregation of platelets normally released when platelets adhere to collagen. Platelet aggregation is the first step in the formation of a thrombus. Current interest is to determine whether a low dose of aspirin, taken on a chronic basis, will decrease the incidence of stroke and myocardial infarction, two events associated with inappropriate thrombus formation.

**INDICATIONS** **Mild pain** Aspirin is effective in relieving a wide spectrum of painful states, including headache, pain from irritation of nerves, joints, and muscle, postpartum, dental, and visceral pain. In addition to being an effective analgesic by itself, aspirin is combined with many other drugs as an analgesic agent (see Table 47-1). **Fever. Arthritis** In high doses, aspirin is the first-line drug for the treatment of rheumatoid arthritis. **Stroke, transient ischemic attack** Aspirin has been shown to be effective in preventing recurrence in men.

*Antipyretic; antiinflammatory; antiplatelet.

**CONTRAINDICATIONS**  **Bleeding ulcers** In addition, caution should be used when patients have gastritis or peptic ulcers.  **Hemorrhagic disorders, hemophilia** In addition, caution should be used when patients are anemic, have impaired liver function, hypoprothrombinemia, or other conditions that compromise blood clotting.  **Severe renal function impairment** Salicylates are excreted via the kidney. In addition, caution should be used with patients prone to fluid retention, as in hypertension and congestive heart failure.

**DOSAGE**  **Pain and fever:** *PO:*  **ADULTS AND CHILDREN OVER 12 YEARS OLD:** 650 mg, repeated up to four times a day. Larger doses do not give any more relief and are generally as effective as an equivalent dose of acetaminophen or 30 to 60 mg of codeine. Should not be used as self-medication for more than 10 days without consulting a physician.  **CHILDREN:** 2 to 11 years old, 1.5 $g/M^2$ or 65 mg/kg, divided into four to six doses. Alternatively, pediatric tablets are 81 mg each: 2 to 3 years old, 160 mg (two tablets); 4 to 5 years old, 240 mg (three tablets); 6 to 8 years old, 325 mg (four tablets or one adult tablet); 9 to 10 years old, 400 mg (five tablets); 11 years old, 480 mg (six tablets). No more than five doses in any 24 hour period.  **Rheumatoid arthritis:** *PO:*  **ADULTS:** Initially, 2.4 to 3.6 g daily in divided doses. Increase weekly. Usual maintenance dose is 3.6 to 5.4 g daily.  **CHILDREN:** Initially, in divided doses, 60 to 90 mg/kg daily for children under 25 kg; 2.4 to 3.6 g daily for children over 25 kg. Increase at weekly intervals if necessary. The dose should not exceed 130 mg/kg daily. Toxicity is frequent at doses above 90 mg/kg.  **Rheumatic fever:** *PO:*  **ADULTS:** 4.9 to 7.8 g daily in divided doses for suppression of acute inflammation.  **CHILDREN:** 90 to 130 mg/kg daily in divided doses for suppression of acute inflammation.  **Transient ischemic attack:** *PO:*  **ADULTS:** As prophylaxis against recurrence, 1.3 g daily in two or four doses.  **Antiplatelet:** *PO:*  **ADULTS:** Optimal dosage not established. Dosages of 300 mg to 1.5 g daily have been used. Current practice favors 80 to 150 mg every 1 or 2 days.  *Special patient populations:*  **CHILDREN:** Pediatric doses are given above. In children given aspirin for varicella infections or influenzalike symptoms, there seems to be an increased risk for the development of Reye's syndrome, although a causal relationship has not been established. Because of this concern, acetaminophen is preferred as an antipyretic for these symptoms.  **PREGNANCY:** Salicylates readily cross the placenta. Fetal abnormalities have been demonstrated with high salicylate concentrations in animal studies. Taken chronically in high doses, salicylates may prolong gestation and increase the risk of maternal or fetal hemorrhage.

**PREPARATIONS**  *Capsules:* 325 mg; *capsules (enteric-coated):* 325 or 500 mg; *tablets:* 324, 325, 500, or 650 mg; *tablets (chewable):* 65 or 81 mg; *tablets (chewing gum):* 227 mg; *tablets (enteric-coated):* 324, 325, 500, 650, or 975 mg; *tablets (extended-release):* 650 or 800 mg; *tablets (film-coated):* 325 or 500 mg; *suppositories:* 60, 65, 120, 125, 130, 195, 200, 300, 325, 600, 650 mg, or 1.2 g.

**DRUG INTERACTIONS**  **Salicylates** may potentiate protein-bound drugs, anticoagulants, oral hypoglycemic drugs, methotrexate, and anticonvulsants.  **Salicylates** may interfere with uricosuric drugs, or loop diuretics.  **Urine acidifying agents** depress excretion of salicylates. Toxic levels of salicylate may accumulate. See entry for drug class for more complete information on drug interactions with salicylates.

**DIAGNOSTIC TEST INTERFERENCE**  **Salicylates** may interfere with several urine tests, including those for sugar, aceto-acetic acid, and vanillylmandelic acid. See the entry for drug class (p. 870).

**FATE**  Aspirin is rapidly hydrolyzed in the blood, releasing salicylic acid, which is also active. In an acidic urine, salicylic acid is uncharged and therefore diffuses back into the blood. In an alkaline urine, salicylic acid is charged and therefore stays in the urine and is excreted. Salicylate is metabolized to inactive salicyluric acid by the liver, however, a single 325 mg aspirin tablet will saturate this liver inactivation system. This means that the liver cannot readily metabolize large doses of aspirin, and the *duration of action* is greatly increased.

### ☙ NURSING CONSIDERATIONS

#### Side effects, toxicities, and associated nursing actions

**CNS** Tinnitus (ringing in the ears) is the most frequent sign of salicylism (mild aspirin toxicity). Hyperventilation can result from the stimulation of the respiratory center by salicylate.

• Question patients about the presence of tinnitus if toxicity is suspected or if patient is using aspirin on a chronic basis.

- Monitor rate and characteristics of respirations.

**CV** Bleeding.

**GI** Bleeding.

**Hematologic** Decreased thrombus formation; hypoprothrombinemia from the inhibition of blood clotting factor synthesis.

- Inspect patients on chronic therapy for the appearance of unexplained bruising or bleeding.
- Check the stool for the presence of occult blood.
- Caution patients to report any explained bruising or bleeding.
- GI iritation may be lessened by administering dose with meals, snack, glass of milk, or large volume of water (8 oz). If GI irritation persists, switching to enteric-coated dosage forms, extended-release forms, or a different brand may help.
- Monitor platelet count and hematocrit.
- Administer salicylates cautiously in patients receiving other anticoagulant drugs.
- Chronic therapy may increase excretion of vitamin C and decrease blood levels of folic acid; supplemental therapy may be necessary.

**Metabolic** An overdose can create acid-base imbalance.

- Monitor arterial blood gases if overdose is suspected.

**Allergic** Hypersensitivity to salicylates.

- Observe for allergic response. If severe, notify the physician.
- Caution patients with allergy to aspirin or other salicylates to wear a medical identification tag or bracelet noting their allergy.
- Patients with a history of asthma or nasal polyps may be more likely to manifest allergic reactions to aspirin.
- Note that patients with allergy to aspirin or other salicylates may be allergic to FD & C yellow dye #5 (tartrazine). This coloring is found in many medications and food products. Alert patients with allergy to aspirin about this possible additional allergy; caution patients to read labels on products carefully to avoid exposure to tartrazine.

### Nursing interventions related to drug administration

- Remind patients to chew the chewable tablet form for several minutes before swallowing or discarding.
- Enteric-coated tablet should not be chewed or crushed.
- Effervescent products containing aspirin may be easier to take and are more rapidly absorbed. They may contain large amounts of sodium and should be avoided by individuals on sodium-restricted diets; instruct patients to read labels carefully.
- Plain aspirin tablets may be crushed and mixed with food or applesauce for administration.

### Patient and family education

- Review with patients the anticipated benefits and possible side effects of drug therapy.
- Caution patients to keep these and all medications out of the reach of children. Children should never be encouraged to take medications by being told they are candy. Caution patients to seek medical help immediately if overdose is suspected.
- Caution patients to read labels of all medications carefully. Many over-the-counter products for pain and for treatment of sinus problems, cold, or menstrual problems contain aspirin or salicylates alone or in combination with other drugs. Caution patients to avoid taking several drugs simultaneously unless absolutely necessary.
- Review with patients the dosages appropriate for children of various sizes and ages. Assist parents in finding a drug form that is easy to administer. Note that absorption from a rectal suppository is variable, and there may be rectal irritation. This route of administration may be the least desirable.
- Remind patients to take this drug only as directed.
- Pain or fever that persists beyond 3 to 5 days may signal a more serious health problem. Instruct patients to seek medical help rather than to self-medicate indefinitely.
- Remind patients to keep all health providers informed of all medications being taken.
- Patients on long-term therapy may find the extended-release preparations helpful, particularly at night; blood levels of the drug may not be so low in the morning.

- Note Contraindications in the Overview of the Class (p. 869). Caution parents to avoid aspirin or salicylates in treating fever or discomfort in children with varicella infections or influenzalike symptoms.
- Caution patients to compare over-the-counter products carefully. Product names may be confusing. For example, Arthritis Strength Bufferin brand contains 486 mg of aspirin per tablet plus buffering agents; Extra Strength Bufferin brand contains 500 mg of aspirin per tablet, plus buffering agents.
- Patients on chronic therapy should avoid the use of alcohol.

## choline salicylate   (KOE-leen)                                        analgesic*

- choline salicylate: Arthropan

**MECHANISM OF ACTION**   Choline salicylate is an inhibitor of prostaglandin synthesis, as are other NSAIDs (see Chapter 48).

**INDICATIONS**   **Mild pain** Salicylates are effective in relieving a wide spectrum of painful states, including headache, pain from irritation of nerves, joints, and muscle, and postpartum, dental, and visceral pain.   **Fever. Arthritis** Choline salicylate is a mint-flavored liquid formulation of salicylate for patients with arthritis.

**CONTRAINDICATIONS**   **Bleeding ulcers** In addition, caution should be used when patients have gastritis or peptic ulcers.   **Hemorrhagic disorders, hemophilia** In addition, caution should be used when patients are anemic, have impaired liver function, hypoprothrombinemia, or other conditions that compromise blood clotting.   **Severe renal function impairment** Salicylates are excreted via the kidney. In addition, caution should be used with patients prone to fluid retention, as in hypertension and congestive heart failure.

**DOSAGE**   **Pain and fever:** *PO:*   **ADULTS AND CHILDREN OVER 12 YEARS OLD:** 435 to 870 mg (2.5 to 5 ml) every 4 hours as needed.   **CHILDREN:** 2 (11.5 ml) $M^2$ daily, divided into four to six doses.   **Rheumatoid arthritis:** *PO:*   **ADULTS:** 4.8 to 7.2 (28 to 41 ml) daily.   **CHILDREN:** 107 to 134 mg (0.6 to 0.8 ml)/kg daily. *Special patient populations:* **CHILDREN:** Pediatric doses are given above. In children given aspirin for varicella infections or influenza-like symptoms, there seems to be an increased risk for the development of Reye's syndrome, although a causal relationship has not been established. Because of this concern, acetaminophen is preferred as an antipyretic for these symptoms over the salicylates.   **PREGNANCY:** Salicylates readily cross the placenta. Fetal abnormalities have been demonstrated with high salicylate concentrations in animal studies. Taken chronically in high doses, salicylates may prolong gestation and increase the risk of maternal or fetal hemorrhage.

**PREPARATIONS**   *Solution:* 870 mg/5 ml.

**DRUG INTERACTIONS**   **Salicylates** may potentiate protein-bound drugs, anticoagulants, oral hypoglycemic drugs, methotrexate, and anticonvulsants.   **Salicylates** may interfere with uricosuric drugs, loop diuretics.   **Urine acidifying agents** depress excretion of salicylates. Toxic levels of salicylate may accumulate. See entry for drug class for more complete information on drug interactions with salicylates.

**DIAGNOSTIC TEST INTERFERENCE**   Salicylates may interfere with several urine tests, including those for sugar, aceto-acetic acid, and vaniltyemandelic acid. See entry for drug class for more complete information on drug interactions with salicylates.

**FATE**   The *onset of action* is about 20 minutes, and the *duration of action* is 4 to 6 hours for the analgesic/antipyretic action. For arthritic swelling and pain, maximum relief may take 2 to 3 weeks to achieve.

In an acidic urine, salicylic acid is uncharged and therefore diffuses back into the blood. In an alkaline urine, salicylic acid is charged and therefore stays in the urine and is excreted. Salicylate is metabolized to inactive salicyluric acid by the liver; however, a single 325 mg dose of salicylate

---

*Antipyretic; antiinflammatory.

saturates this metabolic pathway. This means that the liver cannot readily metabolize large doses of salicylates, and the duration of action is greatly increased.

## ❦ NURSING CONSIDERATIONS

**Side effects, toxicities, and associated nursing actions**   Side effects for all salicylates are the same; see Nursing Considerations for aspirin (p. 871).

**Nursing interventions related to drug administration**

- Choline salicylate should be mixed with fruit juice just before administration; do not mix with antacids.

**Patient and family education**

- Review the anticipated benefits and possible side effects of drug therapy with patients.
- Tell patients to keep these and all medications out of the reach of children. Children should never be encouraged to take medications by being told they are candy. Tell patients to seek medical help immediately if overdose is suspected.
- Instruct patients to read labels of all medications carefully. Many over-the-counter products for pain and for treatment of sinus problems, colds, or menstrual problems contain aspirin or salicylates, alone or in combination with other drugs. Remind patients to avoid taking several drugs simultaneously unless absolutely necessary.
- Remind patients to take this drug only as directed.
- Pain or fever that persists beyond 3 to 5 days may signal a more serious health problem. Instruct patients to seek medical help rather than to self-medicate indefinitely.
- Remind patients to keep all health care providers informed of all medications being taken.
- Note Contraindications in the Overview of the Class (p. 869), and Dosage. Tell parents to avoid aspirin or salicylates in treating fever or discomfort in children with varicella infections or influenzalike symptoms.
- Patients on chronic therapy should avoid the use of alcohol.
- See entry for aspirin (p. 872).

---

## diflunisal   (dye-FLOO-ni-sal)                                        analgesic*

- diflunisal: Dolobid

**MECHANISM OF ACTION**   Diflunisal is an inhibitor of prostaglandin synthesis, as are other NSAIDs (see Chapter 48).

**INDICATIONS**   **Mild pain** Salicylates are effective in relieving a wide spectrum of painful states, including headache, pain from irritation of nerves, joints, and muscle, and postpartum, dental, and visceral pain.   **Arthritis** Diflunisal is used for acute and chronic treatment of rheumatoid arthritis and osteoarthritis.

**CONTRAINDICATIONS**   **Bleeding ulcers** In addition, caution should be used when patients have gastritis or peptic ulcers.   **Hemorrhagic disorders, hemophilia** In addition, caution should be used when patients are anemic, have impaired liver function, hypoprothrombinemia, or other conditions that compromise blood clotting.   **Severe renal function impairment** Salicylates are excreted via the kidney. In addition, caution should be used with patients prone to fluid retention, as in hypertension and congestive heart failure.

**DOSAGE**   **Pain:** *PO:*   **ADULTS AND CHILDREN OVER 12 YEARS OLD:** 1 g followed by a maintenance dose of 500 mg every 12 hours.   **Arthritis:** *PO:*   **ADULTS:** 500 to 1 g daily in two divided doses.   *Special patient populations:*   **CHILDREN:** Not recommended for children under 12 years old.   **PREGNANCY:** Salicylates readily cross the placenta. Fetal abnormalities have been demonstrated with high salicylate concentrations in animal studies. Taken chronically in high doses, salicylates may prolong gestation and increase the risk of maternal or fetal hemorrhage.

**PREPARATIONS**   *Tablets:* 250 or 500 mg.

**DRUG INTERACTIONS**   **Salicylates** may potentiate protein-bound drugs, anticoagulants, oral hypoglycemic drugs, methotrexate, and anticonvulsants.   **Salicylates** may interfere with uricosuric drugs and loop

*Antipyretic; antiinflammatory.

diuretics.   **Urine acidifying agents** depress excretion of salicylates. Toxic levels of salicylate may accumulate. See entry for drug class (p. 870).

**DIAGNOSTIC TEST INTERFERENCE**   Salicylates may interfere with several urine tests, including those for sugar, aceto-acetic acid, and vanilylmandelic acid. See entry for drug class for more complete information on drug interactions with salicylates.

**FATE**   The *onset of action* is about 20 minutes, and the *duration of action* is 4 to 6 hours for the analgesic/antipyretic action. For arthritic swelling and pain, maximum relief may take 2 to 3 weeks to achieve. Diflunisal is rapidly absorbed and highly bound to plasma protein. The *plasma half-life* is 8 to 12 hours. Diflunisal is metabolized in the liver and excreted in the urine.

## ☙ NURSING CONSIDERATIONS

### Side effects, toxicities, and associated nursing actions   Side effects for all salicylates are the same; see Nursing Considerations for aspirin (p. 871).

### Nursing interventions related to drug administration
- Diflunisal tablets should not be crushed or chewed but swallowed whole.

### Patient and family education
- Review the anticipated benefits and possible side effects of drug therapy with patients.
- Tell patients to keep these and all medications out of the reach of children. Children should never be encouraged to take medications by being told they are candy. Tell patients to seek medical help immediately if overdose is suspected.
- Instruct patients to read labels of all medications carefully. Many over-the-counter products for pain and for treatment of sinus problems, colds, or menstrual problems contain aspirin or salicylates, alone or in combination with other drugs. Remind patients to avoid taking several drugs simultaneously unless absolutely necessary.
- Remind patients to take this drug only as directed.
- Pain or fever that persists beyond 3 to 5 days may signal a more serious health problem. Instruct patients to seek medical help rather than to self-medicate indefinitely.
- Remind patients to keep all health care providers informed of all medications being taken.
- Note Contraindications in the Overview of the Drug Class (p. 869) and Dosage. Tell parents to avoid aspirin or salicylates in treating fever or discomfort in children with varicella infections or influenzelike symptoms.
- Patients on chronic therapy should avoid the use of alcohol.
- See entry for aspirin (p. 872).

---

## magnesium salicylate                                              analgesic*

- magnesium salicylate: Doan's Pills, Magan, Analate

**MECHANISM OF ACTION**   Magnesium salicylate is an inhibitor of prostaglandin synthesis as are other NSAIDs (see Chapter 48).

**INDICATIONS**   **Mild pain** Salicylates are effective in relieving a wide spectrum of painful states, including headache, pain from irritation of nerves, joints, and muscle, and postpartum, dental and visceral pain. **Fever. Arthritis.**

**CONTRAINDICATIONS**   **Bleeding ulcers** In addition, caution should be used when patients have gastritis or peptic ulcers.   **Hemorrhagic disorders, hemophilia** In addition, caution should be used when patients are anemnic, have impaired liver function, hypoprothrombinemia, or other conditions that compromise blood clotting.   **Severe renal function impairment** Salicylates are excreted via the kidney. In addition, caution should be used with patients prone to fluid retention, as in hypertension and congestive heart failure. Toxicity from high serum magnesium concentrations is an added problem with the magnesium salt of salicylate is given to a patient with renal impairment.

**DOSAGE**   **Pain and fever:** *PO:*   **ADULTS AND CHILDREN OVER 12 YEARS OLD:** 300 to 600 mg every 4 hours as needed.   **CHILDREN:** 11 years old, 450 mg; 9 to 10 years old, 375 mg; 6 to 8 years old, 300 mg; 4

*Antipyretic; antiinflammatory.

to 5 years old, 225 mg; 2 to 3 years old, 150 mg; administer every 4 hours as needed.    **Arthritis:** *PO:* **ADULTS:** 545 mg to 1.2 g three or four times daily.    *Special patient populations:*    **CHILDREN:** Not recommended for children under 2 years old. In children given aspirin for varicella infections or influenzalike symptoms, there seems to be an increased risk for the development of Reye's syndrome, although a casual relationship has not been established. Because of this concern, acetaminophen is preferred as an antipyretic for these symptoms.    **PREGNANCY:** Salicylates readily cross the placenta. Fetal abnormalities have been demonstrated with high salicylate concentration in animal studies. Taken chronically in high doses, salicylates may prolong gestation and increase the risk of maternal or fetal hemorrhage.

**PREPARATIONS**    *Tablets:* 325, 545, or 600 mg.

**DRUG INTERACTIONS**    **Salicylates** may potentiate protein-bound drugs, anticoagulants, oral hypoglycemic drugs, methotrexate, and anticonvulsants.    **Salicylates** may interfere with uricosuric drugs, and loop diuretics.    **Urine acidifying agents** Toxic levels of salicylate may accumulate. See entry for drug class (p. 870) for more complete information on drug interactions with salicylates.

**LABORATORY TEST INTERFERENCE**    Salicylates may interfere with several urine tests, including those for sugar, acetoacetic acid, and vanillylmandelic acid. See entry for drug class for more complete information on drug interactions with salicylates.

**FATE**    The *onset of action* is about 20 minutes, and the *duration of action* is 4 to 6 hours for the analgesic/antipyretic effect. For arthritic swelling and pain, maximum relief may take 2 to 3 weeks to achieve. In an acidic urine, salicylic acid is uncharged and therefore diffuses back into the blood. In an alkaline urine, salicylic acid is charged and therefore stays in the urine and is excreted. Salicylate is metabolized to inactive salicyluric acid by the liver. however, a single 325 mg dose of salicylate will saturate this liver inactivation system. This means that the liver cannot readily metabolize large doses of salicylates, and the duration of action is greatly increased.

## ❧ NURSING CONSIDERATIONS

### Side effects, toxicities, and associated nursing actions    Side effects for all salicylates are the same; see Nursing Considerations for aspirin (p. 871).

### Nursing interventions related to drug administration

- The choline salicylate and magnesium salicylate combination oral solution should be mixed with fruit juice just before administration; do not mix with antacids.

### Patient and family education

- Review the anticipated benefits and possible side effects of drug therapy with patients.
- Tell patients to keep these and all medications out of the reach of children. Children should never be encouraged to take medications by being told they are candy. Tell patients to seek medical help immediately if overdose is suspected.
- Instruct patients to read labels of all medications carefully. Many over-the-counter products for pain and for treatment of sinus problems, colds, or menstrual problems contain aspirin or salicylates, alone or in combination with other drugs. Remind patients to avoid taking several drugs simultaneously unless absolutely necessary.
- Remind patients to take this drug only as directed.
- Pain or fever that persists beyond 3 to 5 days may signal a more serious health problem. Instruct patients to seek medical help rather than to self-medicate indefinitely.
- Remind patients to keep all health care providers informed of all medications being taken.
- Note Contraindications in the Overview of Drug Class (p. 869) and Dosage. Tell parents to avoid aspirin or salicylates in treating fever or discomfort in children with varicella infections or influenzalike symptoms.
- Patients on chronic therapy should avoid the use of alcohol.
- See entry for aspirin (p. 869).

## salicylamide    (SAL-i-sil-AM-id)                                                                      analgesic, antipyretic

- salicylamide: Uromide

**MECHANISM OF ACTION**  Salicylamide is an inhibitor of prostaglandin synthesis, as are other NSAIDs (see Chapter 48).

**INDICATIONS**  **Mild pain** Salicylates are effective in relieving a wide spectrum of painful states, including headache, pain from irritation of nerves, joints, and muscle, and postpartum, dental, and visceral pain.  **Fever.**

**CONTRAINDICATIONS**  **Salicylamide** is not a true salicylate and is less likely to cause the problems associated with salicylates.

**DOSAGE**  **Pain and fever:** *PO:*  **ADULTS AND CHILDREN OVER 12 YEARS OLD:** 325 to 650 mg three to four times daily.  **CHILDREN:** 65 mg/kg or 1.5 g/$M^2$ given in six doses.  *Special patient populations:* **CHILDREN:** Pediatric doses are given above. In children given aspirin for varicella infections or influenzalike symptoms, there seems to be an increased risk for the development of Reye's syndrome, although a causal relationship has not been established. Because of this concern, acetaminophen is preferred as an antipyretic for these symptoms. It is not clear that salicylamide carries the same risks. **PREGNANCY:** Safe use during pregnancy has not been established.

**PREPARATIONS**  *Tablets:* 325 or 667 mg.

**DRUG INTERACTIONS**  **Salicylate, aspirin, acetaminophen** Salicylamide interferes with the metabolism of these drugs, and they interfere with the metabolism of salicylamide. Salicylamide does not have the drug interaction characteristic of the salicylates.

**FATE**  Salicylamide is well absorbed from the gastrointestinal tract but is metabolized to inactive metabolites. The *plasma half-life* is about 1.5 hours. Salicylamide and its metabolites are excreted in the urine.

## ☙ NURSING CONSIDERATIONS

### Side effects, toxicities, and associated nursing actions

**CNS** Tinnitus (ringing in the ears).
- Question patients about the presence of tinnitus if toxicity is suspected or if patients are using a salicylate on a chronic basis.

**CV** Bleeding.

**GI** Bleeding is not a problem with salicylamide.

**Hematologic** Hypoprothrombinemia from the inhibition of blood clotting factor synthesis.
- Inspect patients on chronic therapy for the appearance of unexplained bruising or bleeding.
- Instruct patients to report any unexplained bruising or bleeding.
- GI irritation may be lessened by administering dose with meals, snack, glass of milk, or large volume of water (8 oz).
- Monitor platelet count and hematocrit.
- Administer salicylates cautiously in patients receiving other anticoagulant drugs.

**Allergic** Apparently, salicylamide does not have cross-sensitivity with salicylates.
- Observe for allergic response. If it is severe, notify the physician.

### Patient and family education
- Review the anticipated benefits and possible side effects of drug therapy with patients.
- Tell patients to keep these and all medications out of the reach of children. Children should never be encouraged to take medications by being told they are candy. Tell patients to seek medical help immediately if overdose is suspected.
- Instruct patients to read labels of all medications carefully. Many over-the-counter products for pain and for treatment of sinus problems, colds, or menstrual problems contain aspirin or salicylates, alone or in combination with other drugs. Remind patients to avoid taking several drugs simultaneously unless absolutely necessary.
- Remind patients to take this drug only as directed.
- Pain or fever that persists beyond 3 to 5 days may signal a more serious health problem. Instruct patients to seek medical help rather than to self-medicate indefinitely.
- Remind patients to keep all health care providers informed of all medications being taken.

- Note Contraindications in the Overview of Drug Class (p. 869) and Dosage. Tell parents to avoid aspirin or salicylates in treating fever or discomfort in children with varicella infections or influenzalike symptoms.
- See entry for aspirin (p. 872).
- Patients on chronic therapy should avoid the use of alcohol.
- Review with patients signs and symptoms of acute overdose: burning of throat or stomach, vomiting, hyperthermia, irritability, confusion, hallucination, seizures, and coma.

---

## salsalate   (SAL-sa-late)                                       antiinflammatory

- salsalate: Disalcid

**MECHANISM OF ACTION**   Salsalate is an inhibitor of prostaglandin synthesis, as are other NSAIDs (see Chapter 48).

**INDICATIONS**   • Arthritis.

**CONTRAINDICATIONS**   **Bleeding ulcers** in addition, caution should be used when patients have gastritis or peptic ulcers.   **Hemorrhagic disorders, hemophilia** In addition, caution should be used when patients are anemic, have impaired liver function, hypoprothrombinemia, or other conditions that compromise blood clotting.   **Severe renal function impairment** Salicylates are excreted via the kidney. In addition, caution should be used with patients prone to fluid retention, as in hypertension and congestive heart failure.

**DOSAGE**   **Rheumatoid arthritis:** *PO:*   **ADULTS:** 3 g daily in two or three divided doses. *Special patient populations:*   **CHILDREN:** Not recommended for children. **PREGNANCY:** Salicylates readily cross the placenta. Fetal abnormalities have been demonstrated with high salicylate concentrations in animal studies. Taken chronically in high doses, salicylates may prolong gestation and increase the risk of maternal or fetal hemorrhage.

**PREPARATIONS**   *Capsules:* 500 mg; *tablets (film-coated):* 500 or 750 mg.

**DRUG INTERACTIONS**   **Salicylates** may potentiate protein-bound drugs, anticoagulants, oral hypoglycemic drugs, methotrexate, and anticonvulsants.   **Salicylates** may interfere with uricosuric drugs and loop diuretics.   **Urine acidifying agents depress excretion of salicylates.** Toxic levels of salicylate may accumulate. See entry for drug class for more complete information on drug interactions with salicylates.

**DIAGNOSTIC TEST INTERFERENCE**   **Salicylates** may interfere with several urine tests, including those for sugar, aceto-acetic acid, and vanillylmandelic acid. See entry for drug class for more complete information on drug interactions with salicylates.

**FATE**   For arthritic swelling and pain, maximum relief may take 2 to 3 weeks to achieve. Salsalate is well absorbed from the gastrointestinal tract and is mostly metabolized to salicylate. In an acidic urine, salicylic acid is uncharged and therefore diffuses back into the blood. In an alkaline urine, salicylic acid is charged and therefore stays in the urine and is excreted. Salicylate is metabolized to inactive salicyluric acid by the liver. However, a single 325 mg dose os salicylate will saturate this liver inactivation system. This means that the liver cannot readily metabolize large doses of salicylates, and the duration of action is greatly increased.

## ✥ NURSING CONSIDERATIONS

### Side effects, toxicities, and associated nursing actions   Side effects for all salicylates are the same; see Nursing Considerations for aspirin (p. 871).

### Nursing interventions related to drug administration
- Film-coated tablets should not be crushed or chewed but swallowed whole.

### Patient and family education
- Review the anticipated benefits and possible side effects of drug therapy with patients.
- Tell patients to keep these and all medications out of the reach of children. Children should never be encouraged to take medications by being told they are candy. Tell patients to seek medical help immediately if overdose is suspected.

- Instruct patients to read labels of all medications carefully. Many over-the-counter products for pain and for treatment of sinus problems, colds, or menstrual problems contain aspirin or salicylates, alone or in combination with other drugs. Remind patients to avoid taking several drugs simultaneously unless absolutely necessary.
- Remind patients to take this drug only as directed.
- Pain or fever that persists beyond 3 to 5 days may signal a more serious health problem. Instruct patients to seek medical help rather than to self-medicate indefinitely.
- Remind patients to keep all health care providers informed of all medications being taken.
- Note Contraindications in the Overview Drug Class (p. 869) and Dosage. Tell parents to avoid aspirin or salicylates in treating fever or discomfort in children with varicella infections or influenzalike symptoms.
- Patients on chronic therapy should avoid the use of alcohol.
- See entry for aspirin (p. 872).

## sodium salicylate   (SAL-i-SIL-ate) or (sah-LIS-i-late)   analgesic*

- sodium salicylate: ♣S-60, Uracel

**MECHANISM OF ACTION**   Sodium salicylate is an inhibitor of prostaglandin synthesis, as are other NSAIDs (see Chapter 48).

**INDICATIONS**   **Mild pain** Salicylates are effective in relieving a wide spectrum of painful states, including headache, pain from irritation of nerves, joints, and muscle, and postpartum, dental, and visceral pain.   **Fever. Arthritis. Skin disorders** Salicylic acid is used in various topical formulations as a peeling and drying agent for the treatment of acne, dandruff, dermatitis, psoriasis, and hyperkaratotic skin disorders. These formulations are not presented below.

**CONTRAINDICATIONS**   **Bleeding ulcers** In addition, caution should be used when patients have gastritis or peptic ulcers.   **Hemorrhagic disorders, hemophilia** In addition, caution should be used when patients are anemic, have impaired liver function, hypoprothrombinemia, or other conditions that compromise blood clotting.   **Severe renal function impairment** Salicylates are excreted via the kidney. In addition, caution should be used with patients prone to fluid retention, as in hypertension and congestive heart failure.

**DOSAGE**   **Pain and fever:** *PO:*   **ADULTS AND CHILDREN OVER 12 YEARS OLD:** 325 to 650 mg every 4 hours as needed.   **CHILDREN:** 11 years old; 480 mg; 9 to 10 years old; 400 mg; 6 to 8 years old; 325 mg; 4 to 5 years old; 240 mg; 2 to 3 years old; 160 mg.   **Rheumatoid arthritis:** *PO:*   **ADULTS:** 3.6 to 5.4 g daily in divided doses.   *Special patient populations:*   **CHILDREN:** Pediatric doses are given above. In children given aspirin for varicella infections or influenza-like symptoms, there seems to be an increased risk for the development of Reye's syndrome, although a causal relationship has not been established. Because of this concern, acetaminophen is preferred as an antipyretic for these symptoms.   **PREGNANCY:** Salicylates readily cross the placenta. Fetal abnormalities have been demonstrated with high salicylate concentrations in animal studies. Taken chronically in high doses, salicylates may prolong gestation and increase the risk of maternal or fetal hemorrhage.

**PREPARATIONS**   *Tablets:* 325 or 650 mg. *tablets (enteric-coated):* 325 or 650 mg. *injection:* 100 mg/ml.

**DRUG INTERACTIONS**   **Salicylates** may potentiate protein-bound drugs, anticoagulants, oral hypoglycemic drugs, methotrexate, and anticonvulsants.   **Salicylates** may interfere with uricosuric drugs and loop diuretics.   **Urine acidifying agents** depress excretion of salicylates. Toxic levels of salicylate may accumulate. See entry for drug class (p. 870) for more complete information on drug interactions with salicylates.

**DIAGNOSTIC TEST INTERFERENCE**   Salicylates may interfere with several urine tests, including those for sugar, acetoacetic acid, and vanillylmandelic acid. See entry for drug class for more complete information on drug interactions with salicylates.

*Antipyretic; antiinflammatory; sclerosing agent.

**FATE**    The *onset of action* is about 20 minutes, and the *duration of action* is 4 to 6 hours for the analgesic/antipyretic effect. For arthritic swelling and pain, maximum relief may take 2 to 3 weeks to achieve. In acidic urine, salicylic acid is uncharged and therefore diffuses back into the blood. In alkaline urine, salicylic acid is charged and therefore stays in the urine and is excreted. Salicylate is metabolized to inactive salicyluric acid by the liver; however, a single 325 mg dose of salicylate will saturate this liver inactivation system. This means that the liver cannot readily metabolize large doses of salicylates, and the duration of action is greatly increased.

## ❦ NURSING CONSIDERATIONS

### Side effects, toxicities, and associated nursing actions    Side effects for all salicylates are the same; see
Nursing Considerations for aspirin (p. 871).

### Nursing interventions related to drug administration
* Enteric-coated tablets should be swallowed whole, not chewed or crushed.
* For IV administration, dilute ordered dose in 1 liter of 0.9% sodium chloride injection of lactated Ringer's injections, and administer over 4 to 8 hours.

### Patient and family education
* Review the anticipated benefits and possible side effects of drug therapy with patients.
* Tell patients to keep these and all medications out of the reach of children. Children should never be encouraged to take medications by being told they are candy. Tell patients to seek medical help immediately if overdose is suspected.
* Instruct patients to read labels of all medications carefully. Many over-the-counter products for pain and for treatment of sinus problems, colds, or menstrual problems contain aspirin or salicylates, alone or in combination with other drugs. Remind patients to avoid taking several drugs simultaneously unless absolutely necessary.
* Remind patients to take this drug only as directed.
* Pain or fever that persists beyond 3 to 5 days may signal a more serious health problem. Instruct patients to seek medical help rather than to self-medicate indefinitely.
* Remind patients to keep all health care providers informed of all medications being taken.
* Note Contraindications in the Overview of Drug Class (p. 869) and Dosage. Tell parents to avoid aspirin or salicylates in treating fever or discomfort in children with varicella infections or influenzalike symptoms.
* Patients on chronic therapy should avoid the use of alcohol.
* See entry for aspirin (p. 872).

---

## sodium thiosalicylate    (thye-oh-sah-LIS-i-late)                                            analgesic*

* sodium thiosalicylate: Arthrolate, Rexolate

**MECHANISM OF ACTION**    Sodium thiosalicylate is an inhibitor of prostaglandin synthesis, as are other NSAIDs (see Chapter 48).

**INDICATIONS**
* Muscular pain. • Rheumatic fever. • Arthritis including osteoarthritis, musculoskeletal disorders, acute gout.

**CONTRAINDICATIONS**    **Bleeding ulcers** In addition, caution should be used when patients have gastritis or peptic ulcers.    **Hemorrhagic disorders, hemophilia** In addition, caution should be used when patients are anemic, have impaired liver function, hypoprothrombinemia, or other conditions that compromise blood clotting.    **Severe renal function impairment** Salicylates are excreted via the kidney. In addition, caution should be used with patients prone to fluid retention, as in hypertension and congestive heart failure.

**DOSAGE**    **Rheumatic fever:** *IM or IV:*    **ADULTS:** 100 to 150 mg every 4 to 6 hours for 3 days, followed by 100 mg twice daily until symptoms disappear.    **Osteoarthritis:** *IM or IV:*    **ADULTS:** 100 mg three times

*Antipyretic; antiinflammatory.

weekly. Musculoskeletal pain:*IM or IV:* ADULTS: 50 to 100 mg once daily or every other day. **Acute gout:** *IM or IV:* ADULTS: 100 mg every 3 to 4 hours for 2 days, then 100 mg daily until symptoms disappear. *Special patient populations:* CHILDREN: Not recommended for children. PREGNANCY: Salicylates readily cross the placenta. Fetal abnormalities have been demonstrated with high salicylate concentrations in animal studies. Taken chronically in high doses, salicylates may prolong gestation and increase the risk of maternal or fetal hemorrhage.

**PREPARATIONS** *Injection:* 50 mg/ml.

**DRUG INTERACTIONS** **Salicylates** may potentiate protein-bound drugs, anticoagulants, oral hypoglycemic drugs, methotrexate, and anticonvulsants. **Salicylates** may interfere with uricosuric drugs and loop diuretics. **Urine acidifying agents** depress excretion of salicylates. Toxic levels of salicylate may accumulate. • See entry for drug class (p. 870) for more complete information on drug interactions with salicylates.

**LABORATORY TEST INTERFERENCE** Salicylates may interfere with several urine tests, including those for sugar, acetoacetic acid, and vanilymandelic acid. See entry for drug class for more complete information on drug interactions with salicylates.

**FATE** For arthritic swelling and pain, maximum relief may take 2 to 3 weeks to achieve. The pharmacokinetics of thiosalicylates are not well characterized.

## 🦋 NURSING CONSIDERATIONS

### Side effects, toxicities, and associated nursing actions
Side effects for all salicylates are the same; see Nursing Considerations for aspirin (p. 871).

### Nursing interventions related to drug administration
- For IM administration, large muscle masses should be used. Record sites and rotate sites.
- For IV administration, administer slowly.

### Patient and family education
- Review the anticipated benefits and possible side effects of drug therapy with patients.
- Tell patients to keep these and all medications out of the reach of children. Children should never be encouraged to take medications by being told they are candy. Tell patients to seek medical help immediately if overdose is suspected.
- Instruct patients to read labels of all medications carefully. Many over-the-counter products for pain and for treatment of sinus problems, colds, or menstrual problems contain aspirin or salicylates, alone or in combination with other drugs. Remind patients to avoid taking several drugs simultaneously unless absolutely necessary.
- Remind patients to take this drug only as directed.
- Pain or fever that persists beyond 3 to 5 days may signal a more serious health problem. Instruct patients to seek medical help rather than to self-medicate indefinitely.
- Remind patients to keep all health care providers informed of all medications being taken.
- Note Contraindications in the Overview of Drug Class and Dosage. Tell parents to avoid aspirin or salicylates in treating fever or discomfort in children with varicella infections or influenzalike symptoms.
- Patients on chronic therapy should avoid the use of alcohol.
- See entry for aspirin (p. 872).

# Chapter Forty-eight

# Nonsteroidal antiinflammatory drugs

| | |
|---|---|
| fenoprofen | naproxen |
| flurbiprofen (See Chapter 61) | oxyphenbutazone |
| ibuprofen | phenylbutazone |
| indomethacin | piroxicam |
| ketoprofen | sulindac |
| meclofenamate | suprofen |
| mefenamic acid | tolmetin |

**OVERVIEW OF THE DRUG CLASS** Nonsteroidal antiinflammatory drugs (NSAIDs) have three major actions: analgesic, antipyretic, and antiinflammatory. Limiting factors to the use of NSAIDs include their tendency to reduce blood clotting and to cause gastrointestinal bleeding. Aspirin is the prototype of the nonsteroidal antiinflammatory drugs. For many years aspirin has been the first drug used to control the pain and inflammation of rheumatoid arthritis. During the past few years several new drugs have been developed that like aspirin, are analgesic, antipyretic, and antiinflammatory. These new drugs are prescription drugs, with the exception of ibuprofen, which is now available as an over-the-counter medication.

**MECHANISM OF ACTION** The primary mechanism of action of the NSAIDs is believed to be the inhibition of the enzyme cyclooxygenase, the enzyme key to the formation of prostaglandins. Prostaglandins are chemical mediators synthesized by most cells from phospholipid components of the membrane. The synthesis of prostaglandins is triggered by other mediators. In turn, the prostaglandins alter a number of physiologic processes. The identity of the prostaglandin formed and the specific receptors of the tissue target determine the physiologic response. In general, prostaglandins affect smooth muscle, leading to contraction or relaxation, depending on the smooth muscle and the specific prostaglandin. However, other responses include inhibition and potentiation of platelet aggregation, increase and decrease in urine formation, and a variety of metabolic and endocrine functions.

Prostaglandins play an important role in inflammation. Prostaglandins are synthesized in response to mechanical, thermal, chemical, bacterial, and other insults, and the subsequent actions of the prostaglandins contribute to the signs and symptoms of inflammation and control of the immunologic response. The antiinflammatory action of the NSAIDs arises from their suppression of prostaglandin synthesis. The NSAIDs also inhibit the early steps in neutrophil activation. Activated neutrophils also release prostaglandins and other products involved in the inflammatory reaction.

**INDICATIONS** **Inflammation** The NSAIDs are prescribed as analgesic antiinflammatory drugs for patients with rheumatoid arthritis who cannot tolerate aspirin. **Pain** NSAIDs are prescribed for patients with painful joint disorders, with or without inflammation, such as osteoarthritis, ankylosing spondylitis, low back pain, and gout. **Dysmenorrhea** Menstrual cramps appear to be due to the overproduction of prostaglandins by the uterus at the time of menstruation. The prostaglandins can cause the uterus to contract to the point of cramping, producing dysmenorrhea. The newer NSAIDs are very effective in eliminating menstrual cramps, particularly if therapy is begun a few days before menses begins.

**CONTRAINDICATIONS** **Peptic ulcer** Prostaglandins protect gastric mucosa and inhibit gastric acid secretion. The gastrointestinal irritation common to aspirin and the other NSAIDs may arise because this protection of gastric mucosa and inhibition of acid secretion is eliminated when these drugs, which are prostaglandin synthesis inhibitors, are present in the stomach. **Hypersensitivity** There is a cross-sensitivity between aspirin and other NSAIDs. Also, asthma may be exacerbated by NSAIDs. **Liver or renal impairment** Most NSAIDs are metabolized by the liver. NSAIDs in high concentrations may cause renal damage.

**DRUG INTERACTIONS** **Protein-bound drugs** In general, the NSAIDs are protein bound and can displace other drugs, especially hydantoins, sulfonamides, sulfonylureas, nifedipine, and verapamil, leading to an increased incidence of the side effects of these drugs. **Acetaminophen** NSAIDs may increase the risk of renal damage if acetaminophen is used concurrently for prolonged periods. **All anticoagulants and thrombolytics, glucocorticoids, alcohol** NSAIDs may increase risk of gastrointestinal side effects, especially ulceration or hemorrhage. **Oral hypoglycemics, insulin** NSAIDs may increase the hypoglycemic effect. Sulfonylureas may also be displaced from binding to plasma proteins, increasing hypoglycemic action. **Diuretics** NSAIDs may decrease their diuretic and antihypertensive effects. The risk of renal failure increases.    **Aspirin or a combination of NSAIDs** Concurrent use increases the incidence of gastrointestinal effects, including ulceration and hemorrhage. Concurrent use of aspirin in general increases the risk of bleeding at all sites.    **Azlocillin, carbenicillin, dextran, dipyridamole, mezlocillin, piperacillin, sulfinpyrazone, ticarcillin, valproic acid** increase the risk of bleeding with NSAIDs because of added inhibition of platelet aggregation.    **Cefamandole, cefoperazone, moxalactam, plicamycin** cause hypoprothrombinemia and decreased platelet aggregation and thereby increase the risk of bleeding when taken in combination with NSAIDs.    **Gold compounds** There is an increased risk of adverse renal effects when taken with NSAIDs.    **Methotrexate** NSAIDs should be discontinued in time to be eliminated from the body before methotrexate is administered. **Probenecid** May decrease the excretion of NSAIDs, causing an increase in the serum concentration of an NSAID.

**DIAGNOSTIC TEST INTERFERENCE**    **Serum potassium concentration** Increased by NSAIDs.    **Serum transaminase concentration** Increased by NSAIDs.

---

## fenoprofen calcium    (fen-oh-PROE-fen)    *antiinflammatory analgesic*

- fenoprofen: Nalfon

**MECHANISM OF ACTION**    Fenoprofen is a nonsteroidal antiinflammatory drug (NSAID). NSAIDs inhibit the enzyme cyclooxygenase and thereby prevent the formation of prostaglandins and thromboxanes. See entry for drug class for more information.

**INDICATIONS**    **Pain and inflammation** Used for rheumatoid arthritis, osteoarthritis, ankylosing spondylitis, acute gouty arthritis.

**CONTRAINDICATIONS**    • Hypersensitivity to fenoprofen or to another NSAID, including aspirin. • Gastrointestinal bleeding or ulcer. • Impaired renal function.

**DOSAGE**    **PO:**   **ADULTS:** 300 to 600 mg, three to four times daily, up to 3.2 g daily.   *Special patient populations:*   **ELDERLY:** Patients over 70 years old generally require only half the usual adult dose. Geriatric patients are more susceptible to the toxic effects of NSAIDs, particularly the gastrointestinal, hepatic, renal, and CNS effects.   **CHILDREN:** Not recommended for children under 12 years old. **PREGNANCY:** Safe use has not been established. Inhibitors of prostaglandin synthesis may have adverse effects on fetal circulation and may interfere with labor and delay parturition.

**PREPARATIONS**    *Capsules:* 200 or 300 mg; *tablets:* 600 mg.

**DRUG INTERACTIONS**    **Protein-bound drugs** In general, the NSAIDs are protein-bound and can displace other drugs, especially hydantoins, sulfonamides, and sulfonylureas.    **Anticoagulant and thrombolytic drugs** may have additive effects with NSAIDs that inhibit platelet aggregation and cause GI bleeding. **Salicylates** tend to compete with other NSAIDs for protein-binding. NSAIDs may be more rapidly metabolized.    **Phenobarbital** may induce liver microsomal enzymes, leading to more rapid degradation of the NSAID. See entry for drug class for a more complete list common to the NSAIDs.

**FATE**    Fenoprofen is well absorbed and highly bound to plasma protein. The *onset of action* is 15 to 30 minutes; the *peak effect* is 2 to 3 hours; and the *duration of action* is 4 to 6 hours. Fenoprofen is metabolized in the liver and excreted in the urine.

### ☙ NURSING CONSIDERATIONS

#### Side effects, toxicities, and associated nursing actions

**CNS** Headache, sleepiness; occasionally, dizziness, tremor, confusion, nervousness, fatigue; paresthesia or weakness.

**Eye** Occasionally, blurred vision.

- Obtain a thorough baseline assessment prior to initiating drug therapy.
- Caution patients to avoid driving or operating hazardous equipment until the effects of the medication can be evaluated.
- Caution patients to notify the physician if visual changes or CNS effects develop.

- Periodic ophthalmologic examinations should be performed on patients on long-term therapy.

**GI** Dyspepsia, constipation, nausea, vomiting; occasionally, abdominal pain, anorexia, diarrhea, flatulence; metallic taste, ulceration of the cheek mucosa.
- Taking doses with meals, snack, antacids, or a large volume of water or milk (240 ml) may lessen gastric irritation.
- Monitor intake, output, and weight if vomiting, diarrhea, or anorexia is severe.
- Monitor stools for occult blood.

**GU** Problems with urination, nephrotic syndrome, renal failure.
- Monitor weight and blood pressure.
- Monitor intake and output, urinalysis, serum electrolytes, BUN, creatinine.

**Hematologic** Anemia, prolongation of bleeding time, easy bruising, thrombocytopenia.
- Monitor complete blood count, differential, platelet count, bleeding time.
- Inspect patient for development of petechiae, unexplained bruising, oozing from gums, nosebleeds, fever, rash, sore throat, stomatitis, malaise.
- Instruct patient to report the development of any unexplained bleeding, oozing from gums, nosebleeds.
- Monitor stools for occult blood.
- Be especially alert to bleeding in persons also receiving anticoagulants.

**Skin** Pruritis, rash, urticaria, sweating.
- Inspect for development of skin changes.

**Metabolic** Hepatic effects, including jaundice, cholestatic hepatitis.
- Monitor liver function tests.
- Assess for the development of jaundice, right upper quadrant abdominal pain, change in color or consistency of stools.

### Nursing interventions related to drug administration
- Tablet may be crushed, or contents of capsule may be mixed with applesauce or other food for ease in taking ordered dose.

### Patient and family education
- Review anticipated benefits and possible side effects of drug therapy with patients. Caution patients to report the development of any unexpected sign or symptom.
- Remind patients to take medications only as ordered.
- Remind patients to keep all health care providers informed of all medications being taken.
- Instruct patients that 2 to 4 weeks of therapy may be necessary before significant improvement is seen in arthritic conditions.

---

## ibuprofen (eye-byoo-PRO-fen)      antiinflammatory analgesic

- ibuprofen: Advil, ♣Apo-Ibuprofen, Motrin, ♣Novoprofen, Nuprin, Rufen

**MECHANISM OF ACTION** Ibuprofen is a nonsteroidal antiinflammatory drug (NSAID). NSAIDs inhibit the enzyme cyclooxygenase and thereby present the formation of prostaglandins and thromboxanes. See entry for drug class for more information.

**INDICATIONS** **Pain** Mild to moderate pain, postpartum, dental, and orthopedic pain, and dysmenorrhea. **Pain and inflammation** Used for rheumatoid arthritis, osteoarthritis, ankylosing spondylitis, acute gouty arthritis.

**CONTRAINDICATIONS** • Hypersensitivity to ibuprofen or to other NSAIDs, including aspirin. • Gastrointestinal bleeding or ulcer.

**DOSAGE** **PO:** **ADULTS:** Pain, fever, dysmenorrhea: 200 to 400 mg every 4 to 6 hours. Arthritis: 400 to 800 mg three or four times daily, not to exceed 3.2 g daily. **CHILDREN:** Arthritis: under 20 kg, 400 mg daily; 20 to 30 kg, 600 mg daily: 30 to 40 kg, 800 mg daily. Larger children receive adult doses. *Special patient populations:* **CHILDREN:** Not recommended for self-medication in children under 12 years old. **PREGNANCY:** Safe use has not been established. Inhibitors of prostaglandin synthesis may have adverse effects on fetal circulation and may interfere with labor and delay parturition.

**PREPARATIONS**   *Tablets:* 200 (OTC strength), or 300, 400, 600, 800 mg; *tablets (film-coated):* 400 or 600 mg.

**DRUG INTERACTIONS**   **Protein-bound drugs** In general, the NSAIDs are protein-bound and can displace other drugs, especially hydantoins, sulfonamides, and sulfonylureas.   **Anticoagulant and thrombolytic drugs** may have additive effects with NSAIDs that inhibit platelet aggregation and cause GI bleeding. **Salicylates** tend to compete with other NSAIDs for protein-binding. NSAID may be more rapidly metabolized. See entry for drug class (p. 882) for a more complete list common to the NSAIDs.

**FATE**   Ibuprofen is rapidly absorbed and highly bound to plasma protein. Ibuprofen is metabolized in the liver and excreted in the urine. The *onset of action* is 30 minutes. The *duration of action* and *plasma half-life* are 2 to 4 hours.

## 🍎 NURSING CONSIDERATIONS

### Side effects, toxicities, and associated nursing actions

**CNS** Dizziness, headache, nervousness, tinnitus.

**Eye** Rarely, blurred vision.

• Obtain a thorough baseline assessment prior to initiating drug therapy.

• Caution patients to avoid driving or operating hazardous equipment until the effects of the medication can be evaluated.

• Caution patients to notify the physician if visual changes or CNS effects develop.

• Periodic ophthalmologic examinations should be performed on patients on long-term therapy.

**CV** Congestive heart failure in patients with compromised cardiac function.

• Monitor weight, blood pressure, intake, output. Assess for jugular venous distention, development of edema.

**GI** Dyspepsia, heartburn, nausea, vomiting, anorexia, diarrhea, constipation, flatulence; rarely, bleeding or ulcer.

• Taking doses with meals, snack, antacids, or a large volume of water or milk (240 ml) may lessen gastric irritation.

• Monitor intake, output, and weight if vomiting, diarrhea, or anorexia is severe.

• Monitor stools for occult blood.

**GU** Acute renal failure in patients with compromised renal function.

• Monitor weight and blood pressure.

• Monitor intake and output, urinalysis, serum electrolytes, BUN, creatinine.

**Hematologic** Prolonged bleeding.

• Monitor complete blood count, differential, platelet count, bleeding time.

• Inspect patient for development of petechiae, unexplained bruising, oozing from gums, nosebleeds, fever, rash, sore throat, stomatitis, malaise.

• Instruct patient to report the development of any unexplained bleeding, oozing from gums, nosebleeds.

• Monitor stools for occult blood.

• Be especially alert to bleeding in persons also receiving anticoagulants.

**Skin** Hypersensitivity.

• Inspect for development of skin changes.

**Metabolic** Rarely, hepatic reactions.

• Monitor liver function tests.

• Assess for the development of jaundice, right upper quadrant abdominal pain, change in color or consistency of stools.

### Nursing interventions related to drug administration

• Tablet may be crushed and mixed with applesauce or other food for ease in taking ordered dose.

### Patient and family education

• Review anticipated benefits and possible side effects of drug therapy with patients. Caution patients to report the development of any unexpected sign or symptom.

• Remind patients to take medications only as ordered.

• Remind patients to keep all health care providers informed of all medications being taken.

• Instruct patients that 2 to 4 weeks of therapy may be necessary before significant improvement is seen in arthritic conditions.

# indomethacin (in-doe-METH-a-sin) antiinflammatory analgesic

- indomethacin sodium trihydrate: Indocin
- indomethacin: ✽Apo-Indomethacin, ✽Indocid, Indameth, Indocin, Indomed, Indo-Lemmon, ✽Novomethacin

**MECHANISM OF ACTION** Indomethacin is a nonsteroidal antiinflammatory drug (NSAID). NSAIDs inhibit the enzyme cyclooxygenase and thereby prevent the formation of prostaglandins and thromboxanes. See entry for drug class for more information (p. 882).

**INDICATIONS** **Arthritis, bursitis** Not for long-term use but for acute flare-ups of rheumatoid arthritis, ankylosing spondylitis, osteoarthritis, bursitis and/or tendonitis, gouty arthritis. **Patent ductus arteriosus** In small, preterm infants, the ductus arteriosus may not close at birth. This causes a shunt of blood from the left to the right side of the heart, leading to congestive heart failure and poor pulmonary function. Treatment with indomethacin causes the duct to close.

**CONTRAINDICATIONS** • Hypersensitivity to indomethacin or to other NSAIDs, including aspirin. • Gastrointestinal bleeding or ulcer.

**DOSAGE** **PO:** **ADULTS:** 25 mg two to four times daily. This may be increased if needed and if tolerated. Sustained-release form: 75 mg daily replaces taking 25 mg three times daily; 75 mg two times daily for daily doses over 150 mg. The sustained-release form should not be used for acute gouty arthritis. **IV:** **NEONATES:** Initially, 0.2 mg/kg. May repeat at 12 to 24 hour intervals if needed for a total dose of 0.6 mg/kg. *Special patient populations:* **ELDERLY:** Patients over 70 years old generally require only half the usual adult dose. Geriatric patients are more suceptible to the toxic effects of NSAIDs, particularly the gastrointestinal, hepatic, renal, and CNS effects. **CHILDREN:** Not recommended for children under 14 years old, except for neonates as described above. **PREGNANCY:** Safe use has not been established. Inhibitors of prostaglandin synthesis may have adverse effects on fetal circulation and may interfere with labor and delay parturition.

**PREPARATIONS** *Capsules:* 25 or 50 mg; *capsules (extended release):* 75 mg; *suspension:* 25 mg/ 5 ml; *suppositories:* 50 mg. *Indomethacin sodium trihydrate, parenteral:* 1 mg. *Incompatibilities:* indomethacin is unstable in an alkaline solution.

**DRUG INTERACTIONS** **Protein-bound drugs** In general, the NSAIDs are protein-bound and can displace other drugs, especially hydantoins, sulfonamides, and sulfonylureas. **Anticoagulant and thrombolytic drugs** may have additive effects with NSAIDs that inhibit platelet aggregation and cause GI bleeding. **Salicylates** tend to compete with other NSAIDs for protein-binding. NSAIDs may be more rapidly metabolized. **Hypotensive drugs and diuretics** Indomethacin can reduce the antihypertensive effects of captopril, furosemide, thiazide diuretics, and beta blockers. **Potassium-increasing agents** Indomethacin may increase serum potassium concentrations. Use cautiously with potassium chloride, triamterene, geriatric patients, neonates. **Lithium** Indomethacin may increase serum lithium concentrations, causing lithium toxicity. **Probenecid** Indomethacin concentrations are increased in patients receiving probenecid. See entry for drug class (p. 882) for a more complete list common to the NSAIDs.

**DIAGNOSTIC TEST INTERFERENCE** **Dexamethasone suppression** Indomethacin may produce false-negative results for this measurement of glucocorticoid suppression in the test for endogenous depression. **5-HIAA** Falsely high levels of urinary 5-hydroxyindoleacetic acid may be measured. See entry for drug class for a more complete list common to the NSAIDs.

**FATE** Indomethacin is well absorbed and highly bound to plasma protein. The *onset* of antigout action is 2 to 4 hours but may take 7 to 14 days for the antirheumatic action. The *peak effect* is 24 to 36 hours for the antigout effect, although the swelling may not subside for 3 to 5 days. The antirheumatic *peak effect* is about 4 weeks. The *plasma half-life* is 3 to 11 hours in adults; in neonates it may be 20 to 28 hours. Geriatric patients also eliminate the drug more slowly. Indomethacin is metabolized in the liver to inactive metabolites and is excreted in the urine and feces.

## ❦ NURSING CONSIDERATIONS
### Side effects, toxicities, and associated nursing actions
**CNS** Headache, tinnitus, incoordination, tremor, dizziness, insomnia.

**Eye** Corneal deposits and retinal disturbances. Retrolental hyperplasia has been reported in 3% to 9% of premature infants.
- Obtain a thorough baseline assessment prior to initiating drug therapy.
- Caution patients to avoid driving or operating hazardous equipment until the effects of the medication can be evaluated.
- Caution patients to notify the physician if visual changes or CNS effects develop.
- Periodic ophthalmologic examinations should be performed on patients on long-term therapy.

**CV** Congestive heart failure and cardiac irregularities are rare side effects.
- Monitor pulse, blood pressure, intake and output, and weight. Observe for development of edema.
- Instruct patient to report weight gain greater than 2 to 5 pounds per week.

**GI** Dyspepsia, nausea, vomiting; GI bleeding occurs in 3% to 9% of neonates.
- Taking doses with meals, snack, antacids, or a large volume of water or milk (240 ml) may lessen gastric irritation.
- Monitor intake, output, and weight if vomiting, diarrhea, or anorexia is severe.

**GU** Hematuria, nephritis, increased serum potassium.
- Inspect urine for signs of hematuria.
- Monitor urinalysis, serum electrolytes, BUN, creatinine.

**Hematologic** Anemia, prolongation of bleeding time.
- Monitor complete blood count, differential, platelet count, bleeding time.
- Inspect patient for development of petechiae, unexplained bruising.
- Instruct patient to report the development of any unexplained bleeding, oozing from gums, nosebleeds.
- Monitor stools for occult blood.
- Be especially alert to bleeding in persons also receiving anticoagulants.

**Skin** Hypersensitivity reactions.
- Visually inspect for development of skin changes.

**Metabolic** Hepatitis.
- Monitor liver function tests.
- Assess for the development of jaundice, right upper quadrant abdominal pain, change in color or consistency of stools.

### Nursing interventions related to drug administration
- Capsules may be opened and contents mixed with food or liquid for ease in taking ordered dose.
- For IV use, dilute sterile powder with 1 or 2 ml of sterile water for injection or 0.9% sodium chloride injection to make a concentration of 1 or 0.5 mg/ml. Do not use diluents containing preservatives. Inject over 5 to 10 seconds. Avoid extravasation.

### Patient and family education
- Review anticipated benefits and possible side effects of drug therapy with patients. Caution patients to report the development of any unexpected sign or symptom.
- Remind patients to take medications only as ordered.
- Remind patients to keep all health care providers informed of all medications being taken.
- Instruct patients that 2 to 4 weeks of therapy may be necessary before significant improvement is seen in arthritic conditions.

---

## ketoprofen    (key-toe-PROE-fen)                                    antiinflammatory analgesic

- ketoprofen: Orudis

**MECHANISM OF ACTION**    Ketoprofen is a nonsteroidal antiinflammatory drug (NSAID). NSAIDs inhibit the enzyme cylcooxygenase and thereby prevent the formation of prostaglandins and thromboxanes. See entry for drug class for more information (p. 882).

**INDICATIONS**    Pain and inflammation Rheumatoid arthritis, osteoarthritis, and ankylosing spondylitis.

**CONTRAINDICATIONS**    • Hypersensitivity to ketoprofen or to other NSAIDs, including aspirin. • Gastrointestinal bleeding or ulcer.

**DOSAGE**    PO:    **ADULTS:** 150 to 300 mg daily divided into three to four doses.    *Special patient populations:* **ELDERLY:** Patients over 70 years old generally require only half the usual adult dose. Geriatric patients are more susceptible to the toxic effects of NSAIDs, particularly the gastrointestinal, hepatic, renal, and CNS effects.    **CHILDREN:** Not recommended for children under 12 years old.    **PREGNANCY:** Safe use has not been established. Inhibitors of prostaglandin synthesis may have adverse effects on fetal circulation and may interfere with labor and delay parturition (FDA pregnancy category C).

**PREPARATIONS**    *Capsules:* 50 or 75 mg.

**DRUG INTERACTIONS**    **Protein-bound drugs** In general, the NSAIDs are protein bound and can displace other drugs, especially hydantoins, sulfonamides, and sulfonylureas.    **Anticoagulant and thrombolytic drugs** may have additive effects with NSAIDs that inhibit platelet aggregation and cause GI bleeding. **Salicylates** tend to compete with other NSAIDs for protein-binding. NSAIDs may be more rapidly metabolized.    **Phenobarbital** may induce liver microsomal enzymes, leading to more rapid degradation of the NSAID. See entry for drug class for a more complete list common to the NSAIDs.

**FATE**    Ketoprofen is well absorbed and highly bound to plasma protein. The *onset of action* is 15 to 30 minutes, and the *duration of action* is 4 to 6 hours. Ketoprofen is metabolized in the liver and excreted in the urine.

## 🐾 NURSING CONSIDERATIONS

### Side effects, toxicities, and associated nursing actions

**CNS** Headache, sleepiness, dizziness, fatigue, tinnitus.

• Obtain a thorough baseline assessment prior to initiating drug therapy.

• Caution patients to avoid driving or operating hazardous equipment until the effects of the medication can be evaluated.

• Caution patients to notify the physician if visual changes or CNS effects develop.

• Periodic ophthalmologic examinations should be performed on patients on long-term therapy.

• Assess for tinnitus. If hearing problems are suspected, refer patient for regular audiometric testing.

**GI** Dyspepsia, constipation, nausea, vomiting; occasionally, abdominal pain, anorexia, diarrhea, flatulence; mouth ulcers, sore tongue.

• Taking doses with meals, snack, antacids, or a large volume of water or milk (240 ml) may lessen gastric irritation.

• Monitor intake, output, and weight if vomiting, diarrhea, or anorexia is severe.

• Monitor stools for occult blood.

**Hematologic** Anemia, prolongation of bleeding time, easy bruising, thrombocytopenia.

• Monitor complete blood count, differential, platelet count, bleeding time.

• Inspect patient for development of petechiae, unexplained bruising, oozing from gums, nosebleeds, fever, rash, sore throat, stomatitis, malaise.

• Instruct patient to report the development of any unexplained bleeding, oozing from gums, nosebleeds.

• Monitor stools for occult blood.

• Be especially alert to bleeding in persons also receiving anticoagulants.

**Skin** Pruritis, rash, urticaria, sweating.

• Inspect for development of skin changes.

**Metabolic** Hepatic effects, including jaundice, cholestatic hepatitis. May give abnormal enzyme levels.

• Monitor liver function tests.

• Assess for the development of jaundice, right upper quadrant abdominal pain, change in color or consistency of stools.

### Nursing interventions related to drug administration

• Contents of capsules may be mixed with applesauce or other food for ease in taking ordered dose.

### Patient and family education

- Review anticipated benefits and possible side effects of drug therapy with patients. Caution patients to report the development of any unexpected sign or symptom.
- Remind patients to take medications only as ordered.
- Remind patients to keep all health care providers informed of all medications being taken.
- Instruct patients that 2 to 4 weeks of therapy may be necessary before significant improvement is seen in arthritic conditions.

---

## meclofenamate sodium (me-kloe-fen-AM-ate) antiinflammatory analgesic

- meclofenamate sodium: Meclomen

**MECHANISM OF ACTION** Meclofenamate is a nonsteroidal antiinflammatory drug (NSAID). NSAIDs inhibit the enzyme cylcooxygenase and thereby prevent the formation of prostaglandins and thromboxanes. See entry for drug class for more information (p. 882).

**INDICATIONS** **Pain and inflammation** Used for rheumatoid arthritis, osteoarthritis.

**CONTRAINDICATIONS** • Hypersensitivity to meclofenamate or to other NSAIDs, including aspirin. • Gastrointestinal bleeding or ulcer.

**DOSAGE** **PO:** **ADULTS:** 200 to 300 daily in four divided doses. *Special patient populations:* **ELDERLY:** Patients over 70 years old generally require only half the usual adult dose. Geriatric patients are more susceptible to the toxic effects of NSAIDs, particularly the gastrointestinal, hepatic, renal, and CNS effects. **CHILDREN:** Not recommended for children under 14 years old. **PREGNANCY:** Safe use has not been established. Inhibitors of prostaglandin synthesis may have adverse effects on fetal circulation and may interfere with labor and delay parturition. Animal studies have demonstrated fetotoxicity from meclofenamate.

**PREPARATIONS** *Capsules:* 50 or 100 mg.

**DRUG INTERACTIONS** **Protein bound drugs** In general, the NSAIDs are protein-bound and can displace other drugs, especially hydantoins, sulfonamides, and sulfonylureas. **Anticoagulant and thrombolytic drugs** may have additive effects with NSAIDs that inhibit platelet aggregation and cause GI bleeding. **Salicylates** tend to compete with other NSAIDs for protein-binding. NSAIDs may be more rapidly metabolized. **Phenobarbital** may induce liver microsomal enzymes, leading to more rapid degradation of the NSAID. See entry for drug class (p. 882) for a more complete list common to the NSAIDs.

**FATE** Meclofenamate is well absorbed and highly bound to plasma protein. The *onset of action* is 30 to 60 minutes, and the *duration of action* is 4 to 6 hours. Meclofenamate is metabolized in the liver and excreted in the urine and feces.

### NURSING CONSIDERATIONS

#### Side effects, toxicities, and associated nursing actions

**CNS** Headache, sleepiness; occasionally, dizziness, tremor, confusion, nervousness, paresthesia, weakness, fatigue; tinnitus.

**Eye** Occasionally, double vision.

- Obtain a thorough baseline assessment prior to initiating drug therapy.
- Caution patients to avoid driving or operating hazardous equipment until the effects of the medication can be evaluated.
- Caution patients to notify the physician if visual changes or CNS effects develop.
- Periodic ophthalmologic examinations should be performed on patients on long-term therapy.
- Assess for hearing changes. If hearing loss is suspected, audiometric testing should be done at regular intervals.

**GI** Diarrhea, dyspepsia, nausea, vomiting; occasionally, abdominal pain, anorexia, flatulence; ulceration of the cheek mucosa.

- Taking doses with meals, snack, antacids, or a large volume of water or milk (240 ml) may lessen gastric irritation.

- Monitor intake, output, and weight if vomiting, diarrhea, or anorexia is severe.

**Hematologic** Anemia, prolongation of bleeding time.

- Monitor complete blood count, differential, platelet count, bleeding time.
- Inspect patient for development of petechiae, unexplained bruising.
- Instruct patient to report the development of any unexplained bleeding, oozing from gums, nose-bleeds.
- Monitor stools for occult blood.
- Be especially alert to bleeding in persons also receiving anticoagulants.

**Skin** Pruritis, rash, urticaria, sweating.

- Inspect for development of skin changes.

**Metabolic** Hepatic effects, including jaundice, cholestatic hepatitis.

- Monitor liver function tests.
- Assess for the development of jaundice, right upper quadrant abdominal pain, change in color or consistency of stools.

### Nursing interventions related to drug administration

- Capsules may be opened and contents mixed with food or liquid for ease in taking ordered dose.

### Patient and family education

- Review anticipated benefits and possible side effects of drug therapy with patients. Caution patients to report the development of any unexpected sign or symptom.
- Remind patients to take medications only as ordered.
- Remind patients to keep all health care providers informed of all medications being taken.
- Instruct patients that 2 to 4 weeks of therapy may be necessary before significant improvement is seen in arthritic conditions.

---

## mefanamic acid  (me-fe-NAM-ik)  antiinflammatory analgesic

- mefanamic acid: Ponstel, ✦Ponstan

**MECHANISM OF ACTION**   Mefanamic acid is a nonsteroidal antiinflammatory drug (NSAID). NSAIDs inhibit the enzyme cylcooxygenase and thereby prevent the formation of prostaglandins and thromboxanes. See entry for drug class for more information (p. 882).

**INDICATIONS**   **Pain and inflammation** Muscular aches and pains, dysmenorrhea, dental and headache pain.

**CONTRAINDICATIONS**   • Hypersensitivity to mefanamic acid or to other NSAIDs including aspirin. • Gastrointestinal bleeding or ulcer.

**DOSAGE**   **PO:**   **ADULTS:** 500 mg initially, then 250 mg every 6 hours as needed.   *Special patient populations:*   **ELDERLY:** Patients over 70 years old generally require only half the usual adult dose. Geriatric patients are more susceptible to the toxic effects of NSAIDs, particularly the gastrointestinal, hepatic, renal, and CNS effects.   **CHILDREN:** Not recommended for children under 14 years old. **PREGNANCY:** Safe use has not been established. Inhibitors of prostaglandin synthesis may have adverse effects on fetal circulation and may interfere with labor and delay parturition.

**PREPARATIONS**   *Capsules:* 250 mg.

**DRUG INTERACTIONS**   **Protein-bound drugs** In general, the NSAIDs are protein-bound and can displace other drugs, especially hydantoins, sulfonamides, and sulfonylureas.   **Anticoagulant and thrombolytic drugs** may have additive effects with NSAIDs that inhibit platelet aggregation and cause GI bleeding. **Salicylates** tend to compete with other NSAIDs for protein-binding. NSAIDs may be more rapidly metabolized.   **Phenobarbital** may induce liver microsomal enzymes, leading to more rapid degradation of the NSAID. See entry for drug class (p. 882) for a more complete list common to the NSAIDs.

**DIAGNOSTIC TEST INTERFERENCE**   **Urinary bile** False-positive test results are possible when using the diazo tablet test.

**FATE**   Mefanamic acid is well absorbed and highly bound to plasma protein. The *onset of action* is 15 to 30 minutes, and the *duration of action* is 4 to 6 hours. Mefanamic acid is metabolized in the liver and excreted in the urine and feces.

## ❦ NURSING CONSIDERATIONS

### Side effects, toxicities, and associated nursing actions

**CNS** Headache, sleepiness; occasionally, dizziness, nervousness.

**Eye** Occasionally, double vision.

- Obtain a thorough baseline assessment prior to initiating drug therapy.
- Caution patients to avoid driving or operating hazardous equipment until the effects of the medication can be evaluated.
- Caution patients to notify the physician if visual changes or CNS effects develop.
- Periodic ophthalmologic examinations should be performed on patients on long-term therapy.

**GI** Diarrhea, dyspepsia, nausea, vomiting; occasionally, abdominal pain, anorexia, flatulence; metallic taste, ulceration of the cheek mucosa.

- Taking doses with meals, snack, antacids, or a large volume of water or milk (240 ml) may lessen gastric irritation.
- Monitor intake, output, and weight if vomiting, diarrhea, or anorexia is severe.

**Hematologic** Anemia, prolongation of bleeding time, easy bruising, thrombocytopenia.

- Monitor complete blood count, differential, platelet count, bleeding time.
- Inspect patient for development of petechiae, unexplained bruising.
- Instruct patient to report the development of any unexplained bleeding, oozing from gums, nosebleeds.
- Monitor stools for occult blood.
- Be especially alert to bleeding in persons also receiving anticoagulants.

**Skin** Pruritis, rash, urticaria, sweating.

- Inspect for development of skin changes.

**Metabolic** Hepatic effects, including altered liver function tests.

- Monitor liver function tests.
- Assess for the development of jaundice, right upper quadrant abdominal pain, change in color or consistency of stools.

### Nursing interventions related to drug administration

- Capsules may be opened and contents mixed with food or liquid for ease in taking ordered dose.

### Patient and family education

- Review anticipated benefits and possible side effects of drug therapy with patients. Caution patients to report the development of any unexpected sign or symptom.
- Remind patients to take medications only as ordered.
- Remind patients to keep all health care providers informed of all medications being taken.
- Instruct patients that 2 to 4 weeks of therapy may be necessary before significant improvement is seen in arthritic conditions.

---

## naproxen  (na-PROX-en)                                          antiinflammatory analgesic

- naproxen: Anaprox, Naprosyn ♣Apo-Naproxen, ♣Naxen, ♣Novonaprox

**MECHANISM OF ACTION**    Naproxen is a nonsteroidal antiinflammatory drug (NSAID). NSAIDs inhibit the enzyme cylcooxygenase and thereby prevent the formation of prostaglandins and thromboxanes. See entry for drug class for more information (p. 882).

**INDICATIONS**   **Pain and inflammation** Used for rheumatoid arthritis, osteoarthritis, ankylosing spondylitis, acute gouty arthritis; also muscular aches and pains, dysmenorrhea, dental and headache pain.

**CONTRAINDICATIONS**    • Hypersensitivity to naproxen or to other NSAIDs, including aspirin. • Gastrointestinal bleeding or ulcer

**DOSAGE**   **PO:**   **ADULTS:** Arthritis: 500 mg daily in divided doses. May increase gradually to 1000 mg if needed. For mild pain, dysmenorrhea: 500 mg initially, then 250 mg every 6 to 8 hours as needed. *Special patient populations:*   **ELDERLY:** Patients over 70 years old generally require only half the usual adult dose. Geriatric patients are more susceptible to the toxic effects of NSAIDs, particularly the gastrointestinal, hepatic, renal, and CNS effects. **CHIIDREN:** Not recommended for children under 14 years old. **PREGNANCY:** Safe use has not been estalbished. Inhibitors of prostaglandin synthesis may have adverse effects on fetal circulation and may interfere with labor and delay parturition (FDA pregnancy category B).

**PREPARATIONS** *Tablets:* 250, 375, or 500 mg. *sodium salt: tablets (film-coated):* 275 mg.

**DRUG INTERACTIONS** **Protein-bound drugs** In general, the NSAIDs are protein bound and can displace other drugs, especially hydantoins, sulfonamides, and sulfonylureas. **Anticoagulant and thrombolytic drugs** may have additive effects with NSAIDs that inhibit platelet aggregation and cause GI bleeding. **Salicylates** tend to compete with other NSAIDs for protein-binding. NSAIDs may be more rapidly metabolized. **Phenobarbital** may induce liver microsomal enzymes, leading to more rapid degradation of the NSAID. See entry for drug class (p. 882) for a more complete list common to the NSAIDs.

**DIAGNOSTIC TEST INTERFERENCE** **5-HIAA** Naproxen may interfere with the determination of urinary 5-hydroxyindoleacetic acid. **Urinary steroids** Naproxen may falsely increase concentrations of 17-ketogenic steroids measured with the m-dinitrobenzene reagent.

**FATE** Naproxen is well absorbed and highly bound to plasma protein. The *onset of action* is 1 to 2 hours, and the *duration of action* is 7 hours. Naproxen is metabolized in the liver and excreted in the urine.

## 🐦 NURSING CONSIDERATIONS

### Side effects, toxicities, and associated nursing actions

**CNS** Headache, sleepiness; occasionally, dizziness, fatigue, tremor, confusion, nervousness; tinnitus. **Eye** Occasionally double vision.
- Obtain a thorough baseline assessment prior to initiating drug therapy.
- Caution patients to avoid driving or operating hazardous equipment until the effects of the medication can be evaluated.
- Caution patients to notify the physician if visual changes or CNS effects develop.
- Periodic ophthalmologic examinations should be performed on patients on long-term therapy.
- Assess for tinnitus. If hearing problems are suspected, refer patient for regular audiometric testing.

**GI** Dyspepsia, constipation, nausea, vomiting; occasionally, abdominal pain, anorexia, diarrhea, flatulence.
- Taking doses with meals, snack, antacids, or a large volume of water or milk (240 ml) may lessen gastric irritation.
- Monitor intake, output, and weight if vomiting, diarrhea, or anorexia is severe.
- Monitor stools for occult blood.

**Hematologic** Anemia, prolongation of bleeding time, easy bruising, thrombocytopenia.
- Monitor complete blood count, differential, platelet count, bleeding time.
- Inspect patient for development of petechiae, unexplained bruising, oozing from gums, nosebleeds, fever, rash, sore throat, stomatitis, malaise.
- Instruct patient to report the development of any unexplained bleeding, oozing from gums, nosebleeds.
- Monitor stools for occult blood.
- Be especially alert to bleeding in persons also receiving anticoagulants.

**Skin** Pruritis, rash, urticaria, sweating.
- Inspect for development of skin changes.

**Metabolic** Hepatic effects, including jaundice, cholestatic hepatitis. May give abnormal enzyme levels.
- Monitor liver function tests.
- Assess for the development of jaundice, right upper quadrant abdominal pain, change in color or consistency of stools.

### Nursing intervenstions related to drug administration
- Tablets may be crushed and mixed with applesauce or other food for ease in taking ordered dose.

### Patient and family education
- Review anticipated benefits and possible side effects of drug therapy with patients. Caution patients to report the development of any unexpected sign or symptom.

- Remind patients to take medications only as ordered.
- Remind patients to keep all health care providers informed of all medications being taken.
- Instruct patients that 2 to 4 weeks of therapy may be necessary before significant improvement is seen in arthritic conditions.

## oxyphenbutazone (ox-i-fen-BYOO-ta-zone)    antiinflammatory analgesic

- oxyphenbutazone: generic; ✤Oxybutazone, ✤Tandearil

**MECHANISM OF ACTION**    Oxyphenbutazone is a nonsteroidal antiinflammatory drug (NSAID). NSAIDs inhibit the enzyme cylcooxygenase and thereby prevent the formation of prostaglandins and thromboxanes. See entry for drug class for more information (p. 882).

**INDICATIONS**    **Pain and inflammation** Used for short-term relief only: rheumatoid arthritis, osteoarthritis, ankylosing spondylitis, acute gouty arthritis.

**CONTRAINDICATIONS**    • Hypersensitivity to oxyphenbutazone or to other NSAIDs, including aspirin. • Gastrointestinal bleeding or ulcer.

**DOSAGE**    **PO:**    **ADULTS:** 300 to 600 mg daily in three or four doses. Improvement should be seen in 3 to 4 days. If no improvement occurs in 1 week, discontinue. *Special patient populations:* **ELDERLY:** Use cautiously in patients over 40 years old, especially in those over 60 years old. Patients over 70 years old generally require only half the usual adult dose. Geriatric patients are more susceptible to the toxic effects of NSAIDs, particularly the gastrointestinal, hepatic, renal, and CNS effects. **CHILDREN:** Not recommended for children under 14 years old. **PREGNANCY:** Safe use has not been established. Inhibitors of prostaglandin synthesis may have adverse effects on fetal circulation and may interfere with labor and delay parturition (FDA pregnancy category C).

**PREPARATIONS**    *Tablets:* 100 mg; *tablets (film-covered):* 100 mg.

**DRUG INTERACTIONS**    **Protein-bound drugs** In general, the NSAIDs are protein-bound and can displace other drugs, especially hydantoins, sulfonamides, and sulfonylureas. **Anticoagulant and thrombolytic drugs** May have additive effects with NSAIDs that inhibit platelet aggregation and cause GI bleeding. **Salicylates** tend to compete with other NSAIDs for protein-binding. NSAIDs may be more rapidly metabolized. **Phenobarbital** may induce liver microsomal enzymes, leading to more rapid degradation of the NSAID. **Phenytoin** Oxyphenbutazone may increase the serum concentration and plasma half-life of phenytoin, leading to phenytoin toxicity. **Methotrexate** Concommitant administration of methotrexate and oxyphenbutazone has caused widespread skin ulcers. **Hypoglycemic drugs** Oxyphenbutazone can displace oral hypoglycemic drugs from plasma protein, causing a hypoglycemic response. See entry for drug class (p. 882) for a more complete list common to the NSAIDs.

**FATE**    Oxyphenbutazone is well absorbed and highly bound to plasma protein. The *plasma half-life* is 50 to 100 hours. Oxyphenbutazone is metabolized in the liver and excreted in the urine.

## 🐦 NURSING CONSIDERATIONS

### Side effects, toxicities, and associated nursing actions

**CNS** Headache, sleepiness; occasionally, dizziness, tremor, confusion, nervousness, paresthesia, weakness, fatigue.

**Eye** Blurred vision, optic neuritis, amblyopia, scotomata, retinal detachment, and hemorrhage.

- Obtain a thorough baseline assessment prior to initiating drug therapy.
- Caution patients to avoid driving or operating hazardous equipment until the effects of the medication can be evaluated.
- Caution patients to notify the physician if visual changes or CNS effects develop.
- Periodic ophthalmologic examinations should be performed on patients on long-term therapy.

**GI** Dyspepsia, constipation, nausea, vomiting; occasionally, abdominal pain, anorexia, diarrhea, flatulence. Serious ulceration may develop, so the patient must be carefully monitored.

- Taking doses with meals, snack, antacids, or large volume of water or milk (240 ml) may lessen gastric irritation.

- Monitor intake, output, and weight if vomiting, diarrhea, or anorexia is severe.
- Monitor stools for occult blood.

**Hematologic** Anemia, prolongation of bleeding time, easy bruising, thrombocytopenia. Bone marrow depression is a serious problem and must be monitored on therapy over 2 weeks' duration.

- Monitor complete blood count, differential, platelet count, bleeding time.
- Inspect patient for development of petechiae, unexplained bruising, oozing from gums, nosebleeds, fever, rash, sore throat, stomatitis, malaise.
- Instruct patient to report the development of any unexplained bleeding, oozing from gums, nosebleeds.
- Monitor stools for occult blood.
- Be especially alert to bleeding in persons also receiving anticoagulants.

**Skin** Pruritis, rash, urticaria, sweating.

- Inspect for development of skin changes.

**Metabolic** Hepatic effects, including jaundice, cholestatic hepatitis. Fatal hepatitis may develop, so the patient must be monitored on therapy over 2 weeks' duration.

- Monitor liver function tests.
- Assess for the development of jaundice, right upper quadrant abdominal pain, change in color or consistency of stools.

**Nursing interventions related to drug administration**

- Capsules may be opened and contents mixed with food or liquid for ease in taking ordered dose.

**Patient and family education**

- Review anticipated benefits and possible side effects of drug therapy with patients. Caution patients to report the development of any unexpected sign or symptom.
- Remind patients to take medications only as ordered.

---

## phenylbutazone  (fen-ill-BYOO-ta-zone)  antiinflammatory analgesic

- phenylbutazone: ✚Apo-Phenylbutazone Azolid, Butagen, Butazolidin, Butazone, ✚Intrabutazone, ✚Neo-Zoline, ✚Novobutazone, ✚Phenbuff

**MECHANISM OF ACTION**  Phenylbutazone is a nonsteroidal antiinflammatory drug (NSAID). NSAIDs inhibit the enzyme cyclo-oxygenase and thereby prevent the formation of prostaglandins and thromboxanes. See entry for drug class (p. 882) for more information.

**INDICATIONS**  **Pain and inflammation** Used for short-term relief only: rheumatoid arthritis, osteoarthritis, ankylosing spondylitis, acute gouty arthritis.

**CONTRAINDICATIONS**  • Hypersensitivity to phenylbutazone or to other NSAIDs, including aspirin. • Gastrointestinal bleeding or ulcer.

**DOSAGE**  **PO:**  **ADULTS:** 300 to 600 mg daily in 3 or 4 doses. Improvement should be seen in 3 to 4 days. If no improvement in 1 week, discontinue.  *Special patient populations:*  **ELDERLY:** Use cautiously in patients over 40 years old and especially those over 60 years old. Patients over 70 years old generally require only half the usual adult dose. Geriatric patients are more susceptible to the toxic effects of NSAIDs, particularly the gastrointestinal, hepatic, renal, and CNS effects.  **CHILDREN:** Not recommended for children under 14 years old.  **PREGNANCY:** Safe use has not been established. Inhibitors of prostaglandin synthesis may have adverse effects on fetal circulation and may interfere with labor and delay parturition (FDA pregnancy category C).

**PREPARATIONS**  *Capsules:* 100 mg; *tablets (film-covered):* 100 mg.

**DRUG INTERACTIONS**  **Protein-bound drugs** In general, the NSAIDs are protein-bound and can displace other drugs, especially hydantoins, sulfonamides, and sulfonylureas.  **Anticoagulant and thrombolytic drugs** may have additive effects with NSAIDs that inhibit platelet aggregation and cause GI bleeding.  **Salicylates** tend to compete with other NSAIDs for protein-binding. NSAIDs may be more rapidly metabolized.  **Phenobarbital** may induce liver microsomal enzymes, leading to more rapid degradation of the NSAID.    **Phenytoin** Phenylbutazone may increase the serum concentration and plasma half-life of phenytoin, leading to phenytoin toxicity.    **Methotrexate** Concommitant administration of methotrexate and phenylbutazone has caused widespread skin ulcers.    **Hypoglycemic drugs** Phenylbutazone can displace oral hypoglycemic drugs from plasma protein, causing a hypoglycemic reaponse. See entry for drug class (p. 882) for a more complete list common to the NSAIDs.

**FATE**    Phenylbutazone is well absorbed and highly bound to plasma protein. The *plasma half-life* is 50 to 100 hours. Phenylbutazone is metabolized in the liver and excreted in the urine.

## 🖑 NURSING CONSIDERATIONS

### Side effects, toxicities, and associated nursing actions

**CNS** Headache, sleepiness; occasionally, dizziness, tremor, confusion, nervousness, paresthesia, weakness, fatigue.

**Eye** Blurred vision, optic neuritis, amblyopia, scotomata, retinal detachment, and hemorrhage.
* Obtain a thorough baseline assessment prior to initiating drug therapy.
* Caution patients to avoid driving or operating hazardous equipment until the effects of the medication can be evaluated.
* Caution patients to notify the physician if visual changes or CNS effects develop.
* Periodic ophthalmologic examinations should be performed on patients on long-term therapy.

**GI** Dyspepsia, constipation, nausea, vomiting; occasionally, abdominal pain, anorexia, diarrhea, flatulence. Serious ulceration may develop, so patients must be carefully monitored.
* Taking doses with meals, snack, antacids, or a large volume of water or milk (240 ml) may lessen gastric irritation.
* Monitor intake, output, and weight if vomiting, diarrhea, or anorexia is severe.
* Monitor stools for occult blood.

**Hematologic** Anemia, prolongation of bleeding time, easy bruising, thrombocytopenia. Bone marrow depression is a serious problem and must be monitored on therapy over 2 weeks' duration.
* Monitor complete blood count, differential, platelet count, bleeding time.
* Inspect patient for development of petechiae, unexplained bruising, oozing from gums, nosebleeds, fever, rash, sore throat, stomatitis, malaise.
* Instruct patient to report the develoment of any unexplained bleeding, oozing from gums, nosebleeds.
* Monitor stools for occult blood.
* Be especially alert to bleeding in persons also receiving anticoagulants.

**Skin** Pruritis, rash, urticaria, sweating.
* Inspect for development of skin changes.

**Metabolic** Hepatic effects, including jaundice, cholestatic hepatitis. The potential for fatal hepatitis is great, so patients on therapy over 2 weeks' duration must be monitored.
* Monitor liver function tests.
* Assess for the development of jaundice, right upper quadrant abdominal pain, change in color or consistency of stools.

### Nursing interventions related to drug administration
* Capsules may be opened and contents mixed with food or liquid for ease in taking ordered dose.

### Patient and family education
* Review anticipated benefits and possible side effects of drug therapy with patients. Caution patients to report the development of any unexpected sign or symptom.
* Remind patients to take medications only as ordered.
* Remind patients to keep all health care providers informed of all medications being taken.
* Instruct patients that 2 to 4 weeks of therapy may be necessary before significant improvement is seen in arthritic conditions.

---

## piroxicam    (peer-OX-i-kam)                                   antiinflammatory analgesic

* piroxicam: Feldene

**MECHANISM OF ACTION** Piroxicam is a nonsteroidal antiinflammatory drug (NSAID). NSAIDs inhibit the enzyme cyclooxygenase and thereby prevent the formation of prostaglandins and thromboxanes. See entry for drug class (p. 882) for more information.

**INDICATIONS** **Pain and inflammation** Used for rheumatoid arthritis and osteoarthritis.

**CONTRAINDICATIONS** • Hypersensitivity to piroxicam or to another NSAID, including aspirin. • Gastrointestinal bleeding or ulcer. • Renal disease: piroxicam can cause renal damage.

**DOSAGE** **PO:** **ADULTS:** 20 mg daily. Occasionally dosages of 30 or 40 mg daily are needed. *Special patient populations:* **ELDERLY:** Patients over 70 years old generally require only half the usual adult dose. Geriatric patients are more susceptible to the toxic effects of NSAIDs, particularly the gastrointestinal, hepatic, renal, and CNS effects. **CHILDREN:** Not recommended for children under 14 years old. **PREGNANCY:** Safe use has not been established. Inhibitors of prostaglandin synthesis may have adverse effects on fetal circulation and may interfere with labor and delay parturition.

**PREPARATIONS** *Capsules:* 10 or 20 mg.

**DRUG INTERACTIONS** **Protein-bound drugs** In general, the NSAIDs are protein-bound and can displace other drugs, especially hydantoins, sulfonamides, and sulfonylureas. **Anticoagulant and thrombolytic drugs** may have additive effects with NSAIDs that inhibit platelet aggregation and cause GI bleeding. **Salicylates** tend to compete with other NSAIDs for protein-binding. NSAIDs may be more rapidly metabolized. **Phenobarbital** may induce liver microsomal enzymes, leading to more rapid degradation of the NSAID. See entry for drug class (p. 882) for a more complete list common to the NSAIDs.

**FATE** Piroxicam is well absorbed and highly bound to plasma protein. The *onset of action* is 15 to 30 minutes. Piroxicam has a very long *plasma half-life,* 30 to 86 hours, and therefore accumulates on daily dosage. Piroxicam is is metabolized slowly in the liver and excreted in the urine and feces.

## 🦫 NURSING CONSIDERATIONS

### Side effects, toxicities, and associated nursing actions

**CNS** Headache, sleepiness; occasionally, dizziness, tremor, confusion, nervousness, fatigue; tinnitus.

**Eye** Occasionally, double vision.

- Obtain a thorough baseline assessment prior to initiating drug therapy.
- Caution patients to avoid driving or operating hazardous equipment until the effects of the medication can be evaluated.
- Caution patients to notify the physician if visual changes or CNS effects develop.
- Periodic ophthalmologic examinations should be performed on patients on long-term therapy.
- Monitor for changes in hearing acuity or development of tinnitus. If hearing changes are suspected, refer for regular audiometric testing.

**GI** About 20% of patients experience significant GI problems, including dyspepsia, constipation, nausea, vomiting; occasionally, abdominal pain, anorexia, diarrhea, flatulence; peptic ulcer with bleeding occurs in about 1% of patients.

- Taking doses with meals, snack, antacids, or a large volume of water or milk (240 ml) may lessen gastric irritation.
- Monitor intake, output, and weight if vomiting, diarrhea, or anorexia is severe.
- Monitor stools for occult blood.

**GU** Nephrotoxicity in about 1% of patients: nephrotic syndrome, renal failure.

- Monitor weight and blood pressure.
- Monitor intake and output, urinalysis, serum electrolytes, BUN, creatinine.

**Hematologic** Anemia, prolongation of bleeding time, easy bruising, thrombocytopenia.

- Monitor complete blood count, differential, platelet count, bleeding time.
- Inspect patient for development of petechiae, unexplained bruising, oozing from gums, nosebleeds, fever, rash, sore throat, stomatitis, malaise.
- Instruct patient to report the development of any unexplained bleeding, oozing from gums, nosebleeds.
- Monitor stools for occult blood.

- Be especially alert to bleeding in persons also receiving anticoagulants.

**Skin** Pruritis, rash, urticaria, sweating.

- Inspect for development of skin changes.

**Metabolic** Hepatic effects, including alterations in liver function tests.

- Monitor liver function tests.
- Assess for the development of jaundice, right upper quadrant abdominal pain, change in color or consistency of stools.

### Nursing interventions related to drug administration

- Capsules may be opened and contents mixed with applesauce or other food for ease in taking ordered dose.

### Patient and family education

- Review anticipated benefits and possible side effects of drug therapy with patients. Caution patients to report the development of any unexpected sign or symptom.
- Remind patients to take medications only as ordered.
- Remind patients to keep all health care providers informed of all medications being taken.
- Instruct patients that 2 to 4 weeks of therapy may be necessary before significant improvement is seen in arthritic conditions.

## sulindac  (sul-IN-dak)                                    antiinflammatory analgesic

- sulindac: Clinoril

**MECHANISM OF ACTION**   Sulindac is a nonsteroidal antiinflammatory drug (NSAID). NSAIDs inhibit the enzyme cyclooxygenase and thereby prevent the formation of prostaglandins and thromboxanes. See entry for drug class for more information (p. 882).

**INDICATIONS**   **Pain and inflammation** Used for rheumatoid arthritis, osteoarthritis, ankylosing spondylitis, acute gouty arthritis, bursitis.

**CONTRAINDICATIONS**   • Hypersensitivity to sulindac or to another NSAID, including aspirin. • Gastrointestinal bleeding or ulcer.

**DOSAGE**   **PO:**   **ADULTS:** Initially, 150 mg two times daily. If needed, may increase to 400 mg daily.   *Special patient populations:*   **ELDERLY:** Patients over 70 years old generally require only half the usual adult dose. Geriatric patients are more susceptible to the toxic effects of NSAIDs, particularly the gastrointestinal, hepatic, renal, and CNS effects.   **CHILDREN:** Not recommended for children under 14 years old.   **PREGNANCY:** Safe use has not been established. Inhibitors of prostaglandin synthesis may have adverse effects on fetal circulation and may interfere with labor and delay parturition.

**PREPARATIONS**   *Tablets:* 150 or 200 mg.

**DRUG INTERACTIONS**   **Protein-bound drugs** In general, the NSAIDs are protein-bound and can displace other drugs, especially hydantoins, sulfonamides, and sulfonylureas.   **Anticoagulant and thrombolytic drugs** may have additive effects with NSAIDs that inhibit platelet aggregation and cause GI bleeding. **Salicylates** tend to compete with other NSAIDs for protein-binding. NSAIDs may be more rapidly metabolized.   **Phenobarbital** may induce liver microsomal enzymes, leading to more rapid degradation of the NSAID.   **Dimethylsulfoxide** may decrease the plasma concentration of sulindac's active sulfide metabolite.   **Probenecid** increases the plasma concentrations of sulindac. See entry for drug class for a more complete list common to the NSAIDs.

**FATE**   Sulindac is well absorbed and highly bound to plasma protein. Sulindac is metabolized to an active sulfide metabolite. Both forms are recirculated through enterohepatic circulation, and metabolites eventually appear in the feces. The *onset* of antirheumatic action may take 7 days, with a *peak* effect in 2 to 3 weeks.

### ❦ NURSING CONSIDERATIONS

#### Side effects, toxicities, and associated nursing actions

**CNS** Headache, dizziness; occasionally, drowsiness, tremor, confusion, nervousness, fatigue; paresthesia, weakness; tinnitus.

**Eye** Occasionally, blurred vision.
- Obtain a thorough baseline assessment prior to initiating drug therapy.
- Caution patients to avoid driving or operating hazardous equipment until the effects of the medication can be evaluated.
- Caution patients to notify the physician if visual changes or CNS effects develop.
- Periodic ophthalmologic examinations should be performed on patients on long-term therapy.
- Monitor for changes in hearing acuity or development of tinnitus. If hearing changes are suspected, refer for regular audiometric testing.

**GI** Dyspepsia, constipation, nausea, vomiting; occasionally, abdominal pain, anorexia, diarrhea, flatulence; ulceration of the cheek mucosa.
- Taking doses with meals, snack, antacids, or a large volume of water or milk (240 ml) may lessen gastric irritation.
- Monitor intake, output, and weight if vomiting, diarrhea, or anorexia is severe.
- Monitor stools for occult blood.

**GU** Problems with urination, nephrotic syndrome, renal failure.
- Monitor weight and blood pressure.
- Monitor intake and output, urinalysis, serum electrolytes, BUN, creatinine.

**Hematologic** Anemia, prolongation of bleeding time, easy bruising, thrombocytopenia.
- Monitor complete blood count, differential, platelet count, bleeding time.
- Inspect patient for development of petechiae, unexplained bruising, oozing from gums, nosebleeds, fever, rash, sore throat, stomatitis, malaise.
- Instruct patient to report the development of any unexplained bleeding, oozing from gums, nosebleeds.
- Monitor stools for occult blood.
- Be especially alert to bleeding in persons also receiving anticoagulants.

**Skin** Pruritis, rash, urticaria, sweating.
- Inspect for development of skin changes.

**Metabolic** Hepatic effects, including jaundice, cholestatic hepatitis.
- Monitor liver function tests.
- Assess for the development of jaundice, right upper quadrant abdominal pain, change in color or consistency of stools.

### Nursing interventions related to drug administration
- Tablets may be crushed and mixed with applesauce or other food for ease in taking ordered dose.

### Patient and family education
- Review anticipated benefits and possible side effects of drug therapy with patients. Caution patients to report the development of any unexpected sign or symptom.
- Remind patients to take medications only as ordered.
- Remind patients to keep all health care providers informed of all medications being taken.
- Instruct patients that 2 to 4 weeks of therapy may be necessary before significant improvement is seen in arthritic conditions.

---

## suprofen   (soo-PROE-fen)                                         antiinflammatory analgesic

- suprofen: Suprol

**MECHANISM OF ACTION**    Suprofen is a nonsteroidal antiinflammatory drug (NSAID). NSAIDs inhibit the enzyme cyclooxygenase and thereby prevent the formation of prostaglandins and thromboxanes. See entry for drug class for more information (p. 882).

**INDICATIONS**   **Pain and inflammation** Used for mild to moderate postoperative pain, including dental and orthopedic surgery, postpartum, muscular aches and pains, pain associated with cancer. Dysmenorrhea. Osteoarthritis.

**CONTRAINDICATIONS**   • Hypersensitivity to suprofen or to another NSAID, including aspirin. • Gastrointestinal bleeding or ulcer.

**DOSAGE**   **PO:**   **ADULTS:** 200 mg every 4 to 6 hours. For osteoarthritis, 200 mg four times daily.   *Special patient populations:*   **ELDERLY:** Patients over 70 years old generally require only half the usual adult dose. Geriatric patients are more susceptible to the toxic effects of NSAIDs, particularly the gastrointestinal, hepatic, renal, and CNS effects.   **CHILDREN:** Not recommended for children under 14 years old.   **PREGNANCY:** Safe use has not been established. Inhibitors of prostaglandin synthesis may have adverse effects on fetal circulation and may interfere with labor and delay parturition.

**PREPARATIONS**   *Capsules:* 200 mg.

**DRUG INTERACTIONS**   **Protein-bound drugs** In general, the NSAIDs are protein-bound and can displace other drugs, especially hydantoins, sulfonamides, and sulfonylureas.   **Anticoagulant and thrombolytic drugs** may have additive effects with NSAIDs that inhibit platelet aggregation and cause GI bleeding. **Salicylates** tend to compete with other NSAIDs for protein-binding. NSAIDs may be more rapidly metabolized.   **Phenobarbital** may induce liver microsomal enzymes, leading to more rapid degradation of the NSAID. See entry for drug class for a more complete list common to the NSAIDs.

**FATE**   Suprofen is well absorbed and highly bound to plasma protein. The *onset of action* is 15 to 30 minutes, and the *duration of action* is 4 to 6 hours. Suprofen is metabolized in the liver and excreted in the urine.

## 🐦 NURSING CONSIDERATIONS

### Side effects, toxicities, and associated nursing actions

**CNS** Headache, sleepiness; occasionally, dizziness, tremor, confusion, nervousness, fatigue, paresthesia, weakness; tinnitus.

**Eye** Occasionally, blurred vision.
- Obtain a thorough baseline assessment prior to initiating drug therapy.
- Caution patients to avoid driving or operating hazardous equipment until the effects of the medication can be evaluated.
- Caution patients to notify the physician if visual changes or CNS effects develop.
- Periodic ophthalmologic examinations should be performed on patients on long-term therapy.
- Monitor for changes in hearing acuity or development of tinnitus. If hearing changes are suspected, refer for regular audiometric testing.

**GI** Dyspepsia, constipation, nausea, vomiting; occasionally, abdominal pain, anorexia, diarrhea, flatulence.
- Taking doses with meals, snack, antacids, or a large volume of water or milk (240 ml) may lessen gastric irritation.
- Monitor intake, output, and weight if vomiting, diarrhea, or anorexia is severe.
- Monitor stools for occult blood.

**GU** Problems with urination, nephrotic syndrome, renal failure.
- Monitor weight and blood pressure.
- Monitor intake and output, urinalysis, serum electrolytes, BUN, creatinine.

**Hematologic** Anemia, prolongation of bleeding time, easy bruising, thrombocytopenia.
- Monitor complete blood count, differential, platelet count, bleeding time.
- Inspect patient for development of petechiae, unexplained bruising, oozing from gums, nosebleeds, fever, rash, sore throat, stomatitis, malaise.
- Instruct patient to report the development of any unexplained bleeding, oozing from gums, nosebleeds.
- Monitor stools for occult blood.
- Be especially alert to bleeding in persons also receiving anticoagulants.

**Skin** Pruritis, rash, urticaria, sweating.
- Inspect for development of skin changes.

**Metabolic** Hepatic effects, including jaundice, cholestatic hepatitis.
- Monitor liver function tests.
- Assess for the development of jaundice, right upper quadrant abdominal pain, change in color or consistency of stools.

### Nursing interventions related to drug administration
- Contents of capsule may be mixed with applesauce or other food for ease in taking ordered dose.

### Patient and family education
- Review anticipated benefits and possible side effects of drug therapy with patients.
- Caution patients to report the development of any unexpected sign or symptom.
- Remind patients to take medications only as ordered.
- Remind patients to keep all health care providers informed of all medications being taken.
- Instruct patients that 2 to 4 weeks of therapy may be necessary before significant improvement is seen in arthritic conditions.

---

## tolmetin sodium    (TOLE-met-in)                                   antiinflammatory analgesic

- tolmetin sodium: Tolectin

**MECHANISM OF ACTION**    Tolmetin is a nonsteroidal antiinflammatory drug (NSAID). NSAIDs inhibit the enzyme cyclooxygenase and thereby prevent the formation of prostaglandins and thromboxanes. See entry for drug class for more information (p. 882).

**INDICATIONS**    **Pain and inflammation** Used for rheumatoid arthritis, osteoarthritis.

**CONTRAINDICATIONS**    • Hypersensitivity to tolmetin or to another NSAID, including aspirin. • Gastrointestinal bleeding or ulcer.

**DOSAGE**    **PO:**    **ADULTS:** Initially, 400 mg three times a day. Adjust as needed, but no more than 2 g daily for rheumatoid arthritis, 1.6 g daily for osteoarthritis.    **CHILDREN:** 20 mg/kg divided into three or four doses. Adjust dose as needed, but no more than 30 mg/kg daily.    *Special patient populations:* **ELDERLY:** Patients over 70 years old generally require only half the usual adult dose. Geriatric patients are more susceptible to the toxic effects of NSAIDs, particularly the gastrointestinal, hepatic, renal and CNS effects.    **CHILDREN:** Not recommended for children under 2 years old.    **PREGNANCY:** Safe use has not been established. Inhibitors of prostaglandin synthesis may have adverse effects on fetal circulation and may interfere with labor and delay parturition (FDA pregnancy category C).

**PREPARATIONS**    *Capsules:* 400 mg; *tablets:* 200 mg.

**DRUG INTERACTIONS**    **Protein-bound drugs** In general, the NSAIDs are protein-bound and can displace other drugs, especially hyantoins, sulfonamides, and sulfonylureas.    **Anticoagulant and thrombolytic drugs** may have additive effects with NSAIDs that inhibit platelet aggregation and cause GI bleeding.    **Salicylates** tend to compete with other NSAIDs for protein-binding. NSAIDs may be more rapidly metabolized.    **Phenobarbital** may induce liver microsomal enzymes, leading to more rapid degradation of the NSAID. See entry for drug class for a more complete list common to the NSAIDs.

**FATE**    Tolmetin is well absorbed and highly bound to plasma protein. The *onset of action* is 15 to 30 minutes, and the *duration of action* is 4 to 6 hours. Tolmetin is metabolized in the liver and excreted in the urine.

### ☙ NURSING CONSIDERATIONS
#### Side effects, toxicities, and associated nursing actions
**CNS** Headache, sleepiness; occasionally, dizziness, tremor, confusion, nervousness, paresthesia, weakness, fatigue, tinnitus.

**Eye** Occasionally, blurred vision.
- Obtain a thorough baseline assessment prior to initiating drug therapy.
- Caution patients to avoid driving or operating hazardous equipment until the effects of the medication can be evaluated.
- Caution patients to notify the physician if visual changes or CNS effects develop.
- Periodic ophthalmologic examinations should be performed on patients on long-term therapy.
- Assess for tinnitus. If hearing problems are suspected, refer patient for regular audiometric testing.

**GI** Dyspepsia, constipation, nausea, vomiting; occasionally, abdominal pain, anorexia, diarrhea, flatulence; ulceration of the cheek mucosa.

- Taking doses with meals, snack, antacids, or a large volume of water or milk (240 ml) may lessen gastric irritation.
- Monitor intake, output, and weight if vomiting, diarrhea, or anorexia is severe.
- Monitor stools for occult blood.

**GU** Problems with urination, nephrotic syndrome, renal failure.

- Monitor weight and blood pressure.
- Monitor intake and output, urinalysis, serum electrolytes, BUN, creatinine.

**Hematologic** Anemia, prolongation of bleeding time, easy bruising, thrombocytopenia.

- Monitor complete blood count, differential, platelet count, bleeding time.
- Inspect patient for development of petechiae, unexplained bruising, oozing from gums, nosebleeds, fever, rash, sore throat, stomatitis, malaise.
- Instruct patient to report the development of any unexplained bleeding, oozing from gums, nosebleeds.
- Monitor stools for occult blood.
- Be especially alert to bleeding in persons also receiving anticoagulants.

**Skin** Pruritis, rash, urticaria, sweating.

- Inspect for development of skin changes.

**Metabolic** Hepatic effects, including alterations in liver function tests, jaundice, cholestatic hepatitis.

- Monitor liver function tests.
- Assess for the development of jaundice, right upper quadrant abdominal pain, change in color consistency of stools.

### Nursing Interventions related to drug administration

- Tablet may be crushed or contents of capsules may be mixed with applesauce or other food for ease in taking ordered dose.

### Patient and family education

- Review anticipated benefits and possible side effects of drug therapy with patients. Caution patients to report the development of any unexpected sign or symptom.
- Remind patients to take medications only as ordered.
- Remind patients to keep all health care providers informed of all medications being taken.
- Instruct patients that 2 to 4 weeks of therapy may be necessary before significant improvement is seen in arthritic conditions.

# Chapter Forty-nine

# Drugs for rheumatoid arthritis

auranofin
aurothioglucose
gold sodium thiomalate
hydroxychloroquine
penicillamine

**OVERVIEW OF THE DRUG CLASS**  Rheumatoid arthritis is an autoimmune disease with a highly variable disease process. It frequently goes into remission for months or years. In early rheumatoid arthritis the synovial membranes are only inflamed, causing a painful swelling. In this situation aspirin and the other nonsteroidal antiinflammatory drugs may be effective in reducing the inflammation. This effect added to the analgesic effect will ease the pain and help to increase the mobility of the affected joint. In mild cases of rheumatoid arthritis, the nonsteroidal antiinflammatory drugs may be sufficient to control symptoms. These drugs do not affect the progression of rheumatoid arthritis, however, which is marked by erosion of the bone at the joint and eventual bone deformation. Drugs that may be effective in altering the progression of joint erosion include gold therapy, hydroxychloroquine, penicillamine, and the immunosuppresive drugs, tried in that order. All of these antirheumatic drugs have potentially serious side effects, which must be monitored carefully.

---

## auranofin   (au-RAN-oh-fin)                                     antirheumatoid

- auranofin: Ridaura

**MECHANISM OF ACTION**   Auranofin is an orally active gold compound used in the treatment of rheumatoid arthritis. The exact antirheumatic mechanisms are not known but are believed to include immuno-modulating effects and a decrease in lysosomal enzyme release.

**INDICATIONS**   **Rheumatiod arthritis** Gold compounds are used when nonsteroidal antiinflammatory drugs are no longer effective in bringing relief and inducing remissions.

**CONTRAINDICATIONS**   **Coexisting severe systemic disease,** including renal disease, hepatic dysfunction or history of infection hepatitis, marked hypertension, heart failure, systemic lupus erythematosus, agranulocytosis or hemorrhagic disease, radiation therapy, eczema, colitis, uncontrolled diabetes, severe debilitation, previous history of toxic reaction to gold therapy.   **Pregnancy.**

**DOSAGE**   **PO:**   **ADULTS:** 6 mg daily in a single dose or divided into two doses. A response should be seen after 6 months of therapy. If the response is inadequate, the dose may be raised to 9 mg daily. After 3 months at 9 mg, if the response is still not adequate, therapy with gold should be discontinued. *Special patient populations:*   **CHILDREN:** Safety for use in children under 16 years of age has not been established.   **PREGNANCY:** Not for use during pregnancy. Teratogenic effects have been demonstrated in test animals.

**PREPARATIONS**   *Capsules:* 3 mg.

**DRUG INTERACTIONS**   None documented.

**DIAGNOSTIC TEST INTERFERENCE**   **Tuberculin skin test** Response may be enhanced by auranofin therapy.

**FATE**   Auranofin is the only gold compound administered orally. About 25% is absorbed from the GI tract. In plasma it is highly bound to plasma protein. The plasma *half-life* is very long, initially being 17 days and with continued therapy lengthening to 26 days. Excretion is primarily in the feces.

**❦ NURSING CONSIDERATIONS**

### Side effects, toxicities, and associated nursing actions

**GI** Diarrhea occurs in about half the patients treated and may be intolerable with oral gold therapy; anorexia, nausea, vomiting, cramps.

- If symptoms are severe or persistent, it may be necessary to switch drugs; consult the physician.

- Monitor intake, output, and weight.
- If diarrhea is severe, monitor electrolytes.

**Hematologic** Anemia, agranulocytosis, leukopenia, thrombocytopenia.

- Monitor complete blood count, white blood cell differential, and platelet count.
- Visually inspect patients for signs of petechiae, bruising.
- Caution patients to report the development of any unexplained bleeding, malaise, fatigue, sore throat.

**Skin** Dermatitis and skin eruptions are common, although less so than with parenteral gold therapy. Any pruritic eruption should be considered a symptom of gold toxicity. May progress to exfoliative dermatitis. Mucous membranes may develop shallow ulcers, especially in the mouth. Metallic taste may be a warning signal.

- Visually inspect skin and mucous membranes prior to initiating therapy; inspect skin carefully on each return visit.
- Instruct patient to report the development of skin or mucous membrane changes.
- Skin changes may be aggravated by sunlight. Caution patients to avoid exposure to the sun or other sources of ultraviolet light. When in the sun, patients should wear a hat, long sleeves, keep legs covered, and use maximum-protection sunscreen on exposed areas.
- Inspect mouth and gums carefully prior to initiating therapy. Instruct patients in regular oral hygiene program: brushing, flossing, avoiding mouthwashes containing alcohol, which may be drying or irritating.

**Metabolic** Changes in hepatic function tests; nephrotic syndrome.

- Monitor weight.
- Assess for jaundice, right upper quadrant abdominal pain, change in color or consistency of stools.
- Monitor serum creatinine, BUN, liver function tests, urinalysis for proteinuria, hematuria.

**Other** Peripheral neuropathy.

- Assess for this side effect.

### Nursing interventions related to drug administration

- To help ensure that patients will return for follow-up, auranofin may be prescribed in sufficient quantities for only 2 weeks of treatment at a time. Emphasize to patients the need to return for regular medical supervision.

### Patient and family education

- Review with patients the anticipated benefits and possible side effects of therapy. Instruct the patient to report the development of any unexpected sign or symptom.
- Caution the patient that several weeks or longer of therapy may be necessary before improvement is seen. At the same time, caution the patient that side effects can develop at any time and should be reported.
- Women of childbearing age may wish to use some form of birth control while on gold therapy; discuss prior to initiating gold therapy.
- Review with patients the importance of continuing all aspects of the treatment program: exercise, judicious use of analgesics and antiinflammatory agents, application of heat, good nutrition, maintenance of ideal body weight, physical therapy, and so forth.

## aurothioglucose (aur-oh-thye-oh-GLOO-kose) antirheumatoid

- aurothioglucose: Solganol

**MECHANISM OF ACTION** Aurothioglucose is an injectable gold compound used in the treatment of rheumatoid arthritis. The exact antirheumatic mechanisms are not known but are believed to include immunomodulating effects and a decrease in lysosomal enzyme release.

**INDICATIONS**   **Rheumatoid arthritis** Gold compounds are used when nonsteroidal antiinflammatory drugs are no longer effective in bringing relief and inducing remissions.

**CONTRAINDICATIONS**   **Coexisting severe systemic disease,** including renal disease, hepatic dysfuntion or history of infection hepatitis, marked hypertension, heart failure, systemic lupus erythematosus, agranulocytosis or hemorrhagic disease, radiation therapy, eczema, colitis, uncontrolled diabetes, severe debilitation, previous history of toxic reaction to gold therapy.   **Pregnancy.**

**DOSAGE**   IM:   ADULTS: 10 mg the first week, 25 mg weeks 2 and 3, then 50 mg weekly until a total dose of 0.8 to 1 g has been administered. If the patient shows improvement and shows no toxicity, therapy is continued with 25 to 50 mg every 3 to 4 weeks. If there is no improvement, therapy is discontinued after 1 g has been administered.   CHILDREN One-fourth the adult dose.   *Special patient populations:*   PREGNANCY: Not for use during pregnancy. Teratogenic effects have been demonstrated in test animals.

**PREPARATIONS**   *Suspension:* 50 mg/ml.

**DRUG INTERACTIONS**   None documented.

**DIAGNOSTIC TEST INTERFERENCE**   **Protein-bound iodide** IM gold therapy interferes with this determination.

**FATE**   Parenteral gold is slowly absorbed and after absorption is highly bound to plasma protein. The biologic *half-life* varies over a wide range and increases with the length of therapy; it can be up to 170 days after 3 months of therapy. Parenteral gold is eventually excreted in the urine and feces.

## ❦ NURSING CONSIDERATIONS

### Side effects, toxicities, and associated nursing actions

**CNS** Headache
- Assess for this side effect. If it is severe or persistent, it may be necessary to discontinue medication or to change to a lower dose; notify the physician.

**Eye** Rarely, conjunctivitis, iritis, corneal ulcers.
- Inspect patient's eyes for signs of irritation.
- Tell patient to report the development of vision or eye problems.

**GI** Anorexia, nausea, vomiting, diarrhea, cramps.
- If symptoms are severe or persistent, it may be necessary to switch drugs; consult the physician.
- Monitor intake, output, and weight.
- If diarrhea is severe, monitor electrolytes.

**Hematologic** Aplastic anemia, agranulocytosis, leukopenia, thrombocytopenia.
- Monitor complete blood count, white blood cell differential, and platelet count.
- Inspect patients for signs of petechiae, bruising.
- Caution patients to report the development of any unexplained bleeding, malaise, fatique, sore throat.

**Skin** Reactions of the skin and mucous membranes are the most frequent adverse effects of parenteral gold therapy. Itching is considered the first symptom, and therapy should be discontinued when it occurs. Severe dermatitis may ensue and may include loss of hair and nails. Mucous membranes at all orifices can swell or ulcerate.
- Inspect skin and mucous membranes prior to initiating therapy; inspect skin carefully on each return visit.
- Instruct patient to report the development of skin or mucous membrane changes.
- Skin changes may be aggravated by sunlight. Caution patients to avoid exposure to the sun or other sources of ultraviolet light. When in the sun, patients should wear a hat, long sleeves, keep legs covered, and use maximum-protection sunscreen on exposed areas.
- Inspect mouth and gums carefully prior to initiating therapy. Instruct patients in regular oral hygiene program: brushing, flossing, avoiding mouthwashes containing alcohol, which may be drying or irritating.

**Lung** Pulmonary infiltration.
- Monitor respiratory rate. Auscultate lung sounds.

**Metabolic** Renal or liver damage; these organs should be monitored.

- Monitor weight.
- Assess for jaundice, right upper quadrant abdominal pain, change in color or consistency of stools.
- Monitor serum creatinine, BUN, liver function tests, urinalysis for proteinuria, hematuria.

**Other** Peripheral neuritis.

- Assess for this side effect.

### Nursing interventions related to drug administration

- Aurothioglucose is an oil-based suspension. Prior to administering, warm vial under warm running water, then rotate betwen hands to resuspend the medication. Prepare dose and administer while medication is still warm.
- Use anatomic landmarks to choose IM injection sites. Use large muscle masses such as the dorso-gluteal site or the rectus femoris muscle in adults or the vastus lateralis in small children. Administer deep IM; aspirate before injecting medication to avoid inadvertent IV administration. Record site and rotate sites.
- Keep patient recumbent and observe carefully for at least 15 minutes after administering dose. Monitor blood pressure, pulse. Have drugs (corticosteroids, epinephrine, antihistamines) and equipment available for treatment of acute allergic-type reactions in settings where parenteral gold is administered.

### Patient and family education

- Review anticipated benefits and possible side effects of therapy with patient. Instruct patient to report the development of any unexpected sign or symptoms.
- Caution the patient that several weeks or longer of therapy may be necessary before improvement is seen. At the same time, caution the patient that side effects can develop at any time and should be reported.
- Women of childbearing age may wish to use some form of birth control while on gold therapy; discuss prior to initiating gold therapy.
- Warn patient that there may be increased joint pain for the first few days after an injection, but this should subside.
- Review with patients the importance of continuing all aspects of the treatment program: exercise, judicious use of analgesics and antiinflammatory agents, application of heat, good nutrition, maintenance of ideal body weight, physical therapy, and so forth.

---

## gold sodium thiomalate (thye-oh-MAH-late)    antirheumatoid

- gold sodium thiomalate: Myochrysine

**MECHANISM OF ACTION**  Gold sodium thiomalate is an injectable gold compound used in the treatment of rheumatoid arthritis. The exact antirheumatic mechanisms are not known but are believed to include immunomodulating effects and a decrease in lysosomal enzyme release.

**INDICATIONS**  **Rheumatoid arthritis** Gold compounds are used when nonsteroidal antiinflammatory drugs are no longer effective in bringing relief and inducing remissions.

**CONTRAINDICATIONS**  **Coexisting severe systemic disease** including renal disease, hepatic dysfunction or history of infection hepatitis, marked hypertension, heart failure, systemic lupus erythematosus, agranulocytosis or hemorrhagic disease, radiation therapy, eczema, colitis, uncontrolled diabetes, severe debilitation, previous history of toxic reaction to gold therapy. **Pregnancy.**

**DOSAGE**  **IM:**  **ADULTS:** 10 mg the first week, 25 mg weeks 2 and 3, then 50 mg weekly until a total dose of 0.8 to 1 g has been administered. If the patient shows improvement and shows no toxicity, therapy is continued with 25 to 50 mg every 2 weeks for 2 to 20 weeks. Thereafter, 25 to 50 mg is given every 3 to 4 weeks as long as the patient maintains improvement. If there is no improvement, therapy is discontinued after 1 g has been administered. **CHILDREN:** the initial test dose is 10 mg. Thereafter, the dose is 1 mg/kg administered according to the schedule above. *Special patient populations:* **PREGNANCY:** Not for use during pregnancy. Teratogenic effects have been demonstrated in test animals.

**PREPARATIONS** *Injection:* 10, 25, or 50 mg/ml.

**DRUG INTERACTIONS** None documented.

**DIAGNOSTIC TEST INTERFERENCE** **Protein-bound iodide** IM gold therapy interferes with this determination.

**FATE** Parenteral gold is slowly absorbed and after absorption is highly bound to plasma protein. The biologic *half-life* varies over a wide range and increases with the length of therapy; it can be up to 170 days after 3 months of therapy. Parenteral gold is eventually excreted in the urine and feces.

☙ **NURSING CONSIDERATIONS**

**Side effects, toxicities, and associated nursing actions**

**CNS** Headache.
- Assess for this side effect. If it is severe or persistent, it may be necessary to discontinue medication or change to a lower dose; notify the physician.

**Eye** Rarely, conjunctivitis, iritis, corneal ulcers.
- Inspect patient's eyes for signs of irritation.
- Tell patient to report the development of vision or eye problems.

**GI** Anorexia, nausea, vomiting, diarrhea, cramps.
- If symptoms are severe or persistent, it may be necessary to switch drugs; consult the physician.
- Monitor intake, output, and weight.
- If diarrhea is severe, monitor electrolytes.

**Hematologic** Aplastic anemia, agranulocytosis, leukopenia, thrombocytopenia.
- Monitor complete blood count, white blood cell differential, and platelet count.
- Inspect patients for signs of petechiae, bruising.
- Caution patients to report the development of any unexplained bleeding, malaise, fatigue, sore throat.

**Skin** Reactions of the skin and mucous membranes are the most frequent adverse effects of parenteral gold therapy. Itching is considered the first symptom, and therapy should be discontinued if it occurs. Severe dermatitis may ensue and may include loss of hair and nails. Mucous membranes at all orifices can swell or ulcerate.
- Inspect skin and mucous membranes prior to initiating therapy; inspect skin carefully on each return visit.
- Instruct patient to report the development of skin or mucous membrane changes.
- Skin changes may be aggravated by sunlight. Caution patients to avoid exposure to the sun or other sources of ultraviolet light. When in the sun, patients should wear a hat, long sleeves, keep legs covered, and use maximum-protection sunscreen on exposed areas.
- Inspect mouth and gums carefully prior to initiating therapy. Instruct patients in regular oral hygiene program: brushing, flossing, avoiding mouthwashes containing alcohol, which may be drying or irritating.

**Lung** Pulmonary infiltration.
- Monitor respiratory rate. Auscultate lung sounds.

**Metabolic** Renal or liver damage; these organs shoud be monitored.
- Monitor weight.
- Assess for jaundice, right upper quadrant abdominal pain, change in color or consistency of stools.
- Monitor serum creatinine, BUN, liver function tests, urinalysis for proteinuria, hematuria.

**Other** Peripheral neuritis.
- Assess for this side effect.

### Nursing interventions related to drug administration

- Inspect solution prior to preparing dose. If particulate matter or strong discoloration are present, discard. Color should be no darker than pale yellow.
- Use anatomic landmarks to choose IM injection sites. Use large muscle masses such as the dorso-gluteal site or the rectus femoris muscle in adults or the vastus lateralis in small children. Administer deep IM; aspirate before injecting medication to avoid inadvertent IV administration. Record site and rotate sites.
- Keep patient recumbent and observe carefully for at least 15 minutes after administering dose. Monitor blood pressure, pulse. Have drugs (corticosteroids, epinephrine, antihistamines) and equipment available for treatment of acute allergic-type reactions in the settings where parenteral gold is administered.

### Patient and family education

- Review anticipated benefits and possible side effects of therapy with patient. Instruct patient to report the development of any unexpected sign or symptoms.
- Caution the patient that several weeks or longer of therapy may be necessary before improvement is seen. At the same time, caution the patient that side effects can develop at any time and should be reported.
- Women of childbearing age may wish to use some form of birth control while on gold therapy; discuss prior to initiating gold therapy.
- Warn patient that there may be increased joint pain for the first few days after an injection, but this should subside.
- Review with patients the importance of continuing all aspects of the treatment program: exercise, judicious use of analgesics and antiinflammatory agents, application of heat, good nutrition, maintenance of ideal body weight, physical therapy, and so forth.

---

# hydroxychloroquine sulfate
(hye-drox-ee-KLOR-oh-kwin)　　　　　　　　　　　　　　antirheumatoid, antimalarial*

- hydroxychloroquine sulfate: Plaquenil

**MECHANISM OF ACTION**　The mechanism for the antirheumatoid action of hydroxychloroquine is not known. The mechanism is believed to involve inhibition of prostaglandin synthesis and inhibition of chemotaxis of white cells.

**INDICATIONS**　• Rheumatoid arthritis • Lupus erythematosus. • Malaria: drug of choice for prophylaxis.

**CONTRAINDICATIONS**　• Retinal or visual changes. • Hypersensitivity.

**DOSAGE**　**Rheumatoid arthritis:**　**PO:**　**ADULTS:** 400 to 600 mg daily taken with meals. After improvement is noted, usually 4 to 12 weeks, the dose is reduced by 50% and continued.　**Lupus erythematosus: PO:**　**ADULTS:** 400 mg one or two times daily. Maintenance: 200 to 400 mg daily.　**Malaria:**　**PO: ADULTS:** Suppressive therapy is 400 mg every 7 days. Therapeutic doses are 800 mg initially, followed by 400 mg in 6 to 8 hours and 400 mg on days 2 and 3.　**CHILDREN:** Suppressive therapy is 6.4 mg/kg every 7 days. Therapeutic doses are 32 mg/kg administered over 3 days; 12.9 mg/kg initially (maximum 800 mg), followed by 6.4 mg/kg (maximum 400 mg) at 6, 24 and 48 hours. *Special patient populations:*　**CHILDREN:** Toxic effects are more common in children.　**PREGNANCY:** Not recommended for use during pregnancy.

**PREPARATIONS**　*Tablets:* 155 mg.

**DRUG INTERACTIONS**　**Phenylbutazone, gold salts** Hydroxychloroquine increases the incidence of serious skin reactions when administered with these drugs.

**FATE**　Hydroxychloroquine is well absorbed from the GI tract. It concentrates in the liver, spleen, kidney, heart, lung, brain. Hydroxychloroquine is excreted unchanged in the urine.

*See p. 383.

## ❦ NURSING CONSIDERATIONS

### Side effects, toxicities, and associated nursing actions

**CNS** Irritability, nervousness, nightmares, headache, dizziness, incoordination; emotional changes, psychosis, convulsions, nerve deafness.
- Obtain a thorough baseline neurologic and mental status exam prior to intiating therapy and at regular intervals during therapy.
- Caution patients to avoid driving or operating hazardous equipment until the effects of the medication can be evaluated.
- Obtain a baseline audiometric test, and repeat at regular intervals.

**Eye** Blurred vision, edema, changes in the fundus, retinopathy. Eye changes should be carefully monitored during therapy.
- Obtain a complete ophthalmoscopic examination prior to initiating therapy, and repeat at regular intervals.
- Caution patients to report any subjective changes in vision.

**GI** Anorexia, nausea, vomiting, diarrhea, cramps.
- Monitor weight. If vomiting and/or diarrhea occur, monitor intake and output.
- If GI symptoms are severe or persist, notify the physician. It may be necessary to change drug or dose.

**Hematologic** Aplastic anemia, agranulocytosis, leukopenia, thrombocytopenia.
- Inspect patients for signs of petechiae, bruising.
- Caution patients to report the development of any unexplained bleeding, bruising, malaise, fever, sore throat.
- Monitor complete blood count, white blood cell differential, and platelet count.

**Skin** Loss of hair and skin and mucosal pigmentation, skin eruptions.
- Visually inspect patient for skin changes.
- Caution patient to report skin changes. Pruritis and other symptoms may not begin until several hours after patient consumes dose.

**Metabolic** Exacerbation of porphyria.
- Question patients about history of this disorder prior to initiating therapy.
- Assess for symptoms: photosensitivity, abdominal pain, neuropathy, fever, leukocytosis, skin lesions.
- Caution patients to avoid exposure to the sun or other sources of ultraviolet light. Caution patients to wear a hat, long sleeves, and keep legs covered when outside. Instruct patients to use a maximum-protection sunscreen on exposed areas.

**Other** Muscle weakness; loss of deep tendon reflexes.
- Assess muscle strength and deep tendon reflexes, especially knee and ankle reflexes, prior to initiating therapy and at regular intervals.

### Nursing interventions related to drug administration

- Administer doses with a large volume (240 ml) of milk or other liquid to lessen gastric irritation.

### Patient and family education

- Review with patients the anticipated benefits and possible side effects of therapy. Instruct the patient to report the development of any unexpected sign or symptom.
- Caution the patient that several weeks or longer of therapy may be necessary before improvement is seen. At the same time, caution the patient that side effects can develop at any time and should be reported.
- Women of childbearing age may wish to use some form of birth control while on therapy. Discuss prior to initiating drug therapy.
- Review with patients the importance of continuing all aspects of the treatment program for the arthritic condition: exercise, judicious use of analgesics and antiinflammatory agents, application of heat, good nutrition, maintenance of ideal body weight, physical therapy, and so forth.
- Caution patients to keep this and all medications out of the reach of children. Children are especially sensitive to ingestion of hydroxychloroquine, and ingestion of small amounts has been fatal.

## penicillamine    (pen-i-SILL-a-meen)    antirheumatic

- penicillamine: Cuprimine, Depen

**MECHANISM OF ACTION**    The mechanism of action of penicillamine is not known but may be related to inhibition of collagen formation. Penicillamine also chelates copper and other heavy metals.

**INDICATIONS**    **Rheumatoid arthritis** Penicillamine is used after gold therapy fails.    **Wilson's disease** is a metabolic disorder in which copper is not cleared normally. Penicillamine chelates copper and promotes its excretion.

**CONTRAINDICATIONS**    • Sensitivity to penicilin. • Renal function impairment.

**DOSAGE**    **Rheumatoid arthritis:**    *PO:*    **ADULTS:** Initially, 125 to 250 mg daily. May increase at 1 to 3 month intervals depending on response and tolerance. Maximum dose is 1.5g/day, but if no response is obtained at doses of 1g/day, therapy is discontinued. Remissions on penicillamine may last months or years. After 6 months on remission, the dose is decreased to 125 to 250 mg/day.    **Wilson's disease:** *PO:*    **ADULTS:** 250 mg four times daily.    **CHILDREN:** 6 months to 12 years old, 250 mg daily. *Special patient populations:*    **PREGNANCY:** Probably teratogenic in pregnancy.

**PREPARATIONS**    *Capsules:* 125 or 250 mg; *tablets:* 250 mg.

**DRUG INTERACTIONS**    **Gold therapy, hydroxychloroquine, cytotoxic drugs, oxyphenbutazone, phenylbutazone** cause serious hematologic and renal actions similar to those of penicillamine and should not be used together.    **Iron salts, antacids** significantly decrease the absorption of penicillamine.    **Digoxin serum levels** are decreased by penicillamine.

**FATE**    Penicillamine is well absorbed, is metabolized in the liver, and is excreted in the urine and feces.

## 🦠 NURSING CONSIDERATIONS

### Side effects, toxicities, and associated nursing actions

**CNS** Tinnitus.
- Assess patients for development of tinnitus. Assess hearing prior to initiating therapy, and at regular intervals.

**Eye** Neuritis
- Assess for changes in vision.

**GI** Anorexia, nausea, vomiting, diarrhea, altered taste, mouth ulcers, inflammation of mucosal surfaces.
- Monitor weight. If vomiting and/or diarrhea occur, monitor intake and output.
- Assess for alterations in taste; these are usually self-limiting.
- Assess mucosal surfaces of mouth carefully at start of therapy and at regular intervals. Review with patients aspects of good oral hygiene: regular brushing, flossing, avoiding mouthwashes containing alcohol, which might be drying or irritating. If mouth ulcers are severe or persistent, it may be necessary to reduce the dose or change drugs; notify the physician.

**GU** Proteinuria; nephrotic syndrome.
- Monitor weight, blood pressure, urinalysis.
- Assess for development of edema, especially of dependent areas.
- Monitor serum creatinine, BUN.

**Hematologic** Bone marrow depression, leukopenia, thrombocytopenia, phlebitis.
- Visually inspect patients for development of bruising, petechiae.
- Instruct patient to report the development of unexplained bleeding or bruising, malaise, sore throat, fever.
- Monitor complete blood count, white blood cell differential, platelet count.

**Lung** Asthma.
- Auscultate breath sounds at regular intervals.

**Skin** Increasing friability of skin; wrinkling; loss of hair.
- Assess for skin changes. Appearance of skin changes often do not necessitate discontinuation of the drug but this should be evaluated individually. Skin changes may be troubling and may require patient instruction on how to avoid skin injury and on symptomatic treatment.
- Caution patient to report the development of any skin changes.

**Hepatic** Hepatic dysfunction, cholestatic jaundice, pancreatitis.

- Assess for development of jaundice, right upper quadrant abdominal pain, change in color or consistency of stools (signs of hepatic problems), and epigastric pain, vomiting, malaise, fever (signs of pancreatitis).
- Monitor liver function tests and serum amylase if indicated.

**Allergic** About 30% of patients develop allergic reactions, usually a rash that itches.

- Visually inspect patients for development of rashes.
- Instruct patient to report immediately the development of skin changes, especially if they first occur after several months of therapy.
- Instruct patient to report the development of fever, which may signal an allergic reaction.
- Emphasize the need to continue the medication as directed. Sporadic use of the drug may contribute to an increased incidence of allergic reactions.

### Nursing interventions related to drug administration

- Question patient about history of allergy to penicillin prior to administering. Cross-sensitivity between the two drugs is possible, though rare.
- Capsules may be opened and contents mixed with 15 to 30 ml of chilled applesauce, other pureed fruits, or fruit juices for ease in administering.
- For treatment of arthritis, penicillamine should be given 1 hour prior to meals and 1 hour apart from other medications, food, or milk.
- For treatment of Wilson's disease, dose should be 30 to 60 minutes prior to meals and at least 2 hours after the evening meal.
- For cystinuria, encourage patients to maintain a high fluid intake, including consuming 500 ml of water at bedtime and again once during the night.
- If oral iron preparations are also being administered, at least 2 hours should elapse between taking the two drugs.
- Penicillamine increases the body's requirement for pyridoxine, and patients requiring penicillamine may also have restricted or poor nutritional intake. Reversible optic neuritis may also be due to pyridoxine deficiency.
- Avoid multivitamin preparations containing copper in patients with Wilson's disease.

### Patient and family education

- Review with patients the anticipated benefits and possible side effects of therapy. Instruct patients to report the development of any unexpected sign or symptom.
- Caution the patient that several weeks or longer of therapy may be necessary before improvement is seen. At the same time, caution the patient that side effects can develop at any time and should be reported.
- Women of childbearing age may wish to use some form of birth control while on penicillamine therapy; discuss prior to initiating therapy.
- Review with patients the importance of continuing all aspects of the treatment program for arthritis: exercise, judicious use of analgesics and antiinflammatory agents, application of heat, good nutrition, maintenance of ideal body weight, physical therapy, and so forth.
- For patients with Wilson's disease, emphasize the importance of following dietary restrictions.

# Chapter Fifty

# Drugs to treat gout

allopurinol
colchicine
probenecid
sulfinpyrazone

## DRUG COMBINATIONS

- probenecid and penicillin G procaine: Wycillin and Probenecid
- probenecid and ampicillin: Principen with Probenecid, Polycillin-PRB, Probampacin
- probenecid with colchicine: colBENEMID, Proben-C

**OVERVIEW OF THE DRUG CLASS**    Gout is a metabolic disease in which total body pools of uric acid (a product of DNA and RNA degradation) are elevated. The uric acid crystallizes in joints or, less commonly, in tendons or bursae. The joint at the base of the big toe is most commonly affected. In an attack of acute gouty arthritis there is a marked inflammation of the joint accompanied by much pain. This acute attack is treated with the drug colchicine, which acts in an unknown manner to relieve the pain of gouty arthritis, with one of the nonsteroidal antiinflammatory drugs already discussed, or in special circumstances with the hormone ACTH. Some patients develop a tophus in a joint: crystals of uric acid with fibrous tissue grown over them. During an acute gouty attack, the drug colchicine or one of the nonsteroidal antiinflammatory drugs provides relief. Patients with tophi or patients with recurrent attacks of gouty arthritis need to receive long-term treatment, often for the rest of their lives, with drugs that will reduce the uric acid levels in the body. If tophi are present, they will often regress with long-term therapy, thereby restoring the joint to a normal range of function. Two drugs, probenicid and sulfinpyrazone, are available as uricosuric drugs. These drugs increase the renal excretion of uric acid by inhibiting its reabsorption from the proximal kidney tubule. About 25% of patients with gout are found to overproduce uric acid. These patients are treated with the drug allopurinol, which prevents the formation of uric acid from xanthine and hypoxanthine, the purine metabolites of DNA and RNA metabolism.

---

## allopurinol    (al-oh-PURE-i-nole)    antigout

- allopurinol: ✤Alloprin, ✤Apo-Allopurinol, Lopurin, ✤Novopurol, ✤Purinol, ✤Roucol, Zyloprim

**MECHANISM OF ACTION**    Allopurinol inhibits the formation of uric acid from xanthine or hypoxanthine so that these precursors are excreted rather than uric acid.

**INDICATIONS**    **Gout** Allopurinol is effective for patients who produce too much uric acid (more than 600 mg uric acid in a 24 hour urine collection). Allopurinol is *not* effective in relieving an acute gouty attack. **Hyperuricemia** Allopurinol may be used prophylactically to reduce the severity of hyperuricemia secondary to myeloproliferative neoplastic diseases such as leukemia, lymphoma, or osteogenic sarcoma.

**CONTRAINDICATIONS**    • Children and nursing mothers. • Hypersensitivity. • Renal or hepatic impairment: caution must be used.

**DOSAGE**    **Gout:**    *PO:*    **ADULTS:** Initially, 100 mg daily, then increase by 100 mg daily at weekly intervals until the serum urate falls to 6 mg/dl. Maximum daily dosage is 800 mg. Dosages for patients with renal impairment must be reduced. Consult the pharmacist.    **Hyperuricemia:**    *PO:*    **ADULTS:** 200 to 800 mg daily.    **CHILDREN:** Up to 6 years old, 50 mg three times daily; 6 to 10 years old, 300 mg daily in single or divided doses.    *Special patient populations:*    **PREGNANCY:** Not for use by pregnant or nursing mothers.

**PREPARATIONS**    *Tablets:* 100 or 300 mg.

**DRUG INTERACTIONS**   **Antineoplastic drugs** Allopurinol inhibits the metabolism of azathioprine and mercaptopurine.   **Diuretics, pyrazinamide, diazoxide, alcohol, mecamylamine** increase uric acid plasma levels.   **Ampicillin and amoxicillin** A rash is likely if either of these is taken with allopurinol.   **Uricosuric agents** are generally additive with allopurinol.   **Chlorpropamide** Allopurinol inhibits its excretion. A hypoglycemic response may arise from excess chlorpropamide.   **Theophylline and related drugs** Allopurinol decreases the clearance of these drugs so that high plasma concentrations may be reached. The dose of theophylline may have to be decreased.

**DIAGNOSTIC TEST INTERFERENCE**   **BUN, serum creatinine** values may be increased.   **Serum alkaline phosphatase, serum transaminase** values may be increased.

**FATE**   Allopurinol is well absorbed and *peak* plasma concentrations are reached in 2 to 6 hours. Allopurinol is metabolized by the enzyme it inhibits to an active metabolite, oxypurinol. Allopurinol and oxypurinol are excreted in the urine and feces.

## ❦ NURSING CONSIDERATIONS

### Side effects, toxicities, and associated nursing actions

**CNS** Drowsiness, headache; neuritis, peripheral neuropathy.
- Caution patient to avoid driving or operating hazardous equipment until the effects of the medication can be evaluated.

**Eye** Rarely, cataracts.
- Assess patients for changes in vision.
- Recommend that patients obtain regular ophthalmologic examinations, especially if over 60.

**GI** Nausea, vomiting, diarrhea, abdominal pain.
- Monitor weight. If vomiting and/or diarrhea occur, monitor intake and output.
- If GI symptoms are severe or persistent, notify the physician.

**GU** Patients with renal disease can show changes in BUN and other renal problems.
- Monitor serum creatinine, BUN.
- Monitor urinalysis, urine uric acid.

**Hematologic** Rarely, leukopenia, thrombocytopenia; patients with bone marrow suppression were usually also taking other drugs with these hematologic side effects.

**Skin** Pruritic rash, rarely accompanied by loss of hair, fever, malaise.

**Allergic** Rare, usually accompanied by fever, chills, arthralgia, rash, pruritis, depression of blood counts.
- Inspect patients for development of petechiae, bruising, development of rash, skin changes, hair loss.
- Caution patients to report the development of unexplained bruising or bleeding, fever, chills, skin changes, rash, sore throat, malaise.
- Monitor complete blood count, white blood cell differential, and platelet count, serum uric acid.

**Other** Alterations in liver function tests; hepatotoxic reactions.
- Assess patients for development of right upper quadrant abdominal pain, jaundice, change in color or consistency of stools.
- Monitor liver function tests.

### Nursing interventions related to drug administration
- Administer doses after meals.

### Patient and family education
- Review with patients anticipated benefits and possible side effects of therapy. Instruct patients to report the development of any unexpected sign or symptom.
- Instruct patients taking allopurinol to maintain oral intake sufficient to ensure a daily urinary output of at least 2 l; this may require an intake of 3000 ml/day.
- Instruct patients with gout to follow a diet that avoids foods with a high amount of purine. Foods to be avoided include organ meats, roe, sardines, scallops, anchovies, broth and consommé, and mincemeat.
- Instruct patients to limit intake of alcohol.

## colchicine    (KOL-chi-seen)    antigout

- colchicine: generic

**MECHANISM OF ACTION**    Colchicine appears to reduce the inflammatory response to deposition of mono-sodium urate crystals in joint tissues.

**INDICATIONS**    Gout Colchicine provides relief from the pain of an acute attack of gouty arthritis, usually within 24 hours.

**CONTRAINDICATIONS**    • Hypersensitivity. • Serious GI, renal, cardiac, hepatic, or blood disorders.

**DOSAGE**    PO:    ADULTS: To relieve or prevent a gouty attack, 0.5 to 1.2 mg initially, followed by 0.5 to 0.6 mg every 1 to 2 hours or 1 to 1.2 mg every 2 hours until the pain is relieved or until nausea, vomiting, or diarrhea occurs. The total dosage required is usually 4 to 8 mg. Joint pain and swelling usually go down in 12 hours and are gone in 2 to 3 days. Prophylaxis: 0.5 or 0.6 mg one to four times a week. IV:    ADULTS: To relieve a gouty attack: Initially, 2 mg, followed by 0.5 mg every 6 hours until relief is obtained. Alternatively, 1 mg initially, with 0.5 mg subsequently or 3 mg initially. Maximum daily dose is 4 mg.    *Special patient populations:*    PREGNANCY: Safe use has not been established.

**PREPARATIONS**    *Tablets:* 0.5, 0.54, or 0.65 mg; *injection:* 0.5 mg/ml.

**DRUG INTERACTIONS**    **Sympathomimetics, CNS depressants** Colchicine enhances the response to these agents.

**DIAGNOSTIC TEST INTERFERENCE**    **17-hydroxysteroids** Determination of urinary values is unreliable when using the Reddy, Jenkins, and Thorn procedure.

**FATE**    Colchicine is metabolized in the liver. Cholchicine and its metabolites undergo enterohepatic circulation and are eventually excreted in the feces. The *onset of action* is 6 to 12 hours, with *peak action* in 24 to 48 hours.

### ☙ NURSING CONSIDERATIONS

#### Side effects, toxicities, and associated nursing actions

**GI** Nausea, vomiting, diarrhea. These are early signs of colchicine toxicity, and the drug should be discontinued when they occur.
- Instruct patients to report the development of GI symptoms.

**GU** Renal damage, hematuria.
- Monitor serum creatinine, BUN.
- Monitor urinalysis. Instruct patient to report a change in color of urine (may reflect hematuria).

**Hematologic** Bone marrow depression, agranulocytosis, thrombocytopenia, leukopenia, aplastic anemia may occur with prolonged administration.
- Inspect patient for bruising, petechiae.
- Instruct patient to report the development of unexplained bruising or bleeding, fever, sore throat, malaise.
- Monitor complete blood count, white blood cell differential, platelet count.

**Skin** Loss of hair, dermatitis.
- Visually inspect patient for these conditions.
- Instruct patient to report the development of any skin or hair changes.

**Other** Liver damage.
- Assess patient for jaundice, right upper quadrant abdominal pain, change in color or consistency of stools.
- Monitor liver function tests.

#### Nursing interventions related to drug administration
- For IV administration, may be given undiluted or diluted with 0.9% sodium chloride without a bacteriostatic agent. Administer at a rate of 0.5 mg over 1 minute.
- Avoid extravasation or IM administration. Check that IV line is in vein before administering.
- Administer oral preparations with milk or a snack to lessen gastric irritation.

#### Patient and family education
- Review anticipated benefits and possible side effects of therapy with patients. Instruct patients to report the development of any unexpected sign or symptom.

- Instruct patients taking colchicine to maintain oral intake sufficient to ensure a daily urinary output of at least 2 l; this may require an intake of 3000 ml/day.
- Instruct patients with gout to follow a diet that avoids foods with a high amount of purine. Foods to be avoided include organ meats, roe, sardines, scallops, anchovies, broth and consommé, and mincemeat.
- Instruct patients to limit intake of alcohol.

## probenecid   (proe-BEN-e-sid)                                          antigout

- probenecid: Benemid, ✿Benuryl, Probalan, ✿Pro-Biosan, SK-Probenecid

**MECHANISM OF ACTION**   Probenecid inhibits the reabsorption of uric acid in the kidney tubules and thereby promotes the excretion of uric acid in the urine.

**INDICATIONS**   Gout Probenecid is used prophylactically to reduce existing tophi and to prevent recurrence of a gouty attack.

**CONTRAINDICATIONS**   • Hypersensitivity. • Blood dyscrasias. • Uric acid kidney stones. • Moderate to severe renal impairment.

**DOSAGE**   PO:   ADULTS: Initially, 250 mg twice daily during the first week, followed by 500 mg twice daily. The goal is to bring the 24 hour uric acid secretion to under 700 mg. The daily dosage may be increased monthly by 500 mg to a maximum of 3 g daily.   *Special patient populations:*   CHILDREN: Not for use by children under 2 years old.   PREGNANCY: Use during pregnancy has not been associated with any adverse effects.

**PREPARATIONS**   *Tablets:* 500 mg.

**DRUG INTERACTIONS**   Salicylates antagonize the uricosuric action.   Methotrexate, sulfonamides, sulfonylureas, naproxen, indomethacin, rifampin, aminosalicylic acid, dapsone, clofibrate, pantothenic acid Probenecid inhibits the renal excretion of these drugs. They may reach toxic levels.

**DIAGNOSTIC TEST INTERFERENCE**   Urinary glucose False-positive test results with cupric sulfate reagents, as in Benedict's Qualitative Reagent, Clinitest, Fehling's Solution. There is no interference with glucose oxidase reagents: Clinistix, TesTape.

**FATE**   Probenecid is well absorbed, with *peak* plasma concentrations in 2 to 4 hours. The *plasma half-life* is 8 to 10 hours. Probenecid is metabolized to active compounds that are excreted in the urine.

☙ **NURSING CONSIDERATIONS**

**Side effects, toxicities, and associated nursing actions**

**CNS** Dizziness, headache.
- Caution patients to avoid driving or operating hazarous equipment until the effects of the medication can be evaluated.

**CV** Flushing.
- Warn patients to anticipate this side effect.

**GI** Nausea, vomiting, anorexia.
- Monitor weight.
- If GI effects are severe or persistent, it may be necessary to lower dosage or change drugs; notify the physician.
- Taking oral doses with meals may lessen gastric irritation.

**GU** Urinary frequency.
- Caution patient about this side effect. Assess patient carefully to differentiate urinary frequency from urinary tract infection.

**Skin** Dermatitis, pruritis.
- Visually inspect patient for signs of skin changes.
- Instruct patient to report the development of skin changes.

**Metabolic** Renal or liver damage is rare.

- Assess patient for weight gain, right upper qudrant abdominal pain, jaundice, change in color or consistency of stools.
- Monitor liver function test, serum creatinine, BUN.

**Allergic** Rarely, skin rash, fever, sweating, hypotension.

- Assess patient for development of allergic reactions.
- Monitor blood pressure.

### Patient and family education

- Review with patients anticipated benefits and possible side effects of therapy. Instruct patients to report the development of any unexpected sign or symptom.
- Instruct patients taking probenecid to maintain oral intake sufficient to ensure a daily urinary output of at least 2 l; this may require an intake of 3000 ml/day.
- Instruct patients with gout to follow a diet that avoids foods with a high amount of purine. Foods to be avoided include organ meats, roe, sardines, scallops, anchovies, broth and consommé, and mincemeat.
- Instruct patients to limit intake of alcohol.
- Alkalinization of the urine helps prevent crystallization of uric acid. For this reason, sodium bicarbonate, potassium citrate, or other alkalinizing agents may be prescribed concurrently with this drug.
- Note drug interactions. Instruct patients to avoid the use of analgesics containing salicylates without prior approval of the physician.

## sulfinpyrazone   (sul-fin-PEER-a-zone)                                      antigout, antiplatelet

- sulfinpyrazone: ♣Antazone, Anturane, ♣Apo-Sulfinpyrazone, ♣Novopyrazone, ♣Zynol

**MECHANISM OF ACTION**   Sulfinpyrazone inhibits the reabsorption of uric acid in the kidney tubules and thereby promotes the excretion of uric acid in the urine. Sulfinpyrazone also inhibits platelet aggregation.

**INDICATIONS**   **Gout** Sulfinpyrazone is used prophylactically to reduce existing tophi and to prevent recurrence of a gouty attack.   **Thromboembolic disorders** To decrease platelet aggregation.

**CONTRAINDICATIONS**   • Peptic ulcer or GI bleeding. • Salicylate therapy.

**DOSAGE**   **PO:**   **ADULTS:** To reduce hyperuricemia of gout. Initially, 100 to 200 mg twice daily for the first week. Raise if needed to 200 to 400 mg twice daily. To decrease platelet aggregation, 600 to 800 mg daily.   *Special patient populations:*   **PREGNANCY:** Safe use has not been established.

**PREPARATIONS**   *Capsules:* 200 mg *tablets* 100 mg.

**DRUG INTERACTIONS**   **Salicylates** antagonize the action of sulfinpyrazone.   **Sulfonamides** Sulfinpyrazone potentiates the action of these drugs.   **Coumarins** Sulfinpyrazone displaces these from albumin and potentiates their action.   **Cholestyramine** may delay the absorption of sulfinpyrazone. Give sulfinpyrazone 1 hour before or 6 hours after cholestyramine.

**FATE**   Sulfinpyrazone is well absorbed, and *peak* concentrations are measured in 2 hours. The *duration of action* is 4 to 6 hours. Sulfinpyrazone is highly bound to plasma protein. It is metabolized in the liver and excreted in the urine.

### ☕ NURSING CONSIDERATIONS

#### Side effects, toxicities, and associated nursing actions

**CNS** Tinnitus.

- Assess patients at regular intervals for changes in hearing or development of tinnitus.

**GI** Nausea, dyspepsia, GI pain, blood loss, reactivation of peptic ulcer.

- Monitor for GI symptoms.
- Instruct patient to report the development of GI symptoms; if severe or persistent, it may be necessary to doscontinue the drug.
- Taking doses with meals or a snack may lessen gastric irritation.

**Skin** Rash.

- Visually inspect patient for rash.

### Patient and family education

- Review with patients anticipated benefits and possible side effects of therapy. Instruct patients to report the development of any unexpected sign or symptom.
- Instruct patients taking sulfinpyrazone to maintain oral intake sufficient to ensure a daily urinary output of at least 2 liter; this may require an intake of 3000 ml/day.
- Instruct patients with gout to follow a diet that avoids foods with a high amount of purine. Foods to be avoided include organ meats, roe, sardines, scallops, anchovies, broth and consommé, and mincemeat.
- Instruct patients to limit intake of alcohol.
- Note drug interactions. Instruct patients to avoid the use of analgesics containing salicylates without prior approval of the physician.

# DRUGS FOR ALLERGY, ASTHMA, AND RESPIRATORY PROBLEMS

**INTRODUCTION**   This unit reviews the many drugs used to treat problems of the respiratory tract. Antihistamines are widely used to control hayfever and allergies. While many antihistamines are prescription drugs, several antihistamines are also widely available over-the-counter for the relief of colds and allergies and as sleep aids. Various drug classes are used to treat asthma. Several adrenergic bronchodilators have been developed for oral, inhalation, and subcutaneous administration for the relief of severe bronchospasm. Theophylline is the major xanthine used as a bronchodilator, but doses must be highly individualized. Cromolyn sodium is used prophylactically to prevent acute asthma attacks. Several glucocorticoids are available for inhalation administration. Administered in this fashion, glucocorticoids may be useful prophylactically for severe asthma without causing systemic side effects.

Nasal decongestants act by constricting nasal blood vessels so that fluids do not escape. Most of these drugs are available over-the-counter. Table 53-1 lists combination products for the relief of nasal congestion. These products commonly combine an antihistamine and nasal decongestant, and often include an analgesic. Expectorants are drugs that help maintain respiratory fluid to keep a cough productive. Antitussives suppress a cough. Selected expectorants and antitussives are available as over-the-counter agents.

# Chapter Fifty-one

# Antihistamines

azatadine

brompheniramine

carbinoxamine

chlorpheniramine

clemastine

cyproheptadine

diphenhydramine

diphenylpyraline

doxylamine

methdilazine

promethazine

terfenadine

trimeprazine

tripelennamine

triprolidine

**DRUG COMBINATIONS**   Antihistamines are commonly combined with other drugs, especially nasal decongestants. These combination products are listed in Table 53-1 (p. 951).

**OVERVIEW OF THE DRUG CLASS**   Histamine is a naturally occurring amine that is formed from the amino acid histidine. Histamine is found in three major sites. One site is in mast cells, which are numerous in the lung and skin, and basophils, the counterparts of mast cells in the blood. The histamine released from the mast cell causes many of the symptoms associated with allergic reactions. This happens because histamine acts at specific receptors, H-1 receptors. The second site is in the gastrointestinal tract, where histamine is a potent stimulant for the secretion of acid in the stomach. These receptors for histamine are called H-2 receptors. The third site is in certain parts of the brain, where histamine is believed to be a neurotransmitter. These receptor sites have not been fully characterized.

**MECHANISM OF ACTION**   Antihistamines are competitive antagonists for histamine at the H-1 histamine receptors. These drugs block many of the actions of the histamine released in allergic reactions. Recently, competitive antagonists for H-2 receptors in the gastrointestinal system have been introduced. These are used to inhibit gastric acid secretion and are described in Chapter 58.

**INDICATIONS**   **Allergies** Antihistamines are effective in decreasing the discomfort of acute allergic reactions that involve the upper respiratory system, such as hay fever, or the skin, such as hives.   **Nasal congestion** The anticholinergic effect of many antihistamines tends to dry up a runny nose and relieve the symptoms of a cold.   **Insomnia, anxiety** In general, antihistamines have a sedating effect. Pyrilamine, doxylamine, and diphenhydramine are included in many over-the-counter sleep aids. This use is not covered in this section.   **Vomiting** Selected antihistamines are especially effective in preventing the nausea and vomiting of motion sickness. These antihistamines are cyclizine, meclizine, and dimenhydrinate (these are covered in Chapter 55).

**CONTRAINDICATIONS**   **Hypersensitivity to antihistamines. Monoamine oxidase therapy. Acute glaucoma, peptic ulcer, prostatic hypertrophy, asthma attack, bladder neck obstruction, pyloroduodenal obstruction** These conditions are made worse by the anticholinergic action of antihistamines.

**DRUG INTERACTIONS**   **CNS depressants** Antihistamines can have additive depression with CNS depressants, including alcohol.   **Epinephrine** Diphenhydramine, tripelennamine, and chlorpheniramine synergize the effects of epinephrine.   **Monoamine oxidase inhibitors** prolong and intensify the anticholinergic effects of antihistamines.

## ☙ NURSING CONSIDERATIONS

### Side effects, toxicities, and associated nursing actions

**CNS** Drowsiness, sedation, dizziness, incoordination; fatigue, confusion. Excitation and insomnia are paradoxical reactions more common in children than adults.

**Eye** Blurred vision.

- Instruct patients to avoid driving or operating hazardous equipment until the effects of the medication can be evaluated.
- Supervise ambulation, especially of the elderly.
- Keep siderails up, keep nightlight on at night, and supervise smoking.
- Increasing or changing dosages is best done near bedtime if drowsiness is a problem. If excitation or insomnia occur, the last dose of the day should be taken by late afternoon if possible.
- If blurred vision occurs, notify physician.

- Antihistamines are occasionally ordered to be given simultaneously with narcotics to relieve pain. Antihistamines potentiate the central nervous system depression, but do not alleviate pain. If both drugs are given together, it may be necessary to reduce the dose of the antihistamine if excessive sedation occurs.

**CV** Hypotension, headache, palpitations; fast heart rate.
- Monitor blood pressure and pulse.
- Supervise ambulation, especially in the elderly.
- Keep siderails up.

**GU** Urinary frequency, difficulty in urination.
- In hospital, monitor intake and output.
- Assess for urinary complaints of frequency, difficulty initiating urination, feeling that bladder is not emptying.
- If difficulty in urination is present, have patient void before receiving dose of medication.

**GI** Dryness of mouth, nose, and throat. Epigastric distress; loss of appetite, nausea, and vomiting.
- Dry mouth may be aggravated if patient must also mouth-breathe. Encourage patient to take frequent sips of water, perform regular oral hygiene (but avoid drying mouthwashes and gargles), chew sugarless gum, or suck on sugarless candies. If drug therapy is short term, patient may be willing to tolerate discomfort. If drug therapy is long term, and dry mouth is significant, some patients may wish to consider the use of commercially available saliva substitutes.
- If constipation occurs, encourage patient to increase dietary intake of fruits, fruit juices, and fiber; to increase fluid intake to 3000 ml per day; and to increase amount of daily exercise. In rare instances, a stool softener may be prescribed.
- GI side effects may be lessened by taking oral doses with meals or light snack.
- Monitor weight and intake and output if loss of appetite seems significant.

**Hematologic** Hemolytic anemia; thrombocytopenia, leukopenia, and agranulocytosis.
- Monitor complete blood count, white blood cell count and differential, and platelets.
- Assess for subjective complaints of fatigue and malaise.
- Instruct patient to report the development of sore throat, fever, petechiae, bruising, or unexplained bleeding.

**Lung** Thickening of bronchial secretions, wheezing.
- Auscultate breath sounds.
- Encourage patient to maintain hydration through intake of up to 3000 ml per 24 hours.

**Skin** Drug rash, photosensitivity, excessive perspiration.
- If photosensitivity occurs, instruct patient to avoid prolonged exposure to the sun or ultraviolet light; to wear a hat, long sleeves, and long pants when in the sun; and to use maximum-protection sunscreens on exposed skin surfaces.
- Inspect for development of drug rash.

### Nursing interventions related to drug administration
- Read labels carefully when preparing parenteral doses. Some forms are for IM or subcutaneous injection only and should not be used for IV administrations.
- Sustained-release forms should be swallowed whole, not crushed or chewed. Scored tablets may be broken before swallowing. Capsules may be opened and contents poured into soft food for ease in taking.
- Use anatomical landmarks for choosing IM injection sites. Only large muscle masses should be used, such as the dorsogluteal site or the rectus femoris muscle in adults, or the vastus lateralis in infants and small children. Aspirate prior to injecting medication to avoid inadvertent IV injection. Record and rotate injection sites.

### Patient and family education
- Review with patients the expected benefits and possible side effects of drug therapy. Caution patients to report the development of any unexplained sign or symptom.
- Teach patients to avoid the use of alcohol and other medications that depress the central nervous system; examples include sedatives, tranquilizers, sleeping pills, barbiturates, and narcotic analgesics.

- Instruct patient that when the drug is used for motion sickness, it should be taken about 30 minutes prior to exposure to motion.
- Encourage patients with allergies to wear a medical identification tag or bracelet indicating their allergies.
- Caution patients to avoid the use of any over the counter preparations unless first approved by the physician.
- Remind patients to keep these and all medications out of the reach of children.

## azatadine maleate    (a-ZA-ta-deen)                                    antihistamine

- azatadine maleate: Optimine

**MECHANISM OF ACTION**   Antihistamines block H-1 receptors for histamine, thereby preventing many allergic symptoms.

**INDICATIONS**   Allergic rhinitis, chronic urticaria.

**CONTRAINDICATIONS**   Hypersensitivity to antihistamines. Monoamine oxidase therapy. Acute glaucoma, peptic ulcer, prostatic hypertrophy, asthma attack, bladder neck obstruction, pyloroduodenal obstruction These conditions are made worse by the anticholinergic action of antihistamines.

**DOSAGE**   PO:   **ADULTS AND CHILDREN OVER 12 YEARS OLD:** 1 to 2 mg twice daily.   **CHILDREN 6 TO 12 YEARS OLD:** 0.5 to 1 mg twice daily.   *Special patient populations:*   PREGNANCY: Safe use has not been established.

**PREPARATIONS**   *Tablets:* 1 mg.

**DRUG INTERACTIONS**   **CNS depressants** Antihistamines can have additive depression with CNS depressants, including alcohol.   **Epinephrine** Diphenhydramine, tripelennamine, and chlorpheniramine synergize the effects of epinephrine.   **Monoamine oxidase inhibitors** prolong and intensify the anticholinergic effects of antihistamines.

**FATE**   Antihistamines are well absorbed after oral administration. The *onset of action* is generally within 15 to 30 minutes, and the *duration of action* is generally 3 to 6 hours. Antihistamines are metabolized in the liver and excreted in the urine.

❦ **NURSING CONSIDERATIONS**

**Side effects, toxicities, and associated nursing actions**
- See entry for drug class (p. 918).

**Nursing interventions related to drug administration**
- See entry for drug class (p. 919).

**Patient and family education**
- See entry for drug class (p. 919).

## brompheniramine maleate    (brome-fen-IR-a-meen)                        antihistamine

- brompheniramine maleate: ✤Parabromdylamine maleate, Brombay, Bromphen, Dimetane

**MECHANISM OF ACTION**   Antihistamines block H-1 receptors for histamine, thereby preventing many allergic symptoms.

**INDICATIONS**   Allergic rhinitis, nasal congestion, chronic urticaria.

**CONTRAINDICATIONS**   Hypersensitivity to antihistamines. Monoamine oxidase therapy. Acute glaucoma, peptic ulcer, prostatic hypertrophy, asthma attack, bladder neck obstruction, pyloroduodenal obstruction These conditions are made worse by the anticholinergic action of antihistamines.

**DOSAGE**   PO:   **ADULTS AND CHILDREN UNDER 12 YEARS OLD:** 4 mg every 4 to 6 hours.   **CHILDREN 6 TO 12 YEARS OLD:** 2 mg every 4 to 6 hours.   **CHILDREN 1 TO 6 YEARS OLD:** 1 mg every 4 to 6 hours.   *Special patient populations:*   PREGNANCY: Safe use has not been established.

**PREPARATIONS**   *Solution:* 2 mg/5 ml; *tablets:* 4 mg; *tablets (extended release):* 8, 12 mg; *injection:* 10, 100 mg/ml.

**DRUG INTERACTIONS**   **CNS depressants** Antihistamines can have additive depression with CNS depressants, including alcohol.   **Epinephrine** Diphenhydramine, tripelennamine, and chlorpheniramine synergize the effects of epinephrine.   **Monoamine oxidase inhibitors** prolong and intensify the anticholinergic effects of antihistamines.

**FATE**   Antihistamines are well absorbed after oral administration. The *onset of action* is generally within 15 to 30 minutes, and the *duration of action* is generally 3 to 6 hours. Antihistamines are metabolized in the liver and excreted in the urine.

## ☙ NURSING CONSIDERATIONS

### Side effects, toxicities, and associated nursing actions

* See entry for drug class (p. 918).

### Nursing interventions related to drug administration

* IV brompheniramine maleate may be given undiluted or may be added to infusing fluids (normal saline or 5% dextrose). Check with the pharmacist for compatibility with other drugs before mixing this drug with infusing drugs. A single bolus injection should be administered over at least 1 minute.

### Patient and family education

* See entry for drug class (p. 919).

---

## carbinoxamine maleate   (kar-bi-NOX-a-meen)      antihistamine

* carbinoxamine maleate: ✚Paracarbinoxamine Maleate, Clistin, Cardec, Rondec

**MECHANISM OF ACTION**   Antihistamines block H-1 receptors for histamine, thereby preventing many allergic symptoms.

**INDICATIONS**   Allergic rhinitis, chronic urticaria.

**CONTRAINDICATIONS**   Hypersensitivity to antihistamines. Monoamine oxidase therapy. Acute glaucoma, peptic ulcer, prostatic hypertrophy, asthma attack, bladder neck obstruction, pyloroduodenal obstruction These conditions are made worse by the anticholinergic action of antihistamines.

**DOSAGE**   **PO:**   **ADULTS AND CHILDREN:** 4 to 8 mg three or four times daily.   **CHILDREN:** 0.2 to 0.4 mg/kg daily, in 3 or 4 divided doses.   *Special patient populations:*   **PREGNANCY:** Safe use has not been established.

**PREPARATIONS**   *Tablets:* 4 mg.

**DRUG INTERACTIONS**   **CNS depressants** Antihistamines can have additive depression with CNS depressants, including alcohol.   **Epinephrine** Diphenhydramine, tripelennamine, and chlorpheniramine synergize the effects of epinephrine.   **Monoamine oxidase inhibitors** prolong and intensify the anticholinergic effects of antihistamines.

**FATE**   Antihistamines are well absorbed after oral administration. The *onset of action* is generally within 15 to 30 minutes, and the *duration of action* is generally 3 to 6 hours. Antihistamines are metabolized in the liver and excreted in the urine.

## ☙ NURSING CONSIDERATIONS

### Side effects, toxicities, and associated nursing actions

* See entry for drug class (p. 918).

### Nursing interventions related to drug administration

* Clistin-D brand tablets containing acetaminophen 300 mg and phenylephrine 10 mg contain FD & C yellow dye #5 (tartrazine), which may cause an allergic reaction in susceptible individuals. While rare, this side effect is seen more commonly in persons with aspirin hypersensitivity.

### Patient and family education

* See entry for drug class (p. 919).

## chlorpheniramine maleate  (klor-fen-EER-a-meen)  antihistamine

• chlorpheniramine maleate: Dexchlorpheniramine Maleate, Chlor-Trimeton, ✤Polaramine

**MECHANISM OF ACTION**  Antihistamines block H-1 receptors for histamine, thereby preventing many allergic symptoms.

**INDICATIONS**  Allergic rhinitis, chronic urticaria.

**CONTRAINDICATIONS**  Hypersensitivity to antihistamines. Monoamine oxidase therapy. Acute glaucoma, peptic ulcer, prostatic hypertrophy, asthma attack, bladder neck obstruction, pyloroduodenal obstruction These conditions are made worse by the anticholinergic action of antihistamines.

**DOSAGE**  PO, self-administration:  ADULTS AND CHILDREN OVER 12 YEARS OLD: 4 mg every 4 to 6 hours.  CHILDREN 6 TO 12 YEARS OLD: 2 mg every 4 to 6 hours.  CHILDREN 2 TO 6 YEARS OLD: 1 mg every 4 to 6 hours.  SC, IM, IV:  ADULTS: 10 to 20 mg for relief of allergic reactions to blood or plasma. *Dexchlorpheniramine Maleate:* 1/2 above doses.  *Special patient populations:* PREGNANCY Safe use has not been established.

**PREPARATIONS**  *Chlorpheniramine maleate, capsules:* 6, 8, 12 mg; *solution:* 2 mg/5 ml; *tablets:* 4 mg; *tablets (chewable):* 2 mg; *tablets (extended release):* 8, 12 mg; *injection:* 10 mg/ml; *injection (IM, SC only):* 100 mg/ml. *Dexchlorpheniramine Maleate, solution:* 2 mg/5 ml; *tablets:* 2 mg; *tablets (extended release):* 4, 6 mg.

**DRUG INTERACTIONS**  CNS depressants Antihistamines can have additive depression with CNS depressants, including alcohol.  Epinephrine Diphenhydramine, tripelennamine, and chlorpheniramine synergize the effects of epinephrine.  Monoamine oxidase inhibitors prolong and intensify the anticholinergic effects of antihistamines

**FATE**  Antihistamines are well absorbed after oral administration. The *onset of action* is generally within 15 to 30 minutes, and the *duration of action* is generally 3 to 6 hours. Antihistamines are metabolized in the liver and excreted in the urine.

### ☙ NURSING CONSIDERATIONS

#### Side effects, toxicities, and associated nursing actions
• See entry for drug class (p. 918).

#### Nursing interventions related to drug administration
• Only the 10 mg/ml solution may be administered IV. May be given undiluted at a rate of 10 mg or less over 1 minute.
• Covangesic brand combination product contains FD & C yellow dye #5 (tartrazine), which may cause an allergic reaction in susceptible individuals. While rare, this side effect is seen more commonly in persons with aspirin hypersensitivity.

#### Patient and family education
• See entry for drug class (p. 919).

## clemastine fumarate  (KLEM-as-teen)  antihistamine

• clemastine fumarate: Tavist

**MECHANISM OF ACTION**  Antihistamines block H-1 receptors for histamine, thereby preventing many allergic symptoms.

**INDICATIONS**  Allergic rhinitis, chronic urticaria.

**CONTRAINDICATIONS**  Hypersensitivity to antihistamines. Monoamine oxidase therapy. Acute glaucoma, peptic ulcer, prostatic hypertrophy, asthma attack, bladder neck obstruction, pyloroduodenal obstruction These conditions are made worse by the anticholinergic action of antihistamines.

**DOSAGE**  PO:  ADULTS AND CHILDREN OVER 12 YEARS OLD: 1.34 mg twice daily or 2.68 mg one to three times daily.  CHILDREN UNDER 12 YEARS OLD: 0.67 to 1.34 mg twice daily.  *Special patient populations:*  PREGNANCY: Safe use has not been established.

**PREPARATIONS**   *Tablets:* 1.34, 2.68 mg.

**DRUG INTERACTIONS**   **CNS depressants** Antihistamines can have additive depression with CNS depressants, including alcohol.   **Epinephrine** Diphenhydramine, tripelennamine, and chlorpheniramine synergize the effects of epinephrine.   **Monoamine oxidase inhibitors** prolong and intensify the anticholinergic effects of antihistamines.

**FATE**   Antihistamines are well absorbed after oral administration. The *onset of action* is generally within 15 to 30 minutes, and the *duration of action* is generally 3 to 6 hours. Antihistamines are metabolized in the liver and excreted in the urine.

## ❦ NURSING CONSIDERATIONS

### Side effects, toxicities, and associated nursing actions
- See entry for drug class (p. 918).

### Nursing interventions related to drug administration
- See entry for drug class (p. 919).

### Patient and family education
- See entry for drug class (p. 919).

## cyproheptadine hydrochloride   (si-proe-HEP-ta-deen)   antihistamine

- cyproheptadine hydrochloride: Periactin, ✳Vimicon

**MECHANISM OF ACTION**   Antihistamines block H-1 receptors for histamine, thereby preventing many allergic symptoms.

**INDICATIONS**   Allergic rhinitis, chronic urticaria.

**CONTRAINDICATIONS**   Hypersensitivity to antihistamines. Monoamine oxidase therapy. Acute glaucoma, peptic ulcer, prostatic hypertrophy, asthma attack, bladder neck obstruction, pyloroduodenal obstruction These conditions are made worse by the anticholinergic action of antihistamines.

**DOSAGE**   PO:   **ADULTS AND CHILDREN OVER 14 YEARS OLD:** 4 mg three times daily.   **CHILDREN 7 TO 14 YEARS OLD:** 4 mg two or three times daily.   **CHILDREN 2 TO 6 YEARS OLD:** 2 mg two or three times daily.   *Special patient populations:*   **PREGNANCY:** Safe use has not been established.

**PREPARATIONS**   *Solution:* 2 mg/5 ml; *tablets:* 4 mg.

**DRUG INTERACTIONS**   **CNS depressants** Antihistamines can have additive depression with CNS depressants, including alcohol.   **Epinephrine** Diphenhydramine, tripelennamine, and chlorpheniramine synergize the effects of epinephrine.   **Monoamine oxidase inhibitors** prolong and intensify the anticholinergic effects of antihistamines.

**FATE**   Antihistamines are well absorbed after oral administration. The *onset of action* is generally within 15 to 30 minutes, and the *duration of action* is generally 3 to 6 hours. Antihistamines are metabolized in the liver and excreted in the urine.

## ❦ NURSING CONSIDERATIONS

### Side effects, toxicities, and associated nursing actions
- See entry for drug class (p. 918).

### Nursing interventions related to drug administration
- See entry for drug class (p. 919).

### Patient and family education
- See entry for drug class (p. 919).

## diphenhydramine hydrochloride   (dye-fen-HYE-dra-meen)   antihistamine

- diphenhydramine hydrochloride: Bromodiphenhydramine Hydrochloride Benadryl, Benylin

**MECHANISM OF ACTION**    Antihistamines block H-1 receptors for histamine, thereby preventing many allergic symptoms.

**INDICATIONS**    Allergic rhinitis, chronic urticaria. Cough, nasal congestion.

**CONTRAINDICATIONS**    Hypersensitivity to antihistamines. Monoamine oxidase therapy. Acute glaucoma, peptic ulcer, prostatic hypertrophy, asthma attack, bladder neck obstruction, pyloroduodenal obstruction These conditions are made worse by the anticholinergic action of antihistamines.

**DOSAGE**    PO:    ADULTS: 25 to 50 mg three or four times daily.    CHILDREN OVER 20 LB: 12.5 to 25 mg three or four times daily.    CHILDREN UNDER 20 LB: 6.25 to 12.5 mg three or four times daily.    *Special patient populations:*    PREGNANCY: Safe use has not been established.

**PREPARATIONS**    *Capsules:* 25, 50 mg; *elixir:* 12.5 mg/5 ml; *solution:* 12.5, 13.3 mg/5 ml; *tablets:* 25, 50 mg; *injection:* 10, 50 mg/ml; *cream:* 1%, 2%; *lotion:* 1%.

**DRUG INTERACTIONS**    **CNS depressants** Antihistamines can have additive depression with CNS depressants, including alcohol.    **Epinephrine** Diphenhydramine, tripelennamine, and chlorpheniramine synergize the effects of epinephrine.    **Monoamine oxidase inhibitors** prolong and intensify the anticholinergic effects of antihistamines.

**FATE**    Antihistamines are well absorbed after oral administration. The *onset of action* is generally within 15 to 30 minutes, and the *duration of action* is generally 3 to 6 hours. Antihistamines are metabolized in the liver and excreted in the urine.

## ❦ NURSING CONSIDERATIONS

### Side effects, toxicities, and associated nursing actions
- See entry for drug class (p. 918).

### Nursing interventions related to drug administration
- IV diphenhydramine may be administered undiluted. Administer slowly at a rate not exceeding 25 mg/min.

### Patient and family education
- See entry for drug class (p. 919).

---

## diphenylpyraline hydrochloride    (dye-fen-il-PEER-a-leen)    antihistamine

- diphenylpyraline hydrochloride: Hispril, ✺Chemhisdine

**MECHANISM OF ACTION**    Antihistamines block H-1 receptors for histamine, thereby preventing many allergic symptoms.

**INDICATIONS**    Allergic rhinitis, chronic urticaria.

**CONTRAINDICATIONS**    Hypersensitivity to antihistamines. Monoamine oxidase therapy. Acute glaucoma, peptic ulcer, prostatic hypertrophy, asthma attack, bladder neck obstruction, pyloroduodenal obstruction. These conditions are made worse by the anticholinergic action of antihistamines.

**DOSAGE**    PO:    ADULTS AND CHILDREN OVER 12 YEARS OLD: 5 mg every 12 hours.    CHILDREN 6 to 12 YEARS OLD: 5 mg once daily.    *Special patient populations:*    PREGNANCY: Safe use has not been established.

**PREPARATIONS**    *Capsule (extended release):* 5 mg.

**DRUG INTERACTIONS**    **CNS depressants** Antihistamines can have additive depression with CNS depressants, including alcohol.    **Epinephrine** Diphenhydramine, tripelennamine, and chlorpheniramine synergize the effects of epinephrine.    **Monoamine oxidase inhibitors** prolong and intensify the anticholinergic effects of antihistamines.

**FATE**    Antihistamines are well absorbed after oral administration. The *onset of action* is generally within 15 to 30 minutes, and the *duration of action* is generally 3 to 6 hours. Antihistamines are metabolized in the liver and excreted in the urine.

## ❦ NURSING CONSIDERATIONS

### Side effects, toxicities, and associated nursing actions
- See entry for drug class (p. 918).

Nursing interventions related to drug administration
  • See entry for drug class (p. 919).
Patient and family education
  • See entry for drug class (p. 919).

## doxylamine succinate   (dox-IL-a-meen)                          antihistamine

  • doxylamine succinate: Sleep Easy, Unisom, Nighttime Sleep Aid

**MECHANISM OF ACTION**   Antihistamines block H-1 receptors for histamine, thereby preventing many allergic symptoms.
**INDICATIONS**   Insomnia.
**CONTRAINDICATIONS**   Hypersensitivity to antihistamines. Monoamine oxidase therapy. Acute glaucoma, peptic ulcer, prostatic hypertrophy, asthma attack, bladder neck obstruction, pyloroduodenal obstruction These conditions are made worse by the anticholinergic action of antihistamines.
**DOSAGE**   PO:   ADULTS AND CHILDREN OVER 12 YEARS OLD: 25 mg 30 minutes before bedtime. As an antihistamine, 7.5 to 12.5 mg every 4 to 6 hours.   CHILDREN 6 TO 12 YEARS OLD: 3.75 to 6.25 mg every 4 to 6 hours as an antihistamine.   *Special patient populations:*   PREGNANCY: Safe use has not been established.
**PREPARATIONS**   *Tablets:* 25 mg.
**DRUG INTERACTIONS**   CNS depressants Antihistamines can have additive depression with CNS depressants, including alcohol.   **Epinephrine** Diphenhydramine, tripelennamine, and chlorpheniramine synergize the effects of epinephrine.   **Monoamine oxidase inhibitors** prolong and intensify the anticholinergic effects of antihistamines.
**FATE**   Antihistamines are well absorbed after oral administration. The *onset of action* is generally within 15 to 30 minutes, and the *duration of action* is generally 3 to 6 hours. Antihistamines are metabolized in the liver and excreted in the urine.

### ❦ NURSING CONSIDERATIONS
Side effects, toxicities, and associated nursing actions
  • See entry for drug class (p. 918).
Nursing interventions related to drug administration
  • See entry for drug class (p. 919).
Patient and family education
  • See entry for drug class (p. 919).

## methdilazine, methdilazine hydrochloride
(meth-DILL-a-zeen)                                                antihistamine

  • methdilazine, methdilazine hydrochloride: ✿Dilosyn, Tacaryl

**MECHANISM OF ACTION**   Antihistamines block H-1 receptors for histamine, thereby preventing many allergic symptoms.
**INDICATIONS**   Allergic rhinitis, chronic urticaria.
**CONTRAINDICATIONS**   Hypersensitivity to antihistamines. Monoamine oxidase therapy. Acute glaucoma, peptic ulcer, prostatic hypertrophy, asthma attack, bladder neck obstruction, pyloroduodenal obstruction These conditions are made worse by the anticholinergic action of antihistamines.
**DOSAGE**   PO:   ADULTS AND CHILDREN OVER 12 YEARS OLD: 8 mg two to four times daily.   CHILDREN 3 TO 12 YEARS OLD: 4 mg two to four times daily.   *Special patient populations:*   PREGNANCY: Safe use has not been established.
**PREPARATIONS**   *Methdilazine, tablets:* 3.6 mg. *Methdilazine hydrochloride, tablets:* 8 mg; *solution:* 4 mg/5 ml.

**DRUG INTERACTIONS**   **CNS depressants** Antihistamines can have additive depression with CNS depressants, including alcohol.   **Epinephrine** Diphenhydramine, tripelennamine, and chlorpheniramine synergize the effects of epinephrine.   **Monoamine oxidase inhibitors** prolong and intensify the anticholinergic effects of antihistamines.

**FATE**   Antihistamines are well absorbed after oral administration. The *onset of action* is generally within 15 to 30 minutes, and the *duration of action* is generally 3 to 6 hours. Antihistamines are metabolized in the liver and excreted in the urine.

### ❦ NURSING CONSIDERATIONS
#### Side effects, toxicities, and associated nursing actions
- See entry for drug class (p. 918).
#### Nursing interventions related to drug administration
- See entry for drug class (p. 919).
#### Patient and family education
- See entry for drug class (p. 919).

---

## promethazine hydrochloride   (proe-METH-a-zeen)                    antihistamine

- promethazine hydrochloride: ✽Histanil, Phenergan, ✽Rhinaris, ✽Secaris

**MECHANISM OF ACTION**   Antihistamines block H-1 receptors for histamine, thereby preventing many allergic symptoms.

**INDICATIONS**   Allergic rhinitis, chronic urticaria.   Sedative, antiemetic.

**CONTRAINDICATIONS**   Hypersensitivity to antihistamines.   Monoamine oxidase therapy.   Acute glaucoma, peptic ulcer, prostatic hypertrophy, asthma attack, bladder neck obstruction, pyloroduodenal obstruction These conditions are made worse by the anticholinergic action of antihistamines.

**DOSAGE**   PO:   **ADULTS AND CHILDREN:** *Antihistamine:* 25 mg before bedtime. *Motion sickness:* 12.5 to 25 mg 30 to 60 minutes prior to departure.   *Special patient populations:*   PREGNANCY: Safe use has not been established.

**PREPARATIONS**   *Tablets:* 12.5, 25, 50 mg; *solution:* 6.25, 25 mg/5 ml; *injection:* 25 mg/ml; *injection (IM):* 25 mg/ml; *suppositories:* 12.5, 25, 50 mg.

**DRUG INTERACTIONS**   **CNS depressants** Antihistamines can have additive depression with CNS depressants, including alcohol.   **Epinephrine** Diphenhydramine, tripelennamine, and chlorpheniramine synergize the effects of epinephrine.   **Monoamine oxidase inhibitors** prolong and intensify the anticholinergic effects of antihistamines.

**FATE**   Antihistamines are well absorbed after oral administration. The *onset of action* is generally within 15 to 30 minutes, and the *duration of action* is generally 3 to 6 hours. Antihistamines are metabolized in the liver and excreted in the urine.

### ❦ NURSING CONSIDERATIONS
#### Side effects, toxicities, and associated nursing actions
- See entry for drug class (p. 918).
#### Nursing interventions related to drug administration
- For IV use, solutions should never be more concentrated than 25 mg/ml. Dilute the drug with up to 9 ml of normal saline to make a dilution of 2.5 to 5 mg/ml. Rate of administration should not exceed 25 mg per minute. Slightly yellow solutions may be safely used. Highly discolored solutions should be discarded.
#### Patient and family education
- See entry for drug class (p. 919).

---

## terfenadine   (ter-FEN-a-deen)                    antihistamine

- terfenadine: Seldane

**MECHANISM OF ACTION**   Antihistamines block H-1 receptors for histamine, thereby preventing many allergic symptoms.

**INDICATIONS**   Allergic rhinitis, chronic urticaria.

**CONTRAINDICATIONS**   Hypersensitivity to antihistamines.   Monoamine oxidase therapy.   Acute glaucoma, peptic ulcer, prostatic hypertrophy, asthma attack, bladder neck obstruction, pyloroduodenal obstruction These conditions are made worse by the anticholinergic action of antihistamines.

**DOSAGE**   PO:   ADULTS AND CHILDREN OVER 12 YEARS OLD: 60 mg twice daily.   CHILDREN 3 TO 6 YEARS OLD: 15 mg twice daily.   CHILDREN 7 TO 12 YEARS OLD: 30 mg twice daily.   *Special patient populations:*   PREGNANCY: Safe use has not been established.

**PREPARATIONS**   *Tablets:* 60 mg.

**DRUG INTERACTIONS**   **CNS depressants** Antihistamines can have additive depression with CNS depressants, including alcohol.   **Epinephrine** Diphenhydramine, tripelennamine, and chlorpheniramine synergize the effects of epinephrine.   **Monoamine oxidase inhibitors** prolong and intensify the anticholinergic effects of antihistamines.

**FATE**   Antihistamines are well absorbed after oral administration. The *onset of action* is generally within 15 to 30 minutes, and the *duration of action* is generally 3 to 6 hours. Antihistamines are metabolized in the liver and excreted in the urine.

**☙ NURSING CONSIDERATIONS**

**Side effects, toxicities, and associated nursing actions**
- See entry for drug class (p. 918).

**Nursing interventions related to drug administration**
- See entry for drug class (p. 919).

**Patient and family education**
- See entry for drug class (p. 919).

---

## trimeprazine tartrate   (trye-MEP-ra-zeen)   antihistamine

- trimeprazine tartrate: ✲Pancectyl, Temaril

**MECHANISM OF ACTION**   Antihistamines block H-1 receptors for histamine, thereby preventing many allergic symptoms.

**INDICATIONS**   Allergic rhinitis, chronic urticaria.

**CONTRAINDICATIONS**   Hypersensitivity to antihistamines.   Monoamine oxidase therapy.   Acute glaucoma, peptic ulcer, prostatic hypertrophy, asthma attack, bladder neck obstruction, pyloroduodenal obstruction These conditions are made worse by the anticholinergic action of antihistamines.

**DOSAGE**   PO:   ADULTS AND CHILDREN OVER 6 YEARS OLD: 2.5 mg four times daily.   CHILDREN 3 TO 6 YEARS OLD: 2.5 mg three times daily.   CHILDREN 6 MONTHS TO 3 YEARS OLD: 1.25 mg at bedtime or 1.25 mg three times daily.   *Special patient populations:*   PREGNANCY: Safe use has not been established.

**PREPARATIONS**   *Tablets:* 2.5 mg; *capsules (extended release):* 5 mg; *solution:* 2.5 mg/5 ml.

**DRUG INTERACTIONS**   **CNS depressants** Antihistamines can have additive depression with CNS depressants, including alcohol.   **Epinephrine** Diphenhydramine, tripelennamine, and chlorpheniramine synergize the effects of epinephrine.   **Monoamine oxidase inhibitors** prolong and intensify the anticholinergic effects of antihistamines.

**FATE**   Antihistamines are well absorbed after oral administration. The *onset of action* is generally within 15 to 30 minutes, and the *duration of action* is generally 3 to 6 hours. Antihistamines are metabolized in the liver and excreted in the urine.

**☙ NURSING CONSIDERATIONS**

**Side effects, toxicities, and associated nursing actions**
- See entry for drug class (p. 918).

**Nursing interventions related to drug administration**
- See entry for drug class (p. 919).

**Patient and family education**
- See entry for drug class (p. 919).

---

# tripelennamine citrate, tripelennamine hydrochloride
(trye-pel-ENN-a-meen)                                                     antihistamine

- tripelennamine citrate, tripelennamine hydrochloride: PBZ, ✿Pyribenzamine

**MECHANISM OF ACTION**   Antihistamines block H-1 receptors for histamine, thereby preventing many allergic symptoms.

**INDICATIONS**   Allergic rhinitis, chronic urticaria.

**CONTRAINDICATIONS**   Hypersensitivity to antihistamines.   Monoamine oxidase therapy. Acute glaucoma, peptic ulcer, prostatic hypertrophy, asthma attack, bladder neck obstruction, pyloroduodenal obstruction These conditions are made worse by the anticholinergic action of antihistamines.

**DOSAGE**   PO:   ADULTS AND CHILDREN OVER 12 YEARS OLD: 25 to 50 mg every 4 to 6 hours.   CHILDREN: 5 mg/kg in 4 to 6 divided doses.   *Special patient populations:*   PREGNANCY: Safe use has not been established.

**PREPARATIONS**   *Citrate, elixir:* 37.5 mg/5 ml. *Hydrochloride, tablets:* 25, 50 mg; *tablets (extended release):* 100 mg; *cream:* 2%.

**DRUG INTERACTIONS**   **CNS depressants** Antihistamines can have additive depression with CNS depressants, including alcohol.   **Epinephrine** Diphenhydramine, tripelennamine, and chlorpheniramine synergize the effects of epinephrine.   **Monoamine oxidase inhibitors** prolong and intensify the anticholinergic effects of antihistamines.

**FATE**   Antihistamines are well absorbed after oral administration. The *onset of action* is generally within 15 to 30 minutes, and the *duration of action* is generally 3 to 6 hours. Antihistamines are metabolized in the liver and excreted in the urine.

## ❦ NURSING CONSIDERATIONS
**Side effects, toxicities, and associated nursing actions**
- See entry for drug class (p. 918).

**Nursing interventions related to drug administration**
- See entry for drug class (p. 919).

**Patient and family education**
- See entry for drug class (p. 919).

---

# triprolidine hydrochloride   (trye-PROE-li-deen)                        antihistamine

- triprolidine hydrochloride: Actidil

**MECHANISM OF ACTION**   Antihistamines block H-1 receptors for histamine, thereby preventing many allergic symptoms.

**INDICATIONS**   Allergic rhinitis, chronic urticaria.

**CONTRAINDICATIONS**   Hypersensitivity to antihistamines.   Monoamine oxidase therapy.   Acute glaucoma, peptic ulcer, prostatic hypertrophy, asthma attack, bladder neck obstruction, pyloroduodenal obstruction These conditions are made worse by the anticholinergic action of antihistamines.

**DOSAGE**   PO:   ADULTS AND CHILDREN OVER 12 YEARS OLD: 2.5 mg four times daily.   CHILDREN 6 TO 12 YEARS OLD: 1.25 mg four times daily.   CHILDREN 4 TO 6 YEARS OLD: 0.938 mg three or four times daily.   CHILDREN 2 TO 4 YEARS OLD: 0.625 mg three or four times daily.   CHILDREN 4 MONTHS TO 2 YEARS OLD: 0.313 mg three or four times daily.   *Special patient populations:* PREGNANCY: Safe use has not been established.

**PREPARATIONS**   *Tablets:* 2.5 mg; *solution:* 1.25 mg/5 ml.

**DRUG INTERACTIONS**   **CNS depressants** Antihistamines can have additive depression with CNS depressants, including alcohol.   **Epinephrine** Diphenhydramine, tripelennamine, and chlorpheniramine synergize the effects of epinephrine.   **Monoamine oxidase inhibitors** prolong and intensify the anticholinergic effects of antihistamines.

**FATE**   Antihistamines are well absorbed after oral administration. The *onset of action* is generally within 15 to 30 minutes, and the *duration of action* is generally 3 to 6 hours. Antihistamines are metabolized in the liver and excreted in the urine.

## ☙ NURSING CONSIDERATIONS

### Side effects, toxicities, and associated nursing actions
• See entry for drug class (p. 918).

### Nursing interventions related to drug administration
• See entry for drug class (p. 919).

### Patient and family education
• See entry for drug class (p. 919).

# Chapter Fifty-two

# Drugs for asthma

| **Adrenergic bronchodilators** | **Xanthines** |
|---|---|
| albuterol | aminophylline |
| bitolterol | dyphylline |
| ephedrine (see Chapter 5) | oxytriphylline |
| epinephrine (see Chapter 5) | theophylline |
| isoetharine | |
| isoproterenol | **Other drugs for asthma** |
| metaproterenol | beclomethasone |
| terbutaline | cromolyn |
| | dexamethasone |
| | flunisolide |
| | triamcinolone |
| | ipratropium |

**INTRODUCTION**     Asthma is a disease of reversible obstruction of the bronchioles. An attack of asthma involves not only constriction of the bronchioles but also edema of the bronchial mucosa and excess secretion of mucus, all of which combine to restrict the caliber of the airway. Asthma is classified as *extrinsic* if an allergic response is the primary stimulus for bronchial constriction. When no such response can be identified, asthma is classified as *intrinsic*.

**Mechanisms in extrinsic asthma**     Extrinsic asthma involves an immunologic mechanism. In patients with extrinsic asthma, the mast cells play a major role in precipitating the attack. In the lung, mast cells are primarily located in the epithelial layer and exposed to the surface. IgE antibodies bind to mast cells, and when an antigen appears it becomes bound to the IgE. The formation of the antigen-antibody complex causes the mast cells to degranulate, releasing several substances, including histamine and leukotrienes C and D, which are chemically related to the prostaglandins. Both histamine and leukotrienes C and D are potent bronchoconstrictors. Histamine also produces vasodilation and increases capillary permeability, which results in the mucosal edema characteristic of asthma.

**Drug therapy for extrinsic asthma**     Drug therapy for extrinsic asthma includes one or more bronchodilator drugs. The bronchodilator drugs include the adrenergic bronchodilators and the xanthine bronchodilators. In addition, cromolyn sodium is a prophylactic agent that prevents the mast cells from degranulating and starting an acute asthma attack. In severe cases of asthma, glucocorticoids may be used to reverse the severe inflammation of the bronchioles. Antihistamines are sometimes used to prevent episodes of mild asthma. Because antihistamines have a drying effect that makes hard plugs of the excess mucus, they are contraindicated for patients with severe asthma. Drugs to antagonize the effects of leukotrienes C and D are under active development.

---

# Adrenergic bronchodilators

albuterol ~ bitolterol ~ ephedrine (see Chapter 5) ~ epinephrine (see Chapter 5) ~ isoetharine ~ isoproterenol ~ metaproterenol ~ terbutaline

**DRUG COMBINATIONS**     Isoetharine and isoproterenol may be combined with cyclopentamine or phenylephrine to prolong bronchodilation (see Table 52-1).

**OVERVIEW OF THE DRUG CLASS**     A number of adrenergic bronchodilators have been developed for oral, inhalation, and subcutaneous administration for the relief of severe bronchospasm. These bronchodilators are compared in Table 52-1. The beta adrenergic system plays a major role in determining the relaxation of bronchial smooth muscle and in inhibiting degranulation of the mast cells. The beta-2 adrenergic receptors mediate both relaxation of bronchial smooth muscle and inhibition of mast cell degranulation. Since beta-1 adrenergic receptors mediate cardiac stimulation, an undesirable action in an antiasthmatic drug, drugs specific for the stimulation of the beta-2 adrenergic receptor, beta-2 agonists, have been introduced in recent years and new ones are under development. In addition to the

**Table 52-1.**

### Adrenergic bronchodilators: onset and duration of action*

| Generic name | Trade name | Administration | Onset (min) | Duration (hr) |
|---|---|---|---|---|
| Albuterol (salbutamol) | Proventil | Inhalation | 30 | 4 to 6 |
| | | Oral | | |
| Bitolterol | Tornalate | Inhalation | 3 | 4 to 8 |
| Ephedrine | Ventolin | Oral | 15 | 2 to 4 |
| Epinephrine hydrochloride | | Subcutaneous | 5 | 1 to 3 |
| | | Inhalation | 2 | 2 to 3 |
| Epinephrine suspension | Sus-Phrine | Subcutaneous | 15 | Up to 8 |
| Isoetharine | Bronkometer | Inhalation | 2 | 1 |
| | Bronkosol | | | |
| | Dilabron | | | |
| Isoetharine and phenylephrine | Bronkosol-2 | Inhalation | 2 | 2 |
| Isoproterenol | Isuprel | Inhalation | 2 | ½ to 2 |
| | Vapo-Iso | | | |
| Isoproterenol and cyclopentamine | Aerolone Compound | Inhalation | 2 | 3½ |
| | Aludrine | | | |
| Isoproterenol and phenylephrine | Nebu-Prel | Inhalation | 2 | 3½ |
| Metaproterenol | Alupent | Inhalation | 2 | 2 to 4 |
| | Metaprel | Oral | 15 | 3 to 4 |
| Terbutaline | Bricanyl Sulfate | Oral | 10 | 4 to 7 |
| | | Subcutaneous | 15 | 2 to 4 |

*From Clark, JB, Queener, SF, and Karb, VB: Pharmacological Basis of Nursing Practice, ed. 2, St. Louis, 1986, The C.V. Mosby Co.

beta adrenergic drugs, the alpha adrenergic drugs cyclopentamine and phenylephrine are included with some formulations of isoetharine and isoproterenol. The alpha adrenergic drug decreases bronchial congestion and slows the systemic absorption of the beta adrenergic drug, thereby increasing the duration of action. Table 52-2 summarizes the alpha and beta activities of sympathomimetic bronchodilators.

**MECHANISM OF ACTION**   Activation of the beta-2 receptor stimulates an enzyme, adenylate cyclase, to synthesize more cyclic adenosine 3', 5'-monophosphate (cyclic AMP), which is the second messenger for the beta-2 receptor. Cyclic AMP activates intracellular pathways that result in (1) the relaxation of smooth muscle, (2) the inhibition of mast cell degranulation, and (3) the stimulation of the ciliary apparatus to remove secretions more effectively. This means that drugs that increase cyclic AMP are bronchodilators as well as inhibitors of mast cell degranulation and promoters of secretion flow in the bronchioles.

**INDICATIONS**   **Bronchospasm** To relieve the bronchospasm of asthma, chronic bronchitis, or status asthmaticus.

**CONTRAINDICATIONS**   **Cardiac arrhythmias or fast heart rate (tachycardia)** Those bronchodilators with significant beta-1 activity (ephedrine, epinephrine, isoproterenol) will cause undue cardiac stress.

**DRUG INTERACTIONS**   **Monoamine oxidase inhibitors** inhibit the degradation of catecholamines and thereby potentiate catecholamines.   **Tricyclic antidepressants, sodium levothyroxine** potentiate adrenergic drugs.   **Guanethidine's** antihypertensive effect will be reduced by adrenergic drugs.   **Other sympathomimetic drugs** have additive cardiac effects.   Halogenated hydrocarbon anesthetics potentiate the arrhythmic effects of sympathomimetics.   **Beta adrenergic blockers** The cardiostimulatory effects of the sympathomimetics antagonize the effects of the beta blockers.

## ⚘ NURSING CONSIDERATIONS
### Side effects, toxicities, and associated nursing actions
**CNS** Nervousness, hyperactivity, excitement, insomnia, emotional lability, dizziness, fatigue.

| Table 52-2. | Sympathomimetic bronchodilators' adrenergic receptor specificity* | | |
|---|---|---|---|
| **Drug** | **Alpha effects** | **Beta-1 effects** | **Beta-2 effects** |
| Albuterol/salbutamol | 0 | 0 | + |
| Bitolterol | 0 | 0 | + |
| Cyclopentamine | + | 0 | 0 |
| Ephedrine | + | + | + |
| Epinephrine | + | + | + |
| Isoetharine | 0 | 0 | + |
| Isoproterenol | 0 | + | + |
| Metaproterenol | 0 | (±) | + |
| Phenylephrine | + | 0 | 0 |
| Terbutaline | 0 | 0 | + |

Alpha effects
Vasoconstriction—
1. Systemic: increased blood pressure.
2. Inhaled: Decreased bronchial congestion, increased duration of action for co-administered beta-2 drug.
Beta-1 effects
1. Stimulation of heart, increasing rate, force of contraction, and rate of repolarization. Overstimulation causes palpitations, arrhythmias.
2. Increased lipolysis (breakdown of fat).
3. Relaxation of gastrointestinal tract.
Beta-2 effects
1. Bronchiole dilation.
2. Stimulation of skeletal muscle to cause a tremulous or shaky feeling.
3. Vasodilation (mainly in blood vessels supplying muscle).
4. Glycogenolysis (breakdown of stored glucose).
Central nervous system effects
Stimulation, causing nervousness, anxiety, insomnia, irritability, dizziness, sweating.

*0, No stimulation; +, stimulation; (±), modest stimulation.
From Clark, JB, Queener, SF, and Karb, VB: Pharmacological Basis of Nursing Practice, ed. 2, St. Louis, 1986, The C.V. Mosby Co.

- Obtain careful baseline history, then assess for CNS effects after starting drug therapy. If CNS effects are pronounced, adjustment of dose or dosing frequency may help.
- Since many of the side effects are dose related, caution patients not to increase dose or frequency without direction from the physician.
- Anxiety may contribute to air hunger, which may contribute to anxiety. Maintain a calm, reassuring appearance to patient. Do not leave acutely ill individuals unattended.
- Monitor respiratory rate.
**CV** At high doses, tachycardia (fast heart rate), palpitation, peripheral vasodilation, changes in blood pressure, pallor.
- Monitor blood pressure, pulse.
- If postural hypotension occurs, caution patients to move slowly from lying to sitting or standing. If dizziness occurs, instruct patients to sit or lie down. Hypotension may be aggravated by prolonged periods of standing or hot showers or baths.
- Acutely ill individuals may need continuous cardiac monitoring.
**GI** Nausea, vomiting, change in appetite, cough, dry mouth.
- Taking oral preparations with meals or snack may lessen gastric irritation.
- Rinse mouth after taking dose or using spray to lessen dry mouth. Instruct patients to increase fluid intake (if not contraindicated by other medical problems), to suck on ice chips, or to suck on

sugarless hard candy for dry mouth. Some patients may wish to use a commercially available saliva substitute.
- Monitor weight. If weight loss occurs secondary to loss of appetite, notify physician.

**GU** Difficulty in urination.
- Monitor intake and output.
- Have patients void before administering next dose.
- Assess patients regularly for difficulty in voiding. For some patients, this is severe enough to warrant discontinuing the drug; for others, it is merely inconvenient.

**Lung** Rarely, paradoxical bronchospasm. More commonly, a symptom of overusage.
- Auscultate breath sounds, monitor respiratory rate.
- Caution patients to use only as ordered.

**Allergic** Rarely, hypersensitivity.
- Monitor for allergic reaction.
- Have available drugs and equipment for an acute allergic response: epinephrine, antihistamines, steroids.

### Nursing interventions related to drug administration
- For medications administered by inhalation, ascertain that patient can self-administer correctly prior to permitting self-management at home.

### Patient and family education
- Review with patients anticipated benefits and possible side effects of drug therapy. Caution patients to report the development of any unusual sign or symptom.
- If prescribed drugs begin to be less effective to patient, caution patient to consult with physician.
- For inhalation medications, instruct patient to exhale deeply, then place lips firmly around mouthpiece, making a tight seal. As patient depresses cannister or activates inhaler, instruct patient to take a slow, deep breath. Have patient hold breath as long as possible, then exhale slowly. Remove mouthpiece.
- Instruct patient to wash the mouthpiece and dry it thoroughly at least once a day.
- If more than one medication is administered via inhalation, adrenergic bronchodilator should be used first to allow bronchodilation to occur. After 5 minutes, the second medication, such as beclomethasone, should be administered.
- Instruct patients to obtain patient information sheets from pharmacists for these drugs.
- Diabetic patients may need to monitor blood sugar more often and may need adjustment of insulin or oral hypoglycemic agent. Caution diabetic patients about this.
- Teach patients to check the expiration dates of medications. Outdated medications should be discarded; flush outdated oral forms down the toilet.
- Teach patients to store oral forms in a dry place. Storing oral forms of adrenergic bronchodilators in the bathroom may allow humidity to cause the drug to decompose or breakdown.
- Caution patients to avoid the use of over-the-counter medications without prior approval from the physician.
- Caution patients to keep all health care providers informed of all medication being taken.
- Caution patients to avoid food items containing caffeine if tachycardia is significant. Examples include coffee, tea, and caffeinated cola beverages.
- The management of asthma and related conditions must be individualized. Emphasize to patient the need to follow medication regimens, as well as to avoid identified irritants, avoid exposure to individuals with known respiratory infections, perform regular exercise within parameters defined by physician, and incorporate periods of rest into daily activities.
- Caution patients to keep these and all medications out of the reach of children.

## albuterol (salbutamol), albuterol sulfate
(al-BYOO-ter-ole)                                                          bronchodilator

- albuterol (salbutamol), albuteral sulfate: Proventil, Ventolin

**MECHANISM OF ACTION**   Albuterol is a beta agonist with relative specificity for the beta-2 adrenergic receptor. For more information, see entry for drug class (p. 931).

**INDICATIONS**   Bronchospasm Effective administered orally or by oral inhalation.

**CONTRAINDICATIONS**   **Excessive use of bronchodilators.   Diabetes mellitus, hyperthyroidism, cardiovascular disorders** Bronchodilators must be used with caution in patients with one of these conditions.

**DOSAGE**   Inhalation:   ADULTS AND CHILDREN OVER 12 YEARS OLD: 180 μg (2 inhalations) every 4 to 6 hours. A dose may be taken prophylactically 15 minutes prior to exercise to prevent exercise-induced bronchospasm.   CHILDREN 6 TO 11 YEARS OLD: 1 or 2 inhalations four times daily.   PO: ADULTS AND CHILDREN OVER 12 YEARS OLD: 2 or 4 mg three or four times daily.   CHILDREN 6 TO 11 YEARS OLD: 2 mg three or four times daily.   CHILDREN 2 TO 5 YEARS OLD: 0.1 mg/kg three times daily.   *Special patient populations:*   ELDERLY: Elderly patients are usually started with an oral dose of 2 mg three or four times daily.   PREGNANCY: Safe use has not been established. However, high doses have been teratogenic in test animals.

**PREPARATIONS**   *Aerosol:* 90 μg per metered spray. *Sulfate, solution:* 2 mg/5 ml; *tablets:* 2, 4 mg.

**DRUG INTERACTIONS**   **Monoamine oxidase inhibitors** inhibit the degradation of catecholamines and thereby potentiate catecholamines.   **Tricyclic antidepressants, sodium levothyroxine** potentiate adrenergic drugs.   **Guanethidine's** antihypertensive effect will be reduced by adrenergic drugs.   **Other sympathomimetic drugs** have additive cardiac effects.   **Halogenated hydrocarbon anesthetics** potentiate the arrhythmic effects of sympathomimetics.   **Beta adrenergic blockers** The cardiostimulatory effects of the sympathomimetics antagonize the effects of the beta blockers.

**FATE**   Albuterol is slowly absorbed after inhalation or oral administration. The *onset of action* for bronchodilation is within 5 to 15 minutes after inhalation or 0.5 to 2 hours after oral administration. The *duration of action* is 3 to 4 hours after inhalation and 4 to 6 hours after oral administration. Albuterol is metabolized in the liver and excreted in the urine and feces.

## ❦ NURSING CONSIDERATIONS

### Side effects, toxicities, and associated nursing actions

**CNS** Infrequent: nervousness, hyperactivity, excitement, insomnia, emotional lability, dizziness, fatigue.

• See entry for drug class for a discussion of other side effects (p. 931).

### Nursing interventions related to drug administration

• See entry for drug class (p. 933).

### Patient and family education

• See entry for drug class (p. 933).

---

## bitoterol mesylate   (bye-TOE-ter-ole)                                                   bronchodilator

• bitoterol mesylate: Tornalate

**MECHANISM OF ACTION**   Bitoterol is a beta agonist with relative specificity for the beta-2 adrenergic receptor. For more information, see entry for drug class (p. 931).

**INDICATIONS**   Bronchospasm Prophylactic or symptomatic treatment; administered by oral inhalation.

**CONTRAINDICATIONS**   **Excessive use of bronchodilators.   Diabetes mellitus, hyperthyroidism, cardiovascular disorders** Bronchodilators must be used with caution in patients with one of these conditions.

**DOSAGE**   Inhalation:   ADULTS AND CHILDREN OVER 12 YEARS OLD: 740 μg (2 inhalations) every 8 hours. Not to exceed 3 inhalations every 6 hours or 2 inhalations every 4 hours. *Special patient populations:*   ELDERLY: Elderly patients are usually started with lower doses.   CHILDREN: Not established for use by children under 12 years old.   PREGNANCY: Safe use has not been established. However, high doses have been teratogenic in test animals.

**PREPARATIONS**   *Aerosol:* 370 µg/metered spray.

**DRUG INTERACTIONS**   **Monoamine oxidase inhibitors** inhibit the degradation of catecholamines and thereby potentiate catecholamines.   **Tricyclic antidepressants, sodium levothyroxine** potentiate adrenergic drugs.   **Guanethidine's** antihypertensive effect will be reduced by adrenergic drugs.   **Other sympathomimetic drugs** have additive cardiac effects.   **Halogenated hydrocarbon anesthetics** potentiate the arrhythmic effects of sympathomimetics.   **Beta adrenergic blockers** The cardiostimulatory effects of the sympathomimetics antagonize the effects of the beta blockers.

**FATE**   Bitoterol is rapidly absorbed after inhalation. The *onset of action* for bronchodilation is within 3 to 5 minutes after inhalation. The *duration of action* is 4 to 8 hours. Bitoterol is probably metabolized to an active metabolite, colterol, by tissue esterases. Metabolites of colterol are excreted in the urine.

## 🦉 NURSING CONSIDERATIONS

### Side effects, toxicities, and associated nursing actions

**CNS** Tremor. Infrequent: nervousness, hyperactivity, excitement, insomnia, emotional lability, dizziness, fatigue.

- See entry for drug class (p. 931) for a discussion of other side effects.

### Nursing interventions related to drug administration

- See entry for drug class (p. 933).

### Patient and family education

- See entry for drug class (p. 933).

---

# isoetharine hydrochloride, isoetharine mesylate
(eye-soe-ETH-a-reen)                                                              bronchodilator

- isoetharine hydrochloride, isoetharine mesylate: Arm-a-Med, Bisorine, Bronkometer, Bronkos, Dey-Lute

**MECHANISM OF ACTION**   Isoetharine is a beta agonist with relative specificity for the beta-2 adrenergic receptor. For more information, see entry for drug class (p. 931).

**INDICATIONS**   **Bronchospasm** Symptomatic or prophylactic relief. Administered by oral inhalation.

**CONTRAINDICATIONS**   **Excessive use of bronchodilators. Diabetes mellitus, hyperthyroidism, cardiovascular disorders** Bronchodilators must be used with caution in patients with one of these conditions.

**DOSAGE**   **Inhalation:**   **ADULTS AND CHILDREN:** *Oxygen aerosolization or IPPB:* 0.5 to 1 ml of 0.5% solution of 0.25 to 0.5 ml of 1% diluted 1:3 (equivalent amounts undiluted are 4 ml of 0.125% solution, 2.5 ml 0.2% solution, 2 ml of a 0.25% solution); *hand-bulb nebulizer:* 4 inhalations of 0.5% or 1% solution. Do not repeat more than every 4 hours, five times daily. *Metered aerosol:* 340 or 680 µg (1 to 2 inhalations) every 4 hours.   **CHILDREN 6 TO 11 YEARS OLD:** 1 or 2 inhalations four times daily. *Special patient populations:*   **ELDERLY:** Elderly patients are usually started with lower doses.   **PREGNANCY:** Safe use has not been established. However, high doses of other beta agonists have been teratogenic in test animals.

**PREPARATIONS**   *Hydrochloride, solution (nebulization):* 0.062%, 0.08%, 0.1%, 0.125%, 0.14%, 0.167%, 0.17%, 0.2%, 0.255%, 0.5%, 1%. *Mesylate, aerosol:* 340 µg/metered spray.

**DRUG INTERACTIONS**   **Monoamine oxidase inhibitors** inhibit the degradation of catecholamines and thereby potentiate catecholamines.   **Tricyclic antidepressants, sodium levothyroxine** potentiate adrenergic drugs.   **Guanethidines** antihypertensive effect will be reduced by adrenergic drugs.   **Other sympathomimetic drugs** have additive cardiac effects.   **Halogenated hydrocarbon anesthetics** potentiate the arrhythmic effects of sympathomimetics.   **Beta adrenergic blockers** The cardiostimulatory effects of the sympathomimetics antagonize the effects of the beta blockers.

**FATE**   Isoetharine is rapidly absorbed after inhalation. The *onset of action* for bronchodilation is within 1 to 5 minutes after inhalation. The *duration of action* is 1 to 4 hours. Isoetharine is metabolized by the enzyme catechol-O-methyltransferase in various tissues. Metabolites are conjugated with sulfuric and glucuronic acids in the liver and excreted in the urine.

## ❧ NURSING CONSIDERATIONS

### Side effects, toxicities, and associated nursing actions

**CNS** Infrequent: nervousness, hyperactivity, excitement, insomnia, emotional lability, dizziness, fatigue.
* See entry for drug class (p. 931) for a discussion of other side effects.

### Nursing interventions related to drug administration
* See entry for drug class (p. 933).

### Patient and family education
* See entry for drug class (p. 933).

---

# isoproterenol hydrochloride, isoproterenol sulfate
(eye-soe-pro-TER-e-nole)                                                          *bronchodilator*

* isoproterenol hydrochloride, isoproterenol sulfate: ✿Isoprenaline, ✿Isopropylnoradrenaline, ✿Isopropylarterenol, Isopro, Isuprel, Medihaler-Iso, Norisodrine

**MECHANISM OF ACTION**    Isoproterenol is a beta agonist, active at both beta-1 and beta-2 adrenergic receptors. For more information, see entry for drug class (p. 931).

**INDICATIONS**    **Bronchospasm** For symptomatic relief. Usually inhaled, but also effective by sublingual tablets. Occasionally give IV to children with status asthmaticus.    **Cardiac standstill, cardiac arrhythmias** Indicated when these are due to AV nodal block but not when secondary to digitalis intoxication.    **Shock** Administered IV to produce cardiac stimulation and vasodilation for cardiogenic shock.

**CONTRAINDICATIONS**    **Excessive use of bronchodilators.**    **Diabetes mellitus, hyperthyroidism, cardiovascular disorders** Bronchodilators must be used with caution in patients with one of these conditions.    **Sensitivity to sympathomimetic amines.**

**DOSAGE**    **Bronchospasm:**    *Inhalation:*    **ADULTS AND CHILDREN:** 120 to 262 μg of the hydrochloride spray or 80 to 160 μg of the sulfate spray (1 to 2 inhalations) every 4 to 6 hours; allow 1 to 5 minutes before a second inhalation is taken; no more that 6 inhalations in any hour during a 24-hour period. *For administration with a hand-bulb nebulizer:* 5 to 15 inhalations of a 0.5% solution. This may be repeated once in 5 to 10 minutes if necessary, then every 3 to 4 hours if necessary, with no more than 5 treatments daily. Adults may require a 1% solution. *For administration via IPPB or compressed oxygen:* 2 ml of a 0.125% solution delivered over 10 to 20 minutes, up to five times daily.    **Sublingual:**    **ADULTS:** 10 to 20 mg with daily dosage not to exceed 60 mg.    **CHILDREN:** 5 to 10 mg with daily dosage not to exceed 30 mg.    *IV:*    **ADULTS:** 0.01 to 0.02 mg for acute asthma attacks not responsive to inhalation therapy.    **CHILDREN:** 0.08 to 1.7 μg/kg for status asthmaticus.    **Cardiac standstill, cardiac arrhythmias:**    *IV:*    **ADULTS:** 0.02 to 0.06 mg as a bolus injection or 5 μg/min by infusion.    **CHILDREN:** ½ adult dose.    **Shock:**    *IV:*    **ADULTS AND CHILDREN:** 0.5 to 5 μg/min as an infusion.    *Special patient populations:*    **ELDERLY:** Elderly patients usually receive lower doses.    **PREGNANCY:** Safe use has not been established. However, high doses of other beta agonists have been teratogenic in test animals.

**PREPARATIONS**    *Hydrochloride, aerosol:* 120, 131 μg/metered spray; *solution (nebulization):* 0.031%, 0.062%, o.25%, 0.5%, 1%; *injection:* 0.02, 0.2 mg/ml; *tablets (sublingual):* 10, 15 mg. *Sulfate, aerosol:* 80 μg/metered spray.

**DRUG INTERACTIONS**    **Monoamine oxidase inhibitors** inhibit the degradation of catecholamines and thereby potentiate catecholamines.    **Tricyclic antidepressants, sodium levothyroxine** potentiate adrenergic drugs.    **Guanethidine's** antihypertensive effect will be reduced by adrenergic drugs.    **Other sympathomimetic drugs** have additive cardiac effects.    **Halogenated hydrocarbon anesthetics** potentiate the arrhythmic effects of sympathomimetics.    **Beta adrenergic blockers** The cardiostimulatory effects of the sympathomimetics antagonize the effects of the beta blockers.

**FATE**    Isoproterenol is rapidly absorbed after inhalation. The *onset of action* for bronchodilation is within 2 to 5 minutes, and the *duration of action* is 0.5 to 2 hours. Isoproterenol is rapidly metabolized in the GI tract and other tissues, and metabolites are excreted in the urine.

## ❦ NURSING CONSIDERATIONS

### Side effects, toxicities, and associated nursing actions

**CNS** Nervousness, hyperactivity, excitement, insomnia, emotional lability, dizziness, fear, fatigue.
- See entry for drug class (p. 931) for a discussion of other side effects.

### Nursing interventions related to drug administration

- Ascertain that patients know to dissolve sublingual dosage form under tongue and not to swallow dosage whole.
- For IV administration, read labels carefully to obtain correct dose.
- For IV infusion, microdrip tubing and an electric infusion monitoring device should be used. Dilute as directed in 5% dextrose in water. Dilute 2 mg (10 ml) of 1:5000 solution in 500 ml of diluent to obtain a concentration of 4 μg/ml.
- For direct IV infusion, administer each 1 ml of a 1:50,000 solution over 1 minute. Read labels carefully; solution in 1:50,000 strength may be supplied or may be made by diluting 0.2 mg (1 ml) of a 1:5000 solution with 10 ml of normal saline for injection.
- See entry for drug class (p. 933).

### Patient and family education

- Tell patients using isoproterenol sublingual tablets that their saliva may turn pinkish to red while they are using this medicine.
- See entry for drug class (p. 933).

---

## metaproterenol sulfate    (met-a-proe-TER-e-nole)    bronchodilator

- metaproterenol sulfate: ✦Orciprenaline Sulfate, Alupent, Metaprel

**MECHANISM OF ACTION**    Metaproterenol is a beta agonist with relative specificity for the beta-2 adrenergic receptor. For more information, see entry for drug class (p. 931).

**INDICATIONS**    **Bronchospasm** Effective administered orally or by inhalation.

**CONTRAINDICATIONS**    **Excessive use of bronchodilators.    Diabetes mellitus, hyperthyroidism, cardiovascular disorders** Bronchodilators must be used with caution in patients with these conditions.

**DOSAGE**    **Inhalation:    ADULTS AND CHILDREN OVER 12 YEARS OLD:** *Metered spray,* 1.3 or 1.95 mg (2 or 3 inhalations) every 3 to 4 hours. Allow 2 minutes between inhalations. No more than 12 inhalations in a 24-hour period. *Hand-bulb nebulizer:* 5 to 15 inhalations of a 5% solution.    **PO:    ADULTS AND CHILDREN** over 9 years old (or over 27 kg): 20 mg three or four times daily.    **CHILDREN** 6 to 9 years old (or under 27 kg): 10 mg three or four times daily.    **CHILDREN** under 6 years old: 1.3 to 2.6 mg/kg daily in divided doses.    *Special patient populations:*    **ELDERLY:** Elderly patients are usually started with lower doses.    **PREGNANCY:** Safe use has not been established. However, high doses have been teratogenic in test animals.

**PREPARATIONS**    *Solution (oral):* 10 mg/5 ml; *tablets:* 10, 20 mg; *aerosol:* 0.65 mg/metered spray; *solution (nebulization):* 0.6%, 5%.

**DRUG INTERACTIONS**    **Monoamine oxidase inhibitors** inhibit the degradation of catecholamines and thereby potentiate catecholamines.    **Tricyclic antidepressants, sodium levothyroxine** potentiate adrenergic drugs.    **Guanethidine's** antihypertensive effect will be reduced by adrenergic drugs.    **Other sympathomimetic drugs** have additive cardiac effects.    **Halogenated hydrocarbon anesthetics** potentiate the arrhythmic effects of sympathomimetics.    **Beta adrenergic blockers** The cardiostimulatory effects of the sympathomimetics antagonize the effects of the beta blockers.

**FATE**    Metoproterenol is rapidly absorbed after inhalation or oral administration. The *onset of action* for bronchodilation is within 1 to 5 minutes after inhalation or 15 to 30 minutes after oral administration. The *duration of action* is 3 to 4 hours. Metaproterenol is metabolized in the liver and excreted in the urine as glucuronic acid conjugates.

## ❦ NURSING CONSIDERATIONS

### Side effects, toxicities, and associated nursing actions

**CNS** Infrequent: nervousness, hyperactivity, excitement, insomnia, emotional lability, dizziness, fatigue.

• See entry for drug class (p. 931) for a discussion of other side effects.
**Nursing interventions related to drug administration**
• See entry for drug class (p. 933).
**Patient and family education**
• See entry for drug class (p. 933).

---

## terbutaline sulfate   (ter-BYOO-te-leen)                    bronchodilator

---

• terbutaline sulfate: Brethine, Brethaire, ♣Bricanyl

**MECHANISM OF ACTION**   Terbutaline is a beta agonist with relative specificity for the beta-2 adrenergic receptor. For more information, see entry for drug class (p. 931).

**INDICATIONS**   Bronchospasm Effective administered orally or subcutaneously.

**CONTRAINDICATIONS**   **Excessive use of bronchodilators.   Diabetes mellitus, hyperthyroidism, cardiovascular disorders** Bronchodilators must be used with caution in patients with one of these conditions. **Sensitivity to catecholamines.**

**DOSAGE**   PO:   **ADULTS AND CHILDREN OVER 15 YEARS OLD:** 5 mg three times daily.   **CHILDREN 12 TO 15 YEARS OLD:** 2.5 mg three times daily.   **SC:   ADULTS:** 0.25 mg. May repeat in 15 to 30 minutes if there is no improvement; no more than 0.5 mg in a 4-hour period.   **CHILDREN:** 3.5 to 5 µg/kg. Inhalation:   **ADULTS AND CHILDREN 12 YEARS AND OLDER:** 400 µg (2 inhalations) every 4 to 6 hours. Allow at least 1 minute between inhalations; 10 to 20 minutes is better. *Special patient populations:*   **ELDERLY:** Elderly patients are usually started with lower doses.   **PREGNANCY:** Safe use has not been established. However, high doses have been teratogenic in test animals.

**PREPARATIONS**   *Tablets:* 2.5, 5 mg; *aerosol:* 200 µg/metered spray; *injection:* 1 mg/ml.

**DRUG INTERACTIONS**   **Monoamine oxidase inhibitors** inhibit the degradation of catecholamines and thereby potentiate catecholamines.   **Tricyclic antidepressants, sodium levothyroxine** potentiate adrenergic drugs.   **Guanethidine's** antihypertensive effect will be reduced by adrenergic drugs.   **Other sympathomimetic drugs** have additive cardiac effects.   **Halogenated hydrocarbon anesthetics** potentiate the arrhythmic effects of sympathomimetics.   **Beta adrenergic blockers** The cardiostimulatory effects of the sympathomimetics antagonize the effects of the beta blockers.

**FATE**   Terbutaline is well absorbed after inhalation, oral, or subcutaneous administration. The *onset of action* for bronchodilation is within 15 minutes after subcutaneous or inhalation administration and 30 minutes after oral administration. The *duration of action* is 1.5 to 4 hours after subcutaneous, 3 to 4 hours after inhalation, and 4 to 8 hours after oral administration. Terbutaline is metabolized in the liver and excreted in the urine and feces.

**❦ NURSING CONSIDERATIONS**
**Side effects, toxicities, and associated nursing actions**
   **CNS** Infrequent: nervousness, hyperactivity, excitement, insomnia, emotional lability, dizziness, fatigue.
• See entry for drug class (p. 931) for a discussion of other side effects.
**Nursing interventions related to drug administration**
• See entry for drug class (p. 933).
**Patient and family education**
• See entry for drug class (p. 933).

---

# Xanthines

aminophylline ~ dyphylline ~ oxtriphylline ~ theophylline

**DRUG COMBINATIONS**   See Table 52-3: Asthma drug combinations.

**OVERVIEW OF THE DRUG CLASS**   The xanthines are orally active bronchodilators. Theophylline is the most widely used of the xanthines. Aminophylline and oxtriphylline are readily metabolized to theophylline ·

**Table 52-3.**

## Prescription combinations including xanthine

| Trade name | Xanthine | Decongestant | Expectorant | Other ingredients |
|---|---|---|---|---|
| Asbron G Elixir, Inlay Tablets | Theophylline | | Guaifenesin | |
| Bronchial Capsules | Theophylline | | Guaifenesin | |
| Brondecon Tablets, Elixir | Oxtriphylline | | Guaifenesin | |
| Co-Xan Syrup, | Theophylline | Ephedrine | Guaifenesin | CO BB (C-V) |
| Dilor-G Tablets, Liquid | Dyphylline | | Guaifenesin | |
| Dyflex-G Tablets | Dyphylline | | Guaifenesin | |
| Dyline-GG Tablets, Liquid | Dyphylline | | Guaifenesin | |
| Elixophyllin GG Liquid | Theophylline | | Guaifenesin | |
| Elixophyllin-Kl Elixir | Theophylline | | Potassium iodide | |
| Glyceryl-T Capsules, Liquid | Theophylline | | Guaifenesin | |
| Guiaphed Elixir | Theophylline | Ephedrine | Guaifenesin | PB |
| Hydrophed DP Syrup, Tablets | Theophylline | Ephedrine | | HZ |
| Isogen Compound Elixir | Theophylline | Ephedrine/Isoproterenol | Potassium iodide | PB |
| Isolate Compound Elixir | Theophylline | Ephedrine/Isoproterenol | Potassium iodide | PB |
| Lanophyllin GG Capsules | Theophylline | | Guaifenesin | |
| Lufyllin-EPG Tablets, Elixir | Dyphylline | Ephedrine | Guaifenesin | PB |
| Lufyllin-GG Tablets, Elixir | Dyphylline | | Guaifenesin | |
| Marax DF Syrup, Tablets | Theophylline | Ephedrine | | HZ |
| Mudrane GG Elixir | Aminophylline | Ephedrine | Guaifenesin | PB |
| Mudrane GG Tablets | Aminophylline | | Guaifenesin | |
| Mudrane Tablets | Aminophylline | Ephedrine | Potassium Iodide | PB |
| Neothylline-GG Tablets | Dyphylline | | Guaifenesin | |
| Quadrinal Tablets | Theophylline | Ephedrine | Potassium Iodide | PB |
| Quiagen Capsules | Theophylline | | Guaifenesin | |
| Quibron Capsules, Liquid | Theophylline | | Guaifenesin | |
| Quibron Plus Capsules, Elixir | Theophylline | Ephedrine | Guaifenesin | BB |
| Slo-Phyllin GG Capsules, Liquid | Theophylline | | Guaifenesin | |
| Synophylate-GG Tablets, Syrup | Theophylline | | Guaifenesin | |
| T.E.H. Compound | Theophylline | Ephedrine | | HZ |
| Theo-Organidin Elixir | Theophylline | | Iodinated Glycerol | |
| Theo-R-Gen Elixir | Theophylline | | Iodinated Glycerol | |
| Theocolate Liquid | Theophylline | | Guaifenesin | |
| Theofedral | Theophylline | Ephedrine | | PB |
| Theolair Plus Tablets, Liquid | Theophylline | | Guaifenesin | |
| Theolate Liquid | Theophylline | | Guaifenesin | |
| Theophenylline Tablets | Theophylline | Ephedrine | | PB |
| Theophylline-Kl Elixir | Theophylline | | Potassium Iodide | |
| Theoral Tablets | Theophylline | Ephedrine | | PB |

KEY: *BB*, Butabarbital; *CO*, codeine; *HZ*, hydroxyzine; *PB*, phenobarbital.

and are active as theophylline. Aminophylline is a combination of theophylline and ethylenediamine; oxtriphylline is a choline salt of theophylline. Dyphylline is a distinct chemical entity but chemically similar to theophylline. In addition to attenuating an acute asthmatic attack, the xanthines are effective prophylactic agents for patients with asthma or reversible bronchospasm.

**MECHANISM OF ACTION**   Theophylline is the prototype of the xanthines used to treat bronchospasm. Like the beta adrenergic agonists, theophylline is thought to act by increasing cellular cyclic AMP concentrations, an action that relaxes bronchial smooth muscle and inhibits mast cell degranulation. Theophylline and the other xanthines accomplish this by inhibiting the degradation of cyclic AMP by the enzyme phosphodiesterase. This action complements that of the beta adrenergic agonists, and the two kinds of agents may both be included in therapy when the effect of either drug alone is insufficient to control bronchospasm.

**INDICATIONS**   Bronchospasm For acute relief or prophylactic treatment of reversible bronchospasm of asthma, emphysema, chronic bronchospasm.

**CONTRAINDICATIONS**   Hypersensitivity to theophylline. Active peptic ulcer.

**DRUG INTERACTIONS**   **Smoking** Cigarette or marijuana smoking induces the hepatic metabolism of theophylline. Smokers may require a 50% to 100% increase in dosage.   **Phenobarbital** may increase the metabolism of theophylline so that larger doses may be required.   **Cimetidine, erythromycin, influenza virus vaccine, troleandomycin** have been reported to increase the serum concentrations of theophylline.   **Furosemide** increases the pharmacologic effects of theophylline.   **Sympathomimetic drugs** may get excessive CNS stimulation with xanthines.   **Digitalis, oral anticoagulants** Theophylline may enhance the sensitivity to these drugs.   **Phenytoin, lithium, nondepolarizine muscle relaxants, beta blockers** Theophylline decreases the effects of these drugs.   **Reserpine** Tachycardia.   **Magnesium-aluminum hydroxides** slow the absorption of theophylline.   **Ketamine, halothane** Increased toxicity (seizures, arrhythmias, respectively).

**DIAGNOSTIC TEST INTERFERENCE**   **Serum uric acid** Theophylline produces false-positive elevations as determined by the colorimetric or Bittner method but not by the uricase method.   **Serum theophylline** Several drugs may interfere with the determination of serum theophylline concentrations, including furosemide, sulfathiazole, phenylbutazone, probenecid, theobromine, caffeine-containing beverages, chocolate, and acetaminophen, unless the determination is made with high-pressure liquid chromatography (HPLC).

---

## theophylline, theophylline sodium glycinate
(thee-OFF-i-lin)                                                                    bronchodilator

- theophylline, theophylline sodium glycinate: Bronkodyl, Elixophyllin, ✿Pulmophyllin, Quibron-T, Somophyllin, Theophyl

**OTHER FORMS OF THEOPHYLLINE**

---

## aminophylline anhydrous, dihydrate   (am-in-OFF-i-lin)   bronchodilator

- aminophylline anhydrous, dihydrate, theophylline ethylenediamine: (theophylline ethylenediamine) Aminophyllin, ✿Corophyllin, ✿Palaron, Phyllocontin, Somophyllin, Truphylline

---

## oxtriphylline   (ox-i-TRY-fi-lin)   bronchodilator

- oxtriphylline: ✿Apo-Oxtriphylline, Choledyl, ✿Chophylline, ✿Novotriphyl

**MECHANISM OF ACTION**   Theophylline relaxes bronchial smooth muscle and depresses mast cell degranulation. For more information, see entry for drug blass (p. 939).

**INDICATIONS**   **Bronchospasm** For acute relief or prophylactic treatment of reversible bronchospasm of asthma, emphysema, chronic bronchospasm.

**CONTRAINDICATIONS**   **Hypersensitivity to theophylline.   Active peptic ulcer.**

**DOSAGE**   The doses given here are also for aminophylline and oxtriphylline. All doses are given as anhydrous theophylline. The theophylline content of theophylline derivatives is:

| Drug | Anhydrous Theophylline content |
|---|---|
| Aminophylline anhydrous | 85.7% |
| Aminophylline hydrous | 78.9% |
| Oxtriphylline | 63.6% |
| Theophylline calcium salicylate | 48.1% |
| Theophylline monohydrate | 90.7% |
| Theophylline sodium glycinate | 45.9% |

The doses below are all given for anhydrous theophylline. To find the theophylline equivalent dose for one of the nonanhydrous forms, divide the theophylline dose by the fractional theophylline content of the other form. For instance, the IV maintenance dose for anhydrous theophylline is given as 0.79 mg/kg hr. The theophylline equivalent dose for aminophylline hydrous is 0.79/0.79 = 1 mg/kg/hr.

**Acute bronchospasm:**   *IV:* If patients are not currently receiving theophylline, a loading dose of 4.7 mg/kg is given, followed by the following maintenance doses:

| Group | Maintenance dosage for the first 12 hr | Maintenance dosage after 12 hr |
|---|---|---|
| Children 6 months to 9 years old | 0.95 mg/kg/hr (1.2 mg/kg/hr) | 0.79 mg/kg pr/hr (1 mg/kg/hr) |
| Children 9 to 16 years old and young adult smokers | 0.79 mg/kg/hr (1 mg/kg/hr) | 0.63 mg/kg/hr (0.8 mg/kg/hr) |
| Healthy, nonsmoking adults | 0.55 mg/kg/hr (0.7 mg/kg/hr) | 0.39 mg/kg/hr (0.5 mg/kg/hr) |
| Older patients and those with cors pulmonale | 0.47 mg/kg/hr (0.6 mg/kg/hr) | 0.24 mg/kg/hr (0.24 mg/kg/hr) |
| Patients with congestive heart failure or liver disease | 0.38 mg/kg/hr (0.5 mg/kg/hr) | 0.08 to 0.16 mg/kg/hr (0.1 to 0.2 mg/kg/hr) |

*PO:* If a patient is not currently receiving theophylline, a loading dose of 6 mg/kg is given, followed by the following maintenance doses:

| Group | Maintenance dosage for the first 12 hr | Maintenance dosage after 12 hr |
|---|---|---|
| Children 6 months to 9 years old | 4 mg/kg every 4 hr × 3 doses | 4 mg/kg every 6 hr |
| Children 9 to 16 years old and young adult smokers | 3 mg/kg every 4 hr × 3 doses | 3 mg/kg every 6 hr |
| Healthy, nonsmoking adults | 3 mg/kg every 6 hr × 2 doses | 3 mg/kg every 8 hr |

*Continued.*

| Group | Maintenance dosage *for the first 12 hr* | Maintenance dosage *after 12 hr* |
|---|---|---|
| Older patients and those with cors pulmonale | 2 mg/kg every 6 hr × 2 doses | 2 mg/kg every 12 hr |
| Patients with congestive heart failure or liver disease | 2 mg/kg every 8 hr × 2 doses | 1 to 2 mg/kg every 12 hr |

**Chronic bronchospasm:**   *PO:* Maximum daily doses are:

| | |
|---|---|
| Children up to 9 years old | 24 mg/kg daily |
| Children 9 to 12 years old | 20 mg/kg daily |
| Children 12 to 16 years old | 18 mg/kg daily |
| Adults 16 years and older | 13 mg/kg or 900 mg daily |

**Adjustment of theophylline dosages:** The therapeutic index for theophylline is low. Serum theophylline concentrations are measured, and dosage adjustments are made accordingly. Desired therapeutic levels are 10 to 20 μg/ml.

| Serum levels | Directions |
|---|---|
| 5 to 7.5 μg/ml | Increase dose 25%, then recheck. |
| 7.5 to 10 μg/ml | Increase dose 25%, then recheck. |
| 10 to 20 μg/ml | Desired level. |
| 20 to 25 μg/ml | Decrease dose by 10%. Recheck after 3 days. |
| 25 to 30 μg/ml | Skip next dose and then decrease dosage 25%. |
| Over 30 μg/ml | Skip next 2 doses and then decrease dosage 50%. |

*Special patient populations:*   **ELDERLY:** Lowered doses are required because the elderly metabolize theophylline slowly.   **CHILDREN:** Pediatric doses are higher because children metabolize theophylline quickly.   **PREGNANCY:** Theophylline has been used during pregnancy without reported adverse effects to the fetus.

**PREPARATIONS**   *Theophylline, anhydrous, capsules:* 100, 200, 250 mg; *capsules (extended release):* 50, 60, 65, 75, 100, 125, 130, 200, 250, 260, 300 mg; *solution:* 27, 50, 53.5 mg/5 ml; *suspension:* 100 mg/5 ml; *tablets:* 100, 125, 200, 225, 250, 300 mg; *tablets (extended release):* 100, 200, 250, 300, 400, 500 mg. *Theophylline, anhydrous, in dextrose, for IV infusion:* 0.4, 0.8, 1.6, 2, 4 mg/ml. *Theophylline, monohydrate: powder. Theophylline sodium glycinate, elixir:* 110 mg/5 ml. *Aminophylline, hydrated, tablets:* 100, 200 mg; *tablets (enteric coated):* 100, 200 mg: *tablets (extended release):* 225 mg; *injection:* 25 mg/ml; *suppositories:* 250, 500 mg. *In sodium chloride, IV infusion:* 1, 2 mg/ml. *Anhydrous, solution:* 105 mg/5 ml; *rectal:* 60 mg/ml. *Oxtryphylline, elixir:* 100 mg/5 ml; *solution:* 50 mg/5 ml; *tablets (enteric coated):* 100, 200 mg; *tablets (extended release):* 400, 600 mg.

**DRUG INTERACTIONS**   **Smoking** Cigarette or marijuana smoking induces the hepatic metabolism of theophylline. Smokers may require a 50% to 100% increase in dosage.   **Phenobarbital** may increase the metabolism of theophylline so that larger doses may be required.   **Cimetidine, erythromycin, influenza virus vaccine, troleandomycin** have been reported to increase the serum concentrations of theophylline.   **Furosemide** increases the pharmacologic effects of theophylline.   **Sympathomimetic drugs** may get excessive CNS stimulation with xanthines.   **Digitalis, oral anticoagulants** Theophylline may enhance the sensitivity to these drugs.   **Phenytoin, lithium, nondepolarizine muscle relaxants, beta blockers** Theophylline decreases the effects of these drugs.   **Reserpine** Tachycardia. **Magnesium-aluminum hydroxides** slow the absorption of theophylline.   **Ketamine, halothane** Increased toxicity (seizures, arrhythmias, respectively).

**DIAGNOSTIC TEST INTERFERENCE**   **Serum uric acid** Theophylline produces false positive elevations as determined by the colorimetric or Bittner method but not by the uricase method.   **Serum theophylline** Several drugs may interfere with the determination of serum theophylline concentrations, including furosemide, sulfathiazole, phenylbutazone, probenecid, theobromine, caffeine-containing beverages, chocolate, and acetaminophen, unless the determination is made with HPLC.

**FATE** The *onset* and *duration of action* depend on the route of administration and formulation. Theophylline is metabolized in the liver and excreted in the urine.

## 🦅 NURSING CONSIDERATIONS

### Side effects, toxicities, and associated nursing actions

**CNS** Irritability, restlessness, dizziness, lightheadedness, vertigo, insomnia, excitability, muscle twitches, stammering speech, mutism.

- Assess for these changes, especially when drug therapy is initiated or dosages are increased.
- If dizziness, lightheadedness, vertigo occur, caution patient to avoid driving or operating hazardous equipment until the effects of the medication wear off or patient is reevaluated by physician.
- Supervise ambulation, keep siderails up, monitor smoking.
- Notify physician for persistent or severe effects.

**CV** Palpitations, tachycardia, hypotension, arrhythmias.

- Monitor blood pressure, pulse, and ECG tracings if available.
- Be alert to CV effects in individuals with known heart conditions.
- Be alert to CV effects of all medications patient is receiving. Adrenergic bronchodilators also can cause these same side effects.
- If postural hypotension occurs, caution patients to move slowly from lying to sitting or standing. Hypotension may be aggravated by prolonged periods of standing, hot showers or baths.

**GI** Nausea, vomiting; loss of appetite, bitter aftertaste, GI distress, diarrhea.

- Monitor intake, output, weight.
- If nausea, vomiting, or diarrhea are severe or persistent, a reduction in dosage or switch to another drug may be necessary; notify physician.
- Anorexia may signal toxicity; monitor serum drug levels.
- Administration of drug after meals, or with full glass of fluids, may lessen GI distress. Use of antacids may help; consult physician.

**GU** Proteinuria, diuresis. In males with prostatic enlargement, urinary retention.

- Monitor urinalysis, intake, and output.
- Monitor for urinary retention, complaints by patients that bladder does not seem to empty, or it is difficult to initiate urination.
- Have patient void prior to administering dose.

**Hematologic** Altered clotting times.

- Monitor PT, PTT, platelets, or other available clotting studies.
- Inspect patient for development of petechiae.
- Instruct patient to report the development of unexplained bleeding, petechiae, or bruising.
- Test stool for occult blood.

**Metabolic** Hyperglycemia, altered liver function tests.

- Monitor blood glucose, liver function tests.
- Instruct diabetic patients to monitor blood glucose levels more closely when medication is started or dosage is changed.
- Caution patient to report the development of jaundice, right upper quadrant abdominal pain, change in color or consistency of stools, malaise.

**Allergic** Dermatitis, pruritis.

- Assess for development of these side effects; notify physician.

### Nursing interventions related to drug administration

- Monitor serum drug levels, if available. If over upper limit of normal, hold dose and notify physician.
- Read orders carefully. Regular oral preparations cannot be interchanged with extended-release formulations without adjustment of dosage or frequency of drug administration.
- For IV administration, microdrip tubing and an electronic infusion device should be used. For acutely ill individuals, it may be appropriate to do cardiac monitoring during IV administration.
- Aminophylline may be administered by direct IV push, but usually should be diluted and administered as an infusion. Rate of administration should not exceed 25 mg/min.

- Aminophylline should not be administered IM.
- Rectal suppository forms are available, but are used only until oral or IV forms may be used. Use only pediatric suppositories for children; do not break or cut adult-dose suppositories for administration to children.

### Patient and family education

- Review with patients the expected benefits and possible side effects associated with drug therapy.
- Caution patients to report the development of any unexpected sign or symptom.
- Extended-release tablets should be swallowed whole, not chewed or crushed. Tablets that are scored may be broken before swallowing. Extended-release capsules may be opened, and the contents mixed with soft food; the food should be swallowed and not chewed. Enteric-coated preparations should be swallowed whole, not chewed or crushed.
- Teach patients to take any missed doses as soon as remembered, unless it is almost time for the next prescribed dose, in which case the patient should omit the forgotten dose and resume the prescribed schedule. Patients should not double up to make up for missed doses.
- Caution patients to avoid over-the-counter preparations unless first approved by the physician.
- In order to maintain consistent blood levels, caution patients to take medication at the same time(s) each day and to always take on either a full or empty stomach. Doses should be taken at regular intervals around the clock.
- Caution patients to avoid smoking cigarettes or marijuana. Patients who do smoke may require an increase in dosage to reach therapeutic serum levels.
- Caution patient to avoid ingestion of charcoal-broiled foods, as the high carbon content may increase drug elimination.
- Caution patients to limit the use of or avoid the use of coffee, tea, chocolate, and other methylxanthines, as they may affect xanthine metabolism.
- Marked day-to-day variations in protein and carbohydrate (CHO) intake may cause fluctuations in drug metabolism. A high CHO, low protein diet is said to increase drug half-life, while a low CHO, high protein diet may shorten drug half-life.
- Remind patients to keep these and all medications out of the reach of children.

## dyphylline    (DYE-fi-lin)                                                    bronchodilator

- dyphylline: Dilor, Dyflex, Lufyllin, Neothylline, ✤Protophylline

**MECHANISM OF ACTION**    Dyphylline relaxes bronchial smooth muscle and depresses mast cell degranulation. For more information, see entry for drug class (p. 939).

**INDICATIONS**    **Bronchospasm** For acute relief or prophylactic treatment of reversible bronchospasm of asthma, emphysema, chronic bronchospasm.

**CONTRAINDICATIONS**    **Hypersensitivity to theophylline. Active peptic ulcer.**

**DOSAGE**    **PO:**    **ADULTS:** Up to 15 mg/kg, four times per day. *Special patient populations:*    **ELDERLY:** Doses must be individualized.    **CHILDREN:** Doses must be individualized.    **PREGNANCY:** Safe use has not been established.

**PREPARATIONS**    *Solution:* 33, 53 mg/5 ml; *tablets:* 200, 400 mg; *injection (IM):* 250 mg/ml.

**DRUG INTERACTIONS**    **Smoking** Cigarette or marijuana smoking induces the hepatic metabolism of theophylline. Smokers may require a 50% to 100% increase in dosage.    **Phenobarbital** may increase the metabolism of theophylline so that larger doses may be required.    **Cimetidine, erythromycin, influenza virus vaccine, troleandomycin** have been reported to increase the serum concentrations of theophylline.    **Sympathomimetic drugs** may get excessive CNS stimulation with xanthines.    **Furosemide** increases the pharmacologic effects of theophylline.    **Digitalis, oral anticoagulants** Theophylline may enhance the sensitivity to these drugs.    **Phenytoin, lithium, nondepolarizine muscle relaxants, beta blockers** Theophylline decreases the effects of these drugs.    **Reserpine** Tachycardia.    **Magnesium-aluminum hydroxides** slow the absorption of theophylline.    **Ketamine, halothane** Increased toxicity (seizures, arrhythmias, respectively).

**DIAGNOSTIC TEST INTERFERENCE**  **Serum uric acid** Theophylline produces false positive elevations as determined by the colorimetric or Bittner method but not by the uricase method.    **Serum theophylline** Several drugs may interfere with the determination of serum theophylline concentrations, including furosemide, sulfathiazole, phenylbutazone, probenecid, theobromine, caffeine-containing beverages, chocolate, and acetaminophen, unless the determination is made with HPLC.

**FATE**  Dyphylline is a derivative of theophylline but is not metabolized to theophylline. Dyphylline is not metabolized and is excreted unchanged in the urine. The plasma *half-life* is 2 hours.

### ❦ NURSING CONSIDERATIONS
#### Side effects, toxicities, and associated nursing actions
- See entry for drug class (p. 943).
#### Nursing interventions related to drug administration
- Monitor serum drug levels, if available. If over upper limit of normal, hold dose and notify physician.
- Dyphylline injection is for IM use only. Choose sites carefully and rotate injection sites.
#### Patient and family education
- See entry for theophylline (p. 943).

---

## Other drugs for asthma

beclomethasone ~ cromolyn ~ dexamethasone ~ flunisolide ~ triamcinolone ~ ipratropium bromide

**OVERVIEW OF THE DRUG CLASS**  The drug classes presented for the treatment of asthma have been bronchodilators: the beta-2 adrenergic agonists and the xanthines. Two additional drug types are used in the treatment of asthma: glucocorticoids and cromolyn. Ipratropium bromide is the first anticholinergic drug available specifically to treat asthma.

**INDICATIONS**  **Asthma** resistant to control with bronchodilators alone. See entries for the individual drugs for information on MECHANISM OF ACTION, CONTRAINDICATIONS, and DRUG ACTIONS.

---

## cromolyn sodium (disodium cromoglycate)                    antiasthmatic

- cromolyn sodium (disodium cromoglycate): ♣Fivent, Intal, ♣Nalcrom, ♣Opticrom, ♣Rynacrom

**MECHANISM OF ACTION**  Cromolyn stabilizes mast cells so that they do not degranulate and release bronchospastic mediators.

**INDICATIONS**  **Asthma** Cromolyn is taken prophylactically.

**CONTRAINDICATIONS**  **Hypersensitivity to cromolyn.**

**DOSAGE**  **Inhalation:** **ADULTS AND CHILDREN OVER 5 YEARS OLD:** 20 mg inhaled four times daily. Cromolyn is a powder packaged in a capsule. It is administered in a special device that punctures the capsule, releasing and dispersing the powder while the patient is inhaling the powder through a special mouthpiece. *Special patient populations:* **CHILDREN:** Children younger than 5 years old cannot generally manage the unique inhaler system. **PREGNANCY:** Safe use has not been established.

**PREPARATIONS**  *Capsule (with powder for inhalation):* 20 mg.

**DRUG INTERACTIONS**  None documented.

**FATE**  Cromolyn is rapidly excreted unchanged in the bile and urine. It is poorly absorbed from the GI tract.

### ❦ NURSING CONSIDERATIONS
#### Side effects, toxicities, and associated nursing actions
**CNS** Drowsiness, dizziness, headache.
- Caution patients to avoid driving and operating hazardous equipment until the effects of medication can be evaluated.
- If drowsiness or dizziness are persistent or severe, notify physician. It may be necessary to change dosage or medication.

**GI** Nausea, stomachache.
* Instruct patient to drink a glass of milk or take a dose of antacid (if approved by the physician) prior to taking dose to lessen GI side effects.

**Lung** Wheezing, bronchospasm; nasal congestion, sneezing, itching, burning, bleeding.
* Instruct patient to drink a glass of milk prior to taking dose to lessen irritation.
* Patient should be supervised closely when first dose is taken to monitor for bronchospasm.
* Auscultate breath sounds before and after dose.

**Allergic** Rash, urticaria; angioedema.
* Monitor for allergic response.
* Have available drugs, personnel, and equipment to treat acute allergic response in settings where cromolyn is prescribed or administered.

**Other** Serum sickness: joint swelling and pain; swollen parotid gland.
* Monitor for this side effect. Instruct patient to report the development of joint discomfort.

### Nursing interventions related to drug administration
* Cromolyn powder for inhalation is administered via a special device called a turbo-inhaler; the trade name for one device is the Spinhaler. Supervise patients carefully to ensure that they can use the device as directed. The drug is supplied as a powder in a capsule. The patient assembles the turbo-inhaler, which pierces the capsule. The patient should exhale, then the mouthpiece should be placed in the mouth. The patient inhales, which causes a small propeller to rotate, aerosolizing the powder. The patient continues to inhale through the mouthpiece until all of the drug is released. The patient should not exhale through the device, since moisture will interfere with the aerosolization. The device should be washed carefully at least weekly. Instructions are provided by the manufacturer and should be reviewed with the patient.
* Cromolyn nasal solution is also administered via a special device. As with the turbo-inhaler, detailed instructions are provided by the manufacturer and should be reviewed with the patient. Tell patients to blow their noses to clear them of nasal drainage before using the nasal solution.
* Cromolyn solution for nebulization can be used with any standard nebulization apparatus.
* When used orally, the contents should be poured out of the capsule and stirred into warm water just before administering.
* An ophthalmic solution is also available. The ophthalmic solution contains benzylkonium chloride, so patients should not wear soft contact lenses during therapy with this eye medication. Review with patients the correct technique for instillation of eye drops. Remind patients that the eye drops must be used at regular intervals (as prescribed) for best effect.

### Patient and family education
* Review with patients the expected benefits and possible side effects of therapy. Caution patients to report the development of any unexpected sign or symptom.
* Unlike many of the other medications for asthma and related disorders, this drug is taken prophylactically and is not used for an acute attack of asthma. Review this point with patients. Patients who develop acute asthma should seek medical assistance.
* Inhalation of cromolyn is difficult for children under the age of 5 to master.
* Patients may find that taking the ordered dose of cromolyn about 15 minutes prior to vigorous exercise may lessen the usual breathing difficulty associated with the exercise.
* Instruct patients not to store cromolyn powder in the bathroom, where humidity or moisture may cause the medicine to break down.
* Teach patients to take missed doses as soon as remembered, then to evenly space any remaining doses for that day. Tell patients not to double up for missed doses.

# beclomethasone dipropionate
(be-kloe-METH-a-sone)                                    *glucocorticoid antiasthmatic*

* beclomethasone dipropionate: Beclovent, Vanceril

# dexamethasone sodium phosphate
(dex-a-METH-a-sone)                                   glucocorticoid antiasthmatic

- dexamethasone sodium phosphate: Decadron Phosphate Respihaler

# flunisolide   (floo-NISS-oh-lide)                   glucocorticoid antiasthmatic

- flunisolide: AeroBid

# triamcinolone   (trye-am-SIN-oh-lone)               glucocorticoid antiasthmatic

- triamcinolone: Azmacort

**MECHANISM OF ACTION**   Glucocorticoids have an antiinflammatory action. The mechanisms by which glucocorticoids specifically act to alleviate asthma are not known, but they do potentiate the action of the bronchodilators. The glucocorticoids presented here are aerosol formulations that can be inhaled daily without systemic absorption to produce adrenal suppression (see Chapter 31 for glucocorticoids and their other uses).

**INDICATIONS**   **Severe asthma**   Glucocorticoids are administered to patients not controlled by bronchodilator therapy.

**CONTRAINDICATIONS**   Systemic fungal infections or sputum cultures positive for *Candida albicans.*

| Dosage | Inhalation | |
|---|---|---|
| Glucocorticoid | Adults | Children |
| Beclomethasone | 2 inhalations 3 or 4 times daily | 1 or 2 inhalations 3 or 4 times daily |
| Dexamethasone | 3 inhalations 3 or 4 times daily | 2 inhalations 3 or 4 times daily |
| Flunisolide | 2 to 4 inhalations 2 times daily | 2 inhalations 2 times daily |
| Triamcinolone | 2 inhalations 3 or 4 times daily | 1 or 2 inhalations 3 or 4 times daily |

*Special patient populations:*   **CHILDREN**: Generally, children under 6 years old cannot inhale the drug.   **PREGNANCY**: Safe use has not been established. Glucocorticoids are teratogens in test animals.

**PREPARATIONS**   *Beclomethasone, aerosol:* 50 μg/metered spray. *Dexamethasone, aerosol:* 84 μg/metered spray. *Flunisolide, aerosol:* 250 μg/metered spray. *Triamcinoline, aerosol:* 100 μm/metered spray.

**DRUG INTERACTIONS**   Generally, the systemic concentration is low. See Chapter 35 for a complete discussion of glucocorticoids.

**FATE**   Glucocorticoids are metabolized in the liver and excreted in the feces.

**☙ NURSING CONSIDERATIONS**

   **Side effects, toxicities, and associated nursing actions**   (See also Chapter 35.)

   **GI** Dry mouth.

   - Instruct patient to gargle and rinse mouth after each dose. This is to help reduce dry mouth and to help reduce fungal infection.

**Metabolic** Adrenal suppression.
- Instruct patient to take as directed and not to increase dose or frequency of dose without physician approval.
- Patients on long-term therapy should have the frequency or dose tapered slowly when discontinuing therapy.
- Monitor blood pressure, weight, general level of energy.

**Other** Hoarseness, localized infections, commonly with *C. albicans* or *Aspergillus niger;* systemic fungal infection.
- Instruct patient to gargle and rinse mouth after each dose.
- Instruct patient to visually inspect mouth and throat for changes at least weekly.
- Instruct patient to report development of fever, malaise, sore throat.

### Nursing interventions related to drug administration
- Instructions for use of the inhalers are provided by the manufacturer and should be reviewed with the patient before use.

### Patient and family education
- Review with patients the expected benefits and possible side effects of therapy. The numerous side effects of long-term steroid therapy are outlined in Chapter 35.
- Tell patients to take this medication only as directed and not to increase dose or frequency of administration.
- Instruct patients to wear a medical identification tag or bracelet noting that patient is receiving glucocorticoid therapy.
- Patients receiving an inhaled bronchodilator and an inhaled glucocorticoid should use the bronchodilator first, then wait several minutes before using the glucocorticoid.
- The inhalation device should be washed and dried after each use, or at least daily.
- Remind patients to keep all medications out of the reach of children.

---

## ipratropium bromide  (i-prah-TROE-pee-um)    bronchodilator

- ipratropium bromide: Atrovent

**MECHANISM OF ACTION**  Ipratropium is an anticholinergic (atropine-like) drug. When inhaled, it relaxes the bronchial smooth muscle.

**INDICATIONS**  Chronic bronchitis and emphysema.

**CONTRAINDICATIONS**  Hypersensitivity.  Acute bronchospasm.  Conditions made worse by anticholinergic action, including narrow angle glaucoma, prostatic hypertrophy, bladder neck obstruction.

**DOSAGE**  Inhalation:  ADULTS: Metered dose, 18 μg/puff.  *Special patient populations:*  CHILDREN: Not recommended for children under 12 years old.  PREGNANCY: Safe use has not been established. Pregnancy category B.

**PREPARATIONS**  *Inhalator, metered dose:* 18 μg/puff.

**DRUG INTERACTIONS**  Anticholinergic drugs have additive anticholinergic (atropine-like) action.

**FATE**  The elimination *half-life* is about 2 hours.

### ☙ NURSING CONSIDERATIONS

#### Side effects, toxicities, and associated nursing actions
**CNS** Nervousness, dizziness, headache.
**CV** Palpitations.
**GI** Nausea.
**Skin** Rash.

**Eye** Blurred vision.
- Instruct patient to avoid driving or operating hazardous equipment if blurred vision develops; notify physician.

## Nursing interventions related to drug administration
- Instructions for use of the inhalers are provided by the manufacturer and should be reviewed with the patient before use.

## Patient and family education
- Review with patients the expected benefits and possible side effects of therapy.
- Tell patients to take this medication only as directed and not to increase the dose or frequency of administration.
- Remind patients to keep all medications out of the reach of children.

# Chapter Fifty-three
# Nasal decongestants

epinephrine (see Chapter 5)
ephedrine (see Chapter 5)
naphazoline
oxymetazoline
phenylephrine
phenylpropanolamine
propylhexedrine
pseudoephedrine
tetrahydrozoline
xylometazoline

**DRUG COMBINATIONS**   See Table 53-1. In addition, many nonprescription combination drugs are available.

**OVERVIEW OF THE DRUG CLASS**   Nasal decongestants are alpha adrenergic agonists, some effective topically, others effective systemically. The *topical* decongestants are applied as drops or sprays. Because these nasal decongestants have an immediate and direct contact with the nasal mucosa, they have a rapid action and provide temporary symptomatic relief by opening up the nasal passages. However, when the effect of the drug wears off, the congestion reappears (rebound congestion). If the nasal decongestant is used with increasing frequency, it has less and less effect. The drug ultimately irritates the nasal passages and causes the congestion to become worse rather than better. For this reason decongestants are most effective when used only occasionally and for no longer than 3 to 5 days.

*Orally* active decongestants are commonly found with other drugs in various cold remedies. Cold remedies are syrups, tablets, or capsules that may also include an antihistamine, analgesic, or other miscellaneous ingredients. These combination products are listed in Table 53-1. Those alpha adrenergic agonists most commonly found in cold remedies include phenylpropanolamine, phenylephrine, and pseudoephedrine.

**MECHANISM OF ACTION**   Nasal congestion results when the blood vessels in the nasal passage become dilated as a result of infection, inflammation, allergy, or emotional upset. This dilation increases capillary permeability and allows fluid to escape into the nasal passage. Drugs that stimulate alpha receptors cause blood vessels to constrict, thereby relieving the congestion. These drugs are alpha adrenergic agonists because they mimic the action of the neurotransmitter norepinephrine.

**INDICATIONS**   **Nasal congestion** Topical sprays or oral formulations relieve congestion associated with the common cold, sinusitis, hay fever, and other respiratory allergies. May provide relief for eustachian tube congestion.   **Conjunctival congestion** Several of the topical nasal decongestants are available in formulations to apply as eye drops.

**CONTRAINDICATIONS**   **Hypersensitivity to sympathomimetic amines.   Severe hypertension or coronary artery disease.** The orally administered drugs can cause an increase in blood pressure and heart rate.

**DRUG INTERACTIONS**   **Monoamine oxidase inhibitors and beta adrenergic blockers** act synergistically with the nasal decongestants.   **Antihypertensive drugs** The effects of methyldopa and reserpine may be reduced by nasal decongestants.   **Isoproterenol and epinephrine** Cardiac effects may be exaggerated by nasal decongestants and lead to cardiac arrhythmias.

---

**⚘ NURSING CONSIDERATIONS**
**Side effects, toxicities, and associated nursing actions**
**CNS** Fear, anxiety, tenseness, restlessness, headache, lightheadedness, tremor, insomnia.
- Assess for these reactions. If they are severe or persistent, it may be necessary to change drugs or discontinue medication; notify the physician.
- If insomnia occurs, take the last dose no later than the evening meal to prevent loss of sleep.
- The appearance of these symptoms after the patient has been using the drug for a period of time may indicate that patient is increasing the frequency or dose; review with patient the recommended

**Table 53-1.**

| Prescription drugs to relieve nasal congestion | | | |
|---|---|---|---|
| **Trade Name** | **Decongestant** | **Antihistamine** | **Other Ingredients*** |
| Aclophen Tablets | Phenylephrine | Chlorpheniramine | AM |
| Actacin Syrup | Pseudoephedrine | Triprolidine | |
| Actagen Syrup | Pseudoephedrine | Triprolidine | |
| Actihist Tablets | Pseudoephedrine | Triprolidine | |
| Aladrine Suspension/Tablets | Ephedrine | | SB |
| Alersule Capsules | Phenylephrine | Chlorpheniramine | |
| Alumadrine Tablets | Phenylpropanolamine | Chlorpheniramine | AM |
| Amaril D Liquid/Spantab | Phenylpropanolamine | Chorpheniramine | PT,PE |
| Anafed Capsules/Syrup | Pseudoephedrine | Chlorpheniramine | |
| Anamine TD Caps | Pseudoephedrine | Chlorpheniramine | |
| Brexin LA Caps | Pseudoephedrine | Chlorpheniramine | |
| Bromfed Syrup/Tablets/PD Capsules | Pseudoephedrine | Brompheniramine | |
| Bromophen Elixir/T.D. Tablets | Phenylpropanolamine | Brompheniramine | PE |
| Brompheril Tablets | Pseudoephedrine | Dexbrompheniramine | |
| Carbodec Syrup | Pseudoephedrine | Carbinoxamine | |
| Cardec-S Syrup | Pseudoephedrine | Carbinoxamine | |
| Cenahist Capsules | Phenylephrine | Chlorpheniramine | MS |
| Chlorafed Half-Strength/Adult Timecelles | Pseudoephedrine | Chlorpheniramine | |
| Codimal LA Cenules | Pseudoephedrine | Chlorpheniramine | |
| Comhist Tablets/LA Capsules | Phenylephrine | Chlorpheniramine | PT |
| Condrin-LA Capsules | Phenylpropanolamine | Chlorpheniramine | |
| Dallergy Capsules/Syrup/Tablets | Phenylephrine | Chlorpheniramine | MS |
| Dallergy Jr. Capsules | Pseudoephedrine | Brompheniramine | |
| Deconade Capsules | Phenylpropanolamine | Chlorpheniramine | |
| Deconamine Syrup/SR Capsules | Pseudoephedrine | Chlorpheniramine | |
| Decongestabs Tablets | Phenylpropanolamine | Chlorpheniramine | PE,PT |
| Dexbrompheniramine w/Pseudo-ephedrine Tablets | Pseudoephedrine | Dexbrompheniramine | |
| Dimaphen S.A. Tablets | Phenylpropanolamine | Brompheniramine | PE |
| Disobrom Tablets | Pseudoephedrine | Dexbrompheniramine | |
| Drize Capsules | Phenylpropanolamine | Chlorpheniramine | |
| Duralex Capsules | Pseudoephedrine | Chlorpheniramine | |
| Dura-Tap/PD Capsules | Pseudoephedrine | Chlorpheniramine | |
| Dura-Vent/A Capsules | Phenylpropanolamine | Chlorpheniramine | |
| Dura-Vent/DA Tablets | Phenylephrine | Chlorpheniramine | MS |
| E-Tapp Elixir | Phenylpropanolamine | Brompheniramine | PE |
| Entafed Capsules | Pseudoephedrine | Chlorpheniramine | |
| Ephedrine and Amyltal Pulvules | Ephedrine | | AB |
| Extendryl JR or SR Capsules/Syrup/Tablets | Phenylephrine | Chlorpheniramine | MS |
| Fedahist Gyrocaps | Pseudoephedrine | Chlorpheniramine | |
| Histabid Duracaps | Phenylpropanolamine | Chlorpheniramine | |
| Histalet Syrup/Forte Tablets | Phenylpropanolamine | Chlorpheniramine | PE,PR |
| Histaminic Capsules/H-S Tablets/Reg or Ped Syrup | Phenylpropanolamine | Chlorpheniramine | PE,PT |
| Histaspan-Plus Caps | Phenylephrine | Chlorpheniramine | |
| Histaspan-D Caps | Phenylephrine | Chlorpheniramine | MS |

*Continued.*

**Table 53-1.**

**Prescription drugs to relieve nasal congestion—cont'd.**

| Trade Name | Decongestant | Antihistamine | Other Ingredients* |
|---|---|---|---|
| Hista-Vadrin Tablets | Phenylpropanolamine | Chlorpheniramine | PE |
| Histor-D Syrup | Phenylephrine | Chlorpheniramine | |
| Histor-D Timecelles | Phenylephrine | Chlorpheniramine | MS |
| Isoclor Timesules | Pseudoephedrine | Chlorpheniramine | |
| Klerist-D Capsules/Tablets | Pseudoephedrine | Chlorpheniramine | |
| Korigesic Tablets | Phenylpropanolamine | Chlorpheniramine | AM,SA,CF |
| Kronofed-A Jr or Regular Kron-ocaps | Pseudoephedrine | Chlorpheniramine | |
| Kronohist Kronocaps | Phenylpropanolamine | Chlorpheniramine | PR |
| Midatapp Elixir | Phenylpropanolamine | Brompheniramine | |
| Naldecon Syrup/Tablets/Pediatric Drops/Syrup | Phenylpropanolamine | Chorpheniramine | PT,PE |
| Naldelate Syrup | Phenylpropanolamine | Chorpheniramine | PT,PE |
| Nalgest Tablets | Phenylpropanolamine | Chorpheniramine | PE,PT |
| Nasahist Capsules | Phenylpropanolamine | Chlorpheniramine | PE |
| Nasec Capsules | Phenylephrine | Chlorpheniramine | |
| ND Clear Capsules | Pseudoephedrine | Chlorpheniramine | |
| ND-Gesic Tablets | Phenylephrine | Chlorpheniramine | AM,PR |
| New-Decongest Tablets/Syrup/Ped Syrup | Phenylpropanolamine | Chlorpheniramine | PE,PT |
| Nolamine Tablets | Phenypropanolamine | Chlorpheniramine | PD |
| Norafed Tablets | Pseudoephedrine | Triprolidine | |
| Norel Plus Capsules | Phenylpropanolamine | Chlorpheniramine | AM,PT |
| Normatane Elixir | Phenylpropanolamine | Brompheniramine | PE |
| Novafed A Capsules | Pseudoephedrine | Chlorpheniramine | |
| Oracap Capsules | Phenylpropanolamine | Chlorpheniramine | |
| Oragest S.R. Capsules | Phenylpropanolamine | Chlorpheniramine | |
| Oraminic Spancaps | Phenylpropanolamine | Chlorpheniramine | |
| Ornade Spancaps | Phenylpropanolamine | Chlorpheniramine | |
| Panadyl Tablets | Phenylpropanolamine | Pyrilamine | PN |
| Phenahist-TR | Phenylpropanolamine | Chlorpheniramine | PE |
| Phenate Tablets | Phenylpropanolamine | Chlorpheniramine | AM |
| Phenergan VC Syrup | Phenylephrine | Promethazine | |
| Phenergan-D Tablets | Pseudoephedrine | Promethazine | |
| Phentox compound Syrup | Phenylpropanolamine | Chlorpheniramine | Pt,PE |
| Pherazine VC Syrup | Phenylephrine | Promethazine | |
| Poly-Histine-D Capsules/Elixir/Ped Capsules | Phenylpropanolamine | Pyrilamine | PN,PT |
| Probahist Capsules | Pseudoephedrine | Chlorpheniramine | |
| Prometh VC Plain Liquid | Phenylephrine | Promethazine | |
| Promethazine VC Syrup | Phenylephrine | Promethazine | |
| Pseudo-Chlor Capsules | Pseudoephedrine | Chlorpheniramine | |
| Pseudo-Hist Capsules | Pseudoephedrine | Chlorpheniramine | |
| Pseudoephedrine and Triprolidine Tablets | Pseudoephedrine | Triprolidine | |
| Resaid S.R. Capsules | Phenylpropanolamine | Chlorpheniramine | |
| Rhinex D Lay Tablets | Phenylpropanolamine | Chlorpheniramine | AM,SA |
| Rhinolar Capsules, Ex Capsules | Phenylpropanolamine | Chlorpheniramine | |
| Rinade B.I.D. Capsules | Pseudoephedrine | Chlorpheniramine | |

**Table 53-1.**

## Prescription drugs to relieve nasal congestion—cont'd.

| Trade Name | Decongestant | Antihistamine | Other Ingredients* |
|---|---|---|---|
| Rondec Syrup/Drops/Tablets/TR Tablets | Pseudoephedrine | Carbinoxamine | |
| Ru-Tuss II Capsules | Phenylpropanolamine | Chlorpheniramine | |
| Rynatan Pediatric Suspension/ Tablets | Phenylephrine | Chlorpheniramine | PR |
| Sinovan Timed Capsules | Phenylephrine | Chlorpheniramine | MS |
| Sinubid Tablets | Phenylpropanolamine | Phenyltoloxamine | AC |
| Sto-Caps Plus Capsules | Phenylephrine | Chlorpheniramine | |
| T-Dry Jr. Capsules | Pseudoephedrine | Chlorpheniramine | |
| Tramine S.R. Tablets | Phenylpropanolamine | Brompheniramine | PE |
| Travist-D Tablets | Phenylpropanolamine | Clemastine | |
| Tri-Phen-Chlor T.B. Tablets | Phenylpropanolamine | Chlorpheniramine | PE,PT |
| Triaminic TR Tablets/Oral Infant Drops | Phenylpropanolamine | Pyrilamine | PN |
| Trifed Tablets | Pseudoephedrine | Triprolidine | |
| Trinaline Repetabs | Pseudophedrine | Azatadine | |
| Triphenyl TD Tablets | Phenylpropanolamine | Pyrilamine | PN |
| Triprolidine w/Pseudoephedrine Syrup | Pseudophedrine | Triprolidine | |
| Tussanil Plain Syrup | Phenylephrine | Chlorpheniramine | |
| Vasominic T.D. Tablets | Phenylpropanolamine | Chlorpheniramine | PE,PT |
| Veltap Elixir | Phenylpropanolamine | Brompheniramine | PE |

AB = Amytal
AC = Ammonium chloride
AM = Acetaminophen
CF = Caffeine
MS = Methscopolamine
PD = Phenindamine

PE = Phenylephrine
PN = Pheniramine
PR = Pyrilamine
PT = Phenyltoloxamine
SA = Salicylamide
SB = Secobarbital

dosage schedule.

**CV** Palpitations, arrhythmias, tachycardia.

• Monitor pulse and blood pressure. Be especially alert to these effects in the elderly or those with preexisting cardiovascular disease or hypertension.

**Eye** Photophobia, irritation, tearing.

• Irritation and tearing are frequent. If the patient can tolerate discomfort, these symptoms may lessen with subsequent doses. If symptoms are severe or persistent, it may be necessary to lower the dose or change drugs.

• If photophobia occurs, instruct the patient to avoid brightly lit areas and to wear sunglasses. Caution that patient that driving after sunset with sunglasses is hazardous and should be avoided.

**GI** Nausea, vomiting.

• Assess for GI symptoms. Persistent or severe symptoms may warrant lowering the dose or changing drugs.

**Skin** Burning, stinging, dryness from topical use.

• Assess for these symptoms. Persistent or severe symptoms may warrant lowering the dose or changing drugs.

### Nursing interventions related to drug administration

• Read labels carefully. Preparations for use in the eye are labeled for ophthalmic use.

• Read orders carefully. Ophthalmic solutions are available in various concentrations.

**Patient and family education**

- Review with patients the expected benefits and possible side effects of therapy. Instruct patients to report the development of any unexpected sign or symptom.
- Review with patients the dosage schedule; not that these drugs should rarely be used for longer than 3 to 4 days (see Dosage). Point out to patients that increasing the frequency or dosage will only tend to foster rebound congestion.
- To prevent contamination, instruct each patient or family member to use a different dropper or spray applicator. Applicators should be wiped off, washed, or rinsed with hot water after each use.
- For best results with topical nasal application, instruct the patient to blow the nose prior to using the medication. After instilling the drops or spray, the patient may blot a runny nose but should avoid blowing the nose for several minutes to allow the maximum amount of medication to be absorbed.
- Instruct the patient to sit upright for applying nasal spray. For applying nasal drops, the patient should have head downward, permitting area or sinus being treated to be in dependent position.
- Since many of these products are available in over-the-counter combination products, instruct patients to read labels carefully. Through oversight, patients may be taking the same drug in several formulations or may be taking drugs in combination products that are not needed or that are contraindicated for that person.
- Many of the ophthalmic preparations contain benzylkonium chloride. Patients who wear soft contact lenses should not wear their lenses during therapy with eye preparations containing benzylkonium chloride or should read labels carefully to obtain a product that does not contain this agent. Consult a pharmacist.
- Remind patients to keep these and all medications out of the reach of children. Only preparations designed for pediatric use should be used with children under the age of 12.

## naphazoline hydrochloride
(naf-AZ-oh-leen)                                            nasal decongestant, ophthalmic decongestant

- naphazoline hydrochloride: Allerest, Clear Eyes, Degest, Naphcon, Privine, VasoClear (OTC)

**MECHANISM OF ACTION**   Nasal decongestants cause blood vessels to constrict, thereby relieving the congestion.

**INDICATIONS**   **Nasal congestion** For the relief of congestion associated with the common cold, sinusitis, hay fever, and other respiratory allergies. May provide relief for eustachian tube congestion.   **Conjunctival congestion** Applied as eye drops.

**CONTRAINDICATIONS**   • Hypersensitivity to sympathomimetic amines. • Severe hypertension or coronary artery disease.

**DOSAGE**   **Intranasal:**   **ADULTS AND CHILDREN OVER 6 YEARS OLD:** Two drops or sprays into each nostril as needed, no more than every 3 hours. Self-administration should be for no more than 3 days. **Ophthalmic:**   **ADULTS AND CHILDREN:** One to three drops of 0.1% solution applied topically to the conjunctiva every 3 to 4 hours as needed. Self-administration should be for no more than 4 days. Lower concentrations of drug provide relief for "blood shot" eyes and minor irritation.   *Special patient populations:*   **CHILDREN:** Not for use by children under 6 years old.   **PREGNANCY:** Safe use has not been established.

**PREPARATIONS**   *Nasal solution:* 0.05%, *ophthalmic solution:* 0.012%, 0.02%, 0.03%, or 0.1%.

**DRUG INTERACTIONS**   **Monoamine oxidase inhibitors and beta adrenergic blockers** act synergistically with the nasal decongestants.   **Antihypertensive drugs** The effects of methyldopa and reserpine may be reduced by nasal decongestants. **Isoproterenol and epinephrine** Cardiac effects may be exaggerated by nasal decongestants and lead to cardiac arrhythmias.

**FATE** The *onset of action* is within 10 minutes, and the *duration of action* is 2 to 6 hours. The drug is not usually absorbed in large enough quantities to cause systemic effects. The metabolism of naphazoline has not been characterized.

## ❦ NURSING CONSIDERATIONS

### Side effects, toxicities, and associated nursing actions
- See entry for drug class (p. 950).

### Nursing interventions related to drug administration
- See entry for drug class (p. 953).

### Patient and family education
- See entry for drug class (p. 954).

---

## oxymetazoline hydrochloride  (ox-i-met-AZ-oh-leen)  nasal decongestant

- oxymetazoline: Afrin, Allerest, Dristan, Duramist, ✽Nafrine, Neo-Synephrine, ✽Ocuclear (OTC)

**MECHANISM OF ACTION**  Nasal decongestants cause blood vessels to constrict, thereby relieving the congestion.

**INDICATIONS**  **Nasal congestion** For the relief of congestion associated with the common cold, sinusitis, hay fever, and other respiratory allergies. May provide relief for eustachian tube congestion.

**CONTRAINDICATIONS**  • Hypersensitivity to sympathomimetic amines. • Severe hypertension or coronary artery disease. • Narrow-angle glaucoma.

**DOSAGE**  **Intranasal**  **ADULTS AND CHILDREN OVER 6 YEARS OLD:** Two or three drops or sprays in each nostril twice daily of the 0.05% solution.  **CHILDREN 2 TO 5 YEARS OLD:** Two or three drops or sprays in each nostril twice daily of the 0.025% solution. Do not self-medicate for more then 3 days. *Special patient populations:*  **PREGNANCY:** Safe use has not been established.

**PREPARATIONS**  *Nasal solution;* 0.05% or 0.025%.

**DRUG INTERACTIONS**  Monoamine oxidase inhibitors and beta-adrenergic blockersact synergistically with the nasal decongestants.  **Antihypertensive drugs** The effects of methyldopa and reserpine may be reduced by nasal decongestants.  **Isoproterenol and epinephrine** Cardiac effects may be exaggerated by nasal decongestants and lead to cardiac arrhythmias.

**FATE** The *onset of action* is 5 to 10 minutes, and the *duration of action* is 6 hours. The drug is usually not absorbed in large enough quantity to produce systemic effects.

## ❦ NURSING CONSIDERATIONS

### Side effects, toxicities, and associated nursing actions
- See entry for drug class (p. 950).

### Nursing interventions related to drug administration
- See entry for drug class (p. 953).

### Patient and family education
- See entry for drug class (p. 954).

---

## phenylephrine hydrochloride
(fen-ill-EF-rin)  nasal decongestant, ophthalmic decongestant

- phenylephrine hydrochloride: Neo-Synephrine, Alcon-Efrin, Coricidin, ✽Prefin Liquifilm, others (OTC)

**MECHANISM OF ACTION**   Nasal decongestants cause blood vessels to constrict, thereby relieving the congestion.

**INDICATIONS**   **Nasal congestion** For the relief of congestion associated with the common cold, sinusitis, hay fever, and other respiratory allergies. May provide relief for eustachian tube congestion.   **Conjunctival congestion** Applied as eye drops.

**CONTRAINDICATIONS**   • Hypersensitivity to sympathomimetic amines. • Severe hypertension or coronary artery disease.

**DOSAGE**   **Intranasal:**   **ADULTS AND CHILDREN OVER 12 YEARS OLD:** Two to three drops or one to two sprays of a 0.25% or 0.5% solution in each nostril, repeated in 4 hours if needed.   **CHILDREN 6 TO 12 YEARS OLD:** Two to three drops or one to two sprays of a 0.25% solution in each nostril, repeated in 4 hours if needed. Do not self-medicate for more than 3 days. **Ophthalmic:**   **ADULTS AND CHILDREN:** One or two drops of a 0.12% to 0.25% ophthalmic solution applied topically every 3 to 4 hours as needed. *Special patient populations:*   **PREGNANCY:** Safe use has not been established.

**PREPARATIONS**   *Nasal solution:* 0.125%, 0.16%, 0.2%, 0.25%, 0.5%, or 1%; *nasal jelly:* 0.5%, *ophthalmic solution:* 0.12% 2.5%, or 10%.

**DRUG INTERACTIONS**   **Monoamine oxidase inhibitors and beta-adrenergic blockers** act synergistically with nasal decongestants.   **Antihypertensive drugs** The effects of methyldopa and reserpine may be reduced by nasal decongestants.   **Isoproterenol and epinephrine** Cardiac effects may be exaggerated by nasal decongestants and lead to cardiac arrhythmias.

**FATE**   The *onset of action* is immediate, and the *duration of action* is 0.5 to 4 hours. The drug is usually not absorbed in large enough quantity to produce systemic effects.

### ☙ NURSING CONSIDERATIONS

#### Side effects, toxicities, and associated nursing actions
- See entry for drug class (p. 950).

#### Nursing interventions related to drug administration
- To use the nasal jelly, instruct patient to blow the nose gently, then place a pea-sized amount of jelly into each nostril, then sniff it well back into the nose. After taking the dose, the patient should wipe tip of tube and replace cap tightly.
- See entry for drug class (p. 953).

#### Patient and family education
- See entry for drug class (p. 954).

---

## phenylpropanolamine hydrochloride
(fen-ill-proe-pa-NOLE-a-meen)                                        nasal decongestant

- phenylpropanolamine hydrochloride: Diadax, Propagest, ✤Propadrine, Sucrets

**MECHANISM OF ACTION**   Nasal decongestants cause blood vessels to constrict, thereby relieving the congestion.

**INDICATIONS**   **Nasal congestion** For the relief of congestion associated with the common cold, sinusitis, hay fever, and other respiratory allergies. May provide relief for eustachian tube congestion.

**CONTRAINDICATIONS**   • Hypersensitivity to sympathomimetic amines. • Severe hypertension or coronary artery disease.

**DOSAGE**   **PO:**   **ADULTS:** 20 to 25 mg every 4 hours, no more than 150 mg daily. Alternatively, 75 mg extended-release capsule twice daily.   **CHILDREN 6 TO 12 YEARS OLD:** 10 to 12.5 mg every 4 hours.   **CHILDREN 2 TO 5 YEARS OLD:** 6.25 mg every 4 hours. Do not self-medicate for more than 3 days. *Special patient populations:*   **ELDERLY:** Individuals over 60 years old are more likely to suffer adverse effects from sympathomimetic drugs.   **PREGNANCY:** Safe use has not been established.

**PREPARATIONS**   *Capsules (extended release):* 37.5, 50, or 75 mg; *lozenges:* 25 mg; *solution (oral):* 12.5 mg/5 ml; *tablets:* 25 or 50 mg; *tablets (extended release):* 75 mg; *tablets (film-coated):* 37.5 mg.

**DRUG INTERACTIONS**   **Monoamine oxidase inhibitors and beta-adrenergic blockers** act synergistically with nasal decongestants.   **Antihypertensive drugs** The effects of methyldopa and reserpine may be reduced by nasal decongestants.   **Isoproterenol and epinephrine** Cardiac effects may be exaggerated by nasal decongestants and lead to cardia arrhythmias.

**FATE**   Phenylpropanolamine is readily absorbed from the GI tract. The *onset of action* is 15 to 30 minutes, and the *duration of action* is 6 hours for regular formulations and 12 hours for extended-release formulations. Phenylpropanolamine is metabolized in the liver to an active metabolite but is excreted largely unchanged in the urine.

❦ **NURSING CONSIDERATIONS**

**Side effects, toxicities, and associated nursing actions**
- See entry for drug class (p. 950).

**Nursing interventions related to drug administration**
- See entry for drug class (p. 953).

**Patient and family education**
- See entry for drug class (p. 954).

---

# propylhexedrine   (proe-pill-HEX-i-dreen)                    nasal decongestant

- propylhexedrine: Benzedrex (OTC)

**MECHANISM OF ACTION**   Nasal decongestants cause blood vessels to constrict, thereby relieving the congestion.

**INDICATIONS**   **Nasal congestion** For the relief of congestion associated with the common cold, sinusitis, hay fever, and other respiratory allergies. May provide relief for eustachian tube congestion.

**CONTRAINDICATIONS**   • Hypersensitivity to sympathomimetic amines. • Severe hypertension or coronary artery disease. • Narrow-angle glaucoma.

**DOSAGE**   **Intranasal:**   **ADULTS AND CHILDREN OVER 6 YEARS OLD:** Two inhalations (0.4 to 0.5 mg) in each nostril no more than every 2 hours. Do not self-medicate for more than 3 days.   *Special patient populations:*   **CHILDREN:** Not recommended for children under 6 years old.   **PREGNANCY:** Safe use has not been established.

**PREPARATIONS**   *Inhalant:* 250 mg.

**DRUG INTERACTIONS**   **Monoamine oxidase inhibitors and beta adrenergic blockers** act synergistically with nasal decongestants.   **Antihypertensive durgs** The effects of methyldopa and reserpine may be reduced by nasal decongestants.   **Isoproterenol and epinephrine** Cardiac effects may be exaggerated by nasal decongestants and lead to cardiac arrhythmias.

**FATE**   The *onset of action* is within minutes, and the *duration of action* is 0.5 to 2 hours. The drug is usually not absorbed in large enough quantity to produce systemic effects.

❦ **NURSING CONSIDERATIONS**

**Side effects, toxicities, and associated nursing actions**
- See entry for drug class (p. 950).

**Nursing interventions related to drug administration**
- This medication is administered with an inhaler. Review manufacturer's instructions with patient and family prior to use.

**Patient and family education**
- See entry for drug class (p. 954).

---

# pseudoephedrine hydrochloride, pseudoephedrine sulfate
(soo-doe-e-FED-rin)                                           nasal decongestant

- pseudoephedrine hydrochloride: Novafed, Sudafed, Sufedrin ✤Pseudofrin, ✤Robidrine (OTC)
- pseudoephedrine sulfate: Afrenol

**MECHANISM OF ACTION**   Nasal decongestants cause blood vessels to constrict, thereby relieving the congestion.

**INDICATIONS**   **Nasal congestion** For the relief of congestion associated with the common cold, sinusitis, hay fever, and other respiratory allergies. May provide relief for eustachian tube congestion.

**CONTRAINDICATIONS**   • Hypersensitivity to sympathomimetic amines. • Severe hypertension or coronary artery disease.

**DOSAGE**   **PO:**   **ADULTS AND CHILDREN OVER 12 YEARS OLD:** 60 mg every 4 to 6 hours; maximum 240 mg daily. Alternatively, 120 mg in an extended-release form every 12 hours.   **CHILDREN 6 TO 11 YEARS OLD:** 30 mg every 4 to 6 hours; maximum 120 mg daily.   **CHILDREN 2 TO 5 YEARS OLD:** 15 mg every 4 to 6 hours, maximum 60 mg daily. Do not self-medicate for more than 3 days. *Special patient populations:*   **ELDERLY:** Individuals over 60 years old are more likely to suffer adverse effects from sympathomimetic drugs.   **PREGNANCY:** Safe use has not been established.

**PREPARATIONS**   *Hydrochloride, capsules (extended release):* 120 mg; *solution:* 15 or 30 mg/ml; 7.5 mg/0.8 ml (drop); *tablets:* 30 or 60 mg. *Sulfate, tablets* (extended release): 120 mg.

**DRUG INTERACTIONS**   **Monoamine oxidase inhibitors and beta adrenergic blockers** act synergistically with the nasal decongestants.   **Antihypertensive drugs** The effects of methyldopa and reserpine may be reduced by nasal decongestants.   **Isoproterenol and epinephrine** Cardiac effects may be exaggerated by nasal decongestants and lead to cardiac arrhythmias.

**FATE**   Pseudoephedrine is well absorbed. The *onset of action* is within 30 minutes, and the *duration of action* is 4 to 6 hours. Pseudoephedrine is metabolized in the liver and excreted unchanged and metabolized in the urine.

**☙ NURSING CONSIDERATIONS**

**Side effects, toxicities, and associated nursing actions**
  • See entry for drug class (p. 950).

**Nursing interventions related to drug administration**
  • See entry for drug class (p. 953).

**Patient and family education**
  • See entry for drug class (p. 954).

---

# tetrahydrozoline hydrochloride
(te-tra-hye-DROZ-a-leen)                    nasal decongestant, ophthalmic decongestant

  • tetrahydrozoline hydrochloride: Murine, Tyzine, Visine, others (OTC)

**MECHANISM OF ACTION**   Nasal decongestants cause blood vessels to constrict, thereby relieving the congestion.

**INDICATIONS**   **Nasal congestion** For the relief of congestion associated with the common cold, sinusitis, hay fever, and other respiratory allergies. May provide relief for eustachian tube congestion.   **Conjunctival congestion** Applied as eye drops.

**CONTRAINDICATIONS**   • Hypersensitivity to sympathomimetic amines. • Severe hypertension or coronary artery disease.

**DOSAGE**   **Intranasal:**   **ADULTS AND CHILDREN OVER 6 YEARS OLD:** two to four drops or sprays of a 0.1% solution in each nostril every 4 to 6 hours.   **CHILDREN 2 TO 5 YEARS OLD:** two to four drops or sprays of a 0.05% solution in each nostril every 4 to 6 hours. Do not self-medicate for more than 3 days.   **Ophthalmic:**   **ADULTS AND CHILDREN:** one or two drops of a 0.05% solution two or three times daily. Do not self-medicate for more than 4 days.   *Special patient populations:*   **CHILDREN:** Pediatric doses are given above.   **PREGNANCY:** Safe use has not been established.

**PREPARATIONS**   *Nasal solution:* 0.05% or 0.1%; *ophthalmic solution:* 0.05%.

**DRUG INTERACTIONS**   **Monoamine oxidase inhibitors and beta adrenergic blockers** act synergistically with nasal decongestants.   **Antihypertensive drugs** The effects of methyldopa and reserpine may be reduced by nasal decongestants.   **Isoproterenol and epinephrine** Cardiac effects may be exaggerated by nasal decongestants and lead to cardiac arrhythmias.

**FATE**    The *onset of action* is within minutes, and the *duration of action* is 4 to 8 hours. The drug is usually not absorbed in large enough quantity to produce systemic effects.

## ❧ NURSING CONSIDERATIONS

### Side effects, toxicities and associated nursing actions
- See entry for drug class (p. 950).

### Nursing interventions related to drug administration
- See entry for drug class (p. 953)

### Patient and family education
- See entry for drug class (p. 954).

---

## xylometazoline hydrochloride    (zye-loe-met-AZ-oh-leen)    nasal decongestant

- xylometazoline hydrochloride: Neo-Synephrine II, Otrivin, others (OTC)

**MECHANISM OF ACTION**    Nasal decongestants cause blood vessels to constrict, thereby relieving the congestion.

**INDICATIONS**    **Nasal congestion** For the relief of congestion associated with the common cold, sinusitis, hay fever, and other respiratory allergies. May provide relief for eustachian tube congestion.    **Conjunctival congestion** Applied as eye drops.

**CONTRAINDICATIONS**    • Hypersensitivity to sympathomimetic amines. • Severe hypertension or coronary artery disease.

**DOSAGE**    **Intranasal:**    **ADULTS AND CHILDREN OVER 12 YEARS OLD:** two or three drops or sprays of the 0.1% solution in each nostril every 8 to 10 hours as needed.    **CHILDREN 6 MONTHS TO 12 YEARS OLD:** two or three drops or sprays of the 0.05% solution in each nostril every 8 to 10 hours as needed. Do not self-medicate for more than 3 days.    *Special patient populations:*    **PREGNANCY:** Safe use has not been established.

**PREPARATIONS**    *Nasal solution:* 0.05% or 0.1%.

**DRUG INTERACTIONS**    **Monoamine oxidase inhibitors and beta adrenergic blockers** act synergistically with the nasal decongestants.    **Antihypertensive drugs** The effects of methyldopa and reserpine may be reduced by nasal decongestants.    **Isoproterenol and epinephrine** Cardiac effects may be exaggerated by nasal decongestants and lead to cardiac arrhythmias.

**FATE**    The *onset of action* is 5 to 10 minutes, and the *duration of action* is 5 to 6 hours. The drug is usually not absorbed in large enough quantity to produce systemic effects.

## ❧ NURSING CONSIDERATIONS

### Side effects, toxicities and associated nursing actions
- See entry for drug class (p. 950).

### Nursing interventions related to drug administration
- See entry for drug class (p. 953).

### Patient and family education
- See entry for drug class (p. 954).

# Chapter Fifty-four

# Expectorants and antitussives

| Expectorants | Antitussives |
|---|---|
| guaifenesin | benzonatate |
| iodide compounds | codeine |
| hydroiodic acid | dextromethorphan |
| iodinated glycerol | diphenhydramine |
| potassium iodide | hydrocodone |
| terpin hydrate | noscapine |

**DRUG COMBINATIONS**    Expectorants and antitussives are commonly combined with each other or with other drugs. Table 54-1 lists prescription combinations to suppress a cough. Table 54-2 lists prescription combinations of expectorants. In addition, many over-the-counter (OTC) preparations are available.

**INTRODUCTION**    Expectorants and antitussives are presented together because they are frequently formulated together. Expectorants promote the output of respiratory tract fluid so that mucus does not dry into plugs in the bronchioles. Antitussives suppress a cough.

---

## Expectorants

guaifenesin ~ iodide compounds ~ hydroiodic acid ~ iodinated glycerol ~ potassium iodide ~ terpin hydrate

**OVERVIEW OF THE DRUG CLASS**    An expectorant is a drug that increases the output of respiratory tract fluid to coat the trachea and bronchi. Having a patient drink plenty of fluids and humidifying the air with a vaporizer are nonpharmacologic but effective ways of maintaining respiratory tract fluid. Although many drugs are used as expectorants, no expectorant has been proven effective. Expectorants formulated alone as well as with other drugs include guaifenesin, hydroiodic acid, iodinated glycerol, potassium iodide, and terpin hydrate. Expectorants found only formulated with other drugs, usually cough suppressants, include calcium iodide and citric acid or its salt, sodium citrate.

**MECHANISM OF ACTION**    • See individual drug.

**INDICATIONS**    • Sore throat, nonproductive cough.

**CONTRAINDICATIONS**    • See individual drug.

**DRUG INTERACTIONS**    • See individual drug.

---

## guaifenesin    (gwye-FEN-e-sin)                                         expectorant

- guaifenesin (glyceryl guaiacolate): Anti-Tuss, ♣Balminil Expectorant, Breonesin, Cremacoat, GG-Cen, Guiatussin Syrup, Hytuss-2X, ♣Neo-Spec, ♣Resyl, Robitussin, others

**MECHANISM OF ACTION**    Guaifenesin stimulates the secretion of respiratory tract fluid. Guaifenesin irritates the stomach when swallowed, initiating a reflex activity of the vagal nerve to stimulate the secretion of respiratory tract fluid.

**INDICATIONS**    • Unproductive cough.

**CONTRAINDICATIONS**    • Hypersensitivity to the drug. • Chronic smokers cough or the cough of asthma or emphysema.

**DOSAGE**    PO:    **ADULTS AND CHILDREN OVER 12 YEARS OLD:** 200 to 400 mg every 4 hours.    **CHILDREN 6 TO 11 YEARS OLD:** 100 to 200 mg every 4 hours.    **CHILDREN 2 TO 5 YEARS OLD:** 50 to 100 mg every 4 hours.    *Special patient populations:*    **PREGNANCY:** Safe use has not been established.

**PREPARATIONS**    *Capsules:* 200 mg; *solution:* 66.7 or 100 mg/5 ml; *tablets:* 100 or 200 mg.

**DRUG INTERACTIONS**    None noted.

Table 54-1.

## Prescription drugs to suppress a cough

| Trade name | Decongestant | Antihistamine | Antitussive | Other Ingredients* | Control Category |
|---|---|---|---|---|---|
| Actagen-C Cough Syrup | Pseudoephedrine | Triprolidine | Codeine | | C-V |
| Actifed w/Codeine Syrup | Pseudoephedrine | Triprolidine | Codeine | | C-V |
| Alamine Expectorant | Pseudoephedrine | | Codeine | GF | C-V |
| Alamine-C Liquid | Pseudoephedrine | Chlorpheniramine | Codeine | | C-V |
| Allerfrin w/Codeine Syrup | Pseudoephedrine | Triprolidine | Codeine | | C-V |
| Ambenyl Syrup | | Bromodiphenhydramine | Codeine | | C-V |
| Anatuss w/Codeine | Phenylpropanolamine | | Codeine | GF,AM | C-III |
| Anatuss w/Codeine Syrup | Phenylpropanolamine | | Codeine | GF | C-V |
| Bromanate DC Cough Syrup | Phenylpropanolamine | Brompheniramine | Codeine | | C-V |
| Bromanyl Syrup | | Bromodiphenhydramine | Codeine | | C-V |
| Bromotuss w/codeine | | Bromodiphenhydramine | Codeine | | C-V |
| Bromphen DC w/Codeine Cough Syrup | Phenylpropanolamine | Brompheniramine | Codeine | | C-V |
| Broncholate CS Syrup | Ephedrine | | Codeine | GF | C-V |
| C-Tussin Expectorant | Pseudoephedrine | | Codeine | GF | C-V |
| Calcidrine Syrup | | | Codeine | CI | C-V |
| Carbodec DM Drops/Syrup | Pseudoephedrine | Carbinoxamine | Dextromethorphan | | |
| Cardec DM Drops/Syrup | Pseudoephedrine | Carbinoxamine | Dextromethorphan | | |
| Cheracol Syrup | | | Codeine | GF | C-V |
| Cheralin Syrup | | | Codeine | PS,AM,AT | C-V |
| Citra Forte Syrup | | Pyrilamine | Hydrocodone | PR,PC | C-III |
| Codafed Expectorant | Pseudoephedrine | | Codeine | GF | C-V |
| Codamine Syrup | Phenylpropanolamine | | Hydrocodone | | C-III |
| Codiclear DH Syrup | | | Hydrocodone | GS | C-III |
| Codimal DH Syrup | Phenylephrine | Pyrilamine | Hydrocodone | | C-III |
| Codimal PH Syrup | Phenylephrine | Pyrilamine | Codeine | | C-V |
| Colrex Compound Capsules | Phenylephrine | Chlorpheniramine | Codeine | AC | C-III |
| Colrex Compound Elixir | Phenylephrine | Chlorpheniramine | Codeine | AC | C-V |
| Conex w/Codeine Syrup | Phenylpropanolamine | | Codeine | GF | C-V |
| Copavin Pulvules | | | Codeine | PV | C-III |
| Detuss Capsules | Phenylpropanolamine | | Caramiphen | | |
| Detussin Expectorant | Pseudoephedrine | | Hydrocodone | GF | C-III |
| Detussin Liquid | Pseudoephedrine | | Hydrocodone | | C-III |
| Dihistine DH Elixir | Pseudoephedrine | Chlorpheniramine | Codeine | | C-V |
| Dihistine Expectorant | Pseudoephedrine | | Codeine | GF | C-V |
| Dilaudid Cough Syrup | | | Hydromorphone | GF | C-II |
| Dimatane-DC Cough Syrup | Phenylpropanolamine | Brompheniramine | Codeine | | C-V |
| Dimatane-DX Cough Syrup | Pseudoephedrine | Brompheniramine | Dextromethorphan | | |

*Continued.*

**Table 54-1.**

## Prescription drugs to suppress a cough—cont'd.

| Trade name | Decongestant | Antihistamine | Antitussive | Other Ingredients* | Control Category |
|---|---|---|---|---|---|
| Donatussin DC Syrup | Phenylephrine | | Hydrocodone | GF | C-III |
| Efricon Expectorant Liquid | Phenylephrine | Chlorpheniramine | Codeine | AC,GS,SC | C-V |
| Entuss Expectorant Syrup | | | Hydrocodone | GS | C-III |
| Entuss Tablets | | | Hydrocodone | GF | C-III |
| Entuss-D Tablets | Pseudoephedrine | | Hydrocodone | GF | C-III |
| Guiamid A.C. Liquid | | | Codeine | GF | C-V |
| Guiatuss DAC Syrup | Pseudoephedrine | | Codeine | GF | C-V |
| Guiatussin w/Codeine Expectorant | | | Codeine | GF | C-V |
| Histadyl E.C. Syrup | Pseudoephedrine | Chlorpheniramine | Codeine | | C-V |
| Histalet DM Syrup | Pseudoephedrine | Chlorpheniramine | Dextromethorphan | | |
| Hycodan Syrup/Tablets | | | Hydrocodone | HA | C-III |
| Hycomine | Phenylephrine | Chlorpheniramine | Hydrocodone | AC,GF | C-III |
| Hycomine Pediatric Syrup | Phenylpropanolamine | | Hydrocodone | | C-III |
| Hycotuss Expectorant | | | Hydrocodone | GF | C-III |
| Hydrocodone Syrup | | | Hydrocodone | HA | C-III |
| Hydropane Syrup | | | Hydrocodone | HA | C-III |
| Hydrophen Pediatric Syrup | Phenylpropanolamine | | Hydrocodone | | C-III |
| Iophen Dm Elixir | | | Dextromethorphan | IG | |
| Iophen-C Liquid | | | Codeine | IG | C-V |
| Isoclor Expectorant | Pseudoephedrine | | Codeine | GF | C-V |
| Kwelcof Liquid | | | Hydrocodone | GF | C-III |
| Mallergan-VC with Codeine Syrup | Phenylephrine | Promethazine | Codeine | | C-V |
| Midahist DH Elixir | Pseudoephedrine | Chlorpheniramine | Codeine | | C-V |
| Midahistine DH Liquid | Pseudoephedrine | Chlorpheniramine | Codeine | | C-V |
| Mybanil Syrup | | Bromodiphenhydramine | Codeine | | C-V |
| Mycadec DM Syrup | Pseudoephedrine | Carbinoxamine | Dextromethorphan | | |
| Mycodone Syrup | | | Hydrocodone | HA | C-III |
| Mycotussin Liquid | Pseudoephedrine | | Hydrocodone | | C-III |
| Myhistine DH Liquid | Pseudoephedrine | Chlorpheniramine | Codeine | | C-V |
| Myhistine Expectorant | Pseudoephedrine | | Codeine | GF | C-V |
| Myhydromine Pediatric Syrup | Phenylpropanolamine | | Hydrocodone | | C-III |
| Myphetane DC Cough Syrup | Phenylpropanolamine | Brompheniramine | Codeine | | C-V |
| Myphetane DX Syrup | Pseudoephedrine | Brompheniramine | Dextromethorphan | | |
| Mytussin AC Expectorant | | | Codeine | GF | C-V |
| Mytussin DAC Syrup | Pseudoephedrine | | Codeine | GF | C-V |
| Naldecon-CX Liquid | Phenylpropanolamine | | Codeine | GF | C-V |
| Normatane DC Syrup | Phenylpropanolamine | Brompheniramine | Codeine | | C-V |
| Nortussin w/Codeine Liquid | | | Codeine | GF | C-V |

| Product | Decongestant | Antihistamine | Antitussive | Other | Schedule |
|---|---|---|---|---|---|
| Novahistine DH Liquid | Pseudoephedrine | Chlorpheniramine | Codeine | | C-V |
| Novahistine Expectorant | Pseudoephedrine | | Codeine | GF | C-V |
| Nucofed Capsules/Syrup | Pseudoephedrine | | Codeine | | C-III |
| Nucofed Expectorant/Pediatric Expectoran | Pseudoephedrine | | Codeine | GF | C-III |
| Pediacof Cough Syrup | Phenylephrine | Chlorpheniramine | Codeine | PI | C-V |
| Pentuss Liquid | | Chlorpheniramine | Codeine | | C-V |
| Phenameth VC w/Codeine Syrup | Phenylephrine | Promethazine | Codeine | | C-V |
| Phenameth w/Codeine | | Promethazine | Codeine | | C-V |
| Phenergan VC with Codeine Syrup | Phenylephrine | Promethazine | Codeine | | C-V |
| Phenergan w/Dextromethorphan Syrup | | Promethazine | Dextromethorphan | | |
| Phenergan with Codeine Syrup | | Promethazine | Codeine | | C-V |
| Pherazine DM Syrup | | Promethazine | Dextromethorphan | | |
| Pherazine VC with Codeine Syrup | Phenylephrine | Promethazine | Codeine | | C-V |
| Poly-Histine CS Syrup | Phenylpropanolamine | Brompheniramine | Codeine | | C-V |
| Prometh VC with Codeine Syrup | Phenylephrine | Promethazine | Codeine | | C-V |
| Prometh w/Codeine Syrup | | Promethazine | Codeine | | C-V |
| Prometh w/Dextromethorphan Syrup | | Promethazine | Dextromethorphan | | |
| Promethazine HC1 w/Codeine Syrup | | Promethazine | Codeine | | C-V |
| Promist Expectorant Liquid | Pseudoephedrine | | Hydrocodone | GF | C-III |
| Promist HD Liquid | Pseudoephedrine | Chlorpheniramine | Hydrocodone | | C-III |
| Prothazine Pediatric Liquid | | Promethazine | Dextromethorphan | | |
| Prothazine-DC Liquid | | Promethazine | Codeine | | C-V |
| Prunicodeine Liquid | | | Codeine | TH | C-V |
| Pseudo-Car DM Syrup | Pseudoephedrine | Carbinoxamine | Dextromethorphan | | |
| PV Tussin | | Phenindamine | Hydrocodone | GF | C-III |
| PV Tussin Syrup | Phenylephrine | Chlorpheniramine | Hydrocodone | PD,PR,AC | C-III |
| Robitussin A-C Syrup | | | Codeine | GF | C-V |
| Robitussin-DAC Syrup | Pseudoephedrine | | Codeine | GF | C-V |
| Rondec-DM Oral Drops/Syrup | Pseudoephedrine | Carbinoxamine | Dextromethorphan | | |
| Ru-Tuss Expectorant | Pseudoephedrine | | Dextromethorphan | GF | |
| Ru-Tuss w/Hydrocodone Liquid | Phenylpropanolamine | Pyrilamine | Hydrocodone | PE,PR | C-III |
| Ryna-C Liquid | Pseudoephedrine | Chlorpheniramine | Codeine | | C-V |
| Ryan-CX Liquid | Pseudoephedrine | | Codeine | GF | C-V |
| Rynatuss Pediatric Suspension | Ephedrine | Chlorpheniramine | Carbetapentane | PE | |
| Rynatuss Tablets | Phenylephrine | Chlorpheniramine | Carbetapentane | EP | |
| SRC Expectorant | Pseudoephedrine | | Hydrocodone | GF | C-III |
| S-T Forte Syrup and Liquid | Phenylpropanolamine | Pheniramine | Hydrocodone | PE,GF | C-III |
| Terpin Hydrate and Codeine Elixir | | | Codeine | TH | C-V |
| T-Koff Syrup | Phenylpropanolamine | Chlorpheniramine | Codeine | PE | C-V |
| Tolu-Sed Cough Syrup | | | Codeine | GF | C-V |
| Torganic-DM Liquid | | | Dextromethorphan | IG | |
| Triacin C Cough Syrup | Pseudoephedrine | Triprolidine | Codeine | | C-V |

*Continued.*

**Table 54-1.** Prescription drugs to suppress a cough—cont'd.

| Trade name | Decongestant | Antihistamine | Antitussive | Other Ingredients* | Control Category |
|---|---|---|---|---|---|
| Triaminic Expectorant DH | Phenylpropanolamine | Pyrilamine | Hydrocodone | PR,GF | C-III |
| Triaminic Expectorant w/Codeine | Phenylpropanolamine | | Codeine | GF | C-V |
| Tricodene Syrup | | Pyrilamine | Codeine | Th | C-V |
| Tricomine Expectorant | Pseudoephedrine | Carbinoxamine | Dextromethorphan | | |
| Trifed-C Cough Syrup | Pseudoephedrine | Triprolidine | Codeine | | C-V |
| Tusquelin Syrup | Phenylpropanolamine | Chlorpheniramine | Dextromethorphan | PE | |
| Tuss Alergine Modified T.D. Capsules | Phenylpropanolamine | | Caramiphen | | |
| Tussadon Liquid | Phenylpropanolamine | | Dextromethorphan | | |
| Tussafed Drops/Syrup | Pseudoephedrine | Carbinoxamine | Dextromethorphan | | |
| Tussafin Expectorant | Pseudoephedrine | | Hydrocodone | GF | C-III |
| Tussanil DH Syrup | Phenylephrine | Chlorpheniramine | Hydrocodone | | C-III |
| Tussanil DH Tablets | Phenylpropanolamine | | Hydrocodone | GF,SA | C-III |
| Tuss-Genade Modified Capsules | Phenylpropanolamine | | Caramiphen | | |
| Tuss-Ornade Liquid/Spansules | Phenylpropanolamine | | Caramiphen | | |
| Tussar SF Cough Syrup/-2 Cough Syrup | | Chlorpheniramine | Codeine | PC,GF,SC | C-V |
| Tussend Expectorant | Pseudoephedrine | | Hydrocodone | GF | C-III |
| Tussend Liquid/Tablets | Pseudoephedrine | | Hydrocodone | | C-III |
| Tussi-Organidin DM Liquid | | | Dextromethorphan | IG | |
| Tussi-Organidin Liquid | | | Codeine | IG | C-V |
| Tussi-R-Gen Expectorant | | | Codeine | IG | C-V |
| Tussigon Tablets | | | Hydrocodone | HA | C-III |
| Tussionex Capsules/Tablets/Suspension | | Phenyltoloxamine | Hydrocodone | | C-III |
| Tussirex Sugar Free Liquid/Syrup | Phenylephrine | Pheniramine | Codeine | SC | C-V |
| Tussogest Capsules | Phenylpropanolamine | | Caramiphen | | |

*AC = Ammonium chloride
AM = Acetaminophen
AT = Antimony potassium tartrate
CI = Calcium iodide
EP = ephedrine
GF = Guaifenesin
GS = Potassium guaiacosulfonate
HA = Homatropine
IG = Iodinated glycerol
PC = Potassium citrate

PD = Phenindamine
PE = Phenylephrine
PI = Potassium iodide
PR = Pyrilamine
PS = Potassium sulfonate
PV = Papaverine
SA = Salicylamide
SC = Sodium citrate
TH = Terpin hydrate

Table
54-2.

## Prescription expectorant combinations*†

| Trade name | Decongestant | Antihistamine | Expectorant | Other ingredients |
|---|---|---|---|---|
| Brexin EX Tablets | Pseudoephedrine | | Guaifenesin | |
| Bromphen Expectorant | Phenylpropanolamine | Brompheniramine | Guaifenesin | PE |
| Broncholate Soft Gels | Ephedrine | | Guaifenesin | |
| Broncholate Syrup | Ephedrine | | Guaifenesin | |
| Congess JR Capsules | Pseudoephedrine | | Guaifenesin | |
| Congess SR Capsules | Pseudoephedrine | | Guaifenesin | |
| Congestac Tablets | Pseudoephedrine | | Guaifenesin | |
| Dura-Gest Capsules | Phenylpropanolamine | | Guaifenesin | PE |
| Dura-Vent | Phenylpropanolamine | | Guaifenesin | |
| Entex Capsules | Phenylpropanolamine | | Guaifenesin | PE |
| Entex LA Tablets | Phenylpropanolamine | | Guaifenesin | |
| Entex Liquid | Phenylpropanolamine | | Guaifenesin | PE |
| Guaifed Capsules | Pseudoephedrine | | Guaifenesin | |
| Guaifed-PD Capsules | Pseudoephedrine | | Guaifenesin | |
| Histalet X Syrup | Pseudoephedrine | | Guaifenesin | |
| Histalet X Tablets | Pseudoephedrine | | Guaifenesin | |
| KIE Syrup | Ephedrine | | Potassium Iodide | |
| Norisodrine w/Calcium Iodide Syrup | | | Calcium Iodide | IP |
| Normatane | Phenylpropanolamine | Brompheniramine | Guaifenesin | PE |
| Polaramine Expectorant | Pseudoephedrine | Dexchlorpheniramine | Guaifenesin | |
| Promist LA Tablets | Pseudoephedrine | | Guaifenesin | |
| Pseudo-Bid A Capsules | Pseudoephedrine | Chlorpheniramine | Guaifenesin | |
| Pseudo-Bid Capsules | Pseudoephedrine | | Guaifenesin | |
| Respaire-120 SR Capsules | Pseudoephedrine | | Guaifenesin | |
| Respaire-60 SR Capsules | Pseudoephedrine | | Guaifenesin | |
| Respinol-G Tablets | Pseudoephedrine | | Guaifenesin | |
| Respinol-LA Tablets | Pseudoephedrine | | Guaifenesin | |
| Rymed-JR Capsules | Phenylpropanolamine | | Guaifenesin | PE |
| Rymed-TR Tablets | Phenylpropanolamine | | Guaifenesin | |
| Sinufed Timecelles | Pseudoephedrine | | Guaifenesin | |
| T-Moist Tablets | Pseudoephedrine | | Guaifenesin | |
| Trihista-Phen Liquid | Phenylpropanolamine | Chlorpheniramine | Guaifenesin | PR |
| Utex-S.R. Tablets | Phenylpropanolamine | | Guaifenesin | |
| V-Dec-M Tablets | Pseudoephedrine | | Guaifenesin | |
| Zephrex Tablets | Pseudoephedrine | | Guaifenesin | |
| Zephrex-LA Tablets | Pseudoephedrine | | Guaifenesin | |

†IP = Isoproterenol      PE = Phenylephrine      PR = Pyrilamine      *Combinations of expectorants with antitussives are found in Table 54-1.

**DIAGNOSTIC TEST INTERFERENCE**    May cause a color interference with certain laboratory determinations of 5-hydroxyindoleacetic acid (5-HIAA) and vanillylmandelic acid (VMA).

**FATE**    The metabolic fate of guaifenesin has not been well characterized.

## 🌼 NURSING CONSIDERATIONS

### Side effects, toxicities, and associated nursing actions

**CNS** Drowsiness.

- Caution patients to avoid driving or operating hazardous equipment until the effects of this medication can be evaluated. If the patient must drive or continue working, it may be possible to reserve the use of this medication to after-work hours and to suck on hard candies, chew gum, and stay well hydrated (2500 to 3000 ml/day) to keep respiratory tract moist and help control coughing.

**GI** Nausea, vomiting.

- Instruct the patient to take the dose after a meal or light snack to reduce gastric irritation.

### Patient and family education

- Review with patients the expected benefits and possible side effects of therapy.
- Discuss with patients the difference between an expectorant and an antitussive. Patients may be inadvertently choosing the wrong medication for their problem.
- Instruct patients to read labels carefully with combination products sold over the counter. Patients may be inadvertently taking unnecessary drugs.
- Instruct patients to use a vaporizer or humidifier to keep air moist at work or home. This may lessen discomfort from dry secretions.
- Keep these and all medications out of the reach of children. Only products labeled for pediatric use should be used with children under the age of 12.

## hydroiodic acid    (hye-droe-eye-OH-dik)    iodide expectorant

- hydroiodic acid: generic

## iodinated glycerol    (eye-OH-di-nay-ted GLI-ser-in)    iodide expectorant

- iodinated glycerol: Organidin

## potassium iodide    iodide expectorant

- potassium iodide: generic

**MECHANISM OF ACTION:**    Iodide compounds are presented as one entry. Iodide is believed to stimulate the bronchial glands to secrete more fluid.

**INDICATIONS**    • Symptomatic treatment of chronic pulmonary diseases with tenacious mucus, including asthma, chronic bronchitis, emphysema, cystic fibrosis, and chronic sinusitis.

**CONTRAINDICATIONS**    • Hyperthyroidism. • Hypersensitivity to iodides. • Hyperkalemia. • Acute bronchitis.

**DOSAGE**    **Hydroiodic acid:**  *PO:*  **ADULTS:** 5 ml taken three or four times daily with a glassful of water to avoid injury to the teeth.  **CHILDREN:** Not recommended for children.  **Iodinated glycerol:**  *PO:*  **ADULTS:** 60 mg four times daily.  **CHILDREN:** ½ adult dose.  **Potassium iodide:**  *PO:*  **ADULTS:** 300 to 650 mg three or four times daily.  **CHILDREN:** 60 to 250 mg four times daily.  *Special patient populations:*  **PREGNANCY:** Safe use has not been established.

**PREPARATIONS**    **Hydroiodic acid:** *syrup:* 70 mg/5 ml.  **Iodinated glycerol:** *solution:* 60 mg/5 ml; 50 mg/ml; *tablets:* 30 mg.  **Potassium iodide:** *solution:* 167 or 325 mg/5 ml, 1 g/ml; *tablets:* 300 mg.

**DRUG INTERACTIONS**   **Lithium and antithyroid drugs** Potentiate the hypothyroid and goitrogenic effects of iodide.   **Potassium-containing drugs and potassium-sparing diuretics** Hyperkalemia may result if taken with potassium iodide.

**DIAGNOSTIC TEST INTERFERENCE**   Thyroid function tests may be affected by iodide.

**FATE**   Iodide is taken up by the thyroid.

☙ **NURSING CONSIDERATIONS**

**Side effects, toxicities, and associated nursing actions**   Iodism from chronic iodine poisoning.

**CNS** Severe headache.

**Eye** Swelling of the eyelids.

**GI** Metallic taste, increased salivation, gastric disturbance, nausea, vomiting, diarrhea.

**Lung** Productive cough, sneezing, pulmonary edema.

**Skin** Acneform skin lesions; skin erruptions; sore mouth; mouth ulcer.

**Metabolic** Thyroid adenoma or goiter.

- These side effects usually disappear within a few days of discontinuing therapy.
- Monitor for these, especially in persons on long-term therapy.
- If signs of iodism appear, discontinue medication and notify the physician.
- Monitor serum potassium levels.

**Allergic** Angioedema; cutaneous and mucosal hemorrhages; serum sickness (fever, arthralgia, lymph node enlargement, eosinophilia).

- Monitor white blood cell differential, temperature.
- Visually inspect for hemorrhages.
- Have drugs, equipment, and personnel available for treatment of acute allergic reactions in settings where these agents are administered.

**Nursing interventions related to drug administration**

- Question patients about a history of allergy to iodine or shellfish before administering.
- Enteric-coated tablets should be swallowed whole and not chewed or crushed. Review this with patients using enteric-coated tablets, and instruct them to take tablets with a full glass of liquid.
- To lessen or disguise the salty taste of solutions, dilute the dose in water, milk, or juice.
- Taking doses with meals, milk, or a light snack may reduce gastric irritation.
- Inspect solutions prior to administering. If crystals are present, heat solution under running water to dissolve them. Highly discolored solutions should be discarded.

**Patient and family education**

- Review with patients the expected benefits and possible side effects of therapy.
- Discuss with patient the difference between an expectorant and an antitussive. Patients may be inadvertently choosing the wrong medication for their problem.
- Instruct patients to read labels carefully with combination products sold over the counter. Patients may be inadvertently taking unnecessary drugs. Caution patients to avoid the use of over-the-counter preparations without prior approval of the physician.
- Instruct patients to use a vaporizer or humidifier to keep air moist at work or home. This may lessen discomfort from dry secretions. Increasing fluid intake to 2500 to 3000 ml/day will also help keep secretions moist.
- Keep these and all medications out of the reach of children. Only products labeled for pediatric use should be used with children under the age of 12.

## terpin hydrate   (TER-pin)                                        expectorant

- terpin hydrate: generic

**MECHANISM OF ACTION**   Terpin hydrate is believed to stimulate the lower respiratory tract secretory glands directly.

**INDICATIONS**   **Cough** Usually used with codeine, an antitussive agent.

**CONTRAINDICATIONS**   **Alcoholism** Terpin hydrate is an elixir with high alcohol content.

**DOSAGE**   PO:   ADULTS AND CHILDREN OVER 12 YEARS OLD: 170 mg three or four times daily.   CHILDREN 10 TO 12 YEARS OLD: 85 mg three or four times daily.   CHILDREN 5 TO 9 YEARS OLD: 40 to 45 mg three or four times daily.   CHILDREN 1 TO 4 YEARS OLD: 20 to 25 mg three or four times daily.   *Special patient populations:*   PREGNANCY: Safe use has not been established.

**PREPARATIONS**   Elixir: 85 mg/5 ml.

**DRUG INTERACTIONS**   None noted.

**FATE**   The metabolic fate of terpin hydrate has not been characterized.

### 🦃 NURSING CONSIDERATIONS

#### Side effects, toxicities, and associated nursing actions
- No side effects noted.

#### Patient and family education
- Review with patients the expected benefits and possible side effects of therapy.
- Discuss with patients the difference between an expectorant and an antitussive. Patients may be inadvertently choosing the wrong medication for their problem.
- Instruct patients to read labels carefully with combination products sold over the counter. Patients may be inadvertently taking unnecessary drugs.
- Instruct patients to use a vaporizer or humidifier to keep air moist at work or home. This may lessen discomfort from dry secretions.
- Keep these and all medications out of the reach of children. Only products labeled for pediatric use should be used with children under the age of 12.

---

# Antitussives

benzonatate ~ codeine ~ dextromethorphan ~ diphenhydramine ~ hydrocodone ~ noscapine

**OVERVIEW OF THE DRUG CLASS**   An *antitussive* is a cough suppressant. Codeine and hydrocodone are good antitussives, but they are opiates and therefore capable of producing drug dependence. Hydrocodone has a greater potential for producing drug dependence than codeine. Most preparations containing codeine or hydrocodone are prescription drugs. Some preparations are available as Schedule V drugs and may be obtained by signing for them with a registered pharmacist. However, dextromethorphan and noscapine are excellent nonaddicting opiate antitussives available over the counter. Benzonatate and diphenhydramine are nonopiate antitussives available by prescription.

**MECHANISM OF ACTION**   The opiates suppress a cough by directly inhibiting the medullary center for the cough reflex. The doses required to suppress a cough are less than those to produce analgesia or respiratory depression. Dextromethorphan and noscapine are not opiates but are chemically related and act similarly. Diphenhydramine and benzonatate act by different mechanisms.

**INDICATIONS**   **Nonproductive cough** Cough suppressants provide symptomatic relief.

**CONTRAINDICATIONS**   • Hypersensitivity to the drug.

**DRUG INTERACTIONS**   **CNS depressants** Respiratory depression, hypotension, profound sedation, or coma can result if the opioid or antihistaminic antitussives are combined with other CNS depressants, including alcohol.

---

## benzonatate   (ben-ZOOE-na-tate)                                              antitussive

- benzonatate: Tessalon

**MECHANISM OF ACTION**   Benzonatate has a unique mechanism of action among antitussives. Benzonatate anesthetizes the stretch receptors of vagal afferent fibers in the bronchi, alveoli, and pleura, which mediate the cough reflex.

**INDICATIONS**   • Nonproductive cough.

**CONTRAINDICATIONS**   • Hypersensitivity to the drug.

**DOSAGE    PO:    ADULTS AND CHILDREN OVER 10 YEARS OLD:** 100 mg three times daily, but no more than 600 mg daily.    **CHILDREN 10 YEARS OR YOUNGER:** 8 mg/kg in three to six divided doses. *Special patient populations:*    **PREGNANCY:** Safe use has not been established.

**PREPARATIONS**    *Capsules* 100 mg.

**DRUG INTERACTIONS**    None noted.

**FATE**    Benzonatate has an *onset of action* of 15 to 20 minutes and a *duration of action* of 3 to 8 hours. The metabolic fate of benzonatate has not been well characterized.

## ✿ NURSING CONSIDERATIONS

### Side effects, toxicities, and associated nursing actions

**CNS** Sedation, headache, dizziness.

* Caution patients to avoid driving or operating hazardous equipment until the effects of the medication can be evaluated.
* Keep side rails up, supervise ambulation, and discourage smoking in the hospital setting.

**Eye** Sensation of burning.

* Assess for complaints of this problem. If they persistent or severe, notify the physician.

**GI** Nausea, GI upset, constipation.

* Taking doses with meals or light snack may lessen gastric irritation.
* Keep record of stools. To avoid constipation, increase fluid intake to 2500 to 3000 ml/day, increase dietary intake of fruit, fruit juices, and fiber, and increase level of daily exercise.

**Skin** Pruritis, skin eruptions.

**Other** Sensation of "chilliness"; numbness in the chest.

* Assess for these changes; if present, notify the physician.

**Allergic** Hypersensitivity.

* Question patient about allergy prior to administering dose.
* Have drugs, equipment, and personnel available to treat acute allergic reactions.

### Nursing interventions related to drug administration

* Instruct the patient to swallow capsules whole, without chewing or trying to crush. If broken open in the mouth, the drug may cause temporary anesthesia of mucous membranes.

### Patient and family education

* Review with patients the expected benefits and possible side effects of therapy. Instruct patients to report the development of any unexpected sign or symptom.
* Discuss with patients the difference between an expectorant and an antitussive. Patients may be inadvertently choosing the wrong medication to treat their problem.
* Instruct patients to read labels carefully on combination products sold over the counter. Patients may be inadvertently taking unnecessary drugs. Caution patients to avoid the use of over-the-counter preparations without prior approval of the physician.
* Instruct patients to use a vaporizer or humidifier to keep air moist at work or home. This may lessen discomfort from dry secretions. Increasing fluid intake to 2500 to 3000 ml/day will also help keep secretions moist.
* Keep these and all medications out of the reach of children. Only medications labeled for pediatric use should be used for children under the age of 12, unless specifically prescribed by the physician.

---

## codeine    (COE-deen)                                                                              antitussive

---

## codeine phosphate, codeine sulfate                                              antitussive

* codeine: Generic,
* codeine phosphate: ✽Paveral
* codeine sulfate: Generic

**MECHANISM OF ACTION**   Codeine is an opiate. See entry for drug class (p. 968).

**INDICATIONS**   • Nonproductive cough.

**CONTRAINDICATIONS**   • Hypersensitivity to the drug.

**DOSAGE**   PO:   **ADULTS AND CHILDREN OVER 12 YEARS OLD:** 10 to 20 mg every 4 to 6 hours; maximum, 120 mg daily.   **CHILDREN 5 TO 11 YEARS:** 5 to 10 mg every 4 to 6 hours; maximum, 60 mg daily. **CHILDREN 2 TO 5 YEARS:** 2.5 to 5 mg every 4 to 6 hours; maximum, 30 mg daily.   *Special patient populations:*   PREGNANCY: Safe use has not been established.

**PREPARATIONS**   *Phosphate: tablets:* 15, 30, or 60 mg. *Sulfate: tablets:* 15, 30, or 60 mg.

**DRUG INTERACTIONS**   **CNS depressants** Respiratory depression, hypotension, profound sedation, or coma can result if the opioid or antihistaminic antitussives are combined with other CNS depressants, including alcohol.

**FATE**   Codeine is well absorbed. Antitussive effects are seen in 1 to 2 hours, and the *duration of action* is 4 hours. Codeine is metabolized in the liver and excreted in the urine.

## ❦ NURSING CONSIDERATIONS

### Side effects, toxicities, and associated nursing actions

**CNS** Lightheadedness, dizziness; sedation; euphoria or dysphoria; anxiety.

**Eye** Pinpoint pupils; visual disturbances.

• Instruct patients to avoid driving or operating hazardous equipment until the effects of the medication can be evaluated.

• Keep side rails up, monitor ambulation, and discourage smoking in the hospital setting.

• Be alert to mood changes. Pronounced or persistent changes may require a change in drug or dose; notify the physician.

**CV** Flushing, fast or slow heart rate; hypotension, palpitations.

• Monitor pulse, blood pressure.

**GI** Dry mouth, loss of appetite, constipation; biliary tract spasm; nausea.

• Monitor intake, output, and weight, and keep a record of stools.

• For dry mouth, instruct patient to take frequent sips of water, suck on sugarless candy or chew sugarless gum, perform frequent oral hygiene (but avoid drying mouthwashes or gargles). As an antitussive, this medication is used on a short-term basis, but some patients may wish to consider the use of a commercially available saliva substitute.

• For constipation, instruct the patient to increase daily fluid intake to 2500 to 3000 ml, increase intake of fruit, fruit juices, and fiber, and increase level of daily exercise.

• Taking tablets with meals, light snack, or milk may lessen gastric irritation.

**GU** Urinary retention; spasms of the ureters or sphincters.

• Monitor intake and output.

• Have patient void before administering each dose.

**Skin** Pruritis, rashes.

**Allergic** Rashes, urticaria.

• Visually inspect patient for development of skin changes.

• Have drugs, equipment, and personnel available to treat an acute allergic response.

### Patient and family education

• Review with patients the expected benefits and possible side effects of therapy. Instruct the patient to report the development of any unexpected sign or symptom.

• Because tolerance and physical dependence may occur following prolonged use of this drug, review with patients the need to take the medication only as ordered and not to increase the prescribed dose.

• Instruct patients to read labels carefully on combination products sold over the counter. Patients may be inadvertently taking unnecessary drugs. Caution patients to avoid the use of over-the-counter preparations without prior approval of the physician.

• Instruct patients to use a vaporizer or humidifier to keep air moist at work or home. This may lessen discomfort from dry secretions. Increasing fluid intake to 2500 to 3000 ml/day will also help keep secretions moist.

- Keep these and all medications out of the reach of children. Only medications labeled for pediatric use should be used for children under the age of 12 unless specifically prescribed by the physician.

## dextromethorphan (dex-troe-meth-OR-fan)   antitussive

- dextromethorphan hydrobromide: ✽Anti-Cough Syrup, ✽Balminil D.M. Syrup, ✽Delsym, ✽Romilar, and others

**MECHANISM OF ACTION**   Dextromethorphan has the antitussive properties but not the other properties of opiates. The opiates suppress a cough by directly inhibiting the medullary center for the cough reflex.

**INDICATIONS**   • Nonproductive cough.

**CONTRAINDICATIONS**   • Hypersensitivity to the drug.

**DOSAGE**   PO:   **ADULTS AND CHILDREN 12 YEARS AND OLDER:** 10 to 20 mg every 4 hours or 30 mg every 6 to 8 hours. Maximum daily dosage is 120 mg.   **CHILDREN 6 TO 11 YEARS OLD:** 5 to 10 mg every 4 hours or 15 mg every 6 to 8 hours. Maximum daily dosage is 60 mg.   **CHILDREN 2 TO 5 YEARS OLD:** 2.5 to 5 mg every 4 hours or 7.5 mg every 6 to 8 hours. Maximum daily dosage is 30 mg. *Special patient populations:*   **CHILDREN:** Not recommended for children under 2 years old. **PREGNANCY:** Safe use has not been established.

**PREPARATIONS**   *Lozenges:* 7.5 mg; *pieces (chewable):* 15 mg., *solution:* 2.5, 5, 7.5, 10, or 15 mg/5 ml; *suspension (extended release):* 30 mg/5 ml.

**DRUG INTERACTIONS**   **Monoamine oxidase inhibitors:** Dextromethorphan should not be taken within 14 days of MAO therapy. Concurrent administration may result in nausea, fever, hypotension, coma, death.

**FATE**   Dextromethorphan is rapidly absorbed. The *onset of action* is 15 to 30 minutes, and the *duration of action* is 3 to 6 hours.

## ☙ NURSING CONSIDERATIONS

### Side effects, toxicities, and associated nursing actions

**CNS** Dizziness.

- Instruct patients to avoid driving or operating hazardous equipment until the effects of the medication can be evaluated.
- Supervise ambulation, keep side rails up, and discourage smoking in the hospital setting.

**GI** Nausea.

- Taking dose with meals, light snack, or glass of milk may lessen gastric irritation.

### Patient and family education

- Review with patients the expected benefits and possible side effects of therapy. Instruct patients to report the development of any unexpected sign or symptom.
- Discuss with patients the difference between an expectorant and an antitussive. Patients may be inadvertently choosing the wrong medication to treat their problem.
- Instruct patients to read labels carefully on combination products sold over the counter. Patients may be inadvertently taking unnecessary drugs. Caution patients to avoid the use of over-the-counter preparations without prior approval of the physician.
- Instruct patients to use a vaporizer or humidifier to keep air moist at work or home. This may lessen discomfort from dry secretions. Increasing fluid intake to 2500 to 3000 ml/day will also help keep secretions moist.
- Keep these and all medications out of the reach of children. Only medications labeled for pediatric use should be used for children under 12 unless specifically prescribed by physician.

## hydrocodone bitartrate (hye-droe-KOE-done)   antitussive

- hydrocodone bitartrate: found only in combinations:✽Hycodan, ✽Robidon (C-III)

**MECHANISM OF ACTION**    Hydrocodone is an opiate. The opiates suppress a cough by directly inhibiting the medullary center for the cough reflex. The doses required to suppress a cough are less than those to produce analgesia or respiratory depression.

**INDICATIONS**   • Nonproductive cough.

**CONTRAINDICATIONS**   • Hypersensitivity to the drug. • Asthma, emphysema. Care should be used to avoid precipitating respiratory insufficiency.

**DOSAGE**   PO:   **ADULTS AND CHILDREN OVER 12 YEARS OLD:** 5 to 10 mg every 4 to 6 hours as needed. **CHILDREN:** 0.6 mg/kg daily in three or four divided doses. A single dose should not exceed 10 mg for a child over 12 years old, 5 mg for a child 2 to 12, or 1.25 mg for a child under 2 years old.   *Special patient populations:*   **PREGNANCY:** Safe use has not been established.

**PREPARATIONS**   *As a resin complex: capsules:* 5 mg; *suspension:* 5 mg/5 ml; *tablets:* 5 mg.

**DRUG INTERACTIONS**   **CNS depressants:** Respiratory depression, hypotension, profound sedation, or coma can result if the opioid or antihistaminic antitussives are combined with other CNS depressants, including alcohol.

**FATE**   Hydrocodone is well absorbed. The *duration of action* is 4 to 6 hours. hydrocodone is metabolized in the liver and excreted in the urine.

## ☙ NURSING CONSIDERATIONS

### Side effects, toxicities, and associated nursing actions

**CNS** Lightheadedness, dizziness; sedation, euphoria or dysphoria; anxiety.

**Eye** Pinpoint pupils; visual disturbances.

- Instruct patients to avoid driving or operating hazardous equipment until the effects of the medication can be evaluated.
- Keep side rails up, monitor ambulation, and supervise smoking in the hospital setting.
- Be alert to mood changes. Pronounced or persistent changes may require change in drug or dose; notify the physician.

**CV** Flushing, fast or slow heart rate; hypotension, palpitations.

- Monitor pulse, blood pressure.

**GI** Dry mouth, loss of appetite, constipation: biliary tract spasm; nausea.

- Monitor intake, output, and weight, and keep a record of stools.
- For dry mouth, instruct patient to take frequent sips of water, suck on sugarless candy or chew sugarless gum, perform frequent oral hygiene (but avoid drying mouthwashes or gargles). As an antitussive, this medication is used on a short-term basis, but some patients may wish to consider the use of a commercially available saliva substitute.
- For constipation, instruct patients to increase daily fluid intake to 2500 to 3000 ml, increase intake of fruit, fruit juices, and fiber, and increase level of daily exercise.
- Taking tablets with meals, light snack, or milk may lessen gastric irritation.

**GU** Urinary retention; spasms of the ureters or sphincters.

- Monitor intake and output.
- Have patient void before administering each dose.

**Skin** Puritis, rashes.

**Allergic** Rashes, urticaria.

- Visually inspect patients for development of skin changes.
- Have drugs, equipment, and personnel available to treat an acute allergic response.

### Patient and family education

- Review with patients the expected benefits and possible side effects of therapy. Instruct patients to report the development of any unexpected sign or symptom.
- Because tolerance and physical dependence may occur following prolonged use of this drug, review with patients the need to take the medication only as ordered and not to increase the dose or frequency of self-medicating. Patients who do not receive relief as anticipated should contact a physician.
- Caution patients to avoid the use of alcohol.
- Discuss with patients the difference between an expectorant and an antitussive. Patients may be inadvertently choosing the wrong medication to treat their problem.

- Instruct patients to read labels carefully on combination products sold over the counter. Patients may be inadvertently taking unnecessary drugs. Caution patients to avoid the use of over-the-counter preparations without prior approval of the physician.
- Instruct patients to use a vaporizer or humidifier to keep air moist at work or home. This may lessen discomfort from dry secretions. Increasing fluid intake to 2500 to 3000 ml/day will also help keep secretions moist.
- Keep these and all medications out of the reach of children. Only medications labeled for pediatric use should be used for children under the age of 12, unless specifically prescribed by the physician.

## noscapine  (NOSS-ka-peen)                                    antitussive

- noscapine: found in combinations only (OTC)

**MECHANISM OF ACTION**   Noscapine is a nonaddicting opiate. The opiates suppress a cough by directly inhibiting the medullary center for the cough reflex.

**INDICATIONS**   • Nonproductive cough.

**CONTRAINDICATIONS**   • Hypersensitivity to the drug.

**DOSAGE**   PO:   **ADULTS AND CHILDREN 12 YEARS AND OLDER:** 15 to 30 mg every 4 to 6 hours. Maximum daily dose is 180 mg.   **CHILDREN 6 TO 12 YEARS OLD:** 7.5 to 15 mg every 4 to 6 hours. Maximum daily dose is 90 mg.   **CHILDREN 2 TO 6 YEARS OLD:** 3.25 to 7.5 mg every 4 to 6 hours. Maximum daily dose is 45 mg.   *Special patient populations:*   **CHILDREN:** Not recommended for children under 2 years old.   **PREGNANCY:** Safe use has not been established.

**PREPARATIONS**   Combined with other drugs only.

**DRUG INTERACTIONS**   **CNS depressants** Respiratory depression, hypotension, profound sedation, or coma can result if the opioid or antihistaminic antitussives are combined with other CNS depressants, including alcohol.

**FATE**   Noscapine is well absorbed. The *duration of action* is 4 to 6 hours. The metabolism of noscapine has not been well characterized.

## 🐝 NURSING CONSIDERATIONS

### Side effects, toxicities, and associated nursing actions

**CNS** Dizziness.
- Instruct patients to avoid driving or operating hazardous equipment until the effects of the medication can be evaluated.
- Supervise ambulation, keep side rails up, and supervise smoking in the hospital setting.

**GI** Nausea.
- Taking the dose with meals, light snack, or glass of milk may lessen gastric irritation.

### Patient and family education

- Review with patients the expected benefits and possible side effects of therapy. Instruct patients to report the development of any unexpected sign or symptom.
- Discuss with patients the difference between an expectorant and an antitussive. Patients may be inadvertently choosing the wrong medication to treat their problem.
- Instruct patients to read labels carefully on combination products sold over the counter. Patients may be inadvertently taking unnecessary drugs. Caution patients to avoid the use of over-the-counter preparations without prior approval of the physician.
- Instruct patients to use a vaporizer or humidifier to keep air moist at work or home. This may lessen discomfort from dry secretions. Increasing fluid intake to 2500 to 3000 ml/day will also keep secretions moist.
- Keep these and all medications out of the reach of children. Only medications labeled for pediatric use should be used for children under the age of 12 unless specifically prescribed by the physician.

# AGENTS AFFECTING THE GASTROINTESTINAL SYSTEM

**INTRODUCTION** The gastrointestinal system processes food and water and eliminates undigestible material. The parasympathetic (cholinergic) nervous system acts as a major stimulant of the digestive processes by increasing both digestive secretions and the tone and motility of the smooth muscle of the stomach and intestines. The sympathetic (adrenergic) nervous system plays a minor role in the digestive processes. Although the parasympathetic nervous system acts on all parts of the digestive tract, current research is uncovering a complex system in which activities in each section of the digestive tract are further regulated by a variety of peptide hormones, prostaglandins, and the biogenic amines histamine and serotonin. At the present time the roles of only a few of these factors are well characterized.

This unit focuses on specific conditions affecting the gastrointestinal tract for which there are pharmacologic interventions. Antiemetics are the drugs that control vomiting. These drugs include antagonists of histamine, acetylcholine, and dopamine, as well as drugs with actions not yet determined. A few cholinergic drugs are used to increase gastrointestinal tone and motility, while a large number of drugs have been developed to decrease the tone and motility of the gastrointestinal system and aid in the treatment of irritable and inflammatory bowel diseases. Various drug classes are used to treat ulcers. These drugs include antacids, sucralfate, and the new H-2 receptor antagonists, cimetidine, famotidine, and ranitidine. Agents to control diarrhea include adsorbents like bismuth and kaolin-pectin, as well as codeine and related drugs. Finally, a large variety of drugs are in use to relieve constipation. Many are available over the counter.

**XV**

# Chapter Fifty-five

# Drugs to control vomiting

benzquinamide

buclizine

chlorpromazine (see Chapter 36)

cyclizine

dimenhydrinate

diphenidol

dronabinol

meclizine

nabilone

promethazine (see Chapter 51)

perphenazine (see Chapter 36)

prochlorperazine (see Chapter 26)

scopolamine

thiethylperazine

triflupromazine (see Chapter 36)

trimeprazine (see Chapter 51)

trimethobenzamide

## OVERVIEW OF THE DRUG CLASS

**Origin of nausea and vomiting**  Vomiting (emesis) is an involuntary act of regurgitating the contents of the stomach and is coordinated by an area in the medulla called the vomiting center. Nausea is the unpleasant sensation that usually precedes vomiting. Input from three major neural sites can stimulate the vomiting center. The first input is that controlled by the higher central nervous system functions, with vomiting being secondary to emotion, pain, or disequilibrium (motion sickness). The second pathway is that arising from peripheral stimuli, with vomiting being secondary to injury or disease of a body tissue or organ. In particular, irritation of the mucosa of the gastrointestinal tract or bowel or biliary distention stimulates the vomiting center by way of the autonomic neurons carrying information to the central nervous system (afferent neurons). A third pathway is from the chemoreceptor trigger zone, a medullary center sensitive to stimulation by circulating drugs and toxins.

**Nonmedicinal treatments of nausea and vomiting**  Nausea and vomiting are not necessarily treated with drugs. For instance, the nausea and vomiting of pregnancy is best treated by having the patient sip water or tea and eat small meals, because antiemetic drugs have been shown to cause fetal abnormalities in experimental animals. Many drugs cause nausea and vomiting as side effects because they act directly on the chemoreceptor trigger zone. Examples of such drugs include levodopa, digitalis, opiates (narcotic analgesics), and aminophylline. The effective treatment is to lower the dose of the offending drug or to increase the dose slowly. Drugs may also irritate the gastric mucosa to cause a reflex stimulation of nausea and vomiting. Aspirin is an example of an irritant drug. The effective treatment is to take the drug with a large volume of liquid or with a meal to coat the mucosa and protect from direct contact with the drug.

## MECHANISM OF ACTION
Drugs currently used to prevent nausea and vomiting are covered in this section. These drugs include antagonists of histamine, acetylcholine, and dopamine, as well as drugs with actions not yet determined. Drugs for treating nausea and vomiting are most effective when administered before nausea and vomiting have begun rather than after. The choice of an antiemetic is determined by the cause of the nausea and vomiting. Motion sickness and vertigo are most effectively treated prophylactically with certain antihistamines or the anticholinergic drug scopolamine. These drugs seem to be effective in blocking the action of acetylcholine in the vomiting center that causes nausea. The effective drugs for reducing the vomiting from chemotherapy and radiation therapy of cancer are antagonists of dopamine. Dopamine is the neurotransmitter triggering nausea and vomiting in the chemoreceptor trigger zone. Antidopaminergic drugs widely used as antiemetics include chlorpromazine, perphenazine, promethazine, thiethylperazone, triflupromazine, and trimeprazine. The cannabinoids, dronabinol and nabilone, are the most recently introduced antiemetics for cancer chemotherapy. Benzquinamide acts by a peripheral mechanism.

## INDICATIONS
**Nausea and vomiting** Especially when taken prophylactically prior to surgery or to chemotherapy or radiation therapy.  **Motion sickness** Scopolamine and the antihistamines are especially effective when taken before travel.  **Vertigo** Meclizine, dimenhydrinate, and diphenidol are sometimes effective. See Table 55-1 for a summary of the indications for the antiemetics covered.

## CONTRAINDICATIONS
**Not for uncomplicated vomiting** in children or for vomiting of unknown etiology in children because of the possible association of antiemetics with the development of Reye's syndrome.

**Table 55-1.**

## Indications for antiemetics

| Drug | Mechanism* | Nausea and vomiting | Motion sickness | Vertigo |
|------|-----------|---------------------|-----------------|---------|
| Benzquinamide | AD | + | | |
| Buclizine | AC | + | + | |
| Chlorpromazine | AD | + | | |
| Cyclizine | AD | + | + | |
| Dimenhydrinate | AC | + | + | + |
| Diphenidol | OT | | + | |
| Dronabinol | AD | + | | |
| Meclizine | AC | + | + | + |
| Nabilone | AD | + | | |
| Promethazine | AD | + | | |
| Perphenazine | AD | + | | |
| Prochlorperazine | AD | + | | |
| Scopolamine | AC | | + | |
| Thiethylperazine | AD | + | | |
| Triflupromazine | AD | + | | |
| Trimeprazine | AD | + | | |
| Trimethobenzamide | AD | + | | |

*AC, anticholinergic; AD, antidopaminergic; OT, other.

**DRUG INTERACTIONS**    **CNS depressants** All centrally acting antiemetics are CNS depressants and should be combined only cautiously with other CNS depressants such as sedative-hypnotic drugs, tranquilizers, antipsychotics, and antidepressants. In particular, the treatment of vomiting in acute alcoholism may lead to serious respiratory depression.

## ❦ NURSING CONSIDERATIONS

### Side effects, toxicities, and associated nursing actions

**CNS** Drowsiness, fatigue, insomnia, restlessness, excitement, nervousness, headache.

- Tell the patient to avoid driving or operating hazardous equipment if drowsiness occurs. Tolerance to this may develop over time, but most patients use antiemetics for such a short time that tolerance does not develop.
- Monitor for CNS side effects. Pronounced or persistent side effects may necessitate a change in drug or dose.

**CV** Hypertension, hypotension, dizziness, atrial fibrillation, premature contractions.

- Monitor the blood pressure and pulse.
- Be alert to syncope associated with hypotension, especially in postoperative patients getting up the first time after surgery, in the elderly, and in patients receiving other CNS depressant medications or drugs known to cause hypotension, such as antihypertensives.
- Supervise ambulation.

**GI** Anorexia, nausea, dry mouth, constipation.

- Monitor intake and output, and record frequency of stools. When possible, measure emesis as a part of output.
- Monitor skin turgor; assess mucous membranes for dryness.
- For xerostomia (dry mouth), advise patients to suck on hard candies or chew gum (sugarless, to avoid dental caries and weight gain), drink frequent sips of water, avoid lemon-glycerin swabs or other rinses that are drying or irritating, but perform regular oral hygiene. Some patients may wish to use a commercially available saliva substitute.
- Assess carefully continued complaints of nausea. It may be difficult to discriminate between nausea

due to the underlying problem and nausea due to treatment with antiemetics.
- Monitor anorexia carefully. Weigh patient. Maintain fluid intake even if patient is unable to eat solid food, but avoid overhydration.
- If constipation develops, advise patients to increase fluid intake to 2500 to 3000 ml/day, increase intake of fruits, juices, and fiber, and increase daily exercise. For some patients, it may be necessary for the physician to prescribe a stool softener.

**Eye** Blurred vision.
- If blurred vision occurs, caution patients to avoid driving or operating hazardous equipment until the effects of the medication lessen. Notify the physician.

**GU** Urinary retention.
- Urinary retention is more common in the elderly, the immobilized, and in men with preexisting prostatic hypertrophy. Suggest that patients void prior to taking dose of antiemetics.

**Allergic** Rash, urticaria, hives.
- Visually inspect patients for the development of rash.
- Have medications available in setting where antiemetics are used to treat acute allergic responses: epinephrine, steroids, and antihistamines.

### Nursing interventions related to drug administration
- Avoid the use of antiemetics in children who may be suffering from Reye's syndrome. This syndrome is characterized by an abrupt onset of persistent severe vomiting, lethargy, irrational behavior, progressive encephalopathy, convulsions, coma, and death.
- Keep patients recumbent following parenteral administration; monitor vital signs.
- Use a water-soluble lubricant to lubricate suppositories.
- Administer IM preparations in a large muscle mass such as the dorsogluteal site or rectus femoris muscle in adults, or the vastus lateralis muscle in infants and small children. Use anatomical landmarks to carefully identify sites. Aspirate carefully prior to injecting medication to avoid inadvertent intravenous injection. If blood is aspirated, withdraw needle and prepare fresh dose of medication. Record and rotate injection sites.

### Patient and family education
- Review anticipated benefits and possible side effects of drug therapy with the patient.
- Instruct patients to avoid the use of alcohol.
- Remind patients to avoid the concomitant use of any medications that may depress the central nervous system without prior approval of the physician. These medications include narcotic pain medications, sedatives, sleeping pills, and many cold remedies.
- Instruct patients to report severe or persistent nausea and vomiting to the physician.
- Caution women who suspect they may be pregnant to avoid the use of any medication without first consulting a physician.
- For motion sickness, patients should always try to sit in the front seat of cars, facing forward. Medication for motion sickness should be taken 1 to 2 hours prior to beginning the trip, rather than after the trip has begun. For extended periods, such as cruises, patients may find that tolerance to motion of the boat (or other vehicles) may develop after 2 to 3 days of exposure.

## benzquinamide hydrochloride    (benz-KWIN-a-mide)    antiemetic

- benzquinamide hydrochloride: Emete-Con

**MECHANISM OF ACTION**    Benzquinamide has antihistaminic and anticholinergic activities but is believed to act on the chemoreceptor trigger zone for antiemetic activity.

**INDICATIONS**    Nausea and vomiting associated with anesthesia and surgery.

**CONTRAINDICATIONS**    Cardiovascular disease Benzquinamide can cause a sudden increase in blood pressure and transient cardiac arrhythmias if administered IV but not IM.

**DOSAGE**    IM    ADULTS: 50 mg or 0.5 to 1 mg/kg. May be repeated in 1 hour and then every 3 to 4 hours if needed. Should be administered at least 15 minutes prior to emergence from anesthesia.    *Special* *patient populations:* **CHILDREN:** Not recommended for children under 12 years old. **PREGNAN-CY:** Safe use has not been established.

**PREPARATIONS** *Injection:* 50 mg.

**DRUG INTERACTIONS** **Pressor agents or epinephrine-like drugs** Since benzquinamide can alter blood pressure, it is given in fractions of the normal dose when pressor agents have been administered concurrently.

**FATE** Benzquinamide is well absorbed. The *onset of action* is 15 minutes; the *duration of action* is 3 to 4 hours. Benzquinamide is metabolized by the liver and excreted in the urine.

## ☙ NURSING CONSIDERATIONS

### Side effects, toxicities, and associated nursing actions
- See entry for drug class (p. 977).

**CNS** Drowsiness; fatigue; insomnia, restlessness, excitement, nervousness, headache.

**CV** Hypertension, hypotension, dizziness, atrial fibrillation, premature contractions.

**Eye** Blurred vision.

**GI** Anorexia, nausea.

**Allergic** Rash, urticaria, hives.

**Other** Autonomic (cholinergic) effects including shivering, sweating, flushing, salivation; twitching, shaking, tremors, weakness.
- Monitor vital signs.
- Monitor for these side effects. If severe or persistent, withhold subsequent doses and notify the physician.

### Nursing interventions related to drug administration
- Reconstitute as directed on the vial; sodium chloride should *not* be used.
- See entry for drug class (p. 978).

### Patient and family education
- See entry for drug class (p. 978).

---

## buclizine hydrochloride    (BYOO-kli-zeen)          antiemetic

- buclizine hydrochloride: Bucladin-S Softabs

**MECHANISM OF ACTION** Buclizine is an antihistamine with anticholinergic activity at the vomiting center.

**INDICATIONS** • Motion sickness.

**CONTRAINDICATIONS** • Hypersensitivity to the drug. • Pregnancy.

**DOSAGE** **PO:** **ADULTS:** 50 mg 30 minutes before travel. Repeat in 4 to 6 hours if needed. *Special patient populations:* **CHILDREN:** Not recommended for children. **PREGNANCY:** Contraindicated in pregnancy. Tetratologic effects have been demonstrated in test animals.

**PREPARATIONS** *Tablet (chewable):* 50 mg.

**DRUG INTERACTIONS** **CNS depressants** have additive depression.

**FATE** Buclizine has a *duration of action* of 4 to 6 hours. Its metabolism has not been characterized.

## ☙ NURSING CONSIDERATIONS

### Side effects, toxicities, and associated nursing actions
**CNS** Drowsiness, headache, jitteriness.

**GI** Dry mouth.
- See entry for drug class (p. 977).

### Nursing interventions related to drug administration
- Bucladin-S Softabs brand contains FD & C yellow dye #5 (tartrazine), which may cause an allergic response in susceptible individuals. While rare, this side effects is seen more often in persons with aspirin hypersensitivity.

### Patient and family education
- For motion sickness, the dose is usually administered 30 minutes prior to the start of the trip.

- Instruct patients to chew the tablet rather than swallow it with fluid.
- See entry for drug class (p. 978).

---

## cyclizine hydrochloride, cyclizine lactate    (SYE-kli-zeen)    antiemetic

- cyclizine hydrochloride, cyclizine lactate: Merezine, ❧Marzine

**MECHANISM OF ACTION**    Cyclizine is an antihistamine with anticholinergic activity at the vomiting center.

**INDICATIONS**    • Motion sickness.

**CONTRAINDICATIONS**    • Hypersensitivity to the drug. • Pregnancy.

**DOSAGE**    PO:    ADULTS: 50 mg 30 minutes before travel. Repeat in 4 to 6 hours if needed.    PO:   CHILDREN 6 TO 12 YEARS OLD: 25 mg 30 minutes before travel. Repeat in 4 to 6 hours if needed. *Special patient populations:*   CHILDREN: Not recommended for children under 6 years old. PREGNANCY: Contraindicated in pregnancy. Teratologic effects have been demonstrated in test animals.

**PREPARATIONS**    *Hydrochloride, tablet:* 50 mg. *Lactate, injection:* 50 mg/ml.

**DRUG INTERACTIONS**    **CNS depressants** Additive depression.    **Salicylates, aminoglycosides** Cyclizine may mask ototoxicity.

**FATE**    Cyclizine has a *duration of action* of 4 to 6 hours. Its metabolism has not been characterized.

❧ **NURSING CONSIDERATIONS**

### Side effects, toxicities, and associated nursing actions
  **CNS** Drowsiness, headache, jitteriness.
  **GI** Dry mouth.
  • See entry for drug class (p. 977).

### Nursing interventions related to drug administration
  • See entry for drug class (p. 978).

### Patient and family education
  • See entry for drug class (p. 978).

---

## dimenhydrinate    (dye-men-HYE-dri-nate)    antiemetic

- dimenhydrinate: ❧Apo-Dimenhydrinate, Dramamine, Dimentabs, Dramalin, Dramocen, Dramoject, Dymenate, ❧Gravol, ❧Nauseatol, ❧Novodimenate, ❧PMS-Dimenhydrinate, Reidamine, ❧Travamine, ❧Travel Eze, Wehamine

**MECHANISM OF ACTION**    Dimenhydrinate is an antihistamine with anticholinergic activity at the vomiting center. Dimenhydrinate is a combination of two drugs—diphenhydramine and chlorotheophylline.

**INDICATIONS**    • Motion sickness.

**CONTRAINDICATIONS**    • Hypersensitivity to the drug. • Pregnancy.

**DOSAGE**    PO:    ADULTS: 50 to 100 mg 30 minutes before travel. Repeat in 4 hours if needed.    CHILDREN 6 TO 12 YEARS OLD: 25 to 50 mg up to three times daily.    CHILDREN 2 TO 5 YEARS OLD: 12.5 to 25 mg up to three times daily. *Special patient populations:*   CHILDREN: Not recommended for children under 2 years old.    PREGNANCY: Contraindicated in pregnancy. Teratologic effects have been demonstrated in test animals.

**PREPARATIONS**    *Solution (oral):* 12.5 mg/4 ml; *tablets:* 50 mg; *injection:* 50 mg/ml.

**DRUG INTERACTIONS**    **CNS depressants** Additive depression.    **Anticholinergic drugs** Dimenhydrinate can have additive effects with drugs having anticholinergic activity, including the tricyclic antidepressants.    **Antibiotics with ototoxicity** Dimenhydrinate may mask symptoms so that permanent damage is incurred.

**FATE**   Dimenhydrinate has an *onset of action* of 15 to 30 minutes after oral administration and a *duration of action* of 3 to 6 hours. Its metabolism has not been characterized.

## 🐦 NURSING CONSIDERATIONS

### Side effects, toxicities, and associated nursing actions

- See entry for drug class (p. 977). The following are specific to this drug:

**CNS** Drowsiness, headaches; paradoxical excitement is common in children.

- Caution parents about this possible side effect in children. If excitement occurs, parent should notify physician and avoid subsequent doses.

**CV** Palpitations, hypotension.

**GI** Dry mouth, constipation.

**Ophthalmic** Blurred vision, double vision.

**Lung** Nasal stuffiness: thickening of bronchial secretions.

- Keep patients well hydrated.

**Allergic** Anaphylaxis, photosensitivity, urticaria, rash.

- If photosensitivity develops, caution patients to avoid prolonged exposure to the sun. When patients are in the sun, caution them to wear a wide-brimmed hat, long-sleeve shirt, and long pants. A maximum-protection sunscreen should also be used.

### Nursing interventions related to drug administration

- See entry for drug class (p. 978).
- For IV admininstration, dilute 50 mg (1 ml) in at least 10 ml of sodium chloride injection, and administer each 50 mg over at least 2 minutes.

### Patient and family education

- Taking oral doses with meals may lessen gastric irritation.
- See entry for drug class (p. 978).

---

## diphenidol hydrochloride   (dye-FEN-i-dole)            antiemetic

- diphenidol hydrochloride: Vontrol

**MECHANISM OF ACTION**   Diphenidol controls vomiting by inhibiting the chemoreceptor trigger zone. Diphenidol also has an antivertigo effect through inhibition of conduction in vestibular-cerebellar pathways.

**INDICATIONS**   **Vertigo and motion sickness** Diphenidol is effective in the prevention and control of these conditions. However, because diphenidol can cause hallucinations, use of this drug is generally restricted to a hospital setting.   **Nausea and vomiting** Used in a hospital setting.

**CONTRAINDICATIONS**   **Hypersensitivity to the drug.**   **Anuria** Renal shutdown would lead to drug accumulation, increasing the risk of serious side effects.   **GI obstruction, glaucoma** Although the anticholinergic effects are reported to be weak, diphenidol is used with caution in the presence of conditions made worse by anticholinergic drugs.

**DOSAGE**   **PO:**   **ADULTS:** 25 to 50 mg every 4 hours as needed. Maximum dose is 300 mg daily.   **CHILDREN OVER 6 MONTHS OLD AND WEIGHING AT LEAST 25 LB:** 0.88 mg/kg, repeated in 1 hour if necessary, then every 4 hours as needed.   *Special patient populations:*   **ELDERLY:** Altered doses for the elderly have not been specifically established. However, because of the risk for mental confusion and hallucinations, diphenidol would not be appropriate for elderly patients with impaired mentation.   **CHILDREN:** Pediatric doses are given above.   **PREGNANCY:** Safe use has not been established.

**PREPARATIONS**   *Tablets:* 25 mg.

**DRUG INTERACTIONS**   **Anticholinergic drugs** Diphenidol can act synergistically with these drugs, especially to impair mentation.   **Cardiac glycosides** Diphenidol can mask the toxic symptoms of the cardiac glycosides.

**FATE**  Diphenidol is well absorbed, with a *duration of action* of about 4 hours. Dephenidol is metabolized in the liver and excreted in the urine.

### ❦ NURSING CONSIDERATIONS

#### Side effects, toxicities, and associated nursing actions

- See entry for drug class (p. 977). For side effects specific to this drug see below.

**CNS** Auditory and visual hallucinations, disorientation, confusion.

- These occur in about 0.5% of patients receiving therapeutic doses. Also, drowsiness or overstimulation; mental depression, sleep disturbances.
- Because of the high incidence of CNS side effects, the use of this drug is usually limited to the hospital or other setting where patients can be carefully supervised. Monitor patients carefully. Reorient if confused. Keep bed siderails up and bed in low position. Keep nightlights on. Notify physician if side effects occur.

**Eye** Blurred vision

**GI** Dry mouth, indigestion.

**Skin** Rash.

#### Nursing interventions related to drug administration

- Vontrol brand tablets contain FD & C yellow dye # 5 (tartrazine), which may cause an allergic reaction in susceptible individuals. While rare, this side effect is seen more commonly in persons with aspirin hypersensitivity.
- See entry for drug class (p. 978).

#### Patient and family education

- See entry for drug class (p. 978).

---

## dronabinol  (droe-NAB-i-nole)                                         antiemetic

- dronabinol: Marinol Rx, C-II (Pending)

**MECHANISM OF ACTION**  Dronabinol is delta-9-tetrahydrocannabinol, the major active substance in marijuana. The cannabinoids appear to act at the chemoreceptor trigger zone to prevent nausea and vomiting.

**INDICATIONS**  **Nausea and vomiting** For cancer chemotherapy; seems to be particularly effective when combined with a phenothiazine.

**CONTRAINDICATIONS**  **Epilepsy** May enhance seizure activity.

**DOSAGE**  PO:  **ADULTS:** 5 to 7.5 mg/M$^2$ every 3 to 4 hours. Begin 4 to 12 hours before chemotherapy and continue 8 to 24 hours after. Dose may be increased by 2.5 mg/M$^2$ if necessary.  *Special patient populations:*  **CHILDREN:** Not for use in children.  **PREGNANCY:** Safe use has not been established. FDA pregnancy category B.

**PREPARATIONS**  *Capsules:* 2.5, 5, 10 mg (in sesame oil).

**DRUG INTERACTIONS**  **Phenothiazines** Cannabinoids act synergistically in the control of nausea and vomiting.

**FATE**  Dronabinol is erratically absorbed. The *peak* plasma concentration is generally achieved in 60 to 90 minutes. Dronabinol binds to protein and is stored in fat, so that the drug is slowly metabolized and eliminated. The plasma *half-life* is 19 hours for the parent drug and 48 hours for metabolites.

### ❦ NURSING CONSIDERATIONS

#### Side effects, toxicities, and associated nursing actions

- See entry for drug class (p. 977).

**CNS** Drowsiness, incoordination, anxiety, hallucinations, dysphoria.

**CV** Rarely, tachycardia (fast heart rate), palpitations.

**Eye** Blurred vision.

#### Nursing interventions related to drug administration

- Some patients may be unwilling to take this drug because it has been illegal to possess marijuana. Discuss with patients the expected benefits of therapy. A patient's predisposition toward a drug may interfere with its effectiveness.

- Keep the environment quiet and remain with the patient if psychological side effects are prominent.

**Patient and family education**
- See entry for drug class (p. 978).

---

## meclizine hydrochloride    (MEK-li-zeen)                               antiemetic

- meclizine hydrochloride: Antivert, ♣Bonamine

**MECHANISM OF ACTION**    Meclizine is an antihistamine with anticholinergic activity in the vomiting center.

**INDICATIONS**    • Motion sickness. • Vertigo.

**CONTRAINDICATIONS**    • Hypersensitivity.

**DOSAGE**    PO:    **ADULTS AND CHILDREN OVER 12 YEARS OLD:** *Motion sickness*—25 to 50 mg 1 hour before travel. *Vertigo*—25 to 100 mg daily in divided doses.    *Special patient populations:*    **CHILDREN:** Not recommended for children under 12 years old.    **PREGNANCY:** Safe use has not been established.

**PREPARATIONS**    *Tablets:* 12.5, 25, 50 mg; *tablets (chewable):* 25 mg.

**DRUG INTERACTIONS**    **CNS depressants** Additive depression.

**FATE**    The *onset of action* is 1 hour, and the *duration of action* is 8 to 24 hours. The metabolic fate of meclizine has not been well characterized.

☙ **NURSING CONSIDERATIONS**

**Side effects, toxicities, and associated nursing actions**
- See entry for drug class (p. 977).

**CNS** Drowsiness, headache, jitteriness.

**GI** Dry mouth.

**Nursing interventions related to drug administration**
- If the chewable tablet is prescribed, instruct patients to chew the dose for best benefit, rather than swallow it with liquid.

**Patient and family education**
- See entry for drug class (p. 978).

---

## nabilone    (NA-bi-lone)                                              antiemetic

- nabilone: Cesamet

**MECHANISM OF ACTION**    Nabilone is an active cannabinoid. The cannabinoids appear to act at the chemoreceptor trigger zone to prevent nausea and vomiting.

**INDICATIONS**    **Nausea and vomiting** Nabilone reduces the severity and duration of nausea and vomiting from cancer chemotherapy in about 50% to 70% of those patients not helped with other antiemetics. Nabilone is especially effective for low-dose cisplatin therapy.

**CONTRAINDICATIONS**    • Psychotic reactions.

**DOSAGE**    PO:    **ADULTS:** 1 mg twice daily, increasing to 2 mg twice daily if required.    *Special patient populations:*    **CHILDREN:** Not recommended for children.    **PREGNANCY:** Safe use has not been established.

**PREPARATIONS**    *Tablets:* 1 mg.

**DRUG INTERACTIONS**    **Phenothiazines** Cannabinoids act synergistically in the control of nausea and vomiting.

**FATE**    Nabilone has a *peak* effect in 1 to 2 hours. The plasma *half-life* is about 2 hours, but metabolites are active and have a half-life of 35 hours. The drug is excreted in the bile and appears in the feces.

## 🦉 NURSING CONSIDERATIONS

### Side effects, toxicities, and associated nursing actions
* See entry for drug class (p. 977).

**CNS** Drowsiness, incoordination, anxiety, hallucinations, dysphoria.

**CV** Rarely, tachycardia (fast heart rate), palpitations.

**Eye** Blurred vision.

### Nursing interventions related to drug administration
* Some patients may be unwilling to take this drug because it has been illegal to possess marijuana. Discuss with patients the expected benefits of therapy. A patient's predisposition toward a drug may interfere with its effectiveness.
* Keep the environment quiet and remain with the patient if psychological side effects are prominent.

### Patient and family education
* See entry for drug class (p. 978).

---

# scopolamine (hyoscine), scopolamine H, scopolamine hydrobromide (hyoscine hydrobromide) (skoe-POL-a-meen) antiemetic

* scopolamine: Triptone, Transderm Scop, ♣Transderm-V

**MECHANISM OF ACTION** An anticholinergic drug, scopolamine blocks the tramsmission of cholinergic impulses from the vestibular nuclei to higher centers in the CNS and from the reticular formation to the vomiting center.

**INDICATIONS** **Motion sickness** Scopolamine is considered the drug of choice for motion sickness.

**CONTRAINDICATIONS** **Conditions worsened by anticholinergic medication,** including glaucoma, phyloric obstruction, urinary bladder neck obstruction, thyrotoxicosis, paralytic ileum, tachycardia secondary to cardiac insufficiency.

**DOSAGE** **PO:** **ADULTS:** 0.25 mg every 4 hours up to 1 mg daily. **Transdermal:** **ADULTS:** One system is applied behind an ear and delivers 0.5 mg over 72 hours. *Special patient populations:* **CHILDREN:** Dosage forms for pediatric use in treating motion sickness have not been developed. **PREGNANCY:** Safe use has not been established.

**PREPARATIONS** *Scopolamine, topical (transdermal):* 0.5 mg/72 hours. *Scopolamine hydrobromide, capsules:* 0.25 mg.

**DRUG INTERACTIONS** **Drugs with anticholinergic effects** Synergistic anticholinergic activity with phenothiazines, antiparkinsonian drugs, glutethimide, meperidine, tricyclic antidepressants, quinidine, disopyramide, some antihistamines. **Methotrimeprazine** Extrapyramidal symptoms have been reported when methotrimeprazine is combined with scopolamine as a premedication.

**FATE** Taken orally, scopolamine has an *onset of action* of about 30 minutes and a *duration of action* of about 6 hours. The transdermal system has an *onset of action* of 4 hours and a *duration of action* up to 72 hours. Scopolamine is metabolized in the liver and excreted in the urine.

## 🦉 NURSING CONSIDERATIONS

### Side effects, toxicities, and associated nursing actions
* See entry for drug class (p. 977).

**CNS** Drowsiness is common; rarely, disorientation, memory distrubances, dizziness, restlessness, confusion, hallucinations.

**Eye** Blurred vision, dilated pupil.

**GI** Dry mouth is very common.

**GU** Rarely, difficulty in urination.
* Be alert to difficulty in voiding, especially in postoperative patients. Monitor intake and output. Palpate the bladder for distension. Notify physician.

**Allergic** Rashes.

**Nursing interventions related to drug administration.**
- For IV use, dilute ordered dose in at least 10 ml of sterile water for injection. Administer at a rate of 0.6 mg or less over 1 minute. The IM route is the usual parenteral route.

**Patient and family education**
- Advise patients using the transdermal route to obtain a patient instruction sheet which should accompany the filled prescription.
- Before patient uses the transdermal form, the skin behind the ear should be cleaned. Remove the protective strip on the single dose. Press firmly to a nonhairy area behind the ear. The dose should adhere through normal daily activities, including bathing and swimming, but if it comes loose or comes off, it should be replaced at a different spot behind one of the ears. Only one dose should be in place at at time. After stopping the dose (by removing the patch), the skin behind the ear should be washed clean to remove traces of the drug. The patient or anyone else handling the patch and applying it to the patient should wash hands carefully after touching the patch to remove traces of the medication that might be absorbed through the fingertips.
- See entry for drug class (p. 978).

---

# thiethylperazine malate, thiethylperazine maleate
(thye-eth-il-PER-a-zeen) antiemetic

- thiethylperazine malate, thiethylperazine maleate: Torecan

**MECHANISM OF ACTION**   Thiethylperazine is a phenothiazine and exerts its antiemetic action by blocking dopamine in the chemoreceptor trigger zone.

**INDICATIONS**   • Nausea and vomiting.

**CONTRAINDICATIONS**   • Hypersensitivity. • Pregnancy. • Severe CNS depression. Coma.

**DOSAGE**   PO, IM, SC, IV, Rectal:   **ADULTS AND CHILDREN OVER 12 YEARS OLD:** 10 mg, one to three times daily as needed.
*Special patient populations:*   **CHILDREN:** Not recommended for children under 12 years old.
**PREGNANCY:** Contraindicated during pregnancy.

**PREPARATIONS**   *Tablets:* 10 mg; *suppositories:* 10 mg; *injection:* 5 mg/ml.

**DRUG INTERACTIONS**   **CNS depressants (including alcohol)** will produce additive depression.
**Anticholinergic drugs** will produce additive anticholinergic effects.

**FATE**   The *onset of action* is 30 minutes, and the *duration of action* is 4 hours.

☙ **NURSING CONSIDERATIONS**

**Side effects, toxicities, and associated nursing actions**
- See entry for drug class (p. 977).
**CNS** Drowsiness, headache, fever, tinnitus; rarely, extrapyramidal effects, seizures.
- For a description of extrapyramidal effects, see pg. 703.
**Eye** Blurred vision.
**GI** Dry mouth.

**Nursing interventions related to drug administration**
- Torecan brand tablets contain FD & C yellow dye #5 (tartrazine), which may cause an allergic response in susceptible individuals. While rare, this side effect is seen more frequently in persons with aspirin hypersensitivity.
- The IM route of administration is preferred over the SC or IV routes.
- See entry for drug class (p. 978).

**Patient and family education**
- See entry for drug class (p. 978).

## trimethobenzamide hydrochloride (trye-METH-oh-prim) antiemetic

• trimethobenzamide hydrochloride: Tigan

**MECHANISM OF ACTION** Trimethobenzamide has an inhibitory activity at the chemoreceptor trigger zone. Trimethobenzamide is structurally related to the antihistamines but has weak antihistaminic activity.

**INDICATIONS** **Nausea and vomiting** Less effective than the phenothiazines in severe vomiting. However, trimethobenzamide has fewer side effects than the phenothiazines and is preferred for long-term therapy.

**CONTRAINDICATIONS**
• Hypersensitivity.

**DOSAGE** **PO:** **ADULTS:** 250 mg three or four times daily. **CHILDREN WEIGHING 25 TO 100 LB:** 100 to 200 mg three or four times daily. **Rectal:** **ADULTS:** 200 mg three or four times daily. **CHILDREN WEIGHING 25 TO 100 LB:** 100 to 200 mg three or four times daily. **CHILDREN WEIGHING UNDER 25 LB:** 100 mg three or four times daily. **IM:** **ADULTS:** 200 mg three or fours times daily.
*Special patient populations:* **CHILDREN:** Suppositories should not be used in neonates. **PREGNANCY:** Trimethobenzamide has not been teratogenic in test animals, but an increased incidence of stillbirths was noted. Safe use is not considered as established.

**PREPARATIONS** *Capsules:* 100, 250 mg; *injection:* 100 mg/ml; *suppositories:* 100 mg.

**DRUG INTERACTIONS** **CNS depressants** Will have additive depression.

**FATE** The *onset of action* of trimethobenzamide is about 10 to 40 minutes, and the *duration of action* is about 3 to 4 hours after oral administration and 2 to 3 hours after IM administration. Trimethobenzamide is metabolized in the liver. The drug and its metabolites are excreted in the urine and feces.

## ☙ NURSING CONSIDERATIONS

### Side effects, toxicities, and associated nursing actions
• See entry for drug class (p. 977).
**CNS** Occasionally, extrapyramidal effects. Rarely, seizures, coma, depression, disorientation, vertigo, dizziness, drowsiness, headache.
• For a description of extrapyramidal effects, see p. 703.
**CV** Occasionally, hypotension after IM administration.
**Eye** Blurred vision.
**GI** Diarrhea.
**Allergic** Skin rashes.

### Nursing interventions related to drug administration
• See entry for drug class (p. 978).

### Patient and family education
• See entry for drug class (p. 978).

# Chapter Fifty-six

# Drugs to increase tone and motility

bethanechol
metoclopramide
neostigmine

**OVERVIEW OF THE DRUG CLASS**  Cholinomimetic drugs play a minor role in the treatment of gastrointestinal disorders. Occasionally, bethanechol or neostigmine is administered to stimulate an atonic intestine or bladder. Both drugs increase gastrointestinal tone and motility. Metoclopramide is a new drug that stimulates the gastrointestinal tract, but it is not a cholinomimetic drug.

**MECHANISM OF ACTION**  Drugs that mimic the action of acetylcholine act by one of two mechanisms: directly, by mimicking acetylcholine, or indirectly, in inhibiting acetylcholinesterase, the enzyme that degrades acetylcholine. Bethanechol is a direct-acting cholinomimetic, and neostigmine is an indirect-acting cholinomimetic. Both drugs increase gastrointestinal tone and motility. Metoclopramide is a dopamine antagonist that also stimulates the upper gastrointestinal tract.

**INDICATIONS**  **Atonic bladder or gastrointestinal system**  Each of the three drugs discussed has its own indications.

**CONTRAINDICATIONS**  • Peptic ulcer. • Mechanical obstruction of the bowel or urinary tract.

**DRUG INTERACTIONS**  **Atropine and other cholinergic antagonists** will block the peripheral (muscarinic) actions of cholinergic drugs. The muscarinic actions include hypotension, bronchoconstriction, salivation, sweating, heart block. Atropine is administered as an antidote for acute toxicity with cholinergic drugs.

---

## bethanechol chloride  (be-THAN-e-kole)  cholinomimetic

- bethanecol chloride: Urabeth, Duvoid, Urecholine

**MECHANISM OF ACTION**  Bethanechol directly stimulates muscarinic receptors. Since bethanechol is relatively resistant to hydrolysis by cholinesterase, bethanechol has a more prolonged action than acetylcholine.

**INDICATIONS**  **Urinary retention**  For acute postoperative and postpartum nonobstructive urinary retention. Bethanechol can also prevent and treat phenothiazine-induced bladder dysfunction and antagonize the inhibition of the bladder and salivary glands caused by tricyclic antidepressants.  **Atonic gastrointestinal tract**  To stimulate gastrointestinal motility postoperatively, following vagotomy, or to overcome paralytic ileus.

**CONTRAINDICATIONS**  **Mechanical obstruction of the GI or urinary tract. Epilepsy, parkinsonism**  Cholinomimetic drugs can activate seizures.  **Hyperthyroidism, peptic ulcer, asthma** are aggravated by parasympathetic stimulation.  **Pregnancy.**

**DOSAGE**  **PO:**  ADULTS: 10 to 50 mg two to four times daily.  **SC:**  ADULTS: 2.5 to 5 mg. May repeat three or four times daily.  CHILDREN: 0.036 mg/kg for diagnosis of flaccid or atonic neurogenic bladder. *Special patient populations:*  CHILDREN: Pediatric use is primarily for diagnostic purposes. PREGNANCY: Contraindicated in pregnancy.

**PREPARATIONS**  *Tablets:* 5, 10, 25, 50 mg; *injection:* 5 mg/ml.

**DRUG INTERACTIONS**  **Cholinesterase inhibitors** produce additive cholinomimetic effects with bethanechol. **Procainamide, quinidine** antagonize the effects of bethanechol.

**DIAGNOSTIC TEST INTERFERENCE**  **Serum amylase and lipase** may be increased following administration of bethanechol.  **Serum bilirubin, aspartate aminotransferase, and sulfobromophthalein** may be retained.

**FATE**  Bethanechol is poorly absorbed from the GI tract. The *onset of action* is 30 minutes, and the *duration of action* is 1 hour. After SC administration, the *onset of action* is 5 to 15 minutes, and the *duration of action* is 2 hours.

## ❦ NURSING CONSIDERATIONS

### Side effects, toxicities, and associated nursing actions

**CV** Hypotension.
* Monitor pulse and blood pressure every 5 minutes until stable following parenteral administration. Monitor every 2 to 4 hours following oral administration until effects of dosage can be determined.
* Supervise ambulation.

**GI** Abdominal cramps; diarrhea; salivation, nausea and vomiting; substernal pressure.
* Assess for these side effects. If persistent or severe, notify physician.
* Have atropine readily available to treat acute response. Dosage of atropine should be prescribed by physician.

**GU** Urinary urgency.
* Have bedpan or urinal handy. Especially following parenteral administration, patient may be unable to walk the distance to the bathroom without urinating.
* Monitor intake and output.

**Skin** Flushing, sweating.

**Allergic** Rarely, hypersensitivity.
* Be alert to these side effects. In addition to having atropine available, drugs to treat allergic reactions should be available.

### Nursing interventions related to drug administration

* The physician may prescribe a test dose to determine patient response prior to prescribing full dose. Observe patient carefully.
* Parenteral doses are administered subcutaneously. Aspirate for blood prior to injecting medication to avoid inadvertent IV administration. If blood appears in aspirate, withdraw needle, prepare new dose, and administer in a new site.

### Patient and family education

* Review with patient the expected benefits and possible side effects of therapy.
* Advise the patient that taking oral doses on an empty stomach will reduce the likelihood of nausea and vomiting.

---

## metoclopramide hydrochloride    (met-oh-kloe-PRA-mide)    upper GI stimulant

* metoclopromide hydrochloride: Clopra, ✤Emax, ✤Maxeran, Reglan

**MECHANISM OF ACTION**    Metoclopramide is a dopamine antagonist that also stimulates the upper GI tract.

**INDICATIONS**    **GI disorders** Metoclopramide is especially used for gastric stasis secondary to diabetes or surgery, management of gastroesophageal reflux, and to prevent vomiting from cancer chemotherapy.

**CONTRAINDICATIONS**    **Seizure disorders. Mechanical obstruction or perforation of the GI tract. Impaired renal function** Patients need to be monitored carefully.

**DOSAGE**    **PO:**    **ADULTS:** Diabetic stasis—10 mg four times daily.    **IV:**    **ADULTS:** Prevention of vomiting during cancer chemotherapy—2 mg/kg before chemotherapy. Intubation of the small bowel or radiographic examination of the upper GI tract—10 mg is given 10 minutes before the procedure. **CHILDREN 6 TO 14 YEARS OLD:** 2.5 to 5 mg.    **CHILDREN UNDER 6 YEARS OLD:** 0.1 mg/kg. *Special patient populations:*    **CHILDREN:** Children have a higher incidence of extrapyramidal reactions with metoclopramide.    **PREGNANCY:** Animal tests have not revealed adverse effects on fertility or on pregnancy (FDA pregnancy category B).

**PREPARATIONS**    *Solution (oral):* 5 mg/5 ml; *tablets:* 10 mg; *injection:* 5 mg/ml.

**DRUG INTERACTIONS**    **Absorption of drugs** Metoclopramide alters the absorption of drugs. In general, drugs absorbed in the stomach are more poorly absorbed because of the increased motility, while drugs absorbed in the small intestine will be better absorbed. **CNS depressants** Metoclopramide will enhance the depression caused by CNS depressants, including alcohol. **Insulin** Because metoclopramide alters the absorption of food, diabetic control with insulin will be affected. The timing of insulin injections may have to be modified.

**FATE** Metoclopramide is well absorbed. The *onset of action* depends on the route of absorption: 1 to 3 minutes after IV administration, 10 to 15 minutes after IM administration, 30 to 60 minutes after oral administration. The *duration of action* is 1 to 2 hours. Metoclopramide is metabolized in the liver and excreted in the urine.

## ☙ NURSING CONSIDERATIONS

### Side effects, toxicities, and associated nursing actions

**CNS** Sedation, lethargy; extrapyramidal reactions.
- If sedation occurs, caution patients to avoid driving or operating hazardous equipment until the effects of medication wear off.
- For a description of extrapyramidal reactions, see p. 703.

**Metabolic** Stimulates secretion of prolactin, which may cause galactorrhea, amenorrhea, gynecomastia, impotence. Produces transient increases in plasma aldosterone concentrations.
- Question patient carefully about development of metabolic side effects. The age of the patient may influence the significance of these potential side effects to the patient. Metabolic side effects may wear off in 2 to 4 weeks. If metabolic side effects occur and are troublesome to patient, it may be appropriate to change drugs. Consult the physician.

### Nursing interventions related to drug administration
- For IM injection, drug may be administered without further dilution.
- For direct IV push, drug may be administered without further dilution. Administer at a rate of 10 mg per 1 to 2 minutes.
- For IV infusion, dilute appropriate dose in 50 ml of compatible IV solution. Protecting dilution from light is recommended but may not be necessary. Consult pharmacist. Administer over at least 15 minutes. Metoclopramide should not be mixed with other infusing drugs.
- Oral doses should be administered 30 minutes prior to a meal, and at bedtime.

### Patient and family education
- Review with patient the expected benefits and possible side effects of therapy.
- Caution diabetic patients about the possible effects of metoclopramide on diabetic control (see Drug interactions above). Instruct patients to monitor blood glucose carefully. Adjust insulin dose or time of insulin dose administration if needed.
- Instruct patients to limit alcohol intake to 1 to 2 ounces per day.

---

## neostigmine methylsulfate (nee-oh-STIG-meen) cholinomimetic

- neostigmine methylsulfate: Prostigmine

**MECHANISM OF ACTION** Neostigmine is an indirect-acting cholinomimetic. Neostigmine inhibits the enzyme acetylcholinesterase that normally degrades the neurotransmitter acetylcholine. Higher than normal concentrations of acetylcholine lead to pronounced parasympathetic effects.

**INDICATIONS** **Postoperative abdominal distention and urinary retention** Bethanechol is the preferred drug. **Myasthenia gravis** See Chapter 42.

**CONTRAINDICATIONS** • Mechanical obstruction of the GI or urinary tract. • Asthma. • Vagotomy.

**DOSAGE** **Urinary retention:** *IM or SC:* ADULTS: 0.25 mg every 4 to 6 hours for 2 to 3 days. **Myasthenia gravis** See Chapter 42. *Special patient populations:* CHILDREN: Not used for children. PREGNANCY: Safe use has not been established.

**PREPARATIONS** *Injection:* 0.25, 0.5, 1 mg/ml.

**DRUG INTERACTIONS** **Non-depolarizing neuromuscular blocking agents** Neostigmine antagonizes their effect. **Aminoglycoside antibiotics, local anesthetics, antiarrhythmic agents** tend to antagonize the effect of neostigmine.

**FATE**    Neostigmine has a variable absorption. The *onset of action* is 10 to 30 minutes, and the *duration of action* is 2 to 4 hours. Neostigmine is hydrolyzed and metabolized, but about 50% is excreted in the urine unchanged and the remainder as metabolites.

## ❦ NURSING CONSIDERATIONS

### Side effects, toxicities, and associated nursing actions

**CNS** Incoordination.

**Eye** Blurred vision, miosis, lacrimation.

- Assess stability and vision. If incoordination or visual difficulties occur, caution patients to avoid driving and other hazardous activities until the effects of the medication wear off. Supervise ambulation.
- Notify physician if side effects are severe or persistent.

**CV** Hypotension, change in heart rate.

- Monitor pulse and blood pressure for first hour following administration.
- If hypotension is present, caution patient to remain recumbent until blood pressure stabilizes. Keep siderails up. Supervise ambulation.

**GI** Nausea, vomiting, excessive salivation.

**GU** Urinary urgency.

**Skin** Sweating.

- Anticipate an exaggerated response to this drug. Have available emesis basin, and bedpan or urinal.
- Anticipate the patient may be unable to walk to bathroom without voiding.
- Have atropine readily available to treat overdose or toxicity.

**Lung** Increased secretions, bronchospasm.

- Have atropine available to treat excessive response.

### Nursing interventions related to drug administration

- Check pulse prior to administering. If less than 80, withhold dose and notify physician.
- Read orders carefully. Dosage for oral neostigmine bromide (see p. 792) is approximately 30 times as large as the parenteral dosages for neostigmine methylsulfate.
- For the use of neostigmine in the treatment of the patient with myasthenia gravis, see p. 792.
- Aspirate carefully prior to injecting parenteral doses to avoid inadvertent IV administration. If blood is aspirated, withdraw needle and prepare fresh dose.

### Patient and family education

- Review with patient anticipated benefits and possible side effects of therapy.

# Chapter Fifty-seven

# Anticholinergic-antispasmodic drugs

anisotropine

atropine

clidinium

dicyclomine

glycopyrrolate

hexocyclium

homatropine

hyoscyamine

isopropamide

mepenzolate

methantheline

methscopolamine

oxyphencyclimine

oxyphenonium

propantheline

tridihexethyl

## DRUG COMBINATIONS

- atropine sulfate and meperidine HCl: Atropine and Demerol Injection (C-II)
- atropine sulfate and morphine sulfate: Morphine and Atropine Sulfates Injection (C-II)
- atropine sulfate, hyoscyamine sulfate, phenobarbital, and scopolamine HBr: Barbidonna, Bellalphen, Donnatal, Hybephen, Hyosophen, Kinesed
- clidinium bromide and chlordiazepoxide HCl: CDP Plus, chlordinium Sealets, Clindex, Clinoxide, Clipoxide, Librax, Lidox, Lidoxide
- hyoscyamine sulfate and phenobarbital: Levsinex, Levsin with Phenobarbital Elixir
- tridihexethyl Cl and meprobamate: Hexabamate, Milpath, Pathibamate, Premate, Trimate

**OVERVIEW OF THE DRUG CLASS**  Anticholinergic-antispasmodic drugs are used for selected patients who have problems related to excessive intestinal motility or peptic ulcer. The classic cholinergic antagonist, atropine, is the prototype of this drug class. Atropine is the classic muscarinic receptor antagonist, blocking peripheral actions of the parasympathetic nervous system. Atropine also has CNS effects, however, so derivatives were designed to carry a charge that prevented their crossing the blood-brain barrier. Finally, drugs were developed that had antispasmodic effects but no anticholinergic effects. These drugs relax the smooth muscle of the gastrointestinal tract and are used to treat hyperactivity or spasm of the intestine.

**MECHANISM OF ACTION**  Anticholinergic drugs are antagonists of acetylcholine and act by blocking the muscarinic receptors. The muscarinic receptors are those receptors for acetylcholine on the tissues innervated by the postganglionic neurons of the parasympathomimetic nervous system. (The term muscarinic is from muscarine, the mushroom toxin.) Cholinergic actions include stimulation of gastric acid secretion and intestinal motility, so drugs to block these actions are useful in treating ulcers and hypermotility syndromes.

**Atropinelike effects**  Atropine is the prototype muscarinic antagonist. Physiologic functions vary in their sensitivity to muscarinic antagonists. In general, the order of sensitivity (from most to least sensitive) is secretions of the salivary, bronchial, and sweat glands; pupillary dilation, ocular accommodation and heart rate; contraction of the detrusor muscle of the bladder and smooth muscle of the GI tract; and gastric secretion and motility. On a practical level, this means that doses of antimuscarinic drugs that decrease gastric secretions will probably cause dryness of the mouth (xerostomia), blurred vision due to an interference with accommodation and photophobia due to dilated pupils (mydriasis), and urinary retention.

**CNS effects**  Anticholinergic drugs that cross the blood-brain barrier cause CNS effects. At toxic doses, CNS stimulation manifested as restlessness, irritability, disorientation, hallucinations, and delirium. These CNS effects are the common toxic effects of atropine and anticholinergic drugs crossing the blood-brain barrier.

**Ganglionic effects**  Many of the anticholinergic drugs used to treat gastrointestinal disorders are quaternary ammonium compounds carrying a permanent positive charge. As charged compounds, these anticholinergics do not cross the blood-brain barrier to cause CNS effects. Toxic levels of these charged compounds are manifested as ganglionic blockage. The major symptom of ganglionic blockade is orthostatic hypotension.

**INDICATIONS**  **Esophageal spasm** Anticholinergic agents decrease esophageal and gastric motility and relax the lower esophageal sphincter.    **Peptic ulcer** These agents may relieve some of the pain of gastric and duodenal ulcer by inhibiting motility and secretions. However, the H-2 receptor antagonists and antacids are the drugs of choice. **Pancreatitis** Generally, anticholinergics are minimally effective at best in reducing pancreatic secretions. **Irritable bowel syndrome** Anticholinergics are useful, especially when abdominal pain and constipation are prominent. **Inflammatory bowel disease** Anticholinergics, however, must be used with caution. If the colon is rendered unresponsive, a condition called toxic megacolon may result and may be fatal.

**CONTRAINDICATIONS** **GI infections** Toxins may be retained and cause toxic megacolon. **Hypersensitivity.** **Infants** Infants under 6 weeks of age are more prone to react with respiratory distress, seizures, poor muscle tone, and coma. **Geriatric patients** This group is more sensitive to the adverse effects of anticholinergic drugs. **Esophageal reflux** Anticholinergic drugs promote gastric retention and aggravate reflux.

**DRUG INTERACTIONS** **Drugs with anticholinergic effects** These include phenothiazines, amantadine, antiparkinson drugs, glutethimide, meperidine, tricyclic antidepressants, quinidine, disopyramide, and some antihistamines. These give additive anticholinergic activity: dry mouth, blurred vision, and constipation. **GI absorption** Anticholinergics can interfere with or delay the absorption of orally administered drugs. Specifically, levodopa absorption may be decreased and that of digoxin may be increased. **Antacids** decrease the absorption of anticholinergics when taken with them. The anticholinergic should be taken an hour before the antacids. **Potassium chloride** Anticholinergics may delay the absorption of potassium chloride, leading to GI mucosal lesions.

## ☙ NURSING CONSIDERATIONS

### Side effects, toxicities, and associated nursing actions

**CNS** CNS stimulation, manifested as restlessness, irritability, disorientation, hallucinations, and delirium at toxic doses.
- Monitor level of consciousness and level of activity.
- Reorient as needed.
- If CNS symptoms are prominent, supervise the patient carefully. Keep side rails up, keep night lights on, and notify the physician.

**CV** Orthostatic hypotension caused by ganglionic blockade. Caution patients to move slowly from lying to sitting or standing. Postural hypotension may be aggravated by prolonged periods of standing or hot showers. Instruct the patient to sit down if dizzness or lightheadedness occurs. In some patients, the use of elastic support stockings may be helpful.
- Keep side rails up on hospital beds.

**Eye** Blurred vision and photophobia.
- If blurred vision occurs, caution patients to avoid driving or operating hazardous equipment until effects of medication wear off.
- Keep lights in the room dim.
- If photophobia occurs, caution the patient to wear sunglasses. Patients should not wear sunglasses while driving at night or in situations where limited vision could be hazardous. Instruct the patient to notify the physician.

**GI** Dry mouth and constipation
- Instruct patients to chew sugarless hard candy or sugarless gum or to take frequent sips of water. Frequent oral hygiene may increase comfort, but drying mouthwashes and gargles should be avoided. The use of commercially available saliva substitutes may be used by some individuals.
- Keep a record of bowel movements.
- Auscultate bowel sounds on a regular basis.
- For constipation, encourage the patient to increase fluid intake to 2500 to 3000 ml/day, to increase intake of fruit and juices, and to add fiber to the diet if not contraindicated by other dietary requirements. Encourage patients to increase level of activity.

**GU** Urinary retention.
- Monitor intake and output.
- Urinary retention is more frequently encountered in the immobilized and in men with preexisting prostatic hypertrophy. Assess carefully patients who have not voided in 4 hours; palpate the bladder

for distention.
- Have patients void prior to administering each dose of medication.

**Lung** Bronchospasm.
- Be alert to this frightening side effect. Have oxygen available. Notify physician.

**Skin** Flushed, dry.
- Monitor temperature every 4 hours.
- Assess skin turgor, mucous membranes.
- Caution patients to avoid hot settings or strenuous work without frequent periods to cool down.

**Nursing interventions related to drug administration**
- IM preparations should be administered in a large muscle mass such as the dorsogluteal site or rectus femoris muscle in adults or the vastus lateralis muscle in infants and small children. Use anatomical landmarks to carefully identify sites. Aspirate carefully prior to injecting medication to avoid inadvertent intravenous injection. If blood is withdrawn, withdraw needle and prepare fresh dose of medication. Record injection site and rotate sites.
- Oral doses are customarily administered 30 minutes prior to each meal and at bedtime.
- For the use of these drugs for ophthalmic conditions, see p. 1032.

**Patient and family education**
- Review with patients the anticipated benefits and possible side effects of therapy.
- Review with patients dietary requirements for their health problem. Reinforce to patients the need to take medications and observe dietary requirements on a regular basis to hasten healing or prevent recurrences of GI problems.

## anisotropine methylbromide
(an-iss-oh-TROE-peen)                                                    anticholinergic-antispasmodic

- anisotropine methylbromide: ♣Ansaid, Valpin

**MECHANISM OF ACTION**    Anisotropine is a quaternary ammonium anticholinergic compound. • See entry for drug class for a complete discussion (p. 991).

**INDICATIONS**    Peptic ulcer.

**CONTRAINDICATIONS**    **GI infections** Toxins may be retained and cause toxic megacolon.    **Hypersensitivity.**    **Infants** Infants under 6 weeks of age are more prone to react with respiratory distress, seizures, poor muscle tone, and coma.    **Geriatric patients** This group is more sensitive to the adverse effects of anticholinergic drugs.    **Esophageal reflux** Anticholinergic drugs promote gastric retention and aggravate reflux.

**DOSAGE**    **PO:** **ADULTS:** 50 mg three times daily. *Special patient populations:* **ELDERLY:** Geriatric patients are more sensitive to the side effects of anticholinergic drugs. **CHILDREN:** Not recommended for children. **PREGNANCY:** Safe use has not been established. Not recommended for nursing mothers because of possible adverse effects on the infant.

**PREPARATIONS**    *Tablets:* 50 mg.

**DRUG INTERACTIONS**    **Drugs with anticholinergic effects** These include phenothiazines, amantadine, antiparkinson drugs, glutethimide, meperidine, tricyclic antidepressants, quinidine, disopyramide, and some antihistamines. These give additive anticholinergic activity: dry mouth, blurred vision, and constipation.    **GI absorption** Anticholinergics can interfere with or delay the absorption of orally administered drugs. Specifically, levodopa absorption may be decreased and that of digoxin may be increased.    **Antacids** decrease the absorption of anticholinergics when taken with them. The anticholinergics should be taken an hour before the antacids.    **Potassium chloride** Anticholinergics may delay the absorption of potassium chloride, leading to GI mucosal lesions.

**FATE**    Anisotropine is incompletely absorbed from the GI tract. The metabolic fate of anisotropine has not been well characterized.

❦ **NURSING CONSIDERATIONS**
**Side effects, toxicities, and associated nursing actions**
- See entry for drug class (p. 992).

**CV** Orthostatic hypotension secondary to ganglionic blockage.
**Eye** Blurred vision and photophobia.
**GI** Dry mouth and constipation.
**GU** Urinary retention.
**Lung** Bronchospasm.
**Skin** Flushed, dry.

### Nursing interventions related to drug administration
   • See entry for drug class (p. 993).
### Patient and family education
   • See entry for drug class (p. 993).

---

## atropine, atropine sulfate   (A-troe-peen)                     anticholinergic

   • atropine: generic; Dey-Dose, Dey-Lute

**MECHANISM OF ACTION**   Atropine is the prototypic muscarinic antagonist. It is a naturally occurring compound derived from the belladonna plant.
   • See entry for drug class for further information (p. 991).

**INDICATIONS**   **GI disorders** Atropine has generally been replaced by synthetic or semisynthetic anticholinergic drugs.   **Surgery** Atropine has been used preoperatively to inhibit salivation and excessive secretions of the respiratory tract.   **Bronchodilation** Atropine can be administered by oral inhalation for acute bronchospasm associated with asthma.   **Ophthalmic** To cause mydriasis and paralyzed accommodation for examinations. • See Chapter 61.

**CONTRAINDICATIONS**   **GI infections** Toxins may be retained and cause toxic megacolon.   **Hypersensitivity.**
   **Infants** Infants under 6 weeks of age are more prone to react with respiratory distress, seizures, poor muscle tone, and coma.   **Geriatric patients** This group is more sensitive to the adverse effects of anticholinergic drugs.   **Esophageal reflux** Anticholinergic drugs promote gastric retention and aggravate reflux.

**DOSAGE**   **PO, IV, IM, SC:**   ADULTS: 0.4 to 0.6 mg every 4 to 6 hours.   **IV, IM, SC:**   CHILDREN: 0.01 mg/kg, not exceeding 0.4 mg, every 4 to 6 hours as needed.   **Inhalation:**   ADULTS: 0.025 mg/kg via a nebulizer three or four times daily.   CHILDREN: 0.05 mg/kg via a nebulizer three or four times daily.   *Special patient populations:*   ELDERLY: Geriatric patients are more sensitive to the side effects of anticholinergic drugs.   PREGNANCY: Safe use has not been established. Not recommended for nursing mothers because of possible adverse effects on the infant.

**PREPARATIONS**   *Sulfate: tablets:* 0.4 mg; *tablets (soluble):* 0.3, 0.4, or 0.6 mg; *solution (nebulization):* 0.033%, 0.2%, or 0.5%; *injection:* 10 mg; 0.05, 0.1, 0.3, 0.4, 0.5, 0.6, 0.8, 1, or 1.2 mg/ml.

**DRUG INTERACTIONS**   **Drugs with anticholinergic effects** These include phenothiazines, amantadine, antiparkinson drugs, glutethimide, meperidine, tricyclic antidepressants, quinidine, disopyramide, and some antihistamines. These give additive anticholinergic activity: dry mouth, blurred vision, and constipation.   **GI absorption** Anticholinergics can interfere with or delay the absorption of orally administered drugs. Specifically, levodopa absorption may be decreased and that of digoxin may be increased.   **Antacids** decrease the absorption of anticholinergics when taken with them. The anticholinergic should be taken an hour before the antacids.   **Potassium chloride** Anticholinergics may delay the absorption of potassium chloride, leading to GI mucosal lesions.

**FATE**   Atropine is well absorbed from the GI tract. The *onset of action* is 30 to 60 minutes, and the *duration of action* is 4 hours. Atropine is metabolized in the liver and excreted in the urine.

### ☙ NURSING CONSIDERATIONS
#### Side effects, toxicities, and associated nursing actions
   • See entry for drug class (p. 992).
   **CV** Orthostatic hypotension secondary to ganglionic blockade.

**Eye** Blurred vision and photophobia.
**GI** Dry mouth and constipation.
**GU** Urinary retention.
**Lung** Bronchospasm.
**Skin** Flushed, dry.

### Nursing Inverventions related to drug administration

- For IV administration, drug may be given undiluted but may be diluted in at least 10 ml of sterile water. Do not add to infusing fluids or drugs. Administer at a rate of 0.6 mg over at least 1 minute.
- Physostigmine salicylate is the antidote for cardiovascular and CNS toxic effects.
- See entry for drug class (p. 993).

### Patient and family education

- See entry for drug class (p. 993).

---

## clidinium bromide  (kli-DI-nee-um)                                    anticholinergic

- clidinium bromide: Quarzan

**MECHANISM OF ACTION**   Clidinium is a synthetic quaternary ammonium antimuscarinic drug. • See entry for drug class for further information (p. 991).

**INDICATIONS**   **GI disorders** An adjunct for treating peptic ulcer disease and functional bowel disorder.

**CONTRAINDICATIONS**   **GI infections** Toxins may be retained and cause toxic megacolon.   **Hypersensitivity.**
**Infants** Infants under 6 weeks of age are more prone to react with respiratory distress, seizures, poor muscle tone, and coma.   **Geriatric patients** This group is more sensitive to the adverse effects of anticholinergic drugs.   **Esophageal reflux** Anticholinergic drugs promote gastric retention and aggravate reflux.

**DOSAGE**   **PO:**   **ADULTS:** 2.5 to 5 mg three or four times daily.   *Special patient populations:*   **ELDERLY:** Geriatric patients are more sensitive to the side effects of anticholinergic drugs.   **CHILDREN:** Not recommended for children.   **PREGNANCY:** Safe use has not been established. Not recommended for nursing mothers because of possible adverse effects on the infant.

**PREPARATIONS**   *Capsules:* 2.5 or 5 mg.

**DRUG INTERACTIONS**   **Drugs with anticholinergic effects** These include phenothiazines, amantidine, antiparkinson drugs, glutethimide, meperidine, tricyclic antidepressants, quinidine, disopyramide, and some antihistamines. These give additive anticholinergic activity: dry mouth, blurred vision, and constipation.   **GI absorption** Anticholinergics can interfere with or delay the absorption of orally administered drugs. Specifically, levodopa absorption may be decreased and that of digoxin may be increased.   **Antacids** decrease the absorption of anticholinergics when taken with them. The anticholinergic should be taken an hour before the antacids.   **Potassium chloride** Anticholinergics may delay the absorption of potassium chloride, leading to GI mucosal lesions.

**FATE**   Clidinium is incompletely absorbed from the GI tract. The *onset of action* is 1 hour, and the *duration of action* is 3 hours. Clidinium is metabolized in the liver and excreted in the urine and feces.

### ☙ NURSING CONSIDERATIONS

#### Side effects, toxicities, and associated nursing actions

- See entry for drug class (p. 992).
**CV** Slowing of heart rate secondary to vagal stimulation; orthostatic hypotension secondary to ganglionic blockade.
**Eye** Blurred vision, photophobia.
**GI** Dry mouth, constipation.
**GU** Urinary retention.
**Lung** Bronchospasm.

**Skin** Flushed, dry.

**Nursing interventions related to drug administration**
- See entry for drug class (p. 993).

**Patient and family education**
- See entry for drug class (p. 993).

---

# dicyclomine hydrochloride    (dye-SYE-kloe-meen)      antispasmodic

- dicyclomine hydrochloride: A-Spas, Antispas, Bentyl, ✿Bentylol, Byclomine, Di-Spaz, ✿Spasmoban, others

**MECHANISM OF ACTION**    Dicyclomine is a tertiary amine with antispasmodic activity but not anticholinergic activity. See entry for drug class for further information (p. 991).

**INDICATIONS**    Irritable bowel syndrome.

**CONTRAINDICATIONS**    **GI infections** Toxins may be retained and cause toxic megacolon.    **Hypersensitivity.** **Infants** Infants under 6 weeks of age are more prone to react with respiratory distress, seizures, poor muscle tone, and coma.    **Geriatric patients** This group is more sensitive to the adverse effects of anticholinergic drugs.    **Esophageal reflux** Anticholinergic drugs promote gastric retention and aggravate reflux.

**DOSAGE**    **PO:**    **ADULTS:** 10 to 20 mg three to four times daily. *Special patient populations:* **ELDERLY:** Geriatric patients are more sensitive to the side effects of anticholinergic drugs. **CHILDREN:** In the U.S., not recommended for children. **PREGNANCY:** Safe use has not been established. Not recommended for nursing mothers because of possible adverse effects on the infant.

**PREPARATIONS**    *Capsules:* 10 or 20 mg; *solution:* 10 mg/5 mg; *tablets:* 20 mg; injection (IM only): 10 mg/ml. Do not combine in the same syringe with chloramphenicol, diazepam, sodium pentobarbital, or sodium bicarbonate.

**DRUG INTERACTIONS**    **Drugs with anticholinergic effects** These include phenothiazines, amantadine, antiparkinson drugs, glutethimide, meperidine, tricyclic antidepressants, quinidine, disopyramide, and some antihistamines. These give additive anticholinergic activity: dry mouth, blurred vision, and constipation.    **GI absorption** Anticholinergics can interfere with or delay the absorption of orally administered drugs. Specifically, levodopa absorption may be decreased and that of digoxin may be increased.    **Antacids** Decrease the absorption of anticholinergics when taken with them. The anticholinergic should be taken an hour before the antacids.    **Potassium chloride** Anticholinergics may delay the absorption of potassium chloride, leading to GI mucosal lesions.

**FATE**    Dicyclomine is slowly absorbed from the GI tract. Dicyclomine is metabolized in the liver and excreted in the urine and feces.

❦ **NURSING CONSIDERATIONS**

Side effects, toxicities, and associated nursing actions
- See entry for drug class (p. 992).

**CNS** Euphoria, dizziness, drowsiness, headache, and weakness.

**GI** Nausea.

**Nursing interventions related to drug administration**
- See entry for drug class (p. 993).

**Patient and family education**
- See entry for drug class (p. 993).

---

# glycopyrrolate    (glye-koe-PYE-roe-late)      anticholinergic

- glycopyrrolate: Robinul

**MECHANISM OF ACTION**    Glycopyrrolate is a synthetic quaternary ammonium antimuscarinic drug. See entry for drug class for further information (p. 991).

**INDICATIONS**    **Peptic ulcer** Glycopyrrolate is an adjunct in the treatment of peptic ulcer.    **Surgery** Glycopyrrolate is used as a preoperative medication to inhibit salivation and excessive secretions of the respiratory tract.

**CONTRAINDICATIONS**    **GI infections** Toxins may be retained and cause toxic megacolon.    **Hypersensitivity. Infants** Infants under 6 weeks of age are more prone to react with respiratory distress, seizures, poor muscle tone, and coma.    **Geriatric patients** This group is more sensitive to the adverse effects of anticholinergic drugs.    **Esophageal reflux** Anticholinergic drugs promote gastric retention and aggravate reflux.

**DOSAGE**    Peptic ulcer disease: *PO, IM, IV:*    ADULTS: 1 mg three times daily.    **Surgery:** *IM:* ADULTS AND CHILDREN OVER 2 YEARS OLD: 0.0044 mg/kg, 30 to 60 minutes before surgery. *Special patient populations:*    ELDERLY: Geriatric patients are more sensitive to the side effects of anticholinergic drugs.    PREGNANCY: Safe use has not been established. Not recommended for nursing mothers because of possible adverse effects on the infant.

**PREPARATIONS**    *Tablets:* 1 or 2 mg; *injection:* 0.2 mg/ml.

**DRUG INTERACTIONS**    **Drugs with anticholinergic effects** These include phenothiazines, amantadine, antiparkinson drugs, glutethimide, meperidine, tricyclic antidepressants, quinidine, disopyramide, and some antihistamines. These give additive anticholinergic activity: dry mouth, blurred vision, and constipation.    **GI absorption** Anticholinergics can interfere with or delay the absorption of orally administered drugs. Specifically, levodopa absorption may be decreased and that of digoxin may be increased.    **Antacids** decrease the absorption of anticholinergics when taken with them. The anticholinergic should be taken an hour before the antacids.    **Potassium chloride** Anticholinergics may delay the absorption of potassium chloride, leading to GI mucosal lesions.

**FATE**    Glycopyrrolate is incompletely absorbed from the GI tract. The *onset of action* is about 1 minute after IV injection, 15 to 30 minutes after IM or SC injection, and longer after oral administration. The *duration of action* is 8 to 12 hours after oral administration but shorter after parenteral administration. Glycopyrrolate is metabolized in the liver and excreted mainly in the feces.

### 🐾 NURSING CONSIDERATIONS

#### Side effects, toxicities, and associated nursing actions
- See entry for drug class (p. 992).

**CV** Slowing of heart rate secondary to vagal stimulation; orthostatic hypotension secondary to ganglionic blockade.
**Eye** Blurred vision, photophobia.
**GI** Dry mouth, constipation.
**GU** Urinary retention.
**Lung** Bronchospasm.
**Skin** Flushed, dry.

#### Nursing interventions related to drug administration
- IV doses may be given undiluted at a rate of 0.2 mg or less over 1 to 2 minutes.

#### Patient and family education
- See entry for drug class (p. 993).

---

## hexocyclium methylsulfate    (hex-oh-SYE-klee-um)    anticholinergic

- hexocyclium methylsulfate: Tral Filmtab

**MECHANISM OF ACTION**    Hexocyclium is a synthetic quaternary ammonium antimuscarinic drug. See entry for drug class for further information (p. 991).

**INDICATIONS**    **Peptic ulcer** Hexocyclium is adjunct therapy.

**CONTRAINDICATIONS**    **GI infections** Toxins may be retained and cause toxic megacolon.    **Hypersensitivity. Infants** Infants under 6 weeks of age are more prone to react with respiratory distress, seizures, poor muscle tone, and coma.    **Geriatric patients** This group is more sensitive to the adverse effects of anticholinergic drugs.    **Esophageal reflux** Anticholinergic drugs promote gastric retention and aggravate reflux.

**DOSAGE**    **PO:**    **ADULTS:** 25 mg four times daily. Alternatively, 50 mg of the timed-release form is given twice daily at lunch and bedtime.    *Special patient populations:*    **ELDERLY:** Geriatric patients are more sensitive to the side effects of anticholinergic drugs.    **CHILDREN:** Not recommended for children.    **PREGNANCY:** Safe use has not been established. Not recommended for nursing mothers because of possible adverse effects on the infant.

**PREPARATIONS**    *Tablets (film-coated):* 25 mg; *timed-release:* 50 mg.

**DRUG INTERACTIONS**    **Drugs with anticholinergic effects** These include phenothiazines, amantadine, antiparkinson drugs, glutethimide, meperidine, tricyclic antidepressants, quinidine, disopyramide, and some antihistamines. These give additive anticholinergic activity: dry mouth, blurred vision, and constipation.    **GI absorption** Anticholinergics can interfere with or delay the absorption of orally administered drugs. Specifically, levodopa absorption may be decreased and that of digoxin may be increased.    **Antacids** Decrease the absorption of anticholinergics when taken together. The anticholinergic should be taken an hour before the antacids.,    **Potassium chloride** Anticholinergics may delay the absorption of potassium chloride, leading to GI mucosal lesions.

**FATE**    Hexocyclium is poorly absorbed from the GI tract. The *onset of action* is variable, and the *duration of action* is 4 hours. The metabolic fate has not been well characterized, but hexocyclium probably is metabolized in the liver and excreted in the feces.

## ☙ NURSING CONSIDERATIONS

### Side effects, toxicities, and associated nursing actions

- See entry for drug class (p. 992).

**CV** Slowing of heart rate secondary to vagal stimulation; orthostatic hypotension secondary to ganglionic blockade.

**Eye** Blurred vision, photophobia.

**GI** Dry mouth, constipation.

**GU** Urinary retention.

**Lung** Bronchospasm.

**Skin** Flushed, dry.

### Nursing interventions related to drug administration

- Tral Filmtab brand tablets contain FD & C yellow dye #5 (tartrazine), which may cause an allergic response in susceptible individuals. Although rare, this side effect is seen more often in persons with aspirin hypersensitivity.

### Patient and family education

- See entry for drug class (p. 993).

---

## homatropine methylbromide    (hoe-MA-troe-peen)    anticholinergic

- homatropine methylbromide: Homapin, ✤Iso-Homatropine

**MECHANISM OF ACTION**    Homatropine is a semisynthetic derivative of atropine. The methylbromide form is a quaternary ammonium. See entry for drug class for further information (p. 991).

**INDICATIONS**    **Peptic ulcer disease** Homatropine is adjunctive therapy.

**CONTRAINDICATIONS**    **GI infections** Toxins may be retained and cause toxic megacolon.    **Hypersensitivity.**    **Infants** Infants under 6 weeks of age are more prone to react with respiratory distress, seizures, poor muscle tone, and coma.    **Geriatric patients** This group is more sensitive to the adverse effects of anticholinergic drugs.    **Esophageal reflux** Anticholinergic drugs promote gastric retention and aggravate reflux.

**DOSAGE**    **PO:**    **ADULTS:** 5 to 10 mg three or four times daily. Give before meals and at bedtime.    *Special patient populations:*    **ELDERLY:** Geriatric patients are more sensitive to the side effects of anticholinergic drugs.    **CHILDREN:** Not recommended for children.    **PREGNANCY:** Safe use has not been established. Not recommended for nursing mothers because of possible adverse effects on the infant.

**PREPARATIONS**   *Tablets:* 5 or 10 mg.

**DRUG INTERACTIONS**   **Drugs with anticholinergic effects** These include phenothiazines, amantadine, antiparkinson drugs, glutethimide, meperdine, tricyclic antidepressants, quinidine, disopyramide, and some antihistamines. These give additive anticholinergic activity: dry mouth, blurred vision, and constipation.   **GI absorption** Anticholinergics can interfere with or delay the absorption of orally administered drugs. Specifically, levodopa absorption may be decreased and that of digoxin may be increased.   **Antacids** Decrease the absorption of anticholinergics when taken with them. The anticholinergic should be taken an hour before the antacids.   **Potassium chloride** Anticholinergics may delay the absorption of potassium chloride, leading to GI mucosal lesions.

**FATE**   Homatropine is poorly absorbed from the GI tract. The *onset of action* is variable. The metabolic fate of homatropine has not been well characterized.

## ❦ NURSING CONSIDERATIONS

### Side effects, toxicities, and associated nursing actions
- See entry for drug class (p. 992).

**CV** Orthostatic hypotension secondary to ganglionic blockade.

**Eye** Blurred vision, photophobia.

**GI** Dry mouth, constipation.

**GU** Urinary retention.

**Lung** Bronchospasm.

**Skin** Flushed, dry.

### Nursing interventions related to drug administration
- See entry for drug class (p. 993).

### Patient and family education
- See entry for drug class (p. 993).

---

## hyoscyamine, hyoscyamine sulfate   (hye-oh-SYE-a-meen)   anticholinergic

- hyoscyamine, hyoscyamine sulfate: Anaspaz, Cystospaz-M, Levsin, Levsinex Timecaps, Neoques

**MECHANISM OF ACTION**   Hyoscyamine is a naturally occuring tertiary amine, one of the principal components of belladonna and an antimuscarinic agent. See entry for drug class (p. 991) for further information.

**INDICATIONS**   **Peptic ulcer disease and irritable bowel syndrome** Hyoscyamine is adjunctive therapy.   **Genitourinary tract disorders** Hyoscyamine is adjunctive therapy.   **Infant colic** Although hyoscyamine has been used, its effectiveness is doubtful.   **Surgery** Preoperative medication to inhibit salivation and other secretions.

**CONTRAINDICATIONS**   **GI infections** Toxins may be retained and cause toxic megacolon.   **Hypersensitivity.** **Infants** Infants under 6 weeks of age are more prone to react with respiratory distress, seizures, poor muscle tone, and coma.   **Geriatric patients** This group is more sensitive to the adverse effects of anticholinergic drugs.   **Esophageal reflux** Anticholinergic drugs promote gastric retention and aggravate reflux.

**DOSAGE**   **Hyoscyamine:** *PO:*   ADULTS: 0.15 to 0.3 mg, up to four times daily.   **Hyoscyamine sulfate:** *PO, sublingual:*   ADULTS: 0.125 to 0.25 mg. three or four times daily.   CHILDREN: 0.0125 mg for children under 10 pounds, 0.025 mg for children 10 to 15 pounds, 0.05 mg for children 15 to 20 pounds, 0.0625 mg for children 20 to 25 lbs, 0.075 mg for children 25 to 30 lbs. Add increments of 0.025 mg for each 10 lb of body weight, up to 0.125 mg at 80 lb. Dose may be repeated every 4 hours as needed.   *IM, IV, SC:* For GI disorders, give double the oral dose. For adults and children over 2 years old, give 0.005 mg/kg as preoperative medication. *Special patient populations:*   ELDERLY: Geriatric patients are more sensitive to the side effects of anticholinergic drugs.   PREGNANCY: Safe use has not been established. Not recommended for nursing mothers because of possible adverse effects on the infant.

**PREPARATIONS** Hyoscyamine: *tablets:* 0.15 mg. *Hyoscyamine bromide: capsules (extended release):* 0.375 mg; *elixir:* 0.125 mg/5 ml; Solution: 0.125 mg/ml; *tablets:* 0.125 mg; *injection:* 0.5 mg/ml.

**DRUG INTERACTIONS** **Drugs with anticholinergic effects** These include phenothiazines, amantadine, antiparkinson drugs, glutethimide, meperidine, tricyclic antidepressants, quinidine, disopyramide, and some antihistamines. These give additive anticholinergic activity: dry mouth, blurred vision, and constipation. **GI absorption** Anticholinergics can interfere with or delay the absorption of orally administered drugs. Specifically, levodopa absorption may be decreased and that of digoxin may be increased. **Antacids** Decrease the absorption of anticholinergics when taken with them. The anticholinergic should be taken an hour before the antacids. **Potassium chloride** Anticholinergics may delay the absorption of potassium chloride, leading to GI mucosal lesions.

**FATE** Hyoscyamine is well absorbed from the GI tract. The *onset of action* is 20 to 30 minutes, and the *duration of action* is 12 hours. Hyoscyamine is metabolized in the liver and excreted in the urine.

## ☙ NURSING CONSIDERATIONS

### Side effects, toxicities, and associated nursing actions
- See entry for drug class (p. 992).

**CNS** CNS stimulation, manifested as restlessness, irritability, disorientation, hallucinations, and delirium at toxic doses.

**CV** Slowing of heart rate secondary to vagal stimulation.

**Eye** Blurred vision, photophobia.

**GI** Dry mouth, constipation.

**GU** Urinary retention.

**Lung** Bronchospasm.

**Skin** Flushed, dry.

### Nursing interventions related to drug administration
- For IV administration, may be given undiluted. Administer dose over at least 1 minute.

### Patient and family education
- See entry for drug class (p. 993).

---

## isopropamide iodide  (eye-so-PROE-pa-mide)  anticholinergic

- isopropamide iodide: Darbid

**MECHANISM OF ACTION** Isopropamide is a synthetic quaternary amine with antimuscarinic activity. See entry for drug class for further information (p. 991).

**INDICATIONS** **Peptic ulcer disease** Adjunctive therapy.

**CONTRAINDICATIONS** **GI infections** Toxins may be retained and cause toxic megacolon. **Hypersensitivity.** **Infants** Infants under 6 weeks of age are more prone to react with respiratory distress, seizures, poor muscle tone, and coma. **Geriatric patients** This group is more sensitive to the adverse effects of anticholinergic drugs. **Esophageal reflux** Anticholinergic drugs promote gastric retention and aggravate reflux.

**DOSAGE** **PO:** **ADULTS:** 5 mg every 12 hours. *Special patient populations:* **ELDERLY:** Geriatric patients are more sensitive to the side effects of anticholinergic drugs. **CHILDREN:** Not recommended for children. **PREGNANCY:** Safe use has not been established. Not recommended for nursing mothers because of possible adverse effects on the infant.

**PREPARATIONS** *Tablets:* 5 mg.

**DRUG INTERACTIONS** **Drugs with anticholinergic effects** These include phenothiazines, amantadine, antiparkinson drugs, glutethimide, meperidine, tricyclic antidepressants, quinidine, disopyramide, and some antihistamines. These give additive anticholinergic activity: dry mouth, blurred vision, and constipation. **GI absorption** Anticholinergics can interfere with or delay the absorption of orally administered drugs. Specifically, levodopa absorption may be decreased and that of digoxin may be increased.    **Antacids** decrease the absorption of anticholinergics when taken together. The anticholinergic should be taken an hour before the antacids.    **Potassium chloride** Anticholinergics may delay the absorption of potassium chloride, leading to GI mucosal lesions.

**FATE**  Isopropamide is incompletely absorbed from the GI tract. The *duration of action* is 10 to 12 hours. Isopropamide is excreted in the urine and feces.

## ☙ NURSING CONSIDERATIONS

### Side effects, toxicities, and associated nursing actions
- See entry for drug class (p. 992).

**CV** Orthostatic hypotension secondary to ganglionic blockade.

**Eye** Blurred vision, photophobia.

**GI** Dry mouth, constipation.

**GU** Urinary retention.

**Lung** Bronchospasm.

**Skin** Flushed, dry.

### Nursing interventions related to drug administration
- See entry for drug class (p. 993).

### Patient and family education
- See entry for drug class (p. 993).

---

## mepenzolate bromide    (me-PEN-soe-late)    anticholinergic

- mepenzolate bromide: Cantil

**MECHANISM OF ACTION**    Mepenzolate is a synthetic quaternary amine with antimuscarinic activity. See entry for drug class for further information (p. 991).

**INDICATIONS**    **Peptic ulcer disease** Adjunctive therapy.

**CONTRAINDICATIONS**    **GI infections** Toxins may be retained and cause toxic megacolon.    **Hypersensitivity.** **Infants** Infants under 6 weeks of age are more prone to react with respiratory distress, seizures, poor muscle tone, and coma.    **Geriatric patients** This group is more sensitive to the adverse effects of anticholinergic drugs.    **Esophageal reflux** Anticholinergic drugs promote gastric retention and aggravate reflux.

**DOSAGE**    **PO:**  **ADULTS:** 25 or 50 mg three or four times daily.  *Special patient populations:*  **ELDERLY:** Geriatric patients are more sensitive to the side effects of anticholinergic drugs.  **CHILDREN:** Not recommended for children.  **PREGNANCY:** Safe use has not been established. Not recommended for nursing mothers because of possible adverse effects on the infant.

**PREPARATIONS**    *Tablets:* 25 mg.

**DRUG INTERACTIONS**    **Drugs with anticholinergic effects** These include phenothiazines, amantadine, antiparkinson drugs, glutethimide, meperidine, tricyclic antidepressants, quinidine, disopyramide, and some antihistamines. These give additive anticholinergic activity: dry mouth, blurred vision, and constipation.    **GI absorption** Anticholinergics can interfere with or delay the absorption of orally administered drugs. Specifically, levodopa absorption may be decreased and that of digoxin may be increased.    **Antacids** decrease the absorption of anticholinergics when taken with thenm. The anticholinergic should be taken an hour before the antacids.    **Potassium chloride** Anticholinergics may delay the absorption of potassium chloride, leading to GI mucosal lesions.

**FATE**  Mepenzolate is incompletely absorbed from the GI tract. Mepenzolate is excreted in the urine and feces.

## ☙ NURSING CONSIDERATIONS

### Side effects, toxicities, and associated nursing actions
- See entry for drug class (p. 992).

**CV** Orthostatic hypotension secondary to ganglionic blockade.

**Eye** Blurred vision, photophobia.

**GI** Dry mouth, constipation.

**GU** Urinary retention.
**Lung** Bronchospasm.
**Skin** Flushed, dry

### Nursing interventions related to drug administration

• Cantil brand tablets contain FD & C yellow dye #5 (tartrazine), which may cause an allergic response in susceptible individuals. Although rare, this response is seen more frequently in persons with aspirin hypersensitivity.

### Patient and family education

• See entry for drug class (p. 993).

---

## methantheline bromide    (meth-AN-tha-leen)                                   anticholinergic

• methantheline: Banthine

**MECHANISM OF ACTION**    Methantheline is a synthetic quaternary amine with antimuscarinic activity. See entry for drug class for further information (p. 991).

**INDICATIONS**    **Peptic ulcer disease** Adjunctive therapy.    **Uninhibited or reflex neurogenic bladder** To reduce bladder contractions and increase capacity.

**CONTRAINDICATIONS**    **GI infections** Toxins may be retained and cause toxic megacolon.    **Hypersensitivity. Infants** Infants under 6 weeks of age are more prone to react with respiratory distress, seizures, poor muscle tone, and coma.    **Geriatric patients** This group is more sensitive to the adverse effects of anticholinergic drugs.    **Esophageal reflux** Anticholinergic drugs promote gastric retention and aggravate reflux.

**DOSAGE**    **PO:**    **ADULTS:** 50 to 100 mg every 6 hours.    **CHILDREN:** 12.5 mg two to three times daily in neonates to 1 month old; 12.5 to 25 mg four times daily for children ages 1 to 12 months old; 12.5 to 50 mg four times daily in children older than 1 year.    *Special patient populations:*    **ELDERLY:** Geriatric patients are more sensitive to the side effects of anticholinergic drugs.    **PREGNANCY:** Safe use has not been established. Not recommended for nursing mothers because of possible adverse effects on the infant.

**PREPERATIONS**    *Tablets:* 50 mg.

**DRUG INTERACTIONS**    **Drugs with anticholinergic effects** These include phenothiazines, amantadine, antiparkinson drugs, glutethimide, merpidine, tricyclic antidepressants, quinidine, disopyramide, and some antihistamines. These give additive anticholinergic activity: dry mouth, blurred vision, and constipation.    **GI absorption** Anticholinergics can interfere with or delay the absorption of orally administered drugs. Specifically, levodopa absorption may be decreased and that of digoxin may be increased.    **Antacids** decrease the absorption of anticholinergics when taken with them. The anticholinergic should be taken an hour before the antacids.    **Potassium chloride** Anticholinergics may delay the absorption of potassium chlorides, leading to GI mucosal lesions.

**FATE**    Methantheline is incompletely absorbed from the GI tract. Methantheline is excreted in the urine and feces.

### ☙ NURSING CONSIDERATIONS

### Side effects, toxicities, and associated nursing actions

• See entry for drug class (p. 992).
**CV** Orthostatic hypotension secondary to ganglionic blockade.
**Eye** Blurred vision, photophobia.
**GI** Dry mouth, constipation.
**GU** Urinary retention.
**Lung** Bronchospasm.
**Skin** Flushed, dry.

### Nursing interventions related to drug administration

• See entry for drug class (p. 993).

**Patient and family education**
• See entry for drug class (p. 993).

---

## methscopolamine bromide  (meth-skoe-POL-a-meen)          anticholinergic

• methscopolamine bromide: Pamine

**MECHANISM OF ACTION**   Methscopolamine is a synthetic quaternary amine with antimuscarinic activity.
• See entry for drug class for further information (p. 991).

**INDICATIONS**   **Peptic ulcer disease** Adjunctive therapy.

**CONTRAINDICATIONS**   **GI infections** Toxins may be retained and cause toxic megacolon.   **Hypersensitivity. Infants** Infants under 6 weeks of age are more prone to react with respiratory distress, seizures, poor muscle tone, and coma.   **Geriatric patients** This group is more sensitive to the adverse effects of anticholinergic drugs.   **Esophageal reflux** Anticholinergic drugs promote gastric retention and aggravate reflux.

**DOSAGE**   **PO:**   **ADULTS:** 2.5 mg three times daily before meals and 2.5 or 5 mg at bedtime.   **CHILDREN:** 0.2 mg/kg in four divided doses.   *Special patient populations:*   **ELDERLY:** Geriatric patients are more sensitive to the side effects of anticholinergic drugs.   **PREGNANCY:** Safe use has not been established. Not recommended for nursing mothers because of possible adverse effects on the infant.

**PREPARATIONS**   *Tablets:* 2.5 mg.

**DRUG INTERACTIONS**   **Drugs with anticholinergic effects** These include phenothiazines, amantadine, antiparkinson drugs, glutethimide, meperidine, tricyclic antidepressants, quinidine, disopyramide, and some antihistamines. These give additive anticholinergic activity: dry mouth, blurred vision, and constipation.   **GI absorption** Anticholinergics can interfere with or delay the absorption of orally administered drugs. Specifically, levodopa absorption may be decreased and that of digoxin may be increased.   **Antacids** Decrease the absorption of anticholinergics when taken with them. The anticholinergic should be taken an hour before the antacids.   **Potassium chloride** Anticholinergics may delay the absorption of potassium chloride, leading to GI mucosal lesions.

**FATE**   Methscopolamine is incompletely absorbed from the GI tract. Methscopolamine is excreted in the urine and feces.

### ❦ NURSING CONSIDERATIONS

**Side effects, toxicities, and associated nursing actions**
• See entry for drug class (p. 992).
**CV** Orthostatic hypotension secondary to ganglionic blockade.
**Eye** Blurred vision, photophobia.
**GI** Dry mouth, constipation.
**GU** Urinary retention.
**Lung** Bronchospasm.
**Skin** Flushed, dry.

**Nursing interventions related to drug administration**
• See entry for drug class (p. 993).

**Patient and family education**
• See entry for drug class (p. 993).

---

## oxyphencyclimine hydrochloride  (ox-i-fen-SYE-kli-meen)          anticholinergic

• oxyphencyclimine: Daricon

**MECHANISM OF ACTION**   Oxyphencyclimine is a synthetic tertiary amine with antimuscarinic activity. See entry for drug class for further information (p. 991).

**INDICATIONS**  **Peptic ulcer disease** Adjunctive therapy.

**CONTRAINDICATIONS**  **GI infections** Toxins may be retained and cause toxic megacolon.  **Hypersensitivity.**  **Infants** Infants under 6 weeks of age are more prone to react with respiratory distress, seizures, poor muscle tone, and coma.  **Geriatric patients** This group is more sensitive to the adverse effects of anticholinergic drugs.  **Esophageal reflux** Anticholinergic drugs promote gastric retention and aggravate reflux.

**DOSAGE**  **PO:** ADULTS: 10 mg twice daily.  *Special patient populations:*  ELDERLY: Geriatric patients are more sensitive to the side effects of anticholinergic drugs.  CHILDREN: Not recommended for children.  PREGNANCY: Safe use has not been established. Not recommended for nursing mothers because of possible adverse effects on the infant.

**PREPARATIONS**  *Tablets:* 10 mg.

**DRUG INTERACTIONS**  **Drugs with anticholinergic effects** These include phenothiazines, amantadine, antiparkinson drugs, glutethimide, meperidine, tricyclic antidepressants, quinidine, disopyramide, and some antihistamines. These give additive anticholinergic activity: dry mouth, blurred vision, and constipation.  **GI absorption** Anticholinergics can interfere with or delay the absorption of orally administered drugs. Specifically, levodopa absorption may be decreased and that of digoxin may be increased.  **Antacids** decrease the absorption of anticholinergics when taken with them. The anticholinergic should be taken an hour before the antacids.  **Potassium chloride** Anticholinergics may delay the absorption of potassium chloride, leading to GI mucosal lesions.

**FATE**  Oxyphencyclimine is absorbed from the GI tract, and the *duration of action* is 12 hours. The metabolic fate of oxyphencyclimine has not been characterized.

## 🐿 NURSING CONSIDERATIONS

### Side effects, toxicities, and associated nursing actions
- See entry for drug class (p. 992).

**CV** Orthostatic hypotention secondary to ganglionic blockade.

**Eye** Blurred vision, photophobia.

**GI** Dry mouth, constipation.

**GU** Urinary retention.

**Lung** Bronchospasm.

**Skin** Flushed, dry.

### Nursing interventions related to drug administration
- See entry for drug class (p. 993).

### Patient and family education
- See entry for drug class (p. 993).

---

## oxyphenonium bromide  (ox-i-fen-OH-nee-um)  anticholinergic

- oxyphenonium bromide: Antrenyl

**MECHANISM OF ACTION**  Oxyphenonium is a synthetic quaternary amine with antimuscarinic activity. See entry for drug class for further information (p. 991).

**INDICATIONS**  **Peptic ulcer disease** Adjunctive therapy.

**CONTRAINDICATIONS**  **GI infections** Toxins may be retained and cause toxic megacolon.  **Hypersensitivity.**  **Infants** Infants under 6 weeks of age are more prone to react with respiratory distress, seizures, poor muscle tone, and coma.  **Geriatric patients** This group is more sensitive to the adverse effects of anticholinergic drugs.  **Esophageal reflux** Anticholinergic drugs promote gastric retention and aggravate reflux.

**DOSAGE**  **PO:** ADULTS: 10 mg four times daily.  *Special patient populations:*  ELDERLY: Geriatric patients are more sensitive to the side effects of anticholinergic drugs.  CHILDREN: Not recommended for children.  PREGNANCY: Safe use has not been established. Not recommended for nursing mothers because of possible adverse effects on the infant.

**PREPARATIONS**  *Tablets:* 5 mg.

**DRUG INTERACTIONS**   **Drugs with anticholinergic effects** These include phenothiazines, amantadine, antiparkinson drugs, glutethimide, meperidine, tricyclic antidepressants, quinidine, disopyramide, and some antihistamines. These give additive anticholinergic activity: dry mouth, blurred vision, and constipation.   **GI absorption** Anticholinergics can interfere with or delay the absorption of orally administered drugs. Specifically, levodopa absorption may be decreased and that of digoxin may be increased.   **Antacids** decrease the absorption of anticholinergics when taken with them. The anticholinergic should be taken an hour before the antacids.   **Potassium chloride** Anticholinergics may delay the absorption of potassium chloride, leading to GI mucosal lesions.

**FATE**   Oxyphenonium is incompletely absorbed from the GI tract and is excreted in the urine.

**✋ NURSING CONSIDERATIONS**

**Side effects, toxicities, and associated nursing actions**

- See entry for drug class (p. 992).

**CV** Orthostatic hypotension secondary to ganglionic blockade.

**Eye** Blurred vision, photophobia.

**GI** Dry mouth, constipation.

**GU** Urinary retention.

**Lung** Bronchospasm.

**Skin** Flushed, dry.

**Nursing interventions related to drug administration**

- See entry for drug class (p. 993).

**Patient and family education**

- See entry for drug class (p. 993).

---

## propantheline bromide   (proe-PAN-thee-leen)   anticholinergic

- propantheline bromide: ✿Banli, ✿Noropropanthil, Norpanth, Pro-Banthine, ✿Propanthel, Prothine, SK-Propantheline Bromide, Uni Prob

**MECHANISM OF ACTION**   Propantheline is a synthetic quaternary amine with antimuscarinic activity. See entry for drug class for further information.

**INDICATIONS**   **Peptic ulcer disease** Adjunctive therapy.

**CONTRAINDICATIONS**   **GI infections** Toxins may be retained and cause toxic megacolon.   **Hypersensitivity.**   **Infants** Infants under 6 weeks of age are more prone to react with respiratory distress, seizures, poor muscle tone, and coma.   **Geriatric patients** This group is more sensitive to the adverse effects of anticholinergic drugs.   **Esophageal reflux** Anticholinergic drugs promote gastric retention and aggravate reflux.

**DOSAGE**   **PO:**   **ADULTS:** 15 mg three times daily before meals and 30 mg at bedtime.   *Special patient populations:*   **ELDERLY:** The geriatric dose is half the usual adult dose. Geriatric patients are more sensitive to the side effects of anticholinergic drugs.   **CHILDREN:** Not recommended for children.   **PREGNANCY:** Safe use has not been established. Not recommended for nursing mothers because of possible adverse effects on the infant.

**PREPARATIONS**   *Tablets:* 7.5 or 15 mg.

**DRUG INTERACTIONS**   **Drugs with anticholinergic effects** These include phenothiazines, amantadine, antiparkinson drugs, glutethimide, meperidine, tricyclic antidepressants, quinidine, disopyramide, and some antihistamines. These give additive anticholinergic activity: dry mouth, blurred vision, and constipation.   **GI absorption** Anticholinergics can interfere with or delay the absorption of orally administered drugs. Specifically, levodopa absorption may be decreased and that of digoxin may be increased.   **Antacids** decrease the absorption of anticholinergics when taken with them. The anticholinergic should be taken an hour before the antacids.   **Potassium chloride** Anticholinergics may delay the absorption of potassium chloride, leading to GI mucosal lesions.

**FATE**   Propantheline is incompletely absorbed from the GI tract. Propantheline is metabolized in the liver and excreted in the urine.

## ☙ NURSING CONSIDERATIONS

### Side effects, toxicities, and associated nursing actions

- See entry for drug class (p. 992).

**CV** Orthostatic hypotension secondary to ganglionic blockade.

**Eye** Blurred vision, photophobia.

**GI** Dry mouth, constipation.

**GU** Urinary retention.

**Lung** Bronchospasm.

**Skin** Flushed, dry.

### Nursing interventions related to drug administration

- See entry for drug class (p. 993).

### Patient and family education

- See entry for drug class (p. 993).

---

## tridihexethyl chloride   (trye-hex-ETH-ill)                anticholinergic

- tridihexethyl chloride: Pathilon

**MECHANISM OF ACTION**   Tridihexethyl is a synthetic quaternary ammonium compound with antimuscarinic activity. • See entry for drug class for further information (p. 991).

**INDICATIONS**   **Peptic ulcer** Adjunctive therapy.

**CONTRAINDICATIONS**   **GI infections** Toxins may be retained and cause toxic megacolon.   **Hypersensitivity.**   **Infants** Infants under 6 weeks of age are more prone to react with respiratory distress, seizures, poor muscle tone, and coma.   **Geriatric patients** This group is more sensitive to the adverse affects of anticholinergic drugs.   **Esophageal reflux** Anticholinergic drugs promote gastric retention and aggravate reflux.

**DOSAGE**   **PO:**   **ADULTS:** 25 mg three times daily before meals and 50 mg at bedtime.   *Special patient populations:*   **ELDERLY:** Geriatric patients are more sensitive to the side effects of anticholinergic drugs.   **CHILDREN:** Pediatric doses are given above.   **PREGNANCY:** Safe use has not been established. Not recommended for nursing mothers because of possible adverse effects on the infant.

**PREPARATIONS**   *Tablets:* 25 mg.

**DRUG INTERACTIONS**   **Drugs with anticholinergic effects** These include phenothiazines, amantadine, antiparkinson drugs, glutethimide, meperidine, tricyclic antidepressants, quinidine, disopyramide, and some antihistamines. These give additive anticholinergic activity: dry mouth, blurred vision, and constipation.   **GI absorption** Anticholinergics can interfere with or delay the absorption of orally administered drugs. Specifically, levodopa absorption may be decreased and that of digoxin may be increased.   **Antacids** decrease the absorption of anticholinergics when taken with them. The anticholinergic should be taken an hour before the antacids.   **Potassium chloride** Anticholinergics may delay the absorption of potassium chloride, leading to GI mucosal lesions.

**FATE**   Tridihexethyl is poorly absorbed and excreted in the urine and feces.

## ☙ NURSING CONSIDERATIONS

### Side effects, toxicities, and associated nursing actions

- See entry for drug class (p. 992).

**CV** Orthostatic hypotension secondary to ganglionic blockade.

**Eye** Blurred vision, photophobia.

**GI** Dry mouth, constipation.

**GU** Urinary retention.

**Lung** Bronchospasm.

**Skin** Flushed, dry.

### Nursing interventions related to drug administration

- See entry for drug class (p. 993).

### Patient and family education

- See entry for drug class (p. 993).

# Chapter Fifty-eight

# Drugs to treat ulcers

| | |
|---|---|
| antacids | ranitidine |
| cimetidine | sucralfate |
| famotidine | |

**OVERVIEW OF THE DRUG CLASS**   An ulcer is the loss of the skin or mucosal tissue that provides the protective layer of cells normally surrounding an organ. In the gastrointestinal system, an ulcer occurs in the esophagus, stomach, or duodenum when the mucosal barrier is destroyed and underlying tissue is exposed to stomach acid. The goal in treating an ulcer is to depress or to neutralize stomach acid to allow the ulcer to heal and to prevent the recurrence of the ulcer.

It is important for patients with esophageal or duodenal ulcers to learn that the conditions causing the ulcer will always be present and that only preventive therapy will decrease the incidence of recurrence. An esophageal ulcer results when there is reflux of stomach acid up into the esophagus because of a defective esophageal sphincter. A duodenal ulcer results from an overactive secretion of acid in the stomach to the point that the stomach contents cannot be neutralized in the duodenum. The acidic contents then damage the duodenal mucosa. Stomach ulcers are most frequently caused by a tumor, but a nonmalignant cause of stomach ulcers is the reflux of duodenal contents back into the stomach because of a faulty pyloric sphincter. The duodenal contents contain bile acids that disrupt the mucosal barrier normally protecting the stomach from acid and pepsin.

**MECHANISM OF ACTION**   Four classes of drugs are used to treat an ulcer: antacids, anticholinergic drugs, H-2 receptor antagonists, and a drug to coat ulcer craters. Antacids are weak bases that can be ingested to neutralize the hydrochloric acid secreted by the stomach. Anticholinergic drugs are presented in Chapter 57. They are taken before meals so they can then depress the secretion of acid that occurs when eating. H-2 receptor antagonists are new antihistamines specific for the H-2 histamine receptor. The major action of these drugs is to block histamine-induced acid secretion. These drugs have revolutionized the treatment of ulcers and largely replaced the use of anticholinergic drugs. Sucralfate is a new drug that binds to ulcer tissue to prevent further destruction by enzymes.

**INDICATIONS**   • Peptic ulcer.
**CONTRAINDICATIONS**   • See individual drug.
**DRUG INTERACTIONS**   • See individual drug.

## antacids

stomach acid neutralizers

• antacids: See Table 58-1.

**MECHANISM OF ACTION**   Antacids are weak bases that can be ingested to neutralize the hydrochloric acid secreted by the stomach. Those antacids preferred for long-term treatment are the nonsystemic antacids, which include alkaline salts of aluminum, magnesium, and calcium, which neutralize acid but are not readily absorbed into the bloodstream. The aluminum and calcium salts tend to cause constipation, whereas magnesium salts have a laxative effect. For this reason, most antacids are a combination of a magnesium salt or hydroxide and an aluminum or calcium salt or hydroxide.

**INDICATIONS**   **Peptic ulcers** To ease the pain from acid secretion.   **Esophageal reflux** To lower esophageal sphincter pressure by increasing stomach pH.   **Renal failure and renal dialysis** Aluminum hydroxide preparations may be used to bind phosphate in the gut.

**CONTRAINDICATIONS**   **Hypertension** Sodium is frequently a component of antacids. Many preparations now list the sodium content.   **Renal failure** Magnesium salts are contraindicated.

**DOSAGE**   PO:   **ADULTS AND CHILDREN:** Dosing is highly individualized. Antacids are usually taken 1 and 3 hours after a meal and at bedtime. In acute situations, they may be taken hourly.   *Special patient populations:*   PREGNANCY: Safe use has not been established.

**PREPARATIONS**   *Aluminum carbonate: capsules:* 500 mg; *suspension:* 400 or 1000 mg/5 ml; *tablets:* 500 mg. *Aluminum hydroxide: capsules:* 475 or 500 mg; *suspension:* 320, 400, or 600 mg/5 ml; *tablets:* 300 or

| Table 58-1. | Antacids | |
|---|---|---|
| **Generic name** | **Trade name** | |
| Aluminum carbonate | Basaljel | |
| Aluminum hydroxide | AlternaGEL, Alu-Cap, Amphojel, Dialume, Nephrox Suspension | |
| Aluminum phosphate | Phosphaljel | |
| Calcium carbonate | Amitone, Alkamints, Calcilac, Calglycine, Chooz, Dicarbosil, Glycate, Gustalac, Mallamint, Pama No. 1, Titracid, Titralac Liquid, Tums | |
| Dihydroxyaluminum Sodium carbonate | Rolaids Antacid | |
| Magaldrate (aluminum magnesium hydroxide) | Magaldrate Oral Suspension, Riopan | |
| Magnesium hydroxide | Milk of Magnesia | |
| Magnesium oxide | Mag-Ox, Maox, Par-Mag, Uromag | |
| Magnesium trisilicate | Magnesium Trisilicate Tablets | |
| **Antacid combinations** | | |
| Magaldrate and Simethicone | Magaldrate Plus Suspension, Riopan Plus | |
| Aluminum hydroxide and magnesium carbonate | Algicon, Gaviscon Liquid, Magnagel, | |
| Aluminum hydroxide and magnesium hydroxide | Algemol, Aludrox, Alumid, Creamalin, Delcid, Kolantyl, Maalox, Rulox, Wingel | |
| Aluminum hydroxide, magnesium hydroxide, and simethecone | Almacone, Alumid, Di-Gel, Gelusil, Improved Alma-Mag, Maalox Plus, Mygel, Mylanta, Silain-Gel, Simaal Gel, Simeco | |
| Aluminum hydroxide and magnesium trisilicate | Alma-Mag, Gaviscon | |
| Calcium carbonate and magnesium carbonate | Marblen, Spastosed | |
| Calcium carbonate and magnesium hydroxide | Bisodol | |
| Calcium carbonate and magnesium hydroxide simethcone | Di-Gel | |
| Aluminum hydroxide, calcium carbonate, and magnesium hydroxide | Camalox | |
| Aluminum hydroxide, calcium carbonate, magnesium hydroxide, and simethicone | Tempo | |
| Aluminum hydroxide, dihydroxaluminum aminoacetate, and magnesium hydroxide | Tralmag | |
| Aluminum hydroxide, magnesium carbonate, and magnesium trisilicate | Escot, Noralac | |
| Aluminum hydroxide, magnesium hydroxide, and magnesium trisilicate | Magnatril | |
| Calcium carbonate, magnesium carbonate, and magnesium oxide | Alkets | |

600 mg; *tablets (chewable):* 500 mg. *Aluminum phosphate: suspension:* 233 mg/5 ml. *Dihydroxyaluminum sodium carbonate: tablets (chewable):* 334 mg. *Magaldrate (aluminum magnesium hydroxide): suspension:* 540 or 1080 mg/5 ml; *tablets:* 480 mg; *tablets (chewable):* 480 mg. *Calcium carbonate: suspension:* 1000 mg/5 ml; *tablets (chewable):* 300, 350, 420, 500, 650, 750, or 850 mg. *Magnesium hydroxide: suspension:* 77.5 mg/g; *tablets:* 300 or 600 mg. *Magnesium oxide: tablets:* 250, 400, 420, or 500 mg. *Magnesium trisilicate: tablets:* 487.5 mg.

**DRUG INTERACTIONS**    **Drug absorption** Antacids may increase or decrease the rate and extent of absorption of other drugs taken at the same time. This may be because the antacid directly absorbs the drug or because the change in pH brought by the antacid alters the way tablets and capsules disintegrate or the forumations dissolve.   **Tetracyclines, digoxin, indomethacin, iron salts, isoniazid, dicumarol, pseu-doephedrine, diazepam, chlordiazepoxide** Studies have shown the absorption of these drugs to be decreased by antacids.

**FATE**   Antacids pass through the gastrointestinal tract largely unchanged and unabsorbed; however, to a small degree aluminum, calcium, or magnesium is absorbed and during prolonged therapy can cause systemic side effects.

## ❦ NURSING CONSIDERATIONS

### Side effects, toxicities, and associated nursing actions
**GI** Aluminum and calcium salts: constipation; magnesium salts: diarrhea.
- If possible, alternate antacids containing aluminum and calcium salts with ones containing magnesium salts to prevent diarrhea and constipation. Note that renal failure patients may not take magnesium preparations.
- If constipation occurs, instruct the patient to increase fluid intake to 2500 to 3000 ml/day, increase dietary intake of fruits, fruit juices, and fiber, and increase level of activity. Note that renal failure patients cannot increase fluid intake; stool softeners may be necessary.

### Nursing interventions related to drug administration
- Shake suspensions carefully before pouring ordered dose, and instruct patients to do the same.
- Antacid tablets should be chewed before swallowing.
- Antacid tablets should be followed with a glass of water or other liquid approved by the physician to ensure that the dose reaches the stomach. Follow antacid suspensions with 2 ounces of fluid for the same reason.
- Note Drug Interactions. In the hospital it may be necessary to rearrange the usual dosing times of other prescribed medications to ensure that medications are not taken at the same time as antacids.

### Patient and family education
- Review with patients the anticipated benefits and possible side effects of therapy.
- Caution patients to report persistent or severe diarrhea or constipation to the physician.
- Impress on patients the need to take ordered doses of antacids at the prescribed times. An antacid taken just before a meal is not as effective as an antacid taken on an empty stomach between meals. An antacid used to bind phosphate may be prescribed to take with meals.
- Because of the possibility of antacids interfering with the absorption of other medications, instruct patients to take other prescribed drugs 1 hour before or 2 hours after doses of antacids. Remind patients to avoid over-the-counter preparations without prior approval of the physician.
- Patients with ulcer disease should avoid the use of alcohol and avoid smoking.
- Stress to patients the importance of following therapeutic dietary prescriptions as well as drug regime.
- Caution patients to read labels on antacids carefully. Preparations vary in the amount of sodium and other ingredients.

# cimetidine, cimetidine hydrochloride
(sye-MET-i-deen)                                           H-2 receptor antagonist

- cimetidine: ♣Apo-Cimetidine, ♣Peptol, ♣Novocimetine, Tagamet

**MECHANISM OF ACTION**   H-2 receptor antagonists specifically block the H-2 histamine receptors that control the basal and stimulated secretion of hydrochloric acid by the parietal cells of the stomach. When an H-2 receptor antagonist is administered, basal secretion of acid is virtually stopped. Food, insulin, and caffeine become relatively ineffective in stimulating acid secretion.

**INDICATIONS**   **Duodenal ulcer** Used with an active ulcer to promote healing and to prevent recurrence. **Hypersecretory conditions** These include the Zollinger-Ellison syndrome, systemic mastocytosis, and multiple endocrine adenoma.   **Gastric ulcer** Promotes healing.

**CONTRAINDICATIONS**   **Renal impairment** Reduction in dosage is required to avoid accumulation of cimetidine.

**DOSAGE**   **PO:**   ADULTS: 300 mg four times daily. Maximum daily dose is 2.4 g.   **IV:**   ADULTS: 300 mg every 6 hours. Maximum daily dose is 2.4 g.   *Special patient populations:*   ELDERLY: Elderly patients are more likely to experience disorientation and other CNS side effects.   CHILDREN: Not recommended for children under 16 years old.   PREGNANCY: Safe use has not been established.

**PREPARATIONS**   *Cimetidine: tablets:* 200, 300, or 400 mg. *Cimetidine hydrochloride: solution (oral):* 300 mg; *Injection:* 150 mg/ml; 6 mg/ml in 0.9% saline.

**DRUG INTERACTIONS**   **Oral anticoagulants, phenytoin, propranolol, benzodiazepines, lidocaine, theophylline** Cimetidine inhibits the hepatic, micosomal enzyme systems that metabolize these drugs, leading to increased plasma concentrations of these drugs.   **Myelosuppressive drugs** Cimetidine potentiates the myelosuppressive effects of alkylating agents, antimetabolites, and radiation therapy.   **Antacids** These reduce the absorption of cimetidine.

**FATE**   Cimetidine is well absorbed. The *duration of action* is about 4 hours. Cimetidine is metabolized in the liver and excreted in the urine.

### ☙ NURSING CONSIDERATIONS

#### Side effects, toxicities, and associated nursing actions

**CNS** Dizziness, confusion, agitation, psychosis, depression, anxiety, hallucinations, disorientation.
- Be alert to these alterations in mood and mental status. Changes are more common in the elderly and are often attributed erroneously to aging or other causes.
- Reorient as needed. Keep night lights on and side rails up as indicated.
- If dizziness occurs, caution patients to avoid driving or operating hazardous equipment until the effects of medication wear off.

**CV** Rarely, arrhythmias, hypotension.
- Monitor pulse and blood pressure.
- Caution patients to move slowly from lying to sitting or standing positions. Supervise ambulation, especially in the elderly.

**GI** Diarrhea.
- Monitor intake and output.
- If diarrhea is severe or persistent, notify the physician. Maintain adequate hydration. Monitor electrolytes.

**Hematologic** Neutropenia.
- Monitor CBC and white blood cell differential. Neutropenia increases susceptibility to infection; the usual treatment of neutropenia is to discontinue the drug.

**Skin** Rashes, urticaria.
- Inspect patient for the development of skin changes. Notify the physician.

**Other** Gynecomastia, breast soreness.
- Gynecomastia and breast tenderness may diminish and disappear after several weeks. If symptoms are severe or persistent, it may be necessary to discontinue the drug.

#### Nursing interventions related to drug administration
- For direct IV injection, dilute 300 mg in at least 20 ml of normal saline for injection. Administer at a rate of 300 mg or less over 2 minutes.
- For intermittent IV infusion, dilute 300 mg of drug in 100 ml of compatible IV solution. Do not add to continuously infusing fluids. Administer over 15 to 20 minutes.
- There may be discomfort associated with IM injection.
- Read labels carefully. Prefilled syringes are intended for IM use or for diluting for intermittent infusion. Prefilled syringes are *not* for direct IV injection.
- Antacids and oral cimetidine should not be administered simultaneously. When both drugs are ordered in the same patient, administer antacid 1 hour before or after cimetidine in the fasting state or 1 hour after cimetidine is administered with food or meals.

- Oral doses are usually administered with or just before meals.

### Patient and family education

- Review with patients the anticipated benefits and possible side effects of therapy. Instruct patients to report the development of any unexpected sign or symptom.
- Because of possible Drug Interactions (see preceding), work out with patient an appropriate time schedule for taking cimetidine and other prescribed drugs in the home setting.
- Caution patients to avoid the use of over-the-counter preparations without prior clearance from the physician.
- Patients requiring cimetidine for treatment of GI problems may also require dietary modifications. Impress on patients the need to adhere to dietary restrictions as well as medication regimes.
- Caution patients with ulcers or other GI problems to avoid the use of alcohol and avoid smoking.
- Remind patients to keep these and all medications out of the reach of children.

---

## famotidine   (fa-MOE-ti-deen)                    H-2 receptor antagonist

- famotidine: Pepcid

**MECHANISM OF ACTION**   H-2 receptor antagonists specifically block the H-2 histamine receptors that control the basal and stimulated secretion of hydrochloric acid by the parietal cells of the stomach. When an H-2 receptor antagonist is administered, basal secretion of acid is virtually stopped. Food, insulin, and caffeine become relatively ineffective in stimulating acid secretion.

**INDICATIONS**   **Duodenal ulcer** Used with active ulcer to promote healing and to prevent recurrence.   **Gastritis** To control intragastic pH in critically ill patients: improve endoscopic findings.

**CONTRAINDICATIONS**   **Renal impairment** Reduction in dosage is required to avoid accumulation of famotidine.

**DOSAGE**   **Active ulcer:** *PO:*   ADULTS: 40 mg daily, at bedtime, or in two divided doses. Maintenance therapy is 20 mg daily.   *IV:*   ADULTS: 20 mg every 12 hours.   **GI hypersecretory conditions:** *PO, IV:* ADULTS: Doses are individualized. Usual starting dose is 20 mg every 6 hours. Doses as high as 800 mg daily have been administered in unusual circumstances.   *Special patient populations:*   PREGNANCY: Safe use has not been established.

**PREPARATIONS**   *Suspension:* 40 mg/5 ml; *tablets:* 20 or 40 mg; *injection:* 10 mg/ml.

**DRUG INTERACTIONS**   **Antacids** These reduce the absorption of famotidine.

**FATE**   Famotidine is incompletely absorbed after oral administration. *Peak plasma concentrations* are within 20 minutes after an IV dose and 1 to 4 hours after an oral dose. The *plasma half-life* is 2.5 to 4 hours. Elimination is prolonged by renal impairment. Limited metabolism occurs in the liver.

### ❧ NURSING CONSIDERATIONS

#### Side effects, toxicities, and associated nursing actions

**CNS** Headache (5%) and dizziness (1%). Occasionally, weakness, paresthesia, seizures, insomnia, drowsiness, depression, disorientation, confusion, anxiety, decreased libido, hallucinations.

- Warn patients to avoid driving or operating hazardous equipment if drowsiness or dizziness develop; notify the physician.
- Question about history of seizures prior to administering; if seizures have occurred previously, check with the physician.
- Assess for signs of depression: withdrawal, lack of interest in personal appearance, anorexia, insomnia.
- Obtain baseline mental status exam, and repeat at regular intervals. Instruct families and patients to report any new signs or symptoms.

**CV** Occasionally, palpitation, hypertension, flushing.

- Monitor blood pressure and pulse. Question patients about palpitations.

**Eye** Occasionally, conjunctival congestion.
- Inspect eyes for signs of irritation; instruct patients to report any symptoms of eye problems.

**GI** Constipation or diarrhea (1% to 2%). Occasionally, nausea, vomiting, flatulence, anorexia, dry mouth, heartburn.
- Instruct the patient to keep a record of stools.
- Monitor intake, output, and weight if GI symptoms are prominent.

**GU** Occasionally, increases in BUN or serum creatinine concentrations and proteinuria.
- Monitor serum creatinine, BUN, and urinalysis.

**Hematologic** Rarely, depression of white blood cells.
- Assess for signs of infection: fever, sore throat, cough.
- Monitor white blood cell count.

**Metabolic** Occasionally, increases in liver function enzymes.
- Monitor liver function tests.
- Instruct patients to report the development of jaundice, fever, malaise, right upper quadrant abdominal pain, or change in color or consistency of stool.

### Nursing interventions related to drug administration
- For IV administration, dilute 20 mg of famotidine to a total of 5 or 10 ml with 0.9% sodium chloride (dilution of 4 or 2 mg/ml). Administer at a rate of 10 mg or less per minute.
- For intermittent infusion, dilute 20 mg of famotidine in 100 ml of 5% dextrose on water or other compatible solution to provide a solution of 0.2 mg/ml. Administer over 15 to 30 minutes.
- Famotidine and antacids may be administered concomitantly if necessary.

### Patient and family education
- Review anticipated benefits and possible side effects of drug therapy with patients and families. Instruct patients to report the development of any new sign or symptom.
- Remind patients to avoid the use of over-the-counter preparations without prior clearance from the physician.
- Impress upon patients the importance of all aspects of treatment for GI problems, including dietary modification, avoiding the use of alcohol, and avoiding smoking.
- Remind patients to keep these and all medications out of the reach of children.

---

## ranitidine hydrochloride    (ra-NIH-teh-deen)    H-2 receptor antagonist

- ranitidine hydrochloride: Zantac

**MECHANISM OF ACTION**    H-2 receptor antagonists specifically block the H-2 histamine receptors that control the basal and stimulated secretion of hydrochloric acid by the parietal cells of the stomach. When an H-2 receptor antagonist is administered, basal secretion of acid is virtually stopped. Food, insulin, and caffeine become relatively ineffective in stimulating acid secretion.

**INDICATIONS**    **Duodenal ulcer** Used with active ulcer to promote healing and prophylactically to prevent recurrence.    **Hypersecretory conditions** These include the Zollinger-Ellison syndrome, systemic mastocytosis, multiple endocrine adenoma.    **Gastric ulcer** Promotes healing.

**CONTRAINDICATIONS**    **Renal impairment** Reduction in dosage is required to avoid accumulation of ranitidine.

**DOSAGE**    PO:    ADULTS: 150 mg twice daily.    **IM, slow IV:**    ADULTS: 50 mg every 6 to 8 hours. Maximum daily dose is 400 mg. For IV administration, 50 mg is diluted to at least 20 ml.    *Special patient populations:*    CHILDREN: Not recommended for children under 16 years old.    PREGNANCY: Safe use has not been established.

**PREPARATIONS**    *Tablets:* 150 mg; *injection:* 25 mg/ml.

**DRUG INTERACTIONS**    Unlike cimetidine, ranitidine has little effect on the hepatic micosomal enzyme systems that metabolize many drugs. In general, ranitidine does not alter the metabolism of other drugs.

**FATE** Ranitidine is well absorbed. The *duration of action* is about 9 hours. Ranitidine is metabolized in the liver and excreted in the urine.

## ❦ NURSING CONSIDERATIONS

### Side effects, toxicities, and associated nursing actions

**CNS** Dizziness, confusion, agitation, psychosis, depression, anxiety, hallucinations, disorientation.

- Be alert to these alterations in mood and mental status. Changes are more common in the elderly and are often attributed erroneously to aging or other causes.
- Reorient as needed. Keep night lights on and side rails up as indicated.
- If dizziness occurs, caution patients to avoid driving or operating hazardous equipment until the effects of medication wear off.

**CV** Rarely, arrhythmias, hypotension.

- Monitor pulse and blood pressure.
- Caution patients to move slowly from lying to sitting or standing positions. Supervise ambulation, especially in the elderly.

**GI** Diarrhea.

- Monitor intake and output.
- If diarrhea is severe or persistent, notify the physician. Maintain adequate hydration. Monitor electrolytes.

**Hematologic** Neutropenia.

- Monitor CBC and white blood cell differential. Neutropenia increases susceptibility to infection; the usual treatment of neutropenia is to discontinue the drug.

**Skin** Rashes, urticaria.

- Inspect patients for the development of skin changes. Notify the physician.

**Other** Gynecomastia, breast soreness.

- Gynecomastia and breast tenderness may diminish and disappear after several weeks. If symptoms are severe or persistent, it may be necessary to discontinue the drug.

### Nursing interventions related to drug administration

- For direct IV injection, dilute 50 mg of ranitidine in at least 20 ml of compatible IV fluid, and administer dose over at least 5 minutes.
- For intermittent IV infusion, dilute 50 mg in at least 100 ml of compatible IV fluid and administer dose over 15 to 20 minutes.
- Antacids may be administered simultaneously without significantly affecting ranitidine absorption. If in doubt, separate dosage times by 2 hours.

### Patient and family education

- Review with patients the anticipated benefits and possible side effects of therapy. Instruct patients to report the development of any unexpected sign or symptom.
- Because of possible Drug Interactions (see preceding), work out with patients an appropriate time schedule for taking ranitidine and other prescribed drugs in the home setting.
- Caution patients to avoid the use of over-the-counter preparations without prior clearance from the physician.
- Patients requiring ranitidine for treatment of GI problems may also require dietary modifications. Impress on patients the need to adhere to dietary restrictions as well as medication regimes.
- Caution patients with ulcers or other GI problems to avoid the use of alcohol, and avoid smoking.
- Remind patients to keep these and all medications out of the reach of children.

---

## sucralfate (soo-KRAL-fate)                                    ulcer coating

- sucralfate: Carafate, ✸Sulcrate

**MECHANISM OF ACTION**    Sucralfate is a complex of sulfated sucrose and aluminum hydroxide that is changed by stomach acid into a viscous material that binds to proteins in ulcerated tissue. This appears to protect the ulcer from the destructive action of the digestive enzyme pepsin.

**INDICATIONS**    Duodenal ulcer Sulcralfate is used during the first 4 to 8 weeks of therapy.

**CONTRAINDICATIONS**    • None noted.

**DOSAGE**    PO:    ADULTS: 1 g four times daily taken on an empty stomach 1 hour before each meal and at bedtime.    *Special patient populations:*    CHILDREN: Not recommended for children under 18 years old.    PREGNANCY: Safe use has not been established.

**PREPARATIONS**    *Tablets:* 1 g.

**DRUG INTERACTIONS**    **Tetracycline, cimetidine, phenytoin** Sucralfate reduces the absorption of these drugs if taken concurrently.

**FATE**    Sucralfate is not absorbed systemically. It is slowly excreted in the feces.

## ❦ NURSING CONSIDERATIONS

### Side effects, toxicities, and associated nursing actions

**CNS** Dizziness, sleepiness, vertigo.
- If CNS effects develop, caution patients to avoid driving or operating hazardous equipment until the effects of the medication wear off. Notify the physician.
- Monitor hospitalized patients carefully. Supervise ambulation. Keep bed in low position and side rails up.

**GI** Constipation, nausea, discomfort.
- Monitor intake and output. Keep a record of stools.
- If constipation develops, encourage patients to increase fluid intake to 2500 to 3000 ml/day, increase the intake of fruits, fruit juices, and fiber, and increase daily exercise. If constipation is severe or persistent, notify the physician.
- If nausea is severe, it may be necessary to discontinue the medication.

**Skin** Rash.
- Inspect patient for development of rash; notify the physician.

### Nursing interventions related to drug administration
- Sucralfate should be taken on an empty stomach, 1 hour before each meal and at bedtime.
- Antacids, if also ordered, should not be administered within 30 minutes of sucralfate.
- See Drug Interactions. If any of these drugs are also prescribed, they should not be administered within 2 hours of sucralfate.

### Patient and family education
- Review with patients the anticipated benefits and possible side effects of therapy. Instruct patients to report the development of any unexpected sign or symptom.
- Because of possible Drug Interactions (see preceding), work out with patients an appropriate time schedule for taking sucralfate and other prescribed drugs in the home setting.
- Caution patients to avoid the use of over-the-counter preparations without prior clearance from the physician.
- Patients requiring sucralfate for treatment of GI problems may also require dietary modifications. Impress on patients the need to adhere to dietary restrictions as well as medication regimes.
- Caution patients with ulcers or other GI problems to avoid the use of alcohol, and avoid smoking.
- Remind patients to keep these and all medications out of the reach of children.

# Chapter Fifty-nine

# Drugs to control diarrhea

bismuth subsalicylate
codeine (see Chapter 45)
dipenoxylate with atropine
kaolin and pectin
loperamide
opium preparations

## DRUG COMBINATIONS
- kaolin, pectin, and atropine sulfate, hyoscyamine sulfate, and scopolamine Br: Donnagel, Kapectolin Belladonna Mixture, Quiagel
- opium tincture and homatropine methylbromide: Dia-Quel, Parelixir (C-V)
- paregoric, bismuth subsalicylate, calcium carrageenan, pectin, and zinc phenolsulfonate: Infantol Pink (C-V)
- powder opium, bismuth subcarbonate, kaolin, and pectin: KBP/O (C-III)
- powdered opium, atropine sulfate, hyoscyamine sulfate, kaolin, pectin, and scopolamine HBr: Donnagel-PG, Kaodonna-PG, Quiagel PG (C-V)

**OVERVIEW OF THE DRUG CLASS**   Diarrhea has no precise definition but rather refers to bowel movements that are frequent (more than three per day), fluid (unformed stools), or large (greater than 200 g/ day). Acute diarrhea lasts for hours or days, whereas chronic diarrhea lasts more than 3 to 4 weeks. Chronic diarrhea requires a thorough examination to establish a cause, which can then be specifically treated. Acute diarrhea rarely requires treatment beyond maintaining adequate liquid intake and avoiding food.

**MECHANISM OF ACTION**   The most effective nonspecific antidiarrheal agents are the opioids, which decrease the tone of the small and large intestines in a manner that slows the transit of material. The longitudinal contractions propelling the contents (peristalsis) are inhibited by the opioids, but the circular contractions that cause the segmental activity that mixes the intestinal contents are stimulated by the opioids. The treatment of diarrhea with opioids is nonspecific, and when diarrhea is caused by poisons, infections, or bacterial toxins, opioids can make the condition worse by delaying the elimination of these agents. Loperamide is a nonopioid with a direct action on intestinal smooth muscle.

In addition to opioids, the bismuth salts and kaolin and pectin are used to treat diarrhea. They absorb toxins and thus remove the cause of diarrhea.

**INDICATIONS**   • Diarrhea.

**CONTRAINDICATIONS**   • See individual drug.

**DRUG INTERACTIONS**   • See individual drug.

## ☙ NURSING CONSIDERATIONS
**Side effects, toxicities, and associated nursing actions**   GI Diarrhea can lead to severe electrolyte abnormalities. • Monitor intake and output, weight, and blood pressure. • Assess skin turgor and mucous membranes. • Monitor serum electrolytes. • Be alert to hypokalemia, characterized by muscle weakness, fatigue, anorexia, vomiting, drowsiness, irritability, and eventual coma and death. • Be alert to hypochloremia: hypertonic muscles, tetany, and depressed respirations.

**Patient and family education**
- Review with patients the anticipated benefits and possible side effects of therapy.
- Instruct patients to keep a record of consistency and frequency of stools. If diarrhea persists beyond 3 to 5 days after the start of drug therapy or worsens after therapy begins, instruct the patient to notify the physician.
- Encourage patients with diarrhea to switch to a clear liquid diet and to maintain an adequate fluid intake of at least 3000 ml/day in the adult. Fruit juices, which may be irritating to the GI tract, should

be avoided, as well as water supplies that may be contaminated, as might occur in foreign travel.

- Instruct patients about the importance of handwashing and careful personal hygiene in slowing the spread of diarrhea. Crowded living conditions and day care centers, where there are groups of small children, are settings where organisms that cause diarrhea can be easily spread.
- Remind patients to keep these and all medications out of the reach of children.

---

### bismuth subsalicylate    (BIZ-muth sub-sa-LIS-a-late)                     antidiarrheal

- bismuth subsalicylate: Pepto-Bismol (OTC)

**MECHANISM OF ACTION**    Binds bacterial toxins that cause diarrhea.

**INDICATIONS**    **Traveler's diarrhea** Bismuth subsalicylate is effective in controlling diarrhea caused by bacteria.

**CONTRAINDICATIONS**    **Infants and elderly patients** May lead to impacted feces.

**DOSAGE**    PO:    **ADULTS:** 30 ml. Repeat every 30 to 60 minutes as needed, up to eight doses.    **CHILDREN:** 10 to 14 years old, 20 ml; 6 to 10 years old, 10 ml; 3 to 6 years old, 5 ml. Repeat every 30 to 50 minutes as needed, up to eight doses.    *Special patient populations:*    **ELDERLY:** Not recommended for elderly patients.    **CHILDREN:** Not for use in children under 3 years old.    **PREGNANCY:** Use with caution during pregnancy.

**PREPARATIONS**    *Suspension:* 262 mg/15 ml; *tablets (chewable):* 300 mg.

**DRUG INTERACTIONS**    **Drug absorption** May interfere with the absorption of other drugs.

**FATE**    Bismuth subsalicylate passes through the gastrointestinal tract without being absorbed. The feces turn black. Salicylate may be released and reduce intestinal inflammation and hypermotility.

### ☙ NURSING CONSIDERATIONS

#### Side effects, toxicities, and associated nursing actions
- See entry of drug class (p. 1015).
  **GI** Feces turn black.
- Caution patients about this effect of drug therapy. If concerned that change in stool color could indicate blood in stool, examine the stool for occult blood.

#### Nursing interventions related to drug administration
- Tablets should be chewed well before swallowing. Patients who find the suspension unappetizing may prefer tablets.
- Shake suspension well before preparing ordered dose.

#### Patient and family education
- See entry of drug class (p. 1015).
- Caution patients to avoid the use of Pepto-Bismol for longer than 2 to 3 weeks. Prolonged use has been associated with changes in mentation.
- Caution patients to avoid the use of aspirin and other products containing salicylates while taking Pepto-Bismol, as this drug may also release salicylates.
- Caution patients taking anticoagulants to avoid the use of Pepto-Bismol or to use only on physician recommendation because of the salicylate in Pepto-Bismol.

---

### diphenoxylate hydrochloride with atropine sulfate
(dye-fen-OX-i-late)                                                      antidiarrheal

- diphenoxylate hydrochloride with atropine sulfate: Diphenatol, Enoxa, Lofene, Lomotil, Lonox, Lo-Trol, Low-Quel, SK-Diphenoxylate

**MECHANISM OF ACTION**    Diphenoxylate is an opioid with minimal CNS activity, but atropine is added to discourage overdosage. Opioids inhibit GI peristalsis.

**INDICATIONS**    Diarrhea.

**CONTRAINDICATIONS**   **Diarrhea** Reduction of intestinal motility may be harmful when diarrhea results from *Shigella, Salmonella,* and some *Escherichia coli* infections.

**DOSAGE**   **PO:**   **ADULTS:** 5 mg four times daily.   **CHILDREN:** 8 to 12 years old, 2 mg five times daily; 5 to 8 years old, 2 mg four times daily; 2 to 5 years old, 2 mg three times daily.   *Special patient populations:*   **ELDERLY:** Altered doses for the elderly have not been specifically established.   **CHILDREN:** Not recommended for children under 2 years old. In general, children have a variable response to diphenoxylate, and the drug must be used with caution.   **PREGNANCY:** Safe use has not been established. Not recommended for nursing mothers.

**PREPARATIONS**   *Solution:* 2.5 mg/5 ml with 0.025 mg/5 ml atropine sulfate; *tablets:* 2.5 mg with 0.025 mg atropine sulfate.

**DRUG INTRACTIONS**   None described.

**FATE**   Diphenoxylate is well absorbed. The *onset of action* is 45 minutes to 1 hour and the *duration of action* is 3 to 4 hours. Diphenoxylate is metabolized to an active metabolite and excreted primarily in the feces.

### 🐦 NURSING CONSIDERATIONS

#### Side effects, toxicities, and associated nursing actions
**CNS** Sedation, dizziness, restlessness, insomnia, headache, euphoria.
**Eye** Blurred vision.
- If sedation, blurred vision, or dizziness occurs, caution patients to avoid driving or operating hazardous equipment until the effects of the medication wear off.
- CNS effects will disappear when drug is discontinued.

**CV** Fast heart rate.
- Monitor pulse and blood pressure.
- Observe carefully patients with a history of heart disease.

**GI** Dry mouth, nausea, vomiting, abdominal discomfort, paralytic ileus, toxic megacolon.
- Many of these side effects are due to the atropine component.
- For dry mouth, instruct patient to chew sugarless gum, suck on sugarless hard candy, or to take frequent sips of clear water.
- Monitor intake, output, weight. Auscultate bowel sounds on regular basis. Keep record of stools.
- If GI symptoms are severe, persistent, or do not appear until after the start of drug therapy, notify the physician.

**Lung** Respiratory depression.
- Monitor respiratory rate.

**Skin** Urticaria.

**Allergic** Pruritis, angioedema.
- Inspect patient for development of objective changes.
- Have drugs and equipment available to treat an acute allergic response.

**Other** Swelling of the gums, numbness of the extremities.
- Assess for these side effects. If they occur, notify the physician.

#### Nursing interventions related to drug administration
- For liquid preparations, use only the plastic dropper supplied by the manufacturer for measuring ordered dose.
- Be especially alert in administering this drug to children, as effects of the drug are highly variable.

#### Patient and family education
- See entry for drug class (p. 1015).
- Impress on patients the need to take this drug only as ordered, as improper use can lead to serious side effects and perhaps addiction.

---

## kaolin and pectin   (KAY-oh-lin and PEK-tin)                    antidiarrheal

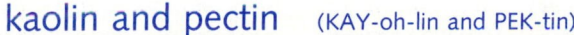

- kaolin and pectin: K-P, Kaopectate (OTC)

**MECHANISM OF ACTION**   Kaolin and pectin absorb bacteria and toxins.

**INDICATIONS**   **Diarrhea** For acute, nonspecific diarrhea.

**CONTRAINDICATIONS**   • None.

**DOSAGE**   **PO:**   **ADULTS:** 60 to 120 ml of the regular-strength suspension or 45 to 90 ml of the concentrated suspension after each loose bowel movement.   **CHILDREN:** 3 to 5 years old, 15 to 30 ml of the regular-strength or 15 ml of the concentrated suspension; 6 to 11 years old, 30 to 60 ml of the regular-strength or 30 ml of the concentrated suspension; 12 years and older, 60 ml of the regular-strength or 45 ml of the concentrated suspension.   *Special patient populations:*   **ELDERLY:** Use with caution.   **CHILDREN:** Use with caution for children under 3 years old.   **PREGNANCY:** Use with caution during pregnancy.

**PREPARATIONS**   *Suspension:* kaolin 0.87 g/5 ml and pectin 43 mg/5 ml; kaolin 0.98 g/5 ml and pectin 21.7 mg/5 ml; kaolin 1.46 g/5 ml and pectin 32.5 mg/5 ml.

**DRUG INTERACTIONS**   **Lincomycin** Kaolin-pectin impairs the absorption of oral lincomycin.

**FATE**   Kaolin and pectin are not absorbed but pass through the GI tract and are excreted in the feces. Pectin may be largely decomposed in the GI tract.

### ☙ NURSING CONSIDERATIONS

#### Side effects, toxicities, and associated nursing actions
**GI** Mild constipation.
- Monitor intake, output, weight, and keep a record of stools.
- If constipation occurs, consider adjusting dose or discontinuing medication (consult the physician). Encourage patient to increase daily fluid intake to 2500 to 3000 ml and to add fruits, fruit juices, and fiber to the diet.

#### Nursing interventions related to drug administration
- Shake suspensions well prior to pouring ordered dose.

#### Patient and family education
- See entry for drug class (p. 1015).

---

## loperamide hydrochloride   (loe-PER-a-mide)   antidiarrheal

- loperamide hydrochloride: Imodium

**MECHANISM OF ACTION**   Loperamide slows intestinal motility through a direct action on the nerve endings and ganglia in the intestinal wall.

**INDICATIONS**   **Diarrhea** Acute or chronic diarrhea secondary to inflammatory bowel disease.   **Ileostomy** Loperamide reduces the volume of discharge.

**CONTRAINDICATIONS**   **Hypersensitivity.** • Diarrhea secondary to infections or pseudomembranous colitis.

**DOSAGE**   **Acute diarrhea:** *PO:*   **ADULTS:** 4 mg initially, followed by 2 mg with the passage of each unformed stool. Maximum dosage is 16 mg daily.   **CHILDREN:** 2 to 5 years old, 1 mg three times daily; 5 to 8 years old, 2 mg twice daily; 8 to 12 years old, 2 mg three times daily. This is the first day dosage. Subsequently, the dosage is 0.1 mg/kg with each unformed stool. Discontinue after 48 hours.   **Chronic diarrhea:** *PO:*   **ADULTS:** 4 to 8 mg daily in single or divided doses.   *Special patient populations:*   **CHILDREN:** Not recommended for children under 2 year olds.   **PREGNANCY:** Use with caution during pregnancy.

**PREPARATIONS**   *Capsules:* 2 mg; *solution:* 0.2 mg/ml.

**DRUG INTERACTIONS**   None described.

**FATE**   Loperamide is slowly absorbed. The drug undergoes enterohepatic circulation and is excreted in the feces.

### ☙ NURSING CONSIDERATIONS

#### Side effects, toxicities, and associated nursing actions
**CNS** Drowsiness, dizziness, fatigue.
- Caution patients to avoid driving or operating hazardous equipment until the effects of medication wear off.

- Assess fatigue carefully. It could also be a result of inadequate hydration or inadequate nutritional intake.

**GI** Nausea and vomiting, dry mouth, constipation, epigastric pain.

- Monitor intake and output, blood pressure, weight. Keep a record of stools. Auscultate bowel sounds. Assess skin turgor and mucous membranes.
- For dry mouth, suggest that patient chew sugarless gum, suck sugarless hard candies, drink frequent sips of water, and perform regular oral hygiene. Caution patients to avoid mouth washes and gargles that are drying. Some patients may wish to use a commercially available saliva substitute.
- For constipation, encourage patients to increase fluid intake to 2500 to 3000 ml/day, increase intake of fruit, fruit juices, and fiber, and increase level of exercise.
- Many of these GI side effects are best treated by adjusting the dose of medication or discontinuing the drug. Consult the physician.

**Allergic** Hypersensitivity.

- Assess history of allergy to medications prior to administering any medication.
- Be alert to unusual responses to drugs.

**Nursing interventions related to drug administration**
- See entry for drug class (p. 1015).

**Patient and family education**
- See entry for drug class (p. 1015).

---

## opium preparations  (OH-pee-um)    antidiarrheal

- opium preparations: Opium tincture, Paregoric (C-III)

**MECHANISM OF ACTION**  Opioids inhibit gastrointestinal motility. See entry for drug class for further information.

**INDICATIONS**  Diarrhea.

**CONTRAINDICATIONS**  Diarrhea caused by poisoning.  Asthma, prostatic hypertrophy, hepatic disease, opioid dependence Use with caution.

**DOSAGE**  Paregoric:  *PO:*  **ADULTS:** 5 to 10 ml one to four times daily.  **CHILDREN:** 0.25 to 0.5 ml/kg one to four times daily.  **Tincture:**  *PO:*  **ADULTS:** 0.6 ml four times daily. Not to exceed 6 ml daily. *Special patient populations:*  **ELDERLY:** The elderly are more sensitive to the constipating effects of drugs.  **CHILDREN:** Tincture should not be used undiluted for children.  **PREGNANCY:** Use with caution during pregnancy.

**PREPARATIONS**  Available as Opium Tincture and Paregoric. Several combinations with bismuth or other compounds are available. See Drug combinations.

**DRUG INTERACTIONS**  At the usual therapeutic doses, interactions are minimal.

**FATE**  Opioids are variably absorbed and metabolized by the liver.

**❦ NURSING CONSIDERATIONS**

**Side effects, toxicities, and associated nursing actions**

**GI** Nausea.

- Assess for nausea. If it is severe or persistent, notify the physician.

**Nursing interventions related to drug administration**
- To administer opium tincture, dilute the ordered dose in 15 to 30 ml of liquid before having the patient try to swallow ordered dose.

**Patient and family education**
- See entry for drug class (p. 1015).

# Chapter Sixty

# Drugs to relieve constipation

**Anthraquinone laxatives**
cascara sagrada
danthron
senna and sennosides

**Bulk-forming laxatives**
karaya
malt soup extract
methylcellulose
psyllium preparations

**Castor oil**

**Diphenylmethane laxatives**
bisacodyl
phenolphthalein

**Hyperosmotic laxatives**
glycerin
sorbitol

**Mineral oil**

**Saline laxatives**
magnesium salts
sodium phosphates

**Stool softeners**
docusate salts

## COMBINATIONS WITH LAXATIVE DRUGS
- cascara sagrada and milk of magnesia: Generic (OTC)
- cascara sagrada and aloe: Nature's Remedy(OTC)
- cascara sagrada and mineral oil: Kondremul with Cascara (OTC)
- danthron and docusate: Dorbantyl, Doxidan, Modane, Unilax, Valax (OTC)
- sennosides and docusate: Gentlax S, Senokap DSS, Senokot S (OTC)
- sennosides and guar gum: Gentlax B Granules (OTC)
- malt soup extract and psyllium: Syllamalt (OTC)
- psyllium and sennosides: Prompt (OTC)
- psyllium and senna: Perdiem (OTC)
- psyllium and wheat bran: Fiberall (OTC)
- phenolphthalein and mineral oil: Petrogalar with Phenolphthalein, Kondremul with Phenol-phthalein, Agoral Marshmallow, Agoral Raspberry (OTC)
- phenolphthalein and docusate: Disolan, Ex-Lax Extra Gentle, Correctol, Feen-A-Mint (OTC)
- mineral oil and milk of magnesia: Haley's M-O (OTC)
- mineral oil and docusate: Milkinol (OTC)

**OVERVIEW OF THE DRUG CLASS** The major muscular activity of the large intestine is a contraction of circular smooth muscle, which decreases the diameter of the segment and kneads the fecal mass without moving it along. About 2 liters of water is removed from the fecal mass in the large intestine. Bulk in the large intestine stimulates stretch receptors to cause a reflex peristalsis, which moves the fecal mass forward. Periodically, usually three to four times daily, strong propulsive contractions occur spontaneously to move the fecal mass through the large intestine. The strongest movements usually occur after the first meal of the day, and the perception of the need to defecate follows the filling of the rectum. The relaxation of the external anal sphincter is a voluntary act, as are the straining movements to expel the feces. The pattern of defecation described implies that defecation is a regular morning event, but the timing of defecation is highly individual and may occur more or less frequently. A normal bowel movement refers to whatever pattern of defecation results in readily passed feces for a given individual. Constipation arises when the frequency of bowel movements decreases and defecation yields hard stools that are difficult to pass.

**MECHANISM OF ACTION** *Laxative, cathartic,* and *purgative* are all terms describing agents that act on the large intestine (colon, bowel) to promote defecation, but these terms have evolved to represent different degrees of action. A laxative promotes soft stools with a minimum incidence of abdominal cramping. A cathartic produces a soft to fluid stool and may also cause abdominal cramping. A purgative produces a watery stool and violent cramping to such an extent that shock and hemorrhaging

| Table 60-1. | Laxatives compared by effect and latency | | |
|---|---|---|---|
| | Softening of formed stool (1 to 3 days) | Soft-semifluid stool (6 to 12 hours) | Watery stool (2 to 6 hours) |
| | Bulk-forming agents<br>  Dietary fiber<br>  Karaya<br>  Malt soup extract<br>  Methylcellulose<br>  Psyllium preparations<br>Docusate salts | Saline laxatives (low-dose)<br>  Milk of magnesia<br>  Magnesium sulfate | Saline laxatives (high-dose)<br>  Milk of magnesia<br>  Magnesium salts<br>  Sodium salts |
| | | Diphenylmethane derivatives<br>  Phenolphthalein<br>  Bisacodyl<br>Anthraquinone derivatives<br>  Senna<br>  Cascara sagrada<br>  Danthron | Castor oil<br>Hyperosmotics<br>  Glycerin<br>  Sorbitol |

may result. Purgatives are no longer used in medical practice, and only some cathartics, also called stimulant cathartics, are commonly used.

Laxatives are classified as (1) bulk-forming, (2) stimulant (irritant) cathartic, (3) saline (osmotic) cathartic, (4) wetting agent (softener), and (5) lubricant. With the exception of lubricants, laxatives act by providing a greater bulk to the fecal mass, primarily by keeping water in the large intestine. The large, hydrated fecal mass can fill the rectum to stimulate defecation, and defecation is accomplished with minimum irritation or strain.

Causes of constipation include poor bowel habits, narcotic analgesics, drugs with anticholinergic side effects, and loss of intestinal muscle tone because of surgery, bed rest, or age. Laxatives are also indicated when straining is painful or risky, such as in women with episiotomies and patients with hemorrhoids, hernias, or aneurysms. Laxatives are also used to clean out the large intestine before surgery or examination.

**INDICATIONS**   Constipation Table 60-1 lists commonly used laxatives by the type of stool formed.

**CONTRAINDICATIONS**   **Presence of nausea and vomiting.   Acute abdominal pain** Laxatives can mask symptoms of appendicitis.   **Intestinal obstruction, fecal impaction, or undiagnosed rectal bleeding. Prolonged use** Use for more than 1 week can lead to dependence on laxatives.

**DRUG INTERACTIONS**   Drug absorption By increasing intestinal motility, all laxatives may decrease transit time of orally administered drugs and thereby decrease their absorption.

**❧ NURSING CONSIDERATIONS**
**Side effects, toxicities, and associated nursing actions**
  **GI** Abdominal cramping.
  • Monitor degree of cramping. This is usually relieved after effects of dose have worn off. However, if severe or persistent, notify physician.
  • Auscultate bowel sounds prior to administering. Drugs to relieve constipation should not be administered if bowel function is absent or questionable.
**Nursing interventions related to drug administration**
  • Oral doses should be administered with 8 ounces of water if possible.
  • Lubricate suppositories with warm water prior to administering. Encourage patient to retain suppositories as long as possible before expelling.
**Patient and family education**
  • Review with patients the anticipated benefits and possible side effects of therapy. Drugs to treat

constipation vary in action, but many patients assume all are the same. For example, patients may assume laxatives and stool softeners may have the same effect and may be expected to produce a stool within the same period of time.
- Impress upon patients the need to use these drugs only as ordered. Chronic use of laxatives can lead to dependence on these drugs.
- Suggest that patients with constipation increase daily fluid intake to 2500 to 3000 ml, add fruit, fruit juices (especially prune juice), and bran to the diet, and increase level of activity.
- Review with patients that normal bowel schedules do not require daily bowel evacuation; every 2 to 4 days may be normal for an individual.
- Review with parents the inadvisability of encouraging laxative dependence in small children.
- Instruct patients taking one or more of these drugs in preparation for GI examination to take the drugs as ordered and to observe prescribed dietary restrictions. A major reason for having to repeat GI examinations is inadequate preparation of the colon or gut.
- Caution pregnant women to consult their physicians prior to self-administering laxatives to treat constipation. Nursing mothers should also avoid laxatives without prior approval of the physician to avoid laxatives being excreted via breast milk, causing diarrhea in the infant.
- Remind patients to keep these and all medications out of the reach of children.

## cascara sagrada  (kas-KARE-a)  anthraquinone laxative

- cascara sagrada: Sold under generic name (OTC)

## danthron  (DAN-thron)  anthraquinone laxative

- danthron: Modane, Dorbane, ✸Dorbantyl, ✸Roydan (OTC)

## senna, sennosides  (SEN-nah)  anthraquinone laxative

- senna, sennosides: Black Draught, Dr. Caldwell's Senna Laxative, Fletcher's Castoria, Gentlax, ✸Glysennid, Nytilax, Senokap, Senokot, ✸X-Prep (OTC)

**MECHANISM OF ACTION**  The anthraquinones are stimulant laxatives derived from plants (senna, cascara sagrada) or synthetics (danthron). These drugs alter fluid and electrolyte absorption, producing net intestinal fluid accumulation. Stimulant laxatives mainly promote evacuation of the colon. Cascara is the mildest and senna is the most potent of the three anthraquinone laxatives.

**INDICATIONS**  **Constipation** Laxatives of this group are available without prescription and are often self-prescribed.

**CONTRAINDICATIONS**  **Prolonged use** Chronic use of stimulant laxatives may produce persistent diarrhea, hypokalemia, loss of essential nutrients, and dehydration.

**DOSAGE**  **Cascara sagrada:**  *PO:*  **ADULTS:** 300 mg to 1 g; *extract:* 200 to 400 mg; *extract fluid:* 0.5 to 1.5 ml.  **CHILDREN:** Ages 2 to 12 receive 1/2 the adult dose and younger children receive 1/4 the adult dose.  **Danthron:**  *PO:*  **ADULTS AND CHILDREN OVER 12 YEARS OLD:** 75 to 150 mg.  **Senna:**  *PO:*  **ADULTS:** 500 mg to 1 g senna, 12 to 36 mg as sennosides.  **CHILDREN:** Ages 6 to 12 years old receive 1/2 the adult dose; ages 1 to 5 receive 1/3 the adult dose; younger children receive 1/4 the adult dose.  *Special patient populations:*  **PREGNANCY:** Use with caution during pregnancy.

**PREPARATIONS**  Cascara sagrada: *Powder;* Aromatic Fluidextract; Fluidextract; extract: *tablets:* 325 mg. Danthron: *solution:* 37.5 mg/5 ml; *tablets:* 37.5, 75 mg. Senna: *leaf powder:* 662 mg/g; *leaf tablets:* 180 mg; *concentrate powder:* 15 mg sennosides/3 g; *tablets:* 8.6 mg sennosides; *suppositories:* 30 mg sennosides; Fluidextract: *solution:* 325, 350 mg/5 ml; Friot ERExtract: *solution:* 7.5 mg sennosides/5 ml; *syrup:* 1 g/5 ml.

**DRUG INTERACTIONS**    **Drug absorption** By increasing intestinal motility, all laxatives potentially decrease the transit time of orally administered drugs and thereby decrease their absorption.

**DIAGNOSTIC TEST INTERFERENCE**    **PSP** Anthroquinone laxatives may discolor the urine, producing an apparent increase in the urinary excretion of phenolsulfonphthalein (PSP).    **Urinary estrogens** False-positive when measured by the Kober procedure.    **Urinary urobilinogen** False-positive.

**FATE**    Danthron is partly absorbed, but the other anthraquinone laxatives are not. Administered orally, the anthraquinones are effective in 6 to 12 hours. As suppositories, they are effective in 30 minutes to 2 hours.

### ❦ NURSING CONSIDERATIONS

#### Side effects, toxicities, and associated nursing actions

**GI** Abdominal discomfort, nausea, mild cramps.
* See entry for drug class (p. 1021).

**GU** Urine may be pink to red to brown.
* Caution patients about this side effect.
* If there is question that a change in the color of urine may be due to blood, the urine should be tested.

#### Nursing interventions related to drug administration
* See entry for drug class (p. 1021).

#### Patient and family education
* See entry for drug class (p. 1021).

---

## karaya    (kar-EYE-ah)    bulk-forming laxative

* karaya: Sold under generic name (OTC)

---

## malt soup extract    bulk-forming laxative

* malt soup extract: Maltsupex (OTC)

---

## methylcellulose    (meth-ill-SELL-yoo-lose)    bulk-forming laxative

* methylcellulose: Cellothyl, Citrucel, Cologel (OTC)

---

## psyllium hydrophilic mucilloid    (SIL-lee-um)    bulk-forming laxative

* psyllium hydrophilic mucilloid: Effersyllium, Hydrocil Instant, ❦Karacil, Konsyl-D, Metamucil, Modane Bulk, Naturacil, Prodiem Plain, Reguloid, Serutan, Siblin Granules, Syllat, V-Lax (OTC)

**MECHANSIM OF ACTION**    Bulk-forming laxatives dissolve or swell in water to form an emollient gel or viscous solution. The resultant bulk is presumed to promote peristalsis and to reduce transit time.

**INDICATIONS**    **Constipation** The laxative of choice for the initial treatment of most cases of simple constipation resulting from a low-fiber or low-fluid diet. Also indicated when straining at defecation should be avoided.

**CONTRAINDICATIONS**   Presence of nausea and vomiting.   **Acute abdominal pain** Laxatives can mask symptoms of appendicitis.   **Intestinal obstruction, fecal impaction, or undiagnosed rectal bleeding. Prolonged use** Use for more than 1 week can lead to dependence on laxatives.

**DOSAGE**   Karaya: *PO:* ADULTS: 5 to 10 g.   **Malt soup extract:** *PO:* ADULTS AND CHILDREN OVER 2 YEARS OLD: 12 to 64 g.   CHILDREN: 1 month to 2 years old—6 to 32 g.   **Methylcellulose:** *PO:* ADULTS: 4 to 6 g;   CHILDREN: 6 to 12 years old—1 to 1.5 g.   **Psyllium hydrophilic mucilloid:** *PO:* ADULTS: 2.5 to 30 g.   CHILDREN 6 TO 12 YEARS OLD: 1.25 to 15 g.   *Special patient populations:* PREGNANCY: Use with moderation during pregnancy.

**PREPARATIONS**   Karaya, *powder.* Malt soup extract, *powder, solution:* 5.3 g/5 ml; *tablets:* 750 mg. Methylcellulose, *powder:* 105 mg/g; *solution:* 450 mg/5 ml; *tablets:* 500 mg. Psyllium hydrophilic mucilloid, *pieces (chewable):* 1.7 g/piece; *powder:* 309 mg to 1 g, read label of each preparation.

**DRUG INTERACTIONS**   **Drug absorption** By increasing intestinal motility, all laxatives may decrease transit time of orally administered drugs and thereby decrease their absorption.

**FATE**   Bulk laxatives are generally not absorbed from the gastrointestinal tract. Malt soup extract may be hydrolyzed in the colon and metabolized in the liver. The laxative effect is generally apparent in 12 to 24 hours, although the full effect may take 2 to 3 days.

## ❦ NURSING CONSIDERATIONS

### Side effects, toxicities, and associated nursing actions
- See entry for drug class (p. 1021).

GI Mild abdominal discomfort.

### Nursing interventions related to drug administration
- Maltsupex brand 750 mg tablets, and Naturacil brand chewable tablets contain FD & C yellow dye #5 (tartrazine), which may cause an allergic response in susceptible individuals. While rare, this side effect is seen more commonly in persons with aspirin hypersensitivity.
- These drugs should be dissolved or diluted as directed by the manufacturer and should be followed with an additional 240 ml of fluid.

### Patient and family education
- See entry for drug class (p. 1021).
- Caution patients to read labels carefully. Patients who must restrict intake of phenylalinine should be warned that some of the bulk-forming laxatives contain aspartame as a sweetener.

---

## castor oil
laxative

- castor oil: Alphamul, Emulsoil, Fleet, Neoloid, ♣Unisoil (OTC)

**MECHANISM OF ACTION**   In the small intestine, castor oil is hydrolyzed to ricinoleic acid, which is the active principal.

**INDICATIONS**   **Constipation** Castor oil is an old remedy and the most potent of the stimulant cathartics, producing a watery stool in 2 to 6 hours. Gas and feces are cleared from the intestine.

**CONTRAINDICATIONS**   Presence of nausea and vomiting.   **Acute abominal pain** Laxatives can mask symptoms of appendicitis.   **Intestinal obstruction, fecal impaction, or undiagnosed rectal bleeding. Prolonged use** Use for more than 1 week can lead to dependence on laxatives.

**DOSAGE**   PO:   ADULTS: 15 ml for constipation, 15 to 60 ml for colonic evacuation.   CHILDREN: For ages 2 to 12 years old, 5 ml for constipation, 5 to 15 ml for colonic evacuation; for ages under 2 years, 1 ml for constipation, 1 to 5 ml for colonic evacuation.   *Special patient populations:* PREGNANCY: Use with caution during pregnancy; may stimulate labor.

**PREPARATIONS**   *Capsules:* 0.62 ml; *suspension:* 36.4%, 60%, 64%, 95%.

**DRUG INTERACTIONS**   **Drug absorption** By increasing intestinal motility, all laxatives may decrease transit time of orally administered drugs and thereby decrease their absorption.

**FATE**   Castor oil is hydrolyzed in the intestine by a lipase and the products metabolized as fatty acids. Loose bowel movements usually occur within 2 to 3 hours after administration.

### 🐾 NURSING CONSIDERATIONS

**Side effects, toxicities, and associated nursing actions**
- See entry for drug class (p. 1021).
- **GI** Abdominal distress, cramping, nausea.

**Nursing interventions related to drug administration**
- Shake emulsions well prior to administering. They may be further diluted in water, milk, fruit juice, or cola before administering.
- Prior to administering castor oil, check with patient to see which juice the patient prefers as a diluent. Some patients may even prefer to take the medication ''straight'' with the juice as a follow-up liquid so the taste of the juice is not ruined by the medication.
- Regular castor oil does not mix with a water-based diluent and sits on top of the juice or fluid. The addition of a small amount of baking soda (less than 1/4 teaspoon) immediately before administering the dose to the patient will cause the mixture to fizz, and the castor oil will be partially suspended in the juice for a minute or two; the patient may be more willing to take the medication in this form. The routine use of the baking soda should be cleared by the pharmacy or physician.

**Patient and family education**
- See entry for drug class (p. 1021).

---

## bisacodyl (bi-sa-KOE-dill)                     diphenylmethane laxative

- bisacodyl: ✽Apo-Bisacodyl, Biscolax, Carter's Little Pils, Deficol, Dulcolax, Fleet Bisacodyl (OTC)

---

## phenolphthalein (fee-noe-THAY-leen)                  diphenylmethane laxative

- phenolphthalein: Correctol, Evac-U-Lax, Evac-U-Gen, Feen-A-Mint, ✽Fructines-Vichy (OTC)

**MECHANISM OF ACTION** Diphenylmethane derivatives are stimulant laxatives. These drugs alter fluid and electrolyte absorption, producing net intestinal fluid accumulation. Stimulant laxatives mainly promote evacuation of the colon.

**INDICATIONS** **Constipation** Laxatives of this group are available without prescription and are often self-prescribed.

**CONTRAINDICATIONS** **Presence of nausea and vomiting.** **Acute abdominal pain** Laxatives can mask symptoms of appendicitis. **Intestinal obstruction, fecal impaction, or undiagnosed rectal bleeding.** **Prolonged use** Use for more than 1 week can lead to dependence on laxatives.

**DOSAGE** **Bisacodyl:** *PO:* ADULTS: 5 to 15 mg. CHILDREN OVER 3 YEARS OLD: 5 to 10 mg or 0.3 mg/kg. *Rectal:* ADULTS AND CHILDREN OVER 2 YEARS OLD: 10 mg. CHILDREN UNDER 2 YEARS OLD: 5 mg. **Phenolphthalein:** *PO:* ADULTS: 30 to 270 mg. CHILDREN OVER 6 YEARS OLD: 30 to 60 mg. CHILDREN 2 TO 5 YEARS OLD: 15 to 20 mg. *Special patient populations:* PREGNANCY: Use with caution during pregnancy.

**PREPARATIONS** *Bisacodyl, tablets (enteric-coated):* 5 mg; *suppositories:* 10 mg; *suspension (rectal):* 0.33 mg/ml. *Phenolphthalein; tablets:* 60 mg; *tablets (chewable):* 60, 64.8, 80, 90, 97.2 mg; *chewing gum:* 97.2 mg; *suspension:* 22 mg/5 ml.

**DRUG INTERACTIONS** **Drug absorption** By increasing intestinal motility, all laxatives may decrease transit time of orally administered drugs and thereby decrease their absorption.

**FATE** Bisacodyl is only minimally absorbed. About 15% of phenolphthalein is absorbed and undergoes enterchepatic circulation and may be active for several days. Following an oral dose effects are seen in 6 to 8 hours. A suppository is effective in 15 to 60 minutes.

## 🦚 NURSING CONSIDERATIONS

### Side effects, toxicities, and associated nursing actions
- See entry for drug class (p. 1021).

**GI** Abdominal cramping.

### Nursing interventions related to drug administration
- Dulcolax brand tablets and Phenolax brand chewable tablets contain FD & C yellow dye #5 (tartrazine), which may cause an allergic response in susceptible individuals. While rare, this side effect is seen more commonly in persons with aspirin hypersensitivity.

### Patient and family education
- See entry for drug class (p. 1021).

---

## glycerin (GLI-ser-in)       hyperosmotic laxatives

- glycerin: Sold under generic name, Fleet Babylax

---

## sorbitol (SOR-bi-tole)       hyperosmotic laxatives

- sorbitol: Sold under generic name

**MECHANISM OF ACTION** Hyperosmotic laxatives are administered rectally. They are poorly absorbed and therefore attract water, increasing the bulk and promoting prompt defecation.

**INDICATIONS** **Constipation** Hyperosmotic laxatives are used to promote prompt evacuation of the colon. They are not used repeatedly.

**CONTRAINDICATIONS** **Presence of nausea and vomiting.** **Acute abdominal pain** Laxatives can mask symptoms of appendicitis. **Intestinal obstruction, fecal impaction, or undiagnosed rectal bleeding.** **Prolonged use** Use for more than 1 week can lead to dependence on laxatives.

**DOSAGE** **Glycerin:** *Rectal:* **ADULTS AND CHILDREN OVER 6 YEARS OLD:** 3 g as a suppository or 5 to 15 ml as an enema. **CHILDREN UNDER 6 YEARS OLD:** 1 to 1.5 g as a suppository or 2 to 5 ml as an enema. **Sorbitol:** *Enema:* **ADULTS AND CHILDREN OVER 2 YEARS OLD:** 120 ml of a 25% to 30% solution. **CHILDREN UNDER 2 YEARS OLD:** 30 to 60 ml. *Special patient populations:* **PREGNANCY:** Use with caution during pregnancy.

**PREPARATIONS** *Glycerin; solution:* 4 ml application; *suppositories, Sorbitol; solution:* 70%.

**DRUG INTERACTIONS** **Drug absorption** By increasing intestinal motility, all laxatives may decrease transit time of orally administered drugs and thereby decrease their absorption.

**FATE** Glycerin and sorbitol are minimally absorbed when administered rectally. Evacuation of the colon is usually achieved within 15 to 30 minutes.

## 🦚 NURSING CONSIDERATIONS

### Side effects, toxicities, and associated nursing actions
- See entry for drug class (p. 1021).

**GI** Abdominal cramping.

### Nursing interventions related to drug administration
- See entry for drug class (p. 1021).

### Patient and family education
- See entry for drug class (p. 1021).

---

## mineral oil       laxative

- mineral oil: Agoral Plain, Kondremul, Neo-Cultol, Petrogalar Plain, Zymenol Emulsion (OTC)

**MECHANISM OF ACTION**   Orally administered mineral oil lubricates fecal material and retards reabsorption of water from the intestinal tract. Rectally administered mineral oil acts as a lubricant.

**INDICATIONS**   **Constipation** Useful in softening fecal impactions.

**CONTRAINDICATIONS**   **Presence of nausea and vomiting. Acute abdominal pain** Laxatives can mask symptoms of appendicitis.   **Intestinal obstruction, fecal impaction, or undiagnosed rectal bleeding. Prolonged use** Use for more than 1 week can lead to dependence on laxatives.

**DOSAGE**   PO:   **ADULTS AND CHILDREN OVER 6 YEARS OLD:** 15 to 45 ml.   **CHILDREN UNDER 6 YEARS OLD:** 10 to 15 ml.   **Enema:**   **ADULTS AND CHILDREN OVER 6 YEARS OLD:** 60 to 150 ml.   **CHILDREN UNDER 6 YEARS OLD:** 30 to 60 ml.   *Special patient populations:*   **PREGNANCY:** Use with caution during pregnancy.

**PREPARATIONS**   *Jelly:* 55% w/w; *suspension:* 1.4, 2.5, 2.75, 3.25 ml/5 ml; *oil.*

**DRUG INTERACTIONS**   **Drug absorption** By increasing intestinal motility, all laxatives may decrease transit time of orally administered drugs and thereby decrease their absorption.   **Fat-soluble drugs and vitamins** Mineral oil impairs the absorption of vitamins A, D, E, K, oral contraceptives, coumarin and indandione anticoagulants, and nonabsorbable sulfonamides.

**FATE**   Mineral oil is minimally absorbed. It is effective 6 to 8 hours after administration.

❦ **NURSING CONSIDERATIONS**

  **Side effects, toxicities, and associated nursing actions**
- See entry for drug class (p. 1021).

  **GI** Abdominal cramping.

  **Lung** Aspiration pneumonitis is possible if some mineral oil is aspirated. This may be a problem in the elderly.
- Caution patient to always sit upright when taking a dose of mineral oil.
- Because of the possibility of aspiration pneumonitis, agents other than mineral oil should be used for long-term therapy.

  **Nursing interventions related to drug administration**
- Avoid using mineral oil or any oil-based substance to lubricate around the nose of elderly or immobilized patients, to avoid the possibility of aspiration.

  **Patient and family education**
- See entry for drug class (p. 1021).
- Regular use of mineral oil may result in leakage of oil or fecal material from the anus. Caution the patient about this. It may be necessary for the patient to wear a perinanal pad to prevent staining of clothing and sheets.

---

## magnesium citrate (citrate of magnesia)   saline laxative

- magnesium citrate (citrate of magnesia): Citroma, ✿ Citro-Mag, Evac-Q-Mag (OTC)

---

## magnesium hydroxide   saline laxative

- magnesium hydroxide: Milk of Magnesia (OTC)

---

## magnesium sulfate (epsom salts)   saline laxative

- magnesium sulfate (epsom salts): Sold under generic name (OTC)

## sodium phosphates

- sodium phosphates: Fleet Phospho Soda, Fleet Enema (OTC)

**MECHANISM OF ACTION**　Saline laxatives are poorly absorbed salts of magnesium or sodium. The concentrated solutions attract water osmotically into the lumen of the large intestine, and the resulting bulk stimulates peristalsis.

**INDICATIONS**　**Constipation** Uses include elimination of parasites after anthelmintic therapy, evacuating the bowel after some poisons have been ingested, or preparation for surgery or colonic examination.

**CONTRAINDICATIONS**　**Presence of nausea and vomiting.　Acute abdominal pain** Laxatives can mask symptoms of appendicitis.　**Intestinal obstruction, fecal impaction, or undiagnosed rectal bleeding. Prolonged use** Use for more than 1 week can lead to dependence on laxatives.

**DOSAGE**　*Magnesium citrate solution:*　**PO:**　**ADULTS:** 100 to 200 ml.　**CHILDREN 6 TO 12 YEARS OLD:** 50 to 100 ml.　**CHILDREN 2 TO 5 YEARS OLD:** 4 to 12 ml. *Magnesium hydroxide:*　**PO:**　**ADULTS:** 30 to 60 ml.　**CHILDREN 6 TO 12 YEARS OLD:** 15 to 30 ml.　**CHILDREN 2 TO 5 YEARS OLD:** 5 to 15 ml. *Magnesium sulfate:*　**PO:**　**ADULTS:** 10 to 30 g.　**CHILDREN 6 TO 12 YEARS OLD:** 5 to 10 g. **CHILDREN 2 TO 5 YEARS OLD:** 2.5 to 5 g. *Sodium phosphates:*　**PO:**　**ADULTS:** 30 to 60 ml. **CHILDREN OVER 10 YEARS OLD:** 50% adult dose.　**CHILDREN 5 TO 10 YEARS OLD:** 25% adult dose.　**Enema:**　**ADULTS:** 120 ml.　**CHILDREN OVER 2 YEARS OLD:** 50% adult dose.　*Special patient populations:*　**PREGNANCY:** Use with caution during pregnancy.

**PREPARATIONS**　*Magnesium citrate: solution, powder. Magnesium hydroxide, suspension:* 77.5 mg/g; *concentrate (3x suspension); tablets:* 300, 600 mg. *Magnesium sulfate: powder, crystals. Sodium phosphates: solution (oral):* dibasic sodium phosphate 900 mg/5 ml with monobasic sodium phosphate 2.4 g/5 ml; *solution (rectal):* dibasic sodium phosphate 60 mg/ml with monobasic sodium phosphate 160 mg/ml.

**DRUG INTERACTIONS**　**Drug absorption** By increasing intestinal motility, all laxatives may decrease transit time of orally administered drugs and thereby decrease their absorption.　**Chlorpromazine, chlordiazepoxide, dicumarol, digoxin, isoniazid** Absorption of these drugs is decreased by magnesium hydroxide.

**FATE**　A variable amount of salts may be absorbed from orally administered saline laxatives, probably less than 20%. Saline laxatives produce a semifluid or watery stool in 3 to 6 hours after oral administration. Enemas are effective in 2 to 5 minutes.

### ❦ NURSING CONSIDERATIONS

#### Side effects, toxicities, and associated nursing actions
- See entry for drug class (p. 1021).
  **GI** Abdominal cramping.

#### Nursing interventions related to drug administration
- Sodium salt preparations should be used with caution in persons with a history of heart disease.

#### Patient and family education
- See entry for drug class (p. 1021).

## docusate calcium　(DOO-ku-sate)

- docusate calcium: Surfak, Dioctocal, Pro-Cal Sof (OTC)

## docusate potassium

- docusate potassium: Dialose, Kasof (OTC)

## docusate sodium

- docusate sodium: Generic, Colace, Diosuccin, Diosul, Disonate, Doss 300, Duosol, Laxinate 100, Modane Soft, ✦Regulex (OTC)

**MECHANISM OF ACTION**   Stool softeners soften fecal material and ease defecation. The softening results from a lowering of the surface tension of the fecal material, allowing water and lipids to penetrate.

**INDICATIONS**   **Constipation** Stool softeners are considered safer to use than mineral oil.

**CONTRAINDICATIONS**   **Presence of nausea and vomiting.**   **Acute abdominal pain** Laxatives can mask symptoms of appendicitis.   **Intestinal obstruction, fecal impaction, or undiagnosed rectal bleeding.**   **Prolonged use** Use for more than 1 week can lead to dependence on laxatives.

**DOSAGE**   **PO:**   **ADULTS AND CHILDREN OVER 12 YEARS OLD:** 50 to 360 mg daily.   **CHILDREN 2 TO 12 YEARS OLD:** 50 to 150 mg daily.   **CHILDREN UNDER 2 YEARS OLD:** 25 mg daily.   *Special patient populations:*   **PREGNANCY:** Use with caution during pregnancy.

**PREPARATIONS**   *Docusate calcium, capsules:* 50, 240 mg. *Docusate potassium, capsules:* 100, 240 mg. *Docusate sodium, capsules:* 50, 100, 240, 250, 300 mg; *solution:* 10, 50 mg/ml, 16.7, 20 mg/5 ml; *tablets:* 50, 100 mg.

**DRUG INTERACTIONS**   **Drug absorption** By increasing intestinal motility, all laxatives may decrease transit time of orally administered drugs and thereby decrease their absorption.

**FATE**   Docusate salts are minimally absorbed. Softning of the feces takes 1 to 3 days.

### ☙ NURSING CONSIDERATIONS

#### Side effects, toxicities, and associated nursing actions
- See entry for drug class (p. 1021).

**GI** Abdominal cramping.

#### Nursing interventions related to drug administration
- See entry for drug class (p. 1021).

#### Patient and family education
- See entry for drug class (p. 1021).
- Stool softeners must usually be taken on a regular basis to achieve desired response. Instruct patients that stool softeners do not act as rapidly as other kinds of drugs for constipation.

# OPHTHALMIC DRUGS

**INTRODUCTION**   The drugs covered in this unit affect the eye by acting through the autonomic nervous system. The details of the physiologic mechanisms are given in the drug sections. Table 61-1 summarizes the pharmacologic mechanisms and uses of autonomic drugs for the eye. These uses include facilitation of an eye examination to allow the measurement of refraction and the treatment of glaucoma.

**XVI**

# Chapter Sixty-one

# Drugs for mydriasis and/or cycloplegia

**Anticholinergic drugs**
atropine
cyclopentolate
homatropine
scopolamine
tropicamide

**Adrenergic drugs**
hydroxamphetamine
phenylephrine

## DRUG COMBINATIONS

- atropine sulfate and prednisolone acetate: Mydrapred
- cyclopentolate hydrochloride and phenylephrine hydrochloride: Cyclomydril
- epinephrine bitartrate and pilocarpine hydrochloride: E-Pilo, PE
- phenylephrine hydrochloride and zinc sulfate: Optised, Phenylzin, Prefrin-Z
- phenylephrine hydrochloride and pyrilamine maleate: Prefrin-A
- phenylephrine hydrochloride and sulfacetamide sodium: Vasosulf
- scopolamine hydrobromide and phenylephrine hydrochloride: Murocoll-2

**OVERVIEW OF THE DRUG CLASS** Examination of the eye requires dilation of the pupil to view the interior of the eye. Mydriasis (dilation of the pupil) can be accomplished with either anticholinergic drugs or with adrenergic drugs. Anticholinergic drugs also produce paralysis of accommodation (cycloplegia).

**MECHANISM OF ACTION** The autonomic nervous system plays a major role in controlling the amount of light entering the eye and in focusing images. The amount of light penetrating the eye is controlled by the size of the pigmented iris, which contains two sets of muscles: the sphincter muscles and the dilator muscles. The sphincter muscles are circular muscles with muscarinic receptors innervated by the parasympathetic nervous system. The pupil is constricted when the sphincter muscles contract so that only a small surface on the eye passes light. The dilator muscles contain alpha receptors innervated by the sympathetic nervous system. As the name indicates, the pupil is dilated when these radial muscles contract after stimulation of the alpha receptors.

*Miosis* is the term that refers to a constricted pupil. Miosis is achieved primarily by stimulating the muscarinic receptors of the sphincter muscles. *Mydriasis* is the term that refers to a dilated pupil and is achieved either by blocking the muscarinic receptors of the sphincter muscles or by stimulating the alpha receptors of the dilator muscles.

The cornea and the lens determine the focus of images onto the retina. The cornea accomplishes the coarse focusing, but the fine focusing for sharp images and near vision is accomplished by the lens. The shape of the lens is controlled by muscarinic receptors of the parasympathetic nervous system. Accommodation for near vision requires the contraction of ciliary muscles to change the shape of the lens. Ligaments normally pull the lens to keep it relatively flat. The contraction of the ciliary muscles relaxes the ligaments so that the lens becomes rounder as required for near vision. *Cycloplegia* refers to the paralysis of the ciliary muscles by drugs that block muscarinic receptors. Cycloplegia causes blurred vision because the shape of the lens can no longer be adjusted for near vision.

**INDICATIONS** • Diagnostic examination of the eye.

**CONTRAINDICATIONS** • See the individual drug.

**DRUG INTERACTIONS** Systemic drug interactions are not common when these drugs are used topically.

### ❦ NURSING CONSIDERATIONS

#### Nursing interventions related to drug administration

- Wash hands carefully prior to administering eye medications.
- Place ordered dose of eye medication in the lower conjunctival sac and never directly on the cornea. Avoid touching any part of the eye with the dropper or applicator. To prevent overflow of medication into nasal and pharyngeal passages and thus reduce systemic absorption, instruct patient to occlude the nasolacrimal duct with one finger for 1 to 2 minutes after the medication has been instilled.
- Each patient should have a separate bottle or tube of medication to avoid accidental cross-contamination.

**Table 61-1.**

## Autonomic drugs affecting the eye

| Mechanism/Drug | Effect | Use |
|---|---|---|
| **PARASYMPATHETIC DRUGS** | | |
| Cholinomimetic drugs | | |
| Carbachol | Constriction | Treatment of glaucoma |
| Demecarium | Improved uptake | |
| Echothiophate | of aqueous humor | |
| Isofluophate | | |
| Physostigmine | | |
| Pilocarpine | | |
| Anticholinergic drugs | | |
| Atropine | Dilation | Eye examination |
| Cyclopentolate | Loss of accomoda- | Measurement of refraction |
| Homatropine | tion | |
| Scopolamine | | |
| Tropicamide | | |
| **SYMPATHETIC DRUGS** | | |
| Alpha receptor agonists | Dilation | Eye examination |
| Hydroxamphetamine | | |
| Phenylephrine | | |
| Alpha and beta agonists | | |
| Dipivefrin | Increased uptake | Treatment of glaucoma |
| Epinephrine | and decreased | |
| | production of | |
| | aqueous humor | |
| Beta blockers | | |
| Levobunolol | Decreased intraocu- | Treatment of glaucoma |
| Timolol | lar pressure | |

### Patient and family education

- Review with patient and family the expected benefits and possible side effects of drug therapy.
- Tell patients to avoid driving or operating hazardous equipment if vision is blurred. Tell adults that they may be unable to drive home following eye examinations during which this medication is used; a friend or family member should drive until the effects of the medication wear off.
- Review with patients and families the correct technique for drug administration, including teaching patients to wash hands prior to administering eye drops. Have patient give a return demonstration to check for understanding and ability of patient to administer drug correctly. Tell patients that bottles or tubes of eye medications should never be shared; each person requiring an eye medication should have a separate, clearly labeled bottle or tube.
- If photophobia occurs, instruct patient to wear sunglasses and avoid bright lights. Sunglasses should not be worn after dusk.
- Instruct patients to administer missed doses as soon as they are remembered, unless within 1 to 2 hours of the next dose. Patients should not double up to make up for missed doses.
- Instruct patients to read labels carefully. Eye medications are often available in a variety of strengths, and patients should use only the strength prescribed to ensure adequate treatment of the eye condition. Remind patients that no medications should be put in the eye unless the medications are clearly labeled for ophthalmic use.
- Remind patients to keep these and all medications out of the reach of children.

## atropine sulfate (A-troe-peen) mydriatic and cycloplegic

- atropine sulfate: Atropisol, Atropair, Atropine-Care, Isopto Atropine Sulfate, ✢SMP Atropine, Ocu-Tropine

**MECHANISM OF ACTION**  Atropine is a muscarinic antagonist, blocking cholinergic receptors of the sphincter and ciliary muscles, thereby causing dilation and loss of accommodation.

**INDICATIONS**  **Eye examination** Atropine produces mydriasis and cycloplegia for examination of the retina and optic disk and accurate measurement of refractive index. Atropine is especially effective in children under 6 years old, a group having active accommodation.  **Inflammatory conditions** Atropine is adjunctive therapy for the management of acute inflammatory conditions.  **Amblyopia (dimness of vision)** Atropine is used to reduce the visual acuity of the unaffected eye to force fixation with the amblyopic eye.

**CONTRAINDICATIONS**  **Glaucoma** Atropine will worsen narrow-angle glaucoma.

**DOSAGE**  **Topical:**  **ADULTS:** 1 drop of a 1% solution 1 hour before examination; alternatively, 0.3 to 0.5 cm of a 1% ointment is placed into the conjunctival sac one to three times the day of examination. **CHILDREN:** 1 to 2 drops of a 0.5% solution in each eye twice daily for 1 to 3 days before examination; alternatively, 0.3 cm of a 1% ointment placed into the conjunctival sac three times daily for 1 to 3 days before the examination.  *Special patient populations:*  **ELDERLY:** Altered doses for the elderly have not been specifically established. Glaucoma should be ruled out before atropine is administered. Elderly patients are also sensitive to the systemic effects of atropine.  **CHILDREN:** Pediatric doses are given above. Because children are treated for 1 or more days, they should be carefully monitored for systemic toxicity.  **PREGNANCY:** Use with caution during pregnancy.

**PREPARATIONS**  *Ointment:* 0.5%, 1%. *Solution:* 0.5%, 1%, 2%, 3%.

**DRUG INTERACTIONS**  Systemic drug interactions are not common when this drug is used topically.

**FATE**  Mydriatic activity peaks in 30 to 40 minutes, but cycloplegic activity is not maximum for several hours. Mydriasis persists for 7 to 12 days and cycloplegia for 2 weeks or more. Atropine sulfate is absorbed through the conjuctiva. Excessive systemic absorption is avoided by applying finger pressure to the lacrimal sac for about 2 minutes following instillation into the eye.

### ❦ NURSING CONSIDERATIONS

#### Side effects, toxicities, and associated nursing actions

**CNS** Mental aberration.
- Assess mental status prior to administering medication. Report any changes in mental status to physician.

**CV** Rapid or irregular pulse.
- Monitor pulse rate in children; instruct adults to report perceived changes in pulse.
- Review administration technique; tachycardia reflects systemic absorption of the drug.

**Eye** Increased intraocular pressure; irritation, hyperemia, edema, follicular conjunctivitis, dermatitis.
- Be certain that glaucoma has been ruled out prior to administering.
- Instruct patients to report any eye irritation that develops during or for up to 2 weeks after use of this medication.

**GI** In infants, abdominal distension.
- Monitor abdominal girth in infants. Monitor bowel sounds and keep a record of patient's bowel movements while on atropine therapy, and for several days after drug is discontinued.

#### Nursing interventions related to drug administration
- See entry for drug class (p. 1032).

#### Patient and family education
- See entry for drug class (p. 1033).

## cyclopentolate hydrochloride    (sye-kloe-PEN-toe-late)   mydriatic and cycloplegic

- cyclopentolate hydrochloride: AK-Pentolate, Cyclogyl, ♣Minims, Ocu-Pentolate, Pentolair

**MECHANISM OF ACTION**   Cyclopentolate is a muscarinic antagonist, blocking cholinergic receptors of the sphincter and ciliary muscles and thereby causing dilation and loss of accommodation.

**INDICATIONS**   Eye examinations Cyclopentolate produces mydriasis and cycloplegia.

**CONTRAINDICATIONS**   • Closed-angle glaucoma.

**DOSAGE**   Topical:   **ADULTS:** 1 drop of a 1% or 2% solution, followed by a second drop in 5 minutes. Apply 40 to 50 minutes before examination. Darkly pigmented eyes require a 2% solution.   **CHILDREN:** 1 drop of a 0.5%, 1%, or 2% solution, followed by a second drop in 5 minutes. Apply 40 to 50 minutes before examination.   *Special patient populations:*   **ELDERLY:** Cyclopentolate should be used with caution in elderly patients because they are predisposed to increased intraocular pressure.   **CHILDREN:** Children are prone to psychotic reactions from systemic absorption.   **PREGNANCY:** Use with caution during pregnancy.

**PREPARATIONS**   *Solution:* 0.5%, 1%, 2%.

**DRUG INTERACTIONS**   Pilocarpine Used to hasten the recovery from mydriasis and cycloplegia. One or 2 drops of a 1% or 2% solution in each eye will reduce the recovery time to 3 to 6 hours.

**FATE**   Cyclopentolate is effective within 60 minutes of instillation into the eye. Systemic absorption may be minimized by applying finger pressure to the lacrimal sac for 2 minutes. Mydriasis and cycloplegia persist for about 24 hours.

### ❧ NURSING CONSIDERATIONS

#### Side effects, toxicities, and associated nursing actions

**CNS** Psychotic reactions and behavioral disturbances in children are associated with systemic absorption. Symptoms seen within an hour include ataxia, incoherent speech, restlessness, wandering, irrelevant talking, hallucinations, disorientation, amnesia.

- Assess mental status prior to administering medication. Report any changes in mental status to physician.

**CV** Tachycardia.

- Monitor pulse rate in children; instruct adults to report perceived changes in pulse.
- Review administration technique; tachycardia reflects systemic absorption of the drug.

**Eye** A transient burning sensation is common; increased intraocular pressure.

- Be certain that glaucoma has been ruled out prior to administering.
- Warn patients about burning sensation prior to administering drug; children may be unable to tolerate burning. If burning is severe or persistent, a lower dose may be necessary. Notify physician.

**Allergic** Reaction is characterized by persistent irritation after instillation of the drug; red, itchy eyes.

- Instruct patients to report any eye irritation that develops during or for up to 2 weeks after use of this medication.

#### Nursing interventions related to drug administration
- See entry for drug class (p. 1032).

#### Patient and family education
- See entry for drug class (p. 1033).

## homatropine hydrobromide    (hoe-MA-troe-peen)    mydriatic and cycloplegic

- homatropine hydrobromide: Ak-Homatropine, Isopto Homatropine

**MECHANISM OF ACTION**   Homatropine is a muscarinic antagonist, blocking cholinergic receptors of the sphincter and ciliary muscles, thereby causing dilation and loss of accomodation.

**INDICATIONS**   • Eye examination. • Management of acute inflammatory conditions of the eye.

**CONTRAINDICATIONS**   • Glaucoma.

**DOSAGE** Topical: ADULTS: 1 or 2 drops of a 2% solution or 1 drop of a 5% solution into each eye immediately before examination and at 5- to 10-minute intervals as needed. CHILDREN: 1 drop of a 2% solution or 1 drop into each eye immediately before examination and at 10-minute intervals as needed. *Special patient populations:* ELDERLY: Homatropine should be used with caution in elderly patients because they are predisposed to increased intraocular pressure. CHILDREN: Pediatric doses are given above. Young children and infants are especially susceptible to adverse systemic antimuscarinic effects. PREGNANCY: Use with caution during pregnancy.

**PREPARATIONS** *Solution:* 2%, 5%.

**DRUG INTERACTIONS** Systemic drug interactions are not common when this drug is used topically.

**FATE** Homatropine is relatively short-acting. The maximum mydriatic effect occurs in 10 to 30 minutes and the maximum cycloplegic effects in 30 to 90 minutes. Excessive systemic absorption is avoided by applying finger pressure to the lacrimal sac for about 2 minutes following instillation into the eye. The *duration of action* for mydriasis ranges from 6 hours to 4 days, and that for cycloplegia is 10 to 48 hours.

## 🦫 NURSING CONSIDERATIONS

### Side effects, toxicities, and associated nursing actions

**CNS** Psychotic reactions and behavioral disturbances in children are associated with systemic absorption. Symptoms seen within an hour include ataxia, incoherent speech, restlessness, wandering, irrelevant talking, hallucinations, disorientation, and amnesia.
- Assess mental status prior to administering medication. Report any changes in mental status to physician.

**CV** Tachycardia.
- Monitor pulse rate in children; instruct adults to report perceived changes in pulse.
- Review administration technique; tachycardia reflects systemic absorption of the drug.

**Eye** A transient burning sensation is common; increased intraocular pressure.
- Be certain that glaucoma has been ruled out prior to administering.
- Warn patients about burning sensation prior to administering drug; children may be unable to tolerate burning. If burning is severe or persistent, a lower dose may be necessary. Notify physician.

**Allergic** Reaction is characterized by persistent irritation after instillation of the drug; red, itchy eyes.
- Instruct patients to report any eye irritation that develops during or for up to 2 weeks after use of this medication.

### Nursing interventions related to drug administration
- See entry for drug class (p. 1032).

### Patient and family education
- See entry for drug class (p. 1033).

---

## scopolamine hydrobromide (skoe-POL-a-meen) mydriatic and cycloplegic

- scopolamine hydrobromide: Isopto Hyoscine

**MECHANISM OF ACTION** Scopolamine (hyoscine) is a muscarinic antagonist, blocking cholinergic receptors of the sphincter and ciliary muscles and thereby causing dilation and loss of accommodation.

**INDICATIONS** Eye examination. **Acute inflammation of the eye** Adjunctive therapy.

**CONTRAINDICATIONS** Glaucoma.

**DOSAGE** Topical: ADULTS: 1 or 2 drops of a 0.25% solution into each eye 1 hour before examination. CHILDREN: 1 drop of a 0.25% solution into each eye twice daily for 2 days before the examination. *Special patient populations:* ELDERLY: Scopolamine should be used with caution in elderly patients because they are predisposed to increased intraocular pressure. CHILDREN: Pediatric doses are given above. Young children and infants are especially susceptible to adverse systemic antimuscarinic effects. PREGNANCY: Use with caution during pregnancy.

**PREPARATIONS** *Solution:* 0.25%

**DRUG INTERACTIONS** Systemic drug interactions are not common when this drug is used topically.

**FATE** The maximum mydriatic effect is in 15 to 30 minutes after application, and the maximum cycloplegic action is in 30 to 45 minutes. The *duration of action* is up to 7 days. Excessive systemic absorption is avoided by applying finger pressure to the lacrimal sac for about 2 minutes following instillation into the eye.

## ✺ NURSING CONSIDERATIONS

### Side effects, toxicities, and associated nursing actions

**CNS** Psychotic reactions and behavioral disturbances in children are associated with systemic absorption. Symptoms seen within an hour include ataxia, incoherent speech, restlessness, wandering, irrelevant talking, hallucinations, disorientation, amnesia.

- Assess mental status prior to administering medication. Report any changes in mental status to physician.

**CV** Tachycardia.

- Monitor pulse rate in children; instruct adults to report perceived changes in pulse.
- Review administration technique; tachycardia reflects systemic absorption of the drug.

**Eye** A transient burning sensation is common; increased intraocular pressure.

- Be certain that glaucoma has been ruled out prior to administering drug.
- Warn patients about burning sensation prior to administering drug; children may be unable to tolerate burning. If burning is severe or persistent, a lower dose may be necessary. Notify physician.

**Allergic** Reaction is characterized by persistent irritation after instillation of the drug; red, itchy eyes.

- Instruct patients to report any eye irritation that develops during or for up to 2 weeks after use of this medication.

### Nursing interventions related to drug administration

- See entry for drug class (p. 1032).

### Patient and family education

- See entry for drug class (p. 1033).

---

## tropicamide  (troe-PIK-a-mide)  mydriatic and cycloplegic

- tropicamide: Mydriacyl, Mydriafair, Ocu-Tropic, Tropicacyl

**MECHANISM OF ACTION** Tropicamide is a muscarinic antagonist, blocking cholinergic receptors of the sphincter and ciliary muscles and thereby causing dilation and loss of accommodation.

**INDICATIONS**   **Eye examination** Not reliable for complete cycloplegia.

**CONTRAINDICATIONS**  Glaucoma.

**DOSAGE**   **Topical:**   **ADULTS AND CHILDREN:** 1 or 2 drops of a 0.5% solution into each eye 15 to 20 minutes before examination produces good mydriasis. For cycloplegia, a 1% solution is necessary and should be repeated in 5 minutes. This must be repeated in 20 to 30 minutes if the examination is not over. *Special patient populations:*   **ELDERLY:** Tropicamide should be used with caution in elderly patients because they are predisposed to increased intraocular pressure.   **CHILDREN:** Pediatric doses are given above. Young children and infants are especially susceptible to adverse systemic antimuscarinic effects.   **PREGNANCY:** Use with caution during pregnancy.

**PREPARATIONS**  *Solution:* 0.5%, 1%.

**DRUG INTERACTIONS**  Systemic drug interactions are not common when this drug is used topically.

**FATE** The maximum mydriatic effect is seen in 20 to 40 minutes, and the maximum cycloplegic effect is in 20 to 35 minutes. Excessive systemic absorption is avoided by applying finger pressure to the lacrimal sac for about 2 minutes following instillation into the eye. Mydriasis persists for about 6 hours and cycloplegia for 1 to 6 hours.

## ✺ NURSING CONSIDERATIONS

### Side effects, toxicities, and associated nursing actions

**CNS** Headache

- Instruct patient to report the development of headache. If severe or persistent, notify physician.

**CV** Tachycardia.
- Monitor pulse rate in children; instruct adults to report perceived changes in pulse.
- Be alert to cardiac effects in persons with a history of heart disease. Monitor blood pressure.
- Review administration technique; cardiac effects reflect systemic absorption of the drug.

**Eye** Stinging, blurred vision.
- Be certain glaucoma has been ruled out prior to administering drug.
- If photophobia occurs, instruct patient to wear sunglasses and avoid bright lights. Sunglasses should not be worn after dusk.
- Tell patients to avoid driving or operating hazardous equipment if vision is blurred. Tell adults that they may be unable to drive home following eye examinations during which this medication is used; a friend or family member should drive until the effects of the medication wear off.
- If stinging is severe or persistent, a lower dose may be necessary; notify physician.

**GI** Dry mouth.
- Review administration technique; dry mouth may reflect systemic absorption of the drug.
- Encourage patients to increase fluid intake, chew sugarless gum or suck on sugarless candy, perform oral hygiene frequently, but avoid drying mouthwashes. Some patients may wish to substitute commercially available saliva substitutes.

**Allergic** Persistent itching and redness of the eye.
- Instruct patients to report any eye irritation that develops during or for up to 2 weeks after use of this medication.

### Nursing interventions related to drug administration
- See entry for drug class (p. 1032).

### Patient and family education
- See entry for drug class (p. 1033).

---

## hydroxamphetamine hydrobromide  (hye-drox-am-FET-a-meen)  mydriatic

- hydroxamphetamine hydrobromide: Paredrine

**MECHANISM OF ACTION**  Hydroxamphetamine is an indirect-acting adrenergic agonist, causing release of norepinephrine from sympathetic nerve endings. The pupil is dilated following contraction of the dilator muscles of the eye.

**INDICATIONS**  **Eye examination** Adrenergic drugs are used when cycloplegia (paralysis of accommodation) is not required for refraction measurements.

**CONTRAINDICATIONS**  **Glaucoma. Hypertension, hyperthyroidism, diabetes mellitus** Patients with these conditions can be made worse by adrenergic drugs.

**DOSAGE**  **Topical:**  **ADULTS AND CHILDREN:** 1 or 2 drops of a 1% solution.  *Special patient populations:*  **ELDERLY:** Elderly patients are more likely to suffer from undetected glaucoma.  **CHILDREN:** Pediatric doses are the same as adult doses.  **PREGNANCY:** Use with caution during pregnancy.

**PREPARATIONS**  *Solution:* 1%.

**DRUG INTERACTIONS**  **Cocaine** blocks the uptake of hydroxamphetamine. Allow at least 2 days between the use of topical cocaine and hydroxamphetamine.  **Guanethedine** blocks the action of hydroxamphetamine.  **Pilocarpine** This cholinergic agonist can be instilled into the eye to counteract excessive mydriasis. Systemic drug interactions are not common when this drug is used topically.

**FATE**  Mydriasis is achieved in about 40 minutes and persists for several hours. Excessive systemic absorption is avoided by applying finger pressure to the lacrimal sac for about 2 minutes following instillation into the eye.

### ☙ NURSING CONSIDERATIONS
#### Side effects, toxicities, and associated nursing actions
**CNS** Headache.
- Instruct patient to report the development of headache. If severe or persistent, notify physician.

**CV** Palpitation, arrhythmias, increased blood pressure, sweating.
* Monitor pulse rate in children; instruct adults to report perceived changes in pulse.
* Be alert to cardiac effects in persons with a history of heart disease. Monitor blood pressure.
* Review administration technique; cardiac effects reflect systemic absorption of the drug.

**Eye** Blurred vision, photophobia.
* Be certain glaucoma has been ruled out prior to administering drug.
* If photophobia occurs, instruct patient to wear sunglasses and avoid bright lights. Sunglasses should not be worn after dusk.
* Tell patients to avoid driving or operating hazardous equipment if vision is blurred. Tell adults that they may be unable to drive home following eye examinations during which this medication is used; a friend or family member should drive until the effects of the medication wear off.

**Nursing interventions related to drug administration**
* See entry for chapter (p. 1032).

**Patient and family education**
* See entry for chapter (p. 1033).

---

## phenylephrine hydrochloride    (fen-il-EF-rin)    mydriatic

* phenylephrine hydrochloride: Ak-Nefrin, Ak-Dilate, Dilitair, Isopto Frin, Mydfrin, Neo-Synephrine, Ocugestrin, OcuPhrin, Prefrin Liquifilm

**MECHANISM OF ACTION**    Phenylephrine is an alpha agonist, dilating the pupil by stimulating contraction of the dilator muscles.

**INDICATIONS**    **Eye examination** Adrenergic drugs are used when cycloplegia (paralysis of accomodation) is not required for refraction measurements.    **Glaucoma** Phenylephrine may decrease intraocular pressure.    **Eye surgery** Phenylephrine not only produces dilation of the pupil but also acts as a vasoconstricter to control bleeding.

**CONTRAINDICATIONS**    **Hypertension, hyperthyroidism, diabetes mellitus** Patients with these conditions can be made worse by adrenergic drugs.

**DOSAGE**    **Topical:**    **ADULTS AND CHILDREN:** For ophthalmoscopy or retinal photography, 1 or 2 drops of a 2.5% or 10% solution 10 to 60 minutes before examination.    *Special patient populations:*    **ELDERLY:** In patients over 50 years old, rebound miosis may occur the day after phenylephrine is used.    **CHILDREN:** Young children may have a severe hypertensive response to phenylephrine. Only the 2.5% solution should be used, particularly with children under 1 year old.    **PREGNANCY:** Use with caution during pregnancy.

**PREPARATIONS**    *Solution:* 0.12%, 2.5%, 10%.

**DRUG INTERACTIONS**    **Cycloplegic drugs** Concomitant use of phenylephrine with one of the anticholinergic ophthalmic drugs will enhance dilation.    **Pilocarpine** This cholinergic agonist can be instilled into the eye to counteract excessive mydriasis.    **Monoamine oxidase inhibitors** may potentiate the response to phenylephrine.    **Guanethedine** will potentiate the response to phenylephrine.

**FATE**    Mydriasis is achieved in 15 to 30 minutes and persists for about 3 hours when the 2.5% solution is used. For the 10% solution, mydriasis takes 10 to 90 minutes and persists for 3 to 7 hours. Excessive systemic absorption is avoided by applying finger pressure to the lacrimal sac for about 2 minutes following instillation into the eye.

### ☙ NURSING CONSIDERATIONS
**Side effects, toxicities, and associated nursing actions**

**CNS** Headache.
* Instruct patient to report the development of headache. If severe or persistent, notify physician.

**CV** Palpitation, arrhythmias, increased blood pressure, sweating.
* Monitor pulse rate in children; instruct adults to report perceived changes in pulse.
* Be alert to cardiac effects in persons with a history of heart disease. Monitor blood pressure.
* Review administration technique; cardiac effects reflect systemic absorption of the drug.

**Eye** Blurred vision, photophobia.
- Be certain glaucoma has been ruled out prior to administering drug.
- If photophobia occurs, instruct patient to wear sunglasses and avoid bright lights. Sunglasses should not be worn after dusk.
- Tell patients to avoid driving or operating hazardous equipment if vision is blurred. Tell adults that they may be unable to drive home following eye examinations during which this medication is used; a friend or family member should drive until the effects of the medication wear off.

## Nursing interventions related to drug administration
- See entry for chapter (p. 1032).

## Patient and family education
- See entry for chapter (p. 1033).

# Chapter Sixty-two
# Drugs to treat glaucoma

**Cholinomimetic drugs**
carbachol
demecarium
echothiophate
isoflurophate
pysostigmine
pilocarpine

**Adrenergic drugs**
dipivefrin
epinephrine
levobunolol
timolol

**INTRODUCTION**   *Glaucoma* is the increase in intraocular pressure resulting from fluid accumulation between the lens and the cornea. The space between the lens and cornea is filled with aqueous humor. Aqueous humor is a protein-poor fluid formed by the ciliary body. This fluid is normally reabsorbed through the trabecular spaces into Schlemm's canal in a special region of the cornea called the anterior chamber. If the aqueous humor cannot be reabsorbed through the anterior chamber, the fluid accumulates and intraocular pressure increases. If the intraocular pressure is not relieved, the optic nerve will become damaged, resulting in blindness.

*Chronic (open-angle) glaucoma* is the more common form of glaucoma and is very gradual in its onset. The defect is a slow degeneration of the anterior chamber so that the uptake of aqueous humor is impaired. Chronic drug therapy is generally effective in controlling the accumulation of aqueous humor and thereby preventing blindness.

The initial treatment for chronic glaucoma is usually the application of a weak cholinomimetic drug to cause constriction of the pupil (miosis). The therapeutic effectiveness is a result of the spread of the trabecular spaces of the anterior chamber when the sphincter muscles contract. The larger area allows improved uptake of the aqueous humor, which relieves intraocular pressure.

The adrenergic drug epinephrine is the alternate drug to initiate therapy, or epinephrine is the next drug added when the miotic drug alone is inadequate. Epinephrine stimulates both alpha and beta receptors, and in the eye, stimulation of alpha receptors reduces resistance to the outflow of aqueous humor, whereas stimulation of the beta receptors decreases production of aqueous humor.

Adrenergic beta blocking drugs have become important in the treatment of chronic glaucoma, either alone or in addition to other drugs. Beta blockers decrease intraocular pressure. The mechanism is not clear but involves reduced production of aqueous humor.

In cases of resistant glaucoma, certain diuretics may be used that have proven effective in decreasing fluid from the eye. These diuretics include carbonic anhydrase inhibitors and osmotic diuretics. Carbonic anhydrase inhibitors such as acetazolamide, dichlorpheramide, and methazolamide have a direct effect that decreases the production of aqeuous humor. Osmotic diuretics such as mannitol and urea draw fluid from the eyeball for an immediate reduction in intraocular pressure. Diuretics are presented in Chapter 3.

*Acute (closed-angle) glaucoma* is characterized by the iris bulging up to shut off access of the aqueous humor to the anterior chamber. This creates an emergency because the build-up of intraocular pressure may become severe rapidly, damaging the optic nerve and causing blindness. Emergency treatment consists of a cholinomimetic drug, a carbonic anhydrase inhibitor, epinephrine, and an osmotic diuretic. This drug regimen is transient treatment while the patient is being prepared for eye surgery in which the iris is cut to allow fluid access to the anterior chamber again.

## ☙ NURSING CONSIDERATIONS
### Nursing interventions related to drug administration
- Wash hands carefully prior to administering eye medications.
- Patient should be supine for administration of this medication or should tilt the head back, in order to diminish systemic absorption of the drug.
- Place ordered dose of eye medication in the lower conjunctival sac and never directly on the cornea. Avoid touching any part of the eye with the dropper or applicator. To prevent overflow of medication into nasal and pharyngeal passages, and thus reduce systemic absorption, instruct patient to occlude

the nasolacrimal duct with one finger for 1 to 2 minutes after the medication has been instilled. Caution the patient not to rub the eyes or tightly close the eyelids. Excess medication may be wiped away with a tissue. Medication that spills onto the hands of the nurse or patient should be immediately washed off.

- Each patient should have a separate bottle or tube of medication to avoid accidental cross-contamination.
- For patients scheduled for surgery, oral medications are often withheld for a period of time prior to surgery. Eye medications should not be withheld unless there is a specific order to do so.

**Patient and family education**

- Review with patient and family the expected benefits and possible side effects of drug therapy.
- Caution patients to avoid driving or operating hazardous equipment if vision is blurred. Caution adults that they may be unable to drive home following eye examinations during which this medication is used; a friend or family member should drive until the effects of the medication wear off.
- Review with patients and families the correct technique for drug administration, including instructing them to wash hands before and after administering drug. Have patient give a return demonstration to indicate ability and knowledge of correct administration technique. Caution patients that bottles or tubes of eye medications should never be shared; each person requiring an eye medication should have a separate, clearly labeled bottle or tube.
- Instruct patients to inspect solution before use. Discolored solutions should be discarded and a new bottle used.
- Instruct patients to administer missed doses as soon as they are remembered, unless within 1 to 2 hours of the next dose. Patients should not double up to make up for missed doses.
- Instruct patients to read labels carefully. Eye medications are often available in a variety of strengths, and patients should use only the strength prescribed to ensure adequate treatment of the eye condition. Remind patients that no medications should be put in the eye unless the medications are clearly marked for ophthalmic use.
- Review with patients being treated for glaucoma the necessity to continue the use of the prescribed drugs even if the patient perceives no difficulty with vision. Glaucoma is a chronic condition that responds best to regular use of prescribed drugs. Encourage patients to return for regular follow-up by the physician.
- Teach the patient that administering the final dose of the day at bedtime may lessen visual changes.
- It is possible that soft contact lenses may absorb eye medications, and preservatives used in eye medications may damage or discolor soft contact lenses. Instruct patients who wear contact lenses to ask the physician about special precautions that should be observed when using this drug.
- Remind patients to keep these and all medications out of the reach of children.

# Cholinomimetic drugs for glaucoma

carbachol ~ demecarium ~ echothiophate ~ isoflurophate ~ pilocarpine

**OVERVIEW OF THE DRUG CLASS**   Cholinomimetic drugs are used in the treatment of chronic glaucoma. The initial treatment for chronic glaucoma is commonly the application of a weak cholinomimetic drug, usually pilocarpine or sometimes carbachol. In resistant cases of glaucoma, a strong cholinomimetic such as demecarium, echothiophate, or isoflurophate may be used.

**MECHANISM OF ACTION**   Drugs that mimic the action of acetylcholine act by one of two mechanisms: directly, by mimicking acetylcholine (these drugs are chemically related to acetylcholine) or indirectly, by inhibiting acetylcholinesterase (these drugs allow acetylcholine to remain intact longer because its degradation is inhibited). In the eye, acetylcholine causes contraction of the sphincter muscles and consequently constriction of the pupil (miosis). The therapeutic effectiveness for glaucoma results from the spread of the trabecular spaces of the anterior chamber when the sphincter muscles contract. The larger area allows improved uptake of the aqueous humor, which relieves intraocular pressure.

**INDICATIONS**     • Glaucoma.

**CONTRAINDICATIONS**     • History of retinal detachment.

**DRUG INTERACTIONS**     **Topical epinephrine, beta blockers, carbonic anhydrase inhibitors** will have additive effects with cholinomimetic drugs in lowering intraocular pressure.     **Systemic cholinesterase inhibitors** may produce additive systemic effects with ophthalmic cholinesterase inhibitors.     **Anesthetic agents** Cholinesterase inhibitors potentiate the effects of halothane.     **Succinylcholine** Even topically applied cholinesterase inhibitors may prevent the hydrolysis of succinylcholine, greatly prolonging the action of succinylcholine.

---

## carbachol     (KAR-ba-kole)                                                     miotic

   • carbachol: Isopto Carbachol, Miostat

**MECHANISM OF ACTION**     Carbachol is a direct-acting cholinomimetic. Miosis results from contraction of the sphincter muscles.

**INDICATIONS**     • Glaucoma.

**CONTRAINDICATIONS**     • Retinal detachment.

**DOSAGE     Topical:     ADULTS:** 1 to 2 drops of a 0.75% to 3% solution to each eye every 4 to 8 hours. Dosage is individualized. Finger pressure should be applied on the lacrimal sac for 1 to 2 minutes following topical instillation to minimize absorption and systemic reactions.     *Special patient populations:* **PREGNANCY:** Safe use has not been established.

**PREPARATIONS**     *Injection:* 0.01%; *solution:* 0.75, 1.5, 2.25, 3%.

**DRUG INTERACTIONS**     **Topical epinephrine, beta blockers, carbonic anhydrase inhibitors** will have additive effects with cholinomimetic drugs in lowering intraocular pressure.     **Systemic cholinesterase inhibitors** may produce additive systemic effects with ophthalmic cholinesterase inhibitors.     **Anesthetic agents** Cholinesterase inhibitors potentiate the effects of halothane.     **Succinylcholine** Even topically applied cholinesterase inhibitors may prevent the hydrolysis of succinylcholine, greatly prolonging the action of succinylcholine.

   **FATE**     After application into the conjunctival sac, miosis occurs in 10 to 20 minutes and persists for 4 to 8 hours. Injection of 0.01% into the anterior chamber of the eye produces miosis in 2 to 5 minutes and persists for 24 hours.

### ☙ NURSING CONSIDERATIONS

#### Side effects, toxicities, and associated nursing actions

   **CNS** Flushing, headache.
   • Forewarn patients about these side effects. If severe or persistent, notify physician, as it may be necessary to lower dose or change drugs.
   • For some patients, analgesics may be necessary to treat headache; consult physician.

   **Eye** Ciliary spasm, temporal or superorbital headaches, conjuctival congestion, myopia.
   • Caution patients to avoid driving or operating hazardous equipment if visual changes occur.
   • Reassure patients that side effects frequently diminish with continued use of the drug.
   • Instruct patients to apply cold compresses to relieve painful spasms.

   **GI** Distress, cramps, diarrhea.
   • If GI symptoms appear, review administration technique, as GI symptoms reflect systemic absorption of the drug.
   • If symptoms are severe or persistent, notify physician.

#### Nursing interventions related to drug administration
   • See entry for chapter (p. 1041).

#### Patient and family education
   • See entry for chapter (p. 1042).

---

## demecarium bromide     (dem-e-KARE-ee-um)                          miotic

   • demecarium bromide: Humorsol

**MECHANISM OF ACTION**   Demecarium is a potent acetylcholinesterase inhibitor and allows prolonged action of acetylcholine to contract the sphincter muscle, causing miosis.

**INDICATIONS**   **Glaucoma** Used for resistant cases.   **Convergent strabismus** May be used in the treatment of crossed eyes in infants.

**CONTRAINDICATIONS**   • Active eye inflammation. • Acute (narrow-angle) glaucoma.

**DOSAGE**   **Topical:**   **ADULTS AND CHILDREN:** 1 to 2 drops for adults, 1 drop for children, in each eye. Adjust dosage after 24 hours to achieve desired response.   *Special patient populations:*   **CHILDREN:** Pediatric doses are generally the lower range of adult doses.   **PREGNANCY:** Safe use has not been established.

**PREPARATIONS**   *Solution:* 0.125%, 0.25%.

**DRUG INTERACTIONS**   **Succinylcholine** Extreme care should be used when giving succinylcholine to a patient receiving even a topical acetylcholinesterase inhibitor.   **Acetylcholinesterase inhibitors** Patients with myasthenia gravis receiving acetylcholinesterase inhibitor therapy may experience additive effects.   **Pesticides** Many pesticides are acetylcholinesterase inhibitors. Farmers, warehouse workers, gardeners, or anyone around areas where pesticides are actively used should exercise extra caution when requiring acetylcholinesterase inhibitor therapy for glaucoma. The severity of side effects of the acetycholinesterase inhibitors may be increased.

**FATE**   Miosis occurs in 15 to 60 minutes and is maximal in 2 to 4 hours. Miosis persists for 3 to 10 days, but may persist for up to 4 weeks. A reduction in intraocular pressure is seen in 24 hours and may persist for up to 9 days.

### ☙ NURSING CONSIDERATIONS

#### Side effects, toxicities, and associated nursing actions

**CV** Irregularities, slow heart rate.
- Monitor heart rate; if bradycardia occurs, notify physician. It may be appropriate for selected patients to monitor and record heart rate on an outpatient basis; consult with physician.
- For this and other side effects, review administration technique, as the appearance of these side effects may reflect systemic absorption.

**Eye** Stinging, burning, tearing, twitching, redness.
- Caution patients to avoid driving or operating hazardous equipment if visual changes occur.
- Reassure patients that side effects frequently diminish with continued use of the drug.
- Instruct patients to apply cold compresses to relieve painful spasms.

**GI** Salivation, nausea, vomiting, cramps, diarrhea.
- If GI symptoms appear, review administration technique, as GI symptoms reflect systemic absorption of the drug.
- If symptoms are severe or persistent, notify physician.

**GU** Incontinence.
- Instruct patient to empty bladder prior to administering medication.
- The development of incontinence may reflect too high a dose; notify physician.

**Lung** Difficulty in breathing.
- Instruct patient to notify physician immediately if difficulty in breathing occurs.
- Have available equipment and personnel to provide ventilatory support in settings where long-acting cholinesterase inhibitors are administered.

#### Nursing interventions related to drug administration
- See entry for chapter (p. 1041).

#### Patient and family education
- See entry for chapter (p. 1042).

## echothiophate iodide   (ek-oh-THYE-oh-fate)      *miotic*

- echothiophate iodide: Phospholine Iodide

**MECHANISM OF ACTION** Echothiophate is a potent acetylcholinesterase inhibitor and allows prolonged action of acetylcholine to contract the sphincter muscle, causing miosis.

**INDICATIONS** **Glaucoma** Used for resistant cases. **Convergent strabismus** May be used in the treatment of crossed eyes in infants.

**CONTRAINDICATIONS** • Active eye inflammation. • Acute (narrow-angle) glaucoma.

**DOSAGE** **Topical:** ADULTS: For glaucoma, dosage is individually adjusted, usually with 2 doses daily. CHILDREN: For convergent strabismus, 1 drop of a 0.125% solution into each eye once daily at bedtime for 2 to 3 weeks. If the eyes become straighter, therapy is continued but at a reduced dosage: 1 drop into each eye every other day or 1 drop of a 0.06% solution daily. Therapy may continue for 1 to 5 years. *Special patient populations:* PREGNANCY: Safe use has not been established.

**PREPARATIONS** 1.5 mg (0.03%), 3 mg (0.06%), 6.25 mg (0.125%), 12.5 mg (0.25%). Available as measured powder with 5 ml diluent.

**DRUG INTERACTIONS** **Succinylcholine** Extreme care should be used when giving succinylcholine to a patient receiving even a topical acetylcholinesterase inhibitor. **Acetylcholinesterase inhibitors** Patients with myasthenia gravis receiving acetylcholinesterase inhibitor therapy may experience additive effects. **Pesticides** Many pesticides are acetylcholinesterase inhibitors. Farmers, warehouse workers, gardeners, or anyone around areas where pesticides are actively used should exercise extra caution when requiring acetylcholinesterase inhibitor therapy for glaucoma. The severity of side effects of the acetylcholinesterase inhibitors may be increased.

**FATE** Miosis occurs in 10 to 30 minutes and is maximum in 30 minutes. Miosis persists for several days, up to 4 weeks. A reduction in intraocular pressure is seen in 24 hours and may persist for up to 4 weeks.

## ☙ NURSING CONSIDERATIONS

### Side effects, toxicities, and associated nursing actions

**CV** Irregularities, slow heart rate.
- Monitor heart rate; if bradycardia occurs, notify physician. It may be appropriate for selected patients to monitor and record heart rate on an outpatient basis; consult with physician.
- For this and other side effects, review administration technique, as the appearance of these side effects may reflect systemic absorption.

**Eye** Stinging, burning, tearing, twitching, redness.
- Caution patients to avoid driving or operating hazardous equipment if visual changes occur.
- Reassure patients that side effects frequently diminish with continued use of the drug.
- Instruct patients to apply cold compresses to relieve painful spasms.

**GI** Salivation, nausea, vomiting, cramps, diarrhea.
- If GI symptoms appear, review administration technique, as GI symptoms reflect systemic absorption of the drug.
- If symptoms are severe or persistent, notify physician.

**GU** Incontinence.
- Instruct patient to empty bladder prior to administering medication.
- The development of incontinence may reflect too high a dose; notify physician.

**Lung** Difficulty in breathing.
- Instruct patient to notify physician immediately if difficulty in breathing occurs.
- Have available equipment and personnel to provide ventilatory support in settings where long-acting cholinesterase inhibitors are administered.

### Nursing interventions related to drug administration
- See entry for chapter (p. 1041).

### Patient and family education
- See entry for chapter (p. 1042).

## isoflurophate (eye-soe-FLOOR-oh-fate)     miotic

- isoflurophate: Floropryl

**MECHANISM OF ACTION**    Isoflurophate is a potent acetylcholinesterase inhibitor and allows prolonged action of acetylcholine to contract the sphincter muscle, causing miosis.

**INDICATIONS**    **Glaucoma** Used for resistant cases.    **Convergent strabismus** May be used in the treatment of crossed eyes in infants.

**CONTRAINDICATIONS**    • Active eye inflammation. • Acute (narrow-angle) glaucoma.

**DOSAGE**    **Topical:**    ADULTS: For glaucoma, 0.5 cm ointment in each eye every 8 to 72 hours for eye. CHILDREN: For convergent strabismus, no more than 0.5 cm ointment in each eye daily or at bedtime for 2 weeks. If the treatment is effective, it is continued, but application is reduced to once every 2 to 7 days. Total treatment time may be 1 to 5 years.    *Special patient populations:*    PREGNANCY: Safe use has not been established.

**PREPARATIONS**    *Ointment:* 0.025%.

**DRUG INTERACTIONS**    **Succinylcholine** Extreme care should be used when giving succinylcholine to a patient receiving even a topical acetylcholinesterase inhibitor.    **Acetylcholinesterase inhibitors** Patients with myasthenia gravis receiving acetylcholinesterase inhibitor therapy may experience additive effects.    **Pesticides** Many pesticides are acetylcholinesterase inhibitors. Farmers, warehouse workers, gardeners, or anyone around areas where pesticides are actively used should exercise extra caution when requiring acetylcholinesterase inhibitor therapy for glaucoma. The severity of side effects of the acetylcholinesterase inhibitors may be increased.

**FATE**    Miosis occurs in 5 to 10 minutes and is maximum in 15 to 20 minutes. Miosis persists for 1 to 4 weeks. A reduction in intraocular pressure is seen in 24 hours and may persist for up to 1 week.

## ☙ NURSING CONSIDERATIONS

### Side effects, toxicities, and associated nursing actions

**CV** Irregularities, slow heart rate.
- Monitor heart rate; if bradycardia occurs, notify physician. It may be appropriate for selected patients to monitor and record heart rate on an outpatient basis; consult with physician.
- For this and other side effects, review administration technique, as the appearance of these side effects may reflect systemic absorption.

**Eye** Stinging, burning, tearing, twitching, redness.
- Caution patients to avoid driving or operating hazardous equipment if visual changes occur.
- Reassure patients that side effects frequently diminish with continued use of the drug.
- Instruct patients to apply cold compresses to relieve painful spasms.

**GI** Salivation, nausea, vomiting, cramps, diarrhea.
- If GI symptoms appear, review administration technique, as GI symptoms reflect systemic absorption of the drug.
- If symptoms are severe or persistent, notify physician.

**GU** Incontinence.
- Instruct patient to empty bladder prior to administering medication.
- The development of incontinence may reflect too high a dose; notify physician.

**Lung** Difficulty in breathing,
- Instruct patient to notify physician immediately if difficulty in breathing occurs.
- Have available equipment and personnel to provide ventilatory support in settings where long-acting cholinesterase inhibitors are administered.

### Nursing interventions related to drug administration
- See entry for drug class (p. 1041).

### Patient and family education
- See entry for drug class (p. 1042).

## physostigmine salicylate, physostigmine sulfate
(fye-zoe-STIG-meen)                                                                                         miotic

- physostigmine salicylate: Isopto Eserine

**MECHANISM OF ACTION** Physostigmine is a short-acting acetylcholinesterase inhibitor and allows prolonged action of acetylcholine to contract the sphincter muscle, causing miosis.

**INDICATIONS** • Glaucoma.

**CONTRAINDICATIONS** • Glaucoma associated with acute inflammatory processes.

**DOSAGE** Topical: ADULTS: Doses must be individualized to achieve a lowering of intraoptic pressure. Generally, therapy is begun with 2 drops of a 0.25% or 0.5% solution up to four times daily. *Special patient populations:* PREGNANCY: Safe use has not been established.

**PREPARATIONS** *Physostigmine salicylate, solution:* 0.25%, 0.5%. *Physostigmine sulfate, ointment:* 0.25%.

**DRUG INTERACTIONS** **Succinylcholine** Extreme care should be used when giving succinylcholine to a patient receiving even a topical acetylcholinesterase inhibitor. **Acetylcholinesterase inhibitors** Patients with myasthenia gravis receiving acetylcholinesterase inhibitor therapy may experience additive effects. **Pesticides** Many pesticides are acetylcholinesterase inhibitors. Farmers, warehouse workers, gardeners, or anyone around areas where pesticides are actively used should exercise extra caution when requiring acetylcholinesterase inhibitor therapy for glaucoma. The severity of side effects of the acetylcholinesterase inhibitors may be increased.

**FATE** Miosis occurs in 10 to 30 minutes and persists for 12 to 48 hours.

☙ **NURSING CONSIDERATIONS**

### Side effects, toxicities, and associated nursing actions

**CV** Irregularities, slow heart rate.
• Monitor heart rate; if bradycardia occurs, notify physician. It may be appropriate for selected patients to monitor and record heart rate on an outpatient basis; consult with physician.
• For this and other side effects, review administration technique, as the appearance of these side effects may reflect systemic absorption.

**Eye** Stinging, burning, tearing, twitching, redness.
• Caution patients to avoid driving or operating hazardous equipment if visual changes occur.
• Reassure patients that side effects frequently diminish with continued use of the drug.
• Instruct patients to apply cold compresses to relieve painful spasms.

**GI** Salivation, nausea, vomiting, cramps, diarrhea.
• If GI symptoms appear, review administration technique, as GI symptoms reflect systemic absorption of the drug.
• If symptoms are severe or persistent, notify physician.

**GU** Incontinence.
• Instruct patient to empty bladder prior to administering medication.
• The development of incontinence may reflect too high a dose; notify physician.

**Lung** Difficulty in breathing.
• Instruct patient to notify physician immediately if difficulty in breathing occurs.
• Have available equipment and personnel to provide ventilatory support in settings where long-acting cholinesterase inhibitors are administered.

### Nursing interventions related to drug administration
• See entry for chapter (p. 1041).

### Patient and family education
• See entry for chapter (p. 1042).

## pilocarpine (pie-loe-KAR-peen)                                    glaucoma

● pilocarpine, pilocarpine hydrochloride, pilocarpine nitrate: Adsorbocarpine, Almocarpine, Akarpine, Isopto Carpine, ✤Minims, ✤Miocarpine, Ocu-Carpine, Ocusert, Pilocar, Pilokair, Pilopine, P.V. Carpine

**MECHANISM OF ACTION**    Pilocarpine is a direct-acting parasympathomimetic agent.

**INDICATIONS**    **Glaucoma** The ocular insert system described below allows controlled release of the drug for the management of chronic (open-angle) glaucoma. May also be used for closed-angle glaucoma to decrease intraocular pressure just before surgery.    **Miosis** To counter the effect of mydriatic and cycloplegic drugs.

**CONTRAINDICATIONS**    • Glaucoma associated with acute inflammatory processes.

**DOSAGE**    **Topically:**    ADULTS: For glaucoma: 1 to 2 drops of a 1% to 4% solution every 4 to 12 hours. To counteract mydriasis: 1 drop of a 1% solution.    **Ocular insert** Pilocarpine ocular inserts are intended for 7-day use. These are inserted into the upper or lower conjunctival sac. The medication diffuses out from the device into the eye in a controlled manner.    *Special patient populations:*    PREGNANCY: Safe use has not been established.

**PREPARATIONS**    *Pilocarpine: ocular system:* 20, 40 µg/hr for 7 days. *Pilocarpine hydrochloride: gel:* 4%; *solution:* 0.25%, 0.5%, 1%, 2%, 3%, 4%, 5%, 6%, 8%, 10%. *Pilocarpine nitrate: solution:* 1%, 2%, 4%.

**DRUG INTERACTIONS**    **Succinylcholine** Extreme care should be used when giving succinylcholine to a patient receiving even a topical acetylcholinesterase inhibitor.    **Acetylcholinesterase inhibitors** Patients with myasthenia gravis receiving acetylcholinesterase inhibitor therapy may experience additive effects.    **Pesticides** Many pesticides are acetylcholinesterase inhibitors. Farmers, warehouse workers, gardeners, or anyone around areas where pesticides are actively used should exercise extra caution when requiring acetylcholinesterase inhibitor therapy for glaucoma. The severity of side effects of the acetylcholinesterase inhibitors may be increased.

**FATE**    *Onset* of miosis is 10 to 30 minutes. The *duration of action* is 4 to 8 hours with a solution. The reduction in intraocular pressure persists for 4 to 14 hours with a solution, 18 to 24 hours with a gel, and 7 days with the Ocusert system in place.

### ☙ NURSING CONSIDERATIONS

#### Side effects, toxicities, and associated nursing actions

**CV** Irregularities, slow heart rate.
- Monitor heart rate; if bradycardia occurs, notify physician. It may be appropriate for selected patients to monitor and record heart rate on an outpatient basis; consult with physician.
- For this and other side effects, review administration technique, as the appearance of these side effects may reflect systemic absorption.

**Eye** Stinging, burning, tearing, twitching, redness.
- Caution patients to avoid driving or operating hazardous equipment if visual changes occur.
- Reassure patients that side effects frequently diminish with continuted use of the drug.
- Instruct patients to apply cold compresses to relieve painful spasms.

**GI** Salivation, nausea, vomiting, cramps, diarrhea.
- If GI symptoms appear, review administration technique, as GI symptoms reflect systemic absorption of the drug.
- If symptoms are severe or persistent, notify physician.

**GU** Incontinence.
- Instruct patient to empty bladder before administering medication.
- The development of incontinence may reflect too high a dose; notify physician.

**Lung** Difficulty in breathing,
- Instruct patient to notify physician immediately if difficulty in breathing occurs.
- Have available equipment and personnel to provide ventilatory support in settings where long-acting cholinesterase inhibitors are administered.

#### Nursing interventions related to drug administration
- For solution or gel, see entry for chapter (p. 1041).
- Gel preparations are usually administered at bedtime. During the night, the gel may crust on the eyelids but can be rinsed off with water.
- For ocular insert system: insert ocular insert into upper or lower conjuctival sac, usually at bedtime. If inserted in the lower sac, it can usually be moved to the upper sac, where it is less likely to fall out,

by gently applying pressure with the finger over the closed eyelid and moving the insert upward. Instruct the patient to check daily to see that the unit is still in place. Replace the unit weekly. If the unit falls out, a new one should be inserted. Instruct patients to review carefully the patient instruction sheet provided by the manufactuer.

**Patient and family education**
- See entry for chapter (p. 1042).

## Adrenergic drugs for glaucoma

dipivefrin ~ epinephrine ~ levobunolol ~ timolol

**OVERVIEW OF THE DRUG CLASS**    Adrenergic drugs and adrenergic blocking drugs both have a role in the treatment of glaucoma.

**MECHANISM OF ACTION**    The adrenergic drugs epinephrine and depivefrin (which is converted to epinephrine) are used either initially or in addition to a cholinomimetic drug in the treatment of chronic glaucoma. Epinephrine stimulates both alpha and beta receptors. Stimulation of alpha receptors reduces resistance to the outflow of aqueous humor, whereas stimulation of the beta receptors decreases production of aqueous humor. The beta blocking drugs timolol and levobunolol are also used either initially or in addition to other drugs in the treatment of chronic glaucoma. The mechanism by which blockade of the beta receptors of the eye decreases intraocular pressure is not clear, particularly since stimulation of the beta receptor also causes reduction of intraocular pressure.

**INDICATIONS**    • Chronic glaucoma.
**CONTRAINDICATIONS**    See individual drug.
**DRUG INTERACTIONS**    See individual drug.

## dipivefrin hydrochloride    (dye-PIH-ve-frin)    glaucoma treatment

- dipivefrin hydrochloride: Propine

**MECHANISM OF ACTION**    Dipivefrin is converted to epinephrine, which stimulates alpha and beta adrenergic receptors. In the eye, stimulation of alpha receptors reduces resistance to the outflow of aqueous humor, whereas stimulation of the beta receptors decreases production of aqueous humor. These actions result in a decrease in intraoptic pressure.

**INDICATIONS**    • Chronic (open-angle) glaucoma.
**CONTRAINDICATIONS**    • Irritation, sensitivity, on use.
**DOSAGE**    Topical:    **ADULTS AND CHILDREN:** 1 drop of a 0.1% solution every 12 hours.    *Special patient populations:*    **PREGNANCY:** Safe use has not been established. Animal studies have not revealed evidence of impaired fertility or harm to the fetus.
**PREPARATIONS**    *Solution:* 0.1%.
**DRUG INTERACTIONS**    Ocular hypotensive agents Dipivefrin usually gives additive reduction in intraocular pressure when used with topical miotics, topical beta adrenergic blocking agents, or systemically administered carbonic anhydrase inhibitors.
**FATE**    Dipivefrin is hydrolyzed to epinephrine by esterases in the cornea, conjunctiva, and aqueous humor. Dipivefrin has greater lipid solubility than epinephrine, and therefore divipefrin penetrates the intact cornea and anterior chamber of the eye much better than does epinephrine. A reduction in intraocular pressure is maximum in 1 hour and persists for 12 hours or more.

### ❦ NURSING CONSIDERATIONS
#### Side effects, toxicities, and associated nursing actions
- Systemic effects of dipivefrin are rare.

**Eye** Conjunctival irritation and discomfort in about 6% of patients. Mydriasis, blurred vision, ocular pain, and headache are occasionally reported.

- Inform patients that side effects usually diminish with continued use of the drug.
- Persistent or severe eye problems may necessitate a change in drug or lowering of dosage; notify the physician.
- Caution patients to avoid driving or operating hazardous equipment if changes in vision occur.

### Nursing interventions related to drug administration
- See entry for chapter (p. 1041).

### Patient and family education
- See entry for chapter (p. 1042).

# epinephrine bitartrate, epinephrine borate,
# epinephrine hydrochloride   (ep-i-NEF-rin)                    mydriatic

- epinephrine bitartrate, epinephrine borate, epinephrine hydrochloride: Epifrim, E-Pilo, Epinal, Eppy/N

**MECHANISM OF ACTION**   Epinephrine is an adrenergic agonist, acting at both alpha and beta adrenergic receptors. Stimulation of alpha receptors reduces resistance to the outflow of aqueous humor, whereas stimulation of the beta receptors decreases production of aqueous humor. Both actions lower intraocular pressure.

**INDICATIONS**   Chronic (open-angle) glaucoma.   **Ocular surgery** Epinephrine causes mydriasis.

**CONTRAINDICATIONS**   Prolonged ocular irritation.

**DOSAGE**   Topical:   **ADULTS AND CHILDREN:** 1 or 2 drops of a 1% or 2% solution once or twice daily is the usual range. Dosage needed may vary from administration once every 2 to 4 days to four times daily. *Special patient populations:*   **PREGNANCY:** Safe use has not been established.

**PREPARATIONS**   *Epinephrine hydrochloride, solution:* 0.1%, 0.25%, 0.5%, 1%, 2%. *Epinephrine bitartrate, solution:* 2%. *Epinephryl borate, solution:* 0.5%, 1%, 2%.

**DRUG INTERACTIONS**   **Miotics and carbonic anhydrase inhibitors** The lowering of intraocular pressure with epinephrine is generally additive when used with these drugs.   **General anesthetics** The halogenated hydrocarbon anesthetics, such as halothane, sensitize the heart to arrhythmias, a tendency exacerbated by epinephrine.   **Digitalis glycosides** These also sensitize the heart to arrhythmias.

**FATE**   The *onset of action* is about 1 hour. Maximum lowering of intraocular pressure takes 4 to 8 hours and persists for 12 to 24 hours. Epinephrine is taken up by sympathetic nerve endings.

## 🐦 NURSING CONSIDERATIONS
### Side effects, toxicities, and associated nursing actions
**CV** Palpitations, tachycardia, extrasystoles, hypertension, headaches, pallor, trembling, faintness. These are rarely seen when epinephrine is applied to the eye.
- Be alert to cardiac side effects in persons with a history of cardiac disease.
- Monitor pulse and blood pressure. In selected individuals, it may be appropriate to teach the patient to monitor and record the pulse on a regular basis in the home.
- Review administration technique with patient if cardiac side effects occur, as these effects may reflect systemic absorption of the drug.

**Eye** Discomfort and irritation, including transient burning or stinging, tearing, ache around the eye. Prolonged use may cause corneal edema.
- Inform patients that side effects usually diminish with continued use of the drug.
- Persistent or severe eye problems may necessitate a change in drug or lowering of dosage; notify the physician.
- Caution patients to avoid driving or operating hazardous equipment if changes in vision occur.

### Nursing interventions related to drug administration
- See entry for chapter (p. 1041).

### Patient and family education
- See entry for chapter (p. 1042).

## levobunolol hydrochloride   (lee-voe-BYOO-noe-lole)   glaucoma treatment

- levobunolol hydrochloride: Betagan

**MECHANISM OF ACTION**   Levobunolol is a beta adrenergic receptor antagonist. Beta receptor blockade results in a lower intraocular pressure, probably because of reduced aqueous humor formation.

**INDICATIONS**   Chronic (open-angle) glaucoma.

**CONTRAINDICATIONS**   Cardiac failure Beta blockers can compromise cardiac function.

**DOSAGE**   Topical:   ADULTS AND CHILDREN: 1 drop of a 0.5% solution once or twice daily.   *Special patient populations:*   PREGNANCY: Safe use has not been established.

**PREPARATIONS**   *Solution:* 0.5%.

**DRUG INTERACTIONS**   Ocular hypotensive agents The effect of levobunolol on lowering intraocular pressure may be additive with that of other drugs used to lower intraocular pressures.   Systemic beta adrenergic blocking drugs An additive effect is possible when topically applied levobunolol is administered concurrently with a systemically administered beta blocker.   Reserpine depletes catecholamines. Topically applied levobunolol may potentiate the side effects, especially hypotension and bradycardia.

**FATE**   The *onset of action* is about 1 hour for lowering of intraocular pressure. The maximum effect is seen in 2 to 6 hours and persists up to 24 hours. Some levobunolol reaches systemic circulation and occasionally gives rise to systemic side effects.

### ❦ NURSING CONSIDERATIONS

#### Side effects, toxicities, and associated nursing actions

CNS Rarely, dizziness, headache.
- Inform patients that side effects often diminish with continued use of the medication.
- Caution patients to avoid driving or operating hazardous equipment if dizziness develops. Notify physician.

CV Bradycardia, arrhythmias, hypotension, and heart block are rare side effects.
- Be alert to cardiac side effects in persons with a history of cardiac disease.
- Monitor pulse and blood pressure. In selected individuals, it may be appropriate to teach the patient to monitor and record the pulse on a regular basis in the home and to notify the physician if the pulse drops below 60.
- Review administration technique with patient if cardiac side effects occur, as these effects may reflect systemic absorption of the drug.

Eye Stinging, discomfort; conjunctivitis, keratitis, blepharoptosis, visual disturbances.
- Inform patients that side effects usually diminish with continued use of the drug.
- Persistent or severe eye problems may necessitate a change in drug or lowering of dosage; notify the physician.
- Caution patients to avoid driving or operating hazardous equipment if changes in vision occur.

Lung Bronchospasm.
- Tell patients to report immediately any difficulty in breathing.

#### Nursing interventions related to drug administration
- See entry for chapter (p. 1041).

#### Patient and family education
- See entry for chapter (p. 1042).

## timolol maleate   (TYE-moe-lole)   glaucoma treatment

- timolol maleate: Timoptic

**MECHANISM OF ACTION**   Timolol is a beta adrenergic receptor antagonist. Beta receptor blockage results in a lower intraocular pressure, probably because of reduced aqueous humor formation.

**INDICATIONS**   Chronic (open-angle) glaucoma Timolol is used topically.   Hypertension, angina, myocardial infarction Timolol is used systemically to treat these conditions. See Chapter 5.

**CONTRAINDICATIONS**    Cardiac failure.

**DOSAGE**    Topically:    ADULTS AND CHILDREN: 1 drop of a 0.25% solution twice daily.    *Special patient populations:*    PREGNANCY: Safe use has not been established.

**PREPARATIONS**    Solution: 0.25%, 0.5%.

**DRUG INTERACTIONS**    **Ocular hypotensive agents** The effect of levobunolol on lowering intraocular pressure may be additive with that of other drugs used to lower intraocular pressures.    **Systemic beta adrenergic blocking drugs** An additive effect is possible when topically applied levobunolol is administered concurrently with a systemically administered beta blocker.    **Reserpine** Reserpine depletes catecholamines. Topically applied levobunolol may potentiate the side effects, especially hypotension and bradycardia.

**FATE**    The *onset of action* is 15 to 30 minutes. The maximum decrease in intraocular pressure is seen in 1 to 5 hours and persists for about 24 hours.

## 🦌 NURSING CONSIDERATIONS

### Side effects, toxicities, and associated nursing actions

**CNS** Rarely, dizziness, headache.
- Inform patients that side effects often diminsh with continued use of the medication.
- Caution patients to avoid driving or operating hazardous equipment if dizziness develops. Notify physician.

**CV** Bradycardia, arrhythmias, hypotension, and heart block are rare side effects.
- Be alert to cardiac side effects in persons with a history of cardiac disease.
- Monitor pulse and blood pressure. In selected individuals, it may be appropriate to teach the patient to monitor and record the pulse on a regular basis in the home and to notify the physician if the pulse drops below 60.
- Review administration technique with patient if cardiac side effects occur, as these effects may reflect systemic absorption of the drug.

**Eye** Stinging, discomfort; conjunctivitis, keratitis, blepharoptosis, visual disturbances.
- Inform patients that side effects usually diminish with continued use of the drug.
- Persistent or severe eye problems may necessitate a change in drug or lowering of dosage; notify the physician.
- Caution patients to avoid driving or operating hazardous equipment if changes in vision occur.

**Lung** Bronchospasm.
- Tell patients to report immediately any difficulty in breathing.

### Nursing interventions related to drug administration
- See entry for chapter (p. 1041).

### Patient and family education
- See entry for chapter (p. 1042).

# Appendix A
# Abbreviations commonly used in pharmacology

| Abbreviation | Meaning |
|---|---|
| A, aa | of each |
| ABG | arterial blood gases |
| a.c. | before meals |
| ACh | acetylcholine |
| ACT | activated clotting time |
| ACTH | adrenocorticotropic hormone |
| a.d. | right ear |
| ad | to, up to |
| ADH | antidiuretic hormone |
| ADL | activities of daily living |
| ad lib | as desired, at pleasure |
| ADR | adverse drug reaction |
| ADT | alternate day therapy |
| a.l. | left ear |
| ALT | alanine aminotransferase (formerly, SGPT) |
| aq | water |
| aq dest. | distilled water |
| AST | aspartate aminotransferase (formerly, SGOT) |
| a.u. | each ear, both ears |
| AV | atrioventricular |
| BBT | basal body temperature |
| b.i.d. | two times daily |
| b.i.n. | two times nightly |
| BMR | basal metabolic rate |
| BP | blood pressure |
| BSP | bromsulphalein |
| BT | bleeding time |
| BUN | blood urea nitrogen |
| C | centigrade, Celsius |
| c | with |
| Ca | calcium |
| Caps | capsule |
| CAT | computerized axial tomography |
| CBC | complete blood count |
| CCr | creatinine clearance |
| CDC | Centers for Disease Control |
| CHF | congestive heart failure |
| Cl | chloride |
| cm | centimeter |
| CNS | central nervous system |
| collyr. | an eyewash |
| COMT | catechol-O-methyltransferase |
| COPD | chronic obstructive pulmonary disease |
| CPK | creatinine phosphokinase |
| CPR | cardiopulmonary resuscitation |
| CSF | cerebrospinal fluid |
| CT | clotting time |
| CTZ | chemoreceptor trigger zone |
| CV | cardiovascular |
| CVA | cerebrovascular accident |
| CVP | central venous pressure |

*Continued.*

## Abbreviations commonly used in pharmacology—cont'd

| Abbreviation | Meaning |
| --- | --- |
| d. | day |
| D&C | dilatation and curettage |
| DERM | dermatologic |
| D., det. | give, let be given |
| DIC | disseminated intravascular clotting |
| dil. | dilute |
| dl | deciliter (100 ml or 0.1 liter) |
| DNA | deoxyribonucleic acid |
| dr. | dram |
| DSD | dry sterile dressing |
| D.t.d. | let such doses be given |
| DTRs | deep tendon reflexes |
| ECG | electrocardiogram |
| ECT | electroconvulsive therapy |
| EEG | electroencephalogram |
| EENT | eye, ear, nose, throat |
| elix | elixir |
| emuls. | emulsion |
| ENT | ear, nose, throat |
| EPS | extrapyramidal symptoms (or syndrome) |
| ER | estrogen receptor |
| ESR | erythrocyte sedimentation rate |
| ext. | extract |
| F | Fahrenheit; fluoride |
| F, Ft. | and make |
| FBS | fasting blood sugar |
| FDA | Food and Drug Administration (USA) |
| Fe | iron |
| FSH | follicle stimulating hormone |
| FUO | fever of unknown origin |
| g, gm, Gm | gram |
| GABA | gamma-aminobutyric acid |
| GFR | glomerular filtration rate |
| GH | growth hormone |
| GI | gastrointestinal |
| G6PD | glucose-6-phosphate dehydrogenase |
| gr | grain |
| gtt | a drop, drops |
| GU | genitourinary |
| h, hr | hour |
| HCG | human chorionic gonadotropin |
| HCl | hydrochloride |
| Hct | hematocrit |
| HDL | high density lipoprotein |
| Hg | mercury |
| Hgb | hemoglobin |
| HIAA | 5-hydroxyindolacetic acid |
| HMG | human menopausal gonadotropin |
| HPA | hypothalamic-pituitary-adrenocortical axis |
| h.s. | at bedtime |
| Hx | history |

| Abbreviation | Meaning |
| --- | --- |
| I | iodine |
| IA | intraarterial |
| IBW | ideal body weight |
| IDDM | insulin dependent diabetes mellitus |
| Ig | immunoglobulin |
| IM | intramuscular |
| I&O | intake and output |
| IOP | intraocular pressure |
| IPPB | intermittent positive pressure breathing |
| IU | international unit |
| IUD | intrauterine device |
| IV | intravenous |
| IVH | intravenous hyperalimentation |
| kg | kilogram |
| KGS | 17-ketogenic steroids |
| KS | 17-ketosteroids |
| KVO | keep vein open |
| l, L | liter |
| lb | pound |
| LDH | lactic dehydrogenase |
| LDL | low density lipoprotein |
| LE | lupus erythematosus |
| LH | luteinizing hormone |
| Li | lithium |
| LVEDP | left ventricular end-diastolic pressure |
| $M^2$ | square meter (of body surface) |
| m. | minim |
| M. | mix |
| MAO(I) | monoamine oxidase (inhibitor) |
| max | maximum |
| MBD | minimal brain dysfunction |
| mcg, μg | microgram |
| mCi, mC | millicurie |
| MDR | minimum daily requirement |
| mEq | milliequivalent |
| Mg | magnesium |
| MI | myocardial infarction |
| MIC | minimum inhibitory concentration |
| mist. | mixture |
| ml | milliliter |
| MRI | magnetic resonance imaging |
| N | nitrogen |
| Na | sodium |
| NAPA | N-acetyl procainamide |
| ng | nanogram (1/1000 of a microgram) |
| NIDDM | non-insulin dependent diabetes mellitus |
| no. | number |
| noct. | night |
| non rep. | do not repeat |
| NPN | non-protein nitrogen |
| NPO | nothing by mouth |
| NSAID | nonsteroidal antiinflammatory drug |
| NSR | normal sinus rhythm |

*Continued.*

## Abbreviations commonly used in pharmacology—cont'd

| Abbreviation | Meaning |
|---|---|
| N&V | nausea and vomiting |
| O | pint |
| o.d. | every day |
| O.D. | right eye |
| o.h. | every hour |
| ol | oil |
| o.m. | every morning |
| o.n. | every night |
| O.S. | left eye |
| os | mouth |
| OTC | over-the-counter |
| o.u. | both eyes |
| oz. | ounce |
| PABA | para-amino-benzoic acid |
| PAWP | pulmonary artery wedge pressure |
| PBI | protein bound iodine |
| p.c. | after meals |
| per | by, through |
| pH | hydrogen ion concentration |
| pil | pill |
| PKU | phenylketonuria |
| PO, p.o. | by mouth |
| PPI | patient packet insert |
| PR | by rectum |
| PRN, p.r.n. | when necessary |
| PT | prothrombin time |
| PTT | partial thromboplastin time |
| PVC | premature ventricular contraction |
| q | every |
| q.d. | every day |
| q.h. | every hour |
| q.i.d. | four times daily |
| q.o.d. | every other day |
| q.s. | as much as required |
| RDA | recommended (daily) dietary allowance |
| REM | rapid eye movement |
| Rept. | let it be repeated |
| RIA | radioimmunoassay |
| RNA | ribonucleic acid |
| ROM | range of motion |
| s | without |
| SA | sinoatrial |
| SC | subcutaneous |
| SGOT | see AST |
| SGPT | see ALT |
| Sig, S. | mark on the label |
| SL | sublingual |
| SLE | systemic lupus erythematosus |
| SMA | sequential multiple analysis |
| SOAP | subjective objective assessment planning |
| s.o.s. | if necessary |
| sp | spirits |

| Abbreviation | Meaning |
| --- | --- |
| SR | sedimentation rate |
| ss | one-half |
| stat | immediately; first dose |
| syr | syrup |
| tab | tablet |
| TCA | tricyclic antidepressant |
| TIA | transient ischemic attack |
| t.i.d. | three times daily |
| t.i.n. | three times nightly |
| TPN | total parenteral nutrition |
| TPR | temperature, pulse, respirations |
| tr | tincture |
| $\mu$ | micron |
| $\mu$Ci | microcurie |
| $\mu$g | microgram |
| ung | ointment |
| URI | urinary tract infection |
| ut dict | as directed |
| VS | vital signs: temperature, pulse, respirations, blood pressure |
| WBC | white blood cell count |
| WBCT | whole blood clotting time |

# Calculations

## Calculating the strength of drug solutions

Calculating the concentration of a drug solution utilizes the following equation:

Concentration = Mass of drug/volume of solution

If you know any two of these quantities, you may solve directly for the third, provided all the quantities are expressed in the same system of units. Therefore as a first step in the solution of any problem, it is frequently necessary to convert units from one system to another, as we see in example 1.

EXAMPLE 1: *Prepare 1 L of a 5% solution.*
You know:
1. Volume of solution (1 L)
2. Concentration (5%)
To solve:
1. Convert all quantities to the same system of units:

5% = 5 g/100 ml; 1 L = 1000 ml (See Appendix E, p. 1064.)

2. Substitute the known quantities into the equation:

5 g/100 ml = Mass of drug/1000 ml

3. Solve for mass of drug:

$$Mass = \frac{1000 \text{ ml} \times 5 \text{ gm}}{100 \text{ ml}} = 50 \text{ gm}$$

EXAMPLE 2: *Prepare 4 oz of a 0.5% solution from tablets gr v each.*
You know:
1. Volume of solution required (4 oz)
2. Concentration of solution (0.5%)
To solve:
1. Convert all quantities to the same system of units:

0.5% = 0.5 g/100 ml
4 oz = 4 x 30 ml = 120 ml
gr v = 5 gr = 0.300 g

2. Substitute the known quantities in the equation:

0.5 g/100 ml = Mass of drug/120 ml

3. Solve for mass of drug:

$$Mass = \frac{120 \text{ ml} \times 0.5 \text{ g}}{100 \text{ ml}} = 0.60 \text{ g}$$

4. Determine the number of tablets required to total 0.60 g:

$$\frac{0.60 \text{ g}}{0.30 \text{ g/tablet}} = 2 \text{ tablets}$$

As shown, 2 tablets would be dissolved in 4 oz to prepare the desired solution.

## Calculating the strength of diluted solutions

The examples just given have all dealt with weight/volume problems. In examining volume/volume problems, the basic equation can be modified slightly and the problems solved in much the same way as before. The equation then becomes:

(Concentration of solution) × (Volume of solution)
= (Concentration of stock) × (Volume of stock)

*Stock* or *stock solution* refers to a concentrated, storage form of a drug, which must ordinarily be diluted before use. Using this equation, calculations are performed much as before, as shown in the following examples.

EXAMPLE 3: *Prepare 1 quart of a 1:5000 solution from a 10% solution.*
You know:
1. Volume of solution (1 qt)
2. Concentration of solution (1:5000)
3. Concentration of stock (10%)
To solve:
1. Convert all quantities to the same system of units:

1 qt ≈ 1L ≈ 1000 ml
1:5000 = 1 g/5000 ml
10% = 10 g/100 ml

2. Substitute in the equation:

1 g/5000 ml × 1000 ml = 10 g/100 ml × Volume of stock

3. Solve for the unknown:

Volume of stock=

$$\frac{1 \text{ g} \times 1000 \text{ ml}}{5000 \text{ ml}} \times \frac{100 \text{ ml}}{10 \text{ g}} = 2 \text{ ml}$$

## Calculating drug dosage

All the examples thus far have dealt with the preparation of a drug for administration. We now turn to the next step: the use of those materials to fulfill the physician's drug order for a patient. The equation is:

Body weight × Dosage =
Volume of drug × Drug concentration

A drug dosage is expressed as units or mass of drug per body weight of patient. For example, 0.1 g of drug/kg body weight is a drug dosage expression, but 0.1 g of drug is not. Occasionally a physician may order a dose of, for example, 500 mg of an antibiotic to be taken every 4 hours. Technically this form does not constitute a drug dosage, but in practice it is understood that 500 mg is the appropriate dose for an average-size patient, that is, the intended dosage is 500 mg/70 kg body weight. More accurate dosages, of course, must be calculated for persons who deviate greatly from the normal weight range or when highly toxic drugs are involved. Common types of problems in drug dosage are presented in the following examples.

EXAMPLE 4: *A 100 kg patient is to receive a dose of 4 units/kg body weight. How many ml of the supplied drug at 100 units/ml will be required?*
You know:

1. Drug dosage (4 units/kg body weight)
2. Patient body weight (100 kg)
3. Concentration of the drug to be administered (100 units/ml)

To solve:

1. Substitute in the equation:

$$100 \text{ kg} \times \frac{4 \text{ units}}{\text{kg}} =$$
$$\text{Volume of drug} \times 100 \text{ units/ml}$$

2. Solve for volume of drug:

$$\text{Volume of drug} = 100 \text{ kg} \times$$
$$\frac{4 \text{ units}}{\text{kg}} \times \frac{\text{ml}}{100 \text{ units}} = 4 \text{ ml}$$

EXAMPLE 5: *The physician orders 0.2 g of drug for a patient. How many capsules at gr iss each will you administer?*
To solve:

1. Convert 0.2 g to 3 gr.
2. Convert gr iss to 1.5 gr.

Therefore

$$\frac{3 \text{gr}}{1.5 \text{ gr/capsule}} = 2 \text{ capsules}$$

## Calculating infusion rates

Many drugs must be administered intravenously by slow infusion rather than as a rapid bolus injection. Large volumes of fluids of various types are also given by intravenous infusion. Disposable infusion sets are available from several manufacturers. These sets are commonly calibrated to deliver 10, 12, 15, 20, 50, or 60 drops/ml of fluid. The nurse in practice can find the calibration, or drop factor, for any particular infusion set by examining the package in which it is supplied. Usually a hospital will have only two sizes available to minimize confusion: one regular, or macrodrip, set of 10, 12, 15 drops/ml (abbreviated gtt/ml), and one pediatric, or microdrip, set of 50 or 60 gtt/ml.

Calculations of infusion rates can be carried out with the following equation:

$$\text{gtt/ml} = \frac{\text{gtt/ml calibration}}{60 \text{ minute/hour}} \times$$
$$\frac{\text{Total ml to be administered}}{\text{Total hours of infusion}}$$

The use of this formula can be illustrated with the following examples:

EXAMPLE 6: *A physician's order reads "3500 ml 5% dextrose in water IV in 24 hours." What is the correct infusion rate if the infusion set delivers 60 gtt/ml?*
You know:

1. gtt/ml calibration = 60 gtt/ml
2. Total ml to be administered = 3500
3. Total hours of infusion = 24

To solve:
Substitute in the equation:

$$\text{gtt/minute} = \frac{60 \text{ gtt/ml}}{60 \text{ minute/hour}} \times$$
$$\frac{3500 \text{ ml}}{24 \text{ hours}} = 145 \text{ to } 146 \text{ gtt/minute}$$

EXAMPLE 7: *To give 50 ml of antibiotic solution IV in 30 minutes, what should the infusion rate be in drops per minute? The infusion set is calibrated for 60 gtt/ml.*
You know:

1. gtt/ml calibration = 60 gtt/ml
2. Total ml to be administered = 50 ml
3. Total hours of infusion = 0.5

To solve:
Substitute in the formula:

$$\text{gtt/minute} = \frac{60 \text{ gtt/ml}}{60 \text{ minute/hour}} \times$$
$$\frac{50 \text{ ml}}{0.5 \text{ hour}} = 100 \text{ gtt/minute}$$

EXAMPLE 8: *If an infusion set calibrated for 15gtt/ml is running at a rate of 45 gtt/minute, how long will be required to infuse 1 L of fluid?*
You know:

1. gtt/ml calibration = 15 gtt/ml
2. Total ml to be administered = 1000 ml (1 L)
3. Flow rate = 45 gtt/minute

To solve:
Substitute in the equation:

$$45 \text{ gtt/minute} = \frac{15 \text{ gtt/ml}}{60 \text{ minute/hour}} \times$$
$$\frac{1000 \text{ ml}}{\text{Hours of infusion}}$$

The formula can be rearranged to solve for the number of hours:

$$\text{Hours of infusion} = \frac{15 \text{ gtt/ml}}{60 \text{ minute/hour}} \times \frac{1000 \text{ ml}}{45 \text{ gtt/minute}} = 5.55 \text{ hours}$$

## Calculating pediatric dosages

Calculation of pediatric dosages requires special knowledge of each drug and how it interacts with the unique metabolism of the infant. Some drugs may be given to children and infants in doses that are in the same proportion to body weight as the doses used in adults. Other drugs must be given in greatly reduced doses because the infant is more sensitive or is incapable of metabolizing the drug as rapidly as an adult. These considerations are taken into account in determining recommended pediatric doses. For many drugs the pediatric doses listed in various drug reference publications will include a statement indicating that the dosage may be calculated for children according to their body weight, for example, but should not exceed a stated upper limit.

Several methods for calculating pediatric dosages exist. Three methods are presented here. The first method, called *Young's rule,* is based on the age of the child and applies to children between 1 and 12 years of age. The equation is:

Child's dose =
$$\frac{\text{Age of child in years}}{\text{Age of child in years} + 12} \times \text{Adult dose}$$

The use of Young's rule is illustrated in the following example.

EXAMPLE 9: *What is the appropriate dose of aspirin for a 3-year-old child? A normal adult dose is gr v.*
You know:
1. Age of the child =3 years
2. Adult dose = gr v
To solve:
Substitute the known quantities in the equation:

$$\text{Child's dose} = \frac{3 \text{ years}}{3 + 12} \times 5 \text{ gr}$$
$$= \frac{1}{5} \times 5 \text{ gr} = 1 \text{ gr, or gr i}$$

A second method for calculating pediatric dosages is based on a comparison of the child's weight to the average weight of an adult. This formula, which applies to all ages of children, is called *Clark's rule.* The equation is:

Child's dose =
$$\frac{\text{Weight of child in pounds}}{150 \text{ lb}} \times \text{Adult dose}$$

The use of Clark's rule is illustrated in the following example.

EXAMPLE 10: *What is the appropriate dose of aspirin for a 30 lb child, if the normal adult dose is gr v?*
You know:
1. Weight of the child = 30 lb
2. Adult dose = 5 gr
To solve:
Substitute the known quantities in the equation:

$$\text{Child's dose} = \frac{30 \text{ lb}}{150 \text{ lb}} \times 5 \text{ gr} = 1 \text{ gr}$$

Note that Clark's rule and Young's rule give the same answer when the child is not greatly lighter or heavier than the normal weight for his or her age. The 3-year- old child used in examples 14 and 15, at 30 lb, is near the normal weight for that age. Clark's rule is considered the more accurate of the two rules, since it will adjust dosage for a child who does deviate from normal weight.

The most accurate method of calculating pediatric dosage is based on the surface area of the child's body relative to that of an adult. Surface area is obviously more difficult to measure than age or weight. Measurements under laboratory conditions show 1.7 square meters ($M^2$) is the average body surface area for an adult. Measurements under similar conditions with children have enabled us to construct charts and nomograms that relate the child's body weight to surface area. An example of such a chart is shown in Appendix F, p. 1065. The equation used for the drug dose calculation is:

Child's dose =
$$\frac{\text{Surface area of child in } M^2}{1.7 \text{ } M^2} \times \text{Adult dose}$$

The use of the formula is illustrated in the following example:

EXAMPLE 11: *What dose of Demerol does a child weighing 10 kg require? The adult dose for Demerol is 50 mg.*
To calculate the dosage on the basis of body surface area, we must first determine the surface area that corresponds to a body weight of 10 kg. That value is 0.46 $M^2$. We may now proceed.
You know:
1. Surface area of child = 0.46 $M^2$
2. Adult dose =50 mg
To solve:
Substitute these values in the equation:

Child's dose
$$= \frac{0.46 \text{ } M^2}{1.7 \text{ } M^2} \times 50 \text{ mg} = 13.5 \text{ mg}$$

# Classification of controlled substances, United States and Canada

## Classification of controlled substances, United States

| Classification | Description | Specific substances |
|---|---|---|
| Schedule I | Drugs that have high potential for abuse and no accepted medical use. Containers are marked C-1. | Heroin, LSD, peyote, marijuana, *NN*-dimethyltryptamine |
| Schedule II | Drugs that have high potential for abuse but have accepted medical use. Dependence may include strong physical and psychological dependence. Containers are marked C-II. | Amobarbital, amphetamine, codeine, dextroamphetamine, meperidine, methadone, hydromorphone, methaqualone, morphine, opium, pentobarbital, phenazocine, methylphenidate, secobarbital |
| Schedule III | Medically accepted drugs that may cause dependence but are less prone to abuse than drugs in Schedules I and II. Containers are marked C-III. | Codeine-containing medications, butabarbital, hexobarbital, paregoric, nalorphine |
| Schedule IV | Medically accepted drugs that may cause mild physical or psychological dependence. Containers are marked C-IV. | Chloral hydrate, chlordiazepoxide, diazepam, meprobamate, phenobarbital |
| Schedule V | Medically accepted drugs with very limited potential for causing mild physical or psychological dependence. Containers are marked C-V. | Drug mixtures containing small quantities of narcotics, such as over-the-counter cough syrups containing codeine |

## Canadian drug classification

| Classification | Description | Specific substances |
|---|---|---|
| **NONPRESCRIPTION DRUGS** | | |
| Proprietary medicines | Drugs that may be widely purchased for self-treatment of symptoms of minor self-limiting diseases; identified by six-digit code preceded by letters *GP*. | Cough drops, medicated shampoos, minor pain relievers |
| Over-the-counter drugs | Drugs available through a pharmacy and used on advice of a health professional for control of symptoms of minor self-limiting diseases; identified by six-digit code preceded by letters *DIN*. | Laxatives, cough syrups, cold remedies, sinus preparations, certain vitamins |
| **PRESCRIPTION DRUGS** | | |
| Schedule F | Over 200 drugs that may not be used except after professional consultation; identified by symbol *Pr* on label. | Hormones, antibiotics, tranquilizers |
| Schedule G | Drugs that affect central nervous system (e.g., stimulants, sedatives); identified by symbol *C* on label. | Amphetamines, barbiturates |
| Narcotics | Drugs used primarily for relief of pain but also possessing significant psychotropic activity; identified by letter *N* on label. | Cannabis (marijuana), cocaine, codeine, morphine, opium, phencyclidine |
| **RESTRICTED DRUGS** | | |
| Schedule H | Drugs with no recognized medical use and significant danger of physiological and psychological side effects; only available to institutions for research. | Lysergic acid diethylamide (LSD), N, N-diethyltryptamine (DET), N, N-dimethyltryptamine (DMT), 4-methyl-2, 5-dimethoxyamphetamine (STP; DOM) |

# Emergency treatment of the poisoned patient*

## Nonspecific antidotes

| Antidote | Trade name | Administration/dosage | Comments |
|---|---|---|---|
| **EMETICS** | | | |
| Ipecac | Ipecac Syrup | ORAL, in 8 oz water: *Children 6 mo-1 yr*—10 ml. *Chidren 1-2 yr*—15 ml. *Adults*—30 ml. Vomiting in 30 min in 90% of patients. May repeat dose after 20-30 min if no vomiting has occurred. | Give only to conscious patients who have gag reflex and are not likely to aspirate vomitus. Do not give when vomitus will itself be injurious (acids, bases, hydrocarbons). Patient should be encouraged to drink water. Water will distend stomach and make it more susceptible to action of ipecac. Walking also helps to induce vomiting. Average return of stomach contents is 20%-60%. Keep vomitus for analysis. |
| Apomorphine | Apomorphine HCl | SUBCUTANEOUS: *Children*—0.066 mg/kg. *Adults*—0.1 mg/kg. | May cause CNS and respiratory depression or protracted vomiting, which are treated with 0.005 mg/kg naloxone HCl. Keep vomitus for analysis. |
| **GASTRIC LAVAGE** | | | |
| Water: 0.45% saline 0.9% saline | | BY GASTRIC TUBE: *Small children*—10 ml/kg. *Adults*—300 ml. | If patient is in deteriorating condition, unconscious, prone to seizures, or lacking a gag reflex, nasotracheal intubation is necessary before lavage to protect airway. Use large-bore (28-40 French Ewald or Burke orogastric lavacutor) tubing to allow aspiration of tablets. Keep first wash for analysis. Continue washings until return is clear (2-20 L). Administering more than recommended volume will distend stomach and may induce vomiting. |
| Activated charcoal | CharcoalantiDote, Liquid-Anti-dose | ORAL OR BY GASTRIC TUBE: *Children*—15-30 g in 4-8 oz water. *Adults*—25-50 g in 8-16 oz water. | Administer as a slurry within first hours of poisoning, after induced vomiting (charcoal will inactivate ipecac) or gastric lavage. Do not use with acetylcysteine in management of acetaminophen poisoning. Do not use magnesium sulfate as cathartic. |
| **CATHARTICS** | | | |
| Sodium sulfate, 10% solution | | ORAL: *Children*—1-2 ml/kg. *Adults*—150-250 ml. | Preferred cathartic for treating poisoned patients. Contraindicated if patient has heart failure or hypertension. |
| Magnesium sulfate (Epsom salts), 10% solution | | ORAL: *Children*—1-2 ml/kg. *Adults*—150-250 ml. | Magnesium salts should not be used if patient has renal failure. |
| Magnesium citrate, 10% solution | | ORAL: *Children*—1-2 ml/kg. *Adults*—150-250ml. | Magnesium salts should not be used if patient has renal failure. Citrate should not be used if activated charcoal has been given. |

*Nonspecific antidotes are used to clear the gastrointestinal tract of ingested poisons. These are the measures most commonly used.

# Equivalents and conversions

## Conversion of units between systems

| Apothecaries' | Metric |
|---|---|
| 15 gr | = 1 g* |
| 1 dr | = 4 g |
| 1 oz | = 32 g |
| 15 m | = 1 ml |
| 1 f dr | = 4 ml |
| 1 f oz | = 30 ml† |

| Household | Metric |
|---|---|
| 1 t | = 5 ml |
| 1 T | = 14 ml |
| 1 pt | = 480 ml (or 500 ml) |
| 1 qt | = 960 ml (or 1000 ml) |
| 1 gal | = 3.84 L (or 4 L) |
| 1 lb (avoirdupois) | = 0.46 kg or 1 kg = 2.2 lb |

*Two factors have been used for converting grains to milligrams. The older conversion factor is 65 mg = 1 gr. This factor is the basis for aspirin and acetaminophen formulations (i.e., a 5 gr aspirin tablet contains 325 mg of aspirin). The newer conversion factor agreed on is 60 mg = 1 gr. This new conversion factor is easier to use for drugs, such as morphine, that are frequently administered in small doses (fractions of grains). For example ¼ gr morphine equals 15 mg, using the new conversion factor. The student should remember that these factors are simply agreed on for ease of calculation. All the sample problems use the conversion 1 g = 60 mg.

†30 ml has been agreed on as the equivalent for 1 f oz. rather than the more exact approximation of 32 ml, since 30 ml is more conveniently and accurately estimated in most clinical glassware.

## Table of equivalents within systems

| System | Equivalents |
|---|---|
| Metric | 1.0 g = 0.001 kg |
| | 1.0 g = 1000 mg |
| | 1.0 L = 1000 ml |
| Apothecaries' | 1.0 gr = ⅟₆₀ dram (dr or ℨ) = ⅟₄₈₀ oz |
| | 60 gr = 1 dr |
| | 8 dr = 1 oz (or ℥) |
| | 1.0 minim (m) = ⅟₆₀ f dr = ⅟₄₈₀ f oz |
| | 60 m = 1 f dr (or ℨ) |
| | 8 f dr = 1 f oz (or ℥) |
| Household | 1.0 lb = 16 oz |
| | 1.0 pt = ½ quart (qt) = ⅛ gallon (gal) |
| | 1.0 pt = 16 f oz = 32 tablespoonsful (T) |
| | 1.0 T = 3 teaspoonsful (t) |

## Interconversion of concentration expressions

| % | Ratio | g/L | mg/ml | mg/dl | μg/ml |
|---|---|---|---|---|---|
| 10.0 | 1:10 | 100 | 100 | 10,000 | 100,000 |
| 1.0 | 1:100 | 10 | 10 | 1,000 | 10,000 |
| 0.1 | 1:1000 | 1.0 | 1.0 | 100 | 1,000 |
| 0.01 | 1:10,000 | 0.1 | 0.1 | 10 | 100 |
| 0.001 | 1:100,000 | 0.01 | 0.01 | 1.0 | 10 |
| 0.0001 | 1:1,000,000 | 0.001 | 0.001 | 0.1 | 0 |

# Appendix F
# Nomogram

**Body surface area as a function of weight**

| Weight | | Surface | Approximate | Weight | | Surface | Approximate |
| kg | lb | area (M²) | age of patient | kg | lb | area (M²) | age of patient |
| --- | --- | --- | --- | --- | --- | --- | --- |
| 4.0 | 8.8 | 0.25 | 3 weeks | 19 | 41 | 0.73 | 5 years |
| 5.7 | 12.5 | 0.29 | 3 months | 21 | 47 | 0.82 | 6 years |
| 7.4 | 16 | 0.36 | 6 months | 24 | 53 | 0.90 | 7 years |
| 10 | 22 | 0.46 | 1 year | 27 | 59 | 0.97 | 8 years |
| 12 | 27 | 0.54 | 2 years | 32 | 71 | 1.12 | 10 years |
| 14 | 31 | 0.60 | 3 years | 39 | 86 | 1.28 | 12 years |
| 16 | 36 | 0.68 | 4 years | 70 | 150 | 1.7 | Adult |

# Appendix G
# FDA pregnancy categories

**A** No risk demonstrated to the fetus in any trimester.
**B** No adverse effects in animals, no human studies available.
**C** Only given after risks to the fetus are considered: animal studies have shown adverse reactions, no human studies available.
**D** Definite fetal risks, may be given in spite of risks if needed in life-threatening conditions.
**X** Absolute fetal abnormalities; not to be used anytime in pregnancy.

# Bibliography

Clark, B, Queener, F, and Karb, V: Pharmacological basis of nursing practice, ed 2, St. Louis, 1986, The CV Mosby Company

Compendium of pharmaceuticals and specialties, Canadian Pharmaceutical Association, Ottawa, 1987

Drug evaluations, ed 6, American Medical Association, Chicago, 1986

Drug information for the health care provider, ed 7, United States Pharmacopeiae Drug Information, Rockville, Md, 1987

Drug information 87, American Hospital Formulary Service, Bethesda, Md, 1987

Skidmore-Roth, L: Mosby's nursing drug reference, St. Louis, 1988, The CV Mosby Company

# Index

Environmental chemicals, drug interactions and, 10
Enzactin, 395*t*
Enzyme induction, 6
E.P. Mycin, 322-323
**ephedrine**, 29*t*, 39-40
  adrenergic receptor specificity of, 932*t*
  in asthma, 930
  as beta-1 adrenergic agonist, 35
  in cough prescriptions, 961*t*, 963*t*
  in expectorants, 965*t*
  in nasal decongestants, 951*t*
  onset and duration of action of, 931*t*
  prescription combinations with, 939*t*
Ephedrine and Amytal Pulvules, 951*t*
**ephedrine hydrochloride**, 39-40
  nasal jelly, 39
**ephedrine sulfate**, 39-40
  extended-release capsules, 39
  nasal solution, 39
  parenteral, 39
Ephedsol, 39
Epidrim, 1050
Epifoam, 601*t*
Epilepsy; *see* Seizures
Epimorph, 845-846
Epinal, 1050
**epinephrine**, 29*t*, 30-32, 1032, 1050
  adrenergic receptor specificity of, 932*t*
  aerosol, 31
  in asthma, 930
  onset and duration of action of, 931*t*
  ophthalmic, 1033*t*, 1049
  suspension, 31, 931*t*
**epinephrine bitartrate**, 1050
  and pilocarpine hydrochloride, 1032
**epinephrine borate**, 1050
**epinephrine hydrochloride**, 31, 1050
  onset and duration of action of, 931*t*
**epinephrine suspension**, 31, 931*t*
EpiPen Jr, 30
Eppy/N, 1050
Epromate, 696
**epsom salts**, 193-194, 1027
Equagesic, 696, 867*t*
Equanil, 705-706
Equazine-M, 696, 867*t*
Eramycin, 332
**ergocalciferol**, 590, 596-597
  clinical summary of, 597*t*
**ergonovine maleate**, 566, 568-569
Ergotrate maleate, 568-569
Ery-Tab, 329
ERYC, 329
Erypar, 332
Erythema nodosum leprosum, clofazimine and, 374
**erythrityl tetranitrate**, 114, 116*t*, 118
Erythrocin, 331-332
Erythrocin stearate, 332
**erythromycin**, 329-332
  clinical summary of, 328
**erythromycin estolate**, 330
  clinical summary of, 328
**erythromycin ethylsuccinate**, 330-331
  clinical summary of, 328
**erythromycin gluceptate**, 331
  clinical summary of, 328

**erythromycin lactobionate**, 331-332
  clinical summary of, 328
**erythromycin stearate**, 332
  clinical summary of, 328
Escot, 1008*t*
Eserdine, 174
Eseridine, 90
Esgic, 867*t*
Esidrix, 172-173
Esimil, 97, 138*t*
Eskabarb, 681-682
Eskalith, 754-756
**esmolol**, 40, 41*t*, 44
Esophageal reflux, antacids in, 1007
Esophageal spasm, anticholinergic-antispas-
  modics in, 991
**esterified estrogens**, 625, 632-633
  combinations of, 650*t*
Estr-Cyp, 630
Estra-L, 630
Estra-Testrin, 650*t*
Estrace, 629-631
**estradiol**, 625, 629-631, 631*t*
  clinical uses of, 630*t*
**estradiol cypionate**, 629-631, 631*t*
  combinations of, 650*t*
  with testosterone cypionate, 630
Estradiol-LA, 630
**estradiol valerate**, 629-631, 631*t*
  combinations of, 650*t*
  with testosterone enanthate, 630
Estradurin, 545-546
Estraguard, 628
**estramustine**, 534*t*, 539-540
Estratab, 632, 632-633
Estratest, 648, 650*t*
Estrofem, 630
Estrogen-responsive breast tumors
  aminoglutethimide in, 535
  diethylstilbestrol in, 537
Estrogenic Substance, 632
Estrogens, 625-633
  clinical uses of, 631*t*
  deficiency of
    chlorotrianisene in, 627
    estrogens in, 625
  as oral contraceptives, 640-641*t*
**estrogens, conjugated**, 625, 631*t*, 631-632
  combinations of, 650*t*
  and meprobamate, 632, 696, 705
  with methyltestosterone, 632
Estroject-LA, 630
**estrone**, 625, 631*t*, 632-633
Estronol, 632
Estronol-LA, 630
**estropipate**, 625, 631*t*, 632-633
**ethacrynate sodium**, 150-152
**ethacrynic acid**, 146, 150-152
  pharmacokinetics of, 166*t*
**ethambutol**, 370*t*, 377-378
**ethambutol hydrochloride**, 370*t*, 377-378
**ethanol**, dextrose solution with, 191*t*
**ethchlorvynol**, 695, 700-701
**ethinamate**, 695, 701-702
**ethinyl estradiol**, 629-631, 631*t*
  combinations of, 650*t*
  with fluoxymesterone, 630
  as oral contraceptive, 640*t*, 641*t*
**ethionamide**, 370*t*, 379-380

Ethon, 174
**ethopropazine hydrochloride**, 815-816
**ethosuximide**, 781*t*, 783-785
**ethoxynaphthamido penicillin sodium**, 266-267
Ethrane, 854*t*
Ethril, 332
**ethylestrenol**, 652
  clinical uses of, 645*t*
**ethynodiol**, 633, 634-635, 638*t*, 640*t*
**ethynodiol diacetate**, 633, 634-635, 638*t*, 640*t*
Etibi, 377-378
**etidocaine**, 859, 862*t*
**etidocaine hydrochloride**, 862*t*
**etomidate**, 855, 857*t*
**etoposide**, 506-508
  indications for, 480*t*
  side effects of, 486*t*
Etra-Testrin, 630
Etrafon, 718
Eudol, 846-847
Euthroid, 584-585, 585*t*
  clinical summary of, 586*t*
Eutonyl Filmtabs, 111-113
Eutron, 138*t*
Eutron Filmtab, 174
Evac-Q-Mag, 1027
Evac-U-Lax, 1025-1026
Ewing's sarcoma, dactinomycin in, 502
Ex-Lax Extra Gentle, 1020
Exna, 170
Exna-R, 138*t*
Expectorants, 960-968
**extended insulin zinc**, 656*t*, 660-661, 661*t*
Extendryl JR or SR Capsules/ Syrup/Tab-
  lets, 951*t*
Extracorporeal circulation, heparin in, 207
Extravasation, cytotoxic agents and, 484-485
Eye examinations
  atropine sulfate in, 1034
  cyclopentolate hydrochloride in, 1035
  hydroxyamphetamine hydrobromide in, 1038
  phenylephrine hydrochloride in, 1039
  scopolamine hydrobromide in, 1036
  tropicamide in, 1037
Eye medications; *see* Ophthalmic drugs
Eye surgery
  epinephrine in, 1050
  phenylephrine hydrochloride in, 1039

**F**

5-F4, 509-510
**factor IX complex**, 220, 223-224
**factor VIII**, 221-223
Factorate, 221-223
FAM, 479*t*
Familial hypophosphatemia
  calcitriol in, 593
  dihydrotachysterol in, 594
  ergocalciferol in, 596
**famotidine**, 1011-1012
Fansidar, 414*t*, 434, 439-440
Fastin, 775
**fat emulsion**, 188-189
FDA pregnancy categories, 25

**gentamicin sulfate**, 308-309
**gentian violet**, 392*t*, 394*t*
Gentlax, 1022-1023
Gentlax B Granules, 1020
Gentlax S, 1020
Geocillin, 260-261
Geopen, 259-260
Geopen Oral, 260-261
Gestational diabetes, insulins in, 655
Gesterol, 635, 638
GFR; *see* Glomerular filtration rate
GG-Cen, 960-966
GH, 557*t*
Giardiasis
furazolidone in, 414*t*, 420
metronidazole in, 414*t*, 425
quinacrine hydrochloride and, 414*t*, 435
Gientran, 185-186
Gitaligin, 62
**gitalin**, 55, 56*t*, 62
Glanders, tetracyclines and, 316
Glaucoma, 1041-1052
acetazolamide in, 141
adrenergic drugs in, 1049-1052
carbonic anhydrase inhibitors in, 136
cholinomimetic drugs in, 1042-1049
demecarium bromide in, 1044
dichlorphenamide in, 143
echothiophate iodide in, 1045
epinephrine and, 30, 1050
isoflurophate in, 1046
levobunolol hydrochloride in, 1051
methazolamide in, 144
phenylephrine hydrochloride in, 1039
pilocarpine in, 1048
timolol maleate in, 47, 1051
**glipizide**, 666, 670*t*, 670-671
Glomerular filtration rate, mannitol and, 156
**glucagon hydrochloride**, 672-673
Glucamide, 669-670
Glucocorticoids, toxic reactions to, 604*t*
Glucose 6-phosphate dehydrogenase deficiency, 22
Glucotrol, 670-671
Glukor, 564-565
**glutethimide**, 695, 702-703
**glyburide**, 666, 670*t*, 671
Glycate, 1008*t*
**glycerin**, 1021*t*, 1026
Glycerites, 12
**glyceryl guaiacolate**, 960-966
Glyceryl-T Capsules, Liquid, 939*t*
**glycopyrrolate**, 996-997
Glysennid, 1022-1023
Goiter, thyroid hormones in, 579
Gold compounds, 902-907
**gold sodium thiomalate**, 905-907
Gonadotropins, 564-566
Gonorrhea; *see Neisseria gonorrhoeae*
**goserelin**, 553-554
Gout, 911-916
allopurinol in, 911
colchicine in, 913
probenicid in, 914
sulfinpyrazone in, 915
Graft rejection, mercaptopurine and, 475
Gram-negative bacteria
amikacin sulfate and, 307
aminoglycosides and, 304

Gram-negative bacteria—cont'd
ampicillin and, 253
azlocillin sodium and, 255
aztreonam and, 280
carbenicillin disodium and, 259
carbenicillin indanyl sodium and, 260
cefamandole nafate and, 283
cefazolin sodium and, 284
cefmenoxime sodium and, 285
cefonicid sodium and, 286
cefoperazone sodium and, 287
ceforanide and, 288
cefotaxime sodium and, 289
cefotetan disodium and, 291
cefoxitin sodium and, 292
ceftazidime pentahydrate and, 294
ceftizoxime sodium and, 295
ceftriaxone sodium and, 296
cefuroxime sodium and, 297
cephalosporins and related beta-lactam
antibiotics and, 277
colistimethate sodium and, 342
gentamicin sulfate and, 308
imipenem with cilastatin sodium and, 301
kanamycin sulfate and, 309
mezlocillin sodium and, 265
moxalactam and, 302
nalidixic acid and, 346
penicillins and, 246
piperacillin sodium and, 271
ticarcillin disodium and, 275
tobramycin sulfate and, 313
Gram-positive bacteria
amoxicillin trihydrate and, 250
ampicillin and, 252
cefaclor in, 281
cefadroxil and, 282
cefamandole nafate and, 283
cefazolin sodium and, 284
cefonicid sodium and, 286
cefoperazone sodium and, 287
ceforanide and, 288
cefotaxime sodium and, 289
cefotetan disodium and, 291
cefoxitin sodium and, 292
ceftazidime pentahydrate and, 294
ceftizoxime sodium and, 295
ceftriaxone sodium and, 296
cefuroxime sodium and, 297
cephalexin and, 298
cephalosporins and related beta-lactam
antibiotics and, 277
cephalothin sodium and, 299
cephradine and, 300
gentamicin sulfate and, 308
imipenem with cilastatin sodium and, 301
kanamycin sulfate and, 309
lincomycin hydrochloride and, 343
moxalactam and, 302
penicillin G and, 269
penicillins and, 246
tetracyclines and, 316
tobramycin sulfate and, 313
troleandomycin and, 333
vancomycin hydrochloride and, 355
Grand mal seizures
carbamazepine in, 780
phenytoin in, 789

Grand mal seizures—cont'd
primidone in, 792
Granulocytopenia, cytotoxic agents and, 480-481
Granuloma inguinale, tetracyclines and, 316
Gravol, 980-981
Grisactin, 399-400
**griseofulvin**, 392*t*, 399-400
Grisovin, 399-400
Growth hormone, 557*t*
insulins in diagnosis of deficiency of, 655
Growth hormones, 561-564
Guaifed Capsules, 965*t*
Guaifed-PD Capsules, 965*t*
**guaifenesin**, 960-966
in cough prescriptions, 961*t*, 962*t*, 963*t*, 964*t*
in expectorants, 965*t*
prescription combinations with, 939*t*
**guanabenz**, 90, 92-93
**guanabenz acetate**, 92-93
**guanadrel**, 97, 99-101
**guanadrel sulfate**, 99-101
**guanethidine**, 97, 101-102
and hydrochlorothiazide, 97, 101
**guanethidine sulfate**, 101-102
and hydrochlorothiazide, 101
**guar gum**, sennosides and, 1020
Guiamid A.C. Liquid, 962*t*
Guiaphed Elixir, 939*t*
Guiatuss DAC Syrup, 962*t*
Guiatussin Syrup, 960-966
Guiatussin w/Codeine Expectorant, 962*t*
Gulfasin, 366-367
Gustalac, 1008*t*
Gyne-Lotrimin, 394*t*, 418-419
Gynecologic infection, ampicillin sodium
with sulbactam sodium in, 254
Gynecort, 601*t*, 618
Gynogen, 630

**H**

H-2 receptor antagonists, 1009-1013
H-BIG, 453
H-H, 138*t*
*Haemophilus influenzae*
cefaclor and, 281
chloramphenicol and, 324
rifampin and, 385
type B vaccine and, 452-453
Hairy cell leukemia, alpha-interferon in, 534
**halazepam**, 683, 690
half-life of, 684*t*
**halcinonide**, 599*t*, 601*t*, 616-617
Halcion, 695
half-life of, 684*t*
Haldol, 728-729
Haldrone, 621
Haley's M-O, 1020
Half-life of drug, 7
Halodrin, 648, 650*t*
Halog, 601*t*, 616-617
**haloperidol**, 728-729
drug class, potency, and side effects of, 719*t*
**haloprogin**, 392*t*, 394*t*
Halotestin, 647-648